D0023456

DIAGNOSTIC MICROBIOLOGY

Bailey and Scott's

DIAGNOSTIC MICROBIOLOGY

SYDNEY M. FINEGOLD, M.D.; SM (AAM); Diplomate, ABMM

Chief, Infectious Disease Section, V.A. Wadsworth Medical Center;
Professor of Medicine, UCLA School of Medicine,
Los Angeles, California

WILLIAM J. MARTIN, Ph.D.; SM(AAM); Diplomate, ABMM

Director, Microbiology Laboratory, Tufts–New England Medical Center;
Professor of Pathology, Tufts University School of Medicine, Boston, Massachusetts;
Formerly Professor of Pathology and of Microbiology and Immunology,
UCLA School of Medicine, Los Angeles, California

SIXTH EDITION

With **193** illustrations and **39** color plates

The C. V. Mosby Company

ST. LOUIS • TORONTO • LONDON   1982

MOSBY

A TRADITION OF PUBLISHING EXCELLENCE

Editor: Don E. Ladig
Manuscript editor: Laura Kaye McNeive
Book design: Susan Trail
Cover design: Diane Beasley
Production: Barbara Merritt, Jeanne A. Gulledge

SIXTH EDITION

Copyright © 1982 by The C.V. Mosby Company

All rights reserved. No part of this book may be reproduced in any manner without written permission of the publisher.

Previous editions copyrighted 1962, 1966, 1970, 1974, 1978

Printed in the United States of America

The C.V. Mosby Company
11830 Westline Industrial Drive, St. Louis, Missouri 63141

Library of Congress Cataloging in Publication Data

Finegold, Sydney M. 1921-
    Diagnostic microbiology.

    Fifth ed.: Bailey and Scott's Diagnostic
microbiology. 1978.
    Bibliography: p.
    Includes index.
    1. Micro-organisms, Pathogenic—Identification.
2. Diagnosis, Laboratory. 3. Medical microbiology—Technique. I. Martin, William Jeffery,
1932-   . II. Bailey, W. Robert (William
Robert), 1917-1974. Diagnostic microbiology.
III. Title. [DNLM: 1. Microbiology—Laboratory
manuals. WQ 25 F495d]
    QR67.F56 1982   616′.01′028   81-14157
    ISBN 0-8016-1577-1   AACR2

TS/VH/VH 9 8 7 6 5 4 3 2   02/C/272

To

Elvyn G. Scott
and
our **wives** and **children**

PREFACE
TO SIXTH EDITION

We were honored and delighted when Elvyn G. Scott invited us to become the new authors of *Bailey and Scott's Diagnostic Microbiology*, which we have long regarded as a classic in its field. We have strived to maintain the high standards of this important work so that it will continue to serve microbiologists and students of medical microbiology. We have made it our aim also to make the book useful to infectious disease clinicians and trainees, clinical pathologists, public health workers, and nurses and nursing students.

The text is changed significantly from the previous edition. There is some reorganization, a great deal of new material is added, and everything is updated. Only medically relevant material is included, and clinical correlations are presented. A new chapter on automation and rapid methods has been added. Almost all of the chapters have been completely rewritten. Among the new topics treated and areas given considerably more attention in this edition are new methods for detection of bacteriuria, the role of *Chlamydia* in disease, the new classification of Enterobacteriaceae, new descriptive material on certain nonfermentative gram-negative bacilli not previously discussed, newly described mycobacteria, new methods for susceptibility testing, an antibiotic removal device for blood cultures, and additional material on noncultural techniques for microbiologic diagnosis, laboratory safety, rapid processing for anaerobes, Legionnaires' disease, *Campylobacter*, *Yersinia*, antimicrobial-induced colitis, *Bacillus cereus*, sexually transmitted diseases, bite infections, bone infections, antibiotic tolerance, toxic shock syndrome, Kawasaki disease, monoclonal antibody, nutritionally variant streptococci, antibiotic-resistant pneumococci, *Vibrio vulnificus*, Actinomycetales, *Lactobacillus*, *Leptotrichia*, *Capnocytophaga*, *Prototheca*, hemotropic bacteria, DF-2, EF-4, HB-5, viral culture, fungi, and certain parasitic agents. It is beyond the scope of this book to discuss the role of the microbiology laboratory in investigations of nosocomial infection outbreaks. Interested readers are referred to an excellent recent article by Goldmann and Macone (Infect. Con. **1**:391-400, 1980).

We acknowledge with gratitude the assistance

of numerous individuals. Particularly, we appreciate the help of George Berlin, Elaine Bixler-Forell, JoAnn Dizikes, Violet Fiacco, Carol Gagne, Janet Hindler, and Daniel Wong. We are particularly grateful to Elvyn G. Scott for his continued advice, assistance, and encouragement. We would like to thank Nobuko Kitamura for the preparation of a number of excellent new illustrations for Chapter 35. We express our deep appreciation to John G. Bartlett, Ann Bjornson, Diane M. Citron, V. R. Dowell, Jr., Paul Edelstein, Violet Fiacco, W. Lance George, Ellie J. C. Goldstein, Theo M. Hawkins, Hannele Jousimies, A. S. Klainer, Irving Krasnow, George Kubica, Martin McHenry, Marjorie Miller, Alan Morgenstein, Maury E. Mulligan, Charles V. Sanders, Elvyn G. Scott, Lakhbir Singh, Alex Sonnenwirth, Vera L. Sutter, Valerie Vargo, Trevor Willis, Analytab Products, Centers for Disease Control, General Diagnostics, The Mayo Clinic, Schering Corporation, and The Upjohn Company, for many of the color photos.

To our wives, Mary and Marcia, we express our thanks for their patience, indulgence, and assistance.

Sydney M. Finegold
William J. Martin

PREFACE
TO FIRST EDITION

Diagnostic Microbiology is the first edition of a new series and not a revision of the former publication *Diagnostic Bacteriology*, the latest edition of which we revised (1958). This new title derives in part from the fact that the new volume includes microorganisms other than bacteria. The reader will note, for example, that the former Society of American Bacteriologists has now become the American Society for Microbiology.

Since this book is designed to be used as a reference text in medical bacteriology laboratories and as a textbook for courses in diagnostic bacteriology at the college level, the material has been consolidated and placed in separate parts and chapters. The selected sequence will be commensurate with the needs of both the diagnostician and the student.

For purposes of orientation in taxonomy and ready reference, an outline of bacterial classification has been included. For the student beginning diagnostic work, some pertinent background information is presented on the cultivation of microorganisms, the microscopic examination of microorganisms, and the proper methods for collecting and handling specimens.

A number of chapters include recommended procedures for the cultivation of both the common and the rare pathogens isolated from clinical material and should serve to familiarize the microbiologist with the wide variety of pathogens that may be encountered. An additional chapter has been devoted to the methods employed in the microbiological examination of surgical tissue and autopsy material.

To effect further consolidation of the book's content, one part has been devoted to a series of chapters which cover the various groups of bacteria of medical importance—their taxonomic position, general characteristics, and procedures for their identification. The chapter on the enteric bacteria introduces the new classification of the family Enterobacteriaceae, outlines the group biochemical characteristics, and discusses the serological aspects. The chapter on the mycobacteria includes a discussion of the increasingly important unclassified (anonymous) acid-fast bacilli, giving the methods for their identification, certain cytochemical tests, and animal inoculation procedures.

The chapter on laboratory diagnosis of viral and rickettsial diseases includes a guide to the collection of specimens and offers recommendations for the appropriate time of collection. In the chapter on laboratory diagnosis of systemic mycotic infections, the biochemical approach in identifying the pathogenic fungi is brought to the reader's attention.

The remainder of the book includes prescribed tests for the susceptibility of bacteria to antibiotics, serological procedures on microorganisms and patients' sera, and a technical section on culture media, stains, reagents, and tests, each in alphabetical sequence.

We would like to express our gratitude to Mrs. Isabelle Schaub and to Sister Marie Judith for committing the continuation of the original publication, *Diagnostic Bacteriology*, to our care and responsibility. We also acknowledge the many kindnesses extended by a number of microbiologists and clinicians in permitting the use of published and unpublished materials.

W. Robert Bailey
Elvyn G. Scott

CONTENTS

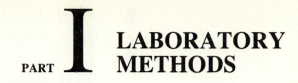

PART I LABORATORY METHODS

1 GENERAL REQUIREMENTS FOR CULTIVATION OF MICROORGANISMS

Great advances relative to the nutritional requirements of bacteria and other microorganisms have been realized during the current century. Consequently, with the exception of a few fastidious forms, most pathogens can be cultivated in the laboratory on artificial media. Emphasis should be placed, therefore, on the proper preparation and selection of culture media in order to isolate and grow the various microbes. The need for quality control should be stressed. A good **culture medium** contains the essential nutrients in the proper concentration, an adequate amount of salt, and an adequate supply of water; is free of inhibitory substances for the organism to be cultured; is of the desired consistency; has the proper reaction (pH) for the metabolism of that organism; and is sterile. It is obvious that such a definition applies only to the preparation of inanimate media, because different requirements exist for obligate parasites.

Additional requirements must also be met, such as those generated by the temperature and oxygen relationships of the culture and by the lack of synthetic ability of certain fastidious pathogens.

Heterotrophic microorganisms, the group to which the pathogens belong, exhibit a wide variety of needs. Despite this, however, numerous dehydrated media that are stable and eminently suitable for use in a diagnostic laboratory are available commercially. This ready supply minimizes concern regarding deterioration of prepared media and reduces storage needs. It is strongly recommended that media makers follow the directions given on the container labels.

PREPARATION OF MEDIA

Clean, detergent-free glassware and equipment are essential to good media preparation. The screw cap, the metal closure, and the plastic plug have virtually replaced the cotton plug in tubes of media, but personnel are cautioned concerning the exclusive use of the push-on metal closure. When tubes of media are stored over a long period, air contamination is likely to occur. Tubes cooling after sterilization take in air—the most likely means of initial contamination.

If a culture medium is to be prepared from its ingredients, the latter should be weighed accurately in a suitable container. Approximately one half of the required amount of water is added first to dissolve the ingredients; then the remainder is added. If it is an agar-containing medium, heat will be necessary to dissolve the agar. Heating on an open flame is **not recommended,** although it is often practiced. The use of a boiling water bath or steam bath is preferred. Complete dissolution of the ingredients of the medium in the required amount of water before sterilization gives a consistent and homogeneous product. Flasks of agar-containing media should be mixed after sterilization to promote a uniform consistency for pouring plates.

For dissolving dehydrated agar media for autoclaving, the use of a microwave oven has been shown to result in a substantial reduction of heat generation and considerable savings in time.[5] The microwave oven has also been used for decontamination procedures in the laboratory.[6]

Media may be **liquid** (broth) or **solid** (containing agar). Sometimes a semisolid consistency is desired, in which case a low concentration of agar is used. Culture media may be also **synthetic,** in which all ingredients are known, or **nonsynthetic,** in which the exact chemical composition is unknown.

The inclusion of small amounts of a carbohydrate, such as glucose, is often recommended for the enhancement of growth in routine plating or broth media. In some instances the presence of such a carbohydrate can lead to a product of fermentation that may alter the characteristic appearance of a reaction produced by a microorganism. Examples are cited later.

Dehydrated media or media prepared according to accepted formulas are now available for the cultivation of anaerobic bacteria. Thioglycollate broth, for example, is useful for biochemical tests on strains of anaerobes that have been previously isolated in pure culture. In the preparation of this medium (which contains peptone, an amino acid, and other ingredients), sodium thioglycollate is added as a reducing agent. This substance possesses sulfhydryl groups (SH—), which tie up molecular oxygen and prevent the formation and accumulation of hydrogen peroxide in the medium.

The cultivation of catalase-negative microorganisms, such as the clostridia, which are unable to break down this toxic substance, becomes possible under these conditions. The addition of thioglycollate or other reducing agents, for example, cysteine or glutathione, to culture media such as nutrient gelatin and milk renders them more suitable for anaerobic or microaerophilic cultivation.

STERILIZATION OF MEDIA

Sterilization may be effected by **heat, filtration,** or **chemical methods.** The method of choice will depend on the medium, its consistency, and its labile constituents. Moist heat rather than dry heat is employed in the sterilization of culture media, and the method of application will vary with the type of medium.

Moist heat
Steam under pressure

The usual application for most media is steam under pressure in an autoclave where temperatures in excess of 100 C are obtained. Although the principle of the autoclave need not be discussed here at length, one important rule about autoclave sterilization must be stressed. In the normal procedure, using 15 pounds of steam for 15 minutes, the autoclave chamber should be flushed **free of air** before the outlet valve is closed. A temperature of 105 C on the chamber thermometer is used as an index of complete live steam content. When this temperature is reached, the outlet valve may be closed, and the pressure allowed to build up to the required level of 15 pounds to attain generally a temperature of 121 C. Automation, however, takes care of such operational needs.

The time of exposure to this temperature and pressure may be allowed to exceed 15 minutes if large volumes of material are being sterilized. It is not recommended that an exposure of more than 30 minutes be used, because overheating can cause a breakdown of nutrient constituents.

At times a lower pressure may be necessary, such as in the heat sterilization of certain carbohydrate solutions. A pressure of 10 to 12 pounds for 10 to 15 minutes will reduce the possibility of hydrolysis.

The temperatures of the autoclave that correspond to the various live steam pressures (above atmospheric) are given in Table 1-1.

It is strongly recommended that the efficiency of the autoclave be checked at regular intervals. This may be conveniently done with the use of filter paper strips impregnated with spores of the thermophile *Bacillus stearothermophilus* and an appropriate amount of dehydrated culture medium with an indicator.

The paper strips,* contained in small enve-

---

*Kilit Sporestrips No. 1, Baltimore Biological Laboratory, Cockeysville, Md.

TABLE 1-1

Autoclave temperatures corresponding to steam pressures in the chamber

Pressure (pounds)	Temperature (° C)	Pressure (pounds)	Temperature (° C)	Pressure (pounds)	Temperature (° C)
1	102.3	10	115.6	15	121.3
3	105.7	11	116.8	16	122.4
5	108.8	12	118.0	17	123.3
7	111.7	13	119.1	18	124.3
9	114.3	14	120.2	20	126.2

lopes, are inserted in the center of a basket of tubes of media or other material to be tested. The basket or material is then placed near the bottom at the front of the autoclave chamber, and the usual sterilizing cycle is carried out. When the cycle is complete, the load is removed from the sterilizer, and the sporestrip envelope is sent to the laboratory.

In the microbiology laboratory the sporestrips are individually removed, using aseptic technique, and are placed directly into tubes containing 12 to 15 ml of sterile distilled water. After dissolution of the medium on the strips, the tubes are gently shaken and placed at 55 C and then observed daily for several days. An unexposed sporestrip is processed in like manner as a control with each sterilization check.

The control is examined after appropriate incubation. This should reveal a change in the color of the indicator, showing that acid (yellow if bromcresol purple is used) has been produced through fermentation of the glucose. If the remainder of the tubes have the same appearance, sterilization has not been effected.

Successful sterilization is indicated by the unchanged appearance of the heated tubes after 7 days' incubation at 55 C. The spores of *B. stearothermophilus* are destroyed when exposed to 121 C for 15 minutes.

A test kit more convenient for use in the microbiology laboratory consists of a sealed glass ampule containing a standardized spore suspension of *B. stearothermophilus*, a culture medium, and an indicator.* The ampule is exposed, incubated, and read as previously described for the sporestrip; an unheated ampule is also included as a positive control. These ampules are for professional use only and are used just once. Because they contain live cultures, they should be handled with care to prevent breakage. Each ampule is destroyed after use, preferably by incineration; unused ampules are stored in a refrigerator at 2 to 10 C.

A third but less reliable alternative is to use adhesive tape on which the word "sterile" is printed invisibly. The word becomes visible if the autoclaving is efficient. The tape may be placed on any suitable container to be autoclaved.

Flowing steam

The flowing steam procedure represents another application of moist heat and may be employed in the sterilization of materials that cannot withstand the elevated temperatures of an autoclave. **Fractional sterilization,** or **tyndallization,** introduced by John Tyndall in 1877, is a procedure involving the use of flowing steam in an Arnold sterilizer.

---

*Kilit ampule, Baltimore Biological Laboratory, Cockeysville, Md.

Material to be so sterilized is exposed for 30 minutes on 3 successive days. After the first and second days the material is placed at room temperature to permit any viable spores present to germinate. Vegetative bacteria are destroyed at flowing steam temperature, whereas their endospores are resistant. This procedure is used for media such as milk that contains an indicator and other media that may be precipitated or changed chemically by the normal autoclave treatment.

Inspissation

A third type of moist heat application is the process known as **inspissation,** or thickening through evaporation. This is used in the sterilization of high-protein-containing media that cannot withstand the high temperatures of the autoclave. The procedure causes coagulation of the material without greatly altering the substance or appearance. Materials such as the Lowenstein-Jensen egg medium, the Loeffler serum medium, and the Dorset egg medium are inspissated.

Modern autoclaves are equipped to allow inspissation procedures. If the Arnold sterilizer or a regular inspissator is used, the tubes containing the medium are placed in a slanted position and are exposed to a temperature of 75 to 80 C for 2 hours on 3 successive days. Precautions should be taken during such treatment to prevent excessive dehydration of the medium.

Manually operated autoclaves may also be used successfully. Tubes of medium are placed in the autoclave chamber in a slanted position in a rack with adequate spacing. The tubes may be closed with a screw cap, loosely fitted initially, when Lowenstein, Loeffler, and Dorset egg media are being prepared. For operation, the exhaust valve of the autoclave is closed, and the door is shut tightly. This traps air in the chamber. The steam is turned on, and the chamber contains an air-steam mixture. The pressure is then raised to 15 pounds and should be rigidly maintained for 10 minutes. The temperature

ranges between 85 and 90 C. After this period, through manipulation of the steam valve and the exhaust valve, the air-steam mixture is replaced with live steam while the pressure is kept **constant** at 15 pounds. When the temperature reaches 105 C, the chamber contains only live steam. The outlet valve is then closed, and an additional 15 minutes at 15 pounds is allowed to effect complete sterilization. During the final phase the chamber temperature rises to 121 C. At the end of this period the pressure should be permitted to subside very slowly. This is achieved by closing the steam valve and keeping the outlet valve tightly closed. The chamber temperature should drop below 60 C before the door is opened. When the tubes of media are cool, their caps should be tightened.

Filtration

Certain materials cannot tolerate the high temperatures used in heat sterilization procedures without deterioration; thus, other methods must be devised. Materials such as urea, certain carbohydrate solutions, serum, plasma, and ascitic fluid must be filter sterilized. Filters made of sintered Pyrex, compressed asbestos, or membranes are employed. These are placed in sidearm flasks, and the entire assembly of filter and flask is sterilized in the autoclave. A test tube of appropriate length may be placed around and under the delivery tube of the filter and may be sterilized with the unit when only a small quantity of filtrate is required. Negative pressure (suction) is applied to draw or positive pressure is applied to force the material through the filter. Membrane filters are preferred to the Seitz asbestos filter for some materials because of the high adsorption capacity of the latter type. The Swinney filter,* consisting of a filter attachment affixed to a hypodermic syringe and needle, is fast and simple for small quantities of material. The nonsterile material is taken up in the syringe, the sterile filter attachment is

---

*Millipore Filter Corp., Bedford, Mass.

affixed, and the material is expressed by positive pressure (exerted by the plunger) into a sterile container. Disposable sterile plastic holders and membrane filters are now being widely used.

Chemical methods

In addition to or in lieu of some of the foregoing, chemical methods may be used. These normally comprise two main types: the use of chemical additives to solutions or treatment with gases. The latter applies primarily to the sterilization of thermolabile plasticware such as Petri dishes, pipets, and syringes, and ethylene oxide may be used. The efficiency of such sterilization may be determined by the use of commercially prepared sporestrips.* As this is not directly concerned with sterilization of media, it will not be discussed here. The use of chemical compounds, such as thymol, a crystalline phenol, as additives to concentrated thermolabile solutions is quite appropriate, however. For example, to sterilize a 20-times-normal concentration of urea or a 20% solution of carbohydrate, approximately 1 g of thymol per 100 ml of medium is added and allowed to stand at room temperature for 24 hours. The dilution serves to nullify any bactericidal effects of the thymol.

SELECTION OF PROPER MEDIA

The number of available media increases annually. Selection of the proper media for specific purposes requires judgment by an experienced person, but for the most part, commercially available media, used in nearly all laboratories today, carry a recommendation based on the broad experience of others in the field. A very important facet in medium selection is the purpose for which the medium is intended. Laboratory personnel are advised to keep their selections to a minimum to avoid duplication of purpose.

Culture media, by virtue of their ingredients, may be selected for general and for specific pur-

poses. The reader will find various terms ascribed to media throughout the literature. For example, terms such as **enrichment, enriched, selective,** and **differential** are very common as applied to media and are found in various sections of this book. These terms are indicative of purpose. Usually the media are special, but for general use a good basic nutrient medium is needed in the preparation of broth and agar media. The choice of such a medium is governed partly by tradition and partly by the experience of the users. In the selection of a basic medium, however, it is generally understood that one that is glucose free tends to give more consistent and reliable results. The presence of small amounts of this carbohydrate in a medium tends to enhance growth; yet fermentation of glucose can result in a pH that is harmful to acid-sensitive organisms. For example, this has been recognized in the cultivation of pneumococci and beta-hemolytic streptococci. The presence of the carbohydrate in a blood agar base medium can lead to the appearance of a green zone around colonies of streptococci, making differentiation between alpha and beta hemolysis extremely difficult.

Trypticase or tryptic soy broth, a pancreatic digest of casein and soybean peptone, is a widely used general medium that will support the growth of many fastidious organisms without further enrichment. Because of its glucose content, however, one should be aware of its limitations in certain areas of application.

Thioglycollate medium, now available in a modified form containing 0.06% glucose, will support the growth of many facultatives, microaerophiles, and anaerobes. In the ensuing chapters of this book, which discuss the isolation and cultivation of various pathogenic microorganisms, recommendations relative to the selection and use of media are made. Chapter 42 gives the formulas and methods of preparation for many of the media in use at the present time.

Valuable information on the choice of media

---

*Attest Biological Indicators, 3M Co., St. Paul, Minn.

and the nutritional requirements of microorganisms may be gained from references 2, 3, and 7 at the end of this chapter.

STORAGE OF MEDIA

Because of the heavy work schedule of most diagnostic laboratories today, bulk preparation of media is often necessary. It should be emphasized that infrequently used media that are subject to deterioration on prolonged storage should be purchased in the smallest available quantity. For example, ¼-pound bottles or smaller packages should be specified in these situations. The average medium should be stored in the refrigerator to avoid deterioration and dehydration. Plating media used for the cultivation of certain fastidious organisms that are sensitive to drying should be kept airtight and refrigerated. Some tubed media, especially those with tightly fitting screw caps, paraffined corks, or rubber stoppers, may be stored for relatively long periods at room temperature. Plates of media that can be readily sealed are available commercially from several companies* and have certain advantages. Such plated media are in wide use in many laboratories and physicians' offices.

---

*Baltimore Biological Laboratory, Cockeysville, Md.; Gibco Diagnostics, Madison, Wisc.; Scott Laboratories, Fiskeville, R.I.; and others.

Refrigeration facilities obviously determine the storage capacity. It is recommended that plated and tubed media be stored in sealed plastic bags. Depending on the media and whether it is plated or tubed, bagged media can be stored for from 2 weeks to 4 months.[1] The laboratory worker is cautioned about the use of media that have been just removed from refrigeration. Plated and tubed media should be allowed to warm to room temperature before use.

REFERENCES

1. Bartlett, R.C.: Medical microbiology: quality, cost and clinical relevance, New York, 1974, John Wiley & Sons, Inc., p. 192.
2. BBL manual of products and laboratory procedures, ed. 5, Cockeysville, Md., 1973, BioQuest, Divison of Becton, Dickinson & Co.
3. Difco manual of dehydrated culture media and reagents for microbiological and clinical laboratory procedures, ed. 9, Detroit, 1953, Difco Laboratories.
4. Difco supplementary literature, Detroit, May 1972, Difco Laboratories.
5. Hanson, C.W., and Martin, W.J.: Microwave oven for melting laboratory media, J. Clin. Microbiol, **7:**401-402, 1978.
6. Latimer, J.M., and Matsen, J.M.: Microwave oven irradiation as a method for bacterial decontamination in a clinical microbiology laboratory, J. Clin. Microbiol. **6:**340-342, 1977.
7. Vera, H.D., and Power D.A.: Media, reagents, and stains. In Lennette, E.H., Balows, A., Hausler, W.J., Jr., and Truant, J.P., editors: Manual of clinical microbiology, ed. 3, Washington, D.C., 1980, American Society for Microbiology.

2 OPTICAL METHODS IN SPECIMEN EXAMINATION

SPECIMEN PREPARATION

Direct microscopic examination of clinical specimens for microorganisms is extremely important. It provides immediate information on the nature and relative numbers of various microbial forms, inflammatory and other host cells, and certain other materials, such as crystals. Data of this type provide information on suitability of the specimen, the likelihood of infection being present, the likely infecting organism(s), and the predominant organism(s) in mixed infections. This information may suggest the desirability of using special media and is very important in quality control in the laboratory.

Specimens received in a laboratory for microbiologic examination can vary widely. They may consist of clinical material, such as blood, urine, pus, cerebrospinal fluid (CSF), or microbial cultures isolated from such material. In examination the laboratory worker or student should consider the nature and possible content of the specimen and be cognizant of the difficulty in cultivating and staining certain microorganisms. Special methods are often needed.

There are two ways in which microbial isolates or microorganisms in certain clinical material may be examined under a microscope: in the **living** state or in the **fixed** state.

Living state

It is often necessary to examine certain microorganisms in the living state, because they are not readily stained or because they cannot be easily cultivated. Also, when they are examined in the living state, morphology is less distorted, and motility and other characteristics may be observed readily.

Two methods—the wet-mount and the hanging-drop techniques—are generally used for such examination.

Wet-mount method

In the wet-mount procedure there are two approaches, the choice being determined by the nature of the specimen: (1) place a loopful of liquid clinical specimen or culture on a clean glass slide, and cover with a coverglass; (2) place a loopful of clean water on the slide, emulsify some nonliquid clinical material or portion of a bacterial colony in it, and add a coverglass. In either case, the coverglass may be ringed with petrolatum to reduce evaporation of the liquid. The preparation may then be examined, either by brightfield or by darkfield microscopy. The latter method may be essential with such microorganisms as the treponeme of syphilis, which is very difficult to stain. This procedure may also be adapted to a wet-mount staining procedure for certain organisms.

Hanging-drop method

A second procedure used in the examination of organisms in the living state is the hanging-drop method. Loopfuls of the specimen may be prepared as with the wet-mount method but on a thin coverglass rather than the slide. The coverglass is then inverted over the concave area of a hollow-ground or well slide to provide the hanging drop. The coverglass can be sealed as in the wet-mount method with petrolatum or a small amount of immersion oil to reduce evaporation. Such a preparation is examined by brightfield microscopy.

Fixed state

Bacteria and other microbes are generally examined in the fixed state and are more readily observed when they are stained. By drying and fixing the organisms on a glass slide, various staining procedures may be carried out. The choice of procedure is determined by the nature of the specimen or the desired result. Staining procedures for bacteria and other microorganisms are discussed in Chapters 3 and 43.

USE AND CARE OF MICROSCOPES

It is assumed that the reader understands the elements of microscopy and is generally familiar with the parts of a microscope. For this reason discussion of the instrument is restricted to a few points that bear emphasis. The lenses of a microscope should be kept clean and free of grease and dust. In using the average compound light microscope equipped with a condenser, only the flat plane or face of the mirror is used. The light source selected should give uniform illumination, such as that provided by a frosted bulb, a fluorescent light, or a special microscope lamp. Most of the new light microscopes have built-in lamps. For routine bacteriologic examination, the condenser of the microscope should be kept almost fully racked up. This position usually provides optimal and uniform illumination of the field. The user of a monocular microscope is strongly advised to keep both eyes open in order to reduce eyestrain.

Since many laboratories are equipped with a variety of microscopes, several instruments are briefly discussed here with some specific advice and information. All light microscopes should be kept covered when not in use, and full attention should be given to protection of the objective lenses. **Immersion oil should never be left on the objective when the instrument is not to be used for some time.** The nosepiece should be rotated so that the low-power objective is in position before the microscope is put away. Repeated use of a solvent such as xylol to remove oil from a lens is discouraged, since this tends to loosen the mounting cement around the lens. **Clean lens paper only** should be used for wiping the objective free of oil. Other commercial tissue is too rough and will scratch the lens.

Brightfield microscope

The brightfield microscope is used for the majority of routine examinations in which stainable microorganisms are to be observed. In brightfield microscopy the organisms appear dark against a bright background.

Darkfield microscope

In contrast with the effect in brightfield microscopy, organisms appear bright against a dark background under the darkfield microscope. This appearance may be produced either by an opaque stop inserted below the condenser or by a stop built into the condenser. This stop permits only peripheral rays of light to enter the condenser. These rays pass through the specimen at an angle such that the field appears unilluminated. Any particles, such as microorganisms in the field, reflect the light and appear bright in the optical system. This type of microscope is particularly adaptable to the examination of microorganisms that are difficult to stain. The treponeme of syphilis in the exudate from a lesion or in other material may be thus examined. Examination is carried out with the living organisms in a wet-mount preparation. Motility is readily determined for other bacteria as well.

In using the conventional darkfield microscope it is essential to use immersion oil on the top of the condenser as well as on the coverglass of the wet-mount preparation to minimize light refraction.

Phase microscope

The phase microscope permits relatively accurate observation of (1) bacteria in tissue sections, (2) parasites in various types of clinical material, (3) Negri or inclusion bodies in virus-infected material, and (4) histologic preparations. A halo of light produced by light passing from the source through an annular diaphragm initiates the effect obtained. Rays of light passing through an area composed of materials varying in refractive index emerge out of phase and give a pattern of bright and dark relief. Objects such as bacteria and inclusion bodies, being of a different refractive index from surrounding tissue, consequently show up in such a microscope, whereas in normal brightfield microscopy these objects must be stained to be observed.

Ultraviolet microscope

The use of ultraviolet light rather than visible white light in microscopy allows for greater resolution. This is because of the shorter wavelength of ultraviolet light. As a result, a magnification can be obtained that is two to three times higher than that possible with visible light. Because of the invisibility of ultraviolet light, a photographic plate is used to record the image, and since glass is impervious to such light, quartz "lenses" rather than glass lenses are employed.

Fluorescence microscope

Fluorescence microscopy has become very popular in a number of laboratories because of its application to the diagnosis of disease. The light source is ultraviolet. The principle involved here is that certain fluorescent chemical complexes have the property of absorbing ultraviolet light and emitting rays of visible light. Microorganisms can be treated with a fluorescent dye or a dye-antibody complex that causes them to fluoresce and become readily distinguishable in a mixed population.

The fluorescent antibody technique has advantages and disadvantages in diagnostic microbiology. Among the former are the time saved by eliminating lengthy cultural study, the sensitivity of the test, the lack of interference from contaminating microorganisms if their staining reactions are known, and the detection of nonviable pathogenic organisms. The disadvantages of the technique are the same as those experienced with most serologic tests: the cross-reactions that inevitably develop between species. Therefore, anyone planning to use the fluorescent antibody technique should be aware of such limitations. Successful results may now be obtained with group A streptococci and other bacteria and in the diagnosis of rabies. The technique has further application in the detection of treponemal antibody (FTA). The reader's attention is directed to Chapter 39, where immunofluorescence is discussed in further detail. The value of this procedure for diagnostic parasitology and mycology is discussed by Cherry.[1]

Electron microscope

The electron microscope has become essential in various fields of research of the biologic sciences; virology presently makes the greatest use of this instrument, but it has also become an invaluable piece of equipment to cytologists.

An electron source is used in lieu of a light source, and magnets are used instead of lenses. Only nonliving material may be examined, and specimens require special preparation. With modern instruments a direct magnification of 200,000 diameters may be obtained. The image may be observed on a fluorescent screen through a window at the base of the evacuated column, or a photographic plate may be inserted to record the image. The result, however, is not a photograph, since photons are not used. The term **electron micrograph** has been in use for some years.

Great advances in the refinement of techniques used in specimen preparation have been made in recent years, and much knowledge has now been amassed relative to the interpretation of electron micrographic images.

REFERENCES

1. Cherry, W.B.: Immunofluorescence techniques. In Lennette, E.H., Balows, A., Hausler, W.J., Jr., and Truant, J.P., editors: Manual of clinical microbiology, ed. 3, Washington, D.C., 1980, American Society for Microbiology.
2. Douglas, S.D.: Microscopy. In Lennette, E.H., Balows, A., Hausler, W.J., Jr., and Truant, J.P., editors: Manual of clinical microbiology, ed. 3, Washington, D.C., 1980, American Society for Microbiology.

3 GENERAL PRINCIPLES IN STAINING PROCEDURES

Bacteria and other microorganisms are usually transparent, which makes the study of morphologic detail difficult when they are examined in the natural state. The early methods of fixing and staining initiated by Paul Ehrlich and Robert Koch allowed the microbiologist to distinguish many structural features not formerly seen.

Unless some specific morphologic feature, dependent on the age of the culture, is to be demonstrated, the microbiologist is advised to use a young culture for routine staining procedures, as old cells lose their affinity for most dyes. Unless one is dealing with organisms that have an unusually long generation time, a 24-hour culture is expected to yield favorable results.

PREPARATION OF A SMEAR

In routine staining procedures the first step is the preparation of a **smear.** A loopful of liquid culture or fluid specimen is spread over an appropriate area of a clean glass slide to make a film, or a section of a colony taken with a needle from a plate or growth from a slant culture is emulsified in a loopful of clean water and spread over the required area. For best results the film should be homogeneous.

In either event the mixing and spreading should never be done vigorously; such treatment is potentially hazardous when working with pathologic material, because it may create aerosols. In addition, harsh treatment will tend to destroy characteristic arrangements of cells, such as chains and clusters.

Ideally, one should always permit a smear to dry in the air and then heat fix it by passing gently through a Bunsen flame to promote adherence of the cells to the slide. Overheating causes distortion and should be avoided. The slide should then be allowed to cool.

When a large number of cultures are to be examined by a routine staining procedure, such as the Gram stain, several small smears can be made on the same slide in areas appropriately marked with a glass-marking pencil.

STAINING OF BACTERIA
Simple stain

1. After fixation of the smear, draw a vertical line on the glass slide about 1 inch from the left or right end using a wax pencil. This will keep the stain away from the fingers when one is holding the slide.
2. Flood the smeared area with the stain to be used (crystal violet, fuchsin, methylene blue, or safranin).
3. Allow the stain to react for the appropriate time (30 seconds to 3 minutes, depending on the stain).
4. Wash off the smear with a gentle stream of cool water. Avoid having the water fall directly on the smear with any force.
5. Blot the smear dry between sheets of bibulous paper, and examine it under the oil-immersion lens.
6. It is good practice to sterilize blotting paper used in this simple procedure involving pathogenic microorganisms. If they are not to be retained for reference, the slides should be placed in disinfectant.

Special staining procedures
Gram stain

The Gram stain ranks among the most important stains for bacteria. Devised by Hans Christian Gram, a Dane, in 1884, it allows one to distinguish broadly between various bacteria that may exhibit a similar morphology. There are various modifications of the technique; the one described in Chapter 43 has been found reliable, even in the hands of a beginner.

On microscopic examination of a gram-stained smear containing a mixed bacterial flora, the differential features of the method become apparent. Many bacteria retain the violet-iodine combination and stain **purple** (gram positive), others stain **red** by the safranin (gram negative). Thus, in using this procedure not only are form, size, and other structural details made visible, but the microorganisms present can be grouped into gram-positive and gram-negative types by their reactions. This is an important diagnostic tool in subsequent identification procedures.

The difference in the staining reaction between gram-positive and gram-negative bacteria can probably be attributed to their different chemical compositions. Gram-negative cell walls have a higher lipid content[2] than do gram-positive cell walls, and although a crystal violet–iodine complex is formed in both kinds of cell, the alcohol removes the lipid from the gram-negative cells, thereby increasing the cell permeability and resulting in the loss of the dye complex. The complex is retained, however, in the gram-positive cells, in which dehydration by the alcohol causes a decrease in permeability.

At times, certain gram-positive organisms appear gram negative. A rapid method to distinguish between gram-positive organisms and gram-negative organisms has been proposed by Gregersen.[1] A colony is stirred into 1 to 2 drops of 3% KOH on a glass slide with a loop. Then the loop is slowly raised. Gram-negative bacteria make the KOH viscous, and a thread of this viscid material follows the loop for 0.5 to 2 cm or more as it is raised. This is thought to be the result of destruction of the cell wall and liberation of the viscid DNA.

Acid-fast stain

Another differential staining technique that depends on the chemical composition of the bacterial cell is the acid-fast stain, which is used in staining tubercle bacilli and other mycobacteria. Since these microorganisms are difficult to stain with the ordinary dyes, basic dyes are used in the presence of controlled amounts of acid and are generally applied with heat. Once stained, the tubercle bacillus is resistant to subsequent treatment with **acid** alcohol, whereas most other bacteria are decolorized. For convenience in viewing, a counterstain of contrasting color is usually applied. The method most commonly employed is that of Ziehl and Neelsen, although the fluorochrome procedure also is recommended. These are described, as used at the Centers for Disease Control (CDC) in Atlanta,[3] in Chapter 43.

Acid-fast organisms are difficult to stain, and once stained they are not easily decolorized. Many theories have been introduced to account for this property of acid fastness. The most acceptable concept is that acid fastness is determined by the selective permeability of the cytoplasmic membrane. The brilliance of the red color is due to the retention of the dye, carbolfuchsin, in solution within the cell. Should the cell be mechanically disrupted, its acid-fast property is lost. That this may not be a precise explanation of the reaction does not invalidate the usefulness of the technique for detecting fundamental differences in bacterial genera.

Capsule stain

The capsule of bacteria does not have the same affinity for dyes as do other cell components, which necessitates the use of special staining procedures. Some are designed to stain the cell and its background but not the capsule, so that the surrounding envelope is seen by contrast, as in the Anthony method. Other procedures produce a differential staining effect wherein the capsule will take a counterstain, as in the Muir method. Another procedure involves the negative stain principle in which the capsule shows up as a clear halo against a dark background, as in the India ink method.

The various procedures are given in Chapter 43.

Flagella stain

Flagella are fragile, heat-labile appendages and require careful handling and staining by special procedures to observe them. Success in staining depends on the freshness and effectiveness of a mordant. Since flagella are beyond the resolving power of the ordinary light microscope, their size must be increased to bring them into view. This may be accomplished by coating their surfaces with a precipitate from an unstable colloidal suspension (the mordant). This precipitate then serves as a layer of stainable material, and the threadlike structure of the flagellum shows up when the appropriate stain is applied.

Various methods may be used, but we have found the Gray method very satisfactory (see Fig. 20-5 and Plate 1). The procedure may be found in Chapter 43. West and associates[4] have proposed a simplified silver-plating stain. Forbes (J. Clin. Microbiol. **13:**807-809, 1981) has recently described a rapid, simple modification of the Leifson stain.

Staining of metachromatic granules

Various methods for staining metachromatic granules have been devised. Some are preferred to others. We have found that two stains yield highly satisfactory results. One of these is the methylene blue stain, and the other is Albert's stain (see Fig. 26-1). Both procedures are outlined in Chapter 43.

Spore stain

Spores are relatively resistant to physical and chemical agents and are not easily stained. In routine staining procedures, such as the Gram stain, they may appear as unstained refractile bodies. Heat is usually required during a special procedure for staining to promote penetration of the stain into the spores. Spores may be detected by darkfield examination.

The Dorner method or a modification thereof gives good results. The procedure is given in Chapter 43.

Relief staining

Relief staining does not stain microbial cells but produces an opaque or darkened background against which the cells stand out in sharp relief as white or light objects. It simulates darkfield microscopy and allows a rapid study of morphology.

Staining of spirochetes

On the whole, spirochetes have a poor affinity for the standard dyes and usually require special stains, such as the silver impregnation method. The Fontana stain usually gives good results. The procedure may be found in standard texts.

Staining of rickettsiae

Although rickettsiae are gram negative, they do not respond well to the Gram stain and are more successfully stained by the Giemsa or Castañeda method. These procedures are found in Chapter 43.

Staining of yeasts and fungi

Fixed smears of yeast can be stained quite readily with crystal violet or methylene blue when these dyes are applied for 30 to 60 seconds or by Gram's method. Wet mounts of yeast can be stained effectively with methylene blue or Gram's iodine. Cells can be emulsified in a drop of either stain and covered with a coverglass. Alternatively, a loopful or small drop of the dye may be placed at the edge of the coverglass covering an unstained suspension (wet mount), and the dye will spread rapidly beneath it. Lactophenol cotton blue is excellent for staining fungi. The procedure is described in Chapter 43.

MOUNTING OF STAINED SMEARS

Microbiologists often want to develop or add to a slide collection for reference and teaching purposes as well as for demonstrations. For such purposes, permanent slides may be prepared by a relatively simple procedure.

If a slide has been examined under oil, blot it with bibulous paper (**do not wipe**), and place a drop of Canada balsam or Permount on a desirable area of the smear. Place a clean coverglass carefully over this to avoid trapping air bubbles. With the butt end of an inoculating loop or needle press on the coverglass to force the mounting material to the sides of the coverglass to completely cover the area beneath.

Place the slides in a horizontal position away from dust to permit proper setting of the balsam. When the slides are completely dry, wipe away excess dye with cheesecloth dampened with xylene and cut away excess balsam with a razor blade. Some persons prefer to add a border of nail polish or other appropriate substance to the coverglass as a protective device. Most permanently mounted slides will last for years without deterioraton.

REFERENCES

1. Gregersen, T.: Rapid method for distinction of Gram-negative from Gram-positive bacteria, Eur. J. Appl. Microbiol. Biotechnol. **5:**123-127, 1978.
2. Salton, M.R.J.: The bacterial cell wall, Amsterdam, 1964, Elsevier Press, Inc.
3. Vestal, A.L.: Procedures for the isolation and identification of mycobacteria, DHEW Pub. No. 75-8230, Atlanta, 1975, Center for Disease Control.
4. West, M., Burdash, N.M., and Freimuth, F.: Simplified silverplating stain for flagella, J. Clin. Microbiol. **6:**414-419, 1977.

4 METHODS OF OBTAINING PURE CULTURES

The importance of **pure cultures** cannot be overemphasized in diagnostic microbiology. They are essential to the accurate determination of colony characteristics, biochemical properties, morphology, staining reaction, immunologic reactions, and susceptibility to antimicrobial agents.

In general, pure cultures are best obtained by using solid media, either in streak plates or in pour plates. Both methods are useful, and each has certain advantages.

STREAK PLATE METHODS

The streak plate method, if properly performed, is probably the most practical and most useful for obtaining discrete colonies and pure cultures. Streaking methods may vary from one laboratory to another, but the following techniques may be used for inoculating any type of agar plate. These plates may be prepared in advance in any desired quantity and stored at room temperature or refrigerated until the time of inoculation. The agar surface should be free of beads of condensation before the streaking is done. One can dry the plate by inverting it and propping it on the lid (Fig. 4-1, *A*).

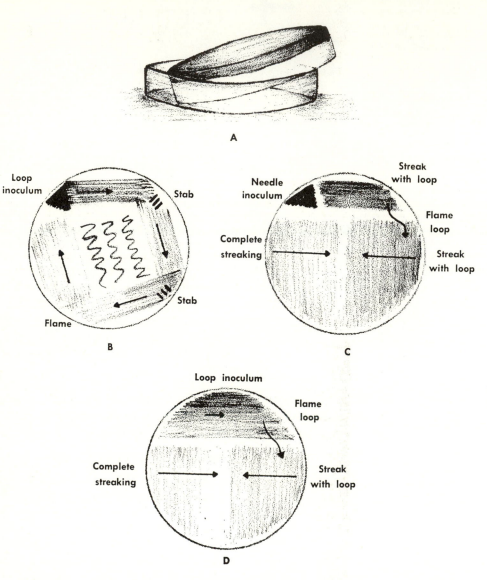

FIG. 4-1
Streak plate technique. **A,** Drying an agar plate in the laboratory. **B,** Method 1. **C,** Method 2.
D, Method 3.

Method 1

Method 1 (Figs. 4-1, *B*, and 4-2), although designed for transfers from broth cultures, may also be used for cultures from agar plates or agar slants. Should either of the latter be used, a reduced amount of inoculum is recommended, and the overlapping should be moderated.

1. Place a loopful of the inoculum near the periphery of the plate as indicated.
2. With the loop spread the inoculum over the top quarter of the plate's surface.
3. Stab the loop into the agar several times and continue streaking, overlapping the previous streak as shown.
4. Stab the loop as before and continue streaking.
5. Flame the loop, allow it to cool, overlap the previous streak, and complete the streaking.
6. Lift the loop, and streak the center of the plate with zigzag motions.

Discrete colonies should be found in the central portion of the plate, whereas additional information on hemolytic activity may be gained from the effect of a reduced oxygen tension on the organisms **stabbed** into the agar. For example, beta-hemolytic streptococci may appear to be alpha hemolytic on the surface.

Method 2

The second method of streaking (Fig. 4-1, *C*) may be used either for cultures growing on solid media (colonies or growth on slants) or for heavy broth cultures. The technique is primarily designed, however, for the former.

1. Select the desired colony from a crowded plate or pick up growth from a slant with a needle. Streak this carefully on a restricted area of the plate as indicated. Flame the needle and put it away.
2. With a sterile, cool loop make one light sweep through the needle-inoculated area

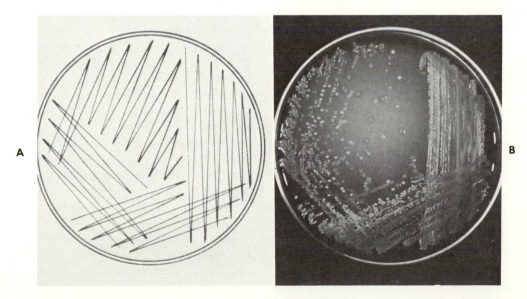

A   B

FIG. 4-2
A, Diagram of procedure for streaking to obtain well-isolated colonies. **B,** Mixed flora separated by technique illustrated in **A.**

and streak the top quarter of the plate's surface with close parallel strokes. Flame the loop and **allow it to cool.**

3. Turn the plate at right angles, make one light sweep with the loop through the lower portion of the second streaked area, and streak, as before, approximately one half of the remaining portion. Do not overlap any of the previously streaked areas.

4. Turn the plate 180 degrees and streak the remainder of the plate with the same loop, avoiding any areas previously streaked.

5. Discrete colonies should appear in the lower portions of the plate.

Method 3

Method 3 (Fig. 4-1, *D*) is the simplest technique and is used largely for broth cultures, but it may also be used for cultures from solid media.

1. Place a loopful of the inoculum near the periphery of the plate and cover approximately one fourth of the plate with close parallel streaks. Flame the loop and allow it to cool.

2. Make one light sweep through the lower portion of this streaked area, turn the plate at right angles, and streak approximately one half of the remaining portion without overlapping previous streaks.

3. Turn the plate 180° and streak the remainder of the plate, avoiding previously streaked areas.

4. The appearance of this plate will resemble that obtained in method 2.

An automated agar plate streaker was found to produce well-separated colonies and to permit accurate colony counts.[2]

POUR PLATE METHODS

Pour plates are generally used in the laboratory as a means of determining the approximate number of viable organisms in a liquid such as water, milk, urine, or broth culture, and data are expressed as the number of **colony-forming units** per milliliter of the substance examined. Pour plates are also used to determine the hemolytic activity of deep colonies of bacteria, such as the streptococci, by using an agar medium containing blood. The pour plate also lends itself to pure culture study when the components of a mixed culture are to be separated. Differences are recognized by size, shape, and color of the colonies.

The pour plate method consists of the preparation of serial dilutions of the specimen in sterile water or other diluent, from which a prescribed volume may be pipetted into tubes of melted agar medium or directly into sterile Petri dishes. The former are then poured into Petri dishes and allowed to set, whereas melted agar medium is added to the latter. After a suitable incubation period, the colonies (surface or subsurface) may be examined for differences in morphology or counted, depending on the exercise. The melted agar medium used should **not** exceed 50 C, and the dilutions should be adequately mixed with the medium. Additional tests on isolates may be carried out as desired.

The usefulness of the pour plate depends to a great extent on the number of colonies developing on the plate. This is particularly important when one is studying organisms for their hemolytic activity or when colonial characteristics aid in the separation of various types. The greatest accuracy in counting is obtained with plates that contain between 30 and 300 colonies. Above this number, counting is difficult, differential characteristics are not readily distinguishable, and colony selection without contamination is almost impossible.

A procedure that may be followed in counting overcrowded plates to estimate numbers present involves the use of a **counting plate.** The agar plate may be placed on the counting plate, which is ruled off in square centimeters. In this way, five or more representative square-centimeter areas may be counted, the average count can be calculated, and this figure then can be multiplied by 62.5 to give the estimated number of colonies per plate. The average Petri dish (inside diameter, 90 mm) has an area of 62.5 sq cm.

If a specimen is suspected of containing a large number of organisms (more than several organisms per microscopic field), an overcrowded pour plate may be avoided by using the following procedure, which is recommended for hemolytic streptococci:

1. Inoculate 8 to 10 ml of broth, sterile buffered saline, or water with one loopful of the original material and mix well.
2. Transfer one loopful of this dilution to a tube of melted agar at about 45 C.
3. Using a sterile pipet, add about 0.5 to 1 ml of sterile defibrinated blood to the inoculated tube, and twirl it between the palms of the hands to thoroughly mix the contents; then pour into a sterile Petri dish. Alternatively, the medium and inoculum may be combined and poured into the dish containing blood, and the entire contents can be mixed by rotating the plate with the lid in place.
4. Allow the medium to gel, then incubate the plate in an inverted position (lid on bottom). This prevents collection of condensation on the agar surface. Unless the surface is dry, it will be difficult to obtain discrete surface colonies.

USE OF ENRICHMENT MEDIA

In the examination of fecal material for the presence of pathogenic bacteria, it is frequently necessary to use an **enrichment** medium (to be differentiated from an enriched medium, which contains a nutritive supplement). These media, because of their chemical composition, inhibit or kill the normal intestinal flora, such as the coliforms (commensals), and permit salmonellae and some shigellae, which may be present only in small numbers, to grow almost unrestricted, thus enriching the population of such forms. After incubation, subcultures from these media must be made to solid plating media to obtain isolated colonies for further study. Tetrathionate broth and selenite broth are examples of enrichment media and are used primarily in enteric bacteriology.

USE OF DIFFERENTIAL AND SELECTIVE MEDIA

Differential media, by virtue of their chemical compositions, characterize certain bacterial genera by their distinctive colonial appearances in culture. Differential media, such as eosin–methylene blue (EMB) agar and MacConkey agar, contain lactose and a dye or indicator in the decolorized state. Bacteria that ferment the lactose with the production of acid or aldehyde produce red colonies or colonies with a metallic sheen, depending on the medium. This distinguishes lactose-fermenting from lactose-nonfermenting organisms.

Selective media are complex plating media that may also serve to differentiate among certain genera but in addition are highly selective in their action on other organisms. Such media as Salmonella-Shigella agar, deoxycholate-citrate agar, and bismuth sulfite agar will inhibit the growth of the majority of coliform bacilli, along with many strains of *Proteus* (those that develop are prevented from swarming), and permit selective isolation of enteric pathogens. The coliform colonies that do develop are readily differentiated from lactose-nonfermenting organisms by color and opacity.

Phenylethyl alcohol blood agar is a selective medium for the isolation of gram-positive cocci in specimens or cultures contaminated with gram-negative organisms, particularly *Proteus* species. Although many gram-negative rods form visible colonies on this medium, spreading or swarming does not occur.* Colonies of gram-positive cocci produced on this medium are similar to those produced on ordinary media, whereas the gram-negative organisms that do

---

*Swarming may also be inhibited by increasing the agar content of the medium to 5%.

grow produce very small colonies. To avoid contamination when selecting colonies, only those that are well separated from the small forms should be used.

Infusion agar containing potassium tellurite and either serum or blood may be used as a selective plating medium for the isolation of members of the genus *Corynebacterium*, particularly in the laboratory diagnosis of diphtheria. On this medium staphylococci and streptococci are usually inhibited.

Pathogenic staphylococci that do develop appear as black colonies on tellurite medium and as golden yellow colonies with yellow halos on mannitol salt agar, a medium containing a high salt concentration (see Chapter 16).

USE OF MEDIA CONTAINING ANTIBIOTICS

Media containing antibiotics are selectively inhibitory and may be effectively used for isolating pathogenic species from a mixed population. Sabouraud dextrose (SAB) agar containing cycloheximide and chloramphenicol supports the growth of dermatophytes and most fungi causing systemic mycoses, although it greatly inhibits the majority of saprophytic fungi and bacteria found in clinical specimens.

An enriched chocolate agar medium containing vancomycin, colistin, nystatin, and trimethoprim lactate has proved effective for the selective isolation of pathogenic *Neisseria* from clinical material.* The antibiotics suppress saprophytic neisseriae, many gram-positive and gram-negative bacteria, and yeast.

OTHER METHODS

The isolation of species of the genus *Clostridium* from clinical material is frequently complicated by the presence of rapidly growing facultative organisms, such as coliforms, *Pseudomo-*

*Modified Thayer-Martin selective medium, Difco Laboratories, Detroit; Baltimore Biological Laboratory, Cockeysville, Md.; Gibco Diagnostics, Madison, Wisc.

nas species, and spreading *Proteus* species. Anaerobic blood agar plates may be overgrown by these organisms, and the isolation of clostridia becomes a difficult task. If the anaerobe produces spores in thioglycollate medium (used in the primary culturing of wound specimens), the heat resistance of these spores ("heat shock" method) may be utilized in the following manner:

1. Inoculate a fresh tube of thioglycollate medium with 0.1 ml of the original culture or specimen containing the suspected species of *Clostridium*.
2. Heat this tube at approximately 80 C for 10 to 15 minutes. This will kill all vegetative forms but will not destroy spores, if present.
3. Incubate the heated culture and an unheated control tube for 24 to 48 hours.
4. Examine daily by making Gram-stained smears; if gram-positive bacilli are found, proceed to step 5.
5. Subculture to two blood agar plates, incubating one aerobically and one anaerobically.

Clostridium perfringens rarely can be recovered successfully by this heating procedure, however, since it fails to sporulate in most media. A method that will aid in the successful isolation of this organism from mixed cultures is as follows:

1. Incubate the thioglycollate medium containing the original mixed culture for a minimum of 48 to 72 hours.
2. Streak several blood agar plates serially from this culture and incubate aerobically and anaerobically.
3. It will be found occasionally that the plates are overgrown with gram-negative organisms. In most cases, however, these will be fewer in number, and isolated colonies of suspected *C. perfringens* will be readily obtained.
4. Transfer such colonies to tubes of thioglycollate medium for subsequent pure-culture study.

Other methods for the isolation of pure cultures, based on physical and chemical alterations, may be used. For example, variation of incubation temperatures, changes in the relative acidity or alkalinity of the medium, or variations in oxygen tension or gas concentration may be employed for the isolation of specific microorganisms. Indeed, in attempting to isolate offending food-poisoning organisms, it may take several of these methods to recover the responsible agent from a food product. Isolation of certain pathogenic bacteria from clinical material frequently may be accomplished more readily by animal inoculation. The techniques of these various methods are more fully described in subsequent chapters. For further information, however, the reader may consult reference 1.

REFERENCES

1. Lennette, E.H., Balows, A., Hausler, W.J., Jr., and Truant, J.P., editors: Manual of clinical microbiology, ed. 3, Washington D.C., 1980, American Society for Microbiology.
2. Tilton, R.C., and Ryan, R.W.: Evaluation of an automated agar plate streaker, J. Clin. Microbiol. 7:298-304, 1978.

PART II RECOMMENDED PROCEDURES WITH CLINICAL SPECIMENS

5 PHILOSOPHY AND GENERAL APPROACH TO CLINICAL SPECIMENS

REJECTION OF SPECIMENS

It is important that criteria be set up for specimen rejection; such criteria are indicated in appropriate places in this book. However, it is an important rule to always talk to the requesting physicians **before** rejecting specimens, since they are primarily responsible for the patients' welfare. They need support and advice. They may know or think they know that an unorthodox specimen may provide useful information. If this is not the case, the microbiologist must explain why it is not and must work with physicians to resolve the dilemma.

Frequently it is necessary and important to do the best possible job on a less than optimal specimen. It may be necessary to educate the clinician, and the best way to do this is to review individual specimens in a friendly and cooperative manner.

EXTENT OF IDENTIFICATION REQUIRED

We lean heavily toward **definitive** identification. For example, speciation of the *Bacteroides fragilis* group may be useful. *B. fragilis* and *B.*

thetaiotaomicron are frequently found as pathogens, whereas recovery of *B. ovatus* may mean contamination of a specimen with normal bowel flora (or, in a blood culture, transient incidental bacteremia).

An outbreak of infantile diarrhea of serious proportion persisted for many months in a large general hospital in the southwestern United States because stool cultures did not reveal any pathogens. Until the *Escherichia coli* isolates were tested for enterotoxin production and found to be positive, all therapeutic and control measures attempted proved futile. Definitive identification of the unusual blood culture isolates from a number of outbreaks—and these were not really recognized initially as outbreaks—finally permitted determination that commercial intravenous fluid bottles were contaminated; this led to definitive control measures.[3] Many cases of bacteremia and many outbreaks across the country were attributable to this source.

Identification of a clostridial blood culture isolate as *Clostridium septicum* will alert the clinician to the possibility of malignancy in a patient because of the strong association between these two events.[1] In a patient without underlying serious disease who is not receiving any antineoplastic or corticosteroid therapy, identification of an *Aspergillus* as *A. fumigatus* makes it more likely to be a clinically significant isolate than if it were another species. Identification of an organism suspected initially of being *B. fragilis* in a patient with bacteremia of unknown source as actually being a *B. splanchnicus* could indicate that the source is probably in the gastrointestinal tract, whereas if it were *B. fragilis* it might also be in the genital tract or even another site.

Precise identification of organisms from a patient with two distinct episodes of infection at an interval of some months might permit establishing that the second infection represents a recurrence rather than a new infection, or it might permit excluding that possibility. Recurrent infection may suggest a foreign body or an abscess from prior surgery; in the absence of prior surgery, it suggests the possibility of malignancy or other underlying process. Definitive identification of an atypical mycobacterium may permit more accurate assessment as to whether the organism is truly involved in the disease, what the source might be, its drug susceptibility pattern, and the likelihood of its responding to the therapeutic regimen chosen.

In the case of certain organisms, especially the anaerobes, incomplete identification may lead to very serious errors in identification, since the anaerobes defy all the usual rules. Things that we learn in our first course of microbiology—that certain organisms produce spores, that some are gram positive and some are gram negative, and so on—do not necessarily help with the anaerobes. It may be very difficult to demonstrate spores in sporulating anaerobes. Gram-positive anaerobes are very commonly decolorized and may appear gram negative, even early in the course of growth. Cocci may be mistaken for bacilli, or, more commonly, bacilli may be mistaken for cocci. It may even be difficult to define what an anaerobe actually is, considering that certain organisms, such as some clostridia (aerotolerant), are capable of relatively good growth under aerobic conditions. There are several outstanding examples in the literature of serious errors of this type in identification. For example, *B. melaninogenicus* has been incorrectly reported as being an anaerobic gram-positive streptococcus, and even such a great anaerobist as Prévot mistakenly classified as a *Fusobacterium* (*F. biacutum*) an organism subsequently shown to be gram positive and a *Clostridium*. Determination of the specific species of a group D *Streptococcus* (e.g., *S. bovis* as opposed to *S. faecalis*)[2] may permit the use of less toxic and less expensive therapeutic remedies. Organisms as diverse as *Listeria monocytogenes* and *Actinomyces viscosus* have been incorrectly identified as diphtheroids (even in reports in the literature) when shortcuts were taken.

Careful bacteriologic studies permit us to define the role of various organisms in different infectious processes, the prognosis associated with these, and so forth. Finally, definitive identification is important in educating clinicians as to the role of various organisms in infectious processes and, perhaps most important, prevents deterioration of the skills and interest of the microbiologist.

At the same time, certain shortcuts and use of limited identification procedures in certain cases is necessary in most clinical laboratories. Careful application of knowledge of the significance of various organisms in these situations and thoughtful use of limited approaches will keep expenses in line and keep the laboratory's workload manageable, while providing for optimum patient care.

QUANTITATION OF RESULTS

The concept of **quantitation** has not been adequately stressed in microbiology except in the case of urine cultures. Quantitation is useful in other situations as well. It may help to distinguish between an organism present as a "contaminant" and an organism actively involved in infection. It is often useful in determining the relative importance of different organisms recovered from mixed infections. Ordinarily, formal quantitation by dilution procedure or even by means of a quantitative loop is not necessary or desirable. Numbers of organisms present can be graded as "many" ("heavy growth"), "moderate numbers," or "few" ("light growth") on the basis of Gram stain appearance and the amount of growth on a plate. For example, does a given colony type extend to the secondary streak, tertiary streak, and so on? The Gram stain is important because differences in amount of growth or rate of growth of different organisms may be related to the fastidiousness of the organism.

EXPEDITING RESULTS

The need for **speed** in identification and susceptibility testing is another crucial area that has been neglected. Few diseases are as dynamic and rapid acting as the infectious diseases. In certain serious infections, such as bacteremia, endocarditis, meningitis, and certain pneumonias, delay of a few hours (or even less in more critical cases) in providing proper therapy may lead to death. It is not always feasible or safe to try to cover all possible types of infecting organisms with antimicrobial therapy. Clearly, the clinician must use this type of empirical approach initially, but the microbiologist must be prepared to assist in choosing a rational approach through knowledge of the role of various organisms in different disease processes and through interpretation of direct smears. In such cases the microbiologist should offer something more than routine daily inspection and subculture so that any necessary or desirable modification of therapy can be made as soon as possible; of course, the clinician must communicate with the laboratory about problem cases. Cultures can be examined at 6- to 12-hour intervals, and the processing can be speeded up considerably for selected cases. Aside from lowering mortality and morbidity, rapid provision of data may shorten hospitalization and thus save money for the patient or the hospital. It may help avoid a surgical procedure.

A limited number of organisms are responsible for the majority of infections. Simple procedures (e.g., Gram stain, colony morphology, catalase, coagulase, bile solubility, oxidase, spot indole, and rapid susceptibility tests) often may provide accurate presumptive identification quickly. Automated rapid procedures can be very helpful.

Somewhat related to this point is the necessity for round-the-clock coverage. Patients do develop pneumonia on Saturdays and Sundays, and they do go into septic shock after 5 PM and even between midnight and 7 AM. In one manner or another, **reliable** (and we emphasize reliable, because many times emergency laboratory technicians know little or no bacteriology) bacteriology must be available at all times. This includes setting up cultures, inspecting cultures set up earlier, and interpreting direct smears. A qualified microbiologist might be on call for problems encountered by the emergency laboratory crew. If available, infectious disease house officers may be able to set up certain special cultures, interpret Gram stains, and so forth.

In conclusion, we acknowledge that the ideal approach to microbiology can and should be modified according to circumstances. A large teaching hospital or clinic will need to do more, and should do more, than is done in smaller hospitals. In a very small community hospital, the services of a qualified consulting microbiologist should be sought. More must be done for the seriously ill patient, and it must be done as quickly as possible. Every patient has the right to optimal medical care, and therefore every hospital either must have all the necessary capabilities or must have access to them and must know when and how to refer specimens or cultures.

INTERACTION WITH THE CLINICIAN

Clinicians, like microbiologists, are human and vary considerably in intelligence, knowledge, character, conscientiousness, personality, and manners. Both clinicians and microbiologists should keep in mind that their primary purpose is to see that the patient is effectively treated. This will be best accomplished by wholehearted collaboration. Unfortunately, some clinicians—like some microbiologists—may be unreasonable at times. As with other interpersonal dealings in life, this may best be handled by a calm, patient, and pleasant attitude on the part of the one "under fire," demonstration of detailed knowledge of the microbiologic features of the case, and expression of a sincere interest in the problem and the patient's welfare. Demand by the physician for inappropriate cultures can often be countered by an explanation of why they would not be helpful (or perhaps might be misleading) and provision of key references from recent literature. In the final analysis, however, it must be remembered that the physician has the primary responsibility for the patient.

The microbiologist is in a position to provide invaluable service to the physician. This includes information on types of specimens that would be most helpful in a given situation, how to collect and transport them, what elements of the normal flora may be encountered, and whether they may be pathogenic under particular circumstances. Also important are interpretation of culture results, likely susceptibility patterns of isolates, and educational services not related to a specific patient.

In communicating with the physician, the microbiologist can avoid confusion and misunderstanding by not using jargon or abbreviations and by providing reports with clear-cut conclusions. Do not assume that the clinician is fully familiar with laboratory procedures or the latest taxonomic schemes. When feasible, provide interpretation on the written report, along with the specific results. However, **never provide only your interpretation** without the actual bacteriologic data (e.g., "Only normal flora isolated").

Monthly newsletters may be used to supplement laboratory manuals in order to provide physicians with such material as details of your procedures, new nomenclature, and changes in usual susceptibility patterns of given organisms in your hospital's setting.

REFERENCES

1. Alpern, R.J., and Dowell, V.R., Jr.: *Clostridium septicum* infections and malignancy, J.A.M.A. **209:**385-388, 1969.
2. Facklam, R.R.: Streptococci and aerococci. In Lennette, E.H., Balows, A., Hausler, W.J., Jr., and Truant, J.P., editors: Manual of clinical microbiology, ed. 3, Washington, D.C., 1980, American Society for Microbiology.
3. Maki, D.G., Rhame, F.S., Goldmann, D.A., and Mandell, G.L.: The infection hazard posed by contaminated intravenous infusion fluid. In Sonnenwirth, A.C., editor: Bacteremia: laboratory and clinical aspects, Springfield, Ill., 1973, Charles C Thomas, Publisher.
4. Neu, H.C.: What should the clinician expect from the microbiology laboratory? Ann. Intern. Med. **89**(Part 2):781-784, 1978.

6 COLLECTION AND TRANSPORT OF SPECIMENS FOR MICROBIOLOGIC EXAMINATION

COLLECTION PROCEDURES

Generally, a report from the bacteriologic laboratory can indicate only what has been found by microscopic and cultural examination. An etiologic diagnosis is thus confirmed or denied. Failure to isolate the causative organism, however, is not necessarily the fault of inadequate technical methods; it is frequently the result of faulty collecting or transport technique. In a busy hospital the collection of specimens is too often relegated to persons who do not understand the requirements and consequences of such procedures. The microbiologist may also deserve criticism on occasion for neglecting to provide adequate supplies or proper instructions, which may result in poorly collected samples. The following are **general considerations** regarding the collection of material for culture. Specific instructions for the handling of a variety of specimens are given in subsequent chapters.

Whenever possible, specimens should be obtained **before antimicrobial agents have been administered.** Often a purulent CSF reveals no bacterial pathogens on smear or culture when an antibiotic has been given within the previous 24 hours. A patient with salmonellosis may have a negative stool culture if the specimen has been collected while he or she was receiving suppressive antibacterial therapy, only to reveal a positive culture several days after therapy has been terminated. If the culture has been taken after initiation of antibacterial therapy, the laboratory should be informed so that specific counteractive measures, such as adding penicillinase or merely diluting the specimen, may be carried out.

It is axiomatic that material should be collected where the suspected organism is **most likely to be found, with as little external contamination as possible.** The skin and all mucosal surfaces are populated with an indigenous flora and may often also acquire a transient flora or even become colonized for extended periods with potential pathogens from the hospital environment. The latter is particularly true of individuals who are quite ill, especially if they are receiving antimicrobial therapy (resistant organisms colonize as normal flora is suppressed). Accordingly, special procedures must be employed to help distinguish between organisms involved in an infectious process and those representing normal flora or "abnormal" colonizers that are not actually causing infection. Four major approaches are utilized to resolve this problem.[8]

1. Cleanse the area with a disinfectant, using enough friction for mechanical cleansing as well. Start centrally and go out in ever enlarging circles. Repeat this several times, using a new swab each time. Alcohol (70%) is satisfactory for skin, but a full 2 minutes of wet contact time is needed. Iodine (2%) and povidone-iodine work more quickly and are effective against spore-forming organisms.
2. Bypass areas of normal flora entirely (e.g., percutaneous transtracheal aspiration rather than coughed sputum).
3. Culture only for a specific pathogen (e.g., group A streptococci in the throat).

4. Quantitate culture results as a means of determining the likelihood of organisms being involved in infection (e.g., quantitative urine culture). Less formal quantitation may also be satisfactory and should **routinely** be used; this may involve grading on a scale of 4+ to 1+, or simply heavy growth, moderate growth, light growth, four colonies, and so forth.

Another factor contributing to the successful isolation of the causative agent is the **stage of the disease** at which the specimen is collected for culture. Enteric pathogens are present in much greater numbers during the **acute,** or diarrheal, stage of intestinal infections and are more likely to be isolated at that time. Viruses responsible for causing meningoencephalitis are isolated from CSF with greater frequency when the fluid is obtained soon after the **onset** of the disease rather than when the symptoms of acute illness have subsided.

There are occasions when patients must participate actively in the collection of a specimen, such as a sputum sample. They should be given full instructions, and cooperation should be encouraged by the ward attendant. Too often a container is placed on the patient's bedside table, with the only instructions being to "spit in this cup."

Specimens should be of a **sufficient quantity** to permit complete examination and should be placed in sterile containers that preclude subsequent contamination of patient, nurse, or ward messenger. A serious danger to the laboratory worker, as well as to all others involved, is the soiled outer surface of a sputum container, a leaking stool sample, or possible contact with blood-containing exudates. The hazard of spreading disease by inadequately trained nonprofessional workers is frequently overlooked. Its control requires continued education and constant vigilance by those in responsible and supervisory positions.

Provision must be made for the **prompt delivery** of specimens to the laboratory if the results of analysis are to be valid. It is difficult, for example, to isolate *Shigella* from a fecal specimen that has remained on the hospital ward too long, permitting overgrowth by commensal organisms and an increasing death rate of the shigellae. In some instances it may be necessary to take culture media and other equipment to the patient's bedside to ensure prompt inoculation of the specimen. This is an unusual circumstance and requires prior arrangements with the laboratory.

Although not a function of specimen collection, it is an essential prerequisite that the **laboratory be given sufficient clinical information** to guide the microbiologist in selection of suitable media and appropriate techniques. Likewise, it is important for the clinician to appreciate the **limitations and potentials** of the bacteriology laboratory and to realize that a negative report does not necessarily invalidate the diagnosis. It is essential that close cooperation and frequent consultation among the clinician, nurse, and microbiologist be the rule rather than the exception.

SPECIMEN CONTAINERS AND THEIR TRANSPORT

In the microbiologic examination of clinical specimens it is essential that the container bearing the specimen does not contribute its own microbial flora. Furthermore, the original flora should neither multiply nor decrease because of prolonged standing on the ward or prolonged refrigeration in the laboratory. In other words, **a sterile container should be used and the specimen should be plated as soon as possible.** Although these are not hard-and-fast rules, any deviation should be the responsibility of the microbiologist.

A variety of containers* have been devised for collecting bacteriologic specimens. Many of these can be used repeatedly after proper sterilization and cleaning, whereas others must be incinerated after use. Apart from the sterile Pyrex Petri dish and its modern counterpart, the

presterilized and disposable plastic dish, the most used (but not necessarily the most desirable) piece of collecting equipment is the cotton–, calcium alginate–, or polyester–tipped wooden applicator stick. These swabs are best prepared by autoclaving the wooden applicator sticks in Sorensen buffer, pH 7.2, for 5 minutes, drying them, and then tipping them with polyester batting,* calcium alginate,† or long-fibered medicinal cotton. One combination packaged as a sterile outfit consists of a Pyrex tube (20×150 mm), either cotton plugged or with a stainless steel or disposable plastic cap,‡ containing the applicator stick, and a small tube (10×75 mm) with several drops of a transport broth (not needed with a polyester tip). This may be used for the collection of material from the throat, nose, eye, ear, wound and operative sites, urogenital orifices, and the rectum, but it is not recommended for optimal recovery of anaerobes (see below). The swab, inoculated with material from the patient, is placed in the inner broth tube to prevent drying out, and the whole outfit is properly labeled and promptly sent to the laboratory.

Another approach uses a sterile disposable culture unit (Culturette)§ consisting of a plastic tube containing a sterile polyester-tipped swab and a small glass ampule of modified[1] Stuart's holding medium. The unit is removed from its sterile envelope, and the swab is used to collect the specimen. It is then returned to the tube, the ampule is crushed, and the swab is forced into the released holding medium. This will provide sufficient moisture for storage up to 72 hours at room temperature.

Some cotton used for applicators may contain fatty acids that may be detrimental to microbial growth.[9] An excellent substitute is calcium algi-

---

*Falcon Plastics, Oxnard, Calif.

*Dacron polyester filling, ½-pound bags, Sears, Roebuck and Co.
†Colab Laboratories, Inc., Chicago Heights, Ill.
‡Morton culture tube closure from Scientific Products, Division of American Hospital Supply Corp., Evanston, Ill.
§Scientific Products, Division of American Hospital Supply Corp., Evanston, Ill.

nate wool, derived from alginic acid, a natural plant product.[5] This silky-fibered material dissolves in certain solutions that are compatible with bacterial preservation (such as dilute Ringer's solution with sodium hexametaphosphate) to form a soluble sodium alginate. Calcium alginate–tipped wooden applicators or flexible aluminum nasopharyngeal swabs, as well as the citrate or hexametaphosphate diluents, are available commercially. Calcium alginate should not be used where herpesvirus is anticipated, as it may inhibit replication of this virus.

A modification of the cotton applicator uses 28-gauge Nichrome or thin aluminum wire in place of the wooden stick. Because of its flexibility, the wire applicator is recommended for collecting specimens from the nasopharynx. To ensure that the small amount of cotton adheres to the wire during passage through the nasal tract, the end of the wire must be bent over and some collodion applied before the wrapping with cotton; otherwise, the outfit remains the same as that previously described. A commercially prepared sterile wire swab also is available.*

A variety of transport media have been devised for prolonging the survival of microorganisms when a significant delay occurs between collection and culturing. Stuart and others[11] advocated a medium that has proved effective in preserving the viability of pathogenic agents in clinical material. The medium consists of buffered semisolid agar devoid of nutrients and containing sodium thioglycollate as a reducing agent and is used in conjunction with cotton swabs. Stuart's medium† maintains a favorable pH and prevents both dehydration of secretions during transport and oxidation and enzymatic self-destruction of the pathogen present. However, the glycerophosphate present permits multiplication of certain organisms.

A report on a transport medium* by Cary and Blair[3] indicates that salmonellae and shigellae can be recovered from fecal specimens for as long as 49 days and *Vibrio cholerae* for 22 days; *Yersinia pestis* survives for at least 75 days. The medium itself remains good after storage at room temperature for longer than 1½ years.

The use of polyester-tipped swabs for delayed recovery of group A streptococci from throat cultures is discussed in Chapter 8. A report by Hosty and co-workers[6] indicates that the incorporation of a small amount of silica gel in the glass tube containing the polyester swab will further maintain the viability of group A streptococci in throat swabs for as long as 3 days before plating.

The collection of specimens for anaerobic culturing poses a special problem in that the conventional methods previously described will not lead to optimal recovery of these air-intolerant microorganisms. A crucial factor in the final success of anaerobic culturing is the transport of clinical specimens: the lethal effect of atmospheric oxygen must be nullified until the specimen has been processed anaerobically in the laboratory.[12] We recommend the use of a double-stoppered collection tube or vial, gassed out with oxygen-free CO_2 or N_2*†; one injects the specimen (pus, body fluid, or other liquid material) through the rubber stopper after first expelling all air from the syringe and needle. In the laboratory, the material is aspirated from the transport container by needle and syringe, inoculated to media, and incubated under anaerobic conditions. If only a swab specimen can be obtained, it may be collected on a swab that has been prepared in a "gassed out" tube* and can

---

*Falcon Plastics, Oxnard, Calif.
†Baltimore Biological Laboratory, Cockeysville, Md.

---

*Available commercially from Scott Laboratories, Inc., Fiskeville, R.I.; Gibco Diagnostics, Madison, Wisc.; and BBL, Cockeysville, Md.
†A convenient type of tube, stopper, and screw cap for laboratories wishing to make their own oxygen-free tubes is the Anaerobic Culture Tube, Hungate type, No. 2047-16125, available from Bellco Glass, Inc., Vineland, N.J.

then be transferred to a rubber-stoppered tube half filled with prereduced and anaerobically sterilized transport medium,* such as the Cary-Blair medium previously described.

An Anaerobic Culturette† generates its own anaerobic atmosphere and contains a small amount of transport medium to prevent drying. The Bio-Bag† offers remarkable flexibility. It is not only suitable for swabs (for short periods; no specific means are incorporated to maintain a moist environment, nor is there a holding medium), but it can also be used to transport specimens in plastic syringes and smaller specimens aspirated (through an attached syringe) into small-gauge sterile plastic tubing. It can also be used for tissue (placed first in a sterile tube or vial). Another versatile apparatus is the Vacutainer Anaerobic Transporter.‡

It is important to note that the materials recommended for anaerobic transport actually constitute ideal **universal transport setups,** since **all** types of microorganisms should survive well in them. It should be stressed that although the swab is the most widely used transport vehicle, it is preferable to submit a larger specimen whenever possible (e.g., a filled syringe or tube). When organisms may be scarce (as in some forms of tuberculosis), the larger the specimen the better. Further details on anaerobic culture techniques are given in Chapters 13 and 27.

Containers for special purposes, such as those used for the collection of 24-hour urine samples, can usually be devised from equipment found around the hospital; or they may be purchased from a surgical supply house.

Although most pathogenic microorganisms are not greatly affected by small changes in temperature, they are generally susceptible to drying out, particularly when on cotton applicator sticks. However, some bacteria, such as the meningococcus in CSF, are quite sensitive to low temperatures and require immediate culturing. On the other hand, clinical material likely to contain abundant microbial flora may in most instances be held at 5 C in a refrigerator for several hours before culturing if it cannot be processed right away. This is particularly true with such specimens as urine, feces, and sputum samples and material on swabs taken from a variety of sources, with the exception of wound cultures, which may contain oxygen-sensitive anaerobes. These should be inoculated promptly. Not only will refrigeration preserve the viability of most pathogens, it will minimize overgrowth of commensal organisms, increased numbers of which could make the isolation of a significant microbe more difficult. Objectively, however, the sooner an organism leaving the sheltered environment of its host is transferred to an appropriate artificial culture medium, the better are the chances of its survival and subsequent multiplication.

On occasion it is necessary to submit specimens to a **reference laboratory** in a distant city, thus requiring transportation by mail or express. If, for example, there is no viral diagnostic service available in the immediate area, it may be necessary to ship specimens at a low temperature to preserve their viability. This is especially true of virus-containing material, such as CSF, throat and rectal swabs, stools, and tissue, which should be refrigerated immediately and shipped in a Styrofoam box with commercial refrigerant packs (e.g., 3M Cryogel). Whole blood is **not** shipped. Rather, the serum is separated and sent in a sterile tube.

If a culture of an isolated organism is to be sent to a reference laboratory (state or public health laboratory), it is not necessary to send it in the frozen state.

In most instances microbiologic specimens can be satisfactorily shipped through the mails, provided that **special precautions** are taken

---

*Available commercially from Scott Laboratories, Inc., Fiskeville, R.I.; Gibco Diagnostics, Madison, Wisc.; and BBL, Cockeysville, Md.
†Marion Scientific Corp., Kansas City, Mo.
‡Becton-Dickinson and Co., Rutherford, N.J.

against breakage and subsequent contamination of the mailing container. According to the Code of Federal Regulations,* a viable organism or its toxin or a diagnostic specimen of a volume less than 50 ml shall be placed in a securely closed, watertight specimen container, which is enclosed in a second durable watertight container. The entire space between the containers should contain sufficient absorbent material to absorb the entire contents in case of breakage or leakage. The containers are then enclosed in an outer shipping container of corrugated fiberboard, cardboard, wood, or such. The outer container shall be labeled with the Etiologic Agents/Biomedical Material red-and-white label (available commercially) (see Chapter 33 and Fig. 33-1).

Double mailing containers must be used when the microbiologist considers the specimen to be of a hazardous nature or thinks it may constitute a definite danger to the person handling the container. This includes clinical specimens, cultures for identification, and so forth.

For the shipment of fecal specimens containing salmonellae or shigellae over long distances, the filter paper method[2] may also be employed. In collecting the specimen by this technique, fresh fecal material must be spread fairly thinly over a strip of filter paper or clean blotting paper and allowed to dry at room temperature. Using forceps, the smeared strip is then folded inward from the ends in such a way that the fecal material is covered. The folded specimen may then be inserted in a plastic envelope (polyethylene is recommended) and placed in a container to conform with postal regulations. It is possible to ship a large number of such specimens in one container through the mail. The pathogens are unaffected by this treatment, whereas the normal intestinal flora dies. On receipt at the laboratory the paper specimen may be cut into three pieces. One piece is placed in physiologic saline for suspension and direct plating, and the remaining pieces are placed in selenite and tet-

rathionate broths, respectively, for enrichment and subsequent plating.

When it is necessary to ship fecal specimens or when such specimens must be held for some time before culturing, it is recommended that they be placed in a preservative solution. The buffered glycerol-saline solution of Sachs[10] has proved satisfactory. (Its final pH should be 7.4; it should be discarded if it becomes acid.) Approximately 1 g of feces is emulsified in not more than 10 ml of preservative, and the preserved specimen is shipped in a heavy glass container (universal type) with a screw cap in the regular double mailing container just described.

A simple gelatin disk method for long-term maintenance of stock cultures and for shipping of cultures has been described by Obara and associates (J. Clin. Microbiol. **14:**61-66, 1981).

HANDLING OF SPECIMENS IN THE LABORATORY

In previous sections of this book the importance of a properly collected specimen was stressed and the responsibility of personnel in its collection was indicated. In the following section the subsequent handling of the specimen in the laboratory is considered. In addition, the responsibility of the laboratory worker is pointed out.

Since it is not always practical for many specimens to be inoculated as soon as they arrive in the laboratory, refrigeration at 4 to 6 C offers a safe and dependable method of storing many clinical samples until they can be conveniently handled. However, some may require immediate plating (such as specimens that might contain gonococci or *Bordetella pertussis*), whereas others must be immediately frozen (e.g., spinal fluid that is to be held for subsequent attempts at virus isolation).

The length of time of refrigeration varies with the type of specimen: swabs from wounds (except for anaerobic cultures), the urogenital tract, throat, and rectum and samples of feces or spu-

---

*Section 72.25 of Part 72, Title 42, amended.

tum can be refrigerated for 2 to 3 hours without appreciable loss of pathogens. Urine specimens for culture may be refrigerated at least 24 hours without affecting the bacterial flora (except the tubercle bacillus, which may be adversely affected by the urine); on the other hand, CSF from a patient with suspected meningitis should be examined **at once.**

Specimens submitted for the isolation of virus should be refrigerated immediately; if they must be held for over 24 hours, they should be frozen (at −70 C if possible). Specimens of clotted blood for virus serology may be refrigerated but never frozen.

Gastric washings and resected lung tissue submitted for culture of *Mycobacterium tuberculosis* should be processed soon after delivery, since tubercle bacilli may die rapidly in either type of specimen.

Pieces of hair or scrapings from the skin and nails submitted for the isolation of fungi may be kept at room temperature (protected from dust) for several days before inoculation. On the other hand, sputum, bronchial secretions, bone marrow, and purulent material from patients suspected of having systemic fungal infection should be inoculated to appropriate media as soon as possible, especially when the diagnosis of histoplasmosis is considered.

REFERENCES

1. Amies, C.R.: A modified formula for the preparation of Stuart's transport medium, Can. J. Public Health, **58:**296-300, 1967.
2. Bailey, W.R., and Bynoe, E.T.: The "filter paper" method for collecting and transporting stools to the laboratory for enteric bacteriological examination, Can. J. Public Health **44:**468-475, 1953.
3. Cary, S.G., and Blair, E.B.: New transport medium for shipment of clinical specimens, J. Bacteriol. **88:**96-98, 1964.
4. Forney, J.E., editor: Collection, handling, and shipment of microbiological specimens, Public Health Serv. Pub. No. 976, Washington D.C., Nov. 1968, U.S. Government Printing Office.
5. Higgins, M.: A comparison of the recovery rate of organisms from cotton-wool and calcium alginate wool swabs, Ministry Health Public Lab. Serv. Bull. 43, 1950.
6. Hosty, T.S., Johnson, M.B., Freear, M.A., Gaddy, R.E., and Hunter, F.R.: Evaluation of the efficiency of four different types of swabs in the recovery of group A streptococci, Health Lab. Sci. **1:**163-169, 1964.
7. Isenberg, H.D., Schoenknecht, F.D., von Graevenitz, A., and Rubin, S.J.: Collection and processing of bacteriological specimens, Cumitech 9, Washington, D.C., 1979, American Society for Microbiology.
8. Matsen, J.M., and Ederer, G.M.: Specimen collection and transport, Hum. Pathol. **7:**297-307, 1976.
9. Pollock, M.R.: Unsaturated fatty acids in cotton plugs, Nature **161:**853, 1948.
10. Sachs, A.: Difficulties associated with bacteriological diagnosis of bacillary dysentery, J. Roy. Army Med. Corps **73:**235-239, 1939.
11. Stuart, R.D., Tosach, S.R., and Patsula, T.M.: The problem of transport of specimens for culture of gonococci, Can. J. Public Health **45:**73-83, 1954.
12. Sutter, V.L., Citron, D.M., and Finegold, S.M.: Wadsworth anaerobic bacteriology manual, ed. 3, St. Louis, 1980, The C.V. Mosby Co.

PART III

CULTIVATION OF PATHOGENIC MICROORGANISMS FROM CLINICAL MATERIAL

7 MICROORGANISMS ENCOUNTERED IN THE BLOOD

The organisms most likely to be found in blood cultures include the following:

Staphylococci (coagulase positive, coagulase negative), micrococci
Coliform bacilli and other enteric organisms
Pseudomonas species
Alpha- and beta-hemolytic streptococci
Pneumococci
Enterococci
Haemophilus influenzae
Clostridium perfringens and related organisms
Bacteroides fragilis, other gram-negative anaerobes
Anaerobic cocci
Diphtheroid bacilli
Opportunistic fungi, such as *Candida* and *Torulopsis*
Legionella species
Neisseria meningitidis
Salmonella species
Brucella species
Francisella tularensis
Listeria monocytogenes
Streptobacillus moniliformis
Leptospira species
Campylobacter fetus and related vibrios

GENERAL CONSIDERATIONS FOR BLOOD CULTURE

Blood for culture is probably the most important single specimen submitted to the microbiology laboratory for examination. It is unique in that it helps provide a clinical diagnosis as well as a specific etiologic diagnosis. The presence of living microorganisms in the patient's blood almost always reflects active and possibly spreading infection in the tissues. The prognosis of such a bacteremia or septicemia may well depend on its prompt recognition by bacteriologic means. Subsequent initiation of specific therapy based on laboratory findings may well prove to be lifesaving. Likewise, a negative culture would prove helpful in ruling out microbial etiology.

It is important to know which infections are likely to show a positive blood culture, and thus further reading on bacteremias is recommended.[30] A **transient bacteremia** frequently occurs during the course of many diseases, including pneumococcal pneumonia, bacterial meningitis, urinary tract infection, typhoid fever, and generalized salmonella infections. Wound infec-

tions caused by a beta-hemolytic streptococcus, by *Staphylococcus aureus*, and by *Bacteroides* species, infections of the gallbladder and biliary tract, osteomyelitis, peritonitis, and puerperal sepsis may be accompanied by bacteremia, which is also a frequent concomitant of operative manipulation in chronically infected areas, as in instrumentation of the urinary tract. It is generally unrewarding, however, to attempt to isolate the causative organism by culturing the blood in cases of tetanus, diphtheria, shigellosis, or tuberculosis.

Although a mild transitory bacteremia is a frequent finding in many infectious diseases, the persistent, continuous, or recurrent type of bacteremia is more serious. When the classic syndrome of a **septicemia** (chills, fever, prostration) caused by the presence of actively multiplying bacteria and their toxins in the bloodstream is found, it is rarely difficult to isolate the causative organism. When localizing signs of infection are notably absent and a persistent positive blood culture is demonstrated, the possibility of a serious intravascular infection, such as bacterial endocarditis, must be considered.

41

In some diseases the probability of obtaining a positive blood culture depends on the **stage of the disease** at which the culture is made. For example, bacteria can be cultured from the blood during the first several days of illness in typhoid fever,* tularemia, plague, and anthrax, but the organisms disappear from the blood during the latter course of the disease. Thus, the early recovery of these bacteria from the blood is important, since it may be the only reliable means available to the clinician for making a diagnosis.

One of the more challenging systemic diseases from the clinical and bacteriologic points of view is **bacterial endocarditis.** Confirmation of the diagnosis is almost entirely dependent on isolation of an organism from the blood. Frequently, the causative bacteria are present only in small numbers.

Furthermore, isolation of the causative organism may be complicated because the patient received prior antibiotic therapy. This may not have been at a drug level high enough to eradicate the microorganism but one that, when carried over in the blood sample, may prove sufficient to inhibit growth in the blood culture bottle.† For this reason it is recommended that a **minimal dilution** of 1 volume of blood in 10 volumes of broth be made as a safeguard against such an eventuality. This dilution also aids in counteracting the bactericidal effect of normal serum. The incorporation of sodium polyanethol sulfonate (SPS) (Liquoid), a synthetic polyanionic agent, in blood culture media makes this degree of dilution unnecessary for this purpose.

Since there is usually a lag period of 1 to 2 hours between the time of entrance of the bacteria into the circulation and the subsequent chill, blood for cultures should be drawn, ideally, **shortly before** the expected temperature rise. The frequency with which blood samples are taken for culture is also important. In patients with suspected bacterial endocarditis who have not received any antibacterial agents, a total of three to four cultures taken during a 24- to 48-hour period should be adequate to establish the diagnosis in most cases, provided that techniques suitable for recovery of anaerobes and other fastidious organisms are included. In endocarditis, the bacteremia is **constant,** so blood cultures may be drawn at any time.

Austrian[8] pointed out that after appropriate antibacterial therapy it is incumbent on the attending physician to obtain negative blood cultures to document the absence of bacteremia. For patients with subacute bacterial endocarditis he recommended blood culture at the termination of therapy and again 2 weeks later, the period during which those patients who will most likely suffer a bacteriologic relapse are observed to do so. It is important to obtain follow-up blood cultures in bacteremic patients even if they become afebrile on antibacterial therapy.

In **brucellosis,** positive blood cultures are usually obtained during exacerbation of symptoms and elevation of temperature, although even during the acute phase isolation of the organism is not regularly successful.

Occasionally, culture of the **bone marrow** has yielded positive results when peripheral blood cultures have been sterile in cases of brucellosis, subacute bacterial endocarditis, histoplasmosis, and, after the first week, typhoid fever. Concurrent bacterial and fungal cultures are recommended when bone marrow biopsies are performed for other diagnostic purposes.

A still more difficult problem for the bacteriologist is the generalized infection caused by a **rarely isolated** organism that requires special methods for its isolation. The causative agents of diseases such as leptospirosis, rat-bite fever, listeriosis, and infection by pasteurellae and

---

*If the results are negative, repeat the procedure weekly for several weeks if the patient continues to be febrile.[26]
†Aberrant forms of bacteria may occur in blood cultures of patients receiving antibiotic therapy.[48]

Legionella require complex culture media, and in some instances animal injection, for their isolation. Some of these special procedures are discussed in a later section.

Blood cultures should be made **immediately** in all cases of unexplained shock, particularly in those following genito-urinary tract manipulation. A single negative blood culture should **never** be depended on to eliminate the possibility of a bacteremia, because a single specimen may be sterile even though the bloodstream as a whole is infected. A minimum of three cultures taken at half-hour intervals is recommended. In patients with **septic shock,** therapy must be begun immediately. Three separate blood cultures may be obtained, one right after another, by three separate venipunctures at different sites and with different syringes. Blood cultures should be made on all patients with **unexplained or persistent fever.** Chills and fever in patients with urinary tract infections, infected burns, soft-tissue infections, postoperative wound sepsis, or indwelling venous catheters make them candidates for having blood cultures taken. Debilitated patients who develop fever while undergoing prolonged therapy with antibiotics, corticosteroids, immunosuppressives, antimetabolites, or parenteral hyperalimentation also should have blood drawn for culture.

The diagnosis of bacteremia can be made only by growing out pathogenic agents from culture media suitably inoculated with adequate amounts of the patient's blood. In the bacteriologic examination of the blood, several important principles must be considered:

1. An acceptable blood collection technique, which minimizes chances of contamination, is mandatory.
2. Enriched **aerobic** and **anaerobic** culture media should be utilized, and conditions of incubation must provide optimal conditions for bacterial growth.
3. Results of presumptively positive findings must be reported **by telephone without delay** to the attending physician.

ROLE OF ANTICOAGULANTS AND OSMOTIC STABILIZERS IN BLOOD CULTURING

As Rosner[66] so aptly observed, the most important attribute of an effective blood culture system is its ability to support rapid growth of a wide variety of microorganisms so that their prompt recovery and identification can be accomplished.

One of these elements would be a means of preventing the blood sample from clotting in the culture bottle, since bacteria become entrapped in clotted blood.[95] Various anticoagulants have been recommended; the most effective one to date appears to be SPS. First reported by Von Haebler and Miles[82] in 1938 as a useful anticoagulant in blood culturing, it is now apparent that SPS* in a concentration of 0.03% will inhibit clotting, neutralize the bactericidal effect of human serum,[50] prevent phagocytosis,[67] and at least partially inactivate certain antibiotics, such as streptomycin, kanamycin, gentamicin, and polymyxin B.[78,80] Furthermore, SPS is stable at autoclave temperatures. It is not recommended, however, for agar pour plate cultures or membrane filter culture systems,[32] and it may be inhibitory to some strains of *Peptostreptococcus anaerobius, Neisseria meningitidis,* and *N. gonorrhoeae*. Sodium amylosulfate (SAS) is less effective in neutralizing serum bactericidal activity,[79] was no better in a clinical blood culture trial, and may be inhibitory to certain gram-negative bacilli (e.g., *K. pneumoniae*).[38]

The inhibitory effect of SPS may be neutralized by adding gelatin (1.2%) to blood culture media.[28,91]

Sodium citrate in a concentration of 0.5% to 1.0% is another anticoagulant. However, it may be inhibitory to gram-positive cocci[60] and is not recommended. Since heparin may exert antimicrobial activity, blood for culture should not be obtained through a heparin lock.[65]

---

*Available in a 5% sterile aqueous solution as Grobax from Roche Diagnostics, Nutley, N.J.

Another factor in the successful recovery of small numbers of circulating microorganisms in the blood is the use of an osmotic stabilizer, such as 10% to 30% sucrose.[67] This is especially true of gram-negative rod bacteremias in patients receiving antimicrobial therapy, where low levels of bacteria (10 colonies/ml or less) can be expected.[31] The sucrose may exert a protective effect on organisms having undergone cell wall damage (preventing osmotic pressure changes).[67] However, hypertonic media also counteract normal bactericidal mechanisms in blood. Most microorganisms with intact cell walls also grow well in enriched hypertonic media.[30] Although a number of studies found benefit in the use of hypertonic sucrose media, better results were obtained without sucrose in the case of fungi[62] and certain bacteria in studies from the Mayo Clinic.[89] It is also difficult to detect growth by macroscopic examination of blood culture bottles when hypertonic media are used.

BLOOD CULTURE PROCEDURES

When blood for culture is drawn, scrupulous care must be exercised in preparing the site for venipuncture. A 2% solution of tincture of iodine is applied to the skin over the area of the selected vein by means of several saturated cotton-tipped applicator sticks or swabs. Start centrally over the planned site of venipuncture and, exerting moderate pressure, move out in concentric circles. The iodine is allowed to dry and then is removed with sponges saturated with 80% isopropyl alcohol. The entire process is repeated, a tourniquet is applied, and 20 ml of blood is withdrawn by a sterile 21-gauge needle on a 20-ml syringe. Many hospitals use 10 ml of blood (two aliquots of 5 ml, each placed into 50 ml of medium). Since bacteremia often involves very small numbers of organisms and cultures may be negative with smaller volumes of blood, the larger blood volume is recommended. In infants and children, volumes of 1 to 5 ml are satisfactory (see the section Blood Cultures on

Newborn Infants and Pediatric Patients). The blood is transferred **immediately** to two small sterile tubes or bottles fitted with rubber stoppers and containing 3.4 ml of 0.35% SPS in sterile physiologic saline.*[27] The blood may be drawn directly into the Vacutainer tubes (this is preferable) if the possibility of backflow into the patient is avoided by keeping the arm dependent. Sterilization of these evacuated blood collection tubes is advised, since some tubes have been found to be contaminated with potential pathogens.[16,88] An alternative method that is preferable is the direct inoculation of blood into culture media at the patient's bedside, employing a transfer set or a needle and syringe. It is then mixed well and promptly transported to the laboratory, where it is immediately incubated. If it is necessary to hold the specimen for a short interval, the blood may be refrigerated for not more than 1 to 2 hours.

For culture, 10 ml of the blood (the contents of one of the Vacutainer tubes) is transferred to a bottle containing 100 ml of brain-heart infusion broth and a brain-heart infusion agar slant (biphasic)[15,63,69] medium, and the remainder is distributed in a bottle containing 100 ml of trypticase soy broth or tryptic soy broth using aseptic technique throughout. This transfer should be effected within 2 to 4 hours after obtaining the blood specimen. The biphasic medium obviates the need for routine subculture and provides increased yield of *Staphylococcus aureus* from blood cultures.[37] In one study,[36] organisms were isolated from tryptic soy broth an average of 0.4 days sooner than from trypticase soy broth. The bottles, available commercially,† should contain 10% CO_2 and a vacuum and 0.025 to 0.03% SPS. One of the two bottles (the

---

*B-D Vacutainer tube No. S3208 XF308, Becton-Dickinson and Co., Rutherford, N.J.

†Among sources of supply are BBL, Cockeysville, Md.; Becton-Dickinson and Co., Rutherford, N.J.; Case Laboratories, Chicago; Difco Laboratories, Detroit; Gibco Laboratories, Madison, Wisc.; and General Diagnostics, Morris Plains, N.J.

trypticase soy broth) may be made hypertonic with sucrose or sorbitol, if desired. After inoculation with the blood, the brain-heart infusion medium bottle is vented. The vent is removed after the vacuum has disappeared; this permits retention of the CO_2. The other (anaerobic) bottle should **not** be vented. Agar pour plates (Plates 3 and 4) may provide more rapid growth and earlier identification than are possible with broth cultures but may not be practical for routine use in the clinical laboratory. A commercially available prereduced medium* in a bottle with a gas-tight stopper proved to be no more effective for recovery of anaerobes than tryptic soy broth or thioglycollate medium.[90] Mangels and co-workers[52] found that the 50-ml PRS-peptone Vacutainer tube inoculated with 5 ml of blood recovered more anaerobes from clinical blood cultures than did either brain-heart infusion broth or Thiol broth and that anaerobes grew more rapidly in the PRS-peptone broth.

An interesting study by Beaman and associates[10] has documented the morphologic and biochemical changes occurring after inoculation of blood into a blood culture medium. Among the interesting observations was the fact that there was a decrease in oxygen pressure (Po_2) in unvented bottles from 44.4 to 8 mm Hg.

Since conventional methods for recovering microorganisms from the blood may require several days for growth and identification, a rapid method using membrane filters was introduced[93] (Fig. 7-1). This procedure proved cumbersome and time consuming and has recently been modified by lysing the blood rather than agglomerating the red cells prior to filtration.[74] This technique requires less time (5 minutes) and a smaller blood sample (10 ml), making it practical for routine clinical usage. It proved very effective in a clinical blood culture trial,[75]

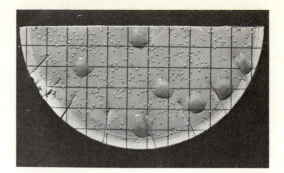

FIG. 7-1
Double bacteremia with *S. aureus* and *K. pneumoniae*. Membrane filter on EMB plate. Small colonies are *S. aureus;* large, mucoid colonies (lactose positive) are *K. pneumoniae*.

yielding distinctly more positives and quicker growth and identification as compared with broth and pour plate techniques. Unfortunately, the disposable filtering apparatus used in these studies was never marketed. Nonetheless, the procedure can be carried out with commercially available reusable apparatus. More recently, another approach that also uses SPS to block antibacterial activity of blood and a technique for lysing erythrocytes and then density gradient centrifugation has been described.[21,22] Still another lysis-filtration system transfers the filter to broth and then uses impedance detection, which can be automated.

A potentially important advance in blood culture technique has recently been introduced. The Antimicrobial Removal Device (ARD)* is a mixed resin system that removes antimicrobial agents and certain other bacterial inhibitors from whole blood.[83] Five to ten milliliters of whole blood is injected aseptically into the ARD bottle, which is then placed on a tumbler specifically designed for rotating the bottle in the appropriate manner. After 15 minutes the ARD bottle is removed from the tumbler, and the blood-saline mixture is aseptically withdrawn

*Brain-heart infusion broth supplemented (with or without Liquoid), prereduced, and anaerobically sterilized, Scott Laboratories, Fiskeville, R.I.

*Marion Laboratories, Kansas City, Mo.

and transferred to a standard blood culture broth and subsequently processed in the usual manner. A clinical evaluation of this device yielded more isolates than did conventional blood cultures and significantly earlier isolation of the agents than was possible by the conventional technique. However, in this study the ARD was compared with conventional blood culture bottles that did not contain SPS. Washington (J.A. Washington II, personal communication) studied 87 patients with bacteremia (28 of whom were receiving antimicrobial agents), comparing the ARD with conventional broth containing SPS. The ARD cultures showed no advantage, except perhaps in *Staphylococcus aureus* bacteremia, and even then the results were probably not better than could be obtained with penicillinase. Gram-negative bacilli (especially *E. coli*, *Pseudomonas*, and *Enterobacter*) were recovered more often in conventional blood cultures than in the ARD cultures.

By the use of the aforementioned techniques and media, most of the common pathogens can be readily cultivated. The latter include streptococci, staphylococci, pneumococci, meningococci, coliform bacilli, anaerobic cocci, and members of the genera *Salmonella*, *Haemophilus*, *Bacteroides*, *Clostridium*, *Acinetobacter*, *Pseudomonas*, *Alcaligenes*, and *Candida*. **Special methods** or special media are necessary for the isolation of *Legionella*, *Actinomyces*, *Brucella*, *Pasteurella*, *Leptospira*, *Listeria*, and *Spirillum*. These are described in subsequent sections.

Blood culture in patients with indwelling intravenous catheters

The problem of bacteremia secondary to indwelling intravenous catheters has been mentioned. With such patients it is common practice on removing the offending catheter to aseptically cut off the indwelling end and drop it into broth for culture. In some institutions such catheter-tip cultures are performed on removal of the catheter even if there has been no suggestion of infection. Maki and co-workers[51] pointed out that it may be difficult to distinguish among true colonization of a catheter site, seeding of the catheter from a distant infected focus, and contamination during the culturing process and that semiquantitative culture (rolling the catheter tip across a blood agar plate and counting colonies subsequently) is helpful in this situation. In cases of catheter-related sepsis, there were always 15 colonies to confluent growth; in other cases, there was no growth or only 1 to 7 colonies.

In another study[18] broth was flushed through catheters that had been removed, and it was then cultured both quantitatively and nonquantitatively. Patients with clinical evidence of bacteremia had at least 1,000 organisms on quantitative culture. *Staphylococcus epidermidis* was much more likely than more virulent organisms to colonize an insert without causing bacteremia. In a majority of patients positive cultures from catheters were from the insertion site rather than from a distant bloodstream focus. These workers found that in patients with clinical bacteremia, nonquantitative culture of the intravascular insert was adequate to incriminate it as the focus of infection for bacteremia. The question also arises in suspected catheter-associated sepsis as to whether to draw blood cultures through the catheter or by separate venipuncture. Studies of this question found a high rate of isolation of *Staphylococcus epidermidis* from catheter-drawn cultures but not from venipuncture cultures. This high rate of false-positive cultures from catheter-drawn cultures indicates that it is preferable to perform venipunctures for blood cultures. On the other hand, comparison of quantitative blood cultures drawn from a peripheral vein with those drawn through catheters may permit determination as to whether the sepsis is related to the intravenous catheter. For a patient studied by Wing and others[92] peripheral venous blood had 25 colonies/ml, whereas blood drawn through the catheter had more than 10,000 colonies/ml.

Other sources of false-positive blood cultures, in addition to contaminated evacuated blood collection tubes previously mentioned, include contaminated benzalkonium solution used for skin disinfection[46] (iodine and alcohol skin preparation avoids this problem), contaminated povidone-iodine solution, and contaminated commercial blood culture media.[57]

Quantitative cultures on blood drawn through a catheter positioned at various sites proximal and distal to heart valves (sometimes in conjunction with dye dilution studies, angiography, and so forth) may permit distinction between bacteremia from a peripheral source and endocarditis and may permit determination of the infected site within the heart in the case of endocarditis;[59] however, this procedure is very difficult technically.

Incubation and examination of cultures

Blood cultures are incubated aerobically at 35 C (except where otherwise indicated) and are examined daily throughout the first week (more frequently when the laboratory is informed that the patient is seriously ill and a specific etiologic diagnosis has not yet been made) for evidence of growth. In the case of biphasic blood culture bottles, the bottles should be tipped daily so as to flow the blood-broth mixture over the surface of the agar slant. When a culture is **positive,** the **broth** may assume one of several appearances. In one type of growth, characteristic of gram-negative rods, the medium above the red cell layer becomes uniformly turbid, and gas bubbles caused by fermentation of glucose may be present. When pneumococci or meningococci are present, a similar although less distinct turbidity is produced, usually accompanied by a greenish tint in the medium. Streptococci grow as "cotton ball" colonies on top of the sedimented red cells, whereas the upper layer of broth may remain clear. This commonly occurs in blood cultures from patients with subacute bacterial endocarditis caused by alpha-hemolytic streptococci. If beta-hemolytic streptococci or other hemolytic organisms are present, marked hemolysis of the blood may be observed, along with turbidity. Pathogenic species of staphylococci will grow out readily and may produce a large jellylike coagulum throughout the broth because of coagulase production. Grossly visible discrete *Staphylococcus* colonies will also develop in the medium and impart turbidity or appear as balls on the surface of the red cell sediment (Plate 7). If the culture is contaminated with *Bacillus* species or a saprophytic fungus, the broth becomes hemolyzed, and a fairly thick pellicle forms on its surface. *Clostridium* species may produce marked hemolysis, an unpleasant odor, and gas under pressure. *Bacteroides* species produce less gas, but a foul odor. Growth of *Haemophilus* does not generally produce any change in the medium and may be detected **only** by subculturing to chocolate agar.

In an **agar slant** (biphasic) bottle, bacterial growth generally appears either as large or small discrete colonies or as confluent growth on the slant, with cloudiness in the broth. Colonies of pneumococci are small, translucent, and difficult to recognize, as are colonies of group A streptococci. *Staphylococcus* colonies, on the other hand, are quite large, opaque, and easily seen, as are those of coliform bacilli, yeasts, and so forth. Growth of clostridia generally appears between the glass side wall and the agar slant and produces large bubbles of gas. *Proteus* and *Pseudomonas** colonies generally appear as a translucent film on the agar slant. Otherwise, growth is similar to that previously described.

A **negative** blood culture usually remains clear, but it may develop cloudiness with continued incubation, sometimes caused by shaking the bottle before making smears, which in this instance will show no bacteria. After prolonged incubation (10 days or more) the bottle may develop a turbidity from fibrin or agar particles. This occurs usually above the red cell layer and

---

Pseudomonas and yeasts may require 3 to 4 days to grow out and are best recovered in an **air-vented** bottle.

may suggest bacterial growth. In either case turbidity alone is not a reliable guide; a smear should be examined to determine the presence of microorganisms.

It is very important that **blind subcultures** be made from blood cultures showing no macroscopic growth. Failure to do this will result in significant delay in identifying bacteremia in many cases. A blind subculture is recommended on the first day of incubation (the day of collection) of a blood culture, preferably after the culture has incubated at least 6 hours. Subcultures are not indicated, of course, in the case of biphasic bottles. Recent studies indicate that there is little or nothing to be gained from routine subculture of macroscopically negative blood cultures after 48 hours of incubation for detection of anaerobic bacteria.[56] For the subculture, an aliquot (a few drops) of broth is aspirated by needle and syringe or is dispensed via a needle subculture unit* and is inoculated to a chocolate agar plate for incubation under 3% to 10% CO_2. Evaluation of the need for routine terminal subculture of blood cultures that appear to be negative before discarding indicates that there is no advantage to such terminal subculture.[14] McCarthy and Senne[54] evaluated the use of acridine orange stain for the detection of microorganisms in blood cultures in lieu of subculture. They found that this stain represented a rapid alternative to conventional subculture techniques for detecting organisms in blood cultures that failed to yield visible evidence of growth after 1 day of incubation.

When growth appears on **any** medium, the culture should be inoculated to two blood agar plates for aerobic and anaerobic incubation and a chocolate agar plate under 3% to 10% CO_2, and a gram-stained smear should be examined. If gram-negative rods are seen in the original bottles, an EMB or MacConkey agar plate should be streaked also. These will permit rapid preliminary identification if the organism is a coliform.

---

*General Diagnostics, Morris Plains, N.J.

In some instances, such as fungemia, failure to hold cultures long enough or to examine them frequently enough may result in a delay in recognizing the presence of pathogenic microorganisms or may even result in their loss of viability. Frequent openings of the culture bottles, on the other hand, may also result in contamination of the contents. The following schedule is offered as a desirable **routine** for the examination of regular blood cultures. Special methods for handling the less common pathogens are described subsequently.

Broth culture procedure

1. On the first day of incubation, shake the nonbiphasic bottle well and subculture (use sterile syringe and needle) a few drops of the blood broth to a chocolate agar plate. Reincubate the blood culture. Examine the blood culture bottle carefully, without agitating it, daily for 7 days.
2. Incubate the plate in 3% to 10% CO_2 and examine it for growth in 24 and 48 hours. Discard thereafter if it is negative.
3. The biphasic blood culture bottle should be tilted daily so that the blood-broth mixture flows over the surface of the agar slant. Prior to tilting each day, both the slant and the broth should be examined carefully for evidence of growth.
4. After 7 days' incubation, discard the broth bottle if there is no growth.
5. In special situations, as in suspected **bacterial endocarditis, fungemia, brucellosis,** or **anaerobic bacteremia** and in referral hospitals it is desirable to hold blood cultures for at least 2 weeks. However, holding routine cultures for more than 7 days merely permits recovery of skin contaminants, such as diphtheroids, which may lead to difficulties in interpretation.

Identification

In line with earlier comments about the seriousness of bacteremia and the importance of instituting specific therapy at the earliest possible moment, it is desirable to determine the identification and antimicrobial susceptibility of organisms from positive blood cultures at the earliest possible moment. The membrane filter system offers real advantages here, in addition to earlier appearance of growth. Growth is present in the form of colonies with typical morphology and reactions on differential media. Availability of colonies permits such rapid tests as the catalase and slide coagulase tests on gram-positive cocci and the oxidase test on gram-negative rods. These same advantages may also be present in pour plate cultures. With broth cultures, subculturing and expeditious use of processing schemes should be carried out. **Direct** or "emergency" inoculation to identification test systems and antimicrobial susceptibility testing should be done on macroscopically positive bottles. These can subsequently be rechecked in the conventional manner. One group[58] has suggested subculturing by means of replica inoculating apparatus to several differential and antibiotic-containing media for assistance in identification and for determination of antimicrobial susceptibility. The first step actually is a Gram stain. It has been determined that the Gram stain is quite reliable in differentiating staphylococci from streptococci in blood cultures that demonstrate gram-positive cocci on smear.[2] A preponderance of clusters was 98% sensitive and 100% specific for identification of staphylococcal species or of *Peptococcus*. In the event of gram-positive cocci one may employ a rapid screening test for *Staphylococcus aureus* that utilizes sensitivity to lysostaphin.[70] In the case of gram-negative rods, one may suspend the organisms in saline and use an API strip or inoculate the Minitek enteric and nonfermenter broth with blood culture fluid and incubate this inoculum for 4 hours before setting up the conventional Minitek system. Of great interest are reports indicating the feasibility of rapid identification of Enterobacteriaceae from blood cultures using the Micro-ID system.[5,23] With conventional blood culture bottles, one may centrifuge the medium for 15 minutes at 4,000 rpm after

removing 10 to 15 ml of this medium aseptically from above the red blood cell layer with a needle and syringe. The supernatant is discarded after centrifugation. A small portion of the pellet may then be used to perform a cytochrome oxidase test, after which 4 ml of sterile saline is added to the tube and adjustment is made as necessary for equivalence with the 0.5 McFarland turbidity standard. One may then add 0.2 ml of this suspension to each of the 15 Micro-ID biochemical tests. Another 0.5 ml may be used to perform a direct antibiotic susceptibility test, and additional amounts may be utilized to inoculate a variety of primary isolation and growth media. This type of technique yielded 96% agreement with conventional identification to the genus and species level. With the Bactec blood culture system there is no separation of red blood cells and culture broth during incubation. However, with two centrifugation steps, one may proceed more or less in the manner just described. A study of direct antimicrobial disk susceptibility testing for bacteria isolated from blood, in comparison with the standard technique, revealed very good reliability for the rapid test.[55] Overall agreement between the two methods was 95%, and the vast majority of disagreements were of a minor variety (shift to or from the intermediate category).

The most frequently isolated skin contaminants include diphtheroid bacilli, which may be microaerophilic. These organisms are strongly catalase-positive, nonmotile, gram-positive rods, which may be confused morphologically with *Listeria monocytogenes*, a distinct pathogen from which they must be differentiated. The reader is referred to Chapter 26 for a discussion of the biochemical reactions of the latter organism.

Conclusion

If all cultures and subcultures are negative, the blood culture may be reported as "**No growth, aerobic or anaerobic, after 7 days' incubation.**"

It is strongly recommended that a stock culture be made, on appropriate media,* of all significant organisms isolated from blood cultures. Such stocks should be maintained for at least several months. This is important for subsequent antimicrobial susceptibility testing by the tube dilution technique or for more extensive studies, such as serologic tests, animal inoculation, or referral to a diagnostic center, which may be indicated on occasion.

PNEUMOCOCCAL AND STREPTOCOCCAL BACTEREMIA

Pneumococcal bacteremia can be demonstrated in about 25% of adult patients with pneumococcal pneumonia,[9] less frequently in infants and children.[12] In many cases, the blood culture may be the **only** specimen from which pneumococci are recovered; it therefore provides the most useful and readily available procedure for confirming a clinical impression of bacteremia or meningitis and should be obtained from **any** patient with a suspected pneumococcal infection.

Although the procedure previously outlined is satisfactory for isolating pneumococci from the blood, certain precautions should be observed in the handling of these cultures. After overnight incubation, gram-stained smears of the broth should be made and examined, regardless of the appearance of the flask. The pneumococci, if present, will have grown out in this period, and longer incubation may result in a loss of the organism through autolysis in a fluid medium. Pneumococci will appear as gram-positive cocci in chains resembling streptococci; some may show the typical lancet-shaped diplococcus with evidence of a capsule.

Whether or not organisms are seen in the smear of the blood broth, a subculture should be made. This demonstrates the presence of

pneumococci in numbers too small to be seen in the smear. Methods for the identification of the pneumococcus may be found in Chapter 18.

Various streptococci may be found in blood cultures as well. Enterococcal bacteremia is associated with manipulation or infection of the genitourinary, biliary, intestinal, or integumentary systems and may also occur in relation to indwelling intravenous catheters. Enterococci may also be found as a cause of septicemia in the newborn. The enterococcus is an important cause of bacterial endocarditis. *Streptococcus bovis* is a nonenterococcal group D streptococcus that is more commonly isolated from the gastrointestinal tract than from the oral cavity. A significant number of patients with *S. bovis* septicemia are found to have carcinoma of the colon. This organism may also cause bacterial endocarditis.

The viridans streptococci are a heterogeneous group of organisms that are still the primary cause of bacterial endocarditis. This group is made up of a variety of species such as *S. mitior*, *S. sanguis*, and *S. mutans*. They are found primarily in the oral cavity of humans but may be found in the gastrointestinal tract as well. These organisms may be found in bacteremia unassociated with endocarditis, with various underlying processes such as liver abscess. A number of reports have dealt with nutritionally deficient streptococci that have been involved in endocarditis. The exact frequency with which these streptococci may be encountered is unknown but they may not be rare. In order to grow these organisms a medium must be supplemented with pyridoxal hydrochloride or pyridoxamine dihydrochloride (the active forms of vitamin B_6), or L-cysteine.[64] These organisms undoubtedly account for a certain number of cases of culture-negative endocarditis. Furthermore, the organisms may grow in broth blood cultures if these are properly supplemented and may even be noted on Gram stain of such blood culture bottles but then fail to grow on subculture. One

---

*CTA medium, Baltimore Biological Laboratory, Cockeysville, Md., is recommended. The culture, after overnight incubation, may be stored in the refrigerator.

may get around this problem by being certain that the medium subcultured to is properly supplemented or by streaking conventional blood agar with a staphylococcus prior to inoculation from the blood culture bottle in order to detect streptococci that satellite about the colonies of staphylococci.

STAPHYLOCOCCAL BACTEREMIA

Staphylococci are also important causes of bacteremia. *Staphylococcus aureus* bacteremia may be associated with pneumonia, abscess formation, or infection of other types throughout the body. It may also be involved in endocarditis. *S. epidermidis* is much less virulent and is found in bacteremia typically only in the case of bacterial endocarditis, which it may cause on occasion, or in association with implanted prosthetic devices such as ventriculoatrial shunts. Both types of staphylococci may be involved in true bacteremia or may be found in blood cultures as contaminants. Statistically, *S. aureus* is much more likely to be associated with true bacteremia. However, it is necessary to take the clinical picture into account and to analyze the nature of the bacteremia more closely. Cultures of patients with definite septicemia caused by either type of staphylococcus characteristically have more than one positive bottle per day if more than one set has been drawn, grow up rather quickly (within 1 to 2 or at most 3 days), and demonstrate positivity in almost all bottles that are eventually positive within 2 days of incubation.[44]

ISOLATION OF NEISSERIA AND HAEMOPHILUS

The isolation of *Neisseria meningitidis* and *Haemophilus influenzae* from the blood culture of all patients with purulent meningitis should be attempted. Through use of the procedures previously described (including the use of gelatin to counteract the inhibition of *Neisseria* by SPS), both organisms may be recovered after 18 to 24 hours' incubation* by subculturing from the broth bottle to a **chocolate agar** plate and following with incubation for 18 to 24 hours in a candle jar. If this subculture shows no growth, the procedure is repeated after incubating the original broth flask for an additional 5 to 10 days. Gram-stained smears of *Neisseria* and *Haemophilus* may be difficult to interpret because of the presence of gram-negative debris and a heavy red background. Consequently, the practice of subculturing the broth flasks routinely may be very valuable. In the case of *N. gonorrhoeae*, CDC's Venereal Disease Control Division (*Criteria and Techniques for the Diagnosis of Gonorrhea*, 1976) recommends culturing blood in an enriched broth, such as trypticase soy broth supplemented with 1% IsoVitaleX, 10% horse serum, and 1% glucose.

H. parainfluenzae has been reported from a number of cases of bacterial endocarditis in recent years and may be a much more important cause of this entity than had been appreciated.[45] The organism is difficult to grow. It prefers aerobic conditions to anaerobic, but an enhanced CO_2 environment is desirable. Since the organism does not grow luxuriantly, the bottles may not be cloudy, so that blind subculturing becomes important. Unless subculturing is carried out on supplemented chocolate agar with incubation in an environment of increased CO_2, subcultures may not grow even when the organism is present. Accordingly, many cases of endocarditis caused by this organism have undoubtedly been overlooked.

Attention is called to a *Haemophilus* species, *H. aphrophilus*, which is an infrequent cause of bacterial endocarditis.[94] The organism is a gram-negative, nonmotile rod that does not require V factor but does require X factor and an increased CO_2 pressure (Pco_2) for its growth (see Chapter 23 for a description of this organism). *H. paraphrophilus* may also be recovered from the blood.

N. gonorrhoeae may require 7 or more days.

SEPTICEMIA AND BACTEREMIC SHOCK CAUSED BY GRAM-NEGATIVE RODS

The association between severe and frequently fatal septicemia caused by gram-negative enteric bacilli and confinement in the hospital is becoming increasingly apparent.[25] In the early antibiotic era the primary concern was for sepsis caused by *Staphylococcus aureus*. More recently, however, many institutions have reported a great increase in infections caused by *Escherichia coli* and members of the genera *Klebsiella*, *Enterobacter*, *Serratia*, *Proteus*, and *Pseudomonas*.[77]

Factors that have played a primary role in initiating these infections include:

1. Those compromising the resistance of the host, such as the use of immunosuppressive agents and antimetabolite drugs
2. The widespread utilization of broad-spectrum antimicrobial agents, which may upset the endogenous flora, with emergence of resistant strains
3. Procedures producing new artifical avenues of infection, such as the use of indwelling bladder and venous catheters, tracheostomies, and mechanical ventilators
4. More extensive surgical procedures
5. The increasing number of chronically debilitated elderly patients admitted to the hospital
6. Nosocomial infections from contaminated intravenous fluids*
7. More prolonged survival of patients with serious, ultimately fatal diseases

Since mortality of 45% to 50% accompanies these gram-negative septicemias,[42] the importance of early diagnosis and the initiation of specific therapy cannot be overemphasized.

---

*See special supplement to vol. 20, no. 9, Morbidity and Mortality Reports, Atlanta, 1971, Center for Disease Control.

ANAEROBIC BACTEREMIA

An increasing interest on the part of both the microbiologist and the clinician in the recovery of anaerobes from clinical material has resulted in numerous reports of the isolation of these bacteria from the blood. In a retrospective study of bacteremia at the Mayo Clinic involving over 3,000 positive blood cultures, Washington[89] found anaerobes in 11%, representing 20% of the patients with bacteremia. Sullivan and co-workers,[73] while studying bacteremia in 300 patients following urologic procedures, found a 31% positive incidence in those having transurethral resections. Although enterococci and *Klebsiella* were isolated most frequently, there were also a relatively large number of anaerobic cocci, *Bacteroides*, and so forth recovered. The authors reported the highest isolation rate in osmotically stabilized broth containing SPS; a membrane filter system also was useful for detecting multiple organism bacteremia (26% in this series).

In papers from the CDC, Felner and Dowell[29] and Alpern and Dowell[4] have reported the isolation of such anaerobes as *Bacteroides fragilis*, fusobacteria (Plates 5 and 6), clostridia (nonhistotoxic), and peptococci from the blood of patients with symptoms of endocarditis, gram-negative rod septicemia, or neonatal sepsis. Alpern and Dowell[3] also studied 27 patients with documented *Clostridium septicum* septicemia associated with malignant disease.

In suspected actinomycosis, freshly prepared brain-heart infusion medium without venting is preferred.

INFECTIONS CAUSED BY SPECIES OF BRUCELLA

The diagnosis of *Brucella* infections in humans is best made by the isolation of the causative organism. *Brucella* is most often found in the bloodstream, particularly in the febrile period, although it is not recovered as readily as the more commonly isolated pneumococcus, streptococcus, or staphylococcus. Two reasons have been advanced for this: (1) the relatively complex nutritional requirements of brucellae and (2) their presence in the blood only in small numbers because of their intracellular proclivity. The first difficulty has been overcome by the introduction of commercially available culture media, such as tryptose, trypticase soy, and Brucella broth and agar,* which will readily support the growth of small inocula. The problem of the small numbers of brucellae can be resolved partly by culturing large quantities of blood (while maintaining a 1:10 blood-broth ratio) or by obtaining numerous cultures over a period of several days. Bone marrow cultures have also proved useful in some instances when blood cultures have been negative.

A simple method for cultivating brucellae and permitting examination of cultures by inoculation of agar has been described by Castañeda-Ruiz[15] and modified by Scott.[69] This method utilizes a bottle containing Brucella or trypticase soy broth and a Brucella or trypticase agar slant, which permits direct observation of colonies developing from the broth culture.† Ten percent CO_2 is incorporated in the atmosphere.

The culture is held for at least 21 days before it is discarded as negative. If growth occurs and consists of small coccoid or short bacillary gram-negative organisms, it may be identified as a species of *Brucella* by agglutination with type-specific antisera, hydrogen sulfide production, and susceptibility to certain dyes. These characteristics are described in Chapter 23.

INFECTIONS CAUSED BY SPECIES OF FRANCISELLA, PASTEURELLA, AND YERSINIA

The organisms comprising this group are non-motile‡ gram-negative rods that usually exhibit polar staining. They are biochemically inactive and moderately to very fastidious in their growth requirements. They are primarily involved in diseases of lower animals, but closely related species can cause bubonic plague and tularemia in humans.

The classification of the genus *Pasteurella* has been altered. *P. tularensis* is now classified as *Francisella tularensis; P. pestis* and *P. pseudotuberculosis* are now in the genus *Yersinia*, which also includes *Y. enterocolitica*.

Tularemia, caused by *F. tularensis*, is a naturally occurring disease in animals such as wild rodents, rabbits, and deer. Human beings contract the disease as a result of handling infected animals (chiefly rabbits) or from the bites of infected deerflies or ticks. The organism will not grow on ordinary media, differing in this respect from *Y. pestis*, the causative agent of plague. It may be cultured on glucose-cysteine agar with thiamine, on chocolate agar, or in heart infusion broth containing glucose, cystine, and hemoglobin. *F. tularensis* is difficult to cultivate from infected material, but successful isolation from the blood, pleural fluid, or pus from unopened skin lesions may be achieved by the following procedure:

1. Inoculate six glucose-cysteine blood agar plates and one plain blood agar control plate with 0.5 to 1 ml of the patient's blood, freshly drawn by venipuncture. Distribute the blood over the plates before it clots, and incubate them inverted aerobically at 35 C. Precautions should be taken to restrict moisture formation, as this is deleterious to the organism.

2. Observe the plates daily for the presence of growth. Minute droplike colonies may appear in 3 to 5 days but can take as long as 10 days to develop.

3. Examine a stained smear of the colony for small gram-negative coccobacilli. If present, the culture may be identified by specific agglutination or fluorescent antibody test.*

---

*Difco Laboratories, Detroit; Baltimore Biological Laboratory, Cockeysville, Md.; General Diagnostics, Morris Plains, N.J.
†Baltimore Biological Laboratory, Cockeysville, Md.
‡*Y. pseudotuberculosis* is motile at 25 C.

---

*The identification is best carried out by a reference laboratory, such as the Centers for Disease Control, Atlanta.

4. Do not report the culture as negative before 3 weeks of incubation.

Note: Great caution is **mandatory** in handling infectious material from patients and cultures! Use syringes or hand-actuated pipets and work in a biologic safety hood.

Guinea pigs can be infected without difficulty, and subcutaneous or intraperitoneal injection of a heavy saline suspension of blood or ground-up tissue is the preferred procedure when only small numbers of organisms may be present. Animals usually survive 5 to 7 days but may die in 2 days; they show enlarged caseous lymph nodes, greatly enlarged spleens, and necrotic foci in the liver and spleen. Accidental laboratory infection is an ever-present hazard; animal injection, therefore, should not be attempted unless the laboratory worker has been previously immunized against tularemia and a safe animal facility (plastic cages with filter tops, vented hoods, and so forth) is available.

Y. pestis infection of humans is most commonly of the **bubonic plague** type, and the bacilli may be cultivated from material obtained from buboes, the spleen, or blood. In the pneumonic type the sputum is most likely to yield the organism. Blood cultures taken during the first 3 days of bubonic disease are positive in most cases. Blood specimens are first cultured in broth and and then subcultured to blood agar plates daily. On this medium after 48 hours the colonies are small (1 mm in diameter), glistening, and transparent, with round granular centers and a notched margin. Cultures are identified by biochemical reactions and specific agglutination, hemagglutination, or bacteriophage lysis. Again, the laboratory worker must use extreme caution in handling specimens, cultures, and animals. Suspected and confirmed cases of plague must be reported to local health departments immediately.

Other members of this group that may infect humans are *P. multocida*, *Y. pseudotuberculosis*, and *Y. enterocolitica*. All are primarily animal pathogens, and humans are accidental hosts. Approximately one half of the cases of *P. multocida* infection in humans result from the bites or scratches of dogs or cats; the remainder are either pulmonary infections resulting from probable animal contact or from miscellaneous causes.[43] Bacteremia is apparently a rare occurrence, although a case of endocarditis caused by *Pasteurella*, nov. sp., following a cat bite was reported. Both *Y. pseudotuberculosis* and *Y. enterocolitica* probably are involved in infection much more commonly than has been appreciated. They may cause septicemia, enteritis or enterocolitis, mesenteric lymphadenitis, and infection in various other parts of the body. Erythema nodosum and arthritis may be part of the clinical picture.

P. multocida grows readily on blood or chocolate agar plates, giving rise to large raised colonies, which show a tendency to become confluent. These organisms are very susceptible to penicillin. Further descriptive bacteriology is found in Chapter 23.

BACTEREMIA CAUSED BY LEPTOSPIRA SPECIES

Human leptospiral infection results principally from contact with an environment that has been contaminated by pathogenic leptospirae from an animal urinary shedder or other reservoir hosts. The organisms enter the body through the abraded skin or the mucosal surfaces of the mouth, nasopharynx, conjunctivae, or genitalia[81]; their principal sources are contaminated waters, soils, vegetation, foodstuffs, and so on. Occupational exposure is a primary factor in leptospirosis; the disease is most frequently associated with such people as farm workers, veterinarians, livestock handlers, abattoir attendants, and sewer workers. The disease is also associated with recreational pursuits such as swimming and camping.

The laboratory diagnosis of leptospirosis depends on isolating the organism from the blood or demonstrating a rise in antibody titer in the serum. Leptospirae may be recovered from the blood and occasionally the spinal fluid during the first week of the initial febrile illness, before circulating antibodies appear. Direct examination of blood by darkfield or stained smear may reveal the characteristic organisms. Cultural methods or the inoculation of young guinea pigs or weanling hamsters may be employed. The organism is readily cultivated on relatively simple media enriched with rabbit serum, such as Fletcher's medium or Stuart's medium.* Blood cultures are made at the patient's bedside or in the laboratory, using venous blood directly from the syringe or defibrinated blood in a sterile bottle. The semisolid medium is dispensed in screw-capped tubes or rubber-stoppered vaccine bottles, and a minimal inoculum of blood is introduced directly into the bottle by puncturing the rubber diaphragm at the patient's bedside.

RAT-BITE FEVER CAUSED BY SPIRILLUM MINOR AND STREPTOBACILLUS MONILIFORMIS

Two kinds of human disease may follow the bite of an infected rat: one, known as **sodoku** in Japan, is caused by a spiral organism presently classified as *Spirillum minor;* the other, more common in the United States, is caused by a highly pleomorphic organism, *Streptobacillus moniliformis*. These diseases present similar symptoms, including a primary ulcer, regional lymphadenopathy, fever, and malaise in addition to a characteristic skin rash. The latter infection may also be accompanied by marked polyarthritis.

A definitive diagnosis of rat-bite fever depends on the demonstration of the causative organism in the blood, lesion exudate, joint fluid, and so forth. In sodoku the presence of spirilla can be demonstrated by injecting 1 to 2 ml of the patient's whole blood intraperitoneally into several white mice or guinea pigs known to be free of naturally occurring spirilla. Mouse peritoneal exudate or the supernate of defibrinated guinea pig blood is obtained and examined

weekly for a period of up to 4 weeks, either by darkfield microscopy or by special stains, for the presence of spirilla.

In rat-bite fever caused by *Streptobacillus*, the blood is cultured in the routine manner. After several days of incubation at 35 C, the organism grows out as "cotton balls" on the surface of the red cell layer in the blood culture bottle. Whether or not growth occurs, the blood culture should be subcultured to fresh tubes of the same medium, using a thin sterile capillary pipet for the transfer. When growth is observed, Gram stains and Wayson stains are made and examined for the presence of pleomorphic gram-negative rods. Coccobacillary, rod-shaped, branching cells and large, swollen, club-shaped cells are seen; special methods may also reveal the presence of cell wall–defective forms, or L forms, of *Streptobacillus*. These are fragile, filterable forms lacking a rigid cell wall; they require a complex medium for growth and are capable of reverting to the parent bacterial cell. Agglutinins are formed against the *Streptobacillus*, and a titer of 1:80 is regarded as diagnostically significant.

INFECTIONS CAUSED BY LISTERIA MONOCYTOGENES

Listeriosis* is a bacterial infection of humans and animals that is being recognized with increasing frequency. The causative organism, *Listeria monocytogenes*, was first isolated from human infection in 1929. Asymptomatic fecal carriage occurs in humans.

Listeriosis is primarily an infection of the infant and the newborn baby, in whom it causes a purulent meningitis or meningoencephalitis or a granulomatous septicemia acquired in utero or during delivery. In the adult it may cause meningitis, abortion, acute septicemia, and other infections.

L. monocytogenes is more frequently isolated

---

*Difco Laboratories, Detroit.

*The reader is referred to an excellent monograph on the subject by Gray and Killinger[35] and also the CDC report on human listeriosis in the United States, 1967-1969.[13]

from the blood and CSF of human patients, although it may be recovered from meconium, vaginal and cervical secretions, discharge from the eye, or tissue collected at autopsy (particularly from the brain, liver, and spleen).

INFECTIONS CAUSED BY CAMPYLOBACTER FETUS

Campylobacter (Vibrio) fetus was first recognized in human infection in the United States by Ward.[85] Human infection is now known to be relatively common.

Since there are no distinctive clinical features of human infection, except for fever, signs of sepsis, and dysentery, a definitive diagnosis must depend on the isolation and identification of *C. fetus* from the blood or other body sites.

C. fetus is readily isolated from blood cultured by the same techniques as those used in cases of suspected brucellosis. The organism grows well in tryptose phosphate or trypticase soy broth. Since the bacterium is a microaerophile, primary incubation in 5% to 10% CO_2 is **essential.** Strains may tend to die out on repeated subculture. See Chapter 24 for a description of the cultural characteristics of this microorganism.

ENDOCARDITIS CAUSED BY COAGULASE-NEGATIVE STAPHYLOCOCCI, MICROCOCCI, AND DIPHTHEROIDS

Although coagulase-negative staphylococci, micrococci, and diphtheroids are generally considered as contaminants when isolated from blood cultures, they can be responsible for serious illness, such as bacterial endocarditis. Until about 1955 the incidence of coagulase-negative staphylococci, for example, in this disease was reported to be around 3%, but a study by Geraci and co-workers[34] in 1968 indicated an incidence of 10% in bacterial endocarditis. The etiologic significance of coagulase-negative staphylococci or micrococci and of diphtheroids from two or more blood cultures, therefore, should not be overlooked. It is recommended that the two iso-

lates be tested simultaneously by biochemical tests and antimicrobial susceptibilities; if results are clearly dissimilar, their probable clinical significance is thereby reduced. Organisms of this type may be especially important in endocarditis on prosthetic valves.

INFECTIONS CAUSED BY MISCELLANEOUS BACTERIA

Although studies to date are limited, it appears that bacteremia is relatively common in the course of Legionnaires' disease. Biphasic blood culture bottles composed of charcoal yeast extract agar slants and a supplemented Mueller-Hinton broth with CO_2 incorporated in the bottle appeared effective in one study for isolating *Legionella pneumophila*.[24] *Legionella pneumophila* was also recovered readily from seeded donor blood using the lysis-centrifugation technique.

A fastidious gram-negative bacillus designated as DF-2 at the CDC has recently been described from bacteremic infections and meningitis in a number of patients, most of whom were immunosuppressed and many of whom had been bitten by dogs.[53] The organism is described further in Chapter 32. In some of these patients the organism had been seen directly on peripheral blood films within the cytoplasm of neutrophils; it may be pleomorphic.

Rothia dentocariosa, an organism of the normal mouth flora that is not often involved in infections, has recently been noted in two patients with endocarditis. In one case the organism grew in vented blood culture bottles. In one of the patients the organism was not detected visibly during a 7-day culture period but grew on routine blind subculture. In the other patient the organism did not cause visible turbidity in the broth but was demonstrable by Gram stain.

An interesting report has described a bloodstream infection in a splenectomized man caused by an unidentified gram-positive rod-shaped bacterium that adhered to the majority of the patient's peripheral blood erythrocytes.[6] The organism was extraerythrocytic and could not be cultivated in vitro; it was also impossible to duplicate the disease in animals that were splenectomized.

INFECTIONS CAUSED BY L FORMS OF BACTERIA AND BY MYCOPLASMA

L forms of microorganisms have been isolated from the blood of patients treated with antibiotic agents, such as penicillin or methicillin, which interfere with cell-wall synthesis.[48] These fragile forms either do not survive or fail to grow in conventional isotonic blood culture media, and the culture remains sterile. However, in an osmotically stabilized medium, such as the previously described hypertonic sucrose broth with SPS, these aberrant forms may revert to their parent organism and subsequently be recovered and identified by conventional means.

Rarely, *Mycoplasma hominis* may be recovered from the blood of women with postpartum fever.

POLYMICROBIAL BACTEREMIA

The finding of two or more different bacterial species in a blood culture is reportedly an uncommon occurrence and may cause concern as to the possibility of contamination. It has been the experience of a number of workers, however, that such findings are not unusual, particularly in patients with gastrointestinal tract, hepatic, or urinary tract abnormalities or with hematologic disorders.[29,40,41] The incidence of two or more isolates from a single culture is generally reported as 6% to 10%; the organisms implicated include the gram-negative enteric bacilli, bacteroides, clostridia, and the gram-positive cocci. In these instances, the key to diagnosis and definitive antibacterial therapy rests with the bacteriology laboratory.

INFECTIONS CAUSED BY FUNGI (FUNGEMIA)

The incidence of bloodstream invasion by fungi, particularly members of the genus *Candida*, has increased significantly. This infection, once considered a rarity, is now a frequent complication in patients requiring therapy with adrenocorticosteroid hormones, cytotoxic agents, irradiation, or multiple antibiotics. Fungemia has also been reported in patients after prolonged venous catheterization[68] or parenteral hyperalimentation[19] and as a postoperative complication of renal transplantation or cardiac valve prosthesis insertion.[17] Candidal endocarditis in heroin addicts is also an increasing problem.[49]

The diagnosis of fungemia depends primarily on isolation of the organism on blood culture, the results of which are not always readily available. Species of *Candida*, particularly *C. albicans* and *C. tropicalis*, may grow in the brain-heart infusion broth–agar slant biphasic bottle previously described within 1 to 4 days, especially if the bottle is vented. Other yeasts, however, such as *C. parapsilosis*, *C. guilliermondii*, and *Torulopsis glabrata* may require 1 to 2 weeks' incubation before growing out. Blood cultures should be held for 21 to 30 days at 30 C in cases of suspected fungemia.[63] The radiometric technique described below detects yeasts more rapidly than does the biphasic bottle technique (Prevost and Bannister: J. Clin. Microbiol. **13:**655-660, 1981).

Sternal marrow or the buffy coat of venous blood may be examined for fungi by methods similar to those used in hematologic studies, using the Giemsa stain or other stain. Cultures should be made of the aspirated material on Sabouraud dextrose (SAB) agar and brain-heart infusion agar without added antibiotics. For best results this is done by transferring 0.5 to 1.0 ml of the specimen directly to several slants of the media at the patient's bedside, using the syringe and needle with which the marrow aspirate was obtained.* These media are incubated at room temperature and at 35 C and are examined for

---

*This procedure may also be used in culturing blood for fungi, especially for prompt isolation of *Candida* species and for *Histoplasma capsulatum* in disseminated disease.[47] Inoculate slants directly with 1 to 2 ml of blood.

the presence of growth at frequent intervals for several weeks.

Appropriate methods for the identification of isolates may be found in Chapter 34.

BLOOD CULTURES ON NEWBORN INFANTS AND PEDIATRIC PATIENTS

Multiple blood cultures (three or more) are preferred for the diagnosis of bacteremias in adults; in newborn infants, however, this becomes impractical for obvious reasons. A retrospective study of single blood cultures taken on infants younger than 28 days was reported by Franciosi and Favara.[33] Approximately 1 to 3 ml of heparinized blood was collected in a bottle containing 5 ml of trypticase soy broth and an agar slant; of 56 patients with positive cultures, 28 were considered to have septicemia, and a single culture was considered satisfactory for diagnosis. Nevertheless, two blood cultures should be obtained when feasible. Since clinical symptoms of neonatal septicemia frequently are minimal, with the possibility of rapid deterioration and death within hours after birth, blood culture is very important in the newborn.

The most frequent isolates from blood cultures from the pediatric population are *Haemophilus influenzae* and *Streptococcus pneumoniae*. Positive blood cultures are more likely with larger volumes of blood. *Haemophilus* is seldom detected visually in broth blood cultures. Recovery of this organism is dependent primarily on blind subculture after 1 day of incubation.

NONCULTURAL TECHNIQUES FOR DETECTION OF BACTEREMIA

As noted earlier, Gram stain of a blood culture bottle may reveal organisms before visible growth can be detected. One may also, on occasion, be able to demonstrate organisms in direct blood smears (Plate 2). This is true, for example, with the DF-2 organism, which frequently causes bacteremia following dog bite or animal contact. Certain organisms such as spirilla and

Borrelia may be demonstrable only in this manner. Gram stain of the buffy coat (white blood cells) may be a worthwhile procedure for critically ill patients, as it may immediately reveal organisms in the blood.[61] It does require the presence of a large number of organisms to be demonstrated in a buffy coat or other direct smear. For the most part, organisms detectable in this manner are gram-positive cocci, usually either staphylococci or pneumococci. Organisms may appear either intracellularly or extracellularly.

A new medium has been proposed that incorporates a tetrazolium dye that is converted from its colorless state to a visible blue color in the course of growth of bacteria that reduce it.[71] Much effort has gone into techniques for the detection of endotoxin in the absence of organisms or prior to the growth of organisms. Problems have related to the presence of inhibitory substances and possible mimicking substances in plasma. Procedures have been proposed to avoid these problems, but at the present time this procedure cannot be considered sufficiently developed for routine use in clinical laboratories. Counterimmunoelectrophoresis (CIE) has been utilized for early detection and rapid identification of *Haemophilus influenzae* type b and *Streptococcus pneumoniae* in blood cultures.[7] Blood culture bottles are first incubated for 18 to 24 hours and then are studied by the CIE technique for detection of antigen of the organisms. In the case of the pneumococcus, visible turbidity was usually present by the time the CIE procedure detected the antigen; however, this was not always true. In the case of *H. influenzae*, none of the cultures showed visible evidence of growth at the time that the antigen could be detected by CIE. Latex particle agglutination was more sensitive and more specific than CIE in detecting *H. influenzae* type b bacteremia. It is inexpensive.

A special method for early detection of bacteremia and fungemia using a radioisotope has been recommended.[20] The method is based on the ability of an organism to release CO_2 from ^{14}C-labeled glucose or other labeled substrate, and the $^{14}CO_2$ formed is detected by sampling the atmosphere above the blood culture by radiometric means. Early detection of positive blood cultures is the major advantage of this procedure, which provides automated sampling of blood culture bottles up to several times per day. Five milliliters of blood is inoculated into each of two bottles—one aerobic and one anaerobic. Various media formulations are available. In a study of children quantitative direct plating of blood yielded earlier diagnosis of *H. influenzae* and *N. meningitidis* bacteremia (but not *S. pneumoniae* bacteremia) than did the radiometric procedure (LaScolea et al.: J. Clin. Microbiol. **13:**478-482, 1981).

Specialized media may be useful in detecting certain groups of organisms such as yeasts and group D and viridans streptococci. On the other hand, *Mycobacterium chelonei* was detected without special media in two patients. Certain organisms, such as pneumococci and enterococci, may be missed without blind subculture. Radiometric detection of organisms may lag behind other evidence of growth (e.g., with pneumococci and *H. influenzae*). In the case of the pneumococcus this may result in false no-growth blood cultures, because by the time the organism can be detected radiometrically it may have already died out.[1] This procedure, it should be noted, offers no clue as to the probable identity of the organism; consequently, conventional procedures must be used thereafter. Terminal subculture is necessary.

Another method makes use of gas chromatography to detect metabolic end products resulting from bacterial growth in blood cultures after a short incubation period. In a limited study, however, it was shown that certain end products, such as volatile fatty acids, were detected, but never before the time that the blood culture was positive by gross inspection.[30] The procedure requires further study of its applicability in the clinical laboratory. In the case of anaerobic bacteremia, several workers have done gas chromatography after the organisms had been detected by visible changes in the broth media or by Gram stain of the blood culture.[96] Detection of specific volatile fatty acids and organic acids permitted rapid presumptive identification of anaerobes in these cases. In one case this procedure was coupled with indirect fluorescent antibody technique to document the presence of *Bacteroides fragilis* that had been detected by Gram stain but that failed to grow in the blood culture.[76] Other procedures that have been proposed for detection of organisms in blood culture but that have not yet been subjected to extensive clinical trials are measurement of changes in electrical impedance, microcalorimetry, and electronic monitoring of stainless steel electrodes implanted in blood culture bottles.

CONTAMINATED BANKED BLOOD AND PLASMA

Of the many complications of blood transfusion, including incompatibility caused by mismatched blood and serum hepatitis, those caused by bacterially contaminated blood are usually the most dangerous to the patient. Not only will severe reactions (chills, fever, and a drop in blood pressure) ensue immediately, but peripheral collapse may occur within 1 hour after the transfusion of massively contaminated blood, and death frequently occurs. It is important, therefore, that the microbiology laboratory offer a procedure for the detection of contamination in preserved blood and its products **before** they are administered to a patient.

The organisms most frequently encountered in fatal transfusion reactions comprise a small group of **psychrophilic gram-negative rods** (often from the donor's skin) that have the ability to multiply in blood stored at refrigerator temperature.[84] These organisms and their optimal temperatures for growth are as follows:

1. *Pseudomonas* species (other than *P. aeruginosa*), which grow slowly at 4 C, rapidly

at room temperature (22 to 25 C), and slowly or not at all at 35 C

2. *Citrobacter* species, which grow best at room temperature and at 35 C
3. Other late lactose-fermenting members of the family Enterobacteriaceae, which multiply at all three temperatures
4. *Achromobacter* species, which grow best at room temperature and at 35 C

These gram-negative organisms are generally found in the air, soil, water, and dust and in the intestinal tract of humans and animals. They can be transferred readily to the skin of humans, where they may become a part of the normal transient flora of that tissue. These organisms multiply in refrigerated blood, autolyze, and release **endotoxins** that may produce a toxic effect when administered in a blood transfusion. The reaction that follows is the result of this phenomenon rather than the effect produced by the introduction of the bacteria into the circulatory system or their multiplication within the patient's tissues.

Contamination of the blood may be caused in various ways: (1) by the use of improperly sterilized equipment and reagents for the collection, (2) by some flaw in aseptic technique during collection, and, most frequently, (3) by the inadequate cleansing and disinfection of the skin over the site of venipuncture. For procedures to obviate these difficulties, the reader is referred to a manual on technical methods and procedures issued by the American Association of Blood Banks.[47]

Sterility test procedure

The following methods for carrying out sterility tests are recommended by the Food and Drug Administration (Code of Federal Regulations, Federal Register, No. 640.2, Washington, D.C., 1976, U.S. Government Printing Office):

a. Sterility tests shall be performed at regular intervals and not less than once monthly. Blood intended for transfusion shall not be tested by a method that entails entering the container. A record shall be kept of the results of sterility tests.

b. Technic of sterility testing: Each month at least one container of normal-appearing blood shall be tested within the 18th to 24th day after collection. The test should be performed by inoculating 10 ml of blood into ten times the volume of fluid thioglycollate medium in a manner that introduces blood throughout the medium without destroying the anaerobic conditions in the lower portions of the broth. The sample should be incubated for 7 to 9 days at 30 to 32 C, or separate samples should be incubated at 18 to 20 C and 35 to 37 C, respectively, and examined every work day for evidence of microbial growth. A subculture of 1 ml inoculated into 10 ml of thioglycollate medium should be made on the third, fourth, or fifth day. The subculture should be incubated for 7 to 9 days as described above and examined daily for evidence of microbial growth.

Culturing plastic packs

Only when blood or plasma is collected in an open system, that is, where the blood container is entered, is it necessary to carry out a periodic sterility check.* After a transfusion reaction, however, it is strongly recommended that the following procedure, described by Walter and associates,[84] be carried out in the culturing of plastic blood packs and plasma packs. To secure a representative sample, the bag should be turned gently end over end to mix the contents; the integral donor tube should also be stripped several times. A 5-inch segment is then sealed with a dielectric sealer and cut free in the center of the seal. Both ends of the segment are then dipped in 70% ethyl alcohol and flamed, and with a pair of scissors similarly flame sterilized, one seal is cut off. This cut end then is held over a tube of thioglycollate medium, the top seal nicked to admit air, and the sample (approximately 1 ml) allowed to run in.

Cultures should be made in duplicate when possible and held for at least 10 days at room temperature and at 35 to 37 C. At the end of the

---

*Public Health Service, Section 73.3004, amended March 25, 1972, Federal Register vol. 37, no. 59.

incubation period a loopful of the culture is streaked on a blood agar plate or placed in another tube of thioglycollate medium and held at the preceding temperatures for 24 hours to confirm sterility. Stained smears of the original cultures also may be examined.

Culture of donor arm bleeding site

In addition to the periodic sterility checks of blood and the equipment and solutions used in its collection, the culture of the venipuncture site before and after the arm "prep" is also recommended as a quality control measure. The following technique may be used:

1. A cotton applicator moistened in 1 ml of pH 7.5 sterile phosphate buffer (see Chapter 44 for preparation) is rubbed vigorously over a 1-inch-square area of the venipuncture site for 1 minute. This is done in duplicate, before and after the "prep."
2. The applicator is then twirled in a tube (15 to 20 ml) of melted and cooled (45 C) soybean-casein digest agar and squeezed out against the inside of the tube.
3. Approximately 1 ml of sterile defibrinated sheep blood is added; the contents are mixed well by inversion and are poured into a sterile Petri dish.
4. The plates are examined after 48 hours' incubation at 35 C, and colony counts are made, together with the identification of significant isolates, if indicated.
5. The number of bacteria per square inch of skin should be reduced almost to zero if an effective degerming has been achieved.

Signs of contamination

Contamination of a bottle of blood often may be suspected from gross examination of the sample. The following changes should be looked for:

1. Change in the color of blood to a bluish black
2. Zone of hemolysis in the lowest portion of the supernatant plasma at the cell-plasma interface
3. Appearance of a large quantity of free hemoglobin in plasma when shaken
4. Appearance of small fibrin clots in a bottle, which had formerly appeared satisfactory, caused by the utilization of citrate by the organisms previously described
5. Turbidity of the supernatant plasma

The transfusion of contaminated blood is followed (usually after the first 50 ml) by a sudden onset of chills, fever, hypotension, and shock. This may progress to convulsions and coma. An immediate Gram stain of blood from the blood container may reveal the presence of organisms; three separate blood cultures from the patient also should be obtained. Residual blood from the container of blood causing the reaction should be cultured at 18 to 20 C and 35 to 37 C. Prompt diagnosis and initiation of specific therapy may be lifesaving.

REFERENCES

1. Adeniyi-Jones, C.C., Stevens, D.L., and Rasquinha, E.S.: False no-growth blood cultures in pneumococcal pneumonia, J. Clin. Microbiol. **12:**572-575, 1980.
2. Agger, W.A., and Maki, D.G.: Efficacy of direct Gram stain in differentiating staphylococci from streptococci in blood cultures positive for gram-positive cocci, J. Clin. Microbiol. **7:**111-113, 1978.
3. Alpern, R.J., and Dowell, V.R., Jr.: *Clostridium septicum* infections and malignancy, J.A.M.A. **209:**385-388, 1969.
4. Alpern, R.J., and Dowell, V.R., Jr.: Nonhistotoxic clostridial bacteremia, Am. J. Clin. Pathol. **55:**717-722, 1971.
5. Appelbaum, P.C., Schick, S.F., and Kellogg, J.A.: Evaluation of the four-hour Micro-ID technique for direct identification of oxidase-negative, gram-negative rods from blood cultures, J. Clin. Microbiol. **12:**533-537, 1980.
6. Archer, G.L., Coleman, P.H., Cole, R.M., Duma, R.J., and Johnston, C.L., Jr.: Human infection from an unidentified erythrocyte-associated bacterium, N. Engl. J. Med. **301:**897-900, 1979.
7. Artman, M., Weiner, M., and Frankl, G.: Counterimmunoelectrophoresis for early detection and rapid identification of *Haemophilus influenzae* type b and *Streptococcus pneumoniae* in blood cultures, J. Clin. Microbiol. **12:**614-616, 1980.

8. Austrian, R.: The role of the microbiological laboratory in the management of bacterial infections, Med. Clin. North Am. **50:**1419-1432, 1966.

9. Austrian, R.: Current status of bacterial pneumonia with special reference to pneumococcal infection, J. Clin. Pathol. **21**(Suppl. 2), 1968.

10. Beaman, K.D., Kasten, B.L., Corlett, C.L., and Gavan, T.L.: Effects of blood on blood culture medium, J. Clin. Microbiol. **10:**488-491, 1979.

11. Bokkenheuser, V.: *Vibrio fetus* infection in man, Am. J. Epidemiol. **91:**400-409, 1970.

12. Burke, J.P., Klein, J.O., Gezon, H.M., and Finland, M.: Pneumococcal bacteremia, Am. J. Dis. Child. **121:**353-359, 1971.

13. Busch, L.A.: Human listeriosis in the United States, 1967-1969, J. Infect. Dis. **123:**328-332, 1971.

14. Campbell, J., and Washington, J.A., II: Evaluation of the necessity for routine terminal subcultures of previously negative blood cultures, J. Clin. Microbiol. **12:**576-578, 1980.

15. Castañeda-Ruiz, M.: Practical method for routine blood cultures in brucellosis, Proc. Soc. Exp. Biol. Med. **64:**114-115, 1947.

16. Center for Disease Control: False-positive blood cultures related to the use of evacuated nonsterile blood-collection tubes, Morbid. Mortal. Rep. **24:**387-388, 1975.

17. Chandhuri, M.R.: Fungal endocarditis after valve replacements, J. Thorac. Cardiovasc. Surg. **60:**207-214, 1970.

18. Cleri, D.J., Corrado, M.L., and Seligman, S.J.: Quantitative culture of intravenous catheters and other intravascular inserts, J. Infect. Dis. **141:**781-786, 1980.

19. Curry, C.R., and Quie, P.G.: Fungal septicemia in patients receiving parenteral hyperalimentation, N. Engl. J. Med. **285:**1221-1225, 1971.

20. DeBlanc, H.J., de Land, F., and Wagner, H.N., Jr.: Automated radiometric detection of bacteria in 2,967 blood cultures, Appl. Microbiol. **22:**846-849, 1971.

21. Dorn, G.L., Haynes, J.R., and Burson, G.G.: Blood culture technique based on centrifugation: Developmental phase, J. Clin. Microbiol. **3:**251-257, 1976; clinical evaluation, **3:**258-263, 1976.

22. Dorn, G.L., Land, G.A., and Wilson, G.E.: Improved blood culture technique based on centrifugation: clinical evaluation, J. Clin. Microbiol. **9:**391-396, 1979.

23. Edberg, S.C., Clare, D., Moore, M.H., and Singer, J.M.: Rapid identification of Enterobacteriaceae from blood cultures with the Micro-ID system, J. Clin. Microbiol. **10:**693-697, 1979.

24. Edelstein, P.H., Meyer, R.D., and Finegold, S.M.: Isolation of *Legionella pneumophila* from blood, Lancet **1:**750-751, 1979.

25. Edmonson, E.B., and Sanford, J.P.: The Klebsiella-Enterobacter (Aerobacter)-Serratia group: a clinical and bacteriological evaluation, Medicine **46:**323-340, 1967.

26. Edwards, P.R., and Ewing, W.H.: Identification of Enterobacteriaceae, ed. 3, Minneapolis, 1972, Burgess Publishing Co.

27. Ellner, P.D.: System for inoculation of blood in the laboratory, Appl. Microbiol. **16:**1892-1894, 1968.

28. Eng, J., and Holten, E.: Gelatin neutralization of the inhibitory effect of sodium polyanethol sulfonate on *Neisseria meningitidis* in blood culture media, J. Clin. Microbiol. **6:**1-3, 1977.

29. Felner, J.M., and Dowell, V.R., Jr.: Anaerobic bacterial endocarditis, N. Engl. J. Med. **283:**1188-1192, 1970.

30. Finegold, S.M.: Early detection of bacteremia. In Sonnenwirth, A.C., editor: Septicemia: laboratory and clinical aspects, Springfield, Ill., 1973, Charles C Thomas, Publisher.

31. Finegold, S.M., White, M.L., Ziment, I., and Winn, W.R.: Rapid diagnosis of bacteremia, Appl. Microbiol. **18:**458-463, 1969.

32. Finegold, S.M., Ziment, I., White, M.L., Winn, W.R., and Carter, W.T.: Evaluation of polyanethol sulfonate (Liquoid) in blood cultures. In Hobby, G.L., editor: Proceedings of the Sixth Interscience Conference on Antimicrobial Agents and Chemotherapy, Washington, D.C., 1968, American Society for Microbiology, pp. 692-696.

33. Franciosi, R.A., and Favara, B.E.: A single blood culture for confirmation of the diagnosis of neonatal septicemia, Am. J. Clin. Pathol. **57:**215-219, 1972.

34. Geraci, J.E., Hanson, K.C., and Giuliani, E.R.: Endocarditis caused by coagulase-negative staphylococci, Mayo Clin. Proc. **43:**420-434, 1968.

35. Gray, M.L., and Killinger, A.H.: *Listeria monocytogenes* and listeric infections, Bacteriol. Rev. **30:**309-382, 1966.

36. Hall, M.M., Ilstrup, D.M., and Washington, J.A., II: Comparison of three blood culture media with tryptic soy broth, J. Clin. Microbiol. **8:**299-301, 1978.

37. Hall, M.M., Mueske, C.A., Ilstrup, D.M., and Washington, J.A., II: Evaluation of a biphasic medium for blood cultures, J. Clin. Microbiol. **10:**673-676, 1979.

38. Hall, M.M., Warren, E., Ilstrup, D.M., and Washington, J.A., II: Comparison of sodium amylosulfate and sodium polyanetholsulfonate in blood culture media, J. Clin. Microbiol. **3:**212-213, 1976.

39. Harkness, J.L., Hall, M., Ilstrup, D.M., and Washington, J.A., II: Effects of atmosphere of incubation and of routine subcultures on detection of bacteremia in vacuum blood culture bottles, J. Clin. Microbiol. **2:**296-299, 1975.

40. Hermans, P.E., and Washington, J.A., II: Polymicrobial bacteremia, Ann. Intern. Med. **73**:387-392, 1970.

41. Hochstein, H.D., Kirkham, W.R., and Young, V.M.: Recovery of more than one organism in septicemias, N. Engl. J. Med. **273**:468-474, 1965.

42. Holloway, W.J., and Scott, E.G.: Gram-negative rod septicemia, Del. Med. J. **40**:181-185, 1968.

43. Holloway, W.J., Scott, E.G., and Adams, Y.B.: *Pasteurella multocida* infection in man, Am. J. Clin. Pathol. **51**:705-708, 1968.

44. Horvitz, R.A., and von Graevenitz, A.: Interpretation of blood cultures yielding *Staphylococcus aureus*, Infection **5**:207-210, 1977.

45. Jemsek, J.G., Greenberg, S.B., Gentry, L.O., Welton, D.E., and Mattox, K.L.: *Haemophilus parainfluenzae* endocarditis: two cases and review of the literature in the past decade, Am. J. Med. **66**:51-56, 1979.

46. Kaslow, R.A., Mackel, D.C., and Mallison, G.F.: Nosocomial pseudobacteremia: positive blood cultures due to contaminated benzalkonium antiseptic, J.A.M.A. **236**:2407-2409, 1976.

47. Koch, M.L.: Bacteriologic problems in blood banking, Bull. Am. Assoc. Blood Banks **12**:397-401, 1959.

48. Lorian, V., and Waluslka, A.: Blood cultures showing aberrant forms of bacteria, Am. J. Clin. Pathol. **57**:406-409, 1972.

49. Louria, D.B., Hensle, T., and Rose, J.: The major medical complications of heroin addiction, Ann. Intern. Med. **67**:1-22, 1967.

50. Lowrance, B.L., and Traub, W.H.: Inactivation of the bactericidal activity of human serum by Liquoid (sodium polyanetholsulfonate), Appl. Microbiol. **17**:839-842, 1969.

51. Maki, D.G., Weise, C.E., and Sarafin, H.W.: A semiquantitative culture method for identifying intravenous-catheter-related infection, N. Engl. J. Med. **296**:1305-1309, 1977.

52. Mangels, J.I., Lindberg, L.H., and Vosti, K.L.: Quantitative evaluation of three commercial blood culture media for growth of anaerobic organisms, J. Clin. Microbiol. **7**:59-62, 1978.

53. Martone, W.J., Zuehl, R.W., Minson, G.E., and Scheld, W.M.: Postsplenectomy sepsis with DF-2: report of a case with isolation of the organism from the patient's dog, Ann. Intern. Med. **93**:457-458, 1980.

54. McCarthy, L.R., and Senne, J.E.: Evaluation of acridine orange stain for detection of microorganisms in blood cultures, J. Clin. Microbiol. **11**:281-285, 1980.

55. Mirrett, S., and Reller, L.B.: Comparison of direct and standard antimicrobial disk susceptibility testing for bacteria isolated from blood, J. Clin. Microbiol. **10**:482-487, 1979.

56. Murray, P.R., and Sondag, J.E.: Evaluation of routine subcultures of macroscopically negative blood cultures for detection of anaerobes, J. Clin. Microbiol. **8**:427-430, 1978.

57. Noble, R.C., and Reeves, S.A.: *Bacillus* species pseudosepsis caused by contaminated commercial blood culture media, J.A.M.A. **230**:1002-1004, 1974.

58. Paisley, J.W., Todd, J.K., and Roe, M.H.: Early detection and preliminary susceptibility testing of positive pediatric blood cultures with the Steers replicator, J. Clin. Microbiol. **6**:367-372, 1977.

59. Pazin, G.J., Peterson, K.L., Griff, F.W., et al.: Determination of site of infection in endocarditis, Ann. Intern. Med. **82**:746-750, 1975.

60. Rammell, C.G.: Inhibition by citrate of the growth of coagulase-positive staphylococci, J. Bacteriol. **84**:1123-1125, 1962.

61. Reik, H., and Rubin, S.J.: Evaluation of the buffy-coat smear for rapid detection of bacteremia, J.A.M.A. **245**:357-359, 1981.

62. Roberts, G.D., Horstmeier, C.D., and Ilstrup, D.M.: Evaluation of a hypertonic sucrose medium for the detection of fungi in blood cultures, J. Clin. Microbiol. **4**:110-111, 1976.

63. Roberts, G.D., and Washington, J.A., II: Detection of fungi in blood cultures, J. Clin. Microbiol. **1**:309-310, 1975.

64. Roberts, R.B., Krieger, A.G., Schiller, N.L., and Gross, K.C.: Viridans streptococcal endocarditis: the role of various species, including pyridoxal-dependent streptococci, Rev. Infect. Dis. **1**:955-966, 1979.

65. Rosett, W., and Hodges, G.R.: Antimicrobial activity of heparin, J. Clin. Microbiol. **11**:30-34, 1980.

66. Rosner, R.: Effect of various anticoagulants and no anticoagulant on ability to isolate bacteria directly from parallel clinical blood specimens, Am. J. Clin. Pathol. **49**:216-219, 1968.

67. Rosner, R.: A quantitative evaluation of three blood culture systems, Am. J. Clin. Pathol. **57**:220-227, 1972.

68. Salter, W., and Zinneman, H.H.: Bacteremia and candida septicemia, Minn. Med. **50**:1489-1499, 1967.

69. Scott, E.G.: A practical blood culture procedure, J. Lab. Clin. Med. **21**:290-294, 1951.

70. Severance, P.J., Kauffman, C.A., and Sheagren, J.N.: Effect of various blood culture media on lysostaphin sensitivity of staphylococci, J. Clin. Microbiol. **12**:709-710, 1980.

71. Shih, C.N., and Balish, E.: New blood culture medium, J. Clin. Microbiol. **6**:249-256, 1977.

72. Sliva, H.S., and Washington, J.A., II: Optimal time for routine early subculture of blood cultures, J. Clin. Microbiol. **12**:445-446, 1980.

73. Sullivan, N.M., Sutter, V.L., Attebery, H.R., and Finegold, S.M.: Bacteremia after genital tract manipulation: bacteriological aspects and evaluation of various blood culture systems, Appl. Microbiol. **23:**1101-1106, 1972.

74. Sullivan, N.M., Sutter, V.L., and Finegold, S.M.: Practical aerobic membrane filtration blood culture technique: development of procedure, J. Clin. Microbiol. **1:**30-36, 1975.

75. Sullivan, N.M., Sutter, V.L., and Finegold, S.M.: Practical aerobic membrane filtration blood culture technique: clinical blood culture trial, J. Clin. Microbiol. **1:**37-43, 1975.

76. Tabaqchali, S., Wills, A.R., Riordan, T., Banim, S.O., and Rees, G.M.: Anaerobic endocarditis: is it missed? Lancet **1:**148-149, 1981.

77. Thoburn, R., Fekety, F.R., Cluff, L.E., and Melvin, V.B.: Infections acquired by hospitalized patients, Arch. Intern. Med. **121:**1-10, 1968.

78. Traub, W.H.: Antagonism of polymyxin B and kanamycin sulfate by Liquoid (sodium polyanetholsulfonate) *in vitro*, Experientia **25:**206-207, 1969.

79. Traub, W.H.: Studies on neutralization of human serum bactericidal activity by sodium amylosulfate, J. Clin. Microbiol. **6:**128-131, 1977.

80. Traub, W.H., and Lowrance, B.L.: Media-dependent antagonism of gentamicin sulfate by Liquoid (sodium polyanetholsulfonate), Experientia **24:**1184-1185, 1969.

81. Turner, L.H.: Leptospirosis, Br. Med. J. **1:**231-235, 1969.

82. Von Haebler, T., and Miles, A.A.: The action of sodium polyanethol sulfonate (Liquoid) on blood cultures, J. Pathol. Bacteriol. **46:**245-252, 1938.

83. Wallis, C., Melnick, J.L., Wende, R.D., and Riely, P.E.: Rapid isolation of bacteria from septicemic patients by use of an antimicrobial agent removal device, J. Clin. Microbiol. **11:**462-464, 1980.

84. Walter, C.W., Kundsin, R.B., and Button, L.N.: New technic for detection of bacterial contamination in a blood bank using plastic equipment, N. Engl. J. Med. **259:**364-369, 1957.

85. Ward, B.R.: The apparent involvement of *Vibrio fetus* in an infection in man, J. Bacteriol. **55:**113-114, 1948.

86. Ward, J.I., Siber, G.R., Scheifele, D.W., and Smith, D.H.: Rapid diagnosis of *Hemophilus influenzae* type b infections by latex particle agglutination and counterimmunoelectrophoresis, J. Pediatr. **93:**37-42, 1978.

87. Washington, J.A., II: Comparison of two commercially available media for detection of bacteremia, Appl. Microbiol. **22:**604-607, 1971.

88. Washington, J.A., II: The microbiology of evacuated blood collection tubes, Ann. Intern. Med. **86:**186-188, 1975.

89. Washington, J.A., II, Hall, M.M., and Warren, E.: Evaluation of blood culture media supplemented with sucrose or with cysteine, J. Clin. Microbiol. **1:**79-81, 1975.

90. Washington, J.A., II, and Martin, W.J.: Comparison of three blood culture media for recovery of anaerobic bacteria, Appl. Microbiol. **25:**70-71, 1973.

91. Wilkins, T.D., and West, S.E.H.: Medium-dependent inhibition of *Peptostreptococcus anaerobius* by sodium polyanethol sulfonate in blood culture media, J. Clin. Microbiol. **3:**393-396, 1976.

92. Wing, E.J., Norden, C.W., Shadduck, R.K., and Winkelstein, A.: Use of quantitative bacteriologic techniques to diagnose catheter-related sepsis, Arch. Intern. Med. **139:**482-483, 1979.

93. Winn, W.R., White, M.L., Carter, W.T., Miller, A.B., and Finegold, S.M.: Rapid diagnosis of bacteremia with quantitative differential-membrane filtration culture, J.A.M.A. **197:**539-548, 1966.

94. Witorsch, P., and Gordon, P.: *Hemophilus aphrophilus* endocarditis, Ann. Intern. Med. **60:**957-961, 1964.

95. Wright, H.D.: The bacteriology of subacute infective endocarditis, J. Pathol. Bacteriol. **28:**541-578, 1925.

96. Wüst, J.: Presumptive diagnosis of anaerobic bacteremia by gas-liquid chromatography of blood cultures, J. Clin. Microbiol. **6:**586-590, 1977.

8 MICROORGANISMS ENCOUNTERED IN RESPIRATORY TRACT INFECTIONS

The pathogens most likely to be found in the upper and lower respiratory tract include the following:

Groups A and B beta-hemolytic streptococci
Corynebacterium diphtheriae
Streptococcus pneumoniae
Haemophilus influenzae
Neisseria meningitidis
Mycobacterium tuberculosis and other mycobacteria
Fungi including *Candida* species, *Histoplasma capsulatum, Coccidioides immitis,* and others
Klebsiella pneumoniae and other coliform bacilli
Pseudomonas aeruginosa and other pseudomonads
Bacteroides melaninogenicus, Fusobacterium nucleatum, and other gram-negative anaerobic rods
Anaerobic and microaerophilic cocci
Bordetella pertussis
Legionella species
Nocardia
Mycoplasma and *chlamydia*
Viruses
Pneumocystis

THROAT AND NASOPHARYNGEAL CULTURES

Throat cultures and nasopharyngeal cultures are important as aids in the diagnosis of certain infections, such as streptococcal sore throat, diphtheria, or candidal infections of the mouth (thrush); in establishing the focus of infection in diseases such as scarlet fever, rheumatic fever, and acute glomerulonephritis; and also in the detection of the carrier state of organisms such as group A beta-hemolytic streptococci, meningococci, *Staphylococcus aureus*, and the diphtheria bacillus.

To obtain the best results it is important that material for a throat culture be obtained **before** antimicrobial therapy and taken in a proper manner. A satisfactory method is as follows:

1. Use a sterile throat culture outfit such as a commercially available disposable unit* that contains a polyester-tipped applicator and an ampule of modified Stuart's transport medium.
2. With the patient's tongue depressed and the throat well exposed and illuminated, rub the swab firmly over the back of the throat (the posterior pharynx), both tonsils or tonsillar fossae, and any areas of inflammation, exudation, or ulceration. Care should be taken to avoid touching the tongue, cheeks, or lips, with the swab.
3. Replace the swab in the inner tube, crush the ampule, force the swab into the released holding medium, and send it to the laboratory immediately, where it should be plated as soon as possible. If it is necessary to hold the culture for more than 1 hour, it should be refrigerated until plates can be streaked.

If diphtheria is suspected, **two** swabs should be taken; one should be inoculated to Loeffler medium immediately and the other handled as described in step 3 above.

*Culturette, Marion Laboratories, Inc., Kansas City, Mo. Special swabs are available for recovery of viruses (viral culturette) and *S. pyogenes* (Strep Culturette).

If a swab has been taken for viral isolation and it is necessary to mail the specimen to a referral laboratory, it should be placed in a sealed plastic bag in a box that contains ice in another sealed plastic bag and that is suitable for shipment of etiologic agents. Specimens for viral culture should never be frozen.

Nasopharyngeal cultures are recommended when attempting the isolation of meningococci, because these organisms are found more commonly in the nasopharynx than in the nose or throat. Nasopharyngeal swabs (Plate 8) also are essential for the recovery of *Neisseria meningitidis* from suspected carriers or *Bordetella pertussis* from suspected cases of whooping cough. Such cultures are best taken on cotton-tipped nichrome or stainless steel wire applicators (B. & S. 28 gauge)* in a sterile tube containing a few drops of broth. With the patient's head firmly held, a nasal speculum is inserted; the wire swab is **gently** inserted (without force) through the nose to the posterior nasopharynx, where it is rotated gently, allowed to remain for 20 to 30 seconds, and then deftly withdrawn. The wire swab may also be bent at a right angle near the cotton tip (bending against the inside of the sterile tube container) and then inserted through the mouth and behind the uvula and soft palate into the nasopharynx. Care must be taken to avoid mouth and throat contamination of the swab. In either case the inoculated swab is returned to the inner tube containing the broth or to the transport medium of a Culturette and is thus transported promptly to the laboratory. A soft rubber catheter inserted in the nasopharynx is an alternative to a swab for diagnosis of pertussis.

Anterior nares cultures are occasionally required, particularly for the study of staphylococ-

*These are cut in 8-inch lengths, and a loop is made at one end to act as a handle. The tip is tightly bent over itself, dipped in collodion, and carefully covered with a tuft of fine eye cotton. An excellent substitute is the calcium alginate swab on a soft flexible aluminum wire, Falcon No. 2050, Oxnard, Calif.

cal or streptococcal nasal carriers. They are taken by introducing a cotton swab moistened with broth about 1 inch into the nares, gently rotating the swab against the nasal mucosa on both sides, and returning it to the broth tube.

ROUTINE PROCEDURES, INCLUDING ISOLATION METHODS FOR HEMOLYTIC STREPTOCOCCI

The throat or nasopharyngeal swab is used for the direct inoculation of blood agar plates, and several methods are available. Since the routine throat culture is taken chiefly to detect the presence of group A **beta-hemolytic streptococci,** the latter's significance will be stressed in the following procedures:

1. If polyester-tipped* swabs are used (as is preferred), direct inoculation of a **moist sheep blood agar** plate (without added glucose, which inhibits characteristic hemolysis) is recommended. Roll the swab firmly over a small portion of the agar surface and streak by using a sterile wire loop. Spread the inoculum over the remainder of the plate to obtain well-isolated colonies. There are many techniques for spreading the inoculum; one is shown in Fig. 4-1. Make a few **stabs** into the agar with the loop for observation of **subsurface hemolysis** by strains producing beta-type hemolysis under reduced oxygen tension. This procedure may be used on either a freshly made culture or on one in which the polyester swab has remained in its original container for several days (must be refrigerated).

2. If an applicator immersed in broth has been used, twirl the swab vigorously against the side of the broth tube to obtain as much material in suspension as possi-

ble. It has been shown that the flora of such a throat swab can be determined better by inoculating a broth suspension than by directly streaking the swab on a blood agar plate.[10] Using a sterile loop, transfer a loopful of the suspension to a blood agar plate and streak as described previously.

3. If a **pour plate** is desired, the cotton-tipped applicator is placed in 2 ml of trypticase soy broth and the suspension prepared as previously described.
   a. Transfer a loopful of this suspension to a 20- × 150-mm screw-capped tube containing approximately 15 ml of melted and **cooled** (45 to 50 C) trypticase soy agar.
   b. Pipet 0.8 ml of sterile defibrinated sheep blood into the agar and mix the entire contents of the tube by inversion. The sheep blood may be conveniently stored in 1-ml amounts in small sterile tubes in a refrigerator, where it will remain stable for 7 to 10 days.
   c. Flame the lip of the tube and pour the agar into a sterile Petri dish; allow it to cool and solidify.

Pour plates are useful in revealing certain strains of group A streptococci that may appear to be nonhemolytic when growing on the surface of blood agar plates, because these strains produce streptolysin O only, which is inactivated by atmospheric oxygen. Most strains of group A streptococci, however, show beta hemolysis around surface colonies because of their production of streptolysin S, which is oxygen stable.

All throat cultures are incubated at 35 C **aerobically**[36] and nasopharyngeal culture plates (for meningococci) are incubated in a candle jar (or 10% CO_2 incubator) for 18 to 24 hours. Some workers recommend incubation under anaerobic conditions.

Incorporation of sulfamethoxazole and trimethoprim in sheep blood agar enhanced recovery of groups A and B streptococci from throat

---

*This fiber appears to prolong the survival of beta-hemolytic streptococci from throat swabs and such swabs may be mailed in an envelope to the laboratory without noticeable loss of streptococci.[34]

cultures according to Gunn and co-workers.[24] Since this medium suppresses many other types of streptococci and since bacitracin disks identify group A beta-hemolytic streptococci with 95% accuracy when used on a pure culture, Kurzynski and associates[33] carried out bacitracin disk susceptibility tests on throat cultures that had been plated on sulfamethoxazole-trimethoprim blood agar plates. Eighty-five percent of group A streptococci could be identified on primary plates of this type within 24 hours as compared with only 26% on conventional sheep blood agar plates. Another interesting approach was employed by Baron and Gates.[3] They utilized side-by-side placement of a 25-μg sulfamethoxazole-trimethoprim disk and a 0.04-unit bacitracin disk in the heavily inoculated area of trypticase soy sheep blood agar plates inoculated with throat cultures. Suppression of normal flora by the sulfamethoxazole-trimethoprim disk permitted visualization of group A streptococci and inhibition of these organisms by the bacitracin disk. This technique would be useful for confirmation of results, particularly in laboratories where fluorescence microscopy is not available or cost effective.

The results obtained from throat cultures on blood agar depend to an extent on the **type of blood** used in preparing the plates. For reasons described in Chapter 17, sheep blood agar plates are recommended for these cultures (horse blood is also acceptable); human blood (either fresh or outdated bank blood) should be used only when sheep blood or horse blood is not available.

Another approach to rapid diagnosis of streptococcal pharyngitis is the use of Gram-stained smears of pharyngeal secretions. This depends on demonstrating polymorphonuclear leukocytes in close association with spherical gram-positive cocci occurring singly or in pairs. However, one may question whether this morphology is truly specific for *Streptococcus pyogenes* in view of the fact that so many streptococci of other types may be found normally in the upper respiratory tract flora.[9] False-negative results are also a problem with this technique in about one fourth of patients.

READING OF PLATES

Blood agar plates inoculated with throat cultures are sometimes confusing to the inexperienced bacteriologist. A knowledge of the **normal flora,** of the organisms that may be significant, and of the colony characteristics of both groups aids in solving the problem. The organisms that may be encountered in the **normal** throat, in order of their predominance, are as follows:

Alpha-hemolytic streptococci
Normal throat species of *Neisseria*, including pigmented forms
Coagulase-negative staphylococci and occasionally *Staphylococcus aureus*
Haemophilus haemolyticus (may be confused with beta-hemolytic streptococci) and *H. influenzae*
Pneumococci
Nonhemolytic (gamma) streptococci
Diphtheroid bacilli
Coliform bacilli (particularly after antimicrobial therapy)
Yeasts, including *Candida albicans*
Beta-hemolytic streptococci other than group A

Microorganisms that may be encountered in an **infected** throat are the following:

Beta-hemolytic streptococci of group A and occasionally groups B, C, and G
Corynebacterium diphtheriae
Meningococcus

Most throat cultures are taken for the detection of group A streptococci. Therefore, either the blood agar streak or pour plate should be carefully examined for the presence of colonies of beta-hemolytic streptococci after overnight incubation. A description of these colonies is detailed in Chapter 17.

Any colony suggestive of **beta-hemolytic streptococci** should be subcultured by stabbing with a straight needle and should be streaked on a sector of a sheep blood agar plate or inoculated to a tube of blood broth. This usually yields a pure culture; if it does not, the process should be repeated. Further identification of these colonies may be carried out by use of the bacitracin disk sensitivity test and confirmed, preferably by the fluorescent antibody procedure or coagglutination. The Phadebact* technique may be utilized for direct serologic grouping of beta-hemolytic streptococci from primary isolation plates.[43] When there are insufficient primary colonies for the direct procedure, the 4-hour or 24-hour procedure may be employed. These procedures are also described in Chapter 17.

BACTERIOLOGIC DIAGNOSIS OF PERTUSSIS

There has been a resurgence in the number of cases of pertussis in recent years. Cases have occurred in adults as well as children.

The diagnosis of **whooping cough** is confirmed by the isolation of *Bordetella pertussis* from the respiratory tract secretions. Nasopharyngeal swabs are used to obtain material for culture, and a special medium, Bordet-Gengou agar containing 15% to 20% sheep blood, is used for cultivating the organism.

Nasopharyngeal swabs are obtained in the following manner. While the child's head is immobilized, the special wire applicator (see discussion of throat and nasopharyngeal cultures elsewhere in this chapter) is carefully passed through the nasal aperture along the nasal floor until it touches the posterior pharyngeal wall. It is left there during several induced coughs before withdrawal, whereupon it is immediately streaked on the surface of the Bordet-Gengou medium, and the inoculum is spread over the plate with a sterile loop or spreader. Penicillin (0.5 unit/ml) may be incorporated in the medium at the time of preparation; this inhibits the growth of penicillin-sensitive organisms normally present in the nasopharynx, usually without affecting the growth of pertussis organisms. The

plates are incubated aerobically at 35 C for 4 or 5 days and are examined with a hand lens for the presence of typical colonies resembling mercury droplets surrounded by a hemolytic zone. *B. pertussis* is identified by staining reaction, fluorescent antibody technique, and agglutination with specific antiserum, as indicated in Chapter 23.

The yield of positive isolations from clinical cases of pertussis varies from 20% to 98%. This variation is apparently related to the procedures used, the stage of the disease, and the prior administration of antibiotics. Using the fluorescent antibody technique, Whitaker and associates[49] were able to confirm the diagnosis in 94% of pertussis cases during the first week of illness. Holwerda and Eldering[29] employed the fluorescent antibody technique in direct staining of early growth from Bordet-Gengou plates* and were able thereby to identify *B. pertussis* 1 day earlier. The fluorescent antibody technique is an aid in diagnosis; however, it should always be used in conjunction with conventional culture procedures.

When laboratory facilities for the culture of *B. pertussis* are not available, one may utilize nasopharyngeal smears for fluorescent antibody detection of the organism.[26] When these smears are treated with 4 or 8 units of aprotinin per milliliter, their fluorescent antibody staining qualities are preserved for at least 3 weeks.

BACTERIOLOGIC DIAGNOSIS OF DIPHTHERIA

The diagnosis of **diphtheria** is a clinical problem, and the responsibility should rest primarily on the attending physician. It is unreasonable and unwise for a clinician to place the responsibility on the bacteriologist and expect a definitive diagnosis within 15 minutes based on the examination of a direct smear of the lesion. Although the appearance of diphtheria bacilli in

---

*Phadebact Streptococcus Test, Pharmacia Inc., Piscataway, N.J.

*This appears to be the chief value of the fluorescent antibody technique in diagnosing pertussis.

stained smears from lesions and membranes is highly characteristic, these organisms cannot be identified by morphology alone, since other nonpathogenic diphtherialike bacilli may be indistinguishable from *Corynebacterium diphtheriae*. The chance of error in either direction is too great when diagnosis is based exclusively on microscopic examination; such a reading should be accepted only as **presumptive** evidence of infection. The identity and type of the organism in question is obtained only after isolating toxigenic *C. diphtheriae* from the patient. Determination of the presence of these organisms requires a careful cultural and microscopic study of several days' duration followed by a virulence test in suitable animals or by an in vitro test.

In primary isolation, *C. diphtheriae* is best cultivated on appropriate media, such as Loeffler medium (three parts animal serum and one part dextrose broth, coagulated as slants) or modified Pai medium, where growth occurs after 18 to 24 hours' incubation at 35 C. Differential and selective media, such as cystine or chocolate-tellurite agar, also give a high proportion of recoveries and should be included in primary inoculation; however, the microscopic morphology of the diphtheria bacillus from chocolate-tellurite agar is not as distinctive as that from Loeffler or Pai medium. These media are described in Chapter 42.

Material received in the laboratory for diphtheria culture is usually sent on swabs taken from the **throat** and **nasopharynx.** These are promptly inoculated to the surface of a Loeffler or Pai slant and streaked on cystine-tellurite agar plates or modified Tinsdale medium. Since severe throat infections caused by beta-hemolytic streptococci may produce lesions simulating diphtheria, it is recommended that sheep blood agar plates be inoculated also and examined for group A streptococci, along with the Loeffler slant and the tellurite plate. After inoculating the media, one can prepare a smear by rolling the swab on a slide, fixing it, and staining it with **methylene blue stain.** It is preferable to have a separate swab for the smear so the other swab may be left on the Loeffler slant after inoculation. The slide should be examined for the presence of irregularly stained gram-positive pleomorphic organisms suggestive of diphtheria bacilli (see below).

The inoculated media are incubated at 35 C. On a Loeffler slant that has been incubated for a short period (2 to 8 hours), *C. diphtheriae* frequently outgrows other organisms present and exhibits a characteristic morphology when stained with **methylene blue.** The bacilli are deeply stained and appear septated, with wedge-shaped ends and tapered points. The cells are often at angles to each other, as in the letters V and Y or Chinese letters, and do not palisade as is seen with some of the diphtheroid bacilli.

If organisms resembling diphtheria bacilli are found in smears from the Loeffler slant but not from the tellurite plate, the growth from the slant is suspended in 1 to 2 ml of sterile broth, and a loopful of this is streaked on a fresh tellurite plate to isolate the organism. All plates should be held and examined for 48 hours before being discarded as negative.

Fluorescent antibody procedures for the detection of *C. diphtheriae* in known or suspected cases of clinical diphtheria have been used as a rapid presumptive diagnostic procedure. The conjugate used cross-reacts with toxigenic strains of *C. ulcerans* (rarely found in the United States) and does not differentiate between toxigenic and nontoxigenic strains of *C. diphtheriae*. It is recommended that the procedure be used in conjunction with conventional culturing procedures to achieve the greatest degree of sensitivity and specificity.

LABORATORY DIAGNOSIS OF VINCENT'S INFECTION ("FUSOSPIROCHETAL DISEASE")

Vincent's gingivitis or stomatitis is a pseudomembranous or ulcerative infection of the gums, mouth, or pharynx. It had been thought to be caused by a gram-negative spirochete, *Borrelia vincentii,* and a straight or slightly curved, anaerobic gram-negative rod with sharply pointed ends, *Fusobacterium nucleatum.* Unusually large spirochetes appear to be specifically associated with this problem, perhaps along with a number of other anaerobes, including *Bacteroides melaninogenicus,* other gram-negative anaerobic rods, and anaerobic cocci. A reduction in local tissue resistance is generally a precursor of the infection.

The pseudomembrane present on tonsillar lesions in Vincent's angina has been mistaken for a similar lesion in diphtheria, and it is important that they be differentiated. One may readily demonstrate fusospirochetal organisms by staining smears with **crystal violet** (that used in Gram stain) for 1 minute and looking for large numbers of the characteristic forms, along with numerous pus cells. Since these organisms are often present in the normal mouth and gums, their presence in smears must be correlated with the clinical findings to be of significance. The key pathogen in Vincent's angina is undoubtedly *Fusobacterium necrophorum,* because when this condition is complicated by sepsis and metastatic infection, *F. necrophorum* is almost always recoverable from blood cultures (Plates 5 and 6) and distant lesions. Cultures are of no diagnostic value and should not be done.

NASOPHARYNGEAL CULTURES FOR MENINGOCOCCI AND HAEMOPHILUS

Nasopharyngeal cultures are important in demonstrating the presence of *Neisseria meningitidis* in cases of suspected meningococcemia and meningococcal meningitis and in the detection of meningococcal carriers. The specimen may be collected through the mouth by passing a wire swab under and beyond the uvula to the posterior wall of the nasopharynx or through the nostril by passing the wire swab along the floor of the nasal passage to the posterior wall. In either case it is desirable to secure á bit of the mucus by gently twirling the swab while in place against the nasopharyngeal wall. It should be noted that *N. meningitidis* can be recovered

from healthy people; carrier rates among population groups experiencing a meningitis outbreak may rise as high as 80%. Under these circumstances it is doubtful that a positive culture is significant. A **negative** culture from a patient convalescing from meningococcal meningitis who may be in contact with younger susceptible persons on returning home is perhaps more meaningful. *N. meningitidis* is extremely sensitive to cold, dehydration, unfavorable pH, or the inhibitory activity of other microflora; therefore, culture material should be inoculated as soon as possible.

Meningococci may be isolated on moist blood agar used in routine throat and nasopharyngeal cultures or modified Thayer-Martin medium (preferred), where they appear after 18 to 24 hours' incubation in a candle jar as small, gray, mucoid, nonhemolytic colonies of gram-negative diplococci.

Like the gonococcus, the meningococcus is **oxidase positive;** this provides a helpful test that can be used for detecting the presence of these colonies in a mixed culture. It must be noted, however, that the nonpathogenic neisseriae of the oropharynx also will give a positive oxidase test. To identify *N. meningitidis,* therefore, it is necessary to carry out a slide agglutination test with a polyvalent antiserum,* fluorescent antibody technique, or a capsular swelling (quellung) reaction test. Fermentation reactions with several carbohydrates are also essential for identification. Refer to Chapter 19 for further information.

Accumulating evidence indicates that *Haemophilus influenzae* carriage may be important in the spread of meningitis. Accordingly, it may be desirable, under certain circumstances, to seek *H. influenzae* in cultures of the nasopharynx or throat. It must be remembered that it is normally found in this location in a small percentage of people. Cotton swabs should be moistened in broth before the sample is taken and should be transported to the laboratory in a transport

---

*Difco Laboratories, Detroit.

medium kept at room temperature. The material should be plated out on chocolate agar or peptic digest agar plates.

THROAT CULTURES FOR SPECIES OF CANDIDA

The yeastlike organism *Candida albicans* may cause an intraoral infection called **thrush** in infants and neonates, diabetics, and individuals receiving antimicrobial or corticosteroid therapy. Material for Gram stain and culture is taken from the whitish, loosely adherent membrane attached to the inner cheek, palate, or other portions of the oral mucosa, using the technique described for throat cultures. On receipt in the laboratory, the swab is inoculated to slants of Sabouraud dextrose agar, with and without added antibiotics (see Chapter 34), and incubated both at room temperature and at 35 C. Primary growth of *Candida* occurs in 2 to 3 days as a yeastlike colony with a characteristic fermentative odor. Identification of *C. albicans* depends on the demonstration of germ tubes or typical chlamydospores on a special medium and other tests. The procedure is described in Chapter 34.

EPIGLOTTITIS AND TRACHEITIS

Epiglottitis is an uncommon but severe life-threatening infection of the epiglottis. The swelling of the epiglottis resulting from the infection may close off the airway, presenting an emergency that requires immediate tracheostomy or endotracheal intubation. It occurs primarily in infants or young children but is seen in adults occasionally. The most common pathogen by far is *Haemophilus influenzae*, with group A streptococci, pneumococci, and staphylococci occasionally responsible. There are reports of isolated cases caused by *H. parainfluenzae* and a beta-lactamase-producing ampicillin-resistant *H. paraphrophilus*.

Blood cultures are frequently positive in epiglottitis, and cultures of the epiglottis yield the offending organism. The epiglottis should not be swabbed or cultured until the airway has been established by means of tracheostomy or endotracheal intubation, as such swabbing may cause reflex laryngospasm and further respiratory tract obstruction.

Jones and associates[31] reported a distinctive illness in infants and young children, with features common to both croup and epiglottitis. The pathology involves marked edema of the mucosa below the glottis. Tracheal suctioning yields copious amounts of mucopurulent material from this area. Cultures yield primarily *Staphylococcus aureus* but also group A streptococcus and *H. influenzae* in other individuals. As in patients with epiglottitis, most of these patients require intubation or tracheostomy.

Bartlett and colleagues[5] have done quantitative studies of the bacteriology and cytology of tracheal secretions in individuals with long-term tracheostomies. It is well established that the trachea rapidly becomes colonized with a variety of bacterial species following tracheostomy. The study of Bartlett and his co-workers indicates that the flora of such tracheostomies is predominantly aerobic, that it is changeable, and that it has little relationship to the flora of the upper respiratory tract in the same individuals. Their data suggest that for these persons neither quantitative cultures nor analysis of the host cellular content of the specimens would help in distinguishing colonization from true infection requiring therapy.

SPUTUM CULTURES

Bacterial pneumonia, pulmonary tuberculosis, and chronic bronchitis constitute a most important group of human diseases. Since specific treatment frequently depends on a bacteriologic diagnosis, the prompt and accurate examination of a properly collected sputum specimen by smear, culture, and antimicrobial susceptibility testing is imperative. This is particularly true for pneumonia caused by *Klebsiella pneumoniae*, other Enterobacteriaceae, *Pseudomonas*, *Legionella*, and *Staphylococcus aureus*, which may be more rapidly fatal than that caused by *Streptococcus pneumoniae*.[1]

Many other organisms of varying types (e.g., *H. influenzae*, *N. meningitidis*, *Nocardia* [Plates 18 and 19], *Yersinia*, *Mycoplasma*, fungi, various mycobacteria [Plate 9], various anaerobes, and viruses) may cause pneumonia, empyema, lung abscess, or other pulmonary infections.

Recovery of an etiologic agent from sputum or other appropriate specimen depends not only on the laboratory methods used but also on the **care taken** in securing the specimen. Too often the culturing of unsuitable material results in misleading information for the clinician because the true infecting agent is missed entirely or because an incidental pathogen is identified. It should require no special courage on the part of the microbiologist to discard a specimen that is obviously saliva as being **unsatisfactory** for bacteriologic examination.

The collection of sputum for culture also requires the cooperation of the patient and should include instructions to obtain material from a deep cough (tracheobronchial sputum), which is expectorated directly into a sterile Petri dish or other satisfactory container.* The volume of the specimen need not be large; 1 to 3 ml of purulent or mucopurulent material is sufficient for most examinations except mycobacteriologic culturing. On receipt in the laboratory the specimen should be examined without delay, especially if histoplasmosis is suspected. However, refrigeration of the specimen for not more than 1 to 3 hours is satisfactory for the recovery of most pathogens if immediate culturing is not feasible.

The organisms most frequently associated with **acute** bacterial infections of the lower respiratory tract are:

Pneumococcus (*Streptococcus pneumoniae*)
Klebsiella pneumoniae
Haemophilus influenzae
Staphylococcus aureus

Coliform bacilli, *Pseudomonas*, and *Proteus* species
Mycoplasma pneumoniae
Legionella species

With the exception of *Mycobacterium tuberculosis* and *Legionella*, it is generally possible to recover the important pulmonary pathogens from the upper respiratory tract of apparently healthy people. The recovery of these organisms, therefore, is not always sufficient evidence of their etiologic role in a particular infection. In acute bacterial pneumonia, however, the pathogen is generally present in large numbers in optimum specimens. **Sputum culture is never satisfactory for diagnosis of anaerobic pulmonary infection.** Sputum should never be cultured anaerobically.

EXAMINATION OF GRAM-STAINED SMEARS

The first step in the examination of sputum is to determine whether the specimen is likely to be reliable. A purulent portion of sputum is carefully selected and transferred to a clean Petri dish. From this a Gram-stained smear is prepared or wet mounts are examined directly by Nomarski interference contrast microscopy.[48] The slide should be scanned at **100×** magnification and the number of squamous epithelial cells and polymorphonuclear leukocytes noted (Plates 10 to 12). Murray and Washington[35] noted that the presence of more than 10 epithelial cells per 100× field correlated with significant oral contamination (on the basis of culture results compared with cultures of transtracheal aspirates); they believed such specimens should be rejected. Van Scoy[45] reviewed their data and decided that cultures yielding viridans streptococci, *S. epidermidis*, *Neisseria* species, *Haemophilus* species, yeast, and *Corynebacterium* (as unlikely causes of pneumonia in adults) could be ignored and that then a more reliable criterion of a valid specimen was the presence of more than 25 leukocytes per low-power field. While *Haemophilus* and *Neisseria* are uncommon causes of pneumonia in adults and most of the

---

*The use of superheated hypertonic saline aerosols for sputum induction is recommended when the cough is not productive. Proper decontamination of the equipment must be carried out when using this procedure.[19]

other organisms rarely, if ever, cause pneumonia, viridans streptococci are not at all uncommon etiologic agents in aspiration pneumonia (often as part of a mixed flora also involving anaerobes). A number of studies validate the concept of screening sputum for epithelial cells and polymorphonuclear leukocytes prior to acceptance for culture. Perhaps the best of these studies is one done by Geckler and associates[22] in which 96 sputum specimens from patients with pneumonia were screened, and the results of cultures of these specimens were compared with cultures of paired transtracheal aspirates. When the sputum specimens had 25 or more leukocytes and fewer than 10 squamous epithelial cells per low-power field, a potential pathogen growing in this specimen was 94% predictive of growth in the transtracheal aspiration. Agreement between sputa with less than 25 squamous epithelial cells and transtracheal aspiration was also good (79%). Careful examination of smears of screened sputum specimens for microorganisms yielded meaningful information to clinicians by correctly predicting culture results in almost 75% of acceptable specimens, according to a study by Heineman and Radano.[27] The most reliable specimen has **less than 10 epithelial cells and more than 25 leukocytes per low-power field.** Also acceptable would be sputum specimens with fewer than 25 epithelial cells and more than 25 leukocytes per low-power field.

It must be remembered that severely leukopenic patients (peripheral white blood cell count of 500/cu mm or less) may not be able to muster sufficient polymorphonuclear leukocytes to meet the above criteria for sputum. Exceptions must be made in such cases. In general, a microbiologist should never discard a specimen outright, except obvious saliva. Rather, problem specimens should be discussed with the clinician responsible for the patient.

An early presumptive diagnosis of bacterial pneumonia can often be made by examining a direct smear of sputum properly stained by the Gram method. The presence of many encapsulated, lancet-shaped cocci occurring singly, in pairs, or in short chains, along with pus cells (Plate 13), may suggest a pneumococcal infection in typical cases. Rein and associates[40] considered a Gram stain positive for pneumococci if a preponderant flora of (or more than 10) gram-positive lancet-shaped diplococci was seen per oil immersion field. A positive smear of this type strongly suggests the presence of pneumococci but misses about one third of specimens that contain pneumococci. The use of Omniserum for the quellung reaction (swelling of capsules on exposure to antiserum) considerably increases the likelihood of accurate identification of pneumococci on direct observation[11] (see Chapter 18). A stained preparation showing great numbers of gram-positive cocci in clusters (Plate 14) is suggestive of staphylococcal pneumonia. Detection of numerous short, fat, encapsulated gram-negative rods (Plate 15) suggests *Klebsiella* infection. Observation of "gram-neutral" bacilli may be a clue to the presence of mycobacteria (Hinson et al.: Am. Rev. Respir. Dis. **123:**365-366, 1981).

However, the **presumptive** aspect of these findings should be emphasized—only by the isolation of pneumococci, staphylococci, pseudomonads, or klebsiellae from cultures of blood, pleural fluid, or perhaps sputum can such an impression be confirmed.

CULTURE FOR PNEUMOCOCCUS

Since *Streptococcus pneumoniae* continues to be the major cause of bacterial pneumonia, the examination of a fresh sputum specimen is the first step in the diagnostic procedure.

Blood-tinged (rust-colored) mucopurulent sputum freshly obtained from patients with lobar pneumonia may be handled in the following manner:

1. Select purulent or bloody flecks and prepare direct smears as follows. Transfer a loopful to a clean slide, press another slide over it, squeeze the slides together, and

then pull them apart. Flame both slides as soon as they are dry. Stain one slide by the Gram method and one by the acid-fast technique.

2. Streak a sheep blood agar plate* with a small loopful of a **selected** portion of the specimen (not saliva). Place the blood plate in a candle jar†; incubate it at 35 C for 18 to 24 hours.

3. If the sputum is unusually tenacious, transfer a mucopurulent mass to a Petri dish containing sterile physiologic saline and swish it around to remove the excess saliva. Transfer to a clean Petri dish, add a small volume of saline, and repeatedly aspirate and expel the specimen in a sterile syringe to emulsify it. **Exercise caution** to avoid aerosols. Use a loopful of this suspension to inoculate the media previously indicated.

4. If after incubation of the blood plate, small, shiny, greenish, transparent, flat colonies with depressed centers and raised edges are seen, they are most likely colonies of pneumococci. These may be cultured and further identified by determining their solubility in bile salts or their susceptibility to Optochin. These tests are described in Chapter 18.

5. Although pneumococci usually predominate in sputum cultures from patients with early lobar pneumonia, the blood plate may also show a large number of colonies of the usual throat flora, consisting of alpha-hemolytic streptococci, nonpathogenic neisseriae, and so forth. Before discarding such a plate as showing only nor-

mal throat flora, it is recommended that a search for pneumococcus colonies be made with a **hand magnifying lens** ($3\times$ to $8\times$). If these colonies are present, an attempt should be made to recover them in pure culture by subculturing to a fresh blood agar plate.

The report that sheep blood agar containing 5 μg of gentamicin per milliliter was distinctly better than sheep blood agar without gentamicin has not been confirmed by Schmid and co-workers.[42] Wu and colleagues[52] also found no benefit from gentamicin-containing sheep blood agar, but they found that anaerobic incubation of sheep blood agar enhanced recovery of pneumococci considerably. This was considered a result of the greater ease of recognition of the larger, more mucoid colonies of S. pneumoniae and the suppression of growth of other organisms present in the respiratory tract secretions.

Pneumococci have been found to survive in sputum for extended periods at room temperature and considerably longer periods at 4 C.[50] Overgrowth of pneumococci by pharyngeal flora occurred significantly more frequently in specimens kept at room temperature than in those kept at 4 C.

QUANTITATIVE SPUTUM CULTURE

Quantitative sputum culturing, by means of liquefying the specimen with a mucolytic agent, homogenizing it, and plating tenfold serial dilutions of it on appropriate solid culture media, has had numerous proponents. Saponin is a stable and rapidly effective mucolytic agent.[12] The technique, however, is cumbersome and time consuming, requires a considerable number of plates, and appears to offer few advantages over conventional methods. N-Acetylcysteine should **not** be used as a liquefying agent, as it has antibacterial activity. A technique employing preliminary washing gives much more reliable information[7] and is worth considering for acutely ill patients in whom transtracheal aspiration is not possible.

---

*The worker is well advised to streak serially two or more blood agar plates and a MacConkey or eosin–methylene blue (EMB) plate (if *Klebsiella* is suspected) to obtain isolated colonies when the bacterial population of the sample is unusually high.

†Austrian and Collins[2] have shown that a small percentage of pneumococci require 3% to 10% CO_2 for recovery on agar plates at the time of primary inoculation.

TRANSTRACHEAL ASPIRATION AND OTHER MEANS TO AVOID UPPER RESPIRATORY TRACT FLORA

Since severe and sometimes fatal necrotizing pneumonia caused by gram-negative enteric bacilli, *S. aureus,* and other pathogens is occurring more frequently and since these same organisms are found not uncommonly in the mouths of hospitalized and nursing home patients[21] (gram-negative bacilli are also common in alcoholics),[20] the reliability of a routine sputum culture (contaminated by mouth flora) has been questioned. In 1959 Pecora[38] proposed transtracheal aspiration, in which a small-gauge catheter is threaded into the trachea through a needle introduced at the cricothyroid membrane as an alternative procedure for obtaining material from the lower respiratory tract, uncontaminated by oropharyngeal microorganisms. The technique has proved safe and the results bacteriologically reliable,[8,28,32] and it is recommended for patients with pneumonia who are unable to raise a satisfactory sputum specimen[25] and for patients with suspected anaerobic pulmonary infection (lung abscess, aspiration pneumonia, bronchiectasis, or Legionnaires' disease).[8] Results of Gram-stained smears of transtracheal aspirates (Plates 16 and 17) correlate much better with their corresponding cultures than do smears of expectorated sputum from the same patient, although a smear from a specimen that shows many polymorphonuclear leukocytes and few squamous epithelial cells on low-power screening is almost as good. The technique is not suitable for individuals with a bleeding tendency or significant ventilation problems or for those who are not able to lie still.

In order to evaluate the possibility of oropharyngeal contamination during transtracheal aspiration, it has been common practice to look for squamous epithelial cells. It has been pointed out that squamous epithelial cells may be found normally in the lower respiratory tract in persons with chronic bronchitis or chronic obstructive pulmonary disease and that it is difficult to distinguish these bronchial squamous epithelial cells from buccal squamous epithelial cells except by electron microscopy.[30] One percent methylene blue nebulized into the oropharynx has served as a reliable marker. Contamination is unlikely in a specimen that is methylene blue negative by spectrophotometry.

With the introduction of the fiberoptic bronchoscope it was hoped that one might be able to obtain lower airway secretions from specific bronchial segments involved with pathology in such a way as to avoid contamination with upper respiratory tract secretions. Early studies, however, indicated that contamination with upper respiratory tract microorganisms was a problem. However, introduction of a double-lumen cannula surrounding a bronchial brush and plugged by polyethylene glycol seemed to provide a system for avoiding this type of contamination. Preliminary results suggest that this technique did work well.[51] However, relatively few patients have been studied. A large clinical study comparing the new fiberoptic bronchoscopy technique with transtracheal aspiration is needed to determine how reliable the bronchoscopy procedure really is. Another technique, used particularly by pediatricians, involves direct lung puncture. This provides an even smaller specimen than can be obtained on the bronchial brush referred to previously. Accordingly, it would be necessary to transport this specimen to the laboratory and set it up in appropriate culture immediately. It seems likely that anaerobes and other delicate organisms might die prior to culture with these latter two procedures.

Of course, when the patient has an empyema along with pneumonia, drainage of the pleural fluid, which is indicated therapeutically, provides an excellent specimen that will accurately reflect the infecting flora of the lung itself.

CULTURE FOR OTHER PATHOGENS

Respiratory tract material from acute or chronic pulmonary infections caused by agents other than pneumococci can vary from a thick, tenacious specimen that reveals species of *Klebsiella* on culture to a foul-smelling purulent aspirate from a patient with a lung abscess, from which species of *Bacteroides* and other anaerobes may be recovered. As a rule, the isolation and identification of klebsiellae pose no problem, although serologic identification by means of capsular swelling test may require the aid of a reference laboratory.* The anaerobes are more difficult to recover and identify; they should be looked for especially in the foul-smelling† material from patients with aspiration pneumonia, lung abscess, bronchiectasis, and empyema. Transtracheal aspirates from these patients should be streaked on two **fresh** blood agar plates and inoculated to two tubes of enriched thioglycollate medium. One set of media is incubated in an **anaerobic jar** subsequently handled as described in Chapter 13; the other set is handled as described for pneumococcus isolation. See Chapter 13 for a description of anaerobic culture procedures.

It should be appreciated that the so-called viridans streptococci are definitely important pathogens in pulmonary infection as well as other serious infections throughout the body. These organisms are often best recovered using anaerobic transport and culture techniques. Since viridans streptococci are so prevalent in the normal oral flora, it is necessary that material for culture for these organisms be obtained in such a way as to preclude contamination from that source.

It should also be appreciated that groups A and B streptococci may cause pneumonia, the latter primarily in newborns. Group C streptococci have also been responsible for pneumonia.[44]

Haemophilus influenzae is an important cause of pneumonia in children and is not a rare cause of pneumonia in adults.[46] Such pneumonia may be complicated by pleural involvement and bacteremia. Encapsulated strains, primarily type b, are the most prevalent. The use of transtracheal aspiration, blood culture, and culture of pleural fluid are all important in diagnosing *H. influenzae* pneumonia. Materials should be cultured on chocolate agar or peptic digest agar. The sputum from patients with cystic fibrosis commonly is overgrown by *Pseudomonas aeruginosa*. This may make it impossible to detect other organisms such as *H. influenzae* that may be important pathogens in infection in these individuals. Roberts and Cole[41] have described an interesting approach to recover *H. influenzae* from sputum containing large numbers of *Pseudomonas* organisms. The specimen is homogenized with pancreatin and streaked onto two plates of a medium containing bacitracin. A V disk is placed in the center of the second set of streaks, and the plates are incubated, one anaerobically and one aerobically. *Pseudomonas* grows poorly or not at all under anaerobic conditions.

Legionella pneumophila and other species of *Legionella* are important causes of a serious type of pneumonia. These organisms stain poorly by the Gram technique but may be demonstrated by the Giménez stain. Direct fluorescent antibody testing of respiratory tract secretions is important when Legionnaires' disease is suspected.[15] Artificial culture techniques have improved to the point that egg yolk sac and guinea pig inoculation are no longer necessary for recovery of organisms from clinical specimens. Buffered charcoal yeast extract agar is the medium of choice.[18,37] Incubation should be at 35 C in humidified air. Transtracheal aspirates and pleural fluid are the best specimens to utilize.[15] The organism may be recovered from sputum by the use of a semiselective medium,[14] but in general the organism is much more easily recovered from specimens normally having no flora. Incubation should be carried out for a period of 2 weeks, although in many cases growth will be noted in 3 or 4 days. All work with these agents

---

*Some antisera are available from Difco Laboratories, Detroit.

†The foul odor is an important clue when present, but it is noted in only about 50% of anaerobic pleuropulmonary infections; thus, absence of such odor does not exclude anaerobic infection.[6]

should be carried out in a biologic safety hood. The CDC should be notified of any suspect isolates; these should be submitted for confirmation if indicated.

The examination of both stained and unstained wet smears prepared directly from the sputum may be informative, particularly when fungus elements can be demonstrated. Darkfield illumination may also be helpful in revealing the presence of spirilla and spirochetes.

Special methods for anaerobes, fungi, chlamydiae, and mycobacteria are described in their respective chapters. See Chapter 14 regarding pleural and pericardial effusions.

NONCULTURAL TECHNIQUES FOR DIAGNOSIS OF RESPIRATORY TRACT INFECTIONS

The use of fluorescent antibody techniques for diagnosis of group A streptococcal pharyngitis and Legionnaires' disease has already been discussed. A fluorescent antibody technique has also been used to demonstrate antibody-coated group A streptococci in throat smears (Sewell et al.: Ann. Clin. Lab. Sci. 11:15-18, 1981). Using a modified nitrous acid extraction microtechnique on tonsillar scrapings, it was found that group A streptococci in the throat could be identified in 30 minutes.[17] Cytopathologic techniques may be helpful in diagnosing certain viral, mycotic, and parasitic infections of the respiratory tract.

CIE can be used to detect pneumococcal polysaccharide in sputum; this is said to correlate better with the presence of pneumococcal pneumonia than recovery of pneumococci by culture.[13] However, this is a relatively expensive procedure, and it is the opinion of some workers that equivalent sensitivity and specificity are available by finding 10 or more lancet-shaped gram-positive diplococci per oil immersion field in a Gram-stained smear of an acceptable sputum specimen. Coagglutination is comparable to CIE in terms of specificity and sensitivity and is actually more sensitive in the case of sputum samples obtained during antibiotic ther-apy.[16] In addition, coagglutination is simpler to perform than CIE and requires much less antiserum. Latex particle agglutination (LPA)* was found to be more sensitive and specific than CIE in the diagnosis of *H. influenzae* type B infections, including epiglottitis and pneumonia.[47] Latex particle agglutination is inexpensive.

---

*Wampole Laboratories, Cranbury, N.J.

REFERENCES

1. Austrian, R.: The role of the microbiology laboratory in the management of bacterial infections, Med. Clin. North Am. **50**:1419-1432, 1966.
2. Austrian, R., and Collins, P.: Importance of carbon dioxide in the isolation of pneumococci, J. Bacteriol. **92**:1281-1284, 1966.
3. Baron, E.J., and Gates, J.W.: Primary plate identification of Group A beta-hemolytic streptococci utilizing a two-disk technique, J. Clin. Microbiol. **10**:80-84, 1979.
4. Bartlett, J.G., Brewer, N.S., and Ryan, K.J. In Washington, J.A., II, editor: Laboratory diagnosis of lower respiratory tract infections, Cumitech 7, Washington, D.C., 1978, American Society for Microbiology.
5. Bartlett, J.G., Faling, L.J., and Willey, S.: Quantitative tracheal bacteriologic and cytologic studies in patients with long-term tracheostomies, Chest **74**:635-639, 1978.
6. Bartlett, J.G., and Finegold, S.M.: Anaerobic infections of the lung and pleural space, Am. Rev. Respir. Dis. **110**:56-77, 1974.
7. Bartlett, J.G., and Finegold, S.M.: Bacteriology of expectorated sputum with quantitative culture and wash technique compared to transtracheal aspirates, Am. Rev. Respir. Dis. **117**:1019-1027, 1978.
8. Bartlett, J.G., Rosenblatt, J.E., and Finegold, S.M.: Percutaneous transtracheal aspiration in the diagnosis of anaerobic pulmonary infection, Ann. Intern. Med. **79**:535-540, 1973.
9. Bisno, A.L.: The diagnosis of streptococcal pharyngitis, Ann. Intern. Med. **90**:426-428, 1979.
10. Committee on Acute Respiratory Diseases: Problems in determining the bacterial flora of the pharynx, Proc. Soc. Exp. Biol. Med. **69**:45-52, 1948.
11. Dilworth, J.A., Stewart, P., Gwaltney, J.M., Jr., Hendley, J.O., and Sande, M.A.: Methods to improve detection of pneumococci in respiratory secretions, J. Clin. Microbiol. **2**:453-455, 1975.

12. Dorn, G.L., Land, G.A., and Smith, K.E.: The compromised host: quantitative sputum analysis with a non-toxic mucolytic agent, Lab. Med. **11**:183-189, 1980.

13. Downes, B.A., and Ellner, P.D.: Comparison of sputum counterimmunoelectrophoresis and culture in diagnosis of pneumococcal pneumonia, J. Clin. Microbiol. **10**:662-665, 1979.

14. Edelstein, P.H., and Finegold, S.M.: Use of a semiselective medium to culture *Legionella pneumophila* from contaminated lung specimens, J. Clin. Microbiol. **10**:141-143, 1979.

15. Edelstein, P.H., Meyer, R.D., and Finegold, S.M.: Laboratory diagnosis of Legionnaires' disease, Am. Rev. Respir. Dis. **121**:317-327, 1980.

16. Edwards, E.A., and Coonrod, J.D.: Coagglutination and counterimmunoelectrophoresis for detection of pneumococcal antigens in the sputum of pneumonia patients, J. Clin. Microbiol. **11**:488-491, 1980.

17. El Kholy, A., Facklam, R., Sabri, G., and Rotta, J.: Serological identification of Group A streptococci from throat scrapings before culture, J. Clin. Microbiol. **8**:725-728, 1978.

18. Feeley, J.C., Gibson, R.J., Gorman, G.W., Langford, N.C., Rasheed, J.K., Mackel, D.C., and Baine, W.B.: Charcoal-yeast extract agar: primary isolation medium for *Legionella pneumophila*, J. Clin. Microbiol. **10**:437-441, 1979.

19. French, M.L.V., Dunlop, S.G., and Wentzler, T.F.: Contamination of sputum induction equipment during patient usage, Appl. Microbiol. **21**:899-902, 1971.

20. Fuxench-López, Z., and Ramirez-Ronda, C.H.: Pharyngeal flora in ambulatory alcoholic patients: prevalence of Gram-negative bacilli, Arch. Intern. Med. **138**:1815-1816, 1978.

21. Garb, J.L., Brown, R.B., Garb, J.R., and Tuthill, R.W.: Differences in etiology of pneumonias in nursing home and community patients, J.A.M.A. **240**:2169-2172, 1978.

22. Geckler, R.W., Gremillion, D.H., McAllister, C.K., and Ellenbogen, C.: Microscopic and bacteriological comparison of paired sputa and transtracheal aspirates, J. Clin. Microbiol. **6**:396-399, 1977.

23. Guckian, J.C., and Christensen, W.D.: Quantitative culture and gram stain of sputum in pneumonia, Am. Rev. Respir. Dis. **118**:997-1005, 1978.

24. Gunn, B.A., Ohashi, D.K., Gaydos, C.A., and Holt, E.S.: Selective and enhanced recovery of Group A and B streptococci from throat cultures with sheep blood agar containing sulfamethoxazole and trimethoprim, J. Clin. Microbiol. **5**:650-655, 1977.

25. Hahn, H.H., and Beaty, H.N.: Transtracheal aspiration in the evaluation of patients with pneumonia, Ann. Intern. Med. **72**:183-187, 1970.

26. Harris, P.P., Thomason, B., and McKinney, R.M.: Preservation of nasopharyngeal smears for fluorescent antibody detection of *Bordetella pertussis*, J. Clin. Microbiol. **12**:799-801, 1980.

27. Heineman, H.S., and Radano, R.R.: Acceptability and cost savings of selective sputum microbiology in a community teaching hospital, J. Clin. Microbiol. **10**:567-573, 1979.

28. Hoeprich, P.D.: Etiologic diagnosis of lower respiratory tract infections, Calif. Med. **112**:1-8, 1970.

29. Holwerda, J., and Eldering, G.: Culture and fluorescent-antibody methods in diagnosis of whooping cough, J. Bacteriol. **86**:449-451, 1963.

30. Irwin, R.S., Demers, R.R., Pratter, M.R., Erickson, A.D., Farrugia, R., and Teplitz, C.: Evaluation of methylene blue and squamous epithelial cells as oropharyngeal markers: a means of identifying oropharyngeal contamination during transtracheal aspiration, J. Infect. Dis. **141**:165-171, 1980.

31. Jones, R., Santos, J.I., Overall, J.C., Jr.: Bacterial tracheitis, J.A.M.A. **242**:721-726, 1979.

32. Kalinske, R.W., Parker, R.H., Brandt, D., and Hoeprich, P.D.: Diagnostic usefulness and safety of transtracheal aspiration, N. Engl. J. Med. **276**:604-608, 1967.

33. Kurzynski, T., Meise, C., Daggs, R., and Helstad, A.: Improved reliability of the primary plate bacitracin test on throat cultures with sulfamethoxazole-trimethoprim blood agar plates, J. Clin. Microbiol. **9**:144-146, 1979.

34. Lattimer, A.D., Siegel, A.C., and DeCelles, J.: Evaluation of the recovery of beta hemolytic streptococci from two mail-in methods, Am. J. Public Health **53**:1594-1602, 1963.

35. Murray, P.R., and Washington, J.A., II: Microscopic and bacteriologic analysis of expectorated sputum, Mayo Clin. Proc. **50**:339-344, 1975.

36. Murray, P.R., Wold, A.D., Schreck, C.A., and Washington, J.A., II: Effects of selective media and atmosphere of incubation on the isolation of group A streptococci, J. Clin. Microbiol. **4**:54-56, 1976.

37. Pasculle, A.W., Feeley, J.C., Gibson, R.J., Cordes, L.G., Myerowitz, R.L., Patton, C.M., Gorman, G.W., Carmack, L.L., Ezzell, J.W., and Dowling, J.N.: Pittsburgh pneumonia agent: direct isolation from human lung tissue, J. Infect. Dis. **141**:727-732, 1980.

38. Pecora, D.V.: A method of securing uncontaminated tracheal secretions for bacterial examination, J. Thorac. Surg. **37**:653, 1959.

39. Pierce, A.K., Edmonson, B., McGee, G., Ketchersid, J., Loudon, R.G., and Sanford, J.P.: An analysis of factors predisposing to gram-negative bacillary necrotizing pneumonia, Am. Rev. Respir. Dis. **94**:309-315, 1966.

40. Rein, M.F., Gwaltney, J.M., Jr., O'Brien, W.M., Jennings, R.H., and Mandell, G.L.: Accuracy of Gram's stain in identifying pneumococci in sputum, J.A.M.A. **239**:2671-2673, 1978.

41. Roberts, D.E., and Cole, P.: Use of selective media in bacteriological investigation of patients with chronic suppurative respiratory infection, Lancet **1**:796-797, 1980.

42. Schmid, R.E., Washington, J.A., II, and Anhalt, J.P.: Gentamicin-blood agar for isolation of *Streptococcus pneumoniae* from respiratory secretions, J. Clin. Microbiol. **7**:426-427, 1978.

43. Slifkin, M., Engwall, C., and Pouchet, G.R.: Direct-plate serological grouping of beta-hemolytic streptococci from primary isolation plates with the Phadebact streptococcus test, J. Clin. Microbiol. **7**:356-360, 1978.

44. Stamm, A.M., and Cobbs, C.G.: Group C streptococcal pneumonia: report of a fatal case and review of the literature, Rev. Infect. Dis. **2**:889-898, 1980.

45. Van Scoy, R.E.: Bacterial sputum cultures: a clinician's viewpoint, Mayo Clin. Proc. **52**:39-41, 1977.

46. Wallace, R.J., Jr., Musher, D.M., and Martin, R.R.: *Hemophilus influenzae* pneumonia in adults, Am. J. Med. **64**:87-93, 1978.

47. Ward, J.I., Siber, G.R., Scheifele, D.W., and Smith, D.H.: Rapid diagnosis of *Hemophilus influenzae* type b infections by latex particle agglutination and counterimmunoelectrophoresis, J. Pediatr. **93**:37-42, 1978.

48. Welch, D.F., and Kelly, M.T.: Sputum screening by Nomarski interference contrast microscopy, J. Clin. Microbiol. **9**:520-524, 1979.

49. Whitaker, J.A., Donaldson, P., and Nelson, J.D.: Diagnosis of pertussis by the fluorescent-antibody method, N. Engl. J. Med. **263**:850-851, 1960.

50. Williams, S.G., and Kauffman, C.A.: Survival of *Streptococcus pneumoniae* in sputum from patients with pneumonia, J. Clin. Microbiol. **7**:3-5, 1978.

51. Wimberly, N., Faling, L.J., and Bartlett, J.G.: A fiberoptic bronchoscopy technique to obtain uncontaminated lower airway secretions for bacterial culture, Am. Rev. Respir. Dis. **119**:337-343, 1979.

52. Wu, T.C., Trask, L.M., and Phee, R.E.: Comparison of media and culture techniques for detection of *Streptococcus pneumoniae* in respiratory secretions, J. Clin. Microbiol. **12**:772-775, 1980.

9 MICROORGANISMS ENCOUNTERED IN THE GASTROINTESTINAL TRACT

Members of the family Enterobacteriaceae make up a large part of the facultatively aerobic microflora of the human intestinal tract. Stool culture may yield these intestinal commensals (the coliforms and species of *Proteus*) as well as enteric pathogens of the *Salmonella, Shigella, Yersinia, Campylobacter,* and *Vibrio* genera and related species, intestinal streptococci (enterococci and others), various yeasts (including *Candida albicans*), and occasionally pathogenic staphylococci. Other organisms that may be sought in stool culture include pathogenic *Escherichia coli, Clostridium difficile, Clostridium perfringens, Clostridium botulinum,* and *Bacillus cereus.* It is rarely necessary to attempt to isolate *Mycobacterium tuberculosis* from fecal material.

Dozens of species of virus have been recovered from the intestinal tract of humans, and the number is constantly increasing. The major viruses of interest in gastroenteritis are the Norwalk agent and the rotavirus.

COLLECTION AND TRANSPORT

1. A clean plastic or waxed container is sufficient if the specimen can be transported promptly to the laboratory.

2. If a delay of over 2 to 3 hours is expected, use Cary-Blair transport medium or 0.033 M phosphate buffer mixed with equal parts of glycerol (pH 7.0) or Amies or Stuart's transport medium. The phosphate buffer–glycerol medium is not satisfactory for *Vibrio parahaemolyticus* or *Campylobacter fetus* ss. *jejuni,* for which Cary-Blair transport medium is recommended.

3. If a delay of many hours is expected or if the specimen is to be sent by mail, use Cary-Blair medium or 0.033 M phosphate buffer with an equal part of glycerol (pH 7.0). For recovery of *Shigella,* buffered glycerol saline was better than Cary-Blair medium, and refrigeration or freezing was better than room temperature storage (Wells and Morris: J. Clin. Microbiol. **13:**789-790, 1981).

4. When stool specimens are not readily obtainable in outbreaks of enteric disease, **rectal swabs** afford the most practical method of securing material for culture, although they should not be relied on for maximum recovery. Rectal swabs are of less value than fecal specimens in the examination of convalescent patients or in carrier surveys. Swabbing mucosal lesions during proctoscopy is preferable to blindly swabbing through the anus.

DIRECT EXAMINATION

Microscopic examination of the stool may be useful on occasion. A fleck of mucus or stool examined with methylene blue stain for pus cells is helpful in indicating the presence of an invasive pathogen. For this procedure one should mix equal amounts of stool and the stain on a microscopic slide using a wooden applicator stick. A coverslip is placed over the mixture, and after 2 or 3 minutes the slide is examined under the high dry objective for the presence of leukocytes. The test is helpful only when there are many leukocytes present since there are often false-positive and false-negative results. A Gram-stained smear may reveal the presence of unique organisms. For example, staphylococci,

in the case of staphylococcal enterocolitis, may be apparent as large numbers of gram-positive cocci that are rather large, perfectly round, and present in clumps (Plate 20). This contrasts with the normally occurring enterococci, which typically are present in pairs that are somewhat elongated and often smaller than staphylococci. The unique comma shape (or the spiral shape that may occur when two or more organisms are joined end-to-end) of *Vibrio* and *Campylobacter* may be apparent on Gram stain (Plate 96). *Clostridium difficile* may be suspected when the predominant flora is rather large gram-positive rods with perfectly parallel walls (Plate 22). These organisms are not as broad as *Clostridium perfringens*. Spores may or may not be evident. Motility of *Vibrio* and *Campylobacter* may be noted in wet mounts. Although it is beyond the scope of the usual clinical laboratory, viruses involved in gastroenteritis, such as the rotavirus, may be demonstrated in stool by electron microscopy or immune electron microscopy. Recently, a simple enzyme immunoassay has become available commercially.*

ISOLATION OF SALMONELLA AND SHIGELLA

Salmonella and *Shigella* are present in the stool in appreciable numbers only during the **acute stage** (first 3 days) of a diarrheal disease; therefore, fecal specimens should be obtained within this period whenever possible. Bits of bloody mucus or epithelium should be selected from the freshly voided specimen for inoculation to appropriate media. In **chronic dysentery,** however, the immediate culturing of material obtained during **proctoscopic examination** offers the best means of obtaining positive *Shigella* isolations. In the aforementioned situations one should remember that rapid proliferation of normal bacterial commensals occurs and that certain forms, particularly *Shigella,* may die off

---

*Rotazyme, Abbott Laboratories, Diagnostics Division, North Chicago, Ill.

rather rapidly after the specimen is collected. These samples, therefore, should be **inoculated to appropriate culture or transport media soon after collection.** Whenever possible, **multiple** stool specimens should be examined; numerous investigations have demonstrated the value of this procedure.[14]

A great variety of culture media have been devised for the isolation of salmonellae and shigellae from fecal specimens. These may be divided into several general groups (discussed in more detail in Chapters 20 and 42) without any sharp division among groups.

1. **Differential mildly selective media,** such as EMB agar, MacConkey agar, and Leifson desoxycholate agar, contain certain carbohydrates, indicators, and chemicals that are inhibitory to many gram-positive bacteria. Differentiation of enteric bacteria is achieved through the incorporation of lactose (and sucrose in some brands of EMB agar), since the organisms that attack lactose will form colored colonies, whereas those that do not ferment lactose will appear as colorless colonies (Plates 52 and 53). Among the latter are found the salmonellae and shigellae, as discussed in Chapter 20.

2. **Differentially moderately selective media,** such as Salmonella-Shigella (SS) agar, xylose lysine desoxycholate (XLD) agar, Hektoen enteric (HE) agar, and desoxycholate citrate agar, and highly selective media, such as Kauffmann brilliant green agar and Wilson-Blair bismuth sulfite agar, are complex combinations of nutrients and chemicals that serve to inhibit many coliforms, especially strains of *Escherichia* and *Proteus,* but they permit the growth of most *Salmonella* and many *Shigella* organisms isolated in the United States. However, not all shigellae do well on SS agar, and these organisms are completely inhibited on brilliant green agar and bismuth sulfite agar; therefore, if one anticipates *Shigella,* less inhibitory media, such as MacConkey agar, should also be used.[17] These pathogens, along with slow or lactose-nonfermenting organisms, generally form colorless colonies,

although some may appear as black (Plate 56) or greenish colonies on certain media (see Chapter 20). The lactose-fermenting organisms that are not inhibited grow as pink, orange, or red colonies on media other than bismuth sulfite agar. Coliforms, if they develop, may appear as small black, brown, or greenish colonies on bismuth sulfite agar.

3. **Selective enrichment media,** such as Leifson selenite-F broth, Mueller tetrathionate broth, and Hajna GN broth, incorporate nutrients and such chemicals as selenium salts, tetrathionate (by oxidation of thiosulfate through addition of iodine just prior to use), and desoxycholate and citrate. Such agents inhibit the growth of gram-positive organisms and temporarily (12 to 18 hours) limit the growth of coliforms and *Proteus,* while encouraging the multiplication of salmonellae and shigellae.

4. **Highly selective media.** It is recognized that selective plating media used for isolating enteric pathogens, by virtue of their inhibitory action on coliforms, may also inhibit less hardy pathogens. Thus, whereas media containing brilliant green, bismuth sulfite, or bile salts and citrate may be excellent for isolation of salmonellae, their value may be limited in the recovery of some *Shigella* species.

XLD agar,* as modified by Taylor,[24] is recommended for general application, but with particular reference to *Shigella* and *Providencia*. The differentiation of the various species is based on xylose fermentation, lysine decarboxylation, and hydrogen sulfide production. In a comparison of the recovery efficiency of various enrichment broths and plating media in a series of more than 1,000 fecal specimens, Taylor and Schelhart[25] concluded that the most successful combination utilized GN or selenite-F enrichment medium, followed by plating on XLD agar. Although shigellae are best isolated by direct inoculation, salmonellae are isolated in greater numbers after

---

*Difco Laboratories, Detroit; Baltimore Biological Laboratory, Cockeysville, Md.

tetrathionate (without brilliant green) enrichment with subsequent culturing to plating medium. A variety of plating media should be used to enhance recovery of a larger number of enteric pathogens. All of the enrichment broths should be subcultured to differential and selective plating media to demonstrate colonies of enteric pathogens.

From the foregoing discussion it should be most apparent that **no single medium can be used for all purposes;** use of a variety of plating and enrichment media results in a higher number of positive isolations than will be obtained with use of only one medium. The following procedures are recommended for culturing stool and rectal specimens for the presence of *Salmonella* and *Shigella*[7]:

1. Using a cotton-tipped swab, **heavily** inoculate with fresh material two or more of the following media, preferably one that is highly selective and one that is moderately selective: SS agar, Hektoen enteric agar, brilliant green agar, XLD agar, and desoxycholate citrate agar. Streak with the swab or a wire spreader to provide good distribution of isolated colonies over a major portion of each plate (see Chapter 4). A suspension of fecal material in enrichment medium also may be used to inoculate these plates (see step 4).

2. At the same time **lightly** inoculate one or more of the following differential media: EMB, MacConkey agar, or desoxycholate agar plate. Then streak as in step 1.

3. Since bismuth sulfite agar is the best medium at present for the isolation of typhoid bacilli, its use is recommended whenever typhoid fever or the carrier state is suspected. **Heavily** streak a bismuth sulfite agar plate as described here. In addition, make two pour plates, using about 0.1 ml and 5 ml of a heavy fecal suspension in broth mixed with the melted and cooled (45 C) agar medium. A hand-operated pipet should be used.

4. Also inoculate **heavily** a tube of selenite enrichment or GN broth with the fecal specimen (usually one part to ten parts). After overnight incubation, and depending on the enrichment broth(s) used, transfer two or three loopfuls from these broth media as follows: selenite to EMB or MacConkey agar and GN to XLD agar.

5. Incubate all media at 35 C for 18 to 24 hours and for 48 hours if indicated (bismuth sulfite plates may require a longer period). Examine the plates in a good light for suspicious colonies.

Salmonellae and shigellae produce typical **colorless** colonies on these media, except on XLD agar, where they appear as **red** colonies, sometimes with black centers. On HE agar, however, coliforms appear as salmon to orange in color, whereas salmonellae and shigellae appear bluish green. *Salmonella typhi* forms **black,** opaque colonies on bismuth sulfite agar. It should be kept in mind that atypical colonies may appear, especially on selective media. With such plates great care must be exercised in picking colonies, since microscopic growth of other inhibited bacteria may be present on or near the ones selected, resulting in mixed cultures. Refer to Chapter 20 and discussion of the Enterobacteriaceae for further identification procedures.

S. typhi may be recovered from the duodenum during acute typhoid fever, using a string capsule device[9]. Selenite enrichment is very helpful with this procedure.[3] The string device is also useful for detecting typhoid carriers.

False-positive *Salmonella* stool cultures related to the use of a colonoscope have been reported (Calif. Morbid. Weekly Rep., July 3, 1981).

ENTEROPATHOGENIC, INVASIVE, AND ENTEROTOXIGENIC ESCHERICHIA COLI

It is now widely accepted that certain toxin-producing invasive or enteropathogenic *Escherichia coli* are responsible for outbreaks and sporadic cases of newborn or infantile diarrhea and diarrhea, including "traveler's diarrhea," in adults.[20] Although the value of serotyping of enteropathogenic *E. coli* has been questioned, the fact that other pathogenic mechanisms are also involved and the disagreement between experts suggest that serotyping should not be totally abandoned at this time particularly in an outbreak involving very young children.

Specimens should be collected early in the course of the illness and before any antibiotics have been administered. Cultures may be obtained from freshly soiled diapers or by means of a rectal swab and must be cultured without delay. Since enteropathogenic or enterotoxigenic *E. coli* organisms are inhibited by the selective media used for the isolation of salmonellae and shigellae (SS agar, desoxycholate citrate agar, and so forth), it is necessary to utilize the less inhibitory media, such as EMB or MacConkey agar, to recover them. Blood agar plates also should be inoculated, because pure cultures are easier to obtain on this medium. It may be necessary to inoculate other media, however, so that the presence of salmonellae and shigellae is not overlooked. Ten colonies, including all different morphotypes, are picked for serotyping, toxin studies, and study of invasive properties. These colonies would need to be sent to a reference laboratory for these studies.

ISOLATION OF CAMPYLOBACTER

Campylobacter fetus ss. *jejuni* has been recognized as a human pathogen since 1947, but only recently has it been associated with infectious diarrhea. Studies from several countries now indicate that *C. fetus* ss. *jejuni* may be isolated from patients with diarrhea at least as frequently as is true for *Salmonella* and *Shigella*.[5,22] Accordingly, it is a major cause of gastroenteritis. Campy BAP* contains 10% sheep blood and a brucella agar base with amphoteri-

cin, cephalothin, vancomycin, polymyxin B, and trimethoprim. This medium seems to be excellent, but comparison studies with other media such as modifications of Skirrow medium are not available. Blaser and colleagues[5] have recommended Campy BAP and believe that it is also desirable to transport or enrich specimens in Campy-Thio. This medium includes the same additives used in Campy BAP. Campy-Thio should be inoculated with five drops of material, or a swab may be immersed in it. The medium is then refrigerated for 8 hours and subcultured to Campy BAP. Campy BAP is inoculated with two drops from Campy-Thio or a swab from a stool specimen. It is streaked for isolation and incubated at **42 C**. *C. fetus* ss. *jejuni* is a strict microaerophile and grows best in an atmosphere containing no more than 6% oxygen. It also requires 5% to 10% CO_2. Some people have achieved this atmosphere using a GasPak hydrogen and CO_2–generator envelope in a GasPak jar with the catalyst removed. However, this should not be done; it is a dangerous practice, since the hydrogen generated may escape into the environment and create a potentially explosive condition. A hydrogen and CO_2–generator envelope with a self-contained catalyst specifically for use for isolation of *Campylobacter* is now available. It is called Campy PAK II.* Alternatively, one may evacuate a jar to 15 to 20 inches of mercury twice and refill each time with 10% CO_2, a mixture of 10% hydrogen and 80% nitrogen, or a mixture of 5% CO_2, 10% hydrogen, and 85% nitrogen.[21] When plates are examined, subcultures should be made immediately, since the organism may lose viability after 72 hours on plating media. Ordinarily, plates should be read at 48 hours. Two types of colonies may be present. Type 1 is flat and grayish with an irregular edge and tends to spread or swarm; type 2 is convex, entire, and glistening and is 1 to 2 mm in diameter (W.L.L. Wang,

---

*Scott Laboratories, Fiskeville, R.I.; BBL Microbiology Systems, Cockeysville, Md.; Remel Laboratories Inc., Lenexa, Kan.; Gibco Diagnostics, Madison, Wisc.

---

*BBL Microbiology Systems, Cockeysville, Md.

personal communication). One may Gram stain colonies to look for *Vibrio*-like forms and may examine motility.

ISOLATION OF YERSINIA ENTEROCOLITICA

Y. enterocolitica may be involved in severe diarrhea as well as other types of infection. The exact incidence of diarrhea caused by this organism is uncertain but in some surveys it has seemed to be as common as that caused by *Salmonella*. There do seem to be regional differences in the frequency of infection with this organism, but the organism is very difficult to isolate at times, and it is likely that we are underestimating the true incidence of this organism's involvement in disease.

Specimens submitted for culture for *Y. enterocolitica* may be refrigerated until culturing, since the organism proliferates at 4 C. Duplicate sets of MacConkey and Salmonella-Shigella agar should be inoculated with one set to be incubated at 35 C and the other at 25 C for a minimum of 48 hours.[21] Plates should be examined with the aid of a stereoscopic microscope under 13× magnification and with oblique illumination. Pinpoint colonies may then be selected for isolation as potential *Y. enterocolitica*. It appears that *Y. enterocolitica* can usually be isolated by direct culture of stool on enteric media from patients with acute diarrhea. Cold enrichment techniques seem to enhance recovery of the organism from convalescent patients and asymptomatic carriers.[11, 26] It is not clear, however, how many of the isolates obtained only by cold enrichment are clinically significant. Some are definitely pathogens, but others are of questionable significance.

The cold enrichment technique employs a swab dipped in feces placed into a test tube containing 5 ml of 0.067 M phosphate buffer (pH 7.6), which is held at 4 to 5 C for 3 weeks.[21] Samples are subcultured onto MacConkey and Salmonella-Shigella agar after 7, 14, and 21 days of cold enrichment. These subcultures are incubated at 25 C for 48 hours. Several selective media appear promising but have not yet been fully evaluated in clinical trials. One of these—cellobiose-arginine-lysine agar—is commercially available as CAL medium.* A new, simplified technique involves mixing one part of stool with two parts of 0.5% KOH for 2 minutes and then plating as described.

On MacConkey agar after 24 hours colonies are 1 to 2 mm in diameter and appear light pink to peach. On Salmonella-Shigella agar colonies are similar in color but are slightly smaller. After 48 hours, colonies are smooth and colorless, resembling *Shigella*. Lactose-negative colonies are picked for further study. It is important to distinguish between *Y. enterocolitica* of the typical variety and two groups of rhamnose-positive strains that have been shown to be separate species. These strains, as well as sucrose-negative strains of *Y. enterocolitica*, do not appear to be enteric pathogens.[21]

ISOLATION OF VIBRIO CHOLERAE AND VIBRIO PARAHAEMOLYTICUS

The most recent pandemic of cholera, which began in 1961 and still continues, spread from Indonesia throughout southeast and south Asia, the Middle East, Africa, portions of Europe, and several Pacific island groups. It has become clear that there is now a low level of endemic cholera in the United States. One case was acquired in Texas in 1973, 11 were acquired in Louisiana in 1978,[4] and a case has been reported from Florida in 1980. In addition, a small number of cases have been imported to the United States by southeast Asian refugees, a smaller number have been imported by United States citizens traveling abroad and returning to the United States, and a small number of cases have been caused by laboratory accidents. The organism has been recovered from Gulf coast waters and from the Chesapeake Bay.[18] Accordingly,

---

*Remel Laboratories Inc., Lenexa, Kan.; Scott Laboratories, Fiskeville, R.I.

attention must be paid in clinical laboratories to the possibility that cholera may be encountered. This would be particularly true, of course, in coastal areas and also in situations in which there was a possibility of imported disease.

Fortunately, an excellent selective and differential medium for *V. cholerae* and *V. parahaemolyticus* is available commercially.[16] This medium is thiosulfate citrate bile salts sucrose agar (TCBS). This medium varies in quality depending on the commercial source, but the medium available from BBL Microbiology Systems is very good.[18] Cary-Blair medium is an excellent transport medium for all the vibrios under discussion.

Stools that are anticipated to have small numbers of organisms (such as from carriers, contacts, or patients receiving antibiotics) should be incubated first in an enrichment broth.[18] Sodium-gelatin-phosphate enrichment broth contains 10 g of NaCl, 30 g of gelatin, and 5 g of K_2HPO_4 per liter of distilled water. Cultures in this broth are incubated overnight and then subcultured to TCBS agar. Enrichment may also be carried out in alkaline peptone water (1.5% peptone and 0.5% NaCl adjusted to pH 9.0 before autoclaving).[21] This broth is incubated at 35 C for 6 to 12 hours and then is subcultured to TCBS agar.

Cultures on TCBS are examined after overnight incubation. Colonies of *V. cholerae* are yellow, flat, and large. There is little growth of normal fecal flora on this medium, although enterococci can form tiny yellow colonies, and *Klebsiella-Enterobacter* can form opaque, heaped-up, dark yellow medium-sized colonies. One should subculture typical colonies of *V. cholerae* to nutrient agar or other noninhibitory media before performing a slide agglutination test. This test is carried out with group antisera. *V. cholerae* O group 1 should agglutinate in the group sera. Confirmatory tests include the "string test," in which a colony is emulsified in 0.5% sodium desoxycholate, and the tip of an inoculating loop is then lifted out of the emul-

sion.[21] This results in a mucuslike string extending up from the emulsion to the tip of the needle. These tests give presumptive identification; in nonendemic areas complete biochemical studies are necessary for definitive identification.

V. cholerae non–O group 1 (formerly called noncholera vibrios or nonagglutinating vibrios) may produce a disease similar to cholera.[12] These organisms may be isolated on TCBS, where they will form either yellow or green colonies. They do not agglutinate in cholera antiserum. Patients with diarrhea caused by non–O group 1 *V. cholerae* may have acquired their illness from raw seafood from a wide range of waters. The most notable recent outbreaks have been in Florida, where the disease has been associated with raw oysters.[6] Bloody diarrhea, which is not usually found in patients with cholera, has been a common occurrence in the cases from Florida.[6]

V. parahaemolyticus is another marine organism that may produce explosive watery diarrhea and abdominal cramps within 24 hours after the ingestion of contaminated seafood. This organism has been isolated from coastal waters throughout the world, including the Pacific, Gulf, and Atlantic coastlines of the United States.[21] It is associated particularly with shellfish of various varieties. Most of the cases in the United States have been identified in the course of outbreaks, but sporadic cases have occurred as well. Fresh stool specimens (or vomitus) may be placed in alkaline peptone water (1% peptone, 3% NaCl, pH 7.4) for 8 hours. Specimens received in transport medium are plated directly. After 24 hours of incubation at 35 C on TCBS, *V. parahaemolyticus* forms colonies 3 to 5 mm in diameter with green-blue centers. The organism should be transferred to a nonselective medium before oxidase testing is done. These organisms are oxidase-positive, curved, gram-negative, motile rods. They do not agglutinate in *V. cholerae* O group 1 antiserum. Other tests are required for confirmation (see Chapter 21).

An alternative to use of TCBS agar for *V. para-haemolyticus* is the addition of 1.5% sodium chloride to xylose lysine desoxycholate agar.[19] The addition of this amount of sodium chloride does not affect the recovery or morphology of other enteric pathogens. This would avoid the need to stock TCBS agar.

See Chapter 21 for other isolation media for *Vibrio* (e.g., TTGA and TGA) and for colonial appearance on these media.

MISCELLANEOUS PATHOGENS

Aeromonas hydrophila has been isolated from children with diarrhea and produces an enterotoxin that is cytotoxic. Its importance in diarrheal disease remains to be established. The organism grows readily on enteric agar media, forming low, convex, usually lactose-negative colonies 1 to 2 mm in diameter.[21] Lactose-positive colonies may resemble *Escherichia coli* but can be distinguished from it because *Aeromonas* is positive on the oxidase test. On TCBS agar *Aeromonas* forms small yellow colonies that may be differentiated from vibrios by the use of *V. cholerae* antiserum, salt tolerance tests, and the decarboxylase reaction.

Other organisms have been believed to be associated with diarrhea in the past, but their etiologic role is open to serious question. These include *Klebsiella*, *Enterobacter*, *Pseudomonas*, and *Plesiomonas*.

COLITIS ASSOCIATED WITH ANTIMICROBIAL AGENTS

This entity is now known to be a bacterial-induced, toxin-mediated process. The majority of cases are caused by toxin-producing strains of *Clostridium difficile*.[1] Cases of pseudomembranous colitis (Plate 21) unrelated to antimicrobial therapy have also been documented to involve *C. difficile*, and this organism is implicated in other types of diarrhea, such as that associated with the use of methotrexate, exacerbations of inflammatory bowel disease, and strangulation obstruction. *C. difficile* is found normally in a significant percentage of newborns and young infants but only in a small percentage of adults. Most of the work done to date has centered about a cytotoxin produced by *C. difficile*, but it has recently been demonstrated that an enterotoxin is produced as well, and this may well be much more important in terms of pathogenesis of the disease. The cytotoxin may be found on occasion, in the absence of disease as well, primarily in newborns and individuals receiving antimicrobial therapy. At the present time there is no ready method for detecting the enterotoxin of *C. difficile* in feces. However, the presence of the cytotoxin generally correlates quite well with the disease, so that clinical laboratory procedures for the diagnosis of pseudomembranous colitis include examination of stools for the presence of *C. difficile* and the cytotoxin. A number of reference laboratories are available for these types of tests.

Specimens for examination for *C. difficile* and the cytotoxin should be fresh or refrigerated. An excellent selective and differential medium is prereduced cycloserine-cefoxitin egg yolk fructose agar (CCFA).* Serial tenfold dilutions of the stool should be made in an anaerobic chamber, and prereduced or reduced CCFA plates should be inoculated in the chamber. Colonies of *C. difficile* on CCFA are 4 to 8 mm in diameter, yellow, of ground glass appearance, circular with a slightly filamentous edge, flat to low umbonate in profile, and lipase and lecithinase negative. Colonies of other bacteria that may appear on this medium and of yeast are rarely larger than 0.5 to 1.5 mm after 48 hours' incubation.

Cytotoxin assay involves dilution of the specimen, centrifugation, membrane filtration of the

---

*Available in prereduced form from Anaerobe Systems, Santa Clara, Calif. Available in dehydrated form (the agar base) with appropriate selective supplement from Oxoid Inc., Columbia, Md.

supernatant, and inoculation of 0.05 to 0.1 ml of the filtrate into a well containing the cell culture monolayer and 1.0 ml of a growth medium. Cytopathic effect is usually evident within 4 to 24 hours. A parallel control test should always be carried out to demonstrate neutralization of the cytopathic effect by *Clostridium sordellii* antitoxin. Further details on the toxin assay are provided in a paper by Bartlett.[1] The cytotoxin may also be demonstrated by CIE.[28]

Staphylococcal pseudomembranous enterocolitis is a syndrome characterized by fever, abdominal pain, and a fulminating diarrhea. Through the use of a selective medium containing a high concentration of sodium chloride, such as Staphylococcus medium 110,* mannitol salt agar,* or other selective media, such as polymyxin Staphylococcus medium, pathogenic staphylococci can be isolated from the stool. By using this technique the carrier rate of coagulase-positive staphylococci found in normal adults may be shown to be as high as 15% to 20%. This figure may be higher in infants or in patients hospitalized for more than several days or in those who have been given antibiotics. A diagnosis of staphylococcal enterocolitis based only on the demonstration of coagulase-positive staphylococci in the stool, therefore, is questionable in light of these findings.

On the other hand, when coagulase-positive staphylococci are isolated in **large numbers** from a stool specimen, and a **Gram stain** of the fecal specimen reveals **large numbers** of gram-positive cocci in clusters, this is likely to be of clinical significance, especially if polymorphonuclear leukocytes are also present. It has recently been shown that staphylococci from patients with pseudomembranous enterocolitis produce a cytopathic toxin that can be distinguished from that produced by *C. difficile*.[2] The toxins from both organisms produce cytotoxic effects in

Walker rat carcinoma cells, but only the *C. difficile* toxin affects fibroblast lines. Furthermore, the *Staphylococcus aureus* toxin is not neutralized by *C. sordellii* antitoxin, nor is it lethal for hamsters by the intraperitoneal route. Accordingly, patients suspected of having staphylococcal pseudomembranous enterocolitis should have stools examined for *S. aureus* by quantitative culture and should have appropriate tests looking for the toxin characteristic of *S. aureus*.

FOOD POISONING

The major causes of foodborne disease in the United States for 1972 to 1978 were as follows (in order): *Salmonella, Staphylococcus, Clostridium perfringens, Shigella, Vibrio parahaemolyticus, Bacillus cereus,* and *Clostridium botulinum*.[23] *Salmonella, Shigella,* and *V. parahaemolyticus* have already been discussed.

Staphylococcal food poisoning results from the ingestion of foods, usually meat or dairy products, in which staphylococci have proliferated and produced heat-stable enterotoxin. The disease is characterized primarily by vomiting, although diarrhea may also occur. The onset of illness is typically within 2 to 6 hours after consumption of the contaminated food, and the disease terminates within 12 to 18 hours. Attempts to isolate staphylococci or demonstrate the toxin should be reserved for recognized outbreaks; ordinarily this is handled by a public health laboratory.

C. perfringens is an important cause of foodborne disease. Type C strains of *C. perfringens* rarely produce a severe necrotizing enteritis. The more common disease involves type A strains of *C. perfringens* and is typically related to inadequate cooking of large pieces of rolled or stuffed meat. The incubation period is 12 to 24 hours; the primary symptom is diarrhea. The disease is typically mild and of short duration. A diagnosis is established by culturing *C. perfringens* from the incriminated food and doing quantitative counts of *C. perfringens* on stool

---

*Difco Laboratories, Detroit; Baltimore Biological Laboratory, Cockeysville, Md.

samples as well. Isolates from the food and stool would have to be examined serologically to distinguish between the infecting organism and strains of *C. perfringens* normally present in the bowel. Again, this is a health department laboratory function.

Bacillus cereus is responsible for two different types of clinical syndromes. One is characterized primarily by vomiting and has a short incubation period (1 to 6 hours). It is associated with ingestion of fried rice. The second form, which is more common, has a longer incubation period (6 to 24 hours) and is characterized primarily by diarrhea. It is associated with the consumption of contaminated meats and vegetables. Isolation of *B. cereus* from the stools alone is of no significance, since the organism may be found there normally. Laboratory diagnosis of *B. cereus* food poisoning is attempted only in the course of an outbreak and is the function of public health officials. Their procedure involves quantitative culture of food for *B. cereus*.

Finally, botulism and infant botulism are problems that demand the attention of highly qualified public health laboratories and do not fall within the province of the usual clinical laboratory.

ISOLATION OF MYCOBACTERIUM TUBERCULOSIS FROM THE STOOL

The examination of fecal specimens for *Mycobacterium tuberculosis* is not routine and is of questionable value when carried out. Tubercle bacilli isolated from intestinal contents probably reflect the presence of pulmonary tuberculosis, because sputum is often swallowed. The method recommended is described by Kubica and Dye[13] and is outlined in Chapter 31.

CANDIDA IN THE STOOL

Candida albicans (and other species of *Candida*) can be found normally on the skin, in the mouth, and in the intestinal tract; intensive use of antibiotics may lead to overgrowth by *Candida* in the colon. It is rare, however, that this is of clinical significance.

VIRUSES

Information on detection of rotavirus has been cited earlier in this chapter. Other information concerning viral gastroenteritis can be found in Chapter 33.

REPORTING

It is important that reports issued from the clinical laboratory accurately reflect the work that was **actually performed.** If a stool specimen was examined only for *Salmonella* and *Shigella*, the report should read "no *Salmonella* or *Shigella* isolated." A report stating "no enteric pathogens isolated" is misleading. It is necessary that the laboratory specifically list those organisms for which culture attempts were made.

REFERENCES

1. Bartlett, J.G.: Antibiotic-associated pseudomembranous colitis, Rev. Infect. Dis. **1:**530-539, 1979.
2. Batts, D.H., Silva, J., and Fekety, R.: Staphylococcal enterocolitis: current chemotherapy and infectious disease. Proceedings of the Eleventh International Congress of Chemotherapy and Nineteenth Interscience Conference on Antimicrobial Agents and Chemotherapy, Washington, D.C., 1980, American Society for Microbiology, pp. 944-945.
3. Benavente, L., Gotuzzo, E., Guerra, J., Grados, O., and Guerra, H.: Diagnosis of *Salmonella typhi* by culture of duodenal string capsule, N. Engl. J. Med. **304:**54, 1981.
4. Blake, P.A., Allegra, D.T., Snyder, J.D., Barrett, T.J., McFarland, L., Caraway, C.T., Feeley, J.C., Craig, J.P., Lee, J.V., Puhr, N.D., and Feldman, R.A.: Cholera: a possible endemic focus in the United States, N. Engl. J. Med. **302:**305-309, 1980.
5. Blaser, M.J., Berkowitz, I.D., LaForce, F.M., Cravens, J., Reller, L.B., and Wang, W.L.: *Campylobacter* enteritis: clinical and epidemiological features, Ann. Intern. Med. **91:**179-185, 1979.
6. Diarrheal illness from uncooked seafood, FDA Drug Bull. **10:**13-14, 1980.
7. Edwards, P.R., and Ewing, W.H.: Identification of enterobacteriaceae, ed. 3, Minneapolis, 1972, Burgess Publishing Co.

8. George, W.L., Sutter, V.L., Citron, D., Finegold, S.M.: Selective and differential medium for isolation of *Clostridium difficile,* J. Clin. Microbiol. **9**:214-219, 1979.

9. Gilman, R.H., and Hornick, R.B.: Duodenal isolation of *Salmonella typhi* by string capsule in acute typhoid fever, J. Clin. Microbiol. **3**:456-457, 1976.

10. Greenwood, J.R., Flanigan, S.M., Pickett, M.J., and Martin, W.J.: Clinical isolation of *Yersinia enterocolitica:* cold temperature enrichment, J. Clin. Microbiol. **2**:559-560, 1975.

11. Hawkins, T.M., and Brenner, D.J.: Isolation and identification of *Yersinia enterocolitica,* Atlanta, 1978, Center for Disease Control.

12. Hughes, J.M., Hollis, D.G., Gangarosa, E.J., and Weaver, R.E.: Non-cholera vibrio infections in the United States, Ann. Intern. Med. **88**:602-606, 1978.

13. Kubica, G.P., and Dye, W.E.: Laboratory methods for clinical and public health mycobacteriology, Public Health Service Pub. No. 1547, Washington, D.C., 1967, U.S. Government Printing Office.

14. McCall, C.E., Martin, W.T., and Boring, J.R.: Efficiency of cultures of rectal swabs and fecal specimens in detecting *Salmonella* carriers: correlation with numbers of salmonellas isolated, J. Hyg. **64**:261-269, 1966.

15. McCormack, W.M., DeWitt, W.E., Bailey, P.E., Morris, G.K., Soeharjono, P., and Gangarosa, E.J.: Evaluation of thiosulfate–citrate–bile salts–sucrose agar, a selective medium for the isolation of *Vibrio cholerae* and other pathogenic vibrios, J. Infect. Dis. **129**:497-500, 1974.

16. Morris, G.K., Merson, M.H., Huq, I., Kibrya, A.K.M.G., and Black, R.: Comparison of four plating media for isolating *Vibrio cholerae,* J. Clin. Microbiol. **9**:79-83, 1979.

17. Rahaman, M.M., Huq, I., and Dey, C.R.: Superiority of MacConkey's agar over Salmonella-Shigella agar for isolation of *Shigella dysenteriae* Type 1, J. Infect. Dis. **131**:700-703, 1975.

18. Rennels, M.B., Levine, M.M., Daya, V., Angle, P., and Young, C.: Selective vs. nonselective media and direct plating vs. enrichment technique in isolation of *Vibrio cholerae:* recommendations for clinical laboratories, J. Infect. Dis. **142**:328-331, 1980.

19. Roland, F.P.: Isolated cases of *Vibrio parahaemolyticus* gastroenteritis, J.A.M.A. **241**:2504, 1979.

20. Sack, R.B.: *Escherichia coli* and acute diarrheal disease, Ann. Intern. Med. **94**:129-130, 1981.

21. Sack, R.B., Tilton, R.C., and Weissfeld, A.S. In Rubin, S.J., editor: Laboratory diagnosis of bacterial diarrhea, Cumitech 12, Washington, D.C., 1980, American Society for Microbiology.

22. Skirrow, M.B.: *Campylobacter* enteritis: a "new" disease. Br. Med. J. **2**:9-11, 1977.

23. Sours, H.E., and Smith, D.G.: Outbreaks of foodborne disease in the United States, 1972-1978, J. Infect. Dis. **142**:122-125, 1980.

24. Taylor, W.I.: Isolation of shigellae; xylose lysine agars; new media for isolation of enteric pathogens, Am. J. Clin. Pathol. **44**:471-475, 1965.

25. Taylor, W.I., and Schelhart, D.; Isolation of *Shigella.* VI. Performance of media with stool specimens, paper M 242, Bacteriol. Proc., p. 107, 1968.

26. Weissfeld, A.S., and Sonnenwirth, A.C.: *Yersinia enterocolitica* in adults with gastrointestinal disturbances: need for cold enrichment, J. Clin. Microbiol. **11**:196-197, 1980.

27. Weissfeld, A.S., and Sonnenwirth, A.C.: Rapid isolation of *Yersinia enterocolitica* from feces. Abstracts of the Eighty-first Annual Meeting of the American Society for Microbiology, March 1981, Abstract C2, p. 263.

28. Welch, D.F., Menge, S.K., and Matsen, J.M.: Identification of toxigenic *Clostridium difficile* by counterimmunoelectrophoresis, J. Clin. Microbiol. **11**:470-473, 1980.

10 MICROORGANISMS ENCOUNTERED IN THE URINARY TRACT

Bacterial infections of the urinary tract affect patients of all age groups and both sexes, and they vary in severity from an unsuspected infection to a condition of severe systemic disease. The clinical diagnosis of pyelonephritis is frequently overlooked because of the absence of urinary tract symptoms and pyuria.[15] The correlation of bacteriuria with unsuspected active pyelonephritis at autopsy has been demonstrated.[21] The role of the indwelling catheter in the development of bacteriuria, frequently accompanied by a gram-negative rod bacteremia, has also been revealed.[11] The demonstration of bacteria by appropriate cultural methods is the only reliable means of making a specific diagnosis. Readers interested in reviews of clinical and other aspects of urinary tract infection are referred to the excellent monographs by Kunin[19] and Stamey[28]; Barry and co-workers[2] present a very good summary of laboratory diagnosis of urinary tract infection.

Urine is an excellent culture medium for the common pathogens of the urinary tract, and when bacteria are deposited in the urine, they multiply readily, often exceeding 1 million/ml.

Since specimens of urine, either clean voided or catheterized, are frequently contaminated on collection, the recovery of organisms, even known pathogens, does not necessarily establish the diagnosis of a urinary tract infection. Studies by Kass, Sanford, MacDonald, Beeson, and others, summarized in an extensive bibliography and review of this topic,[26] indicate that bacterial counts on fresh, voided urine from **infected** patients ordinarily show more than 100,000 (10^5) organisms/ml,* whereas specimens from noninfected or normal persons may be sterile or contain up to 1,000 organisms/ml. It should be pointed out, however, that bacterial counts of less than 10^5/ml may occur in patients who are receiving specific antibacterial therapy or patients who are excessively hydrated, with a consequent dilution of urine. Other factors accounting for low counts despite true infection include fastidious organisms with a slow growth rate (rare) and infection above an obstruction (such as a ureteral stone). To evaluate the clinical significance of a **positive** urine culture, therefore, it is strongly recommended that some means of estimating the number of organisms present in a specimen be part of a routine urine culture.

As indicated by the following lists, the bacterial flora of normal voided urine differs from that of infected specimens. The organisms listed in the first group are most frequently encountered in **normal urine.** These, of course, represent contaminants from the urethra, vagina, and so forth, as bladder urine is normally sterile.

Staphylococci, coagulase negative
Diphtheroid bacilli
Coliform bacilli
Enterococci
Proteus species
Lactobacilli
Alpha- and beta-hemolytic streptococci
Saprophytic yeasts
Bacillus species

---

*This figure is based on first voided urine in the morning; specimens collected later may give lower counts because of hydration and insufficient "incubation time" in the bladder. First morning specimens have had overnight incubation in the bladder.

The flora of **infected urine,** as a rule, includes one or more of the following:

Escherichia coli, Klebsiella, Enterobacter, and *Serratia*

Proteus mirabilis and other *Proteus* species, *Providencia* species, and *Morganella*

Pseudomonas aeruginosa and other *Pseudomonas* species

Enterococci (*Streptococcus faecalis*)

Staphylococci, coagulase positive and coagulase negative (*S. saprophyticus*)

Alcaligenes species

Acinetobacter species

Candida albicans, Torulopsis glabrata, and other yeasts

Gardnerella (Haemophilus) vaginalis

Mycobacterium tuberculosis and other mycobacteria

Beta-hemolytic streptococci, usually groups B and D

Neisseria gonorrhoeae

Salmonella and *Shigella* species

COLLECTION OF SPECIMENS

The distal portions of the human urethra and the perineum are normally colonized with bacteria, particularly in the female. These organisms readily contaminate a normally sterile urine on voiding, but contamination can be prevented by using the "clean catch" technique: the periurethral area (tip of penis, labial folds, vulva) is carefully cleansed with two separate washes with plain soap and water or a mild detergent and **well rinsed** with warmed sterile water to remove the detergent, with the prepuce or labial folds retracted. The urethra is then "flushed" by passage of the first portion of the voiding, which is discarded. The subsequent midstream urine, voided directly into a sterile container, is used for culturing and colony counting.

It is recommended that two successive clean-voided midstream specimens be collected from women to approach a 95% confidence level when using a bacterial count of 10^5/ml as an index of significant bacteriuria,[17] although this is not routinely done in clinical practice unless there is some question about the diagnosis. In the case of males who are able to cooperate, a single urine culture is adequate to establish bacteriuria.[6]

To increase the accuracy of localizing urinary tract infections, Stamey and colleagues[29] recommend the use of suprapubic needle aspiration of the female bladder and a technique of dividing voided urine from the male into urethral, midstream (bladder), and postprostatic massage cultures. In the former procedure, urethral and vaginal contamination is eliminated; in the latter, localization of a lower urinary tract infection to the urethra or prostate gland is facilitated. Another method pertinent to the microbiologist for localizing urinary tract infection is the use of the direct immunofluorescent method to detect bacteria in urine that are coated with antibody. Early studies indicated a very significant correlation between such antibody coating and infection involving the upper urinary tract. More recent experience with this test, however, makes it clear that a number of factors may lead to either false-positive or false-negative results.[9] Mundt and Polk[24] have reviewed the literature on the assessment of the antibody-coated bacteria technique and found that in comparison with bilateral ureteral catheterization or bladder washout, the overall sensitivity of the antibody-coated bacterial assay is 83.1%, and the specificity is 76.7%. Mundt and Polk concluded that this test at present has no role in the management of patients with urinary tract infection. Furthermore, the demonstration that a single dose of an appropriate antimicrobial agent may readily cure bladder infection provides the clinician with a simple and practical way to distinguish between infection of the lower urinary tract and that of the upper urinary tract.[8]

Since urine generally supports the growth of most of the urinary pathogens as well as broth media do, it is absolutely essential for culture purposes that urine be processed within 1 hour of collection or **stored in a refrigerator** at 4 C until it can be cultured. Studies have indicated that such specimens may be kept in the refrigerator for extended periods without significantly reducing their bacterial content,[23] and counts remain stable for at least 24 hours at the refrigerator temperature. Specimens received at various times during a laboratory workday may be placed in a refrigerator as received, then set up in a batch at some designated hour in the afternoon. Another alternative has become available recently in the form of a kit* with a preservative that eliminates the need for refrigeration.[20] This kit contains a boric acid–glycerol–sodium formate preservative. In a study of 1,000 urine specimens in a clinical laboratory, it was found that the commercial kit maintained a stable bacterial population in urine for up to 24 hours as reliably as refrigeration. Furthermore, urine for culture may be collected in a nonsterile container, provided it is promptly aspirated into the transport tube so that contaminants are not allowed to multiply.

CULTURE PROCEDURES

Although anaerobes are involved in urinary tract infection on occasion, voided urine should **never** be cultured anaerobically because of the presence of anaerobes in indigenous flora of the urethra and surrounding areas. In suspected anaerobic urinary tract infection, urine must be obtained by percutaneous suprapubic bladder aspiration or from a nephrostomy tube if one is in place.

A common practice in the past in a number of laboratories has been to centrifuge urine specimens and inoculate either liquid or solid media with the sediment or to inoculate the urine directly into a tube of broth. This should never be done. Centrifugation will concentrate contaminants as well as pathogens; the introduction of only a few contaminating bacteria by directly inoculating broth will invariably result in a positive culture. For these reasons it is strongly recommended that one of the following **quantitative** methods be used for culturing urine specimens.

Calibrated loop–direct streak method

The calibrated loop–direct streak method, first reported by Hoeprich[12] in 1960, uses a calibrated bacteriologic loop to inoculate and streak plates of standard or differential culture media. After proper incubation, the number of colonies present is estimated and reported as a measure of the degree of bacteriuria. Used properly, this technique is reliable for clinical purposes and is simple and rapid. The delivery volume of calibrated loops may change with use; this can be checked by a procedure outlined by Barry and associates.[2]

1. Using a flame-sterilized and cooled platinum loop* calibrated to deliver 0.001 ml, hold the loop **vertically** and immerse it just below the surface of the well-mixed urine specimen. Deliver one loopful to a blood agar plate and an EMB or a MacConkey agar plate.
2. Streak both plates by making a straight line down the center of the plate and then streaking for isolation with a regular loop by a series of very close passes at a 90° angle through the original line (Mayo Clinic technique).
3. Incubate both plates overnight at 35 C and read them the following morning. Examine and count the colonies on both plates; estimate the total count from the blood plate and gram-negative bacterial count from the EMB or MacConkey plate. In each case the colony count is multiplied by 1,000 (0.001 ml used) to give an estimate of the number per milliliter of urine. One hundred colonies would represent 10^5 cells present, for example. If a 0.01-ml

---

*B-D Urine Culture Kit, Becton-Dickinson, Rutherford, N.J.

*Platinum inoculating loop, Cat. No. 7011-J20, Arthur H. Thomas Co., Philadelphia, or Cat. No. N2075-2, Scientific Products, Evanston, Ill.

loop is used, multiply the colony count by 100. After determining the count, proceed with identification of the organisms present* and determine their susceptibility to antimicrobial agents, as described in subsequent sections.

4. If no growth occurs in 24 hours, hold the plates for another day, and if the results are still negative, report as "**No growth after 48 hours.**"

Pour plate method

Although the pour plate method has been criticized as not entirely reflecting the true bacterial count of a urine specimen (clumps of organisms can give rise to single colonies), it remains the most accurate procedure for measuring the degree of bacteriuria. The procedure is as follows:

1. Prepare three tenfold dilutions of well-mixed urine in sterile distilled water in sterile screw-capped tubes as follows:

    1:10 (10^{-1}) = 1.0 ml urine + 9.0 ml water
    1:100 (10^{-2}) = 1.0 ml of 1:10 dilution + 9.0 ml water
    1:1000 (10^{-3}) = 1.0 ml of 1:100 dilution + 9.0 ml water

    Use separate 1-ml serologic pipets for each dilution, with adequate shaking between dilutions.

2. Pipet 1 ml of each of the dilutions into appropriately labeled, sterile Petri dishes.

3. Overlay each dilution with 15 to 20 ml of melted and cooled (50 C) nutrient or infusion agar; mix well by carefully swirling the dishes.

4. When solidified, invert the dishes and incubate overnight at 35 C.

5. Using a Quebec colony counter, enumerate the number of colonies in the plate yielding 30 to 300 colonies; multiply by the dilution to obtain the total number of bacteria per milliliter of urine.

Other methods

Attention has been given to chemical tests for the rapid detection of bacteriuria. These include the reduction of triphenyltetrazolium chloride (TTC) by metabolizing bacteria[27]; the Griess nitrite test, based on the rapid reduction of nitrate by members of the Enterobacteriaceae and staphylococci; the glucose oxidase test, dependent on metabolism of the small amount of glucose present in normal urine by bacteria[18]; and the catalase test, in which rapid gas production from urine reacting with hydrogen peroxide indicates bacteriuria. These tests, however, have been considered unsatisfactory because of substantial numbers of false-negative results and sometimes lack of specificity. Commercial test kits based on these principles have shown correspondingly equivocal results.

A number of **screening culture** tests for bacteriuria have been proposed. In one such method (dip-slide,[4] tube, spoon, paddle, pipet, or cylinder[18]) an agar-coated vehicle is dipped into a freshly voided midstream urine specimen. After overnight incubation, the colonial growth is counted or compared with density photographs of known colony counts and the significance of the culture is determined.* A similar procedure utilizes a filter paper strip that is dipped into the urine specimen, then trans-

---

*Some laboratories consider that a urine culture yielding three or more isolates should be considered a contaminated specimen, and therefore they do not identify the isolates. This is poor practice. Such polymicrobic bacteriuria is not uncommon in individuals with **indwelling catheters**; indeed, such bacteriuria may be of special importance in that it may show a significant association with bacteremia.[7]

---

*Commercial kits utilizing these techniques may be obtained from Smith, Kline & French Laboratories, Philadelphia; Flow Laboratories, Rockville, Md.; Abbott Laboratories, North Chicago, Ill.; Ayerst Laboratories, New York; Baltimore Biological Laboratory, Cockeysville, Md.; and others.

ferred to the surface of either a miniature or a conventional agar plate. After incubation, the number of colonies growing in the inoculum area are counted and their significance is evaluated. Multiple specimens can be cultured on a single conventional agar plate.

These methods—chemical or dip-culture—are not appropriate or offer no advantage for a clinical microbiology laboratory and have their principal value as a screening procedure for bacteriuria in a physician's office or for field surveys. A duplicate urine specimen held in the refrigerator can be submitted for conventional culture and sensitivity testing if the screening test proves to be positive.

Other techniques that have been proposed or utilized as **screening procedures** include measurement of bacterial adenosine triphosphate by luciferase, production of radioactive CO_2 by metabolism of labeled substrates, liberation of unique compounds into headspace gas utilizing specialized substrates and headspace gas chromatography, measurement of the potential generated by growing bacteria using a platinum and a calomel electrode, measurement of heat generated by metabolizing microorganisms using a microcalorimeter, measurement of particle size and distribution by electronic pulse height analysis, and detection of bacteriuria by automated electric impedance monitoring. Particle size distribution analysis proved remarkably effective for rapid screening.[5] With 600 urine specimens the Coulter counter procedure results agreed with routine culture results 98.8% of the time. Results of negative specimens could be obtained in 5 to 10 minutes. There were no false-negative results. It may even prove possible to make a preliminary identification of the infecting species. Impedance screening also seems very promising. The principle of this test is as follows: as bacteria grow and metabolize, the chemical composition of the supporting medium is altered, and metabolic end products are produced. Along with this is a corresponding change in the resistance to the flow of an alter-

nating current when a pair of electrodes are placed in the medium. One can determine how many bacteria must be present to produce a given change in impedance within a given period of time. In a study of more than 1,000 urine specimens by Cady and colleagues[3] it was found that by defining an impedance positive culture as one that gives detectable change within 2.6 hours, 96% of urine cultures tested were correctly classified in terms of having more than or fewer than 10^5 organisms/ml. There were 2.3% false-negative samples and 1.9% false-positive samples; 13.8% of the positive samples were missed. By using a 3.5-hour cutoff, false-negative results were reduced to 1.2% and positive samples missed were reduced to 7.4%, while false-positive samples increased to 4.9%. The *Limulus* amoebocyte lysate test proved remarkably effective as a screen for gram-negative bacteriuria in a small study (Nachum and Shanbrom: J. Clin. Microbiol. **13**:158-162, 1981).

Several items of apparatus are available commercially for rapid screening of urine specimens. These include Abbott's MS-2, Pfizer's Autobac, and Vitek's Automicrobic System (AMS). One of these machines, the Autobac, has undergone a large trial in the clinical microbiology laboratory setting as part of a system of rapid semiautomated screening and processing of urine specimens.[13] This study confirmed and extended the impressive results obtained in an earlier study by Heinze and co-workers.[10]

The Autobac detects positive urine specimens by using light-scatter photometry. At 3 hours 75% of urine specimens that were eventually positive by culture were positive by the Autobac reading. By 6 hours, the Autobac had detected all significant positive specimens. There were 4.6% false-negative samples at 6 hours; however, these comprised specimens from individuals receiving antibiotics, which would not ordinarily be checked by the Autobac in the proposed system, or were positive for slow-growing organisms (probably urethral contaminants). The system proposed by Heinze and associates would exclude from the Autobac screen specimens from the following persons (these specimens would be cultured directly): those receiving antimicrobial agents, those with indwelling urethral catheters, and those whose specimens have been obtained by suprapubic aspiration. Under the system, specimens that are positive by Autobac at 3 hours are put into a 3-hour direct susceptibility test scheme and a 4-hour Micro-ID rapid identification test. Thus, the results from these specimens can be completed within an 8-hour workday. The direct 3-hour susceptibility test and the direct 4-hour identification test were found to be 93% and 94% accurate, as compared with conventional techniques in the aforementioned study. In addition to the specimens that were positive by Autobac at 3 hours and therefore could be worked up within an 8-hour day, an additional number of specimens (73% of the total) were negative by Autobac screen at 6 hours. Heinze and colleagues believed that negative results could be predicted with a high degree of reliability. Accordingly, no further work was required on these specimens. After dropping out cultures that were mixed by Gram stain and that therefore could not be screened rapidly, 82% of all urine specimens screened in this manner by the Autobac procedure were completed within an 8-hour workday. Further details on rapid and automated systems for the clinical microbiology laboratory are presented in Chapter 40.

Quantitation of bacteriuria by the Automicrobic method correlated with culture 99% of the time; yeast counts correlated on 50%. Specimens with two organisms were identified with a 94% correlation. A final report, including identification, was available in 13 hours. At least 30 urine specimen tests per day would be required to pay for the instrument and specimen costs in 1 year.

A simple broth culture screening procedure that appeared to be as sensitive as semiautomated procedures and does not require expensive instruments was described by Murray and Niles

(J. Clin. Microbiol. **13**:85-88, 1981). Another system utilizes a standardized Gram stain for quantitation (Kilbourn: Abstracts of the Third International Symposium on Rapid Methods and Automation in Microbiology, Washington, D.C., May 1981). Positive urine samples are then centrifuged and the sediment used for direct antibiotic susceptibility testing and for inoculation of biochemical tests.

Interpretation of colony counts

Generally, counts of less than 1,000 are suggestive of contamination, whereas urine containing between 1,000 and 10^5 organisms suggests possible infection (and may be an indication for repeat culture), and counts of 10^5 and greater are indicative of infection, although no single concentration of bacteria distinguishes infected from contaminated specimens. Counts in infected patients may be low when the rate of urine flow is rapid, when the patient is receiving suppressive therapy, or occasionally when the urine pH is less than 5 and the specific gravity of the urine is less than 1.003.

Examination of direct smears

The examination of a direct smear of fresh **uncentrifuged** urine has long been used as a screening device to distinguish between true bacteriuria and contamination.[16] It is done by making a smear of the well-mixed urine, allowing the smear to air dry, fixing it with heat, and performing a Gram stain. A positive smear is one showing **one or more bacteria** in the majority of oil-immersion fields.[17]

If 10^5 organisms represent a significant colony count, the correlation of the direct smear has been variously reported as 75% to 95%.[12,16,23] If lower counts are compared with the direct smear (counts between 10^4 and 10^5), the accuracy falls to around 50%.[23] Barbin and others[1] have reported a simplified urine microscopy technique using unspun, unstained urine for rapid detection of significant bacteriuria. A drop of manually agitated, uncentrifuged urine was placed on a glass slide, covered with a glass coverslip, and examined for bacteria under the oil-immersion objective. Demonstration of at least one bacterium per oil field in each of five fields was considered positive. In this study there were 4% false-negative and 4% false-positive samples.

LESS WELL-KNOWN URINARY TRACT PATHOGENS

Evidence increasingly indicates that *Staphylococcus saprophyticus* is an important cause of urinary tract infection. In a study reported by Jordan and associates[14] this organism was found to be the second most common cause of urinary tract infection in young, sexually active, female outpatients without known preexisting kidney disease or preceding manipulation of the urinary tract. Most cases presented as acute cystitis, but pyelonephritis and urinary tract infection in pregnant females were also noted. A simple but adequate identification may be based on resistance to novobiocin by disk diffusion test, absence of hemolysis and coagulase, and intense pigment production (65% of strains yellow, 35% white).

An important study of the acute urethral syndrome in woman by Stamm and co-workers[30] found that in addition to low counts of *Escherichia coli* being documented for many of these women, *Staphylococcus saprophyticus* was occasionally responsible for this picture, and *Chlamydia trachomatis* was not uncommonly involved (probably as a urethritis).

Gardnerella (Haemophilus) vaginalis appears to play a role in urinary tract infection on occasion. In one study[22] more than 15% of 1,000 pregnant patients had specimens obtained by percutanous suprapubic aspiration that yielded this organism on culture. Almost half of these patients had samples that showed the organism consistently. These workers also found *G. vaginalis* in the ureteral urine of a nonpregnant woman with flank pain and ureteral reflux.

A more recent review[31] suggests that mycoplasma may be important in urinary tract infection on occasion. In one study cited in this review *Mycoplasma hominis* was isolated from the upper urinary tracts of 7 of 80 patients with pyelonephritis; 4 of these were in pure culture. Serum and local antibodies were noted in some of the patients. *Ureaplasma urealyticum* was isolated from the upper urinary tracts of five patients, but the isolation rate for the organism in these patients did not differ statistically from that in a control group.

REFERENCES

1. Barbin, G.K., Thorley, J.D., and Reinarz, J.A.: Simplified microscopy for rapid detection of significant bacteriuria in random urine specimens, J. Clin. Microbiol. 7:286-291, 1978.
2. Barry, A.L., Smith, P.B., and Turck, M. (Gavan, T.L., editor): Laboratory diagnosis of urinary tract infections, Cumitech 2, Washington, D.C., 1975, American Society for Microbiology.
3. Cady, P., Dufour, S.W., Lawless, P., Nunke, B., and Kraeger, S.J.: Impedimetric screening for bacteriuria, J. Clin. Microbiol. 7:273-278, 1978.
4. Cohen, S.N., and Kass, E.H.: A simple method for quantitative urine culture, N. Engl. J. Med. 277:176-180, 1969.
5. Dow, C.S, France, A.D., Khan, M.S., and Johnson, T.: Particle size distribution analysis for the rapid detection of microbial infection of urine, J. Clin. Pathol. 32:386-390, 1979.
6. Gleckman, R., Esposito, A., Crowley, M., and Natsios, G.A.: Reliability of a single urine culture in establishing diagnosis of asymptomatic bacteriuria in adult males, J. Clin. Microbiol. 9:596-597, 1979.
7. Gross, P.A., Flower, M., and Barden, G.: Polymicrobic bacteriuria: significant association with bacteremia, J. Clin. Microbiol. 3:246-250, 1976.
8. Harding, G.K.M., Marrie, T.J., Ronald, A.R., Hoban, S., and Muir, P.: Urinary tract infection localization in women, J.A.M.A. 240:1147-1150, 1978.
9. Hawthorne, N.J., Kurtz, S.B., Anhalt, J.P., Segura, J.W.: Accuracy of antibody-coated-bacteria test in recurrent urinary tract infections, Mayo Clin. Proc. 53:651-654, 1978.
10. Heinze, P.A., Thrupp, L.D., and Anselmo, C.R.: A rapid (4-6-hour) urine-culture system for direct identification and direct antimicrobial susceptibility testing, Am. J. Clin. Pathol. 71:177-183, 1979.
11. Hodgin, U.G., and Sanford, J.P.: Gram-negative rod bacteremia, Am. J. Med. 39:952-960, 1965.

12. Hoeprich, P.D.: Culture of the urine, J. Lab. Clin. Med. **56**:899-907, 1960.

13. Jenkins, R.D., Hale, D.C., and Matsen, J.M.: Rapid semiautomated screening and processing of urine specimens, J. Clin. Microbiol. **11**:220-225, 1980.

14. Jordan, P.A., Iravani, A., Richard, G.A., and Baer, H.: Urinary tract infection caused by *Staphylococcus saprophyticus*, J. Infect. Dis. **142**:510-515, 1980.

15. Kaitz, A.L., and Williams, E.J.: Bacteriuria and urinary-tract infection in hospitalized patients, N. Engl. J. Med. **262**:425-430, 1960.

16. Kass, E.H.: Asymptomatic infections of the urinary tract, Trans. Assoc. Am. Physicians **69**:56-64, 1956.

17. Kass, E.H.: Pyelonephritis and bacteriuria: a major problem in preventive medicine, Ann. Intern. Med. **56**:46-53, 1962.

18. Kunin, C.M.: New methods in detecting urinary tract infections, Urol. Clin. North Am. **2**:423-432, 1975.

19. Kunin, C.M.: Detection, prevention and management of urinary tract infections, ed. 3, Philadelphia, 1979, Lea & Febiger.

20. Lauer, B.A., Reller, L.B., and Mirrett, S.: Evaluation of preservative fluid for urine collected for culture, J. Clin. Microbiol. **10**:42-45, 1979.

21. MacDonald, R.A., Levitin, H., Mallory, G.K., and Kass, E.H.: Relation between pyelonephritis and bacterial counts in urine: autopsy study, N. Engl. J. Med. **256**:915-922, 1957.

22. McFadyen, I.R., and Eykyn, S.J.: Suprapubic aspiration of urine in pregnancy, Lancet **1**:1112-1114, 1968.

23. Mou, T.W., and Feldman, H.A.: The enumeration and preservation of bacteria in urine, Am. J. Clin. Pathol. **35**:572-575, 1961.

24. Mundt, K.A., and Polk, B.F.: Identification of site of urinary-tract infections by antibody-coated bacteria assay, Lancet **2**:1172-1175, 1979.

25. Nicholson, D.P., and Koepke, J.A.: The Automicrobic system for urines, J. Clin. Microbiol. **10**:823-833, 1979.

26. Prother, G.C., and Sears, B.R.: In defense of the urethral catheter, J. Urol. **83**:337-344, 1960.

27. Simmons, N.A., and Williams, J.D.: A simple test for significant bacteriuria, Lancet **1**:1377-1378, 1962.

28. Stamey, T.A.: Pathogenesis and treatment of urinary tract infections, Baltimore, 1980, The Williams & Wilkins Co.

29. Stamey, T.A., Gavan, D.E., and Palmer, J.M.: The localization and treatment of urinary tract infections: the role of bactericidal urine levels as opposed to serum levels, Medicine **44**:1-36, 1965.

30. Stamm, W.E., Wagner, K.F., Amsel, R., Alexander, E.R., Turck, M., Counts, G.W., and Holmes, K.K.: Causes of the acute urethral syndrome in women, N. Engl. J. Med. **303**:409-415, 1980.

31. Taylor-Robinson, D., and McCormack, W.M.: The genital mycoplasmas. II, N. Engl. J. Med. **302**:1063-1067, 1980.

11 MICROORGANISMS ENCOUNTERED IN THE GENITAL TRACT

The microbial flora of the normal human genital tract consists chiefly of nonpigmented staphylococci or micrococci and gram-positive rods. In normal females the vaginal flora varies considerably with the pH of the secretions and the amount of glycogen present in the epithelium; these factors in turn depend on ovarian function. In most instances, however, microaerophilic lactobacilli (the Doederlein bacillus[28]) predominate, together with diphtheroids, *Bifidobacterium*, gram-negative enteric bacilli, species of *Bacteroides*, microaerophilic and anaerobic streptococci and cocci, clostridia, enterococci, and coagulase-negative staphylococci.

The normal cervix also has a relatively profuse flora. The organisms present are identical with those found in the upper vagina.

The bacterial flora of the vulva is a mixture of organisms present on the skin of this area, including the acid-fast saprophyte *Mycobacterium smegmatis*, and other bacteria descending from the vagina.

The following organisms are most frequently encountered in the genital tract:

> Coliform bacilli, enterococci, *Bacteroides* species, *Clostridium*, *Peptostreptococcus*, and other organisms indigenous to the genital tract
> Lactobacilli
> *Gardnerella (Haemophilus) vaginalis*
> *Trichomonas vaginalis*

101

Candida albicans, other *Candida* species, and saprophytic yeasts

Beta-hemolytic streptococci of groups A, B, and D

Mycobacterium tuberculosis

Nonpathogenic mycobacteria

Neisseria gonorrhoeae

Treponema pallidum

Haemophilus ducreyi

Mycoplasma species

Chlamydia trachomatis

Herpes simplex virus

ISOLATION OF THE GONOCOCCUS (NEISSERIA GONORRHOEAE)

The importance of gonorrhea is underlined by the fact that it is the most commonly encountered communicable disease in the United States.[48] In 1979 the estimate of reported cases of gonorrhea exceeded 1 million.[16] How many cases go unreported is uncertain.

The laboratory diagnosis of **gonorrhea** depends on the demonstration of intracellular diplococci in smears and on the isolation and identification of *Neisseria gonorrhoeae* by culture procedures. As a rule, gonococci may be found readily in smears of pus from **acute** infections, particularly in the male. In **chronic** infections, especially in the female, the value of the smear findings decreases; cultural methods generally yield a higher percentage of positive results.

Collection of specimens and primary inoculation of media

In the **female,** the best site to obtain a culture is the **cervix,** and this should be collected with care by an experienced professional. A sterile bivalve speculum is moistened with warm water (the usual lubricants contain antibacterial substances that may be lethal to gonococci) and inserted, and the cervical mucus plug is removed with a cotton ball and forceps. The external surface of the cervix is cleansed with a large cotton swab. Gentle compression of the cervix between the speculum blades may produce endocervical exudate. If not, a sterile

alginate or cotton-tipped applicator is then inserted into the endocervical canal and a rotating motion used to force exudate from endocervical glands. Only swabs made of cotton specified as being of low toxicity should be used. The swab is immediately inoculated to a modified Thayer-Martin chocolate agar plate (directions for preparation can be found in Chapter 42) or a Transgrow bottle* (this must be inoculated in an upright position to prevent escape of contained CO_2 gas). The modified Thayer-Martin plate is streaked in a **Z** pattern with the swab and thereafter cross-streaked closely with a sterile bacteriologic loop, preferably in the clinic; the Transgrow bottle is inoculated over the entire agar surface, working from the bottom up, after moistening the swab with excess moisture contained in the bottle. The modified Thayer-Martin plate should be placed in a candle jar (use only white candles) (approximately 3% CO_2) within 1 hour and incubated at 35 C for 20 hours before examination. The Transgrow bottle, used primarily for convenience in a physician's office, VD clinic, or small laboratory, should be incubated at 35 C overnight before shipping; this provides sufficient growth for survival during prolonged transport. It is then sent to the diagnostic facility by mail or other convenient means, avoiding any marked temperature changes.

Anal canal infection is common in the female, so anal cultures are also recommended, especially when the cervical culture is negative, as a follow-up of treatment efficacy. One can easily obtain this specimen without using an anoscope by carefully inserting an alginate or cotton-tipped applicator approximately 1 inch into the anal canal and moving it from side to side to obtain material from the crypts. Obtaining material under direct visualization at anoscopy is preferred when feasible. If the swab shows the

---

*Baltimore Biological Laboratory, Cockeysville, Md.; Difco Laboratories, Detroit; shelf-life at room temperature in excess of 3 months.

presence of fecal material, it is discarded and another swab is used. The swab is inoculated to modified Thayer-Martin medium as previously described. One may inoculate one plate with two cervical specimens (but spaced apart) or one cervical specimen and one anal canal specimen.[29] This provides diagnostic sensitivity equivalent to separate plates and saves considerable cost.

In special situations where a cervical specimen is not indicated (e.g., in children or hysterectomized patients) a urethral or vaginal culture may be substituted. A study of 104 patients who had undergone total hysterectomies yielded the following rates of positivity on culture for *Neisseria gonorrhoeae:* urethral, 100%, vaginal, 41%, and rectal, 12%.[33] Urethral cultures from the female are also recommended in the case of acute symptomatic disease, Bartholin abscess, pelvic inflammatory disease, pharyngitis, or disseminated infection.[30] Repeat cultures are important, as 6% to 8% of infected women have negative cultures at any one visit.[36]

For the **male** with a purulent urethral exudate, the examination of a Gram-stained direct smear (made by **rolling** the swab over the slide to preserve cell morphology) is usually sufficient to confirm a clinical diagnosis of gonorrhea. However, since an appreciable number of males may be asymptomatic and the stained smear probably negative, a **urethral culture** is recommended. This is readily obtained by gently inserting a thin alginate urethrogenital swab* (which may be moistened with sterile water) 2 cm into the urethra, gently rotating it, and then immediately inoculating a modified Thayer-Martin plate or Transgrow bottle as previously described. In addition, anal and pharyngeal specimens should be obtained from homosexuals.

Occasionally, material from other sites may be submitted for gonococcal culture; these include

throat swabs, freshly voided urine, joint fluid, swabs from the eye, and so forth. The swabs and sediments from centrifuged fluids should be immediately inoculated to modified Thayer-Martin medium and to supplemented chocolate agar and handled as indicated above. In patients suspected of disseminated gonococcal infection, blood should be obtained for culture as described in Chapter 7. Culture of uncentrifuged first-voided urine (10 to 20 ml) for *N. gonorrhoeae* in males compares favorably with urethral swab culture and is less expensive and better accepted by patients.[14]

Direct smears for gonococci

To obtain the highest percentage of positive findings in cases of suspected gonorrhea, both **smears and cultures** should be made. In the case of purulent material, slides should be prepared by the examining physician at the time the cultures are taken. Such smears should be carefully prepared by **rolling** the swab over the slide rather than by rubbing it on. All aspects of the swab head should come in contact with the slide. This distributes the pus cells into layers, thereby permitting accurate observation of intracellular organisms. The practice of submitting moist material stuck between two slides is condemned for obvious reasons. Smears of urine and other fluid specimens should be prepared from the centrifuged sediment of these materials. Smears should cover at least 1 sq cm of the slide, if possible. They should be air dried and heat fixed.

Slides must be carefully stained by the Gram method and examined for the presence of characteristic **gram-negative diplococci** with their adjacent sides flattened (coffee-bean shaped). These organisms are generally found inside pus cells in acute gonorrhea (Plate 23), but in very early infections or in chronic gonorrhea they may be found extracellularly only, and frequently as single cocci. It should also be noted that recent administration of a specific antimicrobial agent such as penicillin may either eradicate or

---

*Falcon No. 2050 sterile alginate nasopharyngeal applicator.

alter the morphology and staining reaction of *N. gonorrhoeae*. Care should be taken to distinguish gonococci from bipolar-staining, gram-negative coccobacilli, such as *Moraxella osloensis*, which have been mistaken for neisseriae.[57] Biochemical tests must be carried out to differentiate them with certainty. *N. meningitidis* may also be found rarely in the genitourinary tract and in the anus. Positive smears should be reported as **"Intracellular (extracellular) gram-negative diplococci resembling gonococci found; many (few) pus cells present."** The presence of epithelial cells should also be noted. All elements (bacteria, cells) should be semiquantitated.

In the male the finding of typical gram-negative intracellular diplococci within pus cells of a urethral discharge is sufficient for a laboratory diagnosis.[48] This test ranges in sensitivity from 93% to 99%. In the female the endocervix is the site most often positive for gonococci. Direct smears of exudates from this site are positive in 38% to 69% of patients; thus, a negative smear certainly does not exclude the diagnosis of gonorrhea, and cultures are necessary.[48] The direct smear is both insensitive and nonspecific for pharyngeal gonorrhea. The smear is also not reliable for rectal infection.

Patients whose smears show typical gram-negative diplococci but only in an extracellular location are likely to have nongonococcal urethritis. One study showed that only 10.5% of such patients had cultures positive for *N. gonorrhoeae*.[1]

Limulus lysate test

A nonextracted *Limulus* amoebocyte lysate proved effective in detecting endotoxin in gonococcal urethral exudates. At a dilution breakpoint of 1:1600 the sensitivity of this test was 100% and the specificity 96%.[47] The corresponding sensitivity and specificity for Gram-stained smears from these same patients were 95% and 98%.

Culture media

Many different and complex media have been introduced for the isolation of the gonococcus, but excellent results may be obtained by using the medium introduced by Thayer and Martin[59] in 1964. The original formula, an enriched chocolate agar medium containing the antibiotics ristocetin and polymyxin B, was recommended for the isolation of *N. gonorrhoeae* and *N. meningitidis*. The authors reported that the medium showed an inhibitory action against other neisseriae and most species of mimeae *(Moraxella)* and that it suppressed *Pseudomonas* and *Proteus* species. The removal of ristocetin from the market necessitated a suitable substitute, and Thayer and Martin reported the successful use of vancomycin, sodium colistimethate (colistin), and nystatin[60] (V-C-N inhibitor*). Comparison of the new medium with the original formula showed comparable growth of *N. gonorrhoeae* from both male and female patients, along with a greater inhibition of staphylococci and saprophytic neisseriae.

A further improvement in Thayer-Martin chocolate agar was the incorporation of a chemically defined supplement* that resulted in as good or better recovery of gonococci than was achieved with previous media.[39] The use of Imferon, an iron-dextran complex, as a replacement for ferric nitrate enhanced the growth of both the gonococcus and the meningococcus.[45]

A modification of the Thayer-Martin medium—Transgrow—has been prepared according to the formulation of Martin and Lester.[40] Recommended for transport and growth of pathogenic neisseriae (while maintaining their viability for at least 48 hours at room temperature), the medium suppresses contaminating organisms in a manner similar to that of the original Thayer-Martin formula. The agar content of Transgrow was increased to 2% and the glucose content to

---

*Baltimore Biological Laboratory, Cockeysville, Md.; Difco Laboratories, Detroit.

0.25%; the medium also contains trimethoprim lactate, which is inhibitory to *Proteus* species. It is available commercially,* packaged in a tightly closed flat bottle under a partial CO_2 atmosphere, and has a shelf life of 3 to 4 months. Transgrow medium appears to be superior to other transport media for maintaining the viability of pathogenic neisseriae and can be mailed to the reference laboratory after overnight incubation without appreciable loss of gonococci. The procedure for inoculation of Transgrow bottles has been described previously. Comparative studies with Thayer-Martin medium by CDC's Venereal Disease Research Laboratory have indicated good correlation, both in the laboratory and in field trials.

Martin-Lewis agar, a modification of Thayer-Martin agar, has been introduced for recovery of pathogenic *Neisseria*. Martin-Lewis agar differs from Thayer-Martin agar in that anisomycin (a much more stable compound) is substituted for nystatin, and the concentration of vancomycin is increased from 3 μg/ml to 4 μg/ml.[41] These changes have resulted in improved inhibition of *Candida albicans* and of gram-positive organisms. It should be noted, however, that vancomycin is inhibitory to some strains of *N. gonorrhoeae* even at concentrations of 3 μg/ml.[64]

Another medium that is very good for the isolation of pathogenic *Neisseria* was described in 1973 by Faur and associates.[10,11] Known as New York City (NYC) medium, it consists of a proteose peptone-cornstarch-agar—buffered base containing a supplement of horse plasma and hemoglobin solution, glucose, yeast dialysate, and four antimicrobial agents (vancomycin, colistin, nystatin or amphotericin, and trimethoprim lactate). It is a clear medium that provides 24-hour luxuriant growth of pathogenic *Neisseria* as well as being highly selective.

A modification of NYC medium, which gave good performance as a culture and transport medium without the addition of ambient CO_2, was also reported by Faur and co-workers.[12] The addition to NYC medium of filter-sterilized yeast dialysate provided a carbon source for CO_2 development and release. They found that when it was packaged in an airtight container, it permitted growth of *N. gonorrhoeae* from clinical specimens without provision of ambient CO_2.

The NYC medium has been modified to support the growth of strains of mycoplasma.[20] The modified medium contains lincomycin in place of vancomycin (one of several modifications). This modified NYC medium was compared with Martin-Lewis medium for the recovery of *N. gonorrhoeae* from clinical specimens.[20] There was no statistically significant difference in isolation rate. Granato and colleagues (J. Clin. Microbiol. **13**:963-968, 1981) have reported that the use of an improved NYC (INYC) medium (reduced concentration of vancomycin) markedly enhanced the recovery of *N. gonorrhoeae* from clinical specimens as compared with Martin-Lester medium.

A simplified medium for isolating *N. gonorrhoeae* has been described.[53] This differs from the modified Thayer-Martin medium in that it contains a simplified enrichment and amphotericin B in place of nystatin. It is easy to prepare, and the cost is only one third that of modified Thayer-Martin medium. Although contaminants are found in somewhat greater numbers on this medium, the recovery of *N. gonorrhoeae* is comparable to that of modified Thayer-Martin medium.

Although Transgrow medium has proved to be of value, it appears to have some important deficiencies. The commercial preparations of Transgrow have been found to contain variable CO_2 concentrations.[6] Different batches of the medium vary in ability to support the growth of gonococci. Moisture accumulating inside the

---

*Baltimore Biological Laboratory, Cockeysville, Md.; Difco Laboratories, Detroit; Gibco Diagnostics, Madison, Wisc.; Scott Laboratories, Inc., Fiskeville, RI; and others.

bottles may cause poor visibility and may contribute to the spreading of contaminants and interfere with development of isolated colonies. Furthermore, the narrow bottle neck is inconvenient for inoculation and subculturing of colonies.

Another test system, called Gono-Pak, for growth of *N. gonorrhoeae* has been described by Martin and associates.[38] Consisting of a Petri plate containing modified Thayer-Martin medium, the specimen is inoculated, sealed, and placed in a plastic bag along with a CO_2-generating tablet. Employing modified NYC transport medium,[12] Symington[55] found the Gono-Pak to be suitable for both transportation and incubation of *N. gonorrhoeae*.

An additional development has been that of a rectangular plastic plate that contains a small well to accommodate a CO_2-generating tablet. Known as the Jembec plate,* this plate and a CO_2-generating tablet sealed in a plastic "ziplock" pouch provide a CO_2 environment enclosure. Jembec plates that contain prepoured modified Thayer-Martin medium are known as Neigon plates.†

Carlson and associates[5] evaluated four methods for isolation of *N. gonorrhoeae*. These included a Bio-Bag type C‡ (made up of a ziplock plastic bag containing a Thayer-Martin plate and a crushable CO_2-generating ampule), the Gono-Pak, the Jembec system, and the candle extinction jar. There were no statistically significant differences in isolation rates of the gonococcus from urethral and anal specimens. The Bio-Bag has the advantage of immediate release of CO_2 as compared with the Gono-Pak and Jembec systems, in which CO_2 production is dependent on release of moisture from the medium. A number of other kits for gonococcal isolation and identification are available, including the Isocult-GC, GC-Duet, Gonorette, Unibac-GC, Bullseye plate, Gonocult, and Microcult-GC kits. These are all discussed in a review paper by Lewis and Wiesner.[36] In general, all of the kits for presumptive identification of *N. gonorrhoeae* performed reasonably well, with a sensitivity of 85% to 90%, depending on the particular kit. They offer good reproducibility, convenience, ease of storage, and the saving of time through elimination of the need to prepare and sterilize media. However, the kits are all much more expensive than direct plating of organisms.

In evaluating improved transport systems for *N. gonorrhoeae* in clinical specimens, Symington[56] studied the efficiency of the following: (1) Amies charcoal transport medium, (2) Jembec chambers containing Neigon plates of modified Thayer-Martin medium, and (3) Jembec chambers containing plates of modified NYC transport medium. She found that for up to 2 days in transit, the three systems were not significantly different. However, after 3 days in transit, modified NYC-Jembec chambers were better than the other two (highly significant statistically). The modified NYC-Jembec chambers withstood 241 miles of postal transit during winter months, with 80% of the *N. gonorrhoeae* present in clinical specimens remaining viable from 2 to 5 days under these conditions. The CO_2 generated by the tablet in the Jembec chamber was sufficient to support the growth of *N. gonorrhoeae* if the chambers were incubated at 36 C immediately after inoculation. If delayed in transit, however, the chambers had to be incubated in 5% to 10% CO_2 to promote the growth of *N. gonorrhoeae*.

Jembec plates can be refrigerated for up to 6 weeks, provided the plates are sealed in plastic to prevent drying. Transgrow bottles may be kept under refrigeration for 3 months.[42] All such refrigerated media should be warmed to room temperature before inoculation of specimen material.

---

*Ames Co., Division of Miles Laboratories, Elkhart, Ind.
†Flow Laboratories, Inc., Rockville, Md.
‡Marion Laboratories, Kansas City, Mo.

Handling of specimens in the laboratory

Ideally, specimens for the isolation of gonococci are submitted on modified Thayer-Martin, Martin-Lewis, or NYC medium plates (or in Transgrow bottles) that have been properly inoculated previously and incubated in candle jars overnight. In a hospital situation, however, the specimen for culture is usually received on a swab in holding medium such as the Culturette,* having been obtained from the patient a short time before. Occasionally, one may also receive purulent material from an aspirated joint, a freshly voided urine sample, or other specimens. In any case, the specimen (or sediment following centrifugation) should be inoculated **immediately** to a freshly prepared modified Thayer-Martin or supplemented chocolate agar plate (brought to room temperature), using the **Z** and cross-streaking procedure previously described. Swab specimens should not be left at room temperature unless in Transgrow or other transport medium, and **under no circumstances** in a 35 C incubator; gonococci either die off or are rapidly overgrown by commensal bacteria. However, the swab may be refrigerated at 4 to 6 C for not longer than 3 hours before inoculation without a noticeable reduction in recovery of gonococci (not true of meningococci, which are notably cold sensitive).

Lue and associates[37] have indicated that there is enhanced recovery of *N. gonorrhoeae* from swabs that have been placed in Amies transport medium for selective enrichment for several hours prior to culture. The superiority of this technique over immediate direct plating remains to be determined.

All cultures, including previously inoculated Thayer-Martin plates (or Transgrow bottles received with loosened caps), are placed in a CO$_2$ incubator (5% to 10% CO$_2$) or in a candle jar with a tight-fitting lid† containing a short, thick, white smokeless candle (affixed to a glass slide) that is lighted inside the jar before closing with the lid. This will generate approximately 3% CO$_2$ before extinguishing itself.

The plates or bottles are incubated at **35 C‡** overnight and examined for growth; cultures showing no growth are returned to the incubator for a total period of not less than 48 hours.§ Typical growth of *N. gonorrhoeae* appears as translucent, mucoid, raised colonies of varying size; in Transgrow bottles, colonies may or may not appear typical. The **oxidase test** is used to verify the presence of gonococcus colonies (Plate 51) and, along with the Gram stain of those colonies reacting positively, serves to presumptively identify *N. gonorrhoeae* from a urogenital site. These procedures and further identification tests by carbohydrate fermentation and immunofluorescent and coagglutination techniques are discussed in Chapter 19, along with penicillinase testing and serologic and immunologic diagnosis.

Isolation of gonococci from synovial fluid

CDC's Venereal Disease Control Division (*Criteria and Techniques for the Diagnosis of Gonorrhea,* 1976) recommends that synovial fluid be cultured for gonococci in an enriched broth, such as trypticase soy broth supplemented with 1% IsoVitaleX, 10% horse serum, and 1% glucose.

An interesting paper from Holmes and colleagues[26] concerns the recovery of *N. gonorrhoeae* from "sterile" synovial fluid in gonococcal arthritis by means of a medium developed for the propagation of L forms of those organisms in vitro. The medium was a modification of that

---

*Marion Laboratories, Kansas City, Mo.
†Erno Products Co., Philadelphia; EC jar (clear) 120-mm mouth opening No. C-3118, with metal screw-cap lid. This will hold approximately twelve 90-mm plates and a candle.

‡The incubator should be adjusted to this temperature, because many strains of *N. gonorrhoeae* will not grow well at 37 C.
§Nearly one half of positive cultures require this incubation period.

introduced by Bohnhoff and Page[2] for *N. meningitidis* L forms and consisted of trypticase soy broth supplemented with 10% sucrose and 1.25% agar, to which was added 20% inactivated horse serum, after sterilization. After inoculation, the surface of the medium was overlaid with 0.5 ml of the same medium containing one half the agar concentration, and following 72 hours' incubation, oxidase-positive, reverting L form-type colonies developed. On subculture to chocolate agar, tiny colonies grew and were identified as *N. gonorrhoeae* by fluorescent antibody staining and by carbohydrate fermentation tests. No growth occurred on regular chocolate agar or Thayer-Martin agar inoculated at the same time, after 96 hours' incubation. The authors hypothesized that the gonococci may have existed in the synovial fluid in a cell wall–deficient, osmotically fragile state. A further trial of this medium in patients with suspected gonococcal arthritis is certainly warranted. A stable cell wall–deficient gonococcus has been isolated from a patient with untreated urethritis.[25]

MISCELLANEOUS VENEREAL DISEASES
Syphilis

Although a full discussion of syphilis is not within the scope of this text, mention should be made of the serologic diagnosis of **syphilis** and the methods most frequently used in making this diagnosis. These tests are basically of two types: (1) the **nontreponemal** antibody tests, such as the VDRL and rapid plasma reagin (RPR) flocculation tests and the Kolmer complement fixation test, and (2) the **treponemal** antibody tests, such as the fluorescent treponemal antibody absorption (FTA-ABS) and the microhemagglutination *Treponema pallidum* (MHA-TP) tests. Further discussion of these may be found in Chapter 38.

Mention should be made of **darkfield** microscopy as an aid to the diagnosis of early syphilis. An ample drop of tissue fluid expressed from a primary lesion is placed on a coverglass, which is inverted over a glass slide and pressed to make a thin film. This preparation is then examined microscopically, using the oil immersion objective and a properly adjusted darkfield illumination. The presence of motile treponemes of characteristic morphology in a typical early lesion establishes the diagnosis. Difficulty may be experienced in darkfield examination of oral or rectal lesions, since these sites may contain motile treponemes from the indigenous flora (see Chapter 24).

A fluorescein-labeled *T. pallidum* conjugate* is available for the direct identification of *T. pallidum* by the immunofluorescent technique. Material from the lesion is applied to a slide and air dried; the conjugate is then added, rinsed off, and dried; a coverslip is applied, and the preparation is examined by fluorescent microscopy. Preparations may be made, dried, and examined later, eliminating the necessity of immediate darkfield examination.

Chancroid

Chancroid is a soft chancre of the genitalia of venereal origin, caused by *Haemophilus ducreyi* (Ducrey bacillus), a very small gram-negative rod occurring singly or in small clumps.

Isolation of the organism is difficult. However, *H. ducreyi* can be demonstrated by the following procedure[3]: 10 ml of the patient's blood is distributed in 5-ml amounts in sterile screw-capped tubes. After clotting has occurred, the serum is removed, transferred aseptically to another sterile tube, and inactivated in a 56 C water bath for 30 minutes. After cooling, the serum is inoculated with material obtained from the undermined border of the genital lesion (previously cleansed with saline-moistened gauze) and incubated at 35 C for 48 hours. A Gram-stained smear of the growth is then examined for the presence of coccobacillary gram-negative organisms in tangled chains or in long

---

*Baltimore Biological Laboratory, Cockeysville, Md., Catalog No. 40806.

parallel strands ("schools of fish"), which are diagnostic of *H. ducreyi*.

Hammond and co-workers[23] reported favorable isolation rates of *H. ducreyi* by inoculation of two plates of enriched chocolate agar, one of which contained vancomycin in a concentration of 3 μg/ml. The plates were incubated at 33 C in 5% to 10% CO_2 in a moist atmosphere. Nonmucoid yellow-gray translucent colonies that can be pushed virtually intact across the agar surface appear within 2 to 9 days after inoculation. Gram stain of colonies should reveal organisms with typical morphology. Sottnek and colleagues[54] compared various media for primary isolation of *H. ducreyi* from genital lesions. The organism was isolated on chocolate agar plus vancomycin from 10 of 14 known positive patients, on rabbit blood agar plus vancomycin from 16 of 17 positive patients, and on fetal bovine serum agar plus vancomycin from 9 of 11 patients. Fetal bovine serum was found to support good growth of all strains. CO_2 improved the growth of seven strains.

Smears and cultures prepared from pus aspirated from a bubo are much more likely to yield valid information than is similar material from the base of ulcers. Nevertheless, the smear may be positive in only 50% to 88% of cases.[43] Bubos should be aspirated through normal-appearing skin to prevent fistula formation.

Granuloma inguinale

Granuloma inguinale is an infection of the genital region characterized by a slowly progressive ulceration and caused by *Calymmatobacterium granulomatis*. This organism appears within the cytoplasm of large mononuclear cells as a small (1 to 2 μm), plump, heavily encapsulated coccobacillus (Donovan body) and is best observed in impression smears (stained with Wright stain) of cleansed tissue obtained by punch biopsy or scrapings from the edge of the lesion. A diligent search of smears prepared on several occasions may be necessary to find the organisms.

The organism may be recovered by yolk sac inoculation or cultivation on coagulated egg yolk slants or in a semidefined medium in which the factor in egg yolk is replaced by either lactalbumin hydrolysate or Phytone.* A lowered Eh is necessary for growth. This may be obtained by the use of sodium thioglycollate. The organism morphologically and antigenically resembles members of the genus *Klebsiella*, and, accordingly, some authorities have placed the organism in the family *Enterobacteriaceae*.[43]

Lymphogranuloma venereum

Lymphogranuloma venereum (LGV) is caused by one of a large group of gram-negative intracellular parasites responsible for some important human diseases, including psittacosis and trachoma, the **chlamydiae**.[50] The diagnosis is made by demonstrating delayed skin hypersensitivity to an antigen prepared from infected yolk sacs and by a fourfold rise in complement fixation titer on paired (acute and convalescent) sera, using a similar antigen. A serologic test for syphilis (STS) should also be done on these patients to rule out syphilis.

TRICHOMONAS INFECTION

The most practical method of confirming a diagnosis of *Trichomonas* infection is by the demonstration of **actively motile** flagellates in a saline suspension of vaginal or urethral discharges. The preparation must be examined shortly after collecting, or the characteristic motility and morphology may not be apparent. Cultures of vaginal specimens, semen, urine, and other materials may reveal trichomonads when wet smears are negative. A variety of media are recommended for cultivation of this organism.

CANDIDA INFECTION

The yeastlike fungus *Candida albicans* is also a frequent cause of vaginitis, and it can readily

---

*Baltimore Biological Laboratory, Cockeysville, Md.

be identified by the examination of Gram-stained smears and growth on Sabouraud dextrose agar slants. Methods are described in Chapter 34.

ISOLATION OF GARDNERELLA (HAEMOPHILUS) VAGINALIS

The bacteriologic examination of cases of "nonspecific" vaginitis frequently fails to provide the clinician with any specific agent against which to direct therapy. Gardner and Dukes[15] reported the isolation of a small, pleomorphic, gram-negative bacillus from many of their cases of nonspecific vaginitis, and they named it *Haemophilus vaginalis*. Smears of vaginal discharge in such cases showed epithelial cells covered with these bacilli—the so-called clue cells. The organism grew out on sheep blood agar plates that had been incubated for 24 to 48 hours in a candle jar as colorless, transparent, pinpoint colonies, best seen by oblique illumination, and frequently surrounded by a clear zone of hemolysis. Characteristic "puff ball" colonies appeared in thioglycollate medium enriched with ascitic fluid. Some strains are obligately anaerobic.

Zinnemann and Turner[65] reported the successful cultivation of this organism on a medium that did not contain hemin (X factor), nicotinamide adenine dinucleotide (V factor), or other coenzymes required by members of the genus *Haemophilus*, and they proposed reclassification of it as *Corynebacterium vaginale*. A new genus, *Gardnerella*, has been proposed for this organism, and it is now known as *Gardnerella vaginalis*.[22] Vaginal discharge may be cultured for *G. vaginalis* on V agar.[43] Using the rapid fermentation method of Brown,[4] one may readily identify the organism. It must be remembered that the organism is sometimes seen in the absence of "nonspecific vaginitis." Of greater importance for diagnosis is the addition of 10% KOH to vaginal discharge. This produces a fishy, aminelike odor. This, coupled with the foul odor that is characteristic of this disease,

indicates the likelihood that anaerobic bacteria play a role in this disease.

G. vaginalis is thought to be the cause of nonspecific vaginitis, but this is controversial. There is reason to believe that nonspecific vaginitis may involve *G. vaginalis* and one or more anaerobes.[46] A more recent study from this laboratory (Spiegel et al.: N. Engl. J. Med. **303**:601-607, 1980) concluded that a high ratio of succinate to lactate in vaginal fluid is a useful indicator for the diagnosis of this condition. *G. vaginalis* has also been implicated in puerperal fever and other genitourinary tract infections.

NONGONOCOCCAL (NONSPECIFIC) URETHRITIS AND CERVICITIS

"Nonspecific urethritis" is widespread. For example, it is the most frequently recorded sexually transmitted disease in England. Although it is not a reportable disease in the United States, data obtained from two venereal disease clinics associated with the CDC showed that nonspecific urethritis accounted for 30% of urethritis in black men and up to 70% in white men.[61] The incidence of nonspecific urethritis in women is uncertain, because they generally do not have clinically recognizable symptoms at presentation. So-called postgonococcal urethritis actually represents a dual infection with the gonococcus and an agent of nonspecific urethritis.

The major organism with proven causal relationship to nonspecific urethritis is *Chlamydia trachomatis*.[13] T strains of *Mycoplasma* are probably also important. *Trichomonas vaginalis* and *Herpesvirus hominis* also cause nonspecific urethritis but only account for a small percentage of cases. *Candida albicans* has been claimed to be a cause of occasional cases of this disease, but documentation is lacking. It has also been stated that *Corynebacterium genitalium* type 1 is responsible for a number of cases of nonspecific urethritis. The evidence for this is still not convincing.

The diagnosis of nonspecific urethritis depends on ruling out known causes of urethritis, chiefly gonorrhea, and documenting the presence of polymorphonuclear leukocytes in the urethral exudate. This is done by demonstrating an average of five or more polymorphonuclear leukocytes per field in five high-power (1,000×) fields.[13]

As obligate intracellular organisms, *Chlamydia* are cultured like viruses and are known to be responsible for trachoma, inclusion conjunctivitis, and lymphogranuloma venereum. Besides nonspecific urethritis, *Chlamydia* may cause proctitis, urethral stricture, acute epididymitis, a chronic relapsing urethritis, Reiter's syndrome, hypertrophic erosion of the cervix, purulent cervical mucus, and salpingitis. Mothers infected with *Chlamydia* may transmit to the newborn such diseases as inclusion conjunctivitis, nasopharyngeal infection, otitis media, and subsequently pneumonia. Serotypes D through K of *C. trachomatis* are associated with urethral, cervical, and ocular infections. Other serotypes cause trachoma and lymphogranuloma venereum primarily. The lymphogranuloma venereum immunotypes of *C. trachomatis* are associated with severe proctitis, whereas the other immunotypes produce a mild proctitis (Quinn et al.: N. Engl. J. Med. **305:**195-200, 1981).

Specimens for examination for *Chlamydia* should consist of swabs, scrapings, and small tissue samples. These should be collected in a special transport medium (2SP) consisting of 0.2 M sucrose in 0.02 M phosphate buffer (pH 7.0 to 7.2) with 5% fetal calf serum and added antibiotics.[50] It may be simpler to place the clinical specimen directly into tissue culture growth medium containing streptomycin or gentamicin, vancomycin, and amphotericin B. If the specimen cannot be processed within 24 hours after collection, it can be refrigerated. If this is not possible, the specimen should be frozen at −60 C in the 2SP suspending medium.

Identification of *Chlamydia* in specimens or tissue culture involves demonstration of characteristic intracytoplasmic inclusions by use of

Giemsa stain, iodine stain, other stains, or fluorescent antibody technique. The fluorescent antibody procedure is more sensitive than the others. The technique of culture of *Chlamydia* in irradiated McCoy cells[7,19] provides a more convenient method for testing large numbers of specimens than does the yolk sac inoculation procedure. Based on a count of inclusion bodies, the McCoy cell method is more rapid and allows quantitative measurement of the level of infection.[18] It was also found to be three to four times more sensitive than the detection of inclusions in smears or isolation of the organism in the yolk sac of embryonated eggs.[8,18] Gordon and associates[17] reported that the infectivity of *Chlamydia* was enhanced by centrifugation of the inoculum onto the irradiated cells. Wentworth and Alexander[62] found that 5-iodo-2-deoxyuridine enhanced the susceptibility of McCoy cell cultures to chlamydial infection; elimination of the need for irradiation simplifies the procedure considerably.

Other studies have shown that *Chlamydia* infection can be increased 45 times in DEAE-treated McCoy cells, compared with untreated controls.[49] Moreover, comparative studies with human cervical specimens have shown HeLa 229 cells to be equal to McCoy cells in susceptibility to infection.[35] Wentworth and associates[63] reported that DEAE-dextran increases the level of infectivity of *Chlamydia* 100 times in HeLa cells but less than twice in McCoy cells.

According to Schachter,[50] cycloheximide-treated McCoy cell lines represent the optimum procedure for primary culture and isolation of *Chlamydia*. A microtest (microtiter) procedure developed for isolation of *C. trachomatis* substantially reduces cost and technician time (Yoder et al.: J. Clin. Microbiol. **13:**1036-1039, 1981). In this system also, cycloheximide-treated McCoy cells were superior to IUDR-treated cells. The test is sensitive and rapid.

Dunlop and co-workers[9] reported the isolation of *Chlamydia* from approximately 40% of men with nonspecific urethritis by inserting a swab 2 to 5 cm into the urethra. That these organisms have a significant etiologic role in nongonococcal urethritis in a midwestern community has been reported by Smith and associates.[52] From October 1973 through August 1974, these investigators inoculated 335 genitourinary tract specimens from patients with urethritis into McCoy cell cultures. They obtained 45 *Chlamydia* isolates, 42 of which were recovered when glass vials, rather than plastic microtiter plates, were used as cell culture vessels. Herpes simplex virus was isolated 15 times. *Chlamydia* has also been observed in 30% of women seen in a venereal disease clinic.[44] Furthermore, colonization with this organism was observed in 66% of women who were regular sexual partners of men with *Chlamydia*-associated urethritis, whereas in control groups of men and women isolation rates of less than 5% were obtained. *Chlamydia* may be responsible for clinically manifest cervicitis.

The microorganisms of the *Mycoplasma* group, also called PPLO (pleuropneumonialike organism), are the smallest free-living organisms that can be cultivated on artificial media. They lack a rigid cell wall, require protein-enriched media for growth, and exhibit a characteristic "fried egg" colony when growing on solid media.

Currently, 12 mycoplasmas of human origin have been described.[58] Of these, *M. hominis*, *M. fermentans*, *M. pneumoniae*, and T strains (*Ureaplasma urealyticum*) are found in the human genitourinary tract. T-strain mycoplasmas have been associated with from 60% to more than 90% of cases of nongonococcal urethritis in males, whereas their natural occurrence in a similar group of normal controls ranged from 21% to 26%, as reported by Shepard.[51] It is not established that T strains of mycoplasma play an·important etiologic role in this genital infection, but the data are becoming more convincing that *U. urealyticum* does play a definite role in this disease.

For optimal isolation of mycoplasmas specimens should be inoculated immediately into the growth medium.[58] They should then be maintained at 4 C while being transported to the laboratory as quickly as possible. The basic medium is a beef heart infusion broth available commercially as PPLO broth, supplemented with fresh yeast extract and horse serum. Antibiotics such as penicillin are usually added to inhibit other bacteria. The broth is incubated under normal atmospheric conditions. One may add some of the specimen to a separate vial of broth containing phenol red (0.002%) and urea. *U. urealyticum* possesses a urease that breaks down urea to ammonia, thus raising the pH of the medium. Aliquots of the medium from a culture showing this type of color change are subcultured onto agar media containing urea and a sensitive indicator of ammonia, manganese (II) sulphate. *Ureaplasma* colonies are dark brown on this medium. This technique involving liquid to agar subculture is the most sensitive method for isolation of *Ureaplasma*.[58]

There is no good evidence that mycoplasmas are involved in chronic prostatitis, epididymitis, Reiter's syndrome, or Bartholin abscess.[58] *Mycoplasma hominis* may play a role in some cases of vaginitis, cervicitis, and pelvic inflammatory disease. *Mycoplasma hominis* is a definite cause of postpartum fever.

The usefulness of the modified NYC medium for growth of mycoplasmas, as well as *N. gonorrhoeae*, has already been mentioned.

GENITAL HERPES SIMPLEX INFECTION

Genital herpes simplex infection is a problem of increasing frequency and importance. Moseley and others (J. Clin. Microbiol. **13**:913-918, 1981) compared various diagnostic procedures in 76 patients. Viral isolation was positive in 80%; indirect immunoperoxidase testing was positive in 66%; and direct fluorescent antibody testing was positive in 55%. The latter two tests were positive in nine patients whose viral cultures were negative (subsequently positive in eight of the nine). The two rapid techniques are commercially available.

MICROBIAL AGENTS IN HUMAN ABORTION

Listeria monocytogenes is a cause of septic perinatal infections in the female (some with bacteremia) and purulent meningitis, meningo-encephalitis, or miliary granulomatosis in the neonate. The mother may exhibit flu-like symptoms with a low-grade fever in the last trimester of pregnancy and subsequently may abort or deliver a stillborn baby.[31] Postpartum cultures from the vagina, cervix, or urine may be positive for *L. monocytogenes* from a few days to several weeks, although the patient may appear asymptomatic.[21] In uncontaminated material (blood, CSF), *L. monocytogenes* can be readily isolated by conventional techniques, but contaminated specimens or tissue may require selective media and **cold enrichment** procedures. Refer to Chapter 26 for a further description of these methods.

Although *Campylobacter (Vibrio) fetus* clearly causes abortion in cattle, its role in human abortion is not conclusive. In describing 17 human infections caused by *C. fetus*, King[32] noted that three of these patients (from the French literature) had accompanying problems of pregnancy. Hood and Todd[27] of Charity Hospital in New Orleans reported what is apparently the first human case of *C. fetus* infection involving pregnancy in the western hemisphere. The bacterium was isolated from the placenta of the mother and the brain of the aborted fetus.

A suggested role for *Mycoplasma* in human reproductive failure[34] has not been established, but it appears that *M. hominis* is of etiologic importance in some women with fever following abortion.[58]

The role of *Toxoplasma* infection in abortion must also be considered uncertain.

It is apparent that the clinical microbiologist should be aware of all these agents and, through close communication with the clinician, offer microbiologic aid in their early detection.

REFERENCES

1. Arnold, A.J., and Kleris, G.S.: The "borderline" smear in men with urethritis, J.A.M.A. **244**:157-159, 1980.
2. Bohnhoff, M., and Page, M.I.: Experimental infection with parent and L-phase variants of *Neisseria meningitidis*, J. Bacteriol. **95**:2070-2077, 1968.
3. Borchardt, K.A., and Hoke, A.W.: Simplified laboratory technique for diagnosis of chancroid, Arch. Dermatol. **102**:188-192, 1970.
4. Brown, W.J.: Modification of the rapid fermentation tests for *Neisseria gonorrhoeae*, Appl. Microbiol. **27**:1027-1030, 1974.
5. Carlson, B.L., Haley, M.S., Tisel, N.A., and McCormack, W.M.: Evaluation of four methods for isolation of *Neisseria gonorrhoeae*, J. Clin. Microbiol. **12**:301-303, 1980.
6. Chapel, T., Smeltzen, M., Printz, D., Dassel, R., and Lewis, J.: An evaluation of commercially supplied Transgrow and Amies media for the detection of *Neisseria gonorrhoeae*, Health Lab. Sci. **11**:28-33, 1973.
7. Darougar, S., Kinnison, J.R., and Jones, B.R.: Simplified irradiated McCoy cell culture for isolation of chlamydiae, Excerpta Medica International Congress Series No. 223, 1970, pp. 63-70.
8. Darougar, S., Treharne, J.D., Dwyer, R. St. C., Kinnison, J.R., and Jones, B.R.: Isolation of TRIC agent (*Chlamydia*) in irradiated McCoy cell culture from endemic trachoma in field studies in Iran: comparison with other laboratory tests for detection of *Chlamydia*, Br. J. Ophthalmol. **55**:591-599, 1971.
9. Dunlop, E.M.C., Vaughan-Jackson, J.D., Darougar, S., and Jones, B.R.: Chlamydial infection: incidence in "nonspecific" urethritis, Br. J. Vener. Dis. **48**:425-428, 1972.
10. Faur, Y.C., Weisburd, M.H., Wilson, M.E., and May, P.S.: A new medium for the isolation of pathogenic *Neisseria* (NYC medium). I. Formulation and comparisons with standard media, Health Lab. Sci. **10**:44-54, 1973.
11. Faur, Y.C., Weisburd, M.H., and Wilson, M.E.: A new medium for the isolation of pathogenic *Neisseria* (NYC medium). II. Effect of amphotericin B and trimethoprim lactate on selectivity, Health Lab. Sci. **10**:55-60, 1973.
12. Faur, Y.C., Weisburd, M.H., and Wilson, M.E.: A new medium for the isolation of pathogenic *Neisseria* (NYC medium). III. Performance as a culture and transport medium without addition of ambient carbon dioxide, Health Lab. Sci. **10**:61-74, 1973.

13. Felman, Y.M., and Nikitas, J.A.: Nongonococcal urethritis: a clinical review, J.A.M.A. **245**:381-386, 1981.

14. Feng, W.C., Medeiros, A.A., and Murray, E.S.: Diagnosis of gonorrhea in male patients by culture of uncentrifuged first-voided urine, J.A.M.A. **237**:896-897, 1977.

15. Gardner, H.L., and Dukes, C.D.: *Haemophilus vaginalis* vaginitis, Am. J. Obstet. Gynecol. **69**:962-976, 1955.

16. Gonorrhea: United States, Morbid. Mortal. Weekly Rep. **28**:533-534, 1979.

17. Gordon, F.B., Dressler, H.R., and Quan, A.L.: Relative sensitivity of cell culture and yolk sac for detection of TRIC infection, Am. J. Ophthalmol. **63**(Suppl.):1044-1048, 1967.

18. Gordon, F.B., Harper, I.A., Quan, A.L., Treharne, J.D., Dwyer, R. St. C., and Garland, J.A.: Detection of *Chlamydia (Bedsonia)* in certain infections of man. I. Laboratory procedures: comparison of yolk sac and cell culture for detection and isolation, J. Infect. Dis. **120**:451-462, 1969.

19. Gordon, F.B., and Quan, A.L.: Isolation of the trachoma agent in cell culture, Proc. Soc. Exp. Biol. Med. **118**:354-359, 1965.

20. Granato, P.A., Paepke, J.L., and Weiner, L.B.: Comparison of modified New York City medium with Martin-Lewis medium for recovery of *Neisseria gonorrhoeae* from clinical specimens, J. Clin. Microbiol. **12**:748-752, 1980.

21. Gray, M.L., and Killinger, A.H.: *Listeria monocytogenes* and listeric infections, Bacteriol. Rev. **30**:309-382, 1966.

22. Greenwood, J.R., and Pickett, M.J.: Transfer of *Haemophilus vaginalis* (Gardner and Dukes) to a new genus, *Gardnerella: G. vaginalis* (Gardner and Dukes) comb. nov. Int. J. System. Bacteriol. **30**:170-178, 1980.

23. Hammond, G.W., Lian, C.J., Wilt, J.C., and Ronald, A.R.: Comparison of specimen collection and laboratory techniques for isolation of *Haemophilus ducreyi*, J. Clin. Microbiol. **7**:39-43, 1978.

24. Handsfield, H.H., Holmes, K.K., Wentworth, B.B., Pedersen, A.H.B., Turck, M., and Alexander, E.R.: Etiology and treatment of nongonococcal urethritis. Abstracts of the Twelfth Interscience Conference on Antimicrobial Agents and Chemotherapy [Abstr. 122], Atlantic City, N.J., September 26-29, 1972.

25. Hickman, R.K., and Lawson, J.W.: Isolation of a stable cell wall–defective form of *Neisseria gonorrhoeae* from a case of untreated gonococcal urethritis, J. Clin. Microbiol. **12**:603-605, 1980.

26. Holmes, K.K., Gutman, L.T., Belding, M.E., and Turck, M.: Recovery of *Neisseria gonorrhoeae* from "sterile" synovial fluid in gonococcal arthritis, N. Engl. J. Med. **284**:318-320, 1971.

27. Hood, M., and Todd, J.M.: *Vibrio fetus:* a cause of human abortion, Am. J. Obstet. Gynecol. **80**:506-511, 1960.

28. Hunter, C.A., Jr., Long, K.R., and Schumacher, R.R.: A study of Doderlein's vaginal bacillus, Ann. N.Y. Acad. Sci. **83**:217-226, 1959.

29. Judson, F. N., and Werness, B. A.: Combining cervical and anal-canal specimens for gonorrhea on a single culture plate, J. Clin. Microbiol. **12**:216-219, 1980.

30. Kellogg, D.S., Jr., Holmes, K.K., and Hill, G.A.: Laboratory diagnosis of gonorrhea, Cumitech 4, Washington, D.C., 1976, American Society for Microbiology.

31. Kelly, C.S., and Gibson, J.L.: Listeriosis as a cause of fetal wastage, Obstet. Gynecol. **40**:91-97, 1972.

32. King, E.O: Human infection with *Vibrio fetus* and a closely related vibrio, J. Infect. Dis. **101**:119-128, 1957.

33. Klaus, B.D., Chandler, J.E., and Dans, P.E.: Gonorrhea detection in posthysterectomy patients, J.A.M.A. **240**:1360-1361, 1978.

34. Kundsin, R.B., and Driscoll, S.G.: Mycoplasmas and human reproductive failure, Surg. Gynecol. Obstet. **131**:89-92, 1970.

35. Kuo, C.-C., Wang, S.-P., Wentworth, B.B., and Grayston, J.T.: Primary isolation of TRIC organisms in HeLa 229 cells treated with DEAE-dextran, J. Infect. Dis. **125**:665-668, 1972.

36. Lewis, J.S., and Wiesner, P.J.: Gonorrhea: current laboratory methods, Lab. Management, September 1980, pp. 33-43.

37. Lue, Y.A., Ellner, P.D., and Ellner, D.A.: Improved recovery of *Neisseria gonorrhoeae* from clinical specimens by selective enrichment and detection by immunologic methods, Sex. Trans. Dis. **7**:165-167, 1980.

38. Martin, J.E., Jr., Armstrong, J.H., and Smith, P.B.: A new system for cultivation of *N. gonorrhoeae*, Appl. Microbiol. **27**:802-805, 1974.

39. Martin, J.E., Jr., Billings, T.E., Hackney, J.F., and Thayer, J.D.: Primary isolation of *N. gonorrhoeae* with a new commercial medium, Public Health Rep. **82**:361-363, 1967.

40. Martin, J.E., and Lester, A.: Transgrow: a medium for transport and growth of *Neisseria gonorrhoeae* and *Neisseria meningitidis*, HSMHA Health Reports **86**:30-33, 1971.

41. McTighe, A.H., Patel, C., Smith, L., Cherry, M., Fisher, B., Helman, M., Jones, A., and Weinberg, L.: Laboratory and clinical aspects of infection with *Neisseria gonorrhoeae*, Lab. Med. **11**:524-532, 1980.

42. Morello, J.A., and Bohnhoff, M.: *Neisseria* and *Branhamella*. In Lennette, E.H., Balows, A., Hausler, W.J., Jr., and Truant, J.P., editors: Manual of clinical microbiology, ed. 3, Washington, D.C., 1980, American Society for Microbiology.

43. Morse, S.A.: Sexually transmitted diseases. In Lennette, E.H., Balows, A., Hausler, W.J., Jr., and Truant, J.P., editors: Manual of clinical microbiology, ed. 3, Washington, D.C, 1980, American Society for Microbiology.

44. Oriel, J.D., Reeve, P., Powis, P., Miller, A., and Nicol, C.S.: Chlamydial infection: isolation of *Chlamydia* from patients with non-specific genital infection, Br. J. Vener. Dis. **48:**429-436, 1972.

45. Payne, S.M., and Finkelstein, R.A.: Imferon agar: improved medium for isolation of pathogenic *Neisseria*, J. Clin. Microbiol. **6:**293-297, 1977.

46. Pheifer, T.A., Forsyth, P.S., Durfee, M.A., Pollock, H.M., and Holmes, K.K.: Nonspecific vaginitis: role of *Haemophilus vaginalis* and treatment with metronidazole, N. Engl. J. Med. **298:**1429-1434, 1978.

47. Prior, R.B., and Spagna, V.A.: Response of several *Limulus* amoebocyte lysates to native endotoxin present in gonococcal and nongonococcal urethral exudates from human males, J. Clin. Microbiol. **13:**167-170, 1981.

48. Riccardi, N.B., and Felman, Y.M.: Laboratory diagnosis in the problem of suspected gonococcal infection, J.A.M.A. **242:**2703-2705, 1979.

49. Rota, T.R., and Nichols, R.L.: Infection of cell cultures by trachoma agent: enhancement by DEAE dextran, J. Infect. Dis. **124:**419-421, 1971.

50. Schachter, J.: Chlamydiae (psittacosis–lymphogranuloma venereum–trachoma group). In Lennette, E.H., Balows, A., Hausler, W.J., Jr., and Truant, J.P., editors: Manual of clinical microbiology, ed. 3, Washington, D.C., 1980, American Society for Microbiology.

51. Shepard, M.C.: Nongonococcal urethritis associated with human strains of "T" mycoplasmas, J.A.M.A. **211:**1335-1340, 1970.

52. Smith, T.F., Weed, L.A., Segura, J.W., Pettersen, G.R., and Washington, J.A., II: Isolation of *Chlamydia* from patients with urethritis, Mayo Clin. Proc. **50:**105-110, 1975.

53. Sng, E.H., Rajan, V.S. and Lim, A.L.: Simplified media for isolating *Neisseria gonorrhoeae*, J. Clin. Microbiol. **5:**387-389, 1977.

54. Sottnek, F.O., Biddle, J.W., Kraus, S.J., Weaver, R.E. and Stewart, J.A.: Isolation and identification of *Haemophilus ducreyi* in a clinical study, J. Clin. Microbiol. **12:**170-174, 1980.

55. Symington, D.A.: An evaluation of New York City transport medium for detection of *N. gonorrhoeae* in clinical specimens, Health Lab. Sci. **12:**69-75, 1975.

56. Symington, D.A.: Improved transport system for *Neisseria gonorrhoeae* in clinical specimens, J. Clin. Microbiol. **2:**498-503, 1975.

57. Svihus, R.H., Lucero, E.M., Mikolajczyk, R.J., and Carter, E.E.: Gonorrhea-like syndrome caused by penicillin-resistant Mimeae, J.A.M.A. **177:**121-124, 1961.

58. Taylor-Robinson, D., and McCormack, W.M.: The genital mycoplasmas, N. Engl. J. Med. **302:**1003-1010, 1063-1067, 1980.

59. Thayer, J.D., and Martin, J.E., Jr.: A selective medium for the cultivation of *N. gonorrhoeae* and *N. meningitidis*, Public Health Rep. **79:**49-57, 1964.

60. Thayer, J.D., and Martin, J.E., Jr.: Improved medium selective for cultivation of *N. gonorrhoeae* and *N. meningitidis*, Public Health Rep. **81:**559-562, 1966.

61. Volk, J., and Kraus, S.J.: Nongonococcal urethritis: a venereal disease as prevalent as epidemic gonorrhea, Arch. Intern. Med. **134:**511-514, 1974.

62. Wentworth, B.B., and Alexander, E.R.: Isolation of *Chlamydia trachomatis* by use of 5-iodo-2-deoxyuridine-treated cells, Appl. Microbiol. **27:**912-916, 1974.

63. Wentworth, B.B., Bonin, P., Holmes, K.K., Gutman, L., Wiesner, P., and Alexander, E.R.: Isolation of viruses, bacteria, and other organisms from venereal disease clinic patients: methodology and problems associated with multiple isolations, Health Lab. Sci. **10:**75-81, 1973.

64. Windall, J.J., Hall, M.M., Washington, J.A., II, Douglass, T.J., and Weed, L.A.: Inhibitory effects of vancomycin on *Neisseria gonorrhoeae* in Thayer-Martin medium, J. Infect. Dis. **142:**775, 1980.

65. Zinnemann, K., and Turner, G.C.: The taxonomic position of *"Haemophilus vaginalis" (Corynebacterium vaginale)*, J. Pathol. Bacteriol. **85:**213-219, 1963.

12 MICROORGANISMS ENCOUNTERED IN CEREBROSPINAL FLUID

Bacteriologic examination of the spinal fluid is an essential step in the diagnosis of any case of suspected meningitis. The specimen must be collected under sterile conditions and transported to the laboratory **without delay.**

Acute bacterial meningitis is an infection of the meninges—the membranes covering the brain and spinal cord—and is caused by a variety of gram-positive and gram-negative microorganisms, predominately *Haemophilus influenzae, Neisseria meningitidis,* and *Streptococcus pneumoniae.* Bacterial meningitis also may be secondary to infections in other parts of the body, and *Salmonella* species, coliform bacilli, staphylococci, or mycobacteria may rarely be recovered; in neonatal meningitis, *Escherichia coli* is the most frequent organism isolated, along with group B beta-hemolytic streptococci, an increasingly important pathogen, and *Listeria monocytogenes* (which may also affect adults).

In bacterial meningitis the CSF is usually **purulent,** with an increased white cell count (generally more than 1,000/cu mm), a predominance of polymorphonuclear cells, and a reduced concentration of spinal fluid glucose. Amebic meningoencephalitis may closely simulate bacterial meningitis (see Chapter 33). On the other hand, in meningitis caused by the tubercle bacillus or by nonbacterial agents, such as viruses or fungi, the fluid is usually nonpurulent, with a low cell count of the mononuclear type and a normal or moderately reduced glucose content. However, in early or partially treated bacterial meningitis the cell count may be low and without a polymorphonuclear response, whereas in early tuberculosis or viral meningitis such cells may predominate.

Since it may be difficult or impossible for the clinician to differentiate the meningitides clinically, rapid and accurate means of identifying the etiologic agents must be available in the laboratory. It is therefore strongly recommended that a complete microbiologic workup, including smear and culture, be carried out on all CSF specimens from patients with suspected meningitis, whether the fluid is clear or cloudy.

In a case of suspected meningitis the fluid is generally submitted for chemical and cytologic examination as well as for culturing. Since the amount of fluid provided is usually small, it is suggested that the specimen be centrifuged at 1,500 g for 15 minutes (except when *Cryptococcus neoformans* is suspected) as soon as it is received. The supernatant fluid is then removed with a sterile Pasteur pipet to another tube for chemical or serologic studies, leaving the sediment and a few drops of fluid for culture procedures. In this way the entire specimen may be concentrated by centrifugation, obviating a need for its division into several different tubes for the other examinations. Membrane filtration may also be used, but it is not as effective when antibiotics are present.[26]

Purulent (cloudy) fluids should be examined **immediately** by a Gram-stained smear (using a **sterile** slide), followed by appropriate culturing procedures. In these acute forms of meningitis the etiologic agent frequently can be demonstrated in stained films of the specimen (Plate 24). In some cases, as in *Haemophilus influenzae* and pneumococcus infections, **the organism can be identified immediately by a capsular swelling (quellung) test with specific antiserum.*** Refer to Chapters 18 and 37 for procedures.

---

*Available from Difco Laboratories, Detroit, as pools and some single types. Antisera prepared by Statens Seruminstitut, Copenhagen, Denmark, are also recommended. Particularly useful is **Omni-serum**, a polyvalent pneumococcus antiserum that gives capsular swelling reactions with 84 types.

The following organisms (in approximate order of frequency) are isolated from CSF:

Haemophilus influenzae, type b (infants and children)
Neisseria meningitidis (meningococcus) (most common in Great Britain)
Streptococcus pneumoniae (pneumococcus)
Listeria monocytogenes
Mycobacterium tuberculosis
Staphylococci and streptococci (including group B streptococci and enterococci)
Cryptococcus neoformans
Viruses, other fungi, and other agents
Coliform bacilli and *Pseudomonas* and *Proteus* species
Leptospira species
Anaerobic bacteria
Acinetobacter calcoaceticus

NONCULTURAL TECHNIQUES FOR DEMONSTRATING MICROORGANISMS IN CEREBROSPINAL FLUID

The Gram stain and quellung reaction have already been mentioned in regard to identifying microorganisms in CSF. Other preparations in common use are the acid-fast stain, the India ink preparation, and the acridine orange stain (Lauer et al.: J. Clin. Microbiol. **14**:201-205, 1981).

The radiometric technique described in Chapter 7 may also be used for CSF (and other body fluids). The *Limulus* amoebocyte lysate endotoxin assay may be extremely valuable for rapidly diagnosing gram-negative bacterial meningitis. The results reported by Jorgensen and Lee[21] are impressive. They studied this test in a series of 305 patients, 75 of whom had acute bacterial meningitis. Positive *Limulus* tests were obtained on initial CSF specimens from 84% of patients with culture-proven bacterial meningitis, including all patients with meningitis caused by gram-negative organisms. The initial Gram stain revealed the presence of organisms in only 68% of the patients. One patient with pneumococcal meningitis had a weakly positive *Limulus* assay, whereas all other patients with gram-pos-

itive organisms, those with aseptic meningitis, and those without meningitis had negative tests. The assay may also be used to follow the persistence of endotoxin in the CSF of certain patients during therapy, particularly patients with *H. influenzae* meningitis. In addition to meningitis involving *H. influenzae* and *N. meningitidis*, their series included patients with meningitis caused by *Escherichia coli*, *Klebsiella pneumoniae*, *Alcaligenes*, *Pseudomonas*, *Flavobacterium*, *Acinetobacter*, and *Citrobacter*. Endotoxin has also been detected with the *Limulus* test in the CSF of three patients with plague meningitis.[6] The *Limulus* endotoxin assay provides results in 60 minutes. Drawbacks of the *Limulus* assay are that it does not inform as to which particular gram-negative organism may be involved and that it does not rule out the possibility of meningitis caused by organisms other than gram-negative bacteria.

CIE has been used to detect the soluble polysaccharide antigens of *N. meningitidis*, *Streptococcus pneumoniae*, *H. influenzae*, group B streptococci, and *E. coli* K1. The importance of using antisera with high titers of precipitating antibodies has been stressed. A survey of a number of studies by Finch and Wilkinson[12] revealed that among 779 CSF specimens from patients with meningococcal, pneumococcal, or *H. influenzae* meningitis, the positivity rates by CIE were 75%, 79%, and 84%, respectively. Some cross-reactions were reported. These authors evaluated 76 reference and commercial antisera by CIE. They found that some of the antisera failed to react with the homologous strains. Furthermore, there were several cross-reactions between genera, as well as within species. Accordingly, it is important to be certain that all materials used in CIE tests are of high quality. Although CIE is certainly a valuable adjunct for identification of organisms causing bacterial meningitis, it must be considered a presumptive test and should not be used to replace the Gram stain and culture techniques. Nephelometry was comparable to CIE in detecting *H. influenzae* antigen in CSF (Caceci et al.: J. Clin. Microbiol. **13:**540-547, 1981).

Webb and associates[38] compared a slide coagglutination test using Phadebact streptococcus reagents with CIE for detection of group B streptococcal antigen in CSF from infants with meningitis. Antigen was detected by the coagglutination technique in 83% of infants and by CIE in 87%. Following institution of antimicrobial therapy, antigen could be detected in 11 of 19 infants with group B streptococcal meningitis by coagglutination testing and in only 7 of 18 by CIE. False-positive reactions were noted by coagglutination in one infant with *Streptococcus bovis* meningitis and in another infant with group B streptococcal bacteremia without meningitis. No false-positive reactions were noted with CIE. The commercial availability and simplicity of the slide coagglutination test indicates that this procedure will be useful for early and rapid diagnosis of group B streptococcal meningitis.

Latex particle agglutination* was more sensitive than CIE for the diagnosis of *H. influenzae* type b meningitis.[37] All 25 spinal fluids studied by the latex particle agglutination technique were positive compared to 20 of 24 with CIE. As noted in Chapter 7, latex particle agglutination is more sensitive, more specific, and less expensive than CIE. The latex slide agglutination test for cryptococcal antigen in the CSF is more sensitive than the India ink preparation for diagnosing cryptococcal meningitis. In screening sera for cryptococcal antigen, it is routine practice to use both undiluted serum and serum diluted 1:4. However, dilution of CSF has not generally been practiced or recommended. Stamm and Polt[32] reported a case of cryptococcal meningitis in which a patient's CSF was strongly reactive and consistently required dilution to demonstrate a positive latex slide agglutination test. For patients with a positive India ink examina-

tion and a negative latex test, the test should be repeated with dilution. In cases in which the physician strongly suspects cryptococcal meningitis and the latex test is negative, a repeat test with dilution should be requested, regardless of the results of the India ink examination. It is not warranted for laboratories to routinely do this on all CSF specimens, as the yield would be very low and therefore the cost would not be justified.

Gas-liquid chromatography appears to offer a great deal in terms of early diagnosis of meningitis, although much of the work is still preliminary, and much more experience is needed with clinical specimens. Gas chromatographic estimation of lactate concentrations in the CSF has proven useful in distinguishing persons with bacterial meningitis from those with aseptic meningitis and from normal persons.[2, 14] It may be particularly helpful in partially treated bacterial meningitis, in which bacteriologic studies may be negative. It may also help in cases of bacterial meningitis without cellular response in the CSF.[14] There is some overlap in values between patients with bacterial meningitis and those with aseptic meningitis. Furthermore, it must be appreciated that certain noninfectious disorders of the central nervous system may lead to elevated lactate levels.[14] This seems to be the case particularly with patients with vascular problems of the central nervous system, and may relate to reduced cerebral blood flow and consequent hypoxia of the brain. Nevertheless, lactate levels, when combined with clinical observations and conventional laboratory data, can improve the reliability of rapid diagnosis of bacterial meningitis. LaForce and colleagues[23] have demonstrated the potential usefulness of gas chromatographic measurements of lipid, carbohydrate, and lipolysaccharide components of bacterial cells for the diagnosis of bacterial meningitis. Their studies involved "chemotyping" studies of agents of bacterial meningitis in vitro, experimental meningitis in the dog, and studies of patients with meningitis. Their work

*LPA reagents are available from Wampole Laboratories, Cranbury, N.J.

indicates that this technique has a potential for specific etiologic diagnosis of meningitis. These studies utilized flame ionization detectors. Brooks and colleagues[4] have utilized electron capture detectors in frequency-pulsed gas chromatography to analyze various acids and amines produced by microorganisms commonly involved in meningitis. No clinical studies utilizing these techniques have been published as yet. Other studies involving some members of this group, however, have utilized frequency-pulsed electron capture gas chromatography to analyze large numbers of spinal fluid samples from patients with tuberculous and other forms of lymphocytic meningitis.[3] They are optimistic about the usefulness of their procedures for rapid diagnosis of this type of meningitis.

Enzyme-linked immunosorbent assays for the detection of antigens of *S. pneumoniae* and *H. influenzae* type b in CSF look promising. The pneumococcal antigen assay was evaluated in a rabbit meningitis model,[17] and the *Haemophilus* antigen assay was studied in five cases of human disease.[39] The tests proved specific and considerably more sensitive than CIE. CIE and the rose bengal test were useful in the rapid diagnosis of *Brucella* meningitis in a small group of persons.[9]

ROUTINE CULTURE FOR COMMONLY ISOLATED PATHOGENS

For the cultivation of *H. influenzae*, meningococci, pneumococci, streptococci and other gram-positive cocci, and also the aerobic and anaerobic gram-negative bacilli from CSF, the following procedures are recommended (keep specimens at **35 C** while awaiting examination):

1. Using a loopful of the fluid or sediment obtained by centrifugation, inoculate the following media: two blood agar plates, a chocolate agar plate, a tube of enriched thioglycollate medium and other anaerobic media, if indicated, and a tube of tryptic soy broth.

2. Make a thin smear for Gram staining, an India ink preparation (if appropriate) (described in Chapter 43) for encapsulated *Cryptococcus neoformans,** and an acid-fast stain.

3. Incubate one blood agar plate in an anaerobic Bio-Bag, the other plates in a candle jar, and the fluid media under ordinary conditions at 35 C. Examine all after overnight incubation (and daily thereafter) for the presence of growth. Make a Gram-stained smear of any growth and subculture it to appropriate solid media after reading the smear. It is important to include antimicrobial sensitivity disks on these plates for obvious reasons.

4. Hold all cultures for 72 to 96 hours (5 to 7 days when antibiotics have been given before culture was obtained) before discarding as negative. Anaerobic cultures should be held at least 7 to 10 days.

5. Identify all organisms isolated by the methods described in subsequent sections on the various genera.

Hypertonic culture media have led to recovery of organisms from spinal fluid that could not otherwise be recovered.[25, 29] This was not necessarily related to prior therapy with cell wall–active antibiotics. One of us (SMF) has had very rapid recovery of conventional bacteria from spinal fluid, as compared with routine culture procedures, using a membrane filter procedure.

In all cases of purulent meningitis an attempt should be made to detect the **primary focus** of infection. For this purpose, three blood cultures should be taken and cultures also should be made from underlying foci of infection, such as draining ears or purulent sinusitis, **before** antibacterial therapy is initiated. Petechial rash is common in meningococcal meningitis; the organism can sometimes be demonstrated by smear and culture of the petechiae.

*Artifacts resembling yeast cells have been observed in the spinal fluid of patients who have had recent myelograms.

HAEMOPHILUS INFLUENZAE MENINGITIS

Haemophilus influenzae type **b** (other types may be involved rarely), is the most frequent cause of acute purulent meningitis in children between the neonatal period and 6 years of age and only rarely the cause in adults (probably because of the acquisition of *H. influenzae* antibodies). The organism enters by way of the respiratory tract, where it produces a nasopharyngitis, sinusitis, or middle ear infection. It may reach the bloodstream from these sites and be carried to the meninges, where it produces the characteristic symptoms of acute meningitis.

When morphologically typical, short, slender gram-negative rods appear in sufficient numbers in the CSF (either uncentrifuged or in the sediment), a direct capsular swelling procedure may be carried out using type **b** rabbit antiserum.*

The *Limulus* lysate test for endotoxin is reliable in spinal fluid and almost always is positive in *H. influenzae* and other gram-negative meningitis.[30] Reagents are available commercially.*

The initial culture procedures outlined in the previous section are satisfactory for the isolation of *H. influenzae;* further cultural details can be found in Chapter 23.

MENINGOCOCCAL MENINGITIS

Neisseria meningitidis is the cause of epidemic bacterial meningitis and is involved in sporadic cases as well. All ages may be involved, but cases are seen more frequently among infants and young children. Epidemics may be a special problem in the military. The three stages of meningococcal infection are the local or nasopharyngeal (of no clinical importance to the individual), the invasive or bacteremic stage, and the meningeal phase.

On spinal fluid Gram stain the organisms appear primarily as intracellular gram-negative, coffee bean–shaped diplococci. Capsular swelling tests* may be done successfully when sufficient organisms are present. A slide agglutination test and the fluorescent antibody procedure are also useful. See Chapters 18 and 38 for further details on these procedures and for additional information on cultivation and identification procedures.

PNEUMOCOCCAL MENINGITIS

Streptococcus pneumoniae is the third most common cause of bacterial meningitis. It is seen most often in infants and elderly persons. In infancy, pneumococcal meningitis is usually secondary to otitis media, mastoiditis, and pneumonia. In older persons, the disease is seen most frequently in alcoholics and may accompany extensive pneumococcal pneumonia. Sickle cell disease and previous skull fractures may also predispose to pneumococcal meningitis.

The quellung reaction, CIE and other direct tests, and cultural and identification procedures are discussed in Chapters 18 and 38.

LISTERIA MONOCYTOGENES AS A CAUSE OF MENINGITIS

In recent years attention has been focused on the role of *Listeria monocytogenes* in acute meningitis and meningoencephalitis in human beings. In a study of more than 420 cases of human listeriosis in the United States, Gray and Killinger[16] found that more than 80% occurred as meningitis or meningoencephalitis in neonates or in adults older than 40 years. Fewer than 7% were perinatal infections, with only an influenzalike illness of the mothers but frequently premature delivery of stillborn or acutely ill infants. The organism is also occasionally recovered from the blood or spinal fluid of debilitated patients, alcoholics, or persons undergoing chemotherapy for tumor or leukemia.[24] It has emerged as a

---

*Difco Laboratories, Detroit.

*A variety of antisera are available from Difco Laboratories, Detroit.

significant opportunist pathogen in the immuno-suppressed host. The organism is probably still too often discarded in the laboratory as a contaminating diphtheroid when isolated from CSF, subdural fluid, blood, or other clinical specimens; a high index of suspicion on the part of the microbiologist is the best aid to its recovery. The reader is referred to Chapter 26 on *Listeria*, where identification procedures may be found.

MYCOBACTERIUM TUBERCULOSIS AS A CAUSE OF MENINGITIS

CSF from patients with tuberculous meningitis contains, at best, only a few recoverable tubercle bacilli. Acid-fast stains of the sediment, therefore, rarely reveal their presence. The chance of recovering the organisms increases in proportion to the volume of spinal fluid submitted for examination. About 10 ml is required for an adequate culture.*

Although cultural procedures are preferred for the recovery of tubercle bacilli from CSF, the clinical significance of finding any acid-fast bacilli by smear is obvious. Because of the urgency to discover an etiologic agent, two methods for demonstrating mycobacteria in stained smears are included:

1. Preparations may be made from the pellicle or coagulum ("fibrin web") that forms in some specimens. This formation takes place when the spinal fluid is allowed to stand undisturbed at room temperature or in a refrigerator overnight. Carefully remove the formed coagulum with a **new** loop (a rough, old wire loop is inadequate, since it balls up the material and makes removal difficult). Crush the coagulum by pressure between an albumin-coated slide and a coverglass. Air dry, flame, and then stain the resulting films by the acid-fast or fluorochrome method.

2. Acid-fast bacilli occasionally can be demonstrated in the sediment obtained by centrifuging the CSF at 3,000 rpm or higher for 15 to 30 minutes. Since this method requires the use of the entire sediment and is not always reliable, it is recommended that the sediment be used instead for inoculation of culture media or guinea pig injection. Techniques for these procedures can be found in Chapter 31 on *Mycobacterium tuberculosis*.

CRYPTOCOCCUS NEOFORMANS AS A CAUSE OF MENINGITIS

Cryptococcus neoformans, a yeastlike fungus, has been responsible for a number of meningeal infections in humans, some of which have been diagnosed erroneously as brain tumors or as tuberculous meningitis. Both debilitated and immunosuppressed hosts and normal hosts may be affected. Budding yeast cells with capsules occur in masses in tissue; the CSF, although generally not grossly purulent, may contain numbers of yeast cells as well as variable numbers of lymphocytes. The organisms may be mistaken for lymphocytes in spinal fluid cell counts, since cryptococci resemble them in size and shape; the correct diagnosis may be overlooked unless cultures are made. The organism is heavily encapsulated, however, and one can identify it readily by mixing a loopful of sediment from the centrifuged spinal fluid with a loopful of India ink on a slide, covering with a thin coverglass, scanning under the high dry objective, and confirming under oil immersion.* Large, clear hyaline **capsules** are typically seen surrounding the yeast forms, some of which show single buds. Since the number of cryptococci in CSF may be of the magnitude of only one cell per 15 to 20 ml of fluid, Utz[35] has recommended

---

*Use of the membrane filter culture procedure increases the likelihood of recovery of tubercle bacilli.

*Some authors believe that centrifugation may injure the fragile cryptococcal cells and recommend inoculating the uncentrifuged specimen directly to appropriate culture slants.

that the **entire specimen** be inoculated directly to a series of culture slants. He has frequently made an etiologic diagnosis only after inoculating 40 to 50 ml of fluid collected during encephalography. As in tuberculous meningitis, use of the membrane filter procedure, with as much spinal fluid as possible, increases the likelihood of recovery of fungi. The test for cryptococcal antigen is an especially important and useful diagnostic tool. Gas chromatography may also be useful.[31] Further identification procedures are found in Chapters 34 and 38.

LEPTOSPIRA AS A CAUSE OF MENINGITIS

Human **leptospirosis** is a disease of protean manifestations, varying from a mild and inapparent infection to a severe and sometimes fatal illness with deep jaundice and profound prostration. It is transmitted by contact, either directly or indirectly, with the urine of animal carriers. The central nervous system may be involved in many cases of severe infection, and leptospirae may be recovered from the spinal fluid. In a report by Heath and co-workers[18] of 483 cases of human leptospirosis in the United States, the central nervous system was the organ system most frequently involved (235 cases, or 68%). Because of the diversity of clinical expressions, however, the authors concluded that many human infections, particularly of a mild type, remain undiagnosed in the United States.

Recovery of the organism (see the description of techniques, Chapters 7 and 24) from the CSF or demonstration of a rise in specific antibody may lead to a definitive diagnosis. All suspected cultures should be confirmed by a leptospirosis reference laboratory, such as the CDC.

MENINGITIS CAUSED BY GRAM-NEGATIVE BACTERIA

Meningeal infections caused by coliform bacilli, species of *Pseudomonas* or *Proteus*, and other gram-negative enteric organisms are not common. In a series of 294 cases of bacterial meningitis studied at the Mayo Clinic[11, 15] only 23 (7.7%) were caused by these facultative gram-negative bacilli. In nine of the 23 cases, *Escherichia coli* was the responsible pathogen, causing death in three of four infected newborn infants (newborn infants appear to have a great susceptibility to this organism); other bacterial agents included *Klebsiella*, *Pseudomonas*, *Proteus*, and *Alcaligenes*. An underlying disease process was present in 21 of the patients; the infection was controlled in only 8 of the 23 patients with meningitis. In adults, gram-negative bacillary meningitis may be seen secondary to gram-negative bacteremia, often arising from the urinary tract.

Acinetobacter and Moraxella

A disease simulating meningococcal meningitis, both clinically and bacteriologically, may be produced by a gram-negative coccobacillus previously known as *Mima polymorpha*,[28] and presently classified as *Acinetobacter calcoaceticus*. This organism appears coccoid on solid media and shows both bacillary and coccal forms in liquid media. It stains gram negative, frequently shows bipolar staining, is nonmotile, and does not reduce nitrates.

Moraxella osloensis, formerly classified as a member of de Bord's Mimeae (*M. polymorpha* var. *oxidans*) is similar in morphology and gram reaction to *Neisseria meningitidis* and is also oxidase positive. It has been incriminated in meningitis[36] and is best characterized by biochemical reactions, as described in Chapter 22.

Flavobacterium species

Flavobacterium species are gram-negative bacilli whose natural habitat is the soil and water. They have also been isolated from a variety of other sources, including hospital sink traps, nursery equipment, and water supplies.

A report by Brody and others[1] recorded two outbreaks of meningitis among newborn infants in hospital nurseries in which a gram-negative bacillus was isolated from the spinal fluid of 17 of the 19 infants; there were 15 deaths. The organism, first described in 1944, was studied by King, who found it to be a thin, nonmotile, gram-negative rod, proteolytic and nitrite negative, producing a small amount of indole (tested with Ehrlich reagent) and fermenting carbohydrates in nutrient broth after some delay. After overnight incubation at 35 C, a lavender-green discoloration is seen on blood agar. Another nursery outbreak was described by Cabrera and Davis,[7] who recorded 14 clinical cases of neonatal meningitis, with 10 deaths. The source of this nosocomial epidemic appeared to be a faulty sink trap in the premature nursery, and the organism isolated was similar to that described by King.

Because the organisms satisfy the requirements for inclusion in the genus *Flavobacterium*, King suggested the name *Flavobacterium meningosepticum* for them. For a more complete biochemical and serologic characterization, the reader is referred to King's paper[22] and to Chapter 22.

Pasteurella multocida

The pleomorphic gram-negative coccobacillus *Pasteurella multocida* has been implicated in central nervous system infections, including meningitis.[20] Because of its appearance in stained films of spinal fluid, it has led to incorrect diagnoses of meningococcal, *Haemophilus influenzae,* or "*M. polymorpha*" types of meningitis. Unlike most of the gram-negative rods, *P. multocida* is **very susceptible to penicillin** in vitro (either by the disk technique or by tube dilution). If such an organism is isolated, if it grows poorly or not at all on EMB agar or Mac-Conkey agar, and if it produces no change in the butt of a triple sugar iron (TSI) or Kligler's iron agar (KIA) slant within 24 hours but does produce an acid reaction throughout the medium in 48 to 72 hours, the presence of *P. multocida* should be considered. This may be confirmed biochemically and serologically by sub-

mitting the culture to a reference laboratory. See Chapter 23 for a further description of the organism.

MENINGITIS CAUSED BY ANAEROBIC BACTERIA

Although meningitis involving anaerobes is not common, it has undoubtedly been overlooked many times. Nonetheless, there are well over 200 cases reported in the literature.[13] Anaerobic meningitis is not uncommonly part of a more extensive intracranial infection; brain abscess or subdural or extradural empyema is frequently associated. By far the most common underlying process is otitis media or mastoiditis, usually chronic. *Fusobacterium* and *Bacteroides* species, including *B. fragilis*, and anaerobic (and microaerophilic) cocci are the most commonly encountered anaerobes, but clostridia (chiefly *C. perfringens*) and *Actinomyces* are recovered as well.

Since a number of other agents that cause meningitis grow at least as well, and sometimes better, under anaerobic conditions as aerobically, it is clearly desirable that all spinal fluid be cultured anaerobically as well as by other techniques. Further details on cultivation and identification of anaerobes are given in Chapters 13 and 27 to 30.

CANDIDA MENINGITIS

Candida albicans is a rare cause of meningitis. It may be seen in relation to neurosurgical procedures or head trauma, in patients with foreign bodies such as a CSF shunt,[33] or as part of a generalized infection in immunosuppressed individuals or patients receiving prolonged antimicrobial therapy.

MENINGITIS CAUSED BY MORE THAN ONE BACTERIUM

In the series previously cited, cultures of the CSF of 40 patients (13.6%) revealed two or more organisms isolated simultaneously or at some time during the course of the illness.[11] In some instances the clinical significance of the additional organism was not readily determined.

In a similar study of 534 infants and children conducted at St. Louis Children's Hospital,[19] 20 patients (3.7%) were found to show two different bacterial species in initial CSF cultures. *H. influenzae*, combined variously with *N. meningitidis*, *S. pneumoniae*, *E. coli*, *S. aureus*, *E. aerogenes*, and other *Enterobacter* species, occurred most frequently; the meningococcus or pneumococcus was also accompanied by other bacterial species. The authors pointed out that those having the responsibility for reading CSF cultures should be aware of the possibility of the occurrence of simultaneous mixed bacterial meningeal infections.

ASEPTIC MENINGITIS

Aseptic or nonbacterial meningitis is a **clinical syndrome** rather than a disease of specific etiology. It is generally associated with a viral agent, although approximately one fourth of the cases may remain undiagnosed.

The disease is characterized by rapid onset, with fever and symptoms referable to the central nervous system. In the majority of patients with viral meningitides, the spinal fluid cell count is increased, with lymphocytes predominating (polymorphonuclear cells may appear at the onset). The protein content is generally elevated, while the spinal fluid glucose level is usually normal, an important diagnostic differential from bacterial meningitis, in which the glucose level is depressed.

Aseptic meningitis may be caused by a variety of viral agents, including coxsackievirus group B (occasionally group A), poliovirus, lymphocytic choriomeningitis and arthropod-borne encephalitis viruses, enteroviruses, mumps virus, and herpesvirus. Leptospirosis may also present as a benign aseptic meningitis. The multiplicity of etiologic agents requires a variety of laboratory examinations available only in a diagnostic virology laboratory. These include virus isolation by animal injection or by inoculation of embryonated eggs or tissue cell cultures from specimens of stool, throat washings, and CSF, as well as complement fixation, neutralization tests, and other tests on acute and convalescent sera. Since the only contribution of the bacteriology laboratory in such cases may be the responsibility for the proper collection and transport of the necessary clinical materials, these techniques are considered more fully in Chapter 33.

Aseptic meningitis may also occur after measles, mumps, vaccinia, chickenpox, and smallpox. It may be caused by a parameningeal focus of infection, including brain abscess, and by toxins, neoplasms, and allergens.[34]

EFFECT OF PRIOR ANTIBACTERIAL THERAPY ON RECOVERY OF BACTERIAL PATHOGENS

In a series of 310 cases of bacterial meningitis, Dalton and Allison[8] reported that approximately one half of the patients had received antibacterial drugs before admission to the hospital. This partial treatment reduced the recovery rate of the etiologic agent by approximately 30%, particularly the isolation of *Neisseria meningitidis*, *Streptococcus pneumoniae*, and a miscellaneous group. Elevated spinal fluid lactic acid levels may be very useful in establishing the diagnosis of bacterial meningitis in this situation, but this does not pinpoint the specific infecting agent.[2]

There was also a reduction in the number of positive spinal fluid smears in the treated group, especially in meningococcal meningitis. Gram-positive organisms also tended to appear gram negative. The authors recommended caution in interpreting smears from these treated cases. False-positive Gram stains of spinal fluid may also be a problem caused by organisms in stains and in tubes used to collect or centrifuge the fluid.[27]

REFERENCES

1. Brody, B.H., Moore, H., and King, E.O.: Meningitis caused by an unclassified gram-negative bacterium in newborn infants, J. Dis. Child. **96**:1-5, 1958.
2. Brook, I., Bricknell, K.S., Overturf, G., and Finegold, S.M.: Measurement of lactic acid in cerebrospinal fluid of patients with central nervous system infection, J. Infect. Dis. **137**:384-390, 1978.
3. Brooks, J.B., Edman, D.C., Alley, C.C., Craven, R.B., and Girgis, N.I.: Frequency-pulsed electron capture gas-liquid chromatography and the tryptophan color test for rapid diagnosis of tuberculous and other forms of lymphocytic meningitis, J. Clin. Microbiol. **12**:208-215, 1980.
4. Brooks, J.B., Kellogg, D.S., Jr., Shepherd, M.E., and Alley, C.C.: Rapid differentiation of the major causative agents of bacterial meningitis by use of frequency-pulsed electron capture gas-liquid chromatography: analysis of acids, J. Clin. Microbiol. **11**:45-51, 1980.
5. Brooks, J.B., Kellogg, D.S., Jr., Shepherd, M.E., and Alley, C.C.: Rapid differentiation of the major causative agents of bacterial meningitis by use of frequency-pulsed electron capture gas-liquid chromatography: analysis of amines, J. Clin. Microbiol. **11**:52-58, 1980.
6. Butler, T., Levin, J., Linh, N.N., Chau, D.M., Adickman, M., and Arnold, K.: *Yersinia pestis* infection in Vietnam. II. Quantitative blood cultures and detection of endotoxin in the cerebrospinal fluid of patients with meningitis, J. Infect. Dis. **133**:493-499, 1976.
7. Cabrera, H.A., and Davis, G.H.: Epidemic meningitis of the newborn caused by flavobacteria, J. Dis. Child. **101**:289-295, 1961.
8. Dalton, H.P., and Allison, M.J.: Modification of laboratory results by partial treatment of bacterial meningitis, Am. J. Clin. Pathol. **49**:410-413, 1968.
9. Diaz, R., Maraví-Poma, E., Delgado, G., and Rivero, A.: Rose Bengal plate agglutination and counterimmunoelectrophoresis tests on spinal fluid in the diagnosis of *Brucella* meningitis, J. Clin. Microbiol. **7**:236-237, 1978.
10. Edwards, P.R., and Ewing, W.H.: Identification of Enterobacteriaceae, ed. 3, Minneapolis, 1972, Burgess Publishing Co.
11. Eigler, J.O.C., Wellman, W.E., Rooke, E.D., Keith, H.M., and Svien, H.J.: Bacterial meningitis. I. General review (294 cases), Proc. Staff Meet. Mayo Clin. **36**:357-365, 1961.
12. Finch, C.A., and Wilkinson, H.W.: Practical considerations in using counterimmunoelectrophoresis to identify the principal causative agents of bacterial meningitis, J. Clin. Microbiol. **10**:519-524, 1979.
13. Finegold, S.M.: Anaerobic bacteria in human disease, 1977, New York, Academic Press, Inc.
14. Gästrin B., Briem, H., and Rombo, L.: Rapid diagnosis of meningitis with use of selected clinical data and gas-liquid chromatographic determination of lactate concentration in cerebrospinal fluid, J. Infect. Dis. **139**:529-533, 1979.
15. Gorman, C.A., Wellman, W.E., and Eigler, J.O.C.: Bacterial meningitis. II. Infections caused by certain gram-negative enteric organisms, Proc. Staff Meet. Mayo Clin. **37**:703-712, 1962.
16. Gray, M.L., and Killinger, A.H.: *Listeria monocytogenes* and listeric infections, Bacteriol. Rev. **30**:309-382, 1966.
17. Harding, S.A., Scheld, W.M., McGowan, M.D., and Sande, M.A.: Enzyme-linked immunosorbent assay for detection of *Streptococcus pneumoniae* antigen, J. Clin. Microbiol. **10**:339-342, 1979.
18. Heath, C.W., Jr., Alexander, J.D., and Galton, M.M.: Leptospirosis in the United States, N. Engl. J. Med. **273**:912-922, 1965.
19. Herweg, J.C., Middlekamp, J.N., and Hartmann, A.F., Sr.: Simultaneous mixed bacterial meningitis in children, J. Pediatr. **63**:76-83, 1963.
20. Hubbert, W.T., and Rosen, M.N.: *Pasteurella multocida* infections. II. *Pasteurella multocida* infection in man unrelated to animal bite, Am. J. Public Health **60**:1109-1116, 1970.
21. Jorgensen, J.H., and Lee, J.C.: Rapid diagnosis of gram-negative bacterial meningitis by the *Limulus* endotoxin assay, J. Clin. Microbiol. **7**:12-17, 1978.
22. King, E.O.: Studies on a group of previously unclassified bacteria associated with meningitis in infants, Am. J. Clin. Pathol. **31**:241-247, 1959.
23. LaForce, F.M., Brice, J.L., and Tornabene, T.G.: Diagnosis of bacterial meningitis by gas-liquid chromatography. II. Analysis of spinal fluid, J. Infect. Dis. **140**:453-464, 1979.
24. Louria, D.B., Blevins, A., and Armstrong, D.: *Listeria* infections, Ann. N.Y. Acad. Sci. **174**:545-551, 1970.
25. Louria, D.B., Kaminski, T., Kapila, R., Tecson, F., and Smith, L.: Study on the usefulness of hypertonic culture media, J. Clin. Microbiol. **4**:208-213, 1976.
26. Murray, P.R., and Hampton, C.M.: Recovery of pathogenic bacteria from cerebrospinal fluid, J. Clin. Microbiol. **12**:554-557, 1980.
27. Musher, D.M., and Schell, R.F.: False-positive gram stains of cerebrospinal fluid, Ann. Intern. Med. **79**: 603-604, 1973.
28. Olaffson, M., Lee, Y.C., and Abernathy, T.J.: *Mima polymorpha* meningitis: report of a case and review of the literature, N. Engl. J. Med. **258**:465-470, 1958.
29. Rosner, R.: Comparison of isotonic and radiometric-hypertonic cultures for the recovery of organisms from cerebrospinal, pleural, and synovial fluids, Am. J. Clin. Pathol. **63**:149-152, 1975.

30. Ross, S., et al.: Limulus lysate test for gram-negative bacterial meningitis, J.A.M.A. **233:**1366-1369, 1975.

31. Schlossberg, D., Brooks, J.B., and Shulman, J.A.: Possibility of diagnosing meningitis by gas chromatography: cryptococcal meningitis, J. Clin. Microbiol. **3:**239-245, 1976.

32. Stamm, A.M., and Polt, S.S.: False-negative cryptococcal antigen test, J.A.M.A. **244:**1359, 1980.

33. Sugarman, B., and Massanari, R.M.: *Candida* meningitis in patients with CSF shunts, Arch. Neurol. **37:**180-181, 1980.

34. Swartz, M.N., and Dodge, P.R.: Bacterial meningitis: a review of selected aspects, N. Engl. J. Med. **272:**898-902, 1965.

35. Utz, J.P.: Recognition and current management of the systemic mycoses, Med. Clin. North Am. **51:**519-527, 1967.

36. Waite, C.L., and Kline, A.H.: *Mima polymorpha* meningitis: report of case and review of the literature, J. Dis. Child. **98:**379-384, 1959.

37. Ward, J.I., Siber, G.R., Scheifele, D.W., and Smith, D.H.: Rapid diagnosis of *Hemophilus influenzae* type b infections by latex particle agglutination and counterimmunoelectrophoresis, J. Pediatr. **93:**37-42, 1978.

38. Webb, B.J., Edwards, M.S., and Baker, C.J.: Comparison of slide coagglutination test and countercurrent immunoelectrophoresis for detection of group B streptococcal antigen in cerebrospinal fluid from infants with meningitis, J. Clin. Microbiol. **11:**263-265, 1980.

39. Wetherall, B.L., Hallsworth, P.G., and McDonald, P.J.: Enzyme-linked immunosorbent assay for detection of *Haemophilus influenzae* type b antigen, J. Clin. Microbiol. **11:**573-580, 1980.

13 MICROORGANISMS ENCOUNTERED IN WOUNDS, ABSCESSES, AND BITE INFECTIONS; ANAEROBIC PROCEDURES

Although the microbial flora of infected wounds frequently is varied, the following **organisms are most frequently isolated from wounds and abscesses:**

> *Staphylococcus aureus*
> *Streptococcus pyogenes*
> Coliform bacilli
> *Bacteroides* species and other anaerobic nonsporing gram-negative and gram-positive rods
> *Proteus* species
> *Pseudomonas* species
> *Clostridium* species
> Anaerobic cocci (*Peptococcus, Peptostreptococcus*), microaerophilic streptocci
> Enterococci

Another group, which might be labeled **organisms rarely isolated from wounds and abscesses,** includes the following:

> *Clostridium tetani* and *C. botulinum*
> *Francisella tularensis* and *Pasteurella multocida*
> *Mycobacterium tuberculosis, M. marinum,* and other mycobacteria
> *Corynebacterium diphtheriae*
> *Bacillus anthracis*
> Systemic fungi (*Sporothrix* and so forth)
> *Erysipelothrix insidiosa*
> *Actinomyces* and *Nocardia* species

Since **anaerobic** microorganisms are the predominant microflora of humans and are constantly present in the intestinal, upper respiratory, and genitourinary tracts, it is not unexpected to find them invading both usual and unusual anatomic sites, giving rise to severe (Plate 39) and often fatal infections.[11] Although anaerobes are commonly involved in wounds and abscesses, it should be kept in mind that anaerobes may participate in all varieties of infections and may involve any organ or tissue of the body (Plate 25). Therefore, it seems that anaerobes deserve more attention than they have been given, and it behooves the microbiologist and technologist to familiarize themselves with the techniques for the isolation and identification of these indigenous bacteria.

Although anaerobic procedures are not more difficult to carry out than those used in aerobic bacteriology, only a strict adherence to basic principles and a degree of patience will ensure successful recovery of these pathogens. These principles include the following*: (1) proper

selection of specimens, (2) proper specimen collection, (3) proper specimen transport, (4) use of fresh culture media, and (5) provisions of proper anaerobic environment.

Proper selection of specimens

Certain bacteriologic clues should prompt the microbiologist to carry out anaerobic culturing of selected clinical material. Some of these specimens include:

1. Pus from any deep wound or soft-tissue abscess, especially if it is associated with a **foul or fetid odor** or contains "sulfur granules"
2. Necrotic tissue or debrided material from suspected gas gangrene or less serious gas-forming or necrotizing infections
3. Material from infections close to a mucous membrane
4. Material from abscesses of the brain, lung, liver, or other organ or from intraabdominal, perirectal, subphrenic, or other sites
5. Aspirated fluids from infections of normally sterile sites, including blood and peritoneal, pleural, synovial, or amniotic fluids
6. Material from an infected human or animal bite

*The reader is referred to several excellent anaerobic laboratory manuals,[9, 18, 36] for a more complete discussion of the subject.

7. Exudates with black discoloration or red fluorescence under ultraviolet light
8. Material that, on Gram stain, shows organisms with unique morphology suggestive of anaerobes
9. Food suspected of causing botulism or food poisoning

Proper specimen collection

Since anaerobic organisms are part of the normal flora of body sites such as the skin, oropharynx, intestinal tract, and genitalia, the following are **not** cultured anaerobically:

1. Swabs from the throat, nose, urethra, vagina, cervix, or rectum
2. Expectorated sputum, bronchoscopic specimens, voided or catheterized urine, feces, and gastric contents

Furthermore, all other specimens should be collected so as to preclude or minimize contamination by normal anaerobic microflora. **Collection by needle aspiration rather than by swab is recommended.** This is particularly appropriate in the following clinical situations:

1. Pus from a closed abscess
2. Pleural fluid (by thoracentesis)
3. Urine (by suprapubic bladder aspiration or nephrostomy tube)
4. Pulmonary secretions (by transtracheal aspiration)
5. Peritoneal fluid
6. Sinus tract material (by insertion of a small-gauge pediatric intravenous type of plastic catheter through a decontaminated area and aspiration with a syringe); biopsy of the underlying lesion is preferable when feasible

All air and gas should be expelled from the syringe and needle (Plate 27) and their contents injected directly into a "gassed-out" sterile tube (described later) (Plate 29). If a swab must be used, a two-tube system has been recommended,[36] one tube containing the swab in oxygen-free CO_2, the other containing a prereduced and anaerobically sterilized (PRAS) transport medi-

um, such as Cary-Blair semisolid medium* (Plate 30). After collection, the swab should be inoculated to appropriate culture media as soon as possible. As noted in Chapter 6, the anaerobic Bio-Bag† is excellent for maintaining an anaerobic environment during transport of swabs, small amounts of fluid in plastic catheters, larger specimens in syringes, and so forth.[36] The growth of microorganisms from heparin-containing material may be suppressed.[28]

Proper specimen transport

As indicated previously, once a clinical specimen has left a body site (where the Eh [oxidation-reduction potential] may be as low as or lower than -250 mV),[18] any anaerobes present must be protected from the toxic effect of atmospheric oxygen until the specimen is properly set up anaerobically. While larger volumes of frankly purulent material require little or no protection, it is wise to **routinely** use optimal transport procedures. For this reason the use of a "gassed-out" collection tube is strongly recommended, since it will provide an anaerobic environment during transport to the laboratory. The outfit consists of a tube with a recessed butyl rubber stopper and screw cap; it is prepared with prereduced nonnutritive medium containing cysteine and resazurin indicator, then flushed out with oxygen-free CO_2 and sterilized by autoclaving (Plate 28). The tube can be prepared by hand with a modified Hungate method or in an anaerobic chamber or glove box. Although expensive, it is available commercially.‡ See Chapter 6 regarding the Bellco anaerobic tube, which is very convenient to use. The specimen is injected through the rubber stopper

---

*Scott Laboratories, Fiskeville, R.I.; Gibco, Madison, Wisc.; Baltimore Biological Laboratory, Cockeysville, Md.;

†Marion Scientific Corp., Kansas City, Mo., Catalog No. 26-02-06.

‡Anaport, Scott Laboratories, Fiskeville, R.I.

by syringe and needle and subsequently is removed in the same way in the laboratory. Specimens in tubes of this type maintain anaerobes viable for periods of at least 24 to 48 hours. If the specimens cannot be set up in culture from such tubes within 2 to 3 hours, tubes should be stored at 15 C.[15] This will maintain viability of even cold-sensitive forms such as *Bacteroides fragilis* without permitting growth of *Escherichia coli*. As noted above and in Chapter 6, specimens can be transported effectively in plastic syringes in the anaerobic Bio-Bag. For short periods of transport (up to 20 minutes), the syringe alone is satisfactory. Tissue can be transported in the anaerobic Bio-Bag. Another commercially available transport system is the Vacutainer Anaerobic Transporter* (Plates 31 and 33), which has a self-contained reducing mechanism to reduce oxygen introduced with the swab. The Anaerobic Culturette† generates its own anaerobic atmosphere and contains a small amount of transport medium to prevent drying.

Use of fresh culture media

For the primary inoculation of specimens for anaerobic culturing, all media should be fresh. Storage of plating media under anaerobic conditions is not necessary, but it does extend the effective life of the medium.[16, 27] Availability of a variety of prereduced anaerobic media‡ makes it feasible for even smaller clinical laboratories to use such media. Although prereduced media are not better than nonreduced fresh media for clinical specimens, prereduced media are better for anaerobic culture than many commercially available media that are not prereduced. If anaerobic storage is to be used for longer than 72 hours, the atmosphere should not contain CO_2.[16] Freshly made media may be stored in folded-over Mylar bags (the plastic bags that Petri dishes come in) in the refrigerator for up to 2 weeks.[27]

Provision of a proper anaerobic environment

Numerous methods have been introduced for providing an anaerobic environment, including the PRAS roll-tube method of Hungate, [19] the anaerobic chamber [33] or glove box,[1] and the anaerobic jar.[4] It appears that the use of the anaerobic jar with a catalyst and hydrogen, nitrogen, and 5% to 10% CO_2 offers the most satisfactory and practical method for achieving an anaerobic environment in the clinical laboratory; this is discussed further in the next section. Other methods, including techniques that depend on displacement of oxygen by inert gases alone, by chemical means, or by cultivation in a vacuum, are not recommended in routine clinical practice.

METHODS OF OBTAINING ANAEROBIOSIS
Anaerobic jar method

The simplest method for the cultivation of anaerobes is the use of the **anaerobic jar,** a tightly sealed container in which the oxygen is completely eliminated by various means, including hydrogen and a catalyst. Many modifications of the McIntosh and Fildes jar have been introduced, including the Brewer,* GasPak,* and Torbal jars.*

Brewer and Torbal jars

The Brewer modification of the Brown jar is no longer being sold, but many are still in use. In it the oxygen is removed by means of an electrically heated platinized catalyst with the electrical connection outside the jar (eliminating the danger of explosion). The reaction chamber within the lid is shielded by a heavy wire mesh screen. Details on the use of the Brewer jar may

---

*Becton-Dickinson and Co., Rutherford, N.J.
†Marion Scientific Corp., Kansas City, Mo.
‡Anaerobe systems, Santa Clara, Calif.

---

*Baltimore Biological Laboratory, Cockeysville, Md.; Torsion Balance Co., Clifton, N.J.; Baird & Tatlock, Ltd., London.

be found elsewhere.[12] The Torbal jar is similar but uses a rubber O ring rather than Plasticine and a catalyst active at room temperature (thus no electrical heating is required).

GasPak and similar jars

The introduction by Brewer and Allgeier[3-5] of the GasPak anaerobic jar* (Plate 33) for both 100- and 150-mm plates, a disposable hydrogen and CO_2-generator envelope,* and a disposable anaerobic indicator* makes possible the simplest and most practical system for the cultivation of anaerobes. The polycarbonate plastic anaerobic jar, used with the disposable hydrogen generator, has no external connections, thereby eliminating the need for vacuum pumps, gas tanks, manometers, etc. It uses a room-temperature catalyst (palladium-coated alumina pellets), which obviates the need for an electrical connection to heat the catalyst.

To use this system the inoculated media are placed in the jar, along with one hydrogen and CO_2-generator envelope with a top corner cut off and a methylene blue anaerobic indicator.*[6] After 10 ml of water is introduced with a pipet into the envelope, the jar cover (containing the catalyst in a screened reaction chamber in the lid) is promptly placed in position and the clamps are applied and **screwed only hand tight** (rubber attachments on the clamp provide release of excessive pressure).

As the anaerobic environment is achieved, condensed water appears as a visible mist or fog on the inner wall of the jar (within 10 to 15 minutes), and the lid over the catalyst chamber becomes warm. If this does not occur within 20 to 40 minutes, either the catalyst needs replacing† or the lid was not secured properly. After overnight incubation, the methylene blue indicator should appear colorless, and the jar will be under a slight positive pressure.

Studies by Seip and Evans[30] (unfortunately carried out at 20 to 25 C) give data on oxygen and CO_2 concentrations, catalyst temperature, time of appearance of water condensate, and Eh of various plated culture media in the system. The oxygen concentration was reduced to less than 0.4% in 100 minutes. The Eh of the media reached -100 mV within 60 to 100 minutes and -200 mV within 6 hours. Anaerobic conditions were achieved well before the methylene blue anaerobic indicator became decolorized (longer than 6 hours at 20 to 25 C).

Oxoid has a new anaerobic jar that incorporates a pressure gauge and uses a low-temperature catalyst in a foil matrix. The Almore jar comes with or without a pressure gauge (for use with the evacuation-replacement method of obtaining anaerobiosis) and has a metal lid and certain other interesting features.

It should be pointed out that the disposable hydrogen generator may also be used in the Torbal jar or Brewer jar (see the manufacturer's directions for such use).

Since hydrogen is an **explosive** gas, every precaution must be taken to prevent a laboratory accident when using it:

1. Any open flame in the vicinity must be extinguished.
2. All jars must be inspected for cracks and discarded if they are faulty.
3. The metal screen inside a Brewer jar lid must be intact.
4. A wooden or metal safety shield should be used whenever the catalyst is activated electrically.

---

*Baltimore Biological Laboratory, Cockeysville, Md.

†This should be done **after each use**, since excess moisture and hydrogen sulfide (from H_2S-producing organisms) will inactivate the catalyst. The catalyst may be reactivated by being heated in a 160 C drying oven for 2 hours and subsequently stored in an airtight container with desiccant, such as a discarded antibiotic disc cartridge container.[18] It is convenient to have extra baskets of catalyst for this purpose. These catalysts may be regenerated repeatedly over extended periods of time. Baltimore Biological Laboratory now offers GasPak II, in which the palladium catalyst is included in the disposable hydrogen and CO_2-generator envelope.

Other methods

Other anaerobic methods mentioned previously include the use of PRAS culture media and roll tubes, introduced by Hungate,[19] with modifications by Holdeman and associates,[18] and the anaerobic glove box[1] or chamber.[33]

In the Hungate technique, a closed tube of PRAS medium is inoculated through the rubber stopper by needle and syringe*; in the VPI technique, an open tube of PRAS medium is inoculated in the presence of a continuous stream of oxygen-free gas introduced by a flame-sterilized cannula inserted in the tube.

The anaerobic chamber techniques utilize a plastic glove box or rigid chamber (Plate 36) with attached and sealed gloves, which are used to manipulate the material inside this work area.[20] The chamber is kept continuously anaerobic by a catalyst and hydrogen gas, and material is passed in and out through an interchange, a rigid appurtenance attached by a gastight seal to the chamber. A unique type of chamber is now available commercially.† This chamber permits the use of bare hands within the chamber for better dexterity and comfort and has an adaptor for GasPak jars that permits easy transfer of material between a GasPak jar and the chamber or vice versa.

Several authors[21, 27] have compared the three anaerobic systems—GasPak, glove box, and roll tube—for their effectiveness in the isolation of anaerobic organisms from clinical material and have concluded that recovery of anaerobes is comparable in all three systems and that the GasPak method was as effective as the other more complex methods. The interested reader is referred to the papers cited for further details.

INDICATORS OF ANAEROBIOSIS

The use of an **indicator** of Eh is essential in anaerobic culturing. Among those available, the original Fildes and McIntosh methylene blue indicator is recommended (see Chapter 44 for preparation). The indicator is freshly prepared each time by mixing equal parts of solutions of methylene blue, glucose, and sodium hydroxide in a test tube and boiling until colorless (the methylene blue is reduced to its leuco base). This tube is immediately placed in the previously loaded jar, and the jar is then sealed and charged by the methods described. If anaerobic conditions are secured and maintained throughout the incubation period, the indicator solution will be **colorless.** Should the indicator turn blue, anaerobiosis is not achieved or maintained. A disposable indicator also may be used; it is available commercially‡ in a sealed envelope, which is opened and prepared at the time of use.

Smith[32] recommends the inclusion of a culture of a strict and fastidious anaerobe, such as *Clostridium haemolyticum* or *C. novyi* type b, as a monitor for the adequacy of anaerobic media and methods; if isolated colonies of these organisms are obtained by the procedures used, the techniques are satisfactory for all known anaerobic pathogens.

INOCULATION OF CULTURES

A variety of liquid and solid culture media, including various selective media, are available for primary inoculation of clinical specimens, and many are available commercially.§ A monograph on media for use with anaerobic bacteria is available from the CDC.[10] Murray[25] has presented a detailed study of the growth of anaerobic bacteria on various agar media stored under

---

*A closed system (PRAS II) is available commercially from Scott Laboratories, Fiskeville, R.I. It has a number of unique features.
†Capco, Sunnyvale, Calif.
‡GasPak disposable anaerobic indicator, Baltimore Biological Laboratory, Cockeysville, Md.

§Scott Laboratories, Fiskeville, R.I.; Gibco, Madison, Wisc.; Anaerobe Systems, Santa Clara, Calif.; Nolan Biological Labs, Tucker, Ga.; Carr-Scarborough Microbiologicals Inc., Stone Mountain, Ga. There are also commercially available prereduced plates (Anaerobe Systems, Santa Clara, Calif.)

different conditions, with or without supplements and with or without reduction. The growth of various anaerobes on different blood agar media was variable and a function of both the species tested and the composition of the medium. No single medium was clearly superior for the growth of all anaerobes. The effect of supplementing media with reducing agents and reduction of the media before inoculation was influenced not only by the composition and length of storage of the media but also by the nature of the specific organisms tested. In general, supplementation and reduction seem to be unnecessary and undesirable. A study of different isolation media was carried out by Sondag and co-workers.[34] The three media utilized were Schaedler blood agar as the nonselective medium and colistin–nalidixic acid blood agar and kanamycin-vancomycin-laked blood agar as selective media. Only 77% of the isolates were detected on the nonselective medium, because many anaerobes were overgrown by facultative bacteria such as *Proteus mirabilis*. Most *Bacteroides* were recovered on the kanamycin-vancomycin-laked medium. The colistin–nalidixic acid medium was less satisfactory. The combination of the nonselective medium and the kanamycin-vancomycin-laked medium increased the total detection of anaerobes to 94%. Nineteen percent of the anaerobes were detected after 1 day of incubation and 70% after 2 days of incubation. The remainder were detected between 3 and 7 days of incubation. Livingston and colleagues[23] have described an excellent medium for selection and presumptive identification of the *B. fragilis* group. Treatment of mixed cultures with 50% ethanol for 1 hour proved to be an effective technique for selective isolation of sporeforming bacteria.[22] This procedure resulted in better recovery of *Clostridium* than did heat treatment.

The following media are inoculated as **soon as possible** after collection (methods have been described previously):

1. Swabs (or aspirated material from a syringe or a gassed-out tube) are used to inoculate the following **fresh** solid media*:

    1 trypticase soy blood agar plate (BA)
    1 brucella blood agar plate with vitamin K_1 (10 μg/ml) and hemin (5 μg/ml) (BRBA)
    1 kanamycin-vancomycin-laked blood agar plate (KVLBA) with added vitamin K_1 and hemin[39]
    1 *Bacteroides* bile-esculin agar (BBE)
    1 phenylethanol blood agar (PEA) (optional)

    A direct smear for Gram stain is also prepared (see following section). The plates are streaked, to secure isolated colonies, with a platinum-iridium loop (**not** nichrome, which oxidizes the inoculum).

2. The swab is then placed directly into one or two tubes of enriched thioglycollate medium† (THIO) and gently rotated (avoiding agitation). Optional: freshly boiled and cooled chopped meat–glucose medium (CMG).*

3. If fluid material is submitted, it is inoculated with a capillary pipet; one or more drops are deposited on each of the plates, and several drops are introduced to the bottom of a tube of enriched thioglycollate medium, with as little agitation as possible.

4. If tissue is received, it is promptly transferred to a sterile tissue grinder and ground with sterile alundum or sand and thioglycollate, avoiding aeration (ideally in an anaerobic chamber or under flowing oxygen-free gas). The resulting homogenate is inoculated as a fluid specimen (step 3).

5. If clostridia are suspected, an egg yolk agar plate (EYA)* is also inoculated. One of the

---

*Preparation of these media is described in Chapter 42.
†Freshly prepared, or boiled (10 minutes) and cooled, after which add vitamin K_1 (0.1 μg/ml), sodium bicarbonate (1 mg/ml), and hemin (5 μg/ml). Rabbit or horse serum (10%) or Fildes enrichment (5%) may also be added.[36]

two tubes of THIO may be treated with ethanol[22] or heated and then subcultured onto another EYA. Optional: Nagler egg yolk agar antitoxin plate.* If *Actinomyces* is anticipated, use a brain-heart infusion agar plate also.

In the event of a seriously ill patient, one may set up **duplicate** KVLBA, BBE, and Nagler plates and incubate for 12 to 24 hours (or until growth is visible through the plastic bag) in an anaerobic Bio-Bag (Plate 35). The GasPak jar should not be opened before 48 hours.

EXAMINATION OF DIRECT FILMS

It is important to prepare and examine a Gram-stained film of the original specimen **after** inoculating the media (**before** if the slide has been flame sterilized); usually sufficient residual material remains on the swab. When enough material is present, or if two swabs are submitted, it is desirable to prepare a Gram stain **before** inoculating the media. Examination of this smear may suggest the desirability of including certain selective or other media that would not be used routinely.

The type and approximate number of organisms present are noted, as well as the presence, shape, and location of spores (? clostridia), branching gram-positive elements (? *Actinomyces*), gram-positive cocci in pairs or chains (? staphylococci, streptococci, anaerobic cocci), and gram-negative rods with round or pointed ends (? coliforms, fusobacteria). Pleomorphism and irregularity of staining are also seen with anaerobes. One must be alert to the possibility of false-positive Gram stain smears resulting from the presence of nonviable organisms in commercial culture collection devices or transport media.[17] Acridine orange stains may be easier to read than Gram stains with bloody fluids or thick exudates (Lauer et al.: J. Clin. Microbiol. **14**:201-205, 1981).

---

*Preparation of these media is described in Chapter 42.

A **preliminary report** of these findings should be submitted to the attending physician without delay, since this may aid in the selection of appropriate antimicrobial agents. It also serves as an important quality control feature for the laboratory.

INCUBATION OF CULTURES

Incubate all inoculated media at 35 C in the following manner (based on one culture):

1. The BA plate in a candle jar (approximately 3% CO_2), and the THIO* in air.† These are to be used for routine "aerobic" culture. EMB or MacConkey plates should also be used.

2. The KVLBA, BRBA, BBE, PEA (and EYA or Nagler, if used) plates in a GasPak jar with hydrogen and CO_2 generator, anaerobic indicator, and a paper towel in the bottom of the jar to absorb excess moisture formed during incubation.‡

3. The CO_2 and "aerobic" BA and the EMB or MacConkey plates are examined after overnight incubation, then subcultured; isolates are identified, and antibiotic susceptibility tests are set up, as required by aerobic culture methods delineated in subsequent chapters.

4. The THIO (or CMG) tube is examined after 48 hours. If Gram stain fails to show organisms that seem different from those recovered on solid media, the THIO is discarded. Otherwise, it is subcultured to a BRBA (and any other media that seem indicated) for anaerobic incubation.

---

*This is useful as a "backup" tube and may be examined, when turbid, only when there is no growth on the primary plate (step 2) or there has been failure of anaerobiosis after incubation.

†Some people prefer to incubate the THIO, with loosened cap, in an anaerobic jar.

‡Note that a fresh charge of reactivated catalyst should be used each time a jar is loaded.

5. All of the anaerobic plates are incubated initially for a **minimum of 48 hours** (slow-growing organisms may require up to 7 days); if the jar is opened sooner than 48 hours, some fastidious strains may cease to grow, even if they are reincubated anaerobically.

EXAMINATION OF CULTURES

After appropriate incubation, remove the KVLBA, BRBA, BBE, and PEA (and EYA, if used) plates from the GasPak jar, emptying only one anaerobic jar at a time to avoid undue exposure to air. Examine the growth on each plate, using a hand lens or dissecting microscope. Describe and record on a work sheet the colony types observed; all colony types present on the anaerobic plates are handled as described below:

1. Each different colony type is picked and inoculated to the following:

   A purity BRBA, to be incubated anaerobically
   A one-fourth sector of a chocolate agar plate, to be incubated under CO_2
   A one-fourth sector of BRBA incubated aerobically
   A tube of enriched thioglycollate medium

   The inoculum area of the purity blood plate should be streaked back and forth several times to ensure an even distribution of inoculum, and then it should be streaked for isolation. The following antibiotic disks are placed in the primary area of inoculation: kanamycin (1,000 μg), colistin (10 μg), and vancomycin (5 μg).* Note that with the exception of colistin, the drug concentrations of the disks used in this preliminary grouping are not the same as those used in the Kirby-Bauer susceptibility test and in no way imply susceptibility of an organism for antibiotic therapy. In the area of secondary streaking, one may place a sodium polyanethol sulfonate (SPS) disk for rapid identification of *Peptostrep-*

tococcus anaerobius. A nitrate disk is placed in this area for subsequent determination of nitrate reduction. In all, then, five disks are placed in the area of heaviest inoculum.

The anaerobic BRBA plates, the CO_2 plates, and THIO are incubated for 48 hours, the aerobic plates for 18 to 24 hours. While the above mentioned subculture procedures are being completed, a number of these inoculated plates can be safely held at room temperature in a glass jar under a continuous stream of CO_2 until they are set up anaerobically. The loose-fitting jar top is fabricated of ½-inch-thick Plexiglas and contains a small drill hole to permit escape of the CO_2, which is introduced to the bottom of the jar at a flow rate producing a steady stream of bubbles through a water bottle* (Plate 34). A double-vented jar is also available commercially.†

2. The primary KVLBA and BRBA plates are also examined under ultraviolet light‡ for the presence of colonies of the *Bacteroides melaninogenicus* group, which characteristically exhibit a **brick-red fluorescence** (Plate 107). Growth on KVLBA is presumptive evidence that the organism is a member of the genus *Bacteroides*. Biochemical and other tests for definitive identification are described in Chapter 27.

3. After overnight and 48-hour incubation, respectively, the aerobic plate and the CO_2 plate are examined; if growth occurs, the subculture was probably not an anaerobe.§ If the organism has not previously

---

*Baltimore Biological Laboratory, Cockeysville, Md.

*Procedure adopted from Martin.[24]
†Baltimore Biological Laboratory, Cockeysville, Md.
‡"Blak-Ray" ultraviolet lamp and viewbox, model UVL 56, from Ultra-Violet Products, San Gabriel, Calif.
§Some species of *Clostridium* and occasional other anaerobes are aerotolerant.

been picked up on aerobic plates, it is processed for identification.

4. After 48 hours' incubation, the anaerobic subcultures are examined for growth, hemolysis (Plate 127), pigmentation (Plate 106), pitting of agar (Plate 110), and colonial morphology. If a **pure culture** of an anaerobe is present, a Gram stain (and a repeat THIO subculture if insufficient growth has occurred in THIO [step 1]) is made, examined, and recorded on the work sheet. A rapid method for distinguishing between gram-positive and gram-negative anaerobes based on the disruption of gram-negative cell walls by dilute alkali has been described (Halebian et al.: J. Clin. Microbiol. **13:**444-448, 1981). The special identification disks are read. With the three antibiotic disks, a zone of 10 mm or less is considered resistant, although this cutoff point is not always absolute. *P. anaerobius* will show a zone of 12 to 18 mm around the SPS disk (Plate 124). Most other gram-positive cocci are resistant. Other anaerobes, such as some *Actinomyces* and *Bacteroides*, may also be susceptible to SPS, but this is not a consistent reaction and is not useful for identification. The nitrate disk is removed from the surface of the plate and placed into a clean Petri dish. One drop each of reagents A and B are added. Development of a pink to red color indicates nitrate has been reduced to nitrite. If no color develops in a few minutes, add a small amount of zinc dust and wait 5 minutes. Development of a red color indicates that nitrate was not reduced. If no color develops, nitrate was reduced beyond nitrite (positive test). Motility can be checked in a sealed hanging drop slide from a 4- to 6-hour culture in THIO.

5. The growth in pure culture of the THIO is also Gram stained, examined, and the results noted, with particular attention paid to Gram reaction, cellular morphology, and arrangement of cells.

6. The EYA plate is examined for the presence of lecithinase activity (Plate 128), which is indicated by the formation of an **opaque zone** in the medium around the growth, and for lipase activity (Plate 137), which is indicated by an "oil-on-water" **sheen** on the surface of colonies. This plate can also be used for the detection of catalase by exposing it to air for 30 minutes and then dropping 3% hydrogen peroxide on the colony.[36] If subcultures are required, they should be made before exposing the plate to air. The Nagler reaction is discussed in Chapter 29.

7. Perform the spot indole reaction[35] by smearing a loopful of the growth from the purity blood agar plate on a filter paper saturated with 1% para-dimethylaminocinnamaldehyde in 10% hydrochloric acid.* A blue color indicates a **positive** reaction; no change or a yellow color indicates a **negative** reaction (check with tube test) (Plate 121).

8. Determine the effect of bile (thioglycollate BBL-135C + 2% dehydrated oxgall + 0.1% sodium deoxycholate) by inoculating the above plus a tube of thioglycolate **without** bile and deoxycholate and by observing inhibition or stimulation of the growth.

From the results of the above observations, the group to which the isolate belongs is determined (Tables 13-1 and 13-2), and further tests are then carried out for definitive identification. These procedures are described in the following sections under specific headings, such as anaerobic cocci, Bacteroidaceae, anaerobic spore formers, and so forth.

When gram-positive rods resembling *Actinomyces* have been seen on the original smear or

---

*Stable up to 9 months when stored in a brown bottle at 4 C.

TABLE 13-1

Group identification of gram-negative anaerobes*

Organism	Cellular morphology	Kanamycin† disc (1,000 µg)	Vancomycin† disc (5 µg)	Colistin disc (10 µg)	Pigment	Fluorescence	Pitting	Lipase	Lecithinase	Indole	Catalase	Nitrate reduction	20% bile (growth)	Esculin hydrolysis	Gelatin liquefaction	Motility	Formate-fumarate stimulation
B. fragilis group	B	R	R	R	−	−	−	−	−	V	+⁻	−	+	+	+	−	
Other saccharolytic *Bacteroides*	B CB	R	Rˢ	V	−	−⁺	−	−	−	−	−	−⁺	−	+⁻	V	−	
B. melaninogenicus-B. asaccharolyticus group	B CB	R	Rˢ	Sᴿ	+	+	−	V‡	−	V	−	−	−	+⁻	+	−	
B. ureolyticus	B	S	R	S	−	−	+⁻	−	−	−	−⁺	+⁻	−	−	−	−	+
F. nucleatum	B	S	R	S	−	+⁻	−	−	−	+	−	−	−	−	−	−	
F. necrophorum	B	S	R	S	−	+⁻	−	+⁻	−	+	−	−	−	−	−	−	
F. mortiferum	B	S	R	S	−	−	−	−	−	−	−	−	+	+	−	−	
F. varium	B	S	R	S	−	−	−	−	−	+⁻	−	−	+	−	−	−	
Other *Fusobacterium* sp.	B	S	R	S	−	−⁺	−	−	−	−⁺	−	−	−	V	V	−	
Veillonella	C	S	R	S	−	−⁺	−	−	−	−	V	+	−	−	−	−	
Other gram-negative cocci	C	S	R	S	−	−	−	−	−	−	−	−	−⁺	−	−	−	

From Sutter, Citron, and Finegold.[36]

−, negative reaction; +, positive reaction for majority of strains, includes weak as well as strong acid production from carbohydrates; V, variable reaction; +⁻, most strains positive, reaction helpful if positive; −⁺, most strains negative, some strains positive; S, susceptible; R, resistant; B, bacillus; CB, coccobacillus; C, coccus.

*See also *Clostridium*.

†Available from Baltimore Biological Laboratories.

‡+Lipase indicates *B. melaninogenicus* ss. *intermedius*.

the clinical picture suggests actinomycosis (Plates 40 and 144 to 148), plates should be checked repeatedly with a dissecting microscope for spiderlike or other colonies suggestive of *Actinomyces* or *Arachnia* (Plate 149).

RAPID PROCESSING FOR ANAEROBES

The unique morphology of certain of the anaerobes, notably the gram-negative bacilli and certain clostridia (Plates 37 and 38), may allow one to make reasonable guesses as to the identity of infecting organisms from a Gram stain. Commercially available fluorescent antibody reagents* are available for the *B. fragilis* and *B. melaninogenicus* groups. The *B. melaninogenicus* group reagent (Fluoretec-M) also reacts with *B. bivius* and *B. disiens* (Weissfeld and Sonnenwirth: J. Clin. Microbiol. **13**:798-800, 1981).

*General Diagnostics, Morris Plains, N.J.

TABLE 13-2

Group identification of gram-positive anaerobes*

Organism	Cellular morphology	Spores	Vancomycin disc† (5 µg)	Colistin disc (10 µg)	Kanamycin disc† (1,000 µg)	SPS	Pigment	Fluorescence	Lipase	Lecithinase	Nagler	Indole	Catalase	Nitrate reduction	Gelatin liquefaction	Motility
Peptococcus sp.	C		S	R	V	R	−+	−	−	−		−+	−+	−+	−+	−
P. asaccharolyticus	C		S	R	V	R	−	−	−	−		+	−+	−	−	−
Peptostreptococcus sp.	C		S	R	V	R	−	−	−	−		−	−	−+	−	−
P. anaerobius	C															
	CB		S	R	V	S	−	−	−	−		−	−	−+	−	−
Propionibacterium sp.	B	−	S	R	S		−+	−	−+	−		V	V	V	V	−
P. acnes	B	−	S	R	S		−+	−	−	−		+−	+−	+−	+	−
Eubacterium sp.	B															
	CB	−	S	R	V		−	−	−+	−+		−+	−+	−+	−+	−+
Actinomyces sp.	B	−	S	R	S		−+	−	−+	−		−	−+	+−	−+	−
Lactobacillus sp.	B	−	S^R	R	S^R		−	−	−	−		−	−+	−+		−
Bifidobacterium sp.	B	−	S	R	S^R		−	−	−	−		−	−	−	−	−
C. perfringens	B	−	S	R	S		−	−	−	+	+	−	−	−+	+·	−
Other Nagler-positive *Clostridium* sp.	B	+	S	R	V		−	−	−	+	+	+	−	−+	+−	V
Nagler-negative *Clostridium* sp.	B	+	S^R	R	V		−	V	V	V	−	V	−	V	V	V

From Sutter, Citron, and Finegold.[36]

−, negative reaction; +, positive reaction for majority of strains, includes weak as well as strong acid production from carbohydrates; V, variable reaction; +−, most strains positive, reaction helpful if positive; −+, most strains negative, some strains positive; S, susceptible; R, resistant; B, bacillus; CB, coccobacillus; C, coccus.

*Many *Clostridium* sp. and some nonsporulating gram-positive rods appear gram negative.

†Available from Baltimore Biological Laboratories.

In the case of seriously ill patients, it is important to examine anaerobic plates before the usual 48-hour period. This may be done by setting up duplicate cultures in two different anaerobic jars so that one set may be examined at 12 to 24 hours. A better alternative, however, is to use the Bio-Bag,* which allows one to examine plates at any time without exposing them to air.

*Marion Laboratories, Inc., Kansas City, Mo.

By utilizing selective or differential media in the Bio-Bag (e.g., a BBE plate for the *B. fragilis* group and an egg yolk agar or Nagler plate for clostridia), one may often be able to make a report of the presumptive presence of *B. fragilis* or *C. perfringens* within 24 hours. The preliminary grouping procedures already referred to are very useful in making preliminary or presumptive identification of anaerobes in order to direct therapy while definitive identification is being carried out. Additional clues are given in the *Wadsworth Anaerobic Bacteriology Manual*.[36] Other simple and rapid methods to help in identification include the L-D Presumpto Plate.[10] This is a four-quadrant plate containing esculin agar, 20% bile agar, egg yolk agar, and basal medium for indole. The basal medium contains hemin, so catalase production can also be determined; it is strongest on the esculin quadrant. H_2S production can also be noted. Two additional L-D Presumpto plates have been introduced recently. These permit testing for DNase, starch hydrolysis, milk digestion, gelatin hydrolysis, and fermentation of glucose, mannitol, lactose, and trehalose. Flow Laboratories has introduced an Anaerobe-Tek plate that permits carrying out the same tests available on the three L-D Presumpto plates. A rapid gelatinase test is described in the *Wadsworth Anaerobic Bacteriology Manual*.[36] A spot test for esculin hydrolysis that can be read in 1 hour has been described (Qadri et al.: J. Clin. Microbiol. **13:**459-462, 1981).

QUANTITATION OF BACTERIAL GROWTH

Formal quantitation of growth is not often done in clinical laboratories. At a minimum, however, laboratories ought to give some indication of the quantitative aspects of growth. This might be based on a 1+ to 4+ system (or simply indicating the number of colonies if there are only a few) to light growth, moderate growth, or heavy growth. This is helpful in determining the significance of isolates and the relative importance of various organisms in mixed infections. Quantitation is thought to be important in terms of burn wound sepsis and for determination of receptiveness of a skin graft bed. Some workers feel that quantitative culture is of value in determining the likelihood of surgical wound infection and therefore the decision as to whether to employ primary or delayed closure of a wound. It is of considerable interest, then, that a prom-

ising new technique for quantitative bacteriologic sampling of moist surfaces has been described recently.[8] This has only been studied in vitro and in an artificially contaminated setting. The technique uses a membrane filter paddle with a 5-μm membrane filter. This procedure permitted recovery of *Staphylococcus aureus* from artificially contaminated bovine muscle surface in counts similar to those obtained by quantitative dilutions of biopsied material and significantly better recovery than that with the use of Rodac plates.

BITE INFECTIONS AND OTHER INFECTIONS INVOLVING ORAL FLORA CONTAMINATION (Plates 26 and 89)

Goldstein and co-workers[14] have described the bacteriology of human and animal bite wounds in 73 patients (39 had animal bites and 34 had human bites or clenched fist injuries). In the infected human bites the predominant aerobic and facultative organisms recovered were alpha-hemolytic streptococci, *S. aureus*, group A beta-hemolytic streptococci and *Eikenella corrodens*, in that order. Anaerobes isolated from infected human bite wounds included (in order) anaerobic cocci and streptococci, the *Bacteroides melaninogenicus* group, *Bacteroides ruminicola* ss. *brevis*, and *Fusobacterium nucleatum*. In the infected animal bite wounds, the most commonly encountered aerobic and facultative bacteria were alpha-hemolytic streptococci, *S. aureus*, *Pasteurella multocida* (Plate 90), and *Enterobacter cloacae*. The predominant anaerobes from these infected animal bites were anaerobic cocci and streptococci, *Fusobacterium* species, and *Bacteroides* species.

Bailie and associates[2] studied the oral and nasal fluids of 50 dogs to determine the prevalence of aerobic organisms frequently associated with animal bite wounds. The pathogenic organisms encountered most commonly were IIj, EF-4, *P. multocida*, and *S. aureus*. They also indicated that one of their isolates (designated as unidentified) appeared identical to DF-2. Another study that employed special appropriate techniques noted that *Simonsiella* could be found in the oral cavities of 66 of 67 dogs.[26] This organism is also found in the oral cavity of humans, cats, and other animals (Kuhn and Gregory: Current Microbiol. **1:**11-14, 1978).

The oral flora of snakes contains a variety of gram-negative bacilli including *Pseudomonas, Klebsiella, Proteus,* and *E. coli* (Goldstein et al.: J. Clin. Microbiol. **13:**954-956, 1981). Clostridia may also be recovered from snakebite wounds.

A fastidious gram-negative bacillus designated as DF-2 by the CDC has been responsible for a number of serious infections, including bacteremia, endocarditis, and meningitis.[7,29] Most of the patients have had underlying diseases that impair host defenses, including splenectomy. Several patients were alcoholics, and others had chronic lung disease. Most of the patients had histories of dog bite. The organism is a gram-negative rod that grows slowly on blood or chocolate agar (it does best with a heart infusion base). Growth is enhanced by cultivation with an increased atmosphere of CO_2, and rabbit serum facilitates growth. The organism is oxidase and catalase positive and is fermentative. Other details on this organism are presented in Chapter 32. Three of the seventeen patients reviewed by Butler and colleagues[7] died. Although the organism is a gram-negative bacillus, it is typically resistant to aminoglycosides and is sensitive to penicillin.

Drug addicts transfer oral secretions to sites of self-injection by moistening straining cotton with their tongues, crushing certain pills in their mouths before mixing with water for injection, or licking the needle prior to injection.[31] It is not surprising, then, that "skin poppers" often develop localized infections involving anaerobes from the oral cavity and that *Eikenella corrodens* may be an important pathogen in infections in these individuals.[31]

REFERENCES

1. Aranki, A., Syed, A., Kenney, E.B., and Freter, R.: Isolation of anaerobic bacteria from human gingiva and mouse cecum by means of a simplified glove box procedure, Appl. Microbiol. **17:**568-576, 1969.
2. Bailie, W.E., Stowe, E.C., and Schmitt, A.M.: Aerobic bacterial flora of oral and nasal fluids of canines with reference to bacteria associated with bites. J. Clin. Microbiol. **7:**223-231, 1978.
3. Brewer, J.H., and Allgeier, D.L.: Disposable hydrogen generator, Science **147:**1033-1034, 1965.
4. Brewer, J.H., and Allgeier, D.L.: Safe self-contained carbon dioxide–hydrogen anaerobic system, Appl. Microbiol. **14:**985-988, 1966.
5. Brewer, J.H., and Allgeier, D.L.: A disposable anaerobic system designed for field and laboratory use, Appl. Microbiol. **16:**848-850, 1968.
6. Brewer, J.H., Allgeier, D.L.: and McLaughlin, C.B.: Improved anaerobic indicator, Appl. Microbiol. **14:**135-136, 1966.
7. Butler, T., Weaver, R.E., Ramani, T.K.V., Uyeda, C.T., Bobo, R.A., Ryu, J.S., and Kohler, R.B.: Unidentified Gram-negative rod infection: a new disease of man, Ann. Intern. Med. **86:**1-5, 1977.
8. Craythorn, J.M., et al.: J. Clin. Microbiol. **12:**250-255, 1980.
9. Dowell, V.R., Jr., and Hawkins, T.M.: Laboratory methods in anaerobic bacteriology, CDC Laboratory manual, DHEW Pub. No. (CDC) 74-8272, Washington, D.C., 1974, U.S. Government Printing Office.
10. Dowell, V.R., Jr., Lombard, G.L., Thompson, F.S., and Armfield, A.Y.: Media for isolation, characterization, and identification of obligately anaerobic bacteria, Atlanta, 1977, Public Health Service, Center for Disease Control.
11. Finegold, S.M.: Anaerobic bacteria in human disease, New York, 1977, Academic Press, Inc.
12. Finegold, S.M.: Gram-negative anaerobic rods: Bacteroidaceae. In Sonnenwirth, A.C., and Jarett, L., editors: Gradwohl's clinical laboratory methods and diagnosis, ed. 8, St. Louis, 1980. The C.V. Mosby Co.
13. Finegold, S.M., Shepherd, W.E., and Spaulding, E.H. (Shepherd, W.E., editor): Practical anaerobic bacteriology, Cumitech 5, Washington, D.C., 1977, American Society for Microbiology.
14. Goldstein, E.J.C., Citron, D.M., Wield, B., Blachman, U., Sutter, V.L., Miller, T.A., and Finegold, S.M.: Bacteriology of human and animal bite wounds, J. Clin. Microbiol. **8:**667-672, 1978.
15. Hagen, J.C., Wood, W.S., and Hashimoto, T.: Effect of temperature on survival of *Bacteroides fragilis* subsp. *fragilis* and *Escherichia coli* in pus, J. Clin. Microbiol. **6:**567-570, 1977.

16. Hanson, C.W., and Martin, W.J.: Evaluation of enrichment, storage, and age of blood agar medium in relation to its ability to support growth of anaerobic bacteria, J. Clin. Microbiol. **4:**394-399, 1976.

17. Hoke, C.H., Jr., Batt, J.M., Mirrett, S., Cox, R.L., and Reller, L.B.: False-positive Gram-stained smears, J.A.M.A. **241:**478-480, 1979.

18. Holdeman, L.V., Cato, E.P., and Moore, W.E.C., editors: Anaerobe laboratory manual, ed. 4, Blacksburg, Va., 1977, Virginia Polytechnic Institute and State University.

19. Hungate, R.E.: A roll tube method for cultivation of strict anaerobes. In Methods in microbiology, vol. 3B, New York, 1969, Academic Press, Inc.

20. Jones, G.L., Whaley, D.N., and Dever, S.M.: Use of the flexible anaerobic glove box, Atlanta, 1977, Public Health Service, Center for Disease Control.

21. Killgore, G.E., Starr, S.E., DelBene, V.E., Whaley, D.N., and Dowell, V.R., Jr.: Comparison of three anaerobic systems for the isolation of anaerobic bacteria from clinical specimens, Am. J. Clin. Pathol. **59:**552-559, 1973.

22. Koransky, J.R., Allen, S.D. and Dowell, V.R., Jr.: Use of ethanol for selective isolation of sporeforming microorganisms. Appl. Environ. Microbiol. **35:**762-765, 1978.

23. Livingston, S.J., Kominos, S.D., and Yee, R.B.: New medium for selection and presumptive identification of the *Bacteroides fragilis* group, J. Clin. Microbiol. **7:**448-453, 1978.

24. Martin, W.J.: Practical method for isolation of anaerobic bacteria in the clinical laboratory, Appl. Microbiol. **22:**1168-1171, 1971.

25. Murray, P.R.: Growth of clinical isolates of anaerobic bacteria on agar media: effects of media composition, storage conditions, and reduction under anaerobic conditions, J. Clin. Microbiol. **8:**708-714, 1978.

26. Nyby, M.D., Gregory, D.A., Kuhn, D.A., and Pangborn, J.: Incidence of *Simonsiella* in the oral cavity of dogs, J. Clin. Microbiol. **6:**87-88, 1977.

27. Rosenblatt, J.E., Fallon, A.M., and Finegold, S.M.: Recovery of anaerobes from clinical specimens, Appl. Microbiol. **25:**77-85, 1973.

28. Rosett, W., and Hodges, G.R.: Antimicrobial activity of heparin, J. Clin. Microbiol. **11:**30-34, 1980.

29. Schlossberg, D.: Septicemia caused by DF-2, J. Clin. Microbiol. **9:**297-298, 1979.

30. Seip, W.F., and Evans, G.L.: Atmospheric analysis and redox potentials of culture media in the GasPak system, J. Clin. Microbiol. **11:**226-233, 1980.

31. Silpa, M., and D'Angelo, J.: *Eikenella corrodens* infections in drug abusers, Ann. Intern. Med. **92:**871, 1980.

32. Smith, L.DS.: The pathogenic anaerobic bacteria, ed. 2, Springfield, Ill., 1975, Charles C Thomas, Publisher.

33. Socransky, S., MacDonald, J.B., and Sawyer, S.: The cultivation of *Treponema microdentium* as surface colonies, Arch. Oral Biol. **1:**171-172, 1959.

34. Sondag, J.E., Ali, M., and Murray, P.R.: Relative recovery of anaerobes on different isolation media, J. Clin. Microbiol. **10:**756-757, 1979.

35. Sutter, V.L., and Carter, W.T.: Evaluation of media and reagents for indole-spot tests in anaerobic bacteriology, Am. J. Clin. Pathol. **58:**335-338, 1972.

36. Sutter, V.L., Citron, D.M., and Finegold, S.M.: Wadsworth anaerobic bacteriology manual, ed. 3, St. Louis, 1980, The C.V. Mosby Co.

37. Sutter, V.L., and Finegold, S.M.: Antibiotic disc susceptibility tests for rapid presumptive identification of gram-negative anaerobic bacilli, Appl. Microbiol. **21:**13-20, 1971.

38. Wideman, P.A., Vargo, V.L., Citronbaum, D., and Finegold, S.M.: Evaluation of the sodium polyanethol sulfonate disc test for the identification of *Peptostreptococcus anaerobius*, J. Clin. Microbiol. **4:**330-333, 1976.

39. Wilkins, T.D., Chalgren, S.L., Jiminez-Ulate, F., Drake, C.R., Jr., and Johnson, J.L.: Inhibition of *Bacteroides fragilis* on blood agar plates and reversal of inhibition by added hemin, J. Clin. Microbiol. **3:**359-363, 1976.

14 MICROORGANISMS ENCOUNTERED IN THE EYE, EAR, MASTOID, PARANASAL SINUSES, TEETH, BONE, AND EFFUSIONS

EYE CULTURES

Because of the constant washing activity of tears and their antibacterial constituents, the number of organisms recovered from cultures of many eye infections may be relatively low. Unless the clinical specimen is obviously purulent, it is recommended that a relatively **large inoculum** and a variety of media be used to ensure recovery of an etiologic agent.

The following organisms are **most frequently isolated** from infections of the eye:

Pathogens or potential pathogens
Staphylococcus aureus
Haemophilus species
Streptococcus pneumoniae
Neisseria gonorrhoeae
Alpha- and beta-hemolytic streptococci
Moraxella lacunata
Acinetobacter calcoaceticus
Coliform bacilli and other enteric bacilli
Pseudomonas aeruginosa
Corynebacterium diphtheriae
Viruses and chlamydiae
Fungi (including saprophytes)
Anaerobes
Mycobacterium
Toxoplasma

Nonpathogens, or opportunists

Corynebacterium xerosis, other diphtheroid bacilli, and *Propionibacterium*

Coagulase-negative staphylococci

Micrococci

If a diagnosis of **purulent conjunctivitis** has been made, the purulent material is collected on a sterile cotton swab or surgical instrument (before the local application of antibiotics, irrigating solutions, or other medications) from the surface of the lower conjunctival sac and inner canthus of the eye. This purulent material should be inoculated immediately to blood agar and chocolate agar plates, which should be incubated in a candle jar, to a blood agar plate for anaerobic incubation, and to a tube of enriched thioglycollate broth. All media should be held for at least 48 hours, and any resulting growth should be identified by the appropriate methods. Acute bacterial conjunctivitis is caused most often by *Streptococcus pneumoniae*, group A beta-hemolytic streptococci, *Haemophilus influenzae*, and *Staphylococcus aureus*.[1] It should be appreciated that *S. aureus* may be cultured from the lid margin in at least one third of subjects with normal lids. In the newborn, the three most common types of conjunctivitis in order of frequency are chlamydial, gonococcal, and staphylococcal conjunctivitis.[1] Gonococcal infection usually begins on the third or fourth day of life, chlamydial infection on the fifth to fourteenth day, and staphylococcal conjunctivitis anytime. Chlamydial infection may be diagnosed by the finding of numerous basophilic inclusion bodies in the cytoplasm in a conjunctival scraping stained by the Giemsa technique. Chlamydia and the gonococcus may also cause conjunctivitis in the adult.

The oxidase test may be carried out on the chocolate agar plate to detect colonies of *Neisseria*. Sabouraud dextrose and brain-heart infusion blood agar slants should be inoculated if a mycotic infection is suspected. Whenever possible, a **Gram-stained smear** of the purulent material should also be examined. The results frequently give sufficient information to the physician to confirm a clinical diagnosis and serve as a guide to proper therapy.

S. aureus, Pseudomonas aeruginosa, S. pneumoniae, anaerobic bacteria, and other organisms may cause a severe and damaging corneal infection. All results should be reported without delay to the physician. Trachoma is rare in the United States.

Since potentially pathogenic organisms may be present in an eye without causing disease, it may be very helpful to the clinician, when only one eye is infected, to culture both eyes. Differences in the bacteriology in the two eyes may be significant.

Scrapings of the conjunctivae for the presence of eosinophils or of ulcerative lesions of the cornea for demonstrating viral inclusion bodies must be taken by an ophthalmologist. These scrapings are transferred to a glass slide, dried, and stained by the Wright-Giemsa method.

Moraxella lacunata (Morax-Axenfeld bacillus) is a short, thick, gram-negative diplobacillus that causes a subacute or chronic catarrhal conjunctivitis, which is particularly severe in the outer angle of the eye. The organism is best cultivated on Loeffler medium, where it causes characteristic pitting and proteolysis of the medium, although nonproteolytic strains are being isolated with some frequency. Identification methods are described in Chapter 22.

Haemophilus aegyptius (Koch-Weeks bacillus) is a small gram-negative bacillus closely resembling *H. influenzae;* it is the causative agent of an acute epidemic conjunctivitis commonly called **pinkeye.** The organism grows well on blood agar or chocolate agar plates. (See Chapter 23 for cultural characteristics.)

Corynebacterium diphtheriae may cause a pseudomembranous conjunctivitis; the organism must be demonstrated by culture and proved toxigenic before a diagnosis of diphtheria can be made. The organism may be readily cultivated on Loeffler or Pai medium. Their identifying characteristics and tests for virulence are described in Chapter 26.

The most devastating type of ocular infection

is bacterial endophthalmitis. This infection most often follows cataract surgery, and *S. aureus* is the most common pathogen.[1] An increasing number of isolations of *Staphylococcus epidermidis* are being reported; whether this represents a true role for this organism in this infection or whether it means that some fastidious organism is being overlooked is uncertain.

Viral and fungal infections are discussed in Chapters 33 and 34, respectively.

The interested reader is referred to an excellent monograph, *Laboratory Diagnosis of Ocular Infections*, by Jones et al. (Washington, editor: Cumitech 13, Washington, D.C., 1981, American Society for Microbiology).

EAR CULTURES

The following organisms are encountered **most frequently** from cultures of the ear:

Pathogens or potential pathogens
Pseudomonas aeruginosa
Staphylococcus aureus
Proteus species
Alpha- and beta-hemolytic streptococci
Streptococcus pneumoniae
Haemophilus influenzae
Coliform and other enteric bacilli
Aspergillus fumigatus, Candida albicans, and other fungi
Bacteroides, Fusobacterium, and anaerobic cocci
Nonpathogens, or opportunists
Coagulase-negative staphylococci and micrococci
Diphtheroids
Bacillus species
Saprophytic fungi

The following organisms are **rare or uncommon** pathogens in such cultures:

Corynebacterium diphtheriae
Actinomyces species
Mycobacterium tuberculosis and other mycobacteria
Mycoplasma pneumoniae

Material from the ear, especially that obtained after perforation of the eardrum, is best collected by an otolaryngologist, using sterile equipment and a sterile cotton or polyester swab. Discharges from the ear in **chronic** otitis media usually reveal the presence of pseudomonads and *Proteus* species, but often the major pathogens in chronic otitis media are anaerobes and enteric bacilli.[6] **Acute** or **subacute** otitis usually yields pyogenic cocci *(S. pneumoniae, S. pyogenes, Branhamella catarrhalis)* and *H. influenzae*.

The presence of pneumococcal antigen in middle ear exudates during acute otitis media was studied by latex agglutination, CIE and radioimmunoassay (RIA).[13]

Latex agglutination gave a positive result in 63% and CIE in 76% of samples that cultured *S. pneumoniae*. Using both methods led to detection of antigen in 88% of these samples. In addition, pneumococcal antigen was detected in 15% of samples that grew other pathogens aside from *S. pneumoniae* and in one third of samples in which no pathogenic organisms were recovered. Similar studies should certainly be done to detect antigens of *H. influenzae*. As noted in Chapter 12, *H. influenzae* antigen may also be detected by nephelometry.

Schwartz and associates[17] compared results of cultures of middle ear exudate obtained by tympanocentesis with simultaneous semiquantitative culture of the nasopharynx in 225 children with suppurative otitis media. A 72% prediction rate for middle ear pathogens was obtained from the nasopharyngeal cultures, provided two essentials were observed: (1) the nasopharyngeal culture had to be plated immediately on appropriate solid media, and (2) a semiquantitative method for counting of organisms had to be employed in reading the plates. The technique was most valuable when 25% to 50% or more of the total number of colonies on plates represented a single pathogenic species.

In external otitis the external ear should be cleansed with a 1:1,000 aqueous solution of benzalkonium chloride or other detergent to free the skin of contaminating bacterial flora before a culture is taken, if the results are to be of clinical significance. Otherwise, a variety of nonpathogenic bacteria and saprophytic fungi will be recovered. *P. aeruginosa* and *S. pyogenes* are commonly isolated. Specimens are cultured as described in the preceding section, with the addition of phenylethanol blood agar, to recover other organisms in the presence of spreading *Proteus* species.

MASTOID AND PARANASAL SINUS CULTURES

The widespread use of antimicrobial agents in the treatment of acute infections of the middle ear (otitis media) has resulted in a significant decrease in the incidence of acute mastoiditis, an infection of the mastoid process and surrounding structure. The offending organisms, usually originating from a suppurative otitis, generally are pyogenic cocci (*S. pneumoniae*, *S. aureus*, and group A streptococci).[7] Chronic mastoiditis, like chronic otitis media, commonly involves anaerobic bacteria.[6]

Cultures from the mastoid region are generally taken on a cotton or polyester swab (before antibiotic therapy) and are handled in the laboratory as any other wound culture would be.

Acute suppurative sinusitis may follow a common cold or occur after water is forced into the nose while swimming or diving. The most frequent isolates in this infection include the streptococci, staphylococci, and pneumococci; *Klebsiella*, *Bacteroides*, and *H. influenzae* are occasionally isolated and may give rise to serious complications. In chronic purulent sinusitis, anaerobes again play a more prominent role.[6] The aerobic and anaerobic methods previously described for wound cultures (Chapter 13) are generally satisfactory.

CULTURES OF TEETH AND TOOTH STRUCTURES

The bacterial flora of the normal mouth is made up of a wide variety of microorganisms, including streptococci, filamentous gram-negative and gram-positive anaerobic rods, neisse-

riae, anaerobic cocci, spirochetes, and lactobacilli.[6] The role of anaerobes in Vincent's infection is discussed in Chapter 8.

Effective methods and culture media are available for the bacteriologic examination of root canals, tooth sockets, periapical abscesses, and other dentoalveolar infections.[9,15] Various anaerobes, as well as streptococci, are the predominant pathogens in these infections.[4,6] Specimens are obtained by the dental surgeon, using a rigidly aseptic technique and sterile equipment. The apex of an extracted tooth is cut off with a pair of cutting forceps, and the apical fragment is transferred directly to a tube of enriched medium, such as brucella broth or enriched thioglycollate medium* (penicillinase is added if penicillin has been used). The medium is held at 35 C for several days and observed for growth. Any indication of growth (increase in turbidity) is confirmed by examining a Gram-stained smear, which also serves to guide in the selection of appropriate aerobic and anaerobic media to be used in subculturing. Cultures from sockets or abscesses, obtained either with a sterile curet or cotton applicator, are handled as wound cultures would be.

In culturing root canals, the following method[15] is recommended, using strict asepsis throughout. After a sterile field is established, the seal and previous dressing are removed and discarded. The canal is cleansed of any residual medicament by flushing with about 1 ml of sterile water and is dried by inserting a fresh absorbent point with a wiping motion, then removing and discarding it. Another fresh sterile point is then inserted into the apex and allowed to remain in place for about 1 to 2 minutes, then removed. If the tip appears to be moist with exudate or blood, it is dropped into a tube of culture medium as previously indicated. If the point appears to be dry on removal, it is discarded and

---

*Difco Laboratories, Detroit; Baltimore Biological Laboratory, Cockeysville, Md.; Gibco Laboratories, Madison, Wisc.; Scott Laboratories, Fiskeville, R.I.

a fresh point, aseptically moistened with the culture medium, is inserted into the root canal, left for several minutes, and cultured as before. After 48 hours' incubation at 35 C, the culture tube is examined for the presence of growth, which is evidenced by any increase in turbidity, especially around the tip or surface of the absorbent point. Generally, negative cultures are kept for 1 week, and two consecutive negative cultures are obtained before the root canal is filled.

INFECTION OF BONE

Acute blood-borne osteomyelitis in children involves *S. aureus* in the majority of cases.[18] Blood cultures are positive in about 50% of these cases if they are untreated. In the remainder of the cases direct bone aspiration or surgical biopsy should be strongly considered to establish a specific etiologic diagnosis. Group B streptococci are relatively frequent pathogens in the neonatal period.[18] In chronic osteomyelitis in adults, *S. aureus* is still a major pathogen, but various gram-negative rods in the family Enterobacteriaceae and *Pseudomonas* are important pathogens, along with anaerobes in a percentage of cases. Culture of the sinus tract may not be helpful or may even be misleading. In a comparison of sinus tract cultures and cultures of operative specimens, it was found that when *S. aureus* was present in the sinus tract, it was usually present in the operative specimen as well.[14]. However, fewer than half of the sinus tract cultures obtained from patients with *S. aureus* osteomyelitis contained this organism. Isolation of gram-negative rods from sinus tracts did not correlate well with pathogens isolated from bone.

Osteomyelitis in drug addicts often involves *Pseudomonas* but may involve other gram-negative bacilli, *S. aureus,* and *Candida*. Most of these infections with *Pseudomonas* involve the vertebral column; the next most common site is the pelvic bones. Patients with sickle cell disease or other hemoglobinopathies often have *Salmonella* osteomyelitis. Patients who have impaired host defense mechanisms or who are receiving prolonged intravenous therapy or parenteral nutrition are at risk of developing osteomyelitis caused by *Candida, Aspergillus,* or *Rhizopus*. *Staphylococcus epidermidis* is a rare cause of osteomyelitis overall, but it may be a relatively important pathogen in hemodialysis patients, perhaps as a result of metastatic seeding from the bloodstream by way of indwelling cannulas.[16] *Pseudomonas aeruginosa* is the most common cause of osteomyelitis following puncture wounds of the feet in children.[8]

CULTURES OF EFFUSIONS

All fluids suspected of being exudates should be examined bacteriologically. Clear or slightly cloudy specimens should be centrifuged at 2,500 rpm for 30 minutes, the supernatant fluid removed aseptically, and the sediment examined by means of smears and cultures. Specimens that are grossly purulent should be examined directly by Gram stains of thin films. All specimens should also be inoculated to routine media, including blood and chocolate agar plates, plates for anaerobic incubation, enriched thioglycollate broth, and isolation media for *Mycobacterium tuberculosis* and systemic fungi if indicated. In certain cases, the use of special media may be required. If an anticoagulant is required to prevent clotting of the specimen, SPS (Liquoid) should be used.

One should also examine **synovial, or joint, fluid** for the presence of gonococci by inoculating an enriched broth, such as trypticase soy broth supplemented with 1% IsoVitaleX, 10% horse serum, and 1% glucose, as described in Chapter 11. Joint fluid lactic acid levels are elevated in patients with bacterial arthritis other than that caused by the gonococcus, whereas patients with inflammatory or degenerative joint disease have lower levels.[2] The possibility that acid metabolic products produced in a joint space in the course of bacterial arthritis might be detectable by gas-liquid chromatography and provide a clue to the specific diagnosis remains to be explored further.[3] Septic bursitis almost invariably involves *S. aureus*.[10] Group A beta-hemolytic streptococci and other streptococci may occasionally be involved.

Pleural and pericardial effusions should be centrifuged and the sediment used for inoculation of culture media for mycobacteria and fungi, as well as being set up in routine aerobic and anaerobic culture. In **empyema** the fluid is purulent or seropurulent; it may yield pneumococci, streptococci, coagulase-positive staphylococci, *Haemophilus influenzae*, or various anaerobes (especially *B. melaninogenicus*, *F. nucleatum*, and anaerobic and microaerophilic cocci) on culture. In purulent pericarditis the most common organisms isolated are Enterobacteriaceae and *Pseudomonas* (accounting for 32% of cases), the staphylococcus (22%), streptococci (13%), pneumococci (9%), and *Salmonella*, *Shigella*, and *Neisseria* (7%).[11] Preliminary studies indicate that elevation of pleural fluid lactic acid, as compared with the blood, is indicative of empyema of the pleural space.[5] Mycobacterial infection must always be considered in the case of pleural empyema or purulent pericarditis.

Effusions from patients with **peritonitis** vary in character from the thin cloudy fluid found in tuberculous peritonitis to the foul-smelling purulent specimen from mixed anaerobic-aerobic peritonitis. In one study of 28 episodes of spontaneous bacterial peritonitis, *E. coli* was found to be responsible for 57% of episodes; *S. pneumoniae* and *S. faecalis* were responsible for 11% each; *Klebsiella* species and *S. aureus* were responsible for 7% each; and *Bacteroides fragilis*, group A streptococci, group B streptococci, viridans streptococci, and *Clostridium perfringens* were responsible for one episode each.[19] Peritonitis following peritoneal dialysis, however, most often involves *S. aureus* or coagulase-negative staphylococci and micrococci.[12] Other gram-positive bacteria and Enterobacteriaceae and pseudomonads account for most of the rest of cases. *Candida* is an occasional infecting organism in this situation as well.

In general, the methods for handling these specimens are those described for routine culturing of specimens from wounds (Chapter 13) and should include inoculation of both **aerobic and anaerobic media.** The radiometric method for organism detection may be used for various body fluids as well as for blood cultures.

REFERENCES

1. Baum, J.L.: Ocular infections, N. Engl. J. Med. **299:**28-31, 1978.
2. Brook, I., and Controni, G.: Rapid diagnosis of septic arthritis by quantitative analysis of joint fluid lactic acid with a Monotest lactate kit, J. Clin. Microbiol. **8:**676-679, 1978.
3. Brooks, J.B., and Melton, A.R.: Electron capture gas-liquid chromatographic study of metabolites produced by some arthritic transudate-associated organisms in vitro and in vivo in rabbit models, J. Clin. Microbiol. **8:**402-409, 1978.
4. Burnett, G.W., Scherp, H.W., and Schuster, G.W.: Oral microbiology and infectious disease, ed. 4, Baltimore, 1976, The Williams & Wilkins Co.
5. Chavalittamrong, B., and Angsusingha, K.: Pleural fluid lactic acid as a probable diagnostic aid, J.A.M.A. **244:**768, 1980.
6. Finegold, S.M.: Anaerobic bacteria in human disease, New York, 1977, Academic Press, Inc.
7. Ginsburg, C.M., Rudoy, R., and Nelson, J.D.: Acute mastoiditis in infants and children, Clin. Pediatr. **19:**549-553, 1980.
8. Goldstein, E.J.C., Ahonkhai, V.I., Cristofaro, R.L., Pringle, G.F., and Sierra, M.F.: Source of *Pseudomonas* in osteomyelitis of heels, J. Clin. Microbiol. **12:**711-713, 1980.
9. Grossman, L.I.: Endodontic practice, ed. 8, Philadelphia, 1974, Lea & Febiger.
10. Ho, G., Jr., Tice, A.D., and Kaplan, S.R.: Septic bursitis in the prepatellar and olecranon bursae, Ann. Intern. Med. **89:**21-27, 1978.
11. Klacsmann, P.G., Bulkley, B.H., and Hutchins, G.M.: The changed spectrum of purulent pericarditis, Am. J. Med. **63:**666-673, 1977.
12. Kolmos, H.J., and Andersen, K.E.H.: Peritonitis in peritoneal dialysis, Lancet **1:**1355-1356, 1979.
13. Leinonen, M.K.: Detection of pneumococcal capsular polysaccharide antigens by latex agglutination, counterimmunoelectrophoresis, and radioimmunoassay in middle ear exudates in acute otitis media, J. Clin. Microbiol. **11:**135-140, 1980.

14. Mackowiak, P.A., Jones, S.R., and Smith, J.W.: Diagnostic value of sinus-tract cultures in chronic osteomyelitis, J.A.M.A. **239:**2772-2775, 1978.

15. Nolte, W.A., editor: Oral microbiology, ed. 3, St. Louis, 1977, The C.V. Mosby Co.

16. Parker, M.A., and Tuazon, C.U.: Cervical osteomyelitis. Infection due to *Staphylococcus epidermidis* in hemodialysis patients, J.A.M.A. **240:**50-51, 1978.

17. Schwartz, R., Rodriguez, W.J., Mann, R., Khan, W., and Ross, S.: The nasopharyngeal culture in acute otitis media, J.A.M.A. **241:**2170-2173, 1979.

18. Waldvogel, F.A., and Vasey, H.: Osteomyelitis: the past decade, N. Engl. J. Med. **303:**360-370, 1980.

19. Weinstein, M.P., Iannini, P.B., Stratton, C.W., and Eickhoff, T.C.: Spontaneous bacterial peritonitis. A review of 28 cases with emphasis on improved survival and factors influencing prognosis, Am. J. Med. **64:**592-598, 1978.

15 MICROORGANISMS ENCOUNTERED IN MATERIAL REMOVED AT OPERATION AND NECROPSY

EXAMINATION OF MATERIAL OBTAINED AT OPERATION

Although largely a neglected function of the microbiology laboratory in the past, the current availability of specific antimicrobial agents has made the microbiologic examination of surgical tissue an essential adjunct to the histopathologic diagnosis.

Likewise, the increasing use of more refined techniques in postmortem microbiology has contributed to determination of etiology of infectious processes.

Collection of specimens

To carry out a proper microbiologic examination of excised tissue, a thorough search for aerobic and anaerobic microorganisms, acid-fast bacilli, fungi, viruses, and other pathogenic agents must be made. An **adequate** specimen, therefore, is a prerequisite; the surgeon or pathologist **must** assume the responsibility for obtaining sufficient material at the time of operation.

It is also necessary that a specimen container of **sufficient size** be available to the operator. A sterile, wide-mouthed, screw-capped bottle with a neoprene liner in the lid or a suitable sterile plastic container is recommended. This receptacle should be conveniently placed on the instrument table at the time of surgery so that the operator may deposit material directly into it. This prevents the possibility of accidentally fixing the tissue with formaldehyde or other germicidal agent, and it also avoids any possible contamination by the surgical pathologist. A few drops of sterile saline may be added to prevent drying out of the tissue.

In the collection of material from chronic **draining sinuses** and ulcers, appropriate sterile equipment should be made available to the examining physician. This may include curets, scissors, syringes, needles, medications, dressings, containers, and so forth. With the aid of these instruments, **deep curettage** of the sinus tract may be carried out; it should include the procurement of a portion of the wall of the tract. For collecting material from sinus tracts, an intravenous plastic catheter is introduced into the tract as deeply as possible after appropriate decontamination of the skin site, and material is aspirated with a syringe. This is immediately transferred to a sterile plastic bag, placed in a plastic anaerobic bag transport setup (see Chapter 6), and submitted promptly to the laboratory.

Material obtained from an **ulcer** should contain tissue from the base as well as the edge of the lesion. **Closed abscesses** should be aspirated, using a 15-gauge needle when feasible (to secure necrotic tissue debris that may be present) and a large-caliber syringe, and the material should be transferred to an anaerobic transport tube.[8] When possible, a portion of the abscess wall should be sent for microbiologic study. Some organisms, such as *Nocardia asteroides,* are usually found in the abscess wall; others, such as *Actinomyces israelii,* are more likely to be in the pus itself.[3] Inspection for the presence of **granules** in the aspirated pus and a Gram stain should be a part of every examination, since this may be the first clue to an infection caused by *Actinomyces, Arachnia,* or *Nocardia.*

In some instances, **contaminated** material may be submitted for microbiologic examination. Such specimens as tonsils, autopsy tissue, or similar material may be surface cauterized with an electric soldering iron or heated spatula or blanched by immersing in boiling water for 5 to 10 seconds to reduce surface contamination. The specimen may then be dissected with sterile instruments to permit culturing of the **center** of the specimen, which will not be affected by the heating.

All surgical specimens intended for microbiologic examination should be divided by the operator, using sterile instruments; one half is submitted for histologic examination, and the other half is sent to the microbiology laboratory. A detailed clinical history should accompany the histologic specimen to guide microbiologic studies. Since viable organisms may be few in number in tissue, especially in old chronic lesions, and since they may be irregularly distributed throughout the tissue, it is desirable to secure multiple specimens when the lesion is large enough.[11]

One should keep in mind that surgical specimens differ from other clinical material in that they are frequently obtained at **considerable risk and expense** to the patient. Furthermore, a specimen may represent the entire pathologic process. It is obvious, therefore, that supplementary specimens cannot be obtained with the ease with which similar specimens of blood, urine, or feces can be secured. It is strongly recommended that a portion of the tissue be kept moist in sterile nutrient broth and **refrigerated** (or frozen; this is less desirable) for subsequent studies should preliminary or routine examination prove unproductive.

The routine culturing of all biopsy specimens for fungi has been recommended by Utz.[9] He has obtained positive cultures from the brain, spleen, liver, kidney, prostate gland, epididymis, testis, muscle, skin, synovium, and other tissues, as well as from ulcers of the nose, mouth, epiglottis, and larynx.

Preparation of tissues for culture

In the important step of preparing tissues for culture, it is not enough to merely scrape material from the surface of the specimen with a bacteriologic loop. One must thoroughly **grind** the tissue into a fine suspension, since only a few organisms may be present in the whole sample.*

To prepare this suspension the tissue should first be finely minced with sterile scissors and transferred to a sterile tissue grinder, of which several types are available. A small one is illustrated in Weed's paper[11] on the isolation of fungi from tissue; the use of the ten Broeck tissue grinder† also has proved satisfactory. The tissue is ground to a pasty consistency (10% to 20% suspension), using sterile sand and sterile broth. After settling, the supernatant fluid is transferred to another small tube by use of a sterile capillary or larger pipet. It is then inoculated to culture media, as discussed later, or, when indicated, injected into animals in the same manner as any other biologic fluid. Intraperitoneal or intramuscular injection of guinea pigs and intraperitoneal injection of several mice are recommended. These are examined daily and are cultured at the time of death.

Histologic examination

Although a discussion of histologic techniques is beyond the scope of this text, it should be pointed out that a thorough histologic examination of fixed tissue is an essential part of any pathologic diagnosis. The microscopic study of carefully selected and sectioned tissue, stained by both routine and special methods (such as the Gram, acid-fast, Gomori, Gridley, periodic acid–Schiff methods), serves two useful purposes. First, it demonstrates the histopathology of the lesion—whether it is of a neoplastic, inflammatory, or other nature. If the lesion proves to be of noninflammatory origin, a micro-

---

*Yeastlike fungi, such as *Cryptococcus neoformans*, may be macerated and rendered nonviable by grinding. It is therefore recommended that **minced** tissue be inoculated directly to media for fungi.
†ten Broeck tissue grinder, small size, heavy-walled Pyrex glass, Bellco Glass, Inc., Vineland, N.J.

biologic study may not be necessary. Second, if the appearance suggests infection, it may serve as a guide to the selection of appropriate culture media and isolation techniques. Nonviable gram-positive cocci in the broth added to tissue before grinding led to some misleading results in one report.[1] Granulomatous lesions, whether showing caseation or not, should be cultured for mycobacteria, fungi, *Actinomyces*, and *Brucella*[3] as well as for the usual aerobic and anaerobic pathogens. The use of frozen sections of surgical specimens provides early histopathologic information.

Selection of culture media

In the selection of culture media, one must decide not only whether the tissue specimen contains a mixed or contaminated flora, indicating the need for selective isolation media, but also whether there are **fastidious pathogens** present, which may require special media.

No general rules can be made regarding the particular kinds of media to use; the choice will depend largely on the organisms sought or suspected. It is therefore important that the clinician inform the laboratory personnel as to any suspected organisms. Enriched media, such as blood agar, chocolate agar, heart infusion broth, anaerobic media, and media for the primary isolation of mycobacteria and fungi, must be considered. Incubation under both 3% to 10% CO_2 and anaerobic conditions should be carried out. This is discussed in earlier chapters.

Isolation of some fastidious pathogens

Although the proper techniques for isolation of fastidious pathogens are presented in other parts of the text, a number of items are relevant to the recovery of these microorganisms and are pertinent to this section. In the isolation of **pathogenic fungi** and *Actinomyces* and *Nocardia*, for example, the following points are important:

1. Tissue for mycologic examination should be minced, rather than ground, and trans-

ferred with the knife blade directly to mycologic media (see footnote, p. 152).

2. In severe, disseminated histoplasmosis, cultures of lymph nodes and biopsies of the liver, bone marrow, and upper respiratory tract mucosal ulcers are likely to yield *Histoplasma capsulatum*.

3. Most of the fungi, with the exception of cryptococci, can be isolated on media containing antibiotics. Some require enriched media and may grow at both room and incubator temperatures.

4. *Actinomyces* species are microaerophilic or obligately anaerobic, require enriched media, are inhibited by many antibiotics, and grow best at 35 C in an anaerobic environment.

5. *Nocardia* species, on the other hand, are aerobic and will grow on simple media (including Sabouraud's agar). These organisms are also inhibited by many antimicrobial agents.

It is apparent that no one medium, no specified temperature of incubation, and no single standard technique in handling will be suitable for all microorganisms. Massive inoculation of the tissue should be made to multiple sets of both simple and enriched media and incubated at both room and incubator temperatures for at least 4 weeks before discarding. Specific recommendations are found in Chapter 26.

Acid-fast stains of surgical specimens may be positive in less than one half of those cases subsequently proved to contain pathogenic mycobacteria.[12] A negative stain is thus of little value in ruling out mycobacteria, and a positive smear does **not** always denote tuberculosis; therefore, adequate bacteriologic studies must be made. These methods are considered further in Chapter 31.

The isolation of brucellae from contaminated surgical specimens can be accomplished only by the use of enriched media containing appropriate antibiotics, since routine cultures will generally be overgrown by other microorganisms. A fresh meat extract agar with added glucose* and 5% animal blood has proved satisfactory for the isolation of *Brucella* species from surgical specimens.[10] Moreover, the addition of antibiotics increases the usefulness of this medium for isolating brucellae from clinical material containing a mixed flora.

Lung biopsy and autopsy specimens (and pleural fluid) may be cultured for the agent of Legionnaires' disease on buffered charcoal yeast extract agar. Incubation should be in a moist atmosphere. Growth may not be visible before 3 to 5 days. Work with this agent must be done in a biologic safety hood.

Cultures of most of these fastidious microorganisms should be incubated for 3 to 6 weeks before discarding. Many of the organisms isolated from chronic infections—including *Brucella, Histoplasma, Coccidioides,* and mycobacteria—require long incubation periods before growth becomes apparent. During the first day or so after primary inoculation, the medium should be examined for overgrowth by *Proteus,* pseudomonads, or other presumed contaminants. It is recommended that a portion of the original tissue suspension be stored in a refrigerator until the cultures are obviously free of any contamination. Such material can also be used to set up additional cultures for unusual pathogens if the original conventional cultures are negative. *Listeria monocytogenes* sometimes can be recovered only after cold incubation at 4 C.

Final identification methods should be carried out on all isolates whenever possible. Special procedures involving virulence tests by animal injection, serologic analysis, and definitive identification may not be feasible for the small laboratory. In such cases pure cultures of these isolates should be sent to a reference laboratory for further study. Means for handling and rapid transport of specimens are described in Chapter 6.

EXAMINATION OF MATERIAL OBTAINED AT AUTOPSY

Although postmortem invasion of the bloodstream and organs by commensal organisms can occur, it is now recognized that this does not happen as rapidly as was formerly believed. Earlier studies interpreted the high incidence of positive autopsy cultures as evidence of either antemortem infection or agonal invasion of tissue. On the other hand, O'Toole and co-workers[5] indicate that contamination of tissue by the environment or personnel at the autopsy may be more significant.

The microscopic examination of direct smears stained by the Gram, Ziehl-Neelsen, or other methods, along with a thorough evaluation by culturing blood, tissue, or purulent material from infected areas, may reveal significant data related to the cause of death.

An evaluation of the results of autopsy blood cultures by Wood and associates[13] indicates a good correlation with the results of antemortem cultures or with anatomic data derived at autopsy. A higher degree of correlation is obtained when the blood for culture is obtained close to the time of death. Prior antimicrobial therapy does not necessarily reduce the recovery of pathogens from this source appreciably.

Blood for culture is collected with a sterile syringe and a 14- or 15-gauge needle after searing the heart or one of the great vessels with a soldering iron.* From 10 to 20 ml of blood is inoculated to broths in the manner described in Chapter 7. Small fragments of blood clots may appear, but these do not interfere with the culturing if large-bore needles are used. Some workers believe that culture of aspirated splenic pulp is of greater value in confirming a diagnosis of septicemia than is blood culture.

Cultures of other tissues may be obtained by searing the surface with a soldering iron or hot

---

*Brucella agar (Pfizer Laboratories, Clifton, N.J.) and trypticase soy agar (Baltimore Biological Laboratory, Cockeysville, Md.) can also be used.

---

*Silver and Sonnenwirth[7] indicate that heart blood obtained through the closed chest and before bowel manipulation gives more significant results than do the usual methods.

spatula and passing a needle and syringe, swab, or fine-pointed pipet through the seared area to an unheated and uncontaminated region.

Another method of obtaining autopsy culture material that compares favorably with results obtained by a sterile autopsy technique has been described by de Jongh and associates.[4] In this procedure the tissue surface is seared to dryness with a heated steel spatula, and 1 cu cm of tissue is excised from the center of the seared area using sterile forceps and scissors. Tissue blocks thus obtained are minced and ground as described previously and inoculated to appropriate aerobic and anaerobic media, as indicated by a Gram stain of the homogenate.

In the case of **bacterial endocarditis,** a small portion of the friable vegetation is removed with sterile scissors and forceps and submitted to the laboratory in a Petri dish or preferably in a plastic bag (Bio-Bag) anaerobic transport setup.[8] Here it is gently washed in at least three changes of sterile saline solution and then ground with sterile sand and broth in a tissue grinder, as described previously. A smear is prepared of this suspension, Gram stained, and examined; a portion also is inoculated to blood agar and chocolate agar plates and enriched thioglycollate broth medium. The plates are incubated in a candle jar and also anaerobically at 35 C for 48 hours and examined for the presence of growth. If a delay has occurred in obtaining the specimen (more than 4 hours postmortem), with probable overgrowth of contaminants, it is well to streak the suspension on a phenylethyl alcohol blood agar plate and other media. This is done to better isolate alpha-hemolytic streptococci or other gram-positive cocci that may be overgrown by *Proteus* and other gram-negative bacteria that may be present on the other plates. If indicated, anaerobic subcultures of the thioglycollate broth medium may also be carried out.

It should be emphasized that reliable microbiologic information can often be obtained even when a body has been embalmed.[3] In addition to fungi and mycobacteria, streptococci and various gram-negative bacilli have been recovered from embalmed tissues.

Collection of autopsy specimens for virus isolation*

An effort should be made to obtain postmortem specimens in all fatal cases of central nervous system disease of suspected viral etiology, especially if antemortem studies were not carried out. Using sterile precautions at the time of autopsy, the whole brain is removed and refrigerated but **not** frozen, a 3-inch segment of the descending colon is tied off at both ends, and aliquots of various other tissues are obtained and placed in sealed sterile containers and refrigerated. A blood specimen also should be collected by cardiac puncture; the serum should be separated and then refrigerated. In a fatal case of respiratory disease, lung tissue and a tracheobronchial swab should be collected and refrigerated until shipment; a blood specimen also should be obtained. All specimens thus obtained for virus isolation should be transported **without delay** to the nearest virus reference laboratory; prior arrangements for shipment and handling of such specimens at the laboratory should be made.

Procedures for isolation of Listeria monocytogenes from tissue

The tissues of all fetuses, premature infants, and young babies who have died from an infectious process should be cultured for listeriae for reasons given previously (see discussion of blood cultures). Specimens of the brain, liver, and spleen are most likely to contain the organism. The isolation procedure is given in detail by Seeliger and Cherry.[6]

1. Add 5 to 10 ml of ground tissue to each of two flasks of infusion broth.

---

*Abstracted from the instruction pamphlet by the New Jersey State Department of Health, Dr. Martin Goldfield, Assistant Commissioner.

2. Incubate one flask at 35 C for 24 hours, and inoculate a drop of this to a blood agar plate and a tellurite blood agar plate. Incubate these in a candle jar or CO_2 incubator for at least 48 hours, along with the original broth flask.

3. Store the second flask in a refrigerator at 4 C. If the 35 C subcultures (step 2) are unsuccessful, subculture material from the refrigerated flask at weekly intervals for at least 1 month.

4. *Listeria monocytogenes* is identified by the procedures described in Chapter 26. If the material is likely to be contaminated, inoculate a plate of modified McBride medium with an 18- to 24-hour tryptose broth culture incubated at 35 C (Chapter 26) and incubate at 35 C for 24 hours in a candle jar or CO_2 incubator, along with the original broth tube. Examine and identify as indicated in Chapter 26. If no listeriae are obtained from the 35 C cultures, repeat the process using the 4 C cultures. Subculture these at weekly intervals for 3 months from the original broth culture held in the refrigerator.

REFERENCES

1. Aber, R.C., and Appelbaum, P.C.: Pseudoepidemic of endocarditis in patients undergoing open heart surgery, Infect. Cont. **1**:97-99, 1980.
2. Bearns, R.E., and Girard, K.F.: On the isolation of *Listeria monocytogenes* from biological specimens, Am. J. Med. Technol. **25**:120-126, 1959.
3. Brewer, N.S., and Weed, L.A.: Diagnostic tissue microbiology methods, Human Pathol. **7**:141-149, 1976.
4. De Jongh, D.S., Loftis, J.W., Green, G.S., Shively, J.A., and Minckler, T.M.: Postmortem bacteriology: a practical method for routine use, Am. J. Clin. Pathol. **49**:424-428, 1968.
5. O'Toole, W.F., Saxena, H.M.K., Golden, A., and Ritts, R.E.: Studies of postmortem microbiology using sterile autopsy technique, Arch. Pathol. **80**:540-547, 1965.
6. Seeliger, H.P.R., and Cherry, W.B.: Human listeriosis: its nature and diagnosis, Washington, D.C., 1957, U.S. Government Printing Office.
7. Silver, H., and Sonnenwirth, A.C.: A practical and efficacious method for obtaining significant postmortem blood cultures, Am. J. Clin. Pathol. **52**:433-437, 1969.
8. Sutter, V.L., Citron, D.M., and Finegold, S.M.: Wadsworth anaerobic bacteriology manual, ed. 3, St. Louis, 1980, The C.V. Mosby Co.
9. Utz, J.P.: Recognition and current management of the systemic mycoses, Med. Clin. North Am. **51**:519-527, 1967.
10. Weed, L.A.: Use of a selective medium for isolation of *Brucella* from contaminated surgical specimens, Am. J. Clin. Pathol. **27**:482-485, 1957.
11. Weed, L.A.: Technics for the isolation of fungi from tissues obtained at operation and necropsy, Am. J. Clin. Pathol. **29**:496-502, 1958.
12. Weed, L.A., McDonald, J.R., and Needham, G.M.: The isolation of "saprophytic" acid-fast bacilli from lesions of caseous granulomas, Proc. Staff Meet. Mayo Clin. **31**:246-259, 1956.
13. Wood, W.H., Oldstone, M., and Schultz, R.B.: A reevaluation of blood culture as an autopsy procedure, Am. J. Clin. Pathol. **43**:241-247, 1965.

PART IV METHODS FOR IDENTIFICATION OF PATHOGENIC MICROORGANISMS

16 FACULTATIVE STAPHYLOCOCCI AND MICROCOCCI; TOXIC SHOCK SYNDROME; KAWASAKI DISEASE

Micrococcaceae are ubiquitous and exist as free-living saprophytes, parasites, and pathogenic forms. The great majority of pathogenic "micrococci" fall within the genus *Staphylococcus*, but nonstaphylococci are being isolated from clinical sites with increasing frequency. Collectively, the organisms of the group are **spherical, gram-positive cocci** occurring singly, in pairs, in tetrads, in packets, and in irregular clusters. Most are strongly **catalase positive;** they are nonmotile and may be pigmented. Nitrates are usually reduced to nitrites. They are **aerobic or facultative.**

Despite confusion in the classification of these organisms, clinical laboratories should have few problems in identifying the major pathogens. We will consider the genera *Staphylococcus* and *Micrococcus* in this chapter and *Streptococcus* and *Aerococcus* in Chapters 17 and 18. Anaerobic cocci of all types are covered in Chapter 28.

Although the catalase test is very simple and is widely used, there are occasional pitfalls in using it to differentiate the various groups discussed in the outline below. Some micrococci do not decompose hydrogen peroxide.

CLASSIFICATION OF GRAM-POSITIVE COCCI

Differentiation between *Staphylococcus* and *Micrococcus* can be made in three ways: *Staphylococcus* produces acid from glucose anaerobically, produces acid from glycerol in the presence of erythromycin, and is susceptible to lysis by lysostaphin*; *Micrococcus* is negative in all of these tests (Table 16-1). Ordinary sugar fermentation bases **cannot** be used for the first of these tests (see Chapter 42 for fermentation medium for differentiating *Staphylococcus* and *Micrococcus*). Microorganisms formerly classified as *Micrococcus* subgroups 1 through 4 have now been reclassified on the basis of their DNA homology and guanine plus cytosine content as members of the species *Staphylococcus saprophyticus*.[5] This organism is taxonomically intermediate between *Staphylococcus* and *Micrococcus*. It does not actively produce acid from glucose anaerobically but may slowly produce small amounts of acid. Schleifer and Kloos[26] note that virtually all staphylococci and no micrococci produce acid aerobically from glycerol in the presence of 0.4 µg/ml of erythromycin. Smith's selective medium for corynebacteria, which contains 50 µg/ml of furoxone,* was found to support growth of *Micrococcus* and prevent growth of *Staphylococcus*.[9] Faller and Schleifer (J. Clin. Microbiol. **13**:1031-1035, 1981) recommend two simple and rapid tests for differentiation of these two genera—modified oxidase and benzidine tests. Varaldo and associates[36] propose separating staphylococci from micrococci based on the ability of staphylococci, but not micrococci, to lyse heat-killed cells of *Micrococcus luteus* in a special medium.

GENUS STAPHYLOCOCCUS

Staphylococci are frequently found on the skin, on nasal and other mucous membranes of humans, and in various food products. Three major species are recognized: *S. aureus*, *S. epidermidis*, and *S. saprophyticus*. Three other species, all coagulase negative, have been isolated from 5% to 20% of the infections attributed to coagulase-negative staphylococci. These are *S. hominis*, *S. haemolyticus*, and *S. simulans*.

---

*Schwarz/Mann Research Laboratory, Orangeburg, N.Y.

*Eaton Laboratories, Norwich, N.Y.

TABLE 16-1

Differentiation of *Staphylococcus* and *Micrococcus*

	Staphylococcus	*Micrococcus*
Sensitivity to lyso-staphin,* 200 µg/ml	+	—
Aerobic production of acid from glycerol in presence of 0.4 µg/ml of erythromycin	+	—
Anaerobic acid production from glucose	+†	—

Modified from Baird-Parker.
*Schwartz/Mann Research Laboratory, Orangeburg, N.Y.; Sigma Chemical Co., St. Louis, Mo.
†*S. saprophyticus* and related species grow poorly or not at all under anaerobic conditions.

Reactions for differentiation of the six staphylococcal species of clinical interest are presented in Table 16-2. Details on the media and techniques to be utilized in studying these reactions are presented by Kloos and Smith.[20]

Staphylococcus aureus

Staphylococcus aureus is a **gram-positive, nonmotile coccus** occurring singly, in pairs, in short chains, or in irregular clusters. The last arrangement is probably the most characteristic (Fig. 16-1). The Greek word "staphyle," meaning a bunch of grapes, is used descriptively as the stem of the generic term. In older cultures the cells tend to lose their ability to retain the crystal violet and may appear gram variable or even gram negative. On initial isolation the organism typically produces a golden yellow pigment. This characteristic, however, is variable; white or pale colonies may arise after laboratory cultivation and are not infrequently isolated from clinical sources.

Colonies are usually opaque, circular, smooth, and entire, with a butyrous consistency (Plate 3). The organism grows well on trypticase soy agar or nutrient agar but develops larger colonies on blood agar. The hemolytic activity is variable.

Most strains of *S. aureus* **ferment mannitol,** tolerate relatively high concentrations of salt (7.5% to 10%), grow on phenylethyl alcohol agar medium, and are relatively resistant to polymyxin. These characteristics help promote their isolation from material such as feces, in which a large and varied bacterial flora exists. Polymyxin staphylococcus medium,[13] phenylethyl alcohol agar medium, and mannitol salt agar are recommended for the isolation of *S. aureus* when many other organisms are present. Colonies of salt-tolerant staphylococci appear on mannitol salt agar, surrounded by a yellow halo after 24 to 48 hours, which indicates mannitol fermentation. Mannitol fermentation, among other tests, helps to distinguish *S. aureus* from *S. epidermidis*. *S. saprophyticus* resembles *S. epidermidis* in most properties but may be differentiated from it by its resistance to novobiocin. *S. aureus* and *S. epidermidis* are phosphatase positive; *S. saprophyticus* is negative.

In the differentiation of *S. aureus* from *S. epidermidis*, pigmentation is **not** considered a reliable or valid criterion. Thermostable nuclease activity, on the other hand, agrees well with coagulase activity, but the former test is more difficult to perform, and, therefore, the coagulase test is preferred in most diagnostic laboratories. Production of acid from mannitol and from trehalose aerobically is characteristic of *S. aureus* and *S. saprophyticus*, whereas *S. epidermidis* is negative in this regard.

Bacteriolytic activity has also been used in a system for identification of various staphylococci, as well as for differentiating staphylococci from micrococci.[37] The system requires the use of five different test media and also determination of the phosphatase activity. Varaldo and associates[37] evaluated a micromethod called API STAPH, not yet available in the United States.

TABLE 16-2

Differentiation of human *Staphylococcus* species of some clinical interest

Character	Well-documented clinically important species			Probably clinically important species		
	S. aureus	S. epidermidis	S. saprophyticus	S. hominis	S. haemolyticus	S. simulans
Coagulase*	+†	−	−	−	−	−
Hemolysis	+	− > ±	−	− > ±	+ > ±	±, −
Novobiocin resistance*§	−	−	+	−	−	−
Phosphatase*	+	+	− > ±	− > ±	− > ±	±
Acid, aerobically, from						
D-(+)-Trehalose*	+	−	+	+ > −	+	+ > −
D-Mannitol*	+	−	+ > −	−	+, −	+ > −
Maltose	+	+	+	+	+	− > ±
Sucrose*	+	+	+	+	+	+
D-(+)-Xylose* or L-(+)-arabinose	−	−	−	−	−	−
Xylitol	−	−	+, ± > −	−	−	−
Anaerobic growth in thioglycollate	+‖	+	+ > ± C	−c > ±	±C > ±, +	+
Average colony diameter (mm)¶	7.8	3.7	7.0	4.2	6.5	6.8
Identification accuracy based on the above characters	>95%	>95%	>90%	>80%	>85%	>90%

From Kloos and Smith.[20]
*Characters recommended by the ICSB Subcommittee on the Taxonomy of Staphylococci and Micrococci.
†Reactions: +, positive; ±, weak positive; −, negative.
§Minimal inhibitory concentration ≥ 1.6 μg/ml.
‖Growth in thioglycollate: +, moderate to heavy down tube; ±, weak in lower portion of tube; C denotes large and c denotes very small colonies observed in anaerobic portion of tube; −, no visible growth other than a few scattered colonies.
¶After 3 days at 34 C and 2 days at room temperature.

This micromethod provided very good results.

The best single test for differentiating the staphylococci is the **coagulase tube test,** which demonstrates "free" coagulase. Citrated* rabbit plasma,† 0.5 ml in a small (12- × 100-mm) tube, is inoculated with 0.1 ml of an overnight culture of the organism in BHI broth and incubated at 35 C in a water bath. Complete or partial coagulation in 1 to 4 hours is interpreted as **positive.** A variation of this test may be performed by using a single well-isolated colony from a nonselective medium in plasma. The test may be observed for a period up to 24 hours, but the 4-hour test is much preferred. If a 24-hour test is used, one should be certain that the plasma is sterile, that the inoculum is pure, and that appropriate controls are used. In general, it would be better to confirm the identity of strains requiring a longer clotting period than 4 hours

*Citrated plasma may also be coagulated by organisms other than S. aureus, such as some citrate-utilizing enterococci[9] or gram-negative bacilli, particularly when isolated colonies of staphylococci or overnight incubation are used. The use of EDTA (ethylenediamine tetra-acetate) in place of citrate prevents this problem.
†Dehydrated sterile rabbit plasma is available commercially.

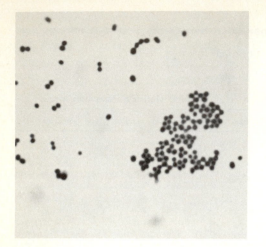

FIG. 16-1
Staphylococcus aureus, showing typical grapelike clusters
(1,000×).

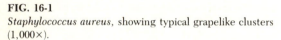

by some other means. Typical strains of *S. epidermidis* and *S. saprophyticus* are coagulase negative, whereas strains of *S. aureus* are coagulase positive.

A word of caution should be offered to those who have adopted the practice of using plasma from outdated human bank blood for this test. Inhibitory factors are found in some human blood, and control tests with known strongly and weakly positive and negative strains should always be included. This should be part of a daily quality control procedure in **all** coagulase testing.

The **coagulase slide test,** which demonstrates "bound" coagulase or "clumping factor," is used by many laboratories and gives results comparable to the tube test. It is performed by emulsifying growth from a typical colony from media **not** containing high concentrations of salt (such as mannitol salt agar) in a drop of distilled water on a slide to make a heavy suspension and adding a drop of plasma. This is mixed thoroughly and observed for clumping **within 10 seconds.** If the reaction is **positive,** easily visible white clumps appear immediately; if no such clumping

appears, the reaction is **negative** and **should be checked by the tube test,** since some strains of *S. aureus* may be negative by slide test. This is an excellent **screening** procedure, however, as most strains of *S. aureus* are positive by the slide test and false-positives do not occur, assuming that proper controls are used and the reaction time is no longer than 10 seconds. Severance and colleagues[28] found that lysostaphin sensitivity was an excellent rapid screening test to differentiate *S. aureus* from other species of staphylococci and micrococci. A 1:10 dilution of the culture is exposed to 2 µg/ml of lysostaphin on a tilting mixer at 37 C for 30 minutes. A reduction of 90% or greater in the number of organisms seen when comparing the pretreatment and posttreatment Gram stains is considered a positive test result. This technique can be used directly from blood culture media of various types, except that Columbia broth yields some false-positive results with *S. epidermidis*.[27]

Some investigators report that a good correlation exists between **phosphatase** production and pathogenicity; yet some coagulase-negative strains are more strongly phosphatase positive than are some coagulase-positive strains.

It is important to recognize that certain naturally occurring variant forms of *S. aureus* may cause infection, even serious infection. Spagna and others[31] described a patient with pneumonia whose cultures showed staphylococci on chocolate agar plates incubated in 5% CO_2 that were considered contaminants because they were not present on blood agar plates incubated in room air. Subsequent careful examination of both types of plates that were incubated in room air revealed the presence of minute clear colonies that apparently had been overlooked initially. Acar and co-workers[1] found that among 1,100 strains of *S. aureus* isolated from clinical material in a period of 1 year, there were 15 isolates that on initial culture grew as dwarf colonies. On their routine media, which was trypticase soy agar with or without horse blood, 8 of the 15 isolates were stable dwarf forms on serial subculture and required thiamine or menadione to grow as normal-appearing staphylococci.

A simple latex slide agglutination test in which the coating material is human plasma detects clumping factor and protein A simultaneously.[12] This has been recommended for rapid, reliable, routine identification of *S. aureus*. No false-positive or false-negative results were obtained. Serologic techniques have also been utilized to detect teichoic acids from *S. aureus* in clinical materials. The techniques used have been CIE, gel diffusion, and ELISA.[2,23] There have been a number of studies seeking antibodies to teichoic acids in patients with deep-seated staphylococcal infection.[23,30] Unfortunately, some patients fail to develop such antibodies; false-positive tests may be obtained from drug addicts. One may also use solid-phase radioimmunoassay for IgG antibody to *S. aureus* to guide therapy.[39] A positive antibody result 14 days after the onset of infection strongly suggests that the patient has endocarditis or complicated bacteremia (a secondary focus or failure to remove a primary focus), as opposed to uncomplicated staphylococcal bacteremia.

Strains of *S. aureus* isolated from human sources can elaborate a variety of metabolites.[11] Some of these are toxic and of pathologic significance; others are either nontoxic or of low toxicity but have some diagnostic significance. Human pathogens produce alpha and delta lysins. Other exotoxins produced by the pathogenic staphylococci are **leukocidin,** which is probably the same as the delta lysin, a **dermonecrotizing toxin,** a **lethal toxin,** a **pyrogenic toxin,** and an **enterotoxin.** Only strains of *S. aureus* that produce enterotoxin cause staphylococcal food poisoning. As noted in Chapter 9, it has been shown recently that staphylococci from patients with pseudomembranous enterocolitis produce a cytopathic toxin that can be distinguished from that produced by *Clostridium difficile,* the more common pathogen in colitis related to antimicrobial therapy.

Alpha hemolysin does not lyse human erythrocytes but does lyse rabbit and sheep red cells. Delta lysin lyses horse erythrocytes. Alpha hemolysin serves as a convenient index of virulence because filtrates of virulent broth cultures usually yield a high titer.

Tests for the dermonecrotizing toxin may be carried out by intradermal injection in a rabbit and tests for lethal toxin by intravenous injection. Tests for enterotoxin are best done by serologic procedures.

Among the nontoxic metabolites produced by the staphylococci are phosphatase and coagulase, to which reference was made previously, hyaluronidase, deoxyribonuclease, staphylokinase, or fibrinolysin, and in addition lipase, gelatinase, and protease. Most, if not all, of these are antigenic.

S. aureus can develop resistance to antibiotics with surprising facility. At least 90% of hospital strains of staphylococci are resistant to penicillin. This resistance to penicillin is mediated by a beta-lactamase or penicillinase. Much less commonly, staphylococci may develop resistance to penicillinase-resistant penicillins such as methicillin. However, in 1980 almost 5% of *S. aureus* strains isolated from nosocomial infections were methicillin resistant, and in 1979 approximately one third of hospitals in the United States had had problems with these organisms (Wenzel et al.: Morbid. Mortal. Weekly Rep. **30:**140-147, 1981). Recently a new type of resistance, restricted to cephalosporins with a specific side chain (necessary for good absorption upon oral administration), has been reported (Lacey and Lord: Lancet **1:**1049-1050, 1981). The pathogenic potential of these strains of *S. aureus* is not known. Staphylococci should be tested for susceptibility to a number of antibiotics by one of the accepted methods. The reader is referred to Chapter 36 for information on methods of antimicrobial susceptibility testing of microorganisms.

The phenomenon of tolerance of *S. aureus* to bactericidal activity of drugs has been described in recent years. In general, beta-lactam antibiotics have been bactericidal for *S. aureus* at concentrations equal to or close to those required for inhibition. In tolerant strains, however, considerably more antibiotic is needed. The minimal bactericidal concentration (MBC) may be more than 100 times the minimal inhibitory concentration (MIC). The usual definition for minimal bactericidal concentration is the concentration of drug that effects a 99.9% or greater decrease in numbers of organisms in a 24-hour period of incubation. Tolerant strains are killed, but more slowly than others. The mechanism of tolerance seems to be lack of autolysin activity. This may be mediated via a bacteriophage. Many studies have shown that one third to two thirds of staphylococcal strains exhibit the phenomenon of tolerance. However, more recent work indicates that every culture of *S. aureus* may contain some tolerant forms. The range of organisms in cultures was from 0.5% to 50%, with an average of 8.6%. At this point there is absolutely no clinical evidence to indicate that tolerance is an important clinical phenomenon, particularly in terms of differences in survival or relapse rates in patients infected with these types of organisms (presumably this means strains in which a great percentage of the bacteria present are tolerant).[19]

Staphylococcus epidermidis

Staphylococcus epidermidis resembles *S. aureus* in microscopic morphology. The colonies are circular, smooth, and usually a pale translucent white. It normally resides on the skin and mucous membranes of humans and other animals. The organism is very salt tolerant, as is *S. aureus*, but differs from that species in being **coagulase negative, thermonuclease negative,** and **mannitol negative.** The organism is basically saprophytic rather than pathogenic. However, it is unquestionably involved in certain clinical syndromes, notably bacterial endocarditis, infection following insertion of surgical prostheses, and infection following bone marrow transplantation[8] or other immunosuppression. It is

also involved in some urinary tract infections.[17] *S. epidermidis* accounts for 2% to 6% of cases of subacute bacterial endocarditis. However, in patients with a prosthetic heart valve, *S. epidermidis* is the most common cause of endocarditis, accounting for 27% of early-onset cases and 10% of late-onset cases.[8] It causes 60% to 95% of infections involving CSF shunts and 14% of peripheral vascular grafts, and it is second only to *S. aureus* in infected total hip replacements.[8] It may also be involved in infection in relation to indwelling intravenous catheters. Urinary tract infections involving *S. epidermidis* usually occur in elderly hospitalized men, particularly after instrumentation. Methicillin-resistant coagulase-negative staphylococci may or may not be resistant to cephalosporins.[3] Typically *S. epidermidis* is more resistant to penicillinase-resistant penicillins and cephalosporins than is *S. aureus*, which is almost always sensitive. One study showed an increase in the incidence of highly methicillin-resistant *S. epidermidis* postoperatively as compared with preoperatively in a survey of skin flora.[3] This is undoubtedly related to use of antimicrobial agents as well as to an increased amount of time spent in the hospital environment. Combinations of various antimicrobial agents may show either synergism or antagonism or neither against *S. epidermidis*.[10,21] However, rifampin commonly shows synergism in vitro[10] and one study showed enhanced killing of organisms in patients when rifampin was added to the usual antibiotic regimens.[4] Vancomycin is generally active against all gram-positive cocci, but *S. epidermidis* may rarely be resistant to it.

Staphylococcus saprophyticus

Staphylococcus saprophyticus, as noted above, resembles *S. epidermidis* closely but is said to be distinctive by virtue of its resistance to novobiocin. It may produce intense yellow pigment. Hovelius and Mårdh[15] found that a nalidixic acid disk diffusion test was more reliable than novobiocin resistance in distinguishing between *S. saprophyticus* and other coagulase-negative staphylococci. *S. saprophyticus* is quite resistant to nalidixic acid. It should be noted that *S. saprophyticus* does not grow reliably on MacConkey agar. Until recent years, urinary isolates of coagulase-negative staphylococci were regarded as "contaminants" or, occasionally, as opportunistic pathogens. Several reports have implicated these organisms as the etiologic agent in a significant number of urinary infections.[16-18,22,38] *S. saprophyticus* subgroup 3, formerly *Micrococcus* subgroup 3, has been noted to have a predilection for the urinary tract. This organism produces not only cystitis but also frank pyelonephritis.[18] It is an occasional cause of the acute urethral syndrome in women.[32] It is rarely found as a contaminant in urine cultures. It has a predilection for epithelial cells of the urinary tract, to which it adheres. Indeed, one may notice a characteristic appearance of urine sediments from patients with urinary tract infection caused by *S. saprophyticus*.[16] One sees aggregates of staphylococcal cells adherent to epithelial cells. In one study cultures from 22% of 787 consecutive female outpatients with signs of bacteriuria yielded *S. saprophyticus*, predominantly in pure culture and in high count.[38] This organism was found in 42% in the age group 16 to 25 years. On the other hand, it is a relatively rare finding in hospitalized women and in men with bacteriuria.

A critical appraisal of the significance of urinary isolates of coagulase-negative Micrococcaceae was given by Williams and associates.[40] Of 16,347 urine cultures submitted to their hospital laboratory, only 68 specimens (0.4%) from 50 patients yielded more than 10^4 coagulase-negative staphylococci per milliliter in pure culture. A total of 62 of the 63 organisms available for their study could be classified as follows: 45 *S. epidermidis* (predominantly subgroup 1), 15 *S. saprophyticus* (subgroup 3), and 2 *S. aureus*. "Probable" urinary infections were noted in only 21 patients; 8 patients had two or more positive urine cultures. All isolates from the same patient

were identical by morphology, antibiotic susceptibility, and hemolytic pattern. Nine (75%) of their 12 isolates of *S. saprophyticus*, which were novobiocin resistant and nonhemolytic on a synergistic hemolysis test, were from patients with probable urinary infection. Eight were young women with acute symptoms and pyuria. Unfortunately, novobiocin resistance could not be relied on to differentiate their isolates of *S. saprophyticus* from *S. epidermidis* (two of 15 strains of *S. saprophyticus* were sensitive). *S. saprophyticus*, in contrast with the other staphylococci discussed, is quite susceptible to most antimicrobial agents except nalidixic acid. It may fail to respond to this agent clinically. A study by John and colleagues[17] of 138 consecutively isolated coagulase-negative staphylococci from the urinary tracts of hospitalized patients found that the most common species was *S. epidermidis* (53%), whereas *S. saprophyticus* made up only 5%. *S. hominis* was found in 12% and *S. haemolyticus* in 10%.

Phage typing of staphylococci

Since the recognition of prevalent hospital phage types is of interest in outbreaks, some laboratories are involved in phage typing of staphylococci. The value of this procedure in epidemiologic studies cannot be questioned, but because of the rather involved and time-consuming procedures that are necessary, it is recommended that typing not be done as a routine.

Phage typing is carried out by the Laboratory Centre for Disease Control (Ottawa), the Cross Infection Laboratory (C.P.H. Laboratory, London), various state public health laboratories, and the Centers for Disease Control (Atlanta).

Diseases caused by staphylococci

The **most common** disorders caused by the pathogenic staphylococci are cellulitis, pustules, boils, carbuncles, impetigo, secondary infection of acne, and postoperative wound infections. One of the most common types of food poisoning is staphylococcal food poisoning, caused by the enterotoxin elaborated in food.

Among the **most serious** staphylococcal infections are septicemia (Plate 7), endocarditis, meningitis, puerperal sepsis, pneumonia (Plate 14), and osteomyelitis. Staphylococcal pseudomembranous enterocolitis (Plate 20) is presently a rare complication of antibiotic therapy.

S. epidermidis is of particular importance clinically in infections such as bacterial endocarditis, particularly after cardiac surgery with valve replacement. Additionally, it is often the cause of a persistent bacteremia following ventriculoatrial shunt for control of hydrocephalus and is involved in infection related to other surgical prostheses.[25] As noted, *S. saprophyticus* and *S. epidermidis* are involved in urinary tract infection.

GENUS MICROCOCCUS

As previously noted, *Micrococcus* is distinguished from *Staphylococcus* primarily by its failure to ferment glucose anaerobically, its failure to produce acid from glycerol in the presence of erythromycin, and its lack of susceptibility to lysis by lysostaphin. *Micrococcus* does have cytochrome enzymes (is benzidine positive). It is usually strongly catalase positive. Speciation is shown in Table 16-3.

TABLE 16-3

Speciation of *Micrococcus*

	M. varians	M. luteus	M. roseus
Pigment	Yellow	Yellow	Pink
Growth in 10% NaCl	+	+	−
Acid aerobically from glucose	+	−	−
Nitrate reduction	+	−	+
Oxidase activity	−	+	− or ±

From Baird-Parker.[5]
+, >80% of strains positive; −, >80% of strains negative; ±, weak.

Members of this genus may cause endocarditis and other infections of the type caused by *S. epidermidis* but are probably much less commonly involved.

TOXIC SHOCK SYNDROME

The toxic shock syndrome was first described as such in 1978, although clearly cases were seen well before that time, in retrospect. Through December 1980, 941 confirmed cases had been reported to CDC, most of them in 1980.[35] Of the cases presented, 99% were in women, and 98% of these women had the onset during a menstrual period. The disease is characterized by sudden onset of fever, diarrhea, vomiting, shock, and a diffuse macular erythematous rash, followed by desquamation of the hands and feet, hyperemia of various mucous membranes, and at times involvement of other organ systems including the liver, kidney, muscular system, gastrointestinal system, cardiopulmonary system, and central nervous system. Most of the women had used tampons and had left them in place for extended periods of time.[29,34] There seems to be a definite association with a particular brand of tampon, Rely, although all other major brands were associated with the disease as well. Not uncommonly, women had recurrences of the syndrome during subsequent menstrual periods. The mortality has been 10% to 15%.

S. aureus was recovered from vaginal cultures in 46 of 48 cases in one study and in 62 of 64 in another.[14,29] In the latter case, only 7 of 71 control vaginal cultures yielded *S. aureus*. A pyrogenic exotoxin has been detected in the blood.[24,33] Cases in men or children were at times associated with staphylococcal infections at various sites. *S. aureus* has also been isolated from the conjunctiva, oral cavity, anterior nose, or stool of patients with the disease.

KAWASAKI DISEASE

Kawasaki disease (mucocutaneous lymph node syndrome) is characterized by fever unresponsive to antibiotics, conjunctival hyperemia, mucosal changes, erythema, and edema of the palms and soles followed by desquamation, a polymorphous rash involving the trunk, and enlarged cervical lymph nodes. Coronary artery involvement with arteritis may occur and may account for a fatal outcome. This disease is of unknown etiology, but it is possible that it is related to the toxic shock syndrome.[14,24] Although most patients with Kawasaki disease are younger than 5 years, there have been 5 cases in young adults, all female, and one had vaginal inflammation from which S. aureus was isolated. Certain features of the toxic shock syndrome are absent from cases of Kawasaki disease, but there are enough similarities that they may well share a common etiology.

REFERENCES

1. Acar, J.F., Goldstein, F.W., and Lagrange, P.: Human infections caused by thiamine- or menadione-requiring *Staphylococcus aureus*, J. Clin. Microbiol. **8:**142-147, 1978.
2. Anhalt, J.P., Kenny, G.E., and Rytel, M.W. (Gavan, T.L., editor): Detection of microbial antigens by counterimmunoelectrophoresis, Cumitech 8, Washington, D.C., 1978, American Society for Microbiology.
3. Archer, G.L., and Tenenbaum, M.J.: Antibiotic-resistant *Staphylococcus epidermidis* in patients undergoing cardiac surgery, Antimicrob. Agents Chemother. **17:**269-272, 1980.
4. Archer, G.L., Tenenbaum, M.J., and Haywood, H.B., III: Rifampin therapy of *Staphylococcus epidermidis*, J.A.M.A. **240:**751-753, 1978.
5. Baird-Parker, A.C.: Methods for identifying staphylococci and micrococci. In Skinner, F.A., and Lovelock, D.W., editors: Identification methods for microbiologists, ed. 2, Technical Series 14, London, 1979, Academic Press, Inc., Ltd., for the Society of Applied Bacteriology.
6. Bayliss, B.G., and Hall, E.R. Plasma coagulation by organisms other than *Staphylococcus aureus*, J. Bacteriol. **89:**101-105, 1965.
7. Bender, J.W., and Hughes, W.T.: Fatal *Staphylococcus epidermidis* sepsis following bone marrow transplantation, Johns Hopkins Med. J. **146:**13-15, 1980.
8. Coagulase-negative staphylococci, Lancet **1:**139-140, 1981.
9. Curry, J.C., and Borovian, G.E.: Selective medium for distinguishing micrococci from staphylococci in the clinical laboratory, J. Clin. Microbiol. **4:**455-457, 1976.
10. Ein, M.E., Smith, N.J., Aruffo, J.F., Heerema, M.S., Bradshaw, M.W., and Williams, T.W., Jr.: Susceptibility and synergy studies of methicillin-resistant *Staphylococcus epidermidis*, Antimicrob. Agents Chemother. **16:**655-659, 1979.
11. Elek, S.D.: *Staphylococcus pyogenes*, London, 1959, E. & S. Livingstone, Ltd.
12. Essers, L., and Radebold, K.: Rapid and reliable identification of *Staphylococcus aureus* by a latex agglutination test, J. Clin. Microbiol. **12:**641-643, 1980.
13. Finegold, S.M., and Sweeney, E.E.: New selective and differential medium for coagulase-positive staphylococci allowing rapid growth and strain differentiation, J. Bacteriol. **81:**636-641, 1961.
14. Glasgow, L.A.: Staphylococcal infection in the toxic-shock syndrome, N. Eng. J. Med. **303:**1473-1475, 1980.
15. Hovelius, B., and Mårdh, P-A.: On the diagnosis of coagulase-negative staphylococci with emphasis on *Staphylococcus saprophyticus*, Acta Path. Microbiol. Scand. Sect. B, **85:**427-434, 1977.
16. Hovelius, B, Mårdh, P-A., and Bygren, P.: Urinary tract infections caused by *Staphylococcus saprophyticus:* recurrences and complications, J. Urol. **122:**645-647, 1979.
17. John, J.F., Jr., Gramling, P.K., and O'Dell, N.M.: Species identification of coagulase-negative staphylococci from urinary tract isolates, J. Clin. Microbiol. **8:**435-437, 1978.
18. Jordan, P.A., Iravani, A., Richard, G.A., and Baer, H.: Urinary tract infection caused by *Staphylococcus saprophyticus*, J. Infect. Dis. **142:**510-515, 1980.
19. Kaye, D.: The clinical significance of tolerance of *Staphylococcus aureus*, Ann. Intern. Med. **93:**924-925, 1980.
20. Kloos, W.E. and Smith, P.B.: Staphylococci. In Lennette, E.H., Balows, A., Hausler, W.J., Jr., and Truant, J.P., editors: Manual of clinical microbiology, ed. 3, Washington, D.C., 1980, American Society for Microbiology.
21. Lowy, F.D., Walsh, J.A., Mayers, M.M., Klein, R.S., and Steigbigel, N.H.: Antibiotic activity in vitro against methicillin-resistant *Staphylococcus epidermidis* and therapy of an experimental infection, Antimicrob. Agents Chemother. **16:**314-321, 1979.
22. Mabeck, C.E.: Significance of coagulase-negative staphylococcal bacteriuria, Lancet **2:**1150-1152, 1969.
23. Mackowiak, P.A., and Smith, J.W.: Teichoic acid antibodies in chronic staphylococcal osteomyelitis, Ann. Intern. Med. **89:**494-496, 1978.
24. McKenna, U.G., Meadows, J.A., Brewer, N.S., Wilson W.R., and Perrault, J.: Toxic shock syndrome, a newly recognized disease entity, Mayo Clin. Proc. **55:**663-672, 1980.

25. Quinn, E.L., Cox, F., and Fisher, M.: The problem of associating coagulase negative staphylococci with disease, Ann. N.Y. Acad. Sci. **128**:428-442, 1965.

26. Schleifer, K.H., and Kloos, W.E.: A simple test system for the separation of staphylococci from micrococci, J. Clin. Microbiol. **1**:337-338, 1975.

27. Severance, P.J., Kauffman, C.A., and Sheagren, J.N.: Effect of various blood culture media on lysostaphin sensitivity of staphylococci, J. Clin. Microbiol. **12**:709-710, 1980.

28. Severance, P.J., Kauffman, C.A., and Sheagren, J.N.: Rapid identification of *Staphylococcus aureus* by using lysostaphin sensitivity, J. Clin. Microbiol. **11**:724-727, 1980.

29. Shands, K.N., Schmid, G.P., Dan, B.B., Blum, D., Guidotti, R.J., Hargrett, N.T., Anderson, R.L., Hill, D.L., Broome, C.V., Band, J.D., and Fraser, D.W.: Toxic-shock syndrome in menstruating women, N. Engl. J. Med. **303**:1436-1442, 1980.

30. Smith, L., Jr., Bogden, J., Wiener, B., Palmieri, C., Smith, L., Minnefor, A., and Oleske, J.: Teichoic acid antibody (TAA) levels in two high risk populations for invasive *S. aureus* infections, Abstract 279, Abstracts of the Nineteenth Interscience Conference on Antibiotics and Chemotherapy, 1979.

31. Spagna, V.A., Fass, R.J., Prior, R.B., and Slama, T.G.: Report of a case of bacterial sepsis caused by a naturally occurring variant form of *Staphylococcus aureus*, J. Infect. Dis. **138**:277-278, 1978.

32. Stamm, W.E., Wagner, K.F., Amsel, R., Alexander, E.R., Turck, M., Counts, G.W., and Holmes, K.K.: Causes of the acute urethral syndrome in women, N. Engl. J. Med. **303**:409-415, 1980.

33. Tofte, R.W., and Crossley, K.B.: Clinical experience with toxic-shock syndrome, N. Engl. J. Med. **303**:1417, 1980.

34. Toxic shock and vaginal tampons, Lancet **2**:1011, 1980.

35. Toxic-shock syndrome: United States, 1970-1980, Morbid. Mortal. Weekly Rep. **30**:25-28,33, 1981.

36. Varaldo, P.E., Grazi, G., Cisani, G., and Satta, G.: Routine separation of staphylococci from micrococci based on bacteriolytic activity production, J. Clin. Microbiol. **9**:147-148, 1979.

37. Varaldo, P.E., Grazi, G., Soro, O., Cisani, G., and Satta, G.: Simplified lyogroup system, a new method for routine identification of staphylococci: description and comparison with three other methods, J. Clin. Microbiol. **12**:63-68, 1980.

38. Wallmark, G., Arremark, I., and Telander, B.: *Staphylococcus saprophyticus*: a frequent cause of acute urinary tract infection among female outpatients, J. Infect. Dis. **138**:791-797, 1978.

39. Wheat, L.J., Kohler, R.B., and White, A.: Solid-phase radioimmunoassay for immunoglobulin G *Staphylococcus aureus* antibody in serious staphylococcal infection, Ann. Intern. Med. **89**:467-472, 1978.

40. Williams, D.N., Lund, M.E., and Blazevic, D.J.: Significance of urinary isolates of coagulase-negative *Micrococcaceae*, J. Clin. Microbiol. **3**:556-559, 1976.

17 FACULTATIVE STREPTOCOCCI AND AEROCOCCI

Members of the genus *Streptococcus* are widely distributed in nature and may be found in milk and dairy products, water, dust, vegetation, and the normal respiratory tract and intestinal tract of various animals, including humans. The majority are probably saprophytic and nonpathogenic, but a number of species are pathogens for humans and animals.

The single streptococcal cell is characteristically spherical but may appear elliptical on occasion. The cells normally occur in **chains** of varying lengths (Plate 47). Cell size varies from 0.5 to 1 μm in diameter, depending on growth conditions and age of culture. Large cells are seen occasionally with normal-sized cells in a chain in an aged culture, whereas undersized cells may appear with normal cells in anaerobic culture.

Liquid cultures normally yield longer chains (Fig. 17-1) than cultures grown on agar. Beta-hemolytic streptococci may exhibit long chains in human infections and in milk from diseased cows.

Streptococci are characteristically **gram positive** but may become gram negative as the cells age. Although a few motile forms have been

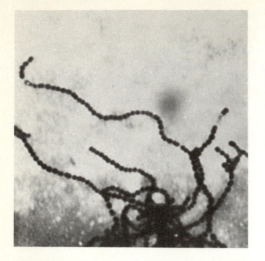

FIG. 17-1
Streptococcus pyogenes, showing chain arrangement
(1,000×).

reported, the streptococci are primarily **nonmotile.** Virulent forms are usually encapsulated and contain an abundance of hyaluronic acid in the capsule. Streptococcal colonies are small, translucent to slightly opaque, circular, generally less than 1 mm in diameter, convex, and appear as minute beads of moisture on a moist agar surface. On drier surfaces, colonies are less moist and almost opaque. By comparison, pneumococcal colonies are flatter and translucent.

Colony variation is quite common, with **mucoid, smooth** or **glossy,** and **matte** or **rough** forms. The mucoid and matte forms contain relatively large amounts of M protein and are virulent, whereas the smooth or glossy forms contain very little of this substance and are usually avirulent.

The organisms grow well on most enriched media and are generally facultative in relation to their oxygen requirements, although some strains are obligately anaerobic (see Chapter 28). They produce quite large amounts of lactic acid, without gas, from fermentable carbohydrates. **Inulin** is usually not fermented, and the organisms are **not soluble** in bile salts. The latter cri-

terion, especially, distinguishes other streptococci from the species *S. pneumoniae* (see Chapter 18). They differ also from the staphylococci and micrococci in being **catalase negative.** The catalase reaction with hydrogen peroxide occasionally presents problems.[12] There are, uncommonly, peroxidase-producing *Streptococcus* and *Aerococcus* strains, and catalase-negative *Micrococcus* and *Staphylococcus* are not differentiated with the relatively simple catalase test. They can be differentiated by means of the benzidine test. A positive benzidine test indicates that the strain contains cytochromes and thus is a member of the Micrococcaceae. A negative reaction indicates that a gram-positive coccus is a member of the Streptococcaceae. It should be noted that benzidine is a potential carcinogen. Accordingly, caution should be used when working with this compound.

CLASSIFICATION OF STREPTOCOCCI

Various classifications for the streptococci have been used over the years. Brown's classification is based on the reactions obtained in **blood agar.**[4] The Lancefield[23] system, based on the antigenic characteristics of **group-specific C substance,** is considered the most reliable. C substance is a cell-wall polysaccharide, which permits the arrangement of the streptococci into a number of antigenic groups identified as Lancefield groups A, B, C, D, and so forth.

Various characteristics useful for differentiating the streptococci and aerococci are given in Table 17-1.

HEMOLYTIC REACTIONS ON BLOOD AGAR

The most useful criterion for the preliminary differentiation of human streptococcal strains is their hemolytic activity on blood agar. As originally postulated by Brown, several types can be observed, particularly in subsurface colonies in pour or stabbed plates.[18]

Alpha (α)—an indistinct zone of partially lysed red cells surrounds the colony, fre-

TABLE 17-1

Characteristics of value for differentiating the major categories of streptococci and aerococci

Category	Most common cellular arrangement	Hemolysis	Streptococcal group antigen	Hydrolysis of bile esculin	Growth in 6.5% NaCl	Bile solubility
Beta-hemolytic "groupable" streptococci	Chains	Beta	A, B, C, F, and G	−	−*	−
Group D streptococci						
Enterococci	Short chains, diplococci	Alpha, beta, none	D	+	+	−
Non-enterococci	Short chains, diplococci	Alpha, none	D	+	−	−
Viridans streptococci	Chains	Alpha, none	None†	−*	−	−
Pneumococci	Diplococci, short chains	Alpha	None	−	−	+
Aerococci	Single cells, tetrads	Alpha, none	None	V	+	−

From Facklam.[12]

+, positive; −, negative; V, variable.

*Occasional exceptions.

†No group B or D antigens present, occasionally group A, C, F, or G antigens present.

quently accompanied by a greenish or brownish discoloration, which is best seen around subsurface colonies (Plate 44).

Beta (β)—a clear, colorless zone surrounds the colony, indicating complete lysis of the red blood cells (Plate 46). This is best seen in deep colonies in a pour plate. Surface colonies, on the other hand, may appear as alpha hemolytic or nonhemolytic because of inactivation of one of the hemolysins, **streptolysin O,** which is **oxygen labile; streptolysin S,** an **oxygen-stable** hemolysin, may be present in only small amounts in these strains showing poor surface hemolysis.

Gamma (γ)—colonies show no apparent hemolysis or discoloration in either surface or subsurface colonies.

Alpha-prime (α′), or wide-zone alpha—a small zone of alpha hemolysis surrounds the colony, with a zone of complete or beta hemolysis extending beyond this zone into the medium (Plate 45). This can be confused with a beta-hemolytic colony when examined only macroscopically.

Hemolysis of mammalian erythrocytes by the streptococci involves a complex system of many variables, including the influence of the basal medium, the production of streptolysins O and S by a given strain, the effect of various types of blood (sheep, horse, rabbit, human), aerobic or anaerobic incubation, and so forth. To begin with, a good basal medium, such as soybean-casein digest agar* without dextrose (the acid produced by carbohydrate fermentation inactivates streptolysin S) at pH 7.3 to 7.4, to which 5% defibrinated sheep blood has been added, is recommended. This medium will support the

---

*BBL trypticase soy agar, Difco tryptic soy agar.

growth of fastidious strains and permit good differentiation of the various types of hemolysis.

Although much has been written about the species of red blood cells and their effect on hemolytic patterns, it appears that this is restricted to the enterococci, of which over 90% show alpha hemolysis on sheep blood agar but are beta hemolytic on other mammalian blood agar media.[38] Sheep blood is recommended, especially for its inhibitory action on the growth of *Haemophilus hemolyticus*, a normal throat commensal whose beta-hemolytic colonies may be confused with those of beta-hemolytic streptococci. When in doubt, the examination of a Gram stain of the suspected colony will rapidly differentiate gram-positive streptococci from gram-negative bacillary forms of *H. hemolyticus*. It should be stressed that outdated human bank blood is *not* recommended for preparation of blood agar, because it may contain inhibitory factors, such as antibacterial substances, antibiotics, or an excess of citrate ion.

Although incubation under increased CO_2 tension (candle jar or CO_2 incubator) for 18 to 24 hours has been recommended for the isolation and recognition of beta-hemolytic streptococci on streaked and stabbed sheep blood agar plates, it should be noted that anaerobic incubation or prolonged aerobic incubation and subsequent overnight refrigeration may increase hemolytic activity of these organisms. However, Murray and associates[28] noted that significantly more non–group A beta-hemolytic streptococci grow in an anaerobic or CO_2 atmosphere. Accordingly, they recommended **aerobic** incubation (with stabbing of the medium) for throat swabs where only group A streptococci are of concern. Aerobic incubation is satisfactory for pour plates.

PREPARATION OF POUR PLATES

The ideal method of identification of hemolytic activity is by the **microscopic examination** of subsurface colonies in a blood agar **pour plate.** Although not always practical, it is not a difficult procedure, and may be carried out as follows:

1. Melt a tube of sterile soy-casein digest agar (15 to 20 ml) and cool to approximately 45 C.
2. Aseptically add 0.6 to 0.8 ml of sterile defibrinated sheep blood.
3. Inoculate this with one **small** loopful (drained against inner wall of tube) of a suspension prepared from the original throat swab suspended in 1 ml of sterile Todd-Hewitt broth.
4. Mix the inoculated medium by rotating the tube between the palms of the hands and pour into a sterile Petri plate. Allow to harden; incubate overnight at 35 C. If desired, one may also streak the surface of the plate with a loopful of the suspension.

When colonies are examined microscopically, the illumination is reduced, and the low-power objective (100× total magnification) is focused on both the colony and the layer of blood cells in approximately the same plane. A colony near the bottom of the plate should be selected for examination to minimize the effect of the intervening agar in focusing on the inverted plate. Surface colonies are examined with the lid of the plate removed.

BETA-HEMOLYTIC STREPTOCOCCI

As previously indicated, beta-hemolytic streptococci produce surface or subsurface colonies surrounded by a clear, cell-free zone of hemolysis. Although seen best in pour plates, beta hemolysis may also be demonstrated by making several stabs with the inoculating loop into the agar at the time of plate streaking. This permits subsurface growth and participation by both streptolysins O and S, if present.

Although beta-hemolytic streptococci of groups A, B, C, D, E, F, G, H, K, L, M, O, and others are found in Lancefield's classification,* **group A strains** (*S. pyogenes*) are most often associated with communicable disease in hu-

*Antisera are available for these and other groups from Difco Laboratories, Detroit, and Burroughs Wellcome Co., Research Triangle Park, N.C.

mans and are the etiologic agents in streptococcal pharyngitis, scarlet fever (*Staphylococcus aureus* may also cause this), epidemic wound infections, erysipelas (Plate 41) and so forth. Group A streptococcal infections are of particular concern because of the sequelae—rheumatic fever and glomerulonephritis. They are subdivided serologically into 44 M types and 26 T agglutination types, depending on type-specific surface antigens.[17] According to Moody and coworkers,[27] more than 90% of group A strains can be typed by a combination of M precipitin and T agglutination procedures.

Human pathogens may also occur among other serologic groups, including groups B and D. Group B strains (*S. agalactiae*) are normally present in the vagina and may be associated with maternal septicemia and neonatal septicemia, pneumonia, and meningitis,[2] as well as other infections in humans[31]; animal strains are involved in bovine mastitis (Plate 42). Group B streptococci are now the major bacterial pathogen in the newborn. Adult males may also develop serious infection with group B streptococci on occasion. The high morbidity and mortality associated with group B streptococcal infection in newborns make rapid, accurate identification of this organism extremely important. Several selective media have been helpful in this regard and for epidemiologic studies.[15,16] Group D strains, including enterococci, are discussed in a subsequent section.

Occasionally, strains of groups C, F, and G have been reported in human infections, including bacteremia, endocarditis, wound infection, abscesses, meningitis, pneumonia, and respiratory and genitourinary tract infection.[10] These strains generally produce beta hemolysis on blood agar. Other beta-hemolytic streptococci are encountered even less commonly but may cause serious infection.[3]

Benzyl penicillin (penicillin G) and other penicillins, including ampicillin, are the drugs of choice in the treatment of infections caused by streptococci of groups A, B, C, F, G, and others. Sulfonamides or erythromycin are sometimes

TABLE 17-2

Differentiation of streptococci found in human infections by serological characteristics

Beta-hemolytic (use group A, B, C, D, F, and G antisera)

Group A	*Streptococcus pyogenes*
Group B	*Streptococcus agalactiae*
Group C*	*Streptococcus equisimilis*, *S. zooepidemicus*, or *S. equi*
Group D	See Table 17-3
Group F	*Streptococcus anginosus*
Group G	Lancefield group G
None	Beta-hemolytic streptococcus, unable to demonstrate group antigen

Non–beta-hemolytic (use group B and D antisera only)

Group B	*Streptococcus agalactiae*
Group D	See Table 17-3

Not group B or D
  Quellung positive† with Omniserum or pooled pneumoccocal antisera
      Streptococcus pneumoniae
  Quellung negative† with Omniserum or pooled pneumoccocal antisera
      Viridans species (see Table 17-3)

From Facklam.[12]
S. equisimilis forms acid in trehalose but not sorbitol broth, *S. zooepidemicus* forms acid in sorbitol but not trehalose broth, and *S equi* does not form acid in either trehalose or sorbitol broth.
†Bile solubility and Optochin susceptibility can be substituted for the quellung test.

used prophylactically against group A streptococcal infections in patients with rheumatic heart disease. Erythromycin is a good therapeutic alternative to penicillin in an individual with hypersensitivity to that drug.

Table 17-2 differentiates the streptococci on the basis of serologic characteristics.

THE BACITRACIN DISK TEST AND OTHER TESTS FOR GROUP A STREPTOCOCCI

A useful **presumptive** test for differentiating group A from other groups of beta-hemolytic streptococci is the bacitracin disk test, first introduced by Maxted[25] and modified by Levinson and Frank.[24] The test depends on the selective inhibition of group A streptococci on a blood agar plate by a paper disk containing 0.04 unit of bacitracin.* (**Caution:** Use the differential disk containing 0.04 unit, not the sensitivity disk containing 10 units.) A high degree of correlation (95%)† between bacitracin and serologic tests with group A streptococci exists if the following conditions are fulfilled[12,18]:

1. A **pure culture** of a beta-hemolytic colony is used—do not use on a primary plate of a mixed culture.
2. A fresh, **moist** blood agar plate must be used—an old, dry plate will reduce diffusion of the bacitracin, giving a false-negative reading.
3. The inoculum size must be such as to ensure **confluent growth**—a light growth of other streptococci may show inhibition zones.
4. The bacitracin disks must be stored in the refrigerator with a desiccant and should be checked biweekly for performance with known group A and non–group A strains. Each new lot of disks obtained also should be checked on receipt.
5. The test should be used only to differentiate **beta**-hemolytic gram-positive streptococci—some alpha strains may show moderate zones of inhibition (8 to 10mm).
6. **Any zone of inhibition,** regardless of size, is positive. In reporting a positive test, the results should be worded "Beta-hemolytic streptococcus (probably group A)" or "Beta-hemolytic streptococcus, presumptively group A by bacitracin test."

Further identification procedures include the use of immunofluorescence techniques and the Lancefield and other serologic procedures, described in Chapters 37 and 39. Nahm and associates[29] have used a monoclonal mouse antibody to streptococcal group A carbohydrate for the Lancefield precipitin test and for immunofluorescence. Both reagents were identically reactive by the precipitin test, but the monoclonal antibody gave the same reactivity in the immunofluorescence test as in the precipitin test, whereas commercial antibodies gave both false-positive and false-negative readings in the fluorescent antibody test. Accordingly, monoclonal reagents appear to be superior to conventional antisera for fluorescent antibody procedures.

OTHER TESTS FOR BETA-HEMOLYTIC STREPTOCOCCI

Gel diffusion technique has been utilized for serologic identification of group B streptococci with favorable results.[9] CIE has been utilized for detection of group B streptococci in specimens containing mixed flora.[14] CIE was used to detect group B streptococci in broths that have been directly inoculated with the clinical sample. After 20 hours of incubation, a positive CIE result was obtained in 54% of specimens that eventually were shown to contain group B streptococci by the Lancefield technique. There were no false-positive CIE results, but a negative result would be considered indeterminate. The CAMP factor is a diffusible, heat-stable extracellular streptococcal protein that acts synergistically with staphylococcal beta hemolysin on sheep or ox erythrocytes. The test is performed by initially streaking a strain of *Staphylococcus* down the center of a blood agar plate. The streptococcal isolate is then streaked perpendicularly to the staphylococcal inoculum without touching it. Group A and group B controls should be included. After overnight incubation at 35 C, the plate is observed for an arrowhead pattern of hemolysis adjacent to the staphylococcal streak—a positive test (Plate 48). A gas chromatographic procedure has been used to analyze carbohydrates of whole cells of various groups of

---

*Available from Baltimore Biological Laboratory (Taxo A); Difco Laboratories (Bacto Differentiation Disc Bacitracin).
†Approximately 0.5% of group A streptococci will be missed by this test, and about 4% of non–group A strains will be incorrectly identified as group A.

beta-hemolytic streptococci as well as group D.[33] A rapid coagglutination method (Plate 244) for identification of group B streptococci in blood cultures has been described.[20]

ALPHA- AND GAMMA-HEMOLYTIC STREPTOCOCCI

Streptococci that generally do not possess group antigens and produce alpha or no hemolysis on blood agar are known collectively as the **viridans streptococcus** group. They are constantly present in the human oropharynx and include such species as *S. salivarius*, *S. mitis*, *S. mutans*, and *S. sanguis*. These organisms are the most frequent cause of subacute bacterial endocarditis, an insidious and fatal infection (if untreated) that usually follows dental or surgical procedures or instrumentation in patients with a previously damaged heart valve or other lesions of the endocardium. These organisms, which often require CO_2 for growth (capnophilic or microaerophilic streptococci), may also play a role in certain other serious infections, such as bacteremia, brain abscess, necrotizing pneumonia, or liver abscess. Biochemical characterization of 153 such strains from clinical material was done by Pulliam and colleagues.[34]

Colonies of alpha-hemolytic streptococci must be distinguished from those of pneumococci or enterococci, both of which also may produce alpha hemolysis on blood agar. Table 17-3 shows some tests that are useful in identifying the alpha-hemolytic (or nonhemolytic) streptococci and group D streptococci; other differential tests are indicated in subsequent sections. Setterstrom and others[36] tested 56 strains of viridans streptococci and obtained excellent overall agreement regarding characterization between the Minitek system and conventional methods provided that (1) all disks were incubated anaerobically for 48 hours, except for esculin and arginine, which required 5 to 7 days; (2) the arginine disks were overlaid with 0.1 ml of sterile mineral oil, even though incubated anaerobically; (3) the Voges-Proskauer tests were performed under

aerobic and anaerobic conditions; and (4) all tests for carbohydrate fermentation, except for raffinose and salicin, were read after the addition of two to three drops of 0.025% phenol red at pH 7.2. Only the starch fermentation test was unreliable. Inulin results were obtained by conventional methods, since this is not available in the Minitek system. Holloway and co-workers[19] also obtained good results with a large number of strains of viridans streptococci with the Minitek system as compared with a conventional system. The API ZYM method was found to be useful in the rapid identification of a number of types of alpha-hemolytic and nonhemolytic streptococci.[39] API now has a system (API 20S Streptococcus system) that uses micromethods for biochemical identification of streptococci and that is said to identify groups A and B streptococci, beta-hemolytic non–A, B, or D streptococci, and D enterococcal and viridans strains. Micromedia has a Strep Combo panel using a prefilled plastic microdilution tray that contains 10 antimicrobial drugs and 15 biochemical reagents. This differentiates streptococci of groups A, B, D, and Q from each other and from staphylococci or micrococci and speciates group D. Formal evaluation of the latter two systems is not yet available.

Penicillin G is the antibiotic of choice in the treatment of streptococcal (nonenterococcal) subacute bacterial endocarditis. It is essential that the organism be isolated promptly from blood cultures (see Chapter 7) and its antimicrobial susceptibility (with bactericidal endpoint) determined.

This antimicrobial agent is also recommended as prophylactic therapy for patients with rheumatic or congenital heart disease who undergo dental or surgical procedures. For penicillin-allergic patients, erythromycin, a cephalosporin, and vancomycin are satisfactory substitutes. Bourgault and colleagues[1] have presented data on antimicrobial susceptibility patterns of 63 strains of viridans streptococci. Penicillin G was the most active agent, with minimal inhibitory

TABLE 17-3

Differentiation of group D and viridans streptococci and aerococci found in human infections

Columns grouped as: Hemolysis (Alpha, Beta, None) and Physiological tests (Bile-esculin through Glucans).

Species	Alpha	Beta	None	Bile-esculin	Growth in 6.5% NaCl	Growth at 10 C	Pyruvate	Arginine	Esculin	Starch	Hippurate	Sucrose	Lactose	Mannitol	Sorbitol	Arabinose	Sorbose	Inulin	Raffinose	Glucans
S. faecalis	+	+	+	+	+	+	+	+*	+	−	V	+*	+*	+	+*	−*	−	−	−*	N
S. faecium	+	−	+	+	+	+	−	+	+	−	V	+	+	+	−	+*	−	+*	+*	N
S. avium	+	−	+	+	+	+	+	−	+	−	−	+	+	+	+	+	+	+	+	N
S. durans	+	−	−*	+	+	+	−	+	+	−	V	−	−	−	−	−	−	−	−*	N
Aerococci	+	+	+	V	+	−	−	−	V	−	+*	+*	+*	V	−	−	−	+*	V	N
S. bovis	−	−	+	+	−	−	−	−	+	+	−	+	+	+	−	−	−	+	+	L
S. mutans	−*	+	+	−*	−	−	−	+*	+*	−	−	+	+	+	+	−	−	+	+	D
S. uberis	+	−	−	−	−*	−	−	−	+	−	+*	+	+	+	−	−*	−	+	+	N
S. MG-intermedius	−*	−	−*	−*	−	−	−	+*	+*	+*	−	+	+	−	−	−	−	−	+*	N*
S. bovis (var.)	−*	−	+	+	−	−	−	−	+	−	−	+	+	−	−	−	−	−	+	N
S. anginosus constel-latus	+	−	+*	−*	−	−	−	+*	+*	−	−	+	+	−	−	−	−	−	−	N
S. equinus	+	−	+	+	−	−	−	−	+	−	−	+	+	−	−	+*	−	−	+*	N
S. sanguis I	+	−	−*	−*	−	−	+*	+	+*	+*	−	+	+	−	+*	−	−	+	−*	D*
S. salivarius	−*	−	+	−*	−	−	−	+	+*	+	−	+	+*	−	−	−	−	+	+*	L*
S. mitis	+	−	+*	−	−	−	−	−	−	−	−	+	+	−	−	−	−	−	−	N*
S. sanguis II	+	−	−*	−	−	−	−	−	−	+*	−	+	+	−	−	−	−	−	+	D*
S. morbillorum	−*	−	+	−	−	−	−	−	−	−*	−	+	+	−	−	−	−	−	−	N
S. acidominimus	+	−	−*	−	−	−	−	−	−	−	+*	+	−	−	−	−	−	−	−	N

From Facklam.[12]

+, positive; −, negative; V, variable reactions; *, occasional exceptions occur. For glucans: D, dextran; L, levans; N, no glucans.

concentrations of 0.06 to 4.0 µg/ml. In general, they found that *S. mitis* and *S. sanguis* type II required higher concentrations of antibiotics for inhibition and killing than did other species of viridans streptococci.

NUTRITIONALLY VARIANT STREPTOCOCCI

As noted in Chapter 7, nutritionally deficient or variant streptococci may be isolated from bacteremia and endocarditis. Although most of the isolates of this type of *Streptococcus* have been from blood cultures, such organisms have also been recovered from a pancreatic abscess and from pleural fluid. These and other observations suggest that the nutritional variants may reside not only in the oral cavity but also in the urogenital and gastrointestinal tracts. Roberts and co-workers[35] studied isolates from consecutive patients with endocarditis caused by viridans streptococci from the periods 1944 to 1955 and 1970 to 1978. Vitamin B_6–dependent streptococci classified as *S. mitior* accounted for 5% to 6% of endocarditis in both time periods. Again as noted in Chapter 7, media must be supplemented with either pyridoxal hydrochloride or pyridoxamine dihydrochloride (the active forms of vitamin B_6) for isolation, for identification, and probably for subsequent susceptibility testing of these agents. The latter point is not established. At least in terms of minimal inhibitory concentrations, according to Cooksey and Swenson,[7] susceptibility results were the same whether or not pyridoxal hydrochloride was added to the test system. Others, however, have noted that isolates may appear susceptible to penicillin G in unsupplemented media but resistant when media are supplemented with pyridoxal hydrochloride. Streptomycin is particularly active against these variants, and it has been suggested that the combination of penicillin G and streptomycin should ordinarily be used to treat endocarditis caused by this type of organism. In studies at CDC over a 2-year period, Cooksey and associates[8] found that the biochemical patterns of the isolates that are nutritionally variant resembled those of five viridans streptococcal species. Two isolates, however, had patterns that did not resemble those of any viridans species.

Washington[40] noted that nutritional variants of streptococci are usually recognized, because they produce turbidity or flocculent growth in broth cultures and resemble streptococci microscopically on Gram stain but fail to grow when subcultured onto ordinary media. He pointed out that there is a definite risk that the microbiologist may presume that these organisms represent nonviable residues of the medium's original sterilization process and that it is imperative for technicians to be aware of the existence of nutritional variants and to do appropriate tests to confirm or rule out their presence. Since these organisms grow as satellite colonies around other organisms such as *Staphylococcus aureus*, this represents a simple first step to check for their presence. The next step would be to subculture to media supplemented with pyridoxal hydrochloride or other appropriate materials. Further complicating the situation is the fact that Sherman and Washington have isolated a **pyridoxine-sensitive viridans streptococcus** from the blood of a patient with endocarditis.

GROUP D STREPTOCOCCI, INCLUDING ENTEROCOCCI

The role of enterococci in bacterial endocarditis is well established. When enterococci are found in bacteremia, the significance is not always clear. A study by Wells and von Graevenitz[41] evaluated the clinical significance of enterococci in blood cultures. They found that persons whose septicemia seemed likely on clinical grounds showed significantly more positive sets of blood cultures and showed two positive bottles in a single set more often than did patients with less likelihood of significant sepsis on clinical grounds. The patients who were likely to have bacteremia from the clinical standpoint also grew cultures with shorter detection times, 90% yielding enterococci within 3 days after collection.

The significant association of *Streptococcus bovis* septicemia with carcinoma of the colon or other intestinal malignancy is important to note.

The streptococci that react serologically with Lancefield group D antisera comprise two different categories. The first contains the **enterococci**, *S. faecalis* and *S. faecium*, of human intestinal origin and important agents in human infections. The second category includes the **nonenterococci** of group D, *S. bovis* and *S. equinus*. Although most human group D clinical isolates are *S. faecalis*, *S. bovis* is being recovered increasingly from patients with subacute bacterial endocarditis and may be found in other infections as well. The differentiation is important, since *S. bovis* is penicillin susceptible and *S. faecalis* is not. It may be that *S. equinus* occurs more commonly than has been appreciated. A study by Bump[5] over a 6-month period revealed that 10% of enterococci from nonrespiratory sources were *S. equinus*. Klein and co-workers[21] reported two cases of *S. equinus* septicemia and cited another report in which seven cases of bacterial endocarditis caused by this organism were reported. The strains isolated from the patients by Klein and associates were very sensitive to penicillin G.

Generally, group D streptococci appear as alpha-hemolytic or nonhemolytic colonies on sheep blood agar; occasional varieties of *S. faecalis* (var. *zymogenes*) will produce wide zones of beta hemolysis. Some group D strains have a distinct buttery odor on the medium. A commercially available sodium chloride plate medium yielded false-negative growth because of the presence of paraffin.[6] Urinary isolates of enterococci that require thymine have been noted to fail to grow on Mueller-Hinton medium used for susceptibility testing, although they grew well on blood agar.[32] Such strains may satellite around *Escherichia coli* and will grow around thymine-impregnated disks. Such thymine-dependent enterococci are resistant to cotrimoxazole.

Traditionally, group D strains have been differentiated from other streptococci by their ability to grow at 45 C and by being thermostable at 60 C for 30 minutes; however, streptococci of other groups may demonstrate these characteristics, especially when standardized test conditions have not been met. The most accurate presumptive test for recognizing group D streptococci is the use of **bile esculin medium** (BEM).[11] Incorporating bile (oxgall) into an agar or broth medium containing esculin* makes the medium selective for the growth of enterococci (also *Listeria monocytogenes* and Enterobacteriaceae) that are capable of hydrolyzing esculin to 6,7-dehydroxycoumarin. This reacts with an iron salt in the medium to form a **dark brown or black** compound (Plate 43). The agar slant or broth is inoculated with a pure culture and examined after 48 hours' incubation at 35 C for the production of a brownish-black color. Plus-minus reactions are read as negative.

Another useful biochemical test for the identification of enterococci is growth in heart infusion broth containing **6.5% sodium chloride** in 18 to 24 hours.

The results of these tests are interpreted as follows[11]:

1. BEM positive, salt tolerance positive—enterococcus
2. BEM positive, salt tolerance negative—group D streptococcus, not enterococcus
3. BEM negative, salt tolerance negative—non–group D streptococcus (serologic grouping suggested)

Enterococci can usually be differentiated from other streptococci by reduction of litmus milk within 4 hours (Schierl and Blazevic: J. Clin. Microbiol. **14:**227-228, 1981). Serologic identification of group D streptococci may be

---

*Several bile esculin media are available: Difco BE agar contains 4% oxgall, Pfizer PSE agar and BBL enterococcus agar contain 1% oxgall plus sodium azide. Some viridans strains may grow and hydrolyze esculin in the latter medium. Accordingly, Facklam[11] recommends the BEM with 4% oxgall. Broth media also are available.

done by the coagglutination technique or by the rapid latex test system. However it is important to supplement these with the bile esculin (BE) and NaCl tests.

The therapy of choice in the treatment of serious enterococcal infections is penicillin (or ampicillin) plus gentamicin or streptomycin (or another aminoglycoside); if penicillin allergy exists, vancomycin may be used. A study of 34 strains of enterococci from clinical specimens revealed that all showed tolerance, although the minimal inhibitory concentrations with penicillin and vancomycin were relatively low.[22] Very high minimal bactericidal concentrations were also seen with four strains of S. *bovis*.

PRESUMPTIVE IDENTIFICATION OF STREPTOCOCCI

Facklam[12] pointed out that several combinations of the tests listed in Table 17-4 can be used to presumptively identify streptococci. The sim-

plest, most convenient, and most accurate combination is bacitracin, sulfamethoxazole and trimethoprim (SXT), CAMP, BE, and the sodium chloride test on agar plates along with the hemolytic reactions. This group of tests should be interpreted as a whole. Facklam then used the following criteria to identify streptococci:

1. Group A streptococci are beta hemolytic, susceptible to bacitracin, resistant to SXT, CAMP reaction negative, and BE negative.
2. Group B streptococci are beta hemolytic, variably susceptible to bacitracin and SXT (mostly resistant to both), CAMP reaction positive, and BE negative. Occasional nonhemolytic group B strains have comparable reaction patterns.
3. Groups C, F, and G streptococci (beta hemolytic, not group A, B, or D) react in three patterns to bacitracin and SXT. All strains are beta hemolytic and react nega-

TABLE 17-4

Presumptive identification of streptococci

Category	Hemolysis	Susceptibility to Bacitracin	SXT	CAMP reaction	Hippurate hydrolysis	Bile esculin reaction	Growth in 6.5% NaCl	Optochin and bile*
Group A	Beta	+	−	−	−	−	−	−
Group B	Beta†	−†	−	+	+	−	+†	−
Beta-hemolytic streptococci, not group A, B, or D	Beta	−†	+	−	−	−	−	−
Group D, enterococcus	Alpha, beta, none	−	−	−	−	+†	+	−
Group D, not enterococcus	Alpha, none	−	+†	−	−	+	−	−
Viridans group	Alpha, none	+†	+	−	−†	−†	−	−
Pneumococcus	Alpha	±	?	−	−	−	−	+

From Facklam.[12]

SXT, Sulfamethoxazole and trimethoprim; +, positive reaction or susceptible; −, negative reaction or resistant.
*Optochin susceptibility and bile solubility.
†Exceptions occasionally occur.

tively in CAMP and BE tests. Most strains are resistant to bacitracin and susceptible to SXT. An appreciable number of these strains may be susceptible to both compounds; a few strains are resistant to both compounds.

4. Group D enterococcal streptococci vary in their hemolytic reaction. Most strains are nonhemolytic, but alpha- and beta-hemolytic strains are common. All strains are resistant to bacitracin and react negatively in CAMP tests. Three patterns of reaction from the SXT, BE, and NaCl tests are characteristic of enterococci. Most strains react positively in BE and NaCl tolerance tests and are resistant to SXT. Some are susceptible to SXT and react positively in BE and NaCl tests. Some are resistant to SXT and tolerant to NaCl (NaCl positive) but are BE negative.

5. Group D nonenterococcal streptococci are alpha hemolytic or nonhemolytic and are usually resistant to bacitracin. However, occasional strains are sensitive, vary in their reactions to SXT disks, are BE positive, and are NaCl intolerant.

6. Viridans streptococci are alpha hemolytic or nonhemolytic and vary in their reaction to bacitracin and SXT. However, most strains are susceptible to SXT and negative in CAMP, BE, and NaCl tolerance tests.

Using this interpretation, 97% of medically important streptococci can be identified presumptively, according to Facklam.[12] Streptococci that do not fit into one of the above reaction patterns should be checked for purity and retested. If the results are still atypical, the streptococci should be serologically grouped and definitively identified in a reference laboratory.

Facklam and associates[13] recommend that the bacitracin, SXT, and CAMP disks be stored at −20 C. They are stable for 1 month at this temperature and may be stable for less than 5 days at 4 C. Any zone of inhibition of growth around either the bacitracin or SXT disks is considered a positive result. The BE plate test is more difficult to interpret than the tube test. Some enterococci react very weakly. Tests should be read against a white background, and any blackening of the medium should be considered a positive reaction, even though this will result in some viridans streptococci being misidentified as group D nonenterococcal streptococci. This error is less dangerous than is misidentifying enterococci, since the antibiotic susceptibilities of the group D nonenterococci are similar to those of the viridans group.

The 6.5% NaCl plates are difficult to interpret. These plates should be carefully inspected immediately after inoculation to be certain that the inoculum is spread so as to not be read as growth.[13]

Various rapid tests for esculin hydrolysis, sodium chloride tolerance, and the CAMP test have been described. There are also various systems for inoculating test media that may facilitate the work in the laboratory. An alpha-toxin–producing strain of *Clostridium perfringens* has been used in place of *S. aureus* in the CAMP test. An alpha-toxin disk test has been described in which group B streptococci completed the hemolysis of sheep erythrocytes partially lysed by the alpha-toxin of *C. perfringens*.[37] The test could be performed satisfactorily on the primary isolation plate of sheep blood agar as well as with the pure culture technique. Ninety-five percent of strains of pure group B streptococci produced positive reactions within 5 hours, and all were positive after overnight incubation. Some workers believe that production of pigment by group B streptococci can be very helpful in characterizing these organisms. In one study[26] pigment was produced in stab cultures in a modified medium by 97% of 297 group B streptococci from clinical specimens. Penicillin is the drug of choice for *S. bovis* and *S. equinus* infections.

Genus Aerococcus

Aerococcus grows primarily in **tetrads** and **clumps,** but occasional single or paired cells are noted. The genus is distinct from *Staphylococ-*

cus and *Micrococcus* by virtue of a **negative** benzidine test. Aerococci may release oxygen from hydrogen peroxide, but this is not catalase mediated. Acid is **not** produced from glucose in anaerobic culture, whereas it usually is by *Streptococcus* (also benzidine negative).

Aerococcus may resemble enterococcal group D streptococci in that most strains tolerate 6.5% sodium chloride and 40% bile, and some strains blacken bile esculin medium. However, *Aerococcus* does not possess the group D antigen, does not grow at 10 or 45 C, and does not hydrolyze arginine.

Aerococcus viridans is alpha hemolytic, but the greening may be delayed until 48 hours of incubation. Hippurate is split by most strains, often slowly.

Aerococcus-like organisms have been isolated from blood cultures of patients with subacute bacterial endocarditis and bacteremia, from urine cultures of patients with urinary tract infection, and, rarely, from empyema and wound infections.[30] The group is apparently much more susceptible to antibiotics than are the enterococci.

REFERENCES

1. Bourgault, A.M., Wilson, W.R., and Washington, J.A., II: Antimicrobial susceptibilities of species of viridans streptococci, J. Infect. Dis. **140**:316-321, 1979.
2. Braunstein, H., Tucker, E.B., and Gibson, B.C.: Identification and significance of *Streptococcus agalactiae*, Am. J. Clin. Pathol. **51**:207-213, 1969.
3. Broome, C.V., Moellering, R.C., Jr., and Watson, B.K.: Clinical significance of Lancefield groups L-T streptococci isolated from blood and cerebrospinal fluid, J. Infect. Dis. **133**:382-392, 1976.
4. Brown, J.H.: Monograph no. 9, New York, 1919, Rockefeller Institute for Medical Research.
5. Bump, C.M.: Isolation of *Streptococcus equinus* from non-respiratory sources in children, J. Clin. Microbiol. **6**:433-434, 1977.
6. Butts, J., and Dees, C.: Inhibition of Lancefield group D enterococci by contamination of a commercial identification medium with paraffins, J. Clin. Microbiol. **12**:802-804, 1980.
7. Cooksey, R.C., and Swenson, J.M.: In vitro antimicrobial inhibition patterns of nutritionally variant streptococci, Antimicrob. Agents Chemother. **16**:514-518, 1979.
8. Cooksey, R.C., Thompson, F.S., and Facklam, R.R.: Physiological characterization of nutritionally variant streptococci, J. Clin. Microbiol. **10**:326-330, 1979.
9. Dillon, H.C., Jr., Pass, M.A., and Buchanan, B.: Modified method for serological identification of group B streptococci, J. Clin. Microbiol. **7**:599-600, 1978.
10. Duma, R.J., Weinbert, R.T., Medrek, T.F., and Kunz, L.J.: Streptococcal infections, Medicine **48**:87-127, 1969.
11. Facklam, R.R.: Comparison of several laboratory media for presumptive identification of enterococci and group D streptococci, Appl. Microbiol. **26**:138-145, 1973.
12. Facklam, R.R.: Streptococci and aerococci. In Lennette, E.H., Balows, A., Hausler, W.J., Jr., and Truant, J.P., editors: Manual of clinical microbiology, ed. 3, Washington, D.C., 1980, American Society for Microbiology.
13. Facklam, R.R., Padula, J.F., Wortham, E.C., Cooksey, R.C., and Rountree, H.A.: Presumptive identification of group A, B, and D streptococci on agar plate media, J. Clin. Microbiol. **9**:665-672, 1979.
14. Fenton, L.J., and Harper, M.H.: Direct use of counterimmunoelectrophoresis in detection of group B streptococci in specimens containing mixed flora, J. Clin. Microbiol. **8**:500-502, 1978.
15. Fenton, L.J., and Harper, M.H.: Evaluation of colistin and nalidixic acid in Todd-Hewitt broth for selective isolation of group B streptococci, J. Clin. Microbiol. **9**:167-169, 1979.
16. Gray, B.M., Pass, M.A., and Dillon, H.C., Jr.: Laboratory and field evaluation of selective media for isolation of group B streptococci, J. Clin. Microbiol. **9**:466-470, 1979.
17. Griffith, F.: The serological classification of *Streptococcus pyogenes*, J. Hygiene **34**:542, 1934.
18. Hall, C.T., In Summary analysis of results for the proficiency testing survey in bacteriology (January 9, 1970), National Communicable Disease Center, May 7, 1970.
19. Holloway, Y., Schaareman, M., and Dankert, J.: Identification of viridans streptococci on the Minitek miniaturised differentiation system, J. Clin. Pathol. **32**:1168-1173, 1979.
20. Holmes, R.L., and Harada, W.A.: Rapid method for identification of group B streptococci in neonatal blood cultures, J. Clin. Microbiol. **13**:279-282, 1981.
21. Klein, R.S., Catalano, M.T., Edberg, S.C., and Casey, J.I.: *Streptococcus equinus* septicemia: report of two cases and review of the literature, Am. J. Med. Sci. **279**:99-103, 1980.
22. Krogstad, D.J., and Parquette, A.R.: Defective killing of enterococci: a common property of antimicrobial agents acting on the cell wall, Antimicrob. Agents Chemother. **17**:965-968, 1980.

23. Lancefield, R.C.: A serological differentiation of human and other groups of hemolytic streptococci, J. Exp. Med. 57:571-595, 1933.
24. Levinson, M.L., and Frank, P.F.: Differentiation of group A from other beta hemolytic streptococci with bacitracin, J. Bacteriol. 69:284-287, 1955.
25. Maxted, W.R.: The use of bacitracin for identifying group A hemolytic streptococci, J. Clin. Pathol. 6:224-226, 1953.
26. Merritt, K., and Jacobs, N.J.: Characterization and incidence of pigment production by human clinical group B streptococci, J. Clin. Microbiol. 8:105-107, 1978.
27. Moody, M.D., Padula, J., Lizana, D., and Hall, C.T.: Epidemiologic characterization of group A streptococci by T agglutination and M precipitation tests in the public health laboratory, Health Lab. Sci. 2:149-162, 1965.
28. Murray, P.R., Wold, A.D., Schreck, C.A., and Washington, J.A., II: Effects of selective media and atmosphere of incubation on the isolation of group A streptococci, J. Clin. Microbiol. 4:54-56, 1976.
29. Nahm, M.H., Murray, P.R., Clevinger, B.L., and Davie, J.M.: Improved diagnostic accuracy using monoclonal antibody to group A streptococcal carbohydrate, J. Clin. Microbiol. 12:506-508, 1980.
30. Parker, M.T., and Ball, L.C.: Streptococci and aerococci associated with systemic infections in man, J. Med. Microbiol. 9:275-302, 1976.
31. Patterson, M.J., and Hafeez, E.B.: Group B streptococci in human disease, Bacteriol. Rev. 40:774-792, 1976.
32. Plorde, J.J., and Bailey, T.: Thymine-requiring enterococci, Ann. Intern. Med. 91:134, 1979.
33. Pritchard, D.G., Coligan, J.E., Speed, S.E., and Gray, B.M.: Carbohydrate fingerprints of streptococcal cells, J. Clin. Microbiol. 13:89-92, 1981.
34. Pulliam, L., Porschen, R.K., and Hadley, W.K.: Biochemical properties of CO_2-dependent streptococci, J. Clin. Microbiol. 12:27-31, 1980.
35. Roberts, R.B., Krieger, A.G., Schiller, N.L., and Gross, K.C.: Viridans streptococcal endocarditis: the role of various species, including pyridoxal-dependent streptococci, Rev. Infect. Dis. 1:955-966, 1979.
36. Setterstrom, J.A., Gross, A., and Stanko, R.S.: Comparison of Minitek and conventional methods for the biochemical characterization of oral streptococci, J. Clin. Microbiol. 10:409-414, 1979.
37. Smith, J.A., and Ngui-Yen, J.H.: Evaluation of a clostridial alpha-toxin disk test for rapid presumptive identification of group B streptococci, J. Clin. Microbiol. 12:18-21, 1980.
38. Updyke, E.L.: Laboratory problems in the diagnosis of streptococcal infections, Public Health Lab. 15:78-80, 1957.
39. Waitkins, S.A., Ball, L.C., and Fraser, C.A.: Use of the API-ZYM system in rapid identification of α and non-haemolytic streptococci, J. Clin. Pathol. 33:53-57, 1980.
40. Washington, J.A., II: Nutritionally variant streptococci, Ann. Intern. Med. 87:793, 1977.
41. Wells, L.D., and von Graevenitz, A.: Clinical significance of enterococci in blood cultures from adult patients, Infection 8:147-151, 1980.

18 PNEUMOCOCCI

STREPTOCOCCUS PNEUMONIAE

The **pneumococcus** is a single species, *Streptococcus (Diplococcus) pneumoniae*. These organisms consist of **gram-positive lanceolate cocci,** characteristically appearing as diplococci but occasionally as short, tight chains or single cocci (Plate 13). In fresh specimens of sputum, spinal fluid, or other exudates, they are frequently surrounded by a capsule. Based on a specific capsular polysaccharide, 83 capsule types have been recognized.

The normal habitat of the pneumococcus is the upper respiratory tract of humans; from there it may invade the lungs and the systemic circulation. The pneumococcus is the most frequent cause of lobar pneumonia in adults. Bacteremia occurs in about one fourth of these patients, usually early in the course of the disease; the organisms also may extend to the pleural cavity or disseminate to the endocardium and pericardium, the meninges, joints, and so forth, with ensuing complications. Pneumococci have also been implicated in infections of the middle ear, mastoid, and eye; they are occasionally isolated from peritoneal fluid, urine, vaginal secretions, wound exudates, and other clinical specimens. Carrier rates in the respiratory tract of healthy adults may vary from 30% to 70%, depending on the season of the year.

Pneumococci require an **enriched** medium for their primary isolation; trypticase or brain-heart infusion agar enriched with 5% defibrinated sheep, horse, or rabbit blood is recommended. Since 5% to 10% of strains require incubation under increased CO_2 tension to grow on primary plate culture, it is necessary to incubate such media in a candle jar or CO_2 incubator. Rare strains of pneumococcus require anaerobic incubation for primary growth.[24]

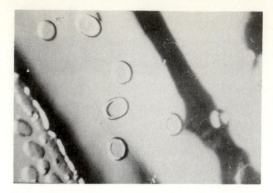

FIG. 18-1
Typical colony morphology of *S. pneumoniae* (20×).

CLINICAL SPECIMENS

The specimens usually submitted for culture include sputum, transtracheal aspirates, blood, CSF, nasopharyngeal swabs (particularly from the pediatric patient), purulent exudates, serous effusions, and so forth. Sputum, if tenacious, may be homogenized by repeated mixing with a small volume of broth in a sterile syringe without a needle attached. Otherwise, a carefully selected portion of purulent or bloody material is teased out with the split halves of a sterile wooden applicator stick, and one portion is inoculated to blood agar. The other portion may be used for preparing a direct smear for Gram staining.

CULTURAL CHARACTERISTICS

After overnight incubation, typical pneumococcal colonies on blood agar are round and glistening with entire edges, **transparent,** mucoid, and about 1 mm in diameter (Plate 49). They are surrounded by an approximate 2-mm zone of alpha hemolysis (beta hemolysis when incubated anaerobically[13]), because of the activity of hyaluronidase (Plate 4). Young colonies are usually dome shaped but on aging become flattened with a raised margin and depressed central portion (Fig. 18-1) or give the appearance of a **checker** or nail head. This is best seen with a dissecting microscope and oblique surface illumination. Alpha-hemolytic streptococci, by contrast, produce small, raised, **opaque** colonies. Colonies of type 3 pneumococcus (occasionally other types) are larger, more mucoid, and more confluent than those already described and resemble droplets of oil on the agar surface. These eventually flatten on drying and exhibit characteristics similar to those of other types.

IDENTIFICATION TESTS FOR PNEUMOCOCCI

In addition to the colony characteristics by which pneumococci may be tentatively identified, certain tests provide a means of differentiating these organisms from the alpha streptococci or other cocci. Among them are the tests for **bile solubility, Optochin susceptibility,** and the **Neufeld (quellung) reaction.**

Bile solubility test

Surface-active agents, such as bile, bile salts (sodium desoxycholate or taurocholate), or sodium dodecyl sulfate ("Dreft"), act on the cell wall of pneumococci and bring about lysis of the cell. In the bile solubility test used at the Mayo Clinic,[22] a few drops of 10% sodium desoxycholate are placed directly onto a 24-hour-old colony on a blood agar plate. The colony typically dissolves if it is a pneumococcus. (Be sure that the colony has not just been floated away by the reagent.) A broth test is described by Facklam.[6] A modification has been used to identify pneumococci in blood cultures.[18]

It should be noted that some strains of pneumococci are insoluble in bile, whereas some strains of alpha-hemolytic streptococci are soluble; the test, therefore, is not absolute.

Optochin susceptibility test

This is currently the most widely used test for differentiating pneumococci from other alpha-hemolytic streptococci. It was first described by Bowers and Jeffries[3] in 1955 and subsequently was modified. The test is carried out by placing a 6-mm or 10-mm absorbent paper disk containing ethylhydrocupreine HCl (Optochin)* on a blood agar plate heavily inoculated with a pure culture of the suspected strain. After overnight incubation in a candle jar or CO_2 incubator at 35 C, pneumococci exhibit zones of inhibition at least 14 or 16 mm in diameter with a 10-mm disk. Zones of 6 to 14 mm with the 6-mm disk and 10 to 16 mm with the 10-mm disk are questionable, and strains giving such zones should be presumptively identified as pneumococci only if they are bile soluble.

The CDC has received cultures of "penicillin-resistant pneumococci" that proved to be alpha streptococci, exhibiting a moderate inhibition zone (10 to 12 mm) to Optochin, especially when light inocula were used.[8]

Note: It is important that each new lot of Optochin disks be checked with known strains of pneumococci and alpha-hemolytic streptococci before use.

Neufeld (quellung) reaction

The **quellung** reaction is the most accurate, reliable, and specific test for the identification of pneumococci and pneumococcal types. Howev-

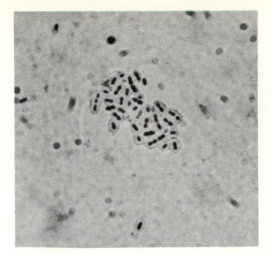

FIG. 18-2
Streptococcus pneumoniae, showing capsular swelling (1,000×).

er, it is used less often than it should be. The procedure, nevertheless, has proved of value in epidemiologic investigations and can be of considerable value in providing rapid, definitive identification of pneumococci in clinical specimens. Typing of penicillin-resistant strains is also important so that resistant types may eventually be incorporated in pneumococcal vaccines. The consensus is that the **capsular "swelling" reaction,** as it is popularly referred to, is not an actual swelling. The phenomenon is probably caused by a change of the refractive properties brought about by the union of the specific antiserum with the capsule (a precipitin reaction), which makes the outline of the capsule more readily visible. Fig. 18-2 and Plate 50 illustrate capsules seen in the quellung reaction. Capsular antisera for the pneumococci are available commercially*; an omnivalent serum, which reacts with all pneumococcal types, has been prepared by Lund and Rasmussen.[15] This "Omniserum"

---

*Taxo P disks, Baltimore Biological Laboratory, Cockeysville, Md.; Optochin disks, Difco Laboratories, Detroit; and others.

*Six pools of 33 types are available from Difco Laboratories, Detroit; Omniserum, 9 pools, and 46 monotypic sera are available from the State Serum Institute, Copenhagen.

has proved very useful as a reliable reagent for the rapid identification of pneumococci in clinical material, such as sputum, cerebrospinal, pleural, or synovial fluid, or in positive blood culture bottles. Not all the type-specific antibodies in Omniserum are in high enough titer to make the capsule visible. They produce agglutination, however, which sometimes must be the sole criterion for a positive reaction.[14]

In addition to the capsular reaction test[10] for identification and typing of pneumococci, one may use CIE,[10] which is less satisfactory, or capillary precipitin typing, which is simpler and as specific as the Neufeld test.[20] Merrill and associates[17] found the direct quellung (Omni) test on sputum smears considerably more accurate than Gram stains when correlated with culture results. There is also a commercially available (Phadebact) coagglutination test for identification of pneumococci.[5]

CIE has been used to detect pneumococcal antigen in sputum[12,21] and nasopharyngeal secretions of children.[4] When used to differentiate pneumococcal pneumonia from other types of pneumonia, CIE of sputum appears to be sensitive and specific. However, it lacks specificity in patients without pneumonia. Furthermore, there is evidence to suggest that sputum Gram stain may correlate as well as CIE with pneumococcal pneumonia.[21] The coagglutination test has also been used to rapidly detect pneumococcal antigens in sputum and blood serum. In one study it appeared to be at least as effective as CIE, and it is simpler.[5]

Directions for performance of the capsular swelling test are given in Chapter 37.

SIGNIFICANCE OF RECOVERY OF PNEUMOCOCCI

Because of the relatively high seasonal carrier rate of pneumococci in the respiratory tract, their recovery from this site may be difficult to interpret. However, isolation, particularly of the recognized virulent strains[2] such as types 1, 3, 4, 7, 8, or 12 from the sputum of a patient with lobar pneumonia is likely to be of clinical significance. Further, isolation of pneumococci from blood or spinal fluid affords definite evidence of a pneumococcal infection, and isolation from spinal fluid suggests a guarded prognosis and has therapeutic implications.

SUSCEPTIBILITY TO ANTIMICROBIAL AGENTS

Pneumococci have typically been highly susceptible to penicillin, which remains the drug of choice in treating infections by this organism; however, recent isolates from South Africa and several other countries, including the United States, have been relatively resistant and occasionally highly resistant. It is clear that these resistant strains may cause serious infections, including meningitis[7] and bacteremia in addition to pneumonia. A number of different serotypes have been involved. Strains of pneumococci may be multiply resistant; in addition to being resistant to penicillin, they may be resistant to cephalosporins, tetracycline, chloramphenicol, gentamicin, clindamycin, erythromycin, and cotrimoxazole. All laboratories must now be on the lookout for strains of pneumococci with increased resistance to penicillin and other antibiotics. Although routine susceptibility testing is not necessary unless resistant organisms have been demonstrated in the community, screening should proceed in all facilities. There is some disagreement as to what procedure to use for screening, assuming that most laboratories use the Kirby-Bauer disk diffusion technique. It is clear that the usual 10-unit penicillin disk is not appropriate for detecting penicillin-insensitive strains whose minimal inhibitory concentrations range from 0.1 to 1.0 µg/ml. The 10-unit disk may be useful in detecting very high degrees of resistance, which occasionally have been demonstrated in pneumococci. Several groups have recommended the use of a 2-unit penicillin disk, preferably along with a 10-unit disk, and also a 1-µg oxacillin disk. Still another group recommends a 5-µg methicillin disk. Breakpoints for susceptibility with the different recommended disks remain to be established. Most workers have chosen zones of less than 35 mm about a 10-unit penicillin disk to indicate resistance or relative resistance. With the 1-μg oxacillin disk, Alexander and Marymont[1] recommend a zone size of less than 12 mm; Maki and co-workers[16] recommend less than 17 mm with this disk. Jacobs and colleagues[11] recommend a zone size of less than 25 mm to indicate resistance to a 5-μg methicillin disk. If there is any question about the results of disk susceptibilities or if the organism appears resistant, quantitative susceptibility tests must certainly be done. Erythromycin is the second-choice agent for the penicillin-allergic patient, but the problem of multiply resistant pneumococci and of pneumococci resistant only to penicillin must be kept in mind.

Since the advent of antibiotics, especially penicillin, the overall mortality of adults with pneumococcal pneumonia has been reduced from 84% to 17%[2] (type 3 infections cause a higher mortality); results in the pediatric group appear to be even better. Pneumococcus types 14, 3, 6, 18, 19, and 23 are isolated most frequently from infections of infants and children.

It should be stressed that pneumococci are usually not recoverable from sputum culture soon after adequate penicillin therapy has been begun. It is therefore imperative that the clinician secure material for culture **before** initiation of any antimicrobial therapy.

REFERENCES

1. Alexander, H., and Marymont, J.H., Jr.: Penicillin resistance in pneumococci, Lab. Med. **11:**727-729, 1980.
2. Austrian, R.: The current status of pneumococcal pneumonia and prospects for prophylaxis, Ninth Annual Infectious Disease Symposium, Delaware Academy of Medicine, May 5, 1972.
3. Bowers, E.F., and Jeffries, L.R.: Optochin in the identification of *Str. pneumoniae,* J. Clin. Pathol. **8:**58, 1955.
4. Congeni, B.L., and Nankervis, G.A.: Diagnosis of pneumonia by counterimmunoelectrophoresis of respiratory secretions, Am. J. Dis. Child. **132:**684-687, 1978.
5. Edwards, E.A., Kilpatrick, M.E., and Hooper, D.: Rapid detection of pneumococcal antigens in sputum and blood serum using a coagglutination test, Milit. Med. **145:**256-258, 1980.
6. Facklam, R.R.: Streptococci and aerococci. In Lennette E.H., Balows, A., Hausler, W.J., Jr., and Truant, J.P., editors: Manual of clinical microbiology, ed. 3, Washington, D.C., 1980, American Society for Microbiology.
7. Gartner, J.C., and Michaels, R.H.: Meningitis from a pneumococcus moderately resistant to penicillin, J.A.M.A. **241:**1707-1709, 1979.
8. Hall, C.T.: Summary analysis of results for the proficiency testing survey in bacteriology (January 9, 1970), National Communicable Disease Center, May 7, 1970.
9. Heffron, R.: Pneumonia, Cambridge, Mass., 1939, The Commonwealth Fund.
10. Henrichsen, J., Berntsson, E., and Kaijser, B.: Comparison of counterimmunoelectrophoresis and the capsular reaction test for typing of pneumococci, J. Clin. Microbiol. **11:**589-592, 1980.
11. Jacobs, M.R., Mithal, Y., Robins-Brown, R.M., Gaspar, M.N., and Koornhof, H.J.: Antimicrobial susceptibility testing of pneumococci: determination of Kirby-Bauer breakpoints for penicillin G, erythromycin, clindamycin, tetracycline, chloramphenicol, and rifampin, Antimicrob. Agents Chemother. **16:**190-197, 1979.
12. Leach, R.P., and Coonrod, J.D.: Detection of pneumococcal antigens in the sputum in pneumococcal pneumonia, Am. Rev. Respir. Dis. **116:**847-851, 1977.
13. Lorian, V., and Popoola, B.: Pneumococci producing beta hemolysis on agar, Appl. Microbiol. **24:**44-47, 1972.
14. Lund, E., and Henrichsen, J.: Laboratory diagnosis, serology, and epidemiology of *Streptococcus pneumoniae.* In Bergan, T., and Norris, J.R., editors: Methods in microbiology, vol. 12, London, 1979, Academic Press.
15. Lund, E., and Rasmussen, P.: Omniserum: a diagnostic pneumococcus serum reacting with the 82 known types of pneumococcus, Acta Pathol. Microbiol. Scand. **68:**458-460, 1966.
16. Maki, D.G., Helstad, A.G., and Kimball, J.L.: Penicillin susceptibility of *Streptococcus pneumoniae* in 1978, Am. J. Clin. Pathol. **73:**177-182, 1980.
17. Merrill, C.W., Gwaltney, J.M., Jr., Hendley, J.W., et al.: Rapid identification of pneumococci. Gram stain vs. the quellung reaction, N. Engl. J. Med. **288:**510-512, 1973.

18. Murray, P.R.: Modification of the bile solubility test for rapid identification of *Streptococcus pneumoniae*, J. Clin. Microbiol. **9:**290-291, 1979.

19. Norrby, S.R., and Pope, K.A.: Pneumococcal pneumonia, J. Infect. **1:**109-120, 1979.

20. Russell, H., Facklam, R.R., Padula, J.F., and Cooksey, R.: Capillary precipitin typing of *Streptococcus pneumoniae*, J. Clin. Microbiol. **8:**355-359, 1978.

21. Schmid, R.E., Anhalt, J.P., Wold, A.D., Keys, T.F., and Washington, J.A., II: Sputum counterimmunoelectrophoresis in the diagnosis of pneumococcal pneumonia, Am. Rev. Respir. Dis. **119:**345-348, 1979.

22. Washington, J.A., II, editor: Laboratory procedures in clinical microbiology, New York, 1981, Springer-Verlag, Inc.

23. White, B.: The biology of pneumococcus, Cambridge, Mass., 1938, The Commonwealth Fund.

24. Yatabe, J.A.H., Baldwin, K.L., and Martin, W.J.: Isolation of an obligately anaerobic *Streptococcus pneumoniae* from blood culture, J. Clin. Microbiol. **6:**181-182, 1977.

19 NEISSERIA AND BRANHAMELLA; MOROCOCCUS

Members of the family Neisseriaceae to be considered in this chapter, *Neisseria* and *Branhamella*, are **gram-negative cocci** occurring in pairs or in masses and are aerobic or facultatively anaerobic. These organisms may be found in the oropharynx or nasopharynx and the genitourinary tract of humans and animals.

Of the six recognized species in the genus *Neisseria*, two are well-established pathogens of humans, as is the one *Branhamella* species. The others are of doubtful pathogenicity, although certain species have been associated with respiratory disorders and central nervous system infections.

NEISSERIA GONORRHOEAE (GONOCOCCUS)

The **gonococcus** is a gram-negative diplococcus in which the paired cells have flattened adjacent walls (Plate 23). The organism is fastidious, requiring enriched media, such as blood agar or chocolate agar, for cultivation. It is an obligate human parasite not found naturally in other animals, and it causes a number of human infections, including urethritis, prostatitis, epididymitis, cervicitis, salpingitis, proctitis, pharyngitis, perihepatitis, septic arthritis, and other complications in adults, vulvovaginitis in children, and ophthalmia in newborns.

The disease is transmitted by sexual intercourse in most instances and causes acute purulent (and sometimes asymptomatic) urethritis in men and cervicitis (frequently asymptomatic) in women. Infection may also occur by extension to other sites, including the joints, rectal crypts, and blood. Less frequently, gonorrheal ophthalmia of the newborn may occur following passage through an infected birth canal; gonorrheal vulvovaginitis in the preadolescent female is usually the result of criminal assault or by contact with an infected fomite. Careful attention to appropriate specimen collection and transport procedures should yield the organism from many of the sites mentioned. When homosexuality or participation in oral or anal sexual acts seems likely, urethral or endocervical swabs should be supplemented by oropharyngeal and anorectal swabs for culture. For obvious reasons, smears obtained from either the rectum or pharynx should not be relied on for diagnosis.

Isolation

Neisseria gonorrhoeae is a fastidious parasite, requiring an enriched culture medium and incubation under increased CO_2 (3% to 10%) for its recovery from clinical material. Luxuriant growth occurs on chocolate agar supplemented with yeast extract or a similar enrichment* or on modified Thayer-Martin (MTM) medium,† a modified chocolate agar made selective for the gonococcus and meningococcus by the addition of certain antibiotics, Martin-Lewis medium, or modified NYC medium. Their use is described in detail in Chapter 11, along with some of the newer developments regarding the transport of specimens and isolation of this organism.

*Available as IsoVitaleX (BBL), Supplement B (Difco).
†Available from Baltimore Biological Laboratory, Cockeysville, Md.; Difco Laboratories, Detroit; and others.

On **moist modified Thayer-Martin** medium after 20 hours' incubation in a candle jar at 35 C,* typical colonies of *N. gonorrhoeae* appear as small (0.5 to 2 mm), translucent, raised, moist grayish white colonies with entire to lobate margins. They are usually mucoid and tend to come off as whole colonies when picked from the agar surface. Colony size varies, depending on the age of the culture or crowding on the plate. Plates without growth should be returned to the incubator for 48 hours' incubation. Cultures should be processed **immediately** after removal from the incubator, as gonococci tend to autolyze in the absence of CO_2.

Kellogg and others[20] observed that gonococci produced four distinct colony types and that these could be correlated with virulence. Viewed through a stereoscopic microscope on a clear medium, types T1 and T2 reflect the light and appear to have bright highlights. T1 colonies are small and raised, and T2 colonies are slightly larger and have an umbonate center.

*Many strains of gonococci do not grow well at 37 C.

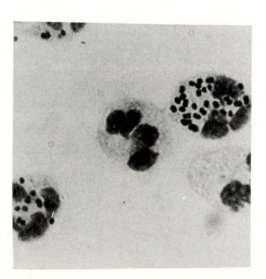

FIG. 19-1
Neisseria gonorrhoeae. Smear of exudate, showing intracellular gonococci (Gram stain, 1,200×).

These two types consist of piliated gonococcal cells and are virulent for humans and animal models. With nonselective subculture these colony forms dissociate to T3 and T4, which are composed of nonpiliated avirulent gonococci. T3 and T4 colonies are larger, flatter, and less opaque and do not reflect the light.

Nutritionally fastidious gonococci that require arginine, hypoxanthine, and uracil (AHU) form small atypical colonies, are very sensitive to penicillin, and are associated with both asymptomatic urethritis and disseminated gonococcal infection.[6] AHU strains also produce colonies of the four types previously referred to, but these are all smaller than those produced by the wild type strains. AHU strains are infrequently isolated from homosexual men (Handsfield et al.: Sex. Transmit. Dis. **1:**1-5, 1980).

Presumptive identification

All members of the genus *Neisseria*, as well as members of other genera (such as *Pseudomonas*, *Moraxella*, and *Aeromonas*) are **oxidase positive.** In the oxidase reaction a bacterial enzyme called **indophenol oxidase** oxidizes a redox dye, which results in a color change in the bacterial colony. In the oxidase test (described in Chapter 44) a freshly prepared or refrigerated (for no longer than 1 week) 1% solution of tetramethyl-p-phenylenediamine dihydrochloride is used. A reagent impregnated filter paper strip* is preferred for the oxidase test. One should use a platinum loop, as nichrome wire may cause a false-positive reaction. A portion of a colony is rubbed on the paper strip; the moist paper where the bacteria are deposited turns dark purple within 10 seconds (Plate 51). Slower reactions are not typical for *Neisseria*. The test should be repeated with an 18-hour culture on blood agar or other medium not containing carbohydrate. If no characteristic colonies are

observed, the agar plate may be flooded with the oxidase reagent to detect inapparent colonies. The oxidase test should not be used directly on Transgrow medium unless it has first been equilibrated to ambient atmosphere.

A thin smear of the oxidase-positive colony is then prepared, Gram stained, and examined microscopically under the oil immersion lens. Typical neisseriae appear as gram-negative diplococci with their **adjacent sides flattened;** the microscopist should note, however, that certain gram-negative diplobacilli (e.g., *Moraxella osloensis*) may resemble gonococci morphologically.

In order to provide physicians with a rapid laboratory diagnosis of gonorrheal infection, the CDC has recommended that material obtained from the genitourinary tract, which has been inoculated to modified Thayer-Martin (or Transgrow) medium and shows growth of typical oxidase-positive colonies consisting of gram-negative diplococci, provides sufficient criteria for the presumptive identification of *N. gonorrhoeae*.[2] This may be reported as: "Presumptive identification—*N. gonorrhoeae*."* Isolation of neisseriae from other sites, such as a pharyngeal culture, or in special social or medicolegal situations, should be identified by the following, more definitive procedure.

Confirmatory identification

A presumptive identification of *N. gonorrhoeae* may be confirmed by carbohydrate degradation reactions or less reliably by direct fluorescent antibody staining. *N. gonorrhoeae* metabolizes **glucose only,** producing acid but no gas (Table 19-1). The recommended base medium—cystine trypticase agar (CTA), pH 7.6—readily supports the growth of **fresh** isolates of gonococci and meningococci, although occasional strains of the former may grow poorly or not at

---

*Pathotec strips, General Diagnostics Division, Warner-Lambert Co., Morris Plains, N.J.

*Approximately 98% of these isolates from urogenital sites are confirmed as *N. gonorrhoeae* by carbohydrate fermentation or fluorescent antibody staining.

TABLE 19-1

Differentiation of selected neisseriae

Organism	Carbohydrate fermentation reactions (CTA base, 1 to 4 days' incubation at 35 C)						Growth	
	Glucose	Maltose	Sucrose	Lactose	Fructose	Mannitol	On MTM	On nutrient agar at 22 C
Branhamella catarrhalis	–	–	–	–	–	–	±	±
Neisseria gonorrhoeae	A*	–	–	–	–	–	+	–
N. meningitidis	A	A	–	–	–	–	+	–
N. sicca	A	A	A	–	A	–	–†	+
N. lactamica	A	A	–	A(slow)	–	–	+	
N. mucosa§	A	A	A	–	A	–		+
N. subflava‖	A	A	–	–	–	–	–†	+
N. flavescens‖	–	–	–	–	–	–	–†	+

Modified from Dr. Charles T. Hall, Licensure and Proficiency Testing Branch, Centers for Disease Control, Atlanta.
*A, acid production (no gas).
†A heavy inoculum can yield growth.
§Not recognized in Bergey's Manual of determinative bacteriology (ed. 8). Reduces nitrate to gas.
‖Bacterial growth shows a yellowish pigmentation on Loeffler's serum medium.

all. Without very careful attention to detail one may get unreliable results with CTA media. Morello and Bohnhoff[27] present an excellent discussion of this test and means for resolving problems that occur with it. The **reagent grade** carbohydrates used (glucose, maltose, sucrose, fructose, and lactose) are added in 1% concentration to the sterilized medium (see Chapter 42 for preparation), which may be stored in the refrigerator.

CTA media are inoculated with a **heavy** suspension prepared from a **subculture** chocolate agar plate 18 to 24 hours old (taken from a **single** colony on the original plate) in about 0.5 ml of saline or trypticase soy broth. One should deposit two to three drops of the suspension on the surface of the medium and then stab into the upper third of its depth using a sterile, cotton-plugged capillary pipet.

The screw caps of the tubes are then **tightened** and incubated without added CO_2 at 35 C. They are examined daily for evidence of growth and production of acid, indicated by turbidity and a **yellow color** of the upper layer of medium. After 24 hours' incubation (occasional strains require 48 to 72 hours incubation), the tubes showing acidity should be checked for purity by microscopic examination of a Gram stain. If only glucose is metabolized, report "*Neisseria gonorrhoeae* isolated." An occasional strain of gonococcus may fail to metabolize glucose on the first attempt; repeat inoculation of CTA medium enriched with 10% ascitic fluid may encourage degradation by these strains. Preferably, one should use the "nongrowth carbohydrate degradation test" described in detail in Cumitech 4 by Kellogg and associates.[19] A rapid carbohydrate degradation test using a barium hydroxide indicator (converted to the white precipitate barium carbonate by CO_2 produced during metabolism) was described by Slifkin and Pouchet.[40] Yong and Prytula[42] have described a rapid microcarbohydrate test for confirmation that utilizes both preformed enzymes and enzymes formed as a result of growth in a small volume of enriched medium. Reliable results are said to be obtained within 4 hours of incubation. The Minitek system* employs paper disks impregnated with high concentrations of carbohydrates and a heavy suspension of organisms. This may be used for the identification of *Neisseria* and provides results within 4 hours as a rule. There is a Bactec *Neisseria* differentiation kit† that consists of three vials containing ^{14}C-labeled dextrose, maltose, and fructose. If the carbohydrates are metabolized, there is a release of radioactive CO_2 into the supernatant gas. The Bactec instrument analyzes the gas for radioactivity and indicates metabolism of that carbohydrate if a given threshold level is exceeded. This test requires incubation of the vials at 35 C for 3 hours. Pizzuto and Washington[36] recommend modifying the nongrowth carbohydrate degradation test by increasing the amount of phenol red indicator and decreasing the concentration of maltose. They compared this modified rapid fermentation test with the Bactec *Neisseria* differentiation kit and the CTA agar method. The rapid fermentation test and the Bactec method accurately identified at least 95% of strains of gonococci (as well as at least 91% of meningococcus strains) within 4 hours. Overall, the CTA method was the most accurate (97%) but required as long as 48 hours of incubation. Another rapid test based on biochemical characteristics involved the use of enzymatic profiles.[7] Ten substrates allowed the separation of gonococci and meningococci from each other and from related species within 4 hours after primary isolation on modified Thayer-Martin medium.

Various serologic techniques have also been proposed for identification of *N. gonorrhoeae*. An antigonococcal lipopolysaccharide hen serum was used in a slide agglutination test for identification of gonococci from primary isolates with good results.[23] There have been several evaluations of the Phadebact gonococcus test (GT),* a slide coagglutination procedure.[1,22] This test performs well when a dense suspension of boiled (5 to 10 minutes) organisms is mixed with the reagents.[1] Positive reactions usually occur within 2 to 3 minutes and confirm the presence of *N. gonorrhoeae*, provided the control test is negative. A small percentage of false-negative tests occur. Also, there may be false-positive results with *Neisseria lactamica*.[1] These can be spotted if one uses, concurrently with the Phadebact test, the O-nitrophenyl-β-D-galactopyranoside (ONPG) test. A lectin slide agglutination test has also been developed for confirmation of *N. gonorrhoeae*.[37] This uses wheat germ lectin as an agglutinin. The test appeared highly sensitive and gave results in 6 to 8 minutes; 1 of 23 isolates of *Neisseria meningitidis* tested (group X) gave a false-positive reaction.

The direct fluorescent antibody staining procedure[31] is a very valuable procedure for confirming colonies of *N. gonorrhoeae*. However, because of cross reactions with group B meningococci and staphylococci, it is less satisfactory for primary cultures and for accurately separating *N. meningitidis* from *N. gonorrhoeae* than are carbohydrate degradation tests. The technique is described in Chapter 39.

A relatively rapid, highly specific identification procedure was described by Bawdon and co-workers.[3] This employs DNA extracted from the culture to be identified (nonviable or mixed cultures or purulent discharge can be used) to transform genetically a uracil- and arginine-deficient auxotroph of *N. gonorrhoeae* to prototrophy.

Serologic evaluation for antigonococcal antibody has been suggested as a means for screening large populations for infection to pick up asymptomatic cases. Even if the test were not specific, it would be satisfactory, since patients

---

*Baltimore Biological Laboratory, Cockeysville, Md.
†Johnston Laboratories Inc., Cockeysville, Md.

*Pharmacia Diagnostics, Piscataway, N.J.

with positive specimens could be checked by appropriate cultures. A variety of techniques have been evaluated for serologic diagnosis of gonococcal infection, but the results have been positive in only 75% to 80% of patients with specimens proved to be culturally positive, and the false-positive reactor rate has been 10% to 15%.[25]

NEISSERIA MENINGITIDIS (MENINGOCOCCUS)

The normal habitat of *N. meningitidis* is the human nasopharynx; many persons may carry the organism for indefinite periods without symptoms. In susceptible persons, however, the meningococcus gains access to the central nervous system primarily via the hematogenous route (with a bacteremic precursor). A suppurative infection of the meninges then occurs, producing the characteristic syndrome of **bacterial meningitis.** The bloodstream invasion may result in an early petechial rash (smears of which may show meningococci) or take the form of septic shock accompanied by disseminated intravascular coagulation, with rapidly fatal outcome (Waterhouse-Friderichsen syndrome). Septic arthritis and endocarditis may also be seen.

The meningococcus is similar to the gonococcus in morphology and staining reactions. The paired cocci have a miniature coffee bean appearance. Some of the cells may be swollen and appear larger. The organism is fastidious in its growth requirements and may be cultivated on enriched media, such as chocolate agar or blood agar, on which it develops relatively large, smooth, raised, nonpigmented colonies. No hemolysis is produced on blood agar. The colonies tend to autolyze fairly rapidly. The colonies may be identified as *Neisseria* by the oxidase test, which shows the same color changes observed with gonococcal colonies (see above).

The organism is **extremely sensitive** to temperature and dehydration; thus, the same facilities provided for the culture of the gonococcus must be accorded the culturing of this species.

Cultivation in a 3% to 10% CO_2 atmosphere greatly enhances growth.

N. meningitidis may be classified serologically into groups A, B, C, D, X, Y, Z, 29E (Z'), and 135 (W135).[12] Groups A and C are encapsulated, whereas group B strains are usually nonencapsulated. The former give rise to larger and more mucoid colonies (often gray) than are observed with strains of group B, in which the colonies are smaller, rougher, and yellowish. Groups 29E and 135 are creamy white in areas of heavy inoculum. Groups A, B, and C strains are generally involved in epidemics of meningitis, whereas all groups except X, Z, and 29E may be isolated from sporadic cases between outbreaks.[4]

Isolation

The organism may be isolated from CSF, the nasopharynx, joint fluid, blood, transtracheal aspirates, skin petechiae, and miscellaneous sites, such as the eye, urethra, endocervix, and anal canal of homosexuals. Material from such sources is streaked on blood or chocolate agar plates or on modified Thayer-Martin (or NYC) medium if a mixed flora is anticipated and incubated in a candle jar at 35 C. Strains of meningococci may grow on blood agar plates incubated in 5% to 10% CO_2. A positive oxidase test on the colonies is presumptive evidence of the presence of the organism. Gram stain indicates the typical morphology. Recognized colonies of the organism may then be transferred to obtain pure cultures for biochemical tests.

Identification

Inoculation of the recommended carbohydrate media—glucose, maltose, lactose, and sucrose—in either CTA or serum or ascitic fluid semisolid agar (see Chapter 42) helps to identify the meningococcus, which ferments only **glucose** and **maltose.** Occasional strains fail to produce acid from either carbohydrate.[14,41] Repeated subculture or use of nongrowth carbohydrate tests[19] (see above) usually lead to typical reactions. Erratic results in carbohydrates may be caused by several factors.[14,27] False-negative reactions may result from nutritional deficiencies in the CTA medium, which fails to support adequate growth of fastidious strains of meningococci. Transient false-negative reactions may occur on initial isolation but often revert to positive after several subcultures. Nonspecific reactions may result from prolonged incubation of the sugars. Impure cultures, of course, may lead to false results, as may carryover of inhibitory agents from selective media. Inasmuch as it is now quite clear that both gonococci and meningococci may occupy similar locations in the body and may produce similar infections, it becomes increasingly important for clinical microbiology laboratories to accurately characterize species of *Neisseria*. True maltose- and glucose-negative variants pose a serious problem for laboratories that depend entirely on carbohydrate utilization for identification of *Neisseria*. It should be noted that the typical colonial morphologies of *N. gonorrhoeae* and *N. meningitidis* are markedly different, so that one may suspect that he or she is dealing with a biochemical variant.

Other types of identification systems have been described in the section on *N. gonorrhoeae*.

The serology of these organisms may be determined by the **capsular swelling** reaction, although it should be noted that only groups A and C possess capsular antigen; group B strains are identified by the agglutination reaction. Only cells from actively growing cultures, or cells directly from clinical material (e.g., sediment from CSF) showing a sufficient number of gram-negative diplococci, should be used for capsular swelling tests. The current method of choice in most diagnostic laboratories, however, is the **slide agglutination test,** using first polyvalent and then monovalent antisera. The reader is cautioned about the limitations of this technique, especially in reference to group B meningococci, since antigenic cross-relationships exist between this organism and other neisseriae. There also appears to be some antigenic cross-

relationship between groups A and C and between *Escherichia coli* and groups B and C.

The direct fluorescent antibody staining procedure also may be used for the identification of meningococci in CSF; fluorescein-labeled antimeningococcal conjugates are available commercially.* The specificity of the fluorescent antibody reaction is a problem. A preparation of antiserum should be absorbed with gonococci to remove cross-reacting antibodies. Nonspecific staining of *Staphylococcus aureus* also occurs. The test should be performed by an experienced microbiologist using appropriate control reagents. The major advantage, of course, of the fluorescent antibody technique is the rapid results that may be achieved for a critically ill patient with meningitis. The direct fluorescent antibody preparation also may be positive when cultures are negative.

CIE may also be used to detect the soluble carbohydrate from the capsule of meningococci in spinal fluid.[27] This works primarily for groups A and C meningococci. Accordingly, meningococcal disease cannot be ruled out if the test is negative. Furthermore, there are some cross-reactions with other bacteria, such as *E. coli*, so that confirmation of results is necessary.

Techniques for capsular swelling and slide agglutination tests are described in Chapter 37; the immunofluorescent procedure is described in Chapter 39.

ANTIBIOTIC SUSCEPTIBILITY OF PATHOGENIC NEISSERIAE

In a comparative study of the susceptibility of gonococci to penicillin in the United States, Martin and co-workers[24] reported that from 1955 to 1965 there was an increase from 0.6% to 42% in cultures requiring more than 0.05 unit/ml of penicillin to inhibit growth. It is clear that penicillin G (or ampicillin) can no longer be

---

*Polyvalent antiserum (groups A through D) from Burroughs Wellcome Co., Research Triangle Park, N.C.; Difco Laboratories, Detroit.

depended on routinely; other drugs that may be useful include spectinomycin, tetracycline, cefoxitin, and cotrimoxazole.

There have been many reports of the failure of penicillin G in the treatment of gonococcal disease related to production of penicillinase by the organism.[33,34] There is no evidence of reduced communicability or invasiveness in these strains. There are reports from various parts of the world of significant increases in the numbers of penicillinase producing gonococci.[18,29,32] In Los Angeles there were 149 cases of infection caused by this organism in a 2½-month period.[32] From March, 1976, when the first organism of this type was identified, through April, 1980, more than 1,000 cases of infection caused by this type of gonococcus have been reported to the CDC.[29] An outbreak in Shreveport, Louisiana, like the Los Angeles outbreak, involved sustained transmission of a penicillinase-producing gonococcus.[29] It is clearly important to obtain posttreatment cultures and to examine these for beta-lactamase production and for antibiotic susceptibility patterns.

Spectinomycin was effective in 21 of 22 patients with such organisms, and certain penicillinase-resistant cephalosporins may also have promise.[33] Beta lactamase–producing strains of N. gonorrhoeae also resistant to spectinomycin have been found but are rare. More recently, there have been disturbing reports of gonococci that are highly resistant to penicillin despite not producing beta-lactamase. Minimal inhibitory concentrations of as high as 50 units/ml have been reported.[39] In the United Kingdom approximately 29% of gonococcal isolates in 1976 were found to have a minimal inhibitory concentration of 0.125 μg/ml or higher, and the upper limit of resistance for non-penicillinase-producing gonococci was 1 μg/ml. Most strains were sensitive to tetracycline. However, a survey of 225 selected strains during 1979 and 1980 revealed that 88 gonococci were resistant to tetracycline, with penicillin minimal inhibitory concentrations being 1 μg/ml or higher.[38] The

organisms are still susceptible to spectinomycin and other drugs.

A simple method for detection of penicillinase-producing gonococci has been described by Hodge and associates.[15] This involves seeding penicillin-sensitive S. aureus on a plate and then placing a penicillin disk on it. Next, a heavy inoculum of the organisms to be tested for penicillinase production are streaked outward from the disk in radial fashion. Strains that produce penicillinase distort the zone of inhibition about the penicillin disk. Congo red agar has been proposed as a means of distinguishing between gonococci and meningococci; meningococci grow on this medium, whereas gonococci typically do not. It was found, however, that certain strains of gonococci do grow on Congo red agar, and these were all penicillin-resistant nonpenicillinase producers.[30]

Present knowledge indicates that penicillin G or ampicillin in high dosage is the drug of choice in the treatment of meningococcal disease but is unsatisfactory for the prophylactic treatment of carriers.[11] Most of these strains can be eliminated by treatment with rifampin[8] or minocycline. Many or most are resistant to sulfadiazine, formerly the agent of choice for carriers.

OTHER NEISSERIA SPECIES AND BRANHAMELLA

Since other neisseriae may be isolated from sputum, the throat, the nasopharynx, and occasionally CSF, they should be recognized and differentiated from the gonococcus and the meningococcus. For these reasons they are included in Table 19-1. N. subflava and N. sicca generally produce small yellowish to greenish colonies that may be smooth or hard and wrinkled and are only rarely involved in infection. N. sicca has caused endocarditis[13] and bacteremia in an immunocompromised patient (Herbert and Ruskin: Am. J. Clin. Pathol. 75:739-743, 1981). N. subflava may produce beta lactamase.[35] N. flavescens and N. lactamica produce colonies similar to those of N. meningitidis but may have a yellowish pigment on primary isolation. These bacteria have been recovered from some pathologic processes, including endocarditis and meningitis.

Although previous authors reported the isolation of **lactose-utilizing** strains of neisseriae,[17,26] little attention was paid until Hollis and co-workers at CDC[16] published results of their study of organisms referred for confirmation as *N. meningitidis*, but which were subsequently found to be lactose positive. This probably reflects those laboratories' not using lactose in their routine biochemical workup for neisseriae.[16] Since then, the species *N. lactamica* has been characterized. *N. lactamica* produces beta-galactosidase, which degrades lactose and ONPG. The majority of strains have been recovered from pharyngeal and nasopharyngeal specimens, but occasionally strains have been recovered from sputum, tracheal aspirates, blood, amniotic fluid, CSF, lung tissue, and so forth. Most studies indicate that *N. lactamica* is only occasionally encountered in infection. It has been most frequently misidentified as *N. meningitidis* or *N. subflava* (Table 19-1).

Branhamella catarrhalis grows as a grayish-white friable colony that is granular and difficult to emulsify. *B. catarrhalis* has been reported from otitis media, maxillary sinusitis, purulent bronchitis,[28] pneumonia, empyema[5] and endocarditis. The organism may be susceptible to penicillin, but the majority of strains produce beta lactamase.[10,35] The organism is usually susceptible to cephalosporins (particularly cefoxitin), erythromycin, tetracycline, chloramphenicol, and cotrimoxazole. It is resistant to clindamycin.

It was previously believed that distinguishing characteristics of this organism were growth on nutrient agar at 22 C and failure to grow on modified Thayer-Martin medium. However, more recent study indicates that the reverse is usually the case in both of the tests.[9] The organism does not demonstrate pigmentation; it reduces nitrate and nitrite.

MOROCOCCUS

Morococcus cerebrosus has been proposed as a name for a gram-negative, oxidase-positive, aggregate-forming coccus isolated from a brain abscess (Long et al.: Int. J. Syst. Bacteriol. **31:**294-301, 1981).

REFERENCES

1. Anand, C.M., and Kadis, E.M.: Evaluation of the Phadebact gonococcus test for confirmation of *Neisseria gonorrhoeae*, J. Clin. Microbiol. **12:**15-17, 1980.
2. Balows, A., and Printz, D.W.: CDC program for diagnosis of gonorrhea, Letter, J.A.M.A. **222:**1557, 1972.
3. Bawdon, R.E., Juni, E., and Britt, E.N.: Identification of *Neisseria gonorrhoeae* by genetic transformation: a clinical laboratory evaluation, J. Clin. Microbiol. **5:**108-109, 1977.
4. Counts, G.W., and Petersdorf, R.G.: "The wheel within a wheel": meningococcal trends, J.A.M.A. **244:**2200-2201, 1980.
5. Cox, P.M., Jr., and Colloff, E.: *Neisseria catarrhalis* empyema in an immunodeficient host, Am. Rev. Respir. Dis. **120:**471-472, 1979.
6. Crawford, G., Knapp, J.S., Hale, J., and Holmes, K.K.: Asymptomatic gonorrhea in men: caused by gonococci with unique nutritional requirements, Science **196:**1352-1353, 1977.
7. D'Amato, R.F., Eriquez, L.A., Tomfohrde, K.M., and Singerman, E.: Rapid identification of *Neisseria gonorrhoeae* and *Neisseria meningitidis* by using enzymatic profiles, J. Clin. Microbiol. **7:**77-81, 1978.
8. Deal, W.G., and Sanders, E.: Efficacy of rifampin in the treatment of meningococcal carriers, N. Engl. J. Med. **281:**641-649, 1969.
9. Doern, G.V., and Morse, S.A.: *Branhamella (Neisseria) catarrhalis:* criteria for laboratory identification, J. Clin. Microbiol. **11:**193-195, 1980.
10. Doern, G.V., Siebers, K.G., Hallick, L.M., and Morse, S.A.: Antibiotic susceptibility of beta-lactamase–producing strains of *Branhamella (Neisseria) catarrhalis*, Antimicrob. Agents Chemother. **17:**24-29, 1980.
11. Dowd, J.M., Blink, D., Miller, C.H., Frank, P.F., and Pierce, W.E.: Antibiotic prophylaxis of carriers of sulfadiazine resistant meningococci, J. Infect. Dis. **116:**473-480, 1966.
12. Galaid, E.I., Cherubin, C.E., Marr, J.S., Schaefler, S., Barone, J., and Lee, W.: Meningococcal disease in New York City, 1973 to 1978, J.A.M.A. **244:**2167-2171, 1980.
13. Gay, R.M. and Sevier, R.E.: *Neisseria sicca* endocarditis: report of a case and review of the literature, J. Clin. Microbiol. **8:**729-732, 1978.

14. Granato, P.A., Howard, R., Wilkinson, B., and Laser, J.: Meningitis caused by maltose-negative variant of *Neisseria meningitidis*, J. Clin. Microbiol. **11**:270-273, 1980.

15. Hodge, W., Ciak, J., and Tramont, E.C.: Simple method for detection of penicillinase-producing *Neisseria gonorrhoeae*, J. Clin. Microbiol. **7**:102-103, 1978.

16. Hollis, D.G., Wiggins, G.T., and Weaver, R.E.: *Neisseria lactamicus* sp. n.: a lactose-fermenting species resembling *Neisseria meningitidis*, Appl. Microbiol. **17**:71-77, 1969.

17. Jensen, J.: Studien uber gramnegative Kokken, Zentralbl. Bakteriol. Parasitenk. Orig. **133**:75-88, 1934.

18. Johnston, N.A., Kolator, B., and Seth, A.D.: A survey of β-lactamase–producing gonococcal isolates reported in the United Kingdom, 1979-1980, Lancet **1**:263-264, 1981.

19. Kellogg, D.S., Jr., Holmes, K.K., and Hill, G.A.: Laboratory diagnosis of gonorrhea, Cumitech 4, Washington, D.C., 1976, American Society for Microbiology.

20. Kellogg, D.S., Jr., Peacock, W.L., Jr., Deacon, W.E., Brown, L., and Pirkle, C.I.: *Neisseria gonorrhoeae*. I. Virulence genetically linked to clonal variation, J. Bacteriol. **85**:1274-1279, 1963.

21. Knapp, J.K., and Holmes, K.K.: Disseminated gonococcal infections caused by *Neisseria gonorrhoeae* with unique nutritional requirements, J. Infect. Dis. **132**:204-208, 1975.

22. Lewis, J.S., and Martin, J.E., Jr.: Evaluation of the Phadebact gonococcus test, a coagglutination procedure for confirmation of *Neisseria gonorrhoeae*, J. Clin. Microbiol. **11**:153-156, 1980.

23. Malysheff, C., Wallace, R., Ashton, F.E., Diena, B.B., and Perry, M.B.: Identification of *Neisseria gonorrhoeae* from primary cultures by a slide agglutination test, J. Clin. Microbiol. **8**:260-261, 1978.

24. Martin, J.E., Jr., Lester, A., Price, E.V., and Schmale, J.D.: Comparative study of gonococcal susceptibility to penicillin in the United States, 1955-1969, Note, J. Infect. Dis. **122**:459-461, 1970.

25. McTighe, A.H., Patel, C., Smith, L., Cherry, M., Fisher, B., Helman, M., Jones, A., and Weinberg, L.: Laboratory and clinical aspects of infection with *Neisseria gonorrhoeae*, Lab. Med. **11**:524-532, 1980.

26. Mitchell, M.S., Rhoden, D.L., and King, E.O.: Lactose-fermenting organisms resembling *Neisseria meningitidis*, J. Bacteriol. **90**:560, 1965.

27. Morello, J.A., and Bohnhoff, M.: *Neisseria* and *Branhamella*. In Lennette, E.H., Balows, A., Hausler, W.J., Jr., and Truant, J.P., editors: Manual of clinical microbiology, ed. 3, Washington, D.C., 1980, American Society for Microbiology.

28. Ninane, G., Joly, J., and Kraytman, M.: Bronchopulmonary infection due to *Branhamella catarrhalis:* 11 cases assessed by transtracheal puncture, Br. Med. J. **1**:276-278, 1978.

29. An outbreak of penicillinase-producing *Neisseria gonorrhoeae*, Shreveport, Louisiana, Morbid. Mortal. Weekly Rep. **29**:241-242, 1980.

30. Payne, S.M., and Finkelstein, R.A.: Growth on Congo Red agar: possible means of identifying penicillin-resistant non-penicillinase-producing gonococci, J. Clin. Microbiol. **6**:534-535, 1977.

31. Peacock, W.L., Welch, B.G., Martin, J.E., Jr., and Thayer, J.D.: Fluorescent antibody technique for identification of presumptively positive gonococcal cultures, Public Health Rep. **83**:337-339, 1968.

32. Penicillinase-producing *Neisseria gonorrhoeae*, Los Angeles, California, Morbid. Mortal. Weekly Rep. **29**:541-543, 1980.

33. Percival, A., Corkill, J.E., Arya, O. P., Rowlands, J., Alergant, C.D., Rees, E., and Annels, E.H.: Penicillinase-producing gonococci in Liverpool, Lancet **2**:1379-1382, 1976.

34. Phillips, I.: β-Lactamase–producing penicillin-resistant gonococcus, Lancet **2**:656-657, 1976.

35. Piot, P., Roberts, M., and Ninane, G.: β-lactamase production in commensal Neisseriaceae, Lancet **1**:619, 1979.

36. Pizzuto, D.J., and Washington, J.A., II: Evaluation of rapid carbohydrate degradation tests for identification of pathogenic *Neisseria*, J. Clin. Microbiol. **11**:394-397, 1980.

37. Schaefer, R.L., Keller, K.F., and Doyle, R.J.: Lectins in diagnostic microbiology: use of wheat germ agglutinin for laboratory identification of *Neisseria gonorrhoeae*, J. Clin. Microbiol. **10**:669-672, 1979.

38. Seth, A.D., and Johnston, N.A.: Penicillin-resistant gonococci, Lancet **2**:531, 1980.

39. Shtibel, R: Non–beta-lactamase producing *Neisseria gonorrhoeae* highly resistant to penicillin, Lancet **2**:39, 1980.

40. Slifkin, M., and Pouchet, G.R.: Rapid carbohydrate fermentation test for confirmation of the pathogenic *Neisseria* using a Ba(OH)$_2$ indicator, J. Clin. Microbiol. **5**:15-19, 1977.

41. Uyeda, C.T., Maruyama, M.M., and Hakes, M.S.: Aberrant strain of group B *Neisseria meningitidis*, J. Clin. Microbiol. **12**:286-287, 1980.

42. Yong, D.C.T., and Prytula, A.: Rapid micro-carbohydrate test for confirmation of *Neisseria gonorrhoeae*, J. Clin. Microbiol. **8**:643-647, 1978.

20 ENTEROBACTERIACEAE

Escherichia

Shigella

Edwardsiella

Salmonella

Arizona

Citrobacter

Klebsiella

Enterobacter

Serratia

Hafnia

Proteus

Providencia

Morganella

Yersinia

Erwinia

Pectobacterium

Kluyvera

Tatumella

Cedecea

The Enterobacteriaceae are by far the most commonly encountered of the aerobic or facultative gram-negative bacilli in clinical specimens. Good perspective is furnished in the study by Blachman and Pickett,[6] in which 768 clinical isolates were analyzed (Fig. 20-1). Of these isolates, 78% were Enterobacteriaceae, 12% nonfermenters, 9% *Haemophilus* species, and 1% "unusual gram-negative bacilli" (*Actinobacillus; Brucella; Campylobacter; Cardiobacterium;* CDC Groups DF-1, DF-2, EF-4, and TM-1; *Eikenella; Haemophilus aphrophilus; Gardnerella (Haemophilus) vaginalis;* and *Streptobacillus*).

With the advent of the eighth edition of *Bergey's Manual of Determinative Bacteriology,*[11] the current classification of the family Enterobacteriaceae has become somewhat clouded, and many clinical microbiologists believe they are faced with something of a dilemma. This situation has been brought about primarily because of the impact the classification system of Edwards and Ewing[23] has had over the years in this country. Without any intent of passing judgment on the different schemes, the classification of Edwards and Ewing as modified by the CDC[9] is used in this book. This classification scheme

199

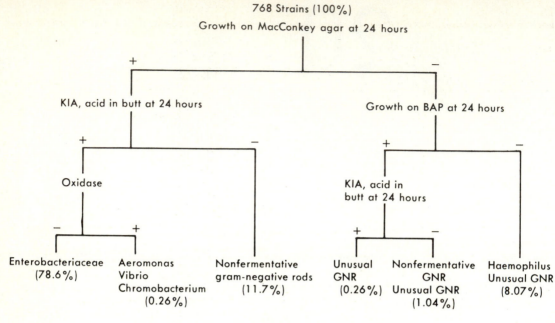

FIG. 20-1

Distribution of aerobic and facultative gram-negative bacilli.

TABLE 20-1

Classification of Enterobacteriaceae

Edwards and Ewing/CDC*	Bergey's Manual (ed. 8)
Family: Enterobacteriaceae	**Family:** Enterobacteriaceae
Tribe I: Escherichieae	Genus I: Escherichia
Genus I: *Escherichia*	Species: *E. coli*
Species: *E. coli*	Genus II: Edwardsiella
Genus II: *Shigella*	Species: *E. tarda*
Species: *S. dysenteriae*	Genus III: Citrobacter
S. flexneri	Species: *C. freundii*
S. boydii	*C. intermedius*
S. sonnei	Genus IV: Salmonella
Tribe II: Edwardsielleae	Species: *S. cholerae-suis*
Genus I: *Edwardsiella*	*S. typhi*
Species: *E. tarda*	*S. enteritidis*
Tribe III: Salmonelleae	*S. arizonae*
Genus I: *Salmonella*	Genus V: Shigella
Species: *S. cholerae-suis*	Species: *S. dysenteriae*
S. typhi	*S. flexneri*
S. enteritidis	*S. boydii*
	S. sonnei

*Modified from Brenner and colleagues.[9]

TABLE 20-1

Classification of Enterobacteriaceae—cont'd

Edwards and Ewing/CDC	Bergey's Manual (ed. 8)
Genus II: *Arizona*	Genus VI: Klebsiella
Species: *A. hinshawii*	Species: *K. pneumoniae*
Genus III: *Citrobacter*	*K. ozaenae*
Species: *C. freundii*	*K. rhinoscleromatis*
C. diversus	Genus VII: Enterobacter
C. amalonaticus	Species: *E. cloacae*
Tribe IV: Klebsielleae	*E. aerogenes*
Genus I: *Klebsiella*	Genus VIII: Hafnia
Species: *K. pneumoniae*	Species: *H. alvei*
K. oxytoca	Genus IX: Serratia
K. ozaenae	Species: *S. marcescens*
K. rhinoscleromatis	Genus X: Proteus
Genus II: *Enterobacter*	Species: *P. vulgaris*
Species: *E. cloacae*	*P. mirabilis*
E. aerogenes	*P. morganii*
E. agglomerans	*P. rettgeri*
E. sakazakii	*P. inconstans*
E. gergoviae	Genus XI: Yersinia
Genus III: *Hafnia*	Species: *Y. enterocolitica*
Species: *H. alvei*	*Y. pseudotuberculosis*
Genus IV: *Serratia*	*Y. pestis*
Species: *S. marcescens*	Genus XII: Erwinia (plant pathogens)
S. liquefaciens	Species: *E. herbicola* (has been considered
S. rubidaec	a human pathogen)
S. plymuthica	
S. odorifera	
S. fonticola	
Tribe V: Proteeae	
Genus I: *Proteus*	
Species: *P. vulgaris*	
P. mirabilis	
Genus II: *Providencia*	
Species: *P. stuartii*	
P. alcalifaciens	
P. rettgeri	
Genus III: *Morganella*	
Species: *M. morganii*	
Tribe VI: Yersineae	
Genus I: *Yersinia*	
Species: *Y. enterocolitica*	
Y. pseudotuberculosis	
Y. pestis	
Y. intermedia	
Y. frederiksenii	
Y. ruckeri	
Tribe VII: Erwinieae (plant pathogens)	
Genus I: *Erwinia*	
Genus II: *Pectobacterium*	

utilizes a polyphasic approach to taxonomy. Members of the family are grouped into genera, species, and biotypes on the basis of their overall morphologic, biochemical, and genetic similarity. The availability of new methods such as new biochemical tests, antibiotic susceptibility patterns, species- or group-specific bacteriophages, DNA-relatedness tests, and computerized identification programs has made this approach a sound one and has helped to eliminate much of the confusion concerning the classification of the Enterobacteriaceae. Of particular importance are the tests for DNA relatedness[8]: genome size, guanine plus cytosine (G + C) content, and DNA-DNA hybridization. These tests most accurately determine the degree to which two organisms are related. Because it is not practical to perform these tests in a clinical setting, the CDC has correlated the results of DNA-DNA hybridization studies with the results of biochemical analyses to determine the biochemical tests that are useful in differentiating and identifying members of Enterobacteriaceae. These are the tests that are routinely used in clinical laboratories for identifying members of the family.

Both systems are presented in Table 20-1. Table 20-2 shows specific changes in nomenclature relating to each classification scheme. The genus *Kluyvera* has been recently proposed by Farmer and associates (J. Clin. Microbiol. **13:**919-933, 1981). Formerly known as Enteric group 8 (API group 1), these bacteria were reported to share the properties of most members of the family Enterobacteriaceae. Three species were defined by DNA-DNA hybridization: *K. ascorbata*, *K. cryocrescens*, and *Kluyvera* species group 3. *K. ascorbata* can be differentiated from *K. cryocrescens* by its positive ascorbate test, inability to grow at 5 C in a refrigerator, and smaller zones of inhibition around carbenicillin and cephalothin disks. The authors believed these bacteria were probably infrequent opportunistic pathogens. Two additional genera have been proposed recently. *Tatumella*

TABLE 20-2

Specific changes in nomenclature

Edwards and Ewing/CDC*	Bergey's Manual (ed. 8)
Citrobacter diversus	*Citrobacter intermedius,* biotype b
Citrobacter amalonaticus	*Citrobacter intermedius,* biotype a
Arizona hinshawii	*Salmonella arizonae*
Klebsiella oxytoca	*Klebsiella pneumoniae,* indole positive or indole positive and gelatin positive
Enterobacter agglomerans	*Erwinia herbicola*
Enterobacter gergoviae	
Enterobacter sakazakii	*Enterobacter cloacae,* yellow pigmented, sorbitol negative, delayed DNase positive
Serratia liquefaciens	*Enterobacter liquefaciens*
Serratia rubidaea	*Serratia marcescens*
Serratia plymuthica	
Serratia odorifera	
Serratia fonticola	
Providencia stuartii	*Proteus inconstans,* subgroup B (*Providencia alcalifaciens,* biogroup 4)†
Providencia stuartii, urea-positive	*Proteus rettgeri,* biogroup 5‡
Providencia alcalifaciens	*Proteus inconstans,* subgroup A
Providencia rettgeri	*Proteus rettgeri,* biogroups 1-4‡
Morganella morganii	*Proteus morganii*
Yersinia intermedia	*Yersinia enterocolitica*
Yersinia frederiksenii	
Yersinia pseudotuberculosis	

*Modified from Brenner and colleagues.[9]

†*Proteus inconstans* subgroup B was later referred to as *Providencia alcalifaciens* biogroup 4 by Edwards and Ewing.[23]

‡Penner and associates[78] divided the strains of *Proteus rettgeri* into five biogroups on the basis of biochemical reactions. Biogroup 5 was subsequently classified as urease-positive *Providencia stuartii*. Biogroups 1 to 4 became *Providencia rettgeri*.

ptyseos (previously group EF-9) has been isolated primarily from sputum (Hollis et al.: J. Clin. Microbiol. **14**:79-88, 1981). It differs from other Enterobacteriaceae by its large zone of inhibition around penicillin, its tendency to die on some media within 7 days, and its small number of flagella. It is susceptible to ampicillin, cephalothin, tetracycline, chloramphenicol, and aminoglycosides. *Cedecea* (named for CDC) is isolated from clinical specimens but is of unknown significance (Grimont et al.: Int. J. Syst. Bacteriol. **31**:317-326, 1981). The organism is lipase positive, resistant to colistin and cephalothin, and negative for DNase, gelatin liquefaction, and utilization of L-arabinose and L-rhamnose. Two species are proposed, *C. davisae* and *C. lapagei*.

FAMILY ENTEROBACTERIACEAE

Members of the Enterobacteriaceae are gram-negative straight rods, most of which are motile, although some strains are nonmotile (*Shigella* and *Klebsiella*), and nonmotile variants of motile species can also occur. The motile species possess **peritrichous** flagella, differing from members of the Pseudomonadaceae, which have polar flagella. Several strains of *Salmonella*, *Shigella*, *Escherichia*, *Klebsiella*, *Enterobacter*, and *Proteus* possess fimbriae or pili.[10] The latter are not organs of locomotion, are considerably smaller than flagella, and bear no antigenic relationship to them.[20] They are readily observed under the electron microscope.

All species ferment glucose. Aerogenic and anaerogenic forms are found. The absence of gas in the fermentation of carbohydrates is characteristic of some genera. Nitrates are usually reduced to nitrites. Indophenol-oxidase is not produced, and alginate is not liquefied. Pectate is liquefied only by members of the genus *Pectobacterium*.

The family is composed of a large and diverse group of organisms varying in antigenic structure and biochemical properties. The genera within the family have been established mainly on the basis of biochemical characteristics, whereas original species—the names of many of which still remain—were established on both biochemical and ecologic bases. The antigenic complexity of these bacteria has led to the development of antigenic schemes, patterned after the Kauffmann-White scheme for *Salmonella*, in which numerous serotypes are listed. Many of these serotypes are biochemically similar and can be distinguished only by serologic procedures.

The organisms are found in the intestine of humans and other animals, in the soil, and on plants. Many are parasites; others are saprophytes. Many species are pathogenic for humans, producing enteric and septicemic infections.

Culturally, these bacteria produce similar growth on blood agar, usually appearing as relatively large, shiny, gray colonies, which may or may not be hemolytic. Species that produce hydrogen sulfide show a definite greening around subsurface colonies in blood agar. On trypticase soy agar, nutrient agar, or meat infusion agar the colonies may vary in size, depending on the genus, but they are usually grayish-white, translucent, and slightly convex. Some colonies are large and mucoid, as in the case of *Klebsiella*, certain types of *Shigella*, and certain variants of *Salmonella*, especially *S. enteritidis* serotype Typhimurium. Colony variation does occur, giving rise to smooth and rough forms. Individual species or type colony characteristics are described under each of the respective genera.

ISOLATION OF ENTEROBACTERIACEAE

Because this book is primarily confined to diagnostic procedures for **pathogenic** microorganisms, emphasis is on the pathogenic members of the family.

The general procedures described in Chapters 6 and 9 for isolation of the gram-negative enteric bacteria should be followed to obtain best results. Since these organisms may be isolated from various clinical sources, their isolation from fecal material, blood, urine, and other body fluids is presented again in this chapter. Laboratory personnel are reminded that clinical specimens may contain relatively few pathogens, and appropriate enrichment procedures are not only highly recommended but often necessary. It should be recalled that enrichment procedures satisfactory for *Salmonella* and *Shigella* are not applicable to coliforms and *Proteus*, since the latter are usually inhibited by their use.

Isolation from stools

A freshly passed stool is the specimen of choice when enteric disease is suspected, and whenever possible multiple specimens should be submitted for culture.[23] Although rectal swabs may be used for collecting adequate specimens from acutely ill persons who are shedding large numbers of organisms, their use cannot be expected to yield the maximal number of positive cultures.[109] The number of pathogenic enteric organisms may decrease during the period between collection and processing in the laboratory. If any delay is anticipated in their arrival at the laboratory, specimens should be preserved by one of the procedures described earlier (see Chapter 9). Specimens from carriers may show very few pathogens, and in certain cases the appearance of these organisms may be only intermittent. Stuart medium[107] is highly recommended as a transport medium for such specimens if they are to be shipped to a diagnostic laboratory. Ewing and co-workers[32] reported excellent recovery of *Salmonella typhi* from stools in transit in this medium after 1 week.

Because of the wide and varied flora present in fecal material, one or more of the following **enrichment media** inhibitory for the normal intestinal flora must be used. The enrichment media normally employed are **GN broth** (Hajna), the **selenite broth** of Leifson, and the **tetrathionate broth** of Muller. Kauffman's modification[53] of tetrathionate contains both bile and

brilliant green and gives excellent recovery of salmonellae but inhibits most shigellae. Tetrathionate broth containing bile salts may be used for general enrichment, since members of salmonellae, including *S. typhi*, are usually greatly increased in this medium. Some shigellae may also be recovered from it. Tetrathionate broth containing brilliant green $(1:10^5)$ is useful only for salmonellae other than *S. typhi*. It is recommended that these enrichment media be inoculated with one part stool specimen to 10 parts broth. If mucus is present, a portion of it should also be placed in the enrichment broth. If preserved diluted specimens are used (see Chapter 6), at least 2 ml should be placed in the enrichment broth. After 18 to 24 hours of incubation at 35 C, appropriate plating media should be streaked for isolation with inoculum from the enrichment broth. It can be beneficial to hold enrichment media for an additional 24 hours and, if the first plates are negative, to inoculate another set of plates.

Cold-temperature enrichment has been used to increase isolation of *Yersinia enterocolitica* from stool specimens. Whereas cold-temperature enrichment significantly increases the isolation of *Y. enterocolitica* from stools of convalescent and asymptomatic patients, it only minimally increased the number of isolates from patients with diarrhea caused by serotype O:3.[71]

Numerous **plating media** are in use today. Some of these are selective, whereas others are differential. Desoxycholate citrate agar, Salmonella-Shigella (SS) agar, Hektoen enteric (HE) agar, bismuth sulfite agar, brilliant green agar (BGA), eosin–methylene blue (EMB) agar (Plate 53), xylose lysine desoxycholate (XLD) agar, and MacConkey agar (Plate 52) are among the most widely used.* Most laboratories prefer to employ one selective medium, such as SS or

---

*To inhibit the spreading of *Proteus* strains on MacConkey or EMB media, the agar concentration may be increased to 5%.

HE agar, and one differential medium, such as MacConkey or EMB agar. Two procedures are followed: (1) the **direct** plating of the specimen on these media, and (2) the **indirect** procedure using enrichment first (see above). Bismuth sulfite is the medium of choice when *S. typhi* is suspected, because it is still the most efficient in the isolation of this pathogen.

To isolate diarrhea-inducing (enterotoxigenic, enteroinvasive, and enteropathogenic) *Escherichia coli*, *Klebsiella*, *Enterobacter*, or *Citrobacter* from fecal material, tetrathionate and selenite enrichment broths are **not** recommended, since both are inhibitory for most strains of these genera. In these instances, the less inhibitory media (either MacConkey or EMB agar) are used for primary isolation by the direct plating procedure. Blood agar also is recommended by some investigators.

Some lactose-fermenting, gram-negative enteric bacteria can tolerate the inhibitory substances present in the enrichment broths and the selective media. These bacteria can be recognized readily by their appearance on selective plates.

Lactose-negative bacteria, such as *Salmonella* and *Shigella*, give rise to small **colorless** colonies in desoxycholate citrate, MacConkey, EMB, XLD, and SS media. On HE agar salmonellae and shigellae appear **bluish-green.** Colonies of *Proteus* may be confused with *Salmonella* and *Shigella*, especially on desoxycholate and also on EMB and MacConkey media containing 5% agar, because of their lactose-negative characteristic. Colonies of **lactose-fermenting** organisms on desoxycholate citrate agar (if not inhibited), MacConkey agar, and SS medium appear **red;** on EMB agar they appear **dark purple** to **black** and often have a **metallic sheen.** On HE agar they appear **salmon** to **orange.**

On bismuth sulfite agar, *S. typhi* gives rise to **black** colonies (Plate 56) with a metallic sheen if the colonies are well separated. A pour plate is recommended in those instances when only a few organisms are likely to be present. In this procedure a relatively large inoculum (3 to 5 ml) of fluid stool or preserved stool specimen is placed in a Petri dish, and approximately 15 ml of the melted medium is added and rotated thoroughly to mix. Subsurface colonies usually have a typical appearance. For example, subsurface colonies of *S. typhi*, if well separated, are circular, **jet black,** and well defined. Only those near the surface exhibit the characteristic metallic sheen. Some strains of salmonellae (*S. enteritidis* and *S. enteritidis* serotype Paratyphi-B), as well as certain other members of Enterobacteriaceae, give rise to black colonies on this medium. Thus, every black colony that appears should not be presumptively identified as *S. typhi*. Generally, salmonellae other than *S. typhi* (bioserotype Paratyphi-A, serotype Typhimurium, and *S. cholerae-suis*) grow as dark green, flat colonies or as colonies with black centers and green peripheries.

Isolation from blood

Blood culture specimens are usually collected from individuals with a febrile disease of unknown etiology, and therefore the media used are generally dictated by the needs of the suspected organism. General methods are discussed in Chapter 7, but if blood cultures are desired for *Salmonella* or *Shigella* **specifically** (shigellae are only rarely found in the blood), approximately 10 ml of blood should be placed in 90 to 100 ml of bile broth and incubated at 35 C. If the culture is negative after 24 hours, incubation should be continued for 10 to 14 days before a negative result is reported.

In **typhoid fever** a positive blood culture is usually obtained during the first or second week after onset. In septicemias produced by other salmonellae, blood cultures* should be taken during the first week and, if negative, should be repeated during the second week and thereafter if considered necessary. Laboratory personnel

---

*Cultures of bone marrow also may be helpful in salmonelloses.

are reminded that in typhoid fever a blood culture may be positive **before** stool cultures become positive. During the first week blood cultures are positive in about 90% of the cases, whereas stool cultures are positive in only about 10% of the cases during this period.

Subculture of blood cultures on the appropriate type of agar medium—bismuth sulfite, EMB, or MacConkey—is carried out as described for stool isolations. Many investigators find that a plate of either EMB or MacConkey agar will suffice at this phase of the procedure.

Isolation from urine

S. typhi may be isolated from urine in about 25% of cases of typhoid fever. Other members of the Enterobacteriaceae may also be isolated from this source, including other species of *Salmonella* and, more commonly, certain members of the genera *Escherichia*, *Klebsiella*, and *Proteus*. Direct plating of the specimen on selective and differential media is recommended. Best results for isolating salmonellae from urine are usually obtained by centrifuging the specimen at 2,500 to 3,000 rpm for 20 to 30 minutes to sediment the bacteria. Several loopfuls of the sediment may then be plated on selective and differential media and the remainder added to enrichment broth. The enrichment procedure aids in the recovery of *S. typhi*. Subculture from the enrichment broth is carried out on the appropriate plating media after 24 or 48 hours. If centrifugation is not employed for specimens from suspected *Salmonella* infections, 2 to 3 ml of the specimen should be added to the enrichment broth.

PRELIMINARY SCREENING OF CULTURES

Colonies of salmonellae and shigellae, the characteristics of which have been discussed earlier in this chapter, may be recognized by their **lactose-negative** appearance on isolation plates. Suspected colonies of these two genera

should be picked carefully with an inoculating needle and transferred to the screening medium. If time permits, it is advisable to select two or three colonies from each plate, since mixed infections are not infrequent. **It is poor technique to touch the agar surrounding a colony to test the temperature of the needle, as members of the inhibited flora may be still present and viable although not visible. Only the center of the colony should be touched, using a cool needle.**

With the inoculating needle a part of the colony should be stabbed first into the butt of a slant of either **triple sugar iron** (TSI) **agar** or **Kligler's iron agar** (KIA) and then streaked in a zigzag fashion over the slanted surface. The tube is always closed with a cotton plug or a **loose** closure, never with a tightly fitting rubber stopper or cork. The latter procedure can lead to a misinterpretation of the results, as is explained in the following section. The formulas for these screening media are given in Chapter 42.

Since all Enterobacteriaceae are indophenol-oxidase negative and most members reduce nitrate to nitrite, much time and effort can be saved if oxidase and nitrate reduction tests are performed early in the identification process. Members of *Erwinia* are nitrate negative, and some biogroups of *E. agglomerans* fail to reduce nitrate to nitrite.

Examination and interpretation of reactions

TSI agar contains the three sugars, glucose, lactose, and sucrose; phenol red indicator to indicate fermentation; and ferrous sulfate to demonstrate hydrogen sulfide production (indicated by blackening in the butt). The glucose concentration is one tenth of the concentration of lactose and sucrose in order that the fermentation of this carbohydrate **alone** may be detected. KIA is exactly like TSI agar, except it lacks the carbohydrate sucrose. The small amount of acid produced by fermentation of glucose is oxidized rapidly in the slant, which will remain or revert to an alkaline pH; in contrast,

TABLE 20-3

Reactions observed in TSI agar

Reaction	Explanation
Acid butt (yellow), alkaline slant (red)	Glucose fermented
Acid throughout medium, butt and slant yellow	Lactose or sucrose or both fermented
Gas bubbles in butt, medium sometimes split	Aerogenic culture
Blackening in butt	Hydrogen sulfide produced
Alkaline slant and butt (medium entirely red)	None of three sugars fermented

the acid reaction is maintained in the butt because it is under lower oxygen tension. To enhance the alkaline condition in the slant, **free exchange of air** must be permitted through the use of a loose closure, as stated earlier. If the tube is tightly closed with a stopper or screw cap, an acid reaction (caused solely by glucose fermentation) will also involve the slant. The reactions in TSI, which is basically **red** when uninoculated, are shown in Table 20-3. **It is to be emphasized that ideally the reactions should be read after 18 to 24 hours, and they cannot be properly interpreted if the slants are incubated for more than 48 hours.**

IDENTIFICATION OF ENTEROBACTERIACEAE

Since some colonies of *Proteus* species can be confused with salmonellae and other lactose-negative enterobacteria on initial isolation, all TSI (or KIA) cultures should be further screened on Christensen **urea agar slants** or in Rustigian and Stuart tubed **urea broth** (weakly buffered). A heavy inoculum is prescribed, and this is spread over the surface of the agar slant or properly emulsified in the urea broth. Urease activity is observed by a change of color (red) in the indicator caused by the production of ammonia. A positive test in 2 to 4 hours in the broth or on urea agar slants at 35 C indicates *Proteus*, urea-positive *P. stuartii*, or *P. rettgeri*. A positive test after 24 hours might indicate a member of the genera *Klebsiella*, *Enterobacter*, *Serratia*, or *Yersinia*.

The reactions observed on TSI agar (or KIA) slants, **together with the effect on urea,** usually indicate the possible genus to which the isolate belongs (see reaction tree in Fig. 20-2). One should not draw premature conclusions, however, because final identification depends on biochemical and serologic confirmation. Many investigators use the growth from TSI agar (or KIA) slants for slide agglutination tests with polyvalent *Salmonella* or *Shigella* antisera. This is justified in cases of outbreaks or when rapid reporting is required. Cultures from these agar slants should be streaked on meat infusion agar, trypticase soy agar, or MacConkey agar for purity. A single colony may then be transferred to a tube of broth for culture, followed by a complete series of tests.

Another medium that has been used with a good deal of success in conjunction with TSI agar or KIA is **lysine-iron-agar** (LIA).[24] Using a straight wire, inoculum is taken carefully from a well-selected colony and transferred to KIA or TSI agar in the usual way, and **without going back** to the colony on the plate, a tube of LIA is inoculated by stabbing the butt of the medium **twice** and then streaking the slant. If the spot where the stab was made in the TSI agar (or KIA) medium is touched with the tip of the wire, a sufficient number of organisms will be obtained for inoculation of the LIA medium.

TABLE 20-4

Interpretation of reactions on TSI agar (see Plates 59 to 66)

Reaction	Carbohydrates fermented	Possible organisms
Acid butt Acid slant Gas in butt No H$_2$S	Glucose with acid and gas Lactose and/or sucrose with acid and gas	*Escherichia** *Klebsiella* or *Enterobacter* *Proteus*†, *Providencia*‡ *Citrobacter*, *Serratia*
Acid butt Alkaline slant Gas in butt H$_2$S produced	Glucose with acid and gas Lactose and sucrose not fermented	*Salmonella* *Proteus* *Arizona* (certain types) *Citrobacter freundii* (certain types) *Edwardsiella*
Acid butt Alkaline slant No gas in butt No H$_2$S	Glucose with acid only Lactose and sucrose not fermented	*Escherichia* (anaerogenic biotypes) *Salmonella*§ *Shigella* *Providencia* *Serratia* *Enterobacter agglomerans* *Yersinia*
Acid butt Acid slant Gas in butt H$_2$S produced	Glucose with acid and gas Lactose and/or sucrose with acid and gas	*Arizona* *Citrobacter freundii*
Alkaline or neutral butt Alkaline slant No H$_2$S	None	*Alcaligenes*‖ *Pseudomonas*‖ *Acinetobacter*‖

*Rarely, a strain is H$_2$S positive.
†Approximately 6% of *Proteus* strains are H$_2$S negative.
‡Only a small percent, 5% or less, of *Providencia* species ferment lactose.
§*Salmonella typhi* produces a small amount of H$_2$S but seldom gas.
‖Included here because colonies of these organisms may be frequently confused with lactose-negative members of Enterobacteriaceae and may be selected from isolation plates.

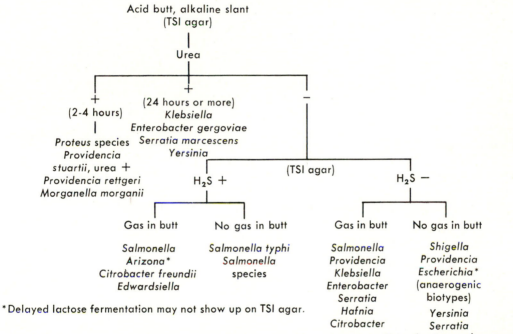

FIG. 20-2
Tentative differentiation of Enterobacteriaceae.

Table 20-5

Typical reaction patterns of Enterobacteriaceae on TSI and LIA (see Plates 59 to 66)

Organism	TSI				LIA		
	Slant	Butt	Gas	H₂S	Slant	Butt	H₂S
Arizona	K or A	A	+	+	K	K	+ or −
Citrobacter							
freundii	A or K	A	+	+	K	A	+ or −
diversus	A or K	A	+	−√	K	A	−
amalonaticus	A or K	A	+	−	K	A	−
*Escherichia coli**	A	A	+ or −	−	K	K or A	−
	K	A	−	−	K	K or A	−
	K	A	−	−	K	K√	−
	K	A	+√	−	K	K or A	−
Edwardsiella†	K	A	+	+	K	K	+
Enterobacter‡							
cloacae	A or K	A	+	−	K	A√	−
aerogenes	A	A	+	−	K	K√	−
agglomerans	K or A	A	− or +	−	K	A	−
sakazakii	A	A	+	−	K	A	−
gergoviae	K or A	A	+	−	K	K or (K)	−
Hafnia alvei	K	A	+	−	K	K	−
Klebsiella	A or K	A	+	−	K	K (or A§)	−
Proteus							
vulgaris	K or A	A	+	+√	R	A	−
mirabilis	K	A	+	+√	R	A	−
Providencia							
alcalifaciens	K	A	+ or −	−	R	A	−
stuartii	K	A	− or +	−	R	A	−
rettgeri	K	A	−	−	R	A	−
Morganella morganii	K	A	+	−√	K‖ or R	A	−
Salmonella							
typhi	K	A	−	+ or −√	K	K¶	+ or −
other	K	A	+	+¶	K	K	+ or −
Serratia	K or A	A	− or +	−	K	K or A	−
Shigella	K	A	−√	−	K	A	−
Yersinia	K	A	−	−	K	A	−

Modified from Washington.[112] A, acidic; K, alkaline; R, red; S, slant; √, key reaction.

*Mucoid colonies with negative motility and ornithine tests should be referred.

†Refer for confirmation.

‡DNase and oxidase tests must be done on all *Enterobacter* patterns. If negative, send out as *Enterobacter*. If DNase is positive, send out as *Serratia marcescens* and refer for confirmation. If oxidase is positive, refer. Any *Enterobacter* pattern with a green sheen must be referred. Refer all K/A TSI and K/K LIA *Enterobacter* patterns without doing DNase or oxidase tests.

§May be reported as *Klebsiella* if colonial morphology is mucoid and oxidase test is negative.

‖Refer for phenylalanine deaminase test.

¶Rare exceptions.

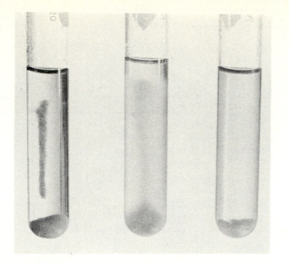

FIG. 20-3
Semisolid motility medium. Tube on left shows *Shigella* (nonmotile). Center tube is *E. coli* (motility results in diffuse growth pattern). Tube on right is uninoculated.

The combinations of reactions obtained by this[23,60] or other screening methods[60,112] yield much useful information relatively early (Table 20-5).

Motility-indole-lysine (MIL) medium is a reliable medium, except for occasional falsely weak or negative indole reactions. Used together with TSI and urea agar, MIL permits reliable early recognition of enteric pathogens of the Enterobacteriaceae[83] (See Fig. 20-3 for the motility test.)

Table 20-6 shows the tests on which differentiation of the Enterobacteriaceae may be made. Tests to which reference is made in Table 20-6 are given in Chapters 42 and 44.

Lactose-fermenting members of Enterobacteriaceae

A large number of organisms within the family Enterobacteriaceae ferment the carbohydrate **lactose,** and those that do so may be tentatively identified by the reactions shown in Fig. 20-4. In recent years lactose-fermenting strains of *S.*

typhi (and other *Salmonella*) have been reported. Such strains are otherwise like *S. typhi* in possessing the Vi, O, and H antigens of this organism (antigenic structure is shown in Table 20-8). Some lactose-positive members of the family ferment the sugar promptly, whereas others exhibit a delayed reaction. In Fig. 20-2 the differentiation between these genera is shown.

The IMViC reaction (Plate 58) is used primarily to distinguish between the coliform bacteria, but it also may be applied advantageously to other organisms in the family. The letters stand for **indole, methyl red, Voges-Proskauer,** and **citrate** reactions (the "i" is inserted for euphony). These may be carried out and interpreted as shown.

Test for indole

Inoculate tryptophan broth. Test after 48 hours by the addition of the Kovacs or Ehrlich reagent (see Chapter 44). A **red** color indicates production of indole from the amino acid.

Methyl red test

Inoculate MR-VP medium (Clark and Lubs dextrose broth medium). Test after 48 to 96 hours by adding 5 drops of methyl red indicator (see Chapter 44 for more rapid procedures). A **red** color is read as positive. A yellow color is read as negative. Read the test immediately after adding the reagent.

Voges-Proskauer test

Inoculate MR-VP medium (same as in previous test) and test for the production of acetylmethylcarbinol after 48 hours of incubation by adding to 1 ml of culture 15 drops of 5% alpha-naphthol in absolute ethyl alcohol and 10 drops of 40% potassium hydroxide (see Chapter 44 for more rapid procedures). The necessary volume of culture may be pipetted to a small tube before the MR test above is performed. A positive test is the development of a **red** color in 15 to 30 minutes. An alternative test is given in Chapter 44.

TABLE 20-6

Differentiation of Enterobacteriaceae by biochemical tests* (see Plates 59 to 66)

Test	Escherichieae Escherichia	Escherichieae Shigella	Edwardsielleae Edwardsiella	Salmonelleae Salmonella	Arizona	Citrobacter freundii	Citrobacter diversus	Citrobacter amalonaticus	Klebsiella pneumoniae	Klebsiella oxytoca	Klebsiella ozaenae	Klebsiella rhinoscleromatis	Enterobacter cloacae	Enterobacter aerogenes	Enterobacter agglomerans	Enterobacter gergoviae	Enterobacter sakazakii	Serratia marcescens	Serratia liquefaciens
Indole	+	−+	+	−	−	−	+	+	−	+	−	−	−	−	−+	−	−	−	−
Methyl red	+	+	+	+	+	+	+	+	−+	−+	+	+	−	−	−+	d	−+	−+	+−
Voges-Proskauer	−	−	−	−	−	−	−	−	+	+	−	−	+	+	+−	+	+	+	−+
Simmons citrate	−	−	−	d	+	+	+	+	+	+	−+	−	+	+	d	+	+	+	+
Hydrogen sulfide (TSI)	−	−	+	+	+	+−	−	−	−	−	−	−	−	−	−	−	−	−	−
Urease	−	−	−	−¶	−	d^w	d^w	d	+	+	−+	−	+−	−	d^w	+	−	d^w	d^w
KCN	−	−	−	−	−	+	−	+	+	+	+−	+	+	+	−+	−	+	+	+
Motility	+−	−	+	+	+	+	+	+	−	−	−	−	+	+	+−	+	+	+	+
Gelatin (22 C)	−	−	−	−	(+)	−	−	d	−	(+)−	−	−	(+)−	−(+)	d	−	−	+(+)	+
Lysine decarboxylase	d	−	+	+	+	−	−	−	+	+	−+	−	−	+	−	+(+)	−	+	+(+)
Arginine dihydrolase	d	d	−	+(+)	+(+)	d	+(+)	+	−	−	−	−	+	−	−	−	+	−	−
Ornithine decarboxylase	d	d#	+	+	+	d	+	+	−	−	−	−	+	+	+	+	+	+	+
Phenylalanine deaminase	−	−	−	−	−	−	−	−	−	−	−	−	−	−	−+	−	−	−	−
Malonate	−	−	−	−	+	−+	−+	−	+	+	−	+−	+−	+−	+−	+	−+	−	−
Gas from glucose	+	−#	+	+	+	+	+	+	+	+	d	−	+	+	−+	+	+	+−**	+−
Lactose	+	−#	−	−	d	(+)+	d	d	+	+	d	d	+(+)	+	d	d	+	−	d
Sucrose	d	−#	−	−	d	−+	d	d	+	+	d	+(+)	+	+	d	+	+	+	+
D-Mannitol	+	+−	−	+	+	+	+	+	+	+	−	+	+	+	+	+	+	+	+
Dulcitol	d	d	−	d††	−	d	+−	−	−+	−+	−	−	−+	−	−+	−	−	−	−
Salicin	d	−	−	−	d	(+)+	(+)	+	+	+	+	+(+)	+	d	+	+	+	+	+
Adonitol	−	−	−	−	−	−	+	−	+−	+−	+	+	−+	+	−	−	−	d	d
Inositol i (meso)	−	−	−	d	−	−	−	−	+	+	d	+	d	+	d	−(+)	d	d	+(+)
D-Sorbitol	d	d	−	+	+	+	+	+	+	+	d	+	+	+	d	−	−	+	+
L-Arabinose	+	d	−+	+††	+	+	+	+	+	+	+	+	+	+	+	+	+	−	+
Raffinose	d	d	−	−	d	−	−	−	+	+	+	+	+	+	d	+	−	−	−
L-Rhamnose	d	d	−	+	+	+	+	+	+	+	d	−+	+	+	+(+)	+	+	−	d

Adapted from Edwards and Ewing.[23]

+, 90% or more positive in 1 or 2 days; −, 90% or more negative; d, different biochemical types [+, (+), −]; (+), delayed positive (decarboxylase reactions, 3 or 4 days); +−, majority of cultures positive; −+, majority negative; w, weakly positive reaction.

*This chart is simply a guide. Users are urged to consult other publications, such as CDC publications entitled "Biochemical Reactions Given by Enterobacteriaceae in Commonly used Tests" and "Differentiation of Enterobacteriaceae by Biochemical Reactions" (W.H. Ewing, 1973), for percentage data, additional tests, and references.

†Adapted from Sonnenwirth.[103]

‡Adapted from Darland and others.[16]

| Klebsielleae | | | | | Proteeae | | | | | | Yersineae | | | | | | | | Erwinieae | |
| Serratia | | | | Hafnia alvei | Proteus | | Providencia | | | Morganella morganii | Yersinia | | | | | | | Erwinia§ | Pectobacterium† | Test |
rubidaea	odorifera	fonticola	plymuthica	Hafnia alvei	vulgaris	mirabilis	rettgeri	alcalifaciens	stuartii	Morganella morganii	pestis†	pseudotuberculosis‡	enterocolitica†	intermedia	frederiksenii	ruckeri	Erwinia§	Pectobacterium†	Test
−	+	−	−	−	+	−	+	+	+	+	−	−	‖	+	+	−	−	−+	Indole
−+	+	+		−+	+	+	+	+	+	+	+	$+^{w}$35 C +25 C	+			+	−	+−	Methyl red
+	+−	−	+−	+−	−	−+	−	−	−		−35 C −25 C	−35 C −25 C	−35 C +−25 C	−35 C −25 C	−35 C −25 C	−35 C −($+^{w}$)25 C	+	−+	Voges-Proskauer
+(+)	(+)−	+	+−	d	d	+(+)	+	+	+		−	−				(+)	+	d 35 C +(+) 25 C	Simmons citrate
−	−	−			+	+										−	−	−	Hydrogen sulfide (TSI)
d^{w}	−	−			+	+	+	−	−+	+	−	+	+	+	+	−	−	d	Urease
−+	−+	+		+	+	+	+	+	+		−	−	−			d	−	+−	KCN
+−	+	+		+	+	+	+	+	+	+−	−35 C −25 C	−35 C (+)+ 25 C	−35 C +25 C			−35 C +− 25 C	+	+−	Motility
+(+)	+	−	+	−	+	+	−	−	−	−	−	−	−	−	−	+(+)	+	+(+)	Gelatin (22 C)
+(+)	+	+	−	+	−	−	−	−	−	−						+(+)	−	−	Lysine decarboxylase
−	−	−	−	d	−	−		−	−	−						−	−	−	Arginine dihydrolase
−	+−	−	+	+	−	+	−	−	−	+			+	+	+	+	−	−	Ornithine decarboxylase
−	−	−			+	+	+	+	+	+						−	−	−	Phenylalanine deaminase
+−	−	+		+−	−	−	−	−	−		−					−	−	−+	Malonate
d	−	+	−+	+	+−	+	−+	+−	−	+−	−	−	−			−+	−	−+ 35 C d 25 C	Gas from glucose
+	(+)+	+		d	−	−	−	−	−	−	−	−	−			−(+)	−	d 35 C +(+) 25 C	Lactose
+	+−	(+)+		d	+	d	d	d	(+)+	−	−	−	+			−	+	+− 35 C + 25 C	Sucrose
+	+	+	+	+	−	−	+−	−	d	−	+	+	+	+	+	+	−	+−	D-Mannitol
−	−	+			−	−	−	−	−	−	−	−	−			−	−	−	Dulcitol
+(+)	+	+		d	d	d	+−	−	−	−	+	(+)	d			−	+	d 35 C + 25 C	Salicin
+(+)	+	+	−		−	−	d	+	−+	−	−	−	−			−	−	−	Adonitol
d	(+)+	+	+		−	−	+	−	+	−			d			−	−	−	Inositol i (meso)
−	+	+		−	−	d	−	d	−		−+	−	+	+	+	−	d	−	D-Sorbitol
+	+	+	+	+	−	−	−	−	−	−	+	+(+)	+			−	d	+− 35 C + 25 C	L-Arabinose
+	+−	+			−	−	−	−	−	−		−+	−			−	+	d 35 C +(+) 25 C	Raffinose
−	+(+)	+−	−	+	−	−	+−	−	−	−	−	+	−	+	+	−	−	d	L-Rhamnose

§Adapted from Buchanan and Gibbons.[11]

‖Majority of strains isolated in the United States are indole positive, whereas most of the strains isolated in Europe have been indole negative.

¶Rare exceptions.

#Certain biotypes of S. flexneri produce gas; cultures of S. sonnei ferment lactose and sucrose slowly and decarboxylate ornithine.

**Gas volume produced by cultures of Serratia, Proteus, and Providencia are small.

††S. typhi, S. cholerae-suis, S. enteritidis bioser. Paratyphi-A and Pullorum and a few others ordinarily do not ferment dulcitol promptly. S. cholerae-suis does not ferment arabinose.

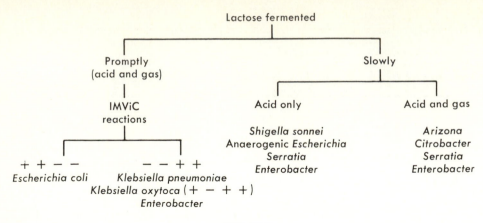

FIG. 20-4
Differentiation of lactose-fermenting Enterobacteriaceae.

Citrate test

Inoculate Simmons citrate agar with a light inoculum. A positive test is indicated by the development of a **Prussian blue color** in the medium, showing that the organism can utilize citrate as a sole source of carbon.

ANTIGENIC COMPLEXITY OF ENTEROBACTERIACEAE

The members of the Enterobacteriaceae exhibit a mosaic of antigens that fall into three main categories as follows:

1. The **K** (from German *Kapsel*), or **envelope,** antigens are those that, by concept, surround the cell. With certain exceptions these are heat labile. In the genus *Klebsiella* the subdivision into capsular types is based on the K antigens. K antigens mask the heat-stable somatic antigens of the cell and cause live cells to be inagglutinable in O antisera. Examples are the Vi antigen of *S. typhi* and the B antigen found in certain types of *E. coli.*

2. The **O** (from German *Ohne Hauch*, nonspreading), or **somatic,** antigens, which are heat stable, are located primarily in the cell wall. Chemically they are polysaccharide in nature. The O complex of antigens determines the somatic subgroup to which the organism belongs, in the genera *Salmonella, Arizona, Citrobacter, Escherichia, Providencia, Serratia,* and others.

3. The **H** (from German *Hauch*, spreading) antigens are the **flagellar** antigens. These are located in the flagella, are protein in nature, and are heat labile. The serotypes within the somatic groups in *Salmonella* and some other genera in the Enterobacteriaceae are determined by the H antigens.

IDENTIFICATION OF GENERA WITHIN THE FAMILY ENTEROBACTERIACEAE
Genus Salmonella

Salmonella cholerae-suis is the type species of the genus. Salmonellae are usually motile, but nonmotile forms do occur.[54] With the exception of *S. typhi* and *S. enteritidis* serotype Gallinarum, they all produce **gas** in glucose. Suspected colonies of salmonellae on isolation media are inoculated to slants of TSI agar (or KIA). Isolates that produce acid, gas, and hydrogen sulfide in the butt and an alkaline slant in this medium and are **urease negative** should be tested with *Salmonella* polyvalent antisera. Pure cultures should be tested for motility and inoculated to

TABLE 20-7

Biochemical reactions of genus *Salmonella* (see Plates 60 and 61)

Test	Reaction	Test	Reaction
Adonitol	−	Methyl red	+
Dulcitol	+	Voges-Proskauer	−
Glucose	+ with gas	Simmons citrate	Variable*
Inositol	Variable	KCN†	−
Lactose	−	Phenylalanine deaminase†	−
Mannitol	+	Sodium malonate†	−
Salicin	−	Lysine decarboxylase	+
Sucrose	−	Arginine dihydrolase†	+
Indole	−	Ornithine decarboxylase†	+

*S. typhi and some other salmonellae are citrate negative.
†Descriptions of these media and procedures for the tests performed may be found in Chapters 42 and 44. Although not used routinely in all laboratories, they aid in group differentiation.

TABLE 20-8

Some examples of the Kauffmann-White or *Salmonella* antigenic scheme

Species, bioserotypes and serotypes	O antigens	H antigens Phase 1	H antigens Phase 2
	Group A		
Paratyphi-A	1, 2, 12	a	—
	Group B		
Tinda	1, 4, 12, 27	a	e, n, z_{15}
Paratyphi-B	1,4, 5, 12	b	1, 2
Typhimurium	1,4, 5, 12	i	1, 2
Heidelberg	4, 5, 12	r	1, 2
	Group C$_1$		
Paratyphi-C	6, 7, Vi	c	1, 5
Thompson	6, 7	k	1, 5
	Group C$_2$		
Newport	6, 8	e, h	1, 2
	Group D		
S. typhi	9, 12, Vi	d	—
S. enteritidis	1, 9, 12	g, m	—
Sendai	1, 9, 12	a	1, 5
	Group E$_1$		
Oxford	3, 10	a	1, 7
London	3, 10	l, v	1, 6

the biochemical media shown in Table 20-7. Typical salmonellae give the reactions shown.

Serologic identification

The Kauffmann-White or *Salmonella* antigenic scheme has a long list of serotypes that are arranged in O, or somatic, subgroups. The H (or flagellar) antigens, as previously stated, determine the type.

Table 20-8 shows an abbreviated example of a Kauffmann-White scheme, but it will help the student and laboratory worker to understand the schematic arrangement of the serotypes. There are more alphabetized somatic groups in the scheme than are shown (i.e., some 1,700 serotypes). The tabulated types shown are not necessarily the most common.

Because approximately 65 different somatic antigens have been recognized, serologic typing with polyvalent O antisera is essential. These sera are commercially available.* They will agglutinate the majority of strains found in the United States and Canada. **Group** identification is determined by O-typing sera, and **type** identification is determined by H-typing antisera. O-grouping sera for subgroups A, B, C_1, C_2, D, and E as well as H-typing sera for flagellar antigens a, b, c, d, i, 1, 2, 3, 5, 6, and 7 are available.* **Vi** antiserum is also available.

The serologic procedure usually employed is the **slide agglutination test,** in which a concentrated suspension of cells in saline is used. Details of the technique may be found in Chapter 37, but the reader's attention at this point is drawn to certain important considerations.

1. The culture to be tested must be **smooth** and not autoagglutinable in saline. A preliminary test with a 0.2% solution of acriflavine in 0.85% saline is an excellent indicator of smoothness. If a loopful of the test suspension, as a control, is mixed **gradually** on a slide with a loopful of acriflavine and cells remain in homogeneous suspension, the culture may be considered smooth.

2. If the culture suspension fails to agglutinate in the O diagnostic sera, heat it at 100 C for 15 to 30 minutes, cool, and retest with the same sera. Some salmonellae possess **K** antigens, previously mentioned, and are inagglutinable in the live or unheated form in O antisera. Examples of envelope antigens are the Vi antigen of *S. typhi* and *S. enteritidis* serotype Paratyphi-C, the 5 antigen in somatic group B, and the M antigen in some serotypes. Vi-containing types will agglutinate in the live or unheated form in Vi antiserum.

3. O-inagglutinable cultures should be sent to a reference laboratory* for identification by complete serologic analysis. **These cultures should be sent through the state or provincial laboratories.**

4. The majority of the salmonellae are **diphasic;** that is, the motile types may exhibit two antigenic forms referred to as phases (see Edwards and Ewing[23] for a complete discussion of this subject). These phases share the same O antigens but possess different H antigens, as seen in Table 20-8, and to identify the serotype it is necessary to identify the specific H antigens in both phases. These may not always be in evidence, and phase-suppression procedures may be necessary to reveal the **latent** phase. This can be accomplished by inoculating the organism into a small Petri dish containing semisolid agar in which is incorporated specific antiserum against the antigen(s) of the one identified phase. The homologous phase will be arrested at the site of inoculation, whereas the other

---

*Lederle Laboratories, Pearl River, N.Y.; Difco Laboratories, Detroit; Baltimore Biological Laboratory, Cockeysville, Md.; Lee Laboratories, Grayson, Ga.

*Enteric Section, Centers for Disease Control, Atlanta; Central Public Health Laboratory, Colindale, London.

phase will develop (or express itself) and may be identified. Such procedures can be carried out only by properly equipped laboratories. It should be noted that some flagellated salmonellae are nonmotile, and special procedures are required for their identification.[3]

5. To completely identify the O antigen and H antigen complexes, the use of absorbed **single factor** typing sera is required. These antisera are prepared by adding a concentrated suspension of cells containing the appropriate antigens to a suitable dilution of the multifactor serum, incubating in a water bath for 2 hours at 50 C, and refrigerating overnight. After centrifugation, the supernate will contain the unabsorbed and desired agglutinating antibodies. Such a procedure is referred to as **agglutinin absorption.**

Characteristics of Salmonella typhi

The typhoid organism exhibits its characteristic biochemical activity in the carbohydrates and produces small amounts of hydrogen sulfide in KIA or TSI agar. The organism is **anaerogenic** and citrate negative, which aids in its identification. A flagella stain of *S. typhi* is shown in Fig. 20-5.

This organism undergoes several different types of variation, among which is **H-to-O** variation, involving the loss of flagella. The H form is motile, and the O form is nonmotile. There are two well-recognized variants of *S. typhi:* H901 (motile) and O901 (nonmotile), which are used widely in the preparation of H and O antigen suspensions, respectively, for the Widal test. The preparation of these antigens and the Widal test are discussed in Chapter 37.

Another type of variation exhibited by the typhoid organism is **V-to-W** variation, involving loss of the Vi antigen. In the **V** form the organism is virulent and inagglutinable in O antiserum. The **W** form readily agglutinates in O antiserum and is avirulent. V colonies on nutrient or

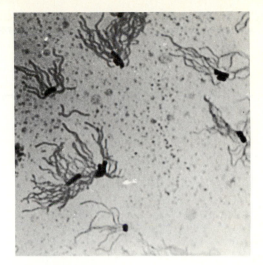

FIG. 20-5
Salmonella typhi, showing peritrichous flagella using Gray's method (1,200×).

starch agar medium appear orange-red by oblique light, whereas W colonies appear greenish-blue. Only the V form is typable by the typhoid Vi phages. If the phage type of the organism is required for epidemiologic purposes, a fresh culture in the V form should be sent to a reference laboratory.

The following criteria may serve to identify the organism. If a gram-negative isolate on TSI agar (or KIA) shows an acid butt, no gas, a small amount of hydrogen sulfide (may resemble a mustache), and an alkaline slant and also agglutinates in Vi typing serum, chances are good that this organism is *S. typhi*. Laboratory personnel should confirm this, however, with further biochemical studies and serology.

The reader is reminded of the existence, although rare, of lactose-positive variants of *S. typhi*.

Genus Arizona

Members of the genus *Arizona* are gram-negative, short, motile rods that show a close relationship to the salmonellae. The type species of the genus is *Arizona hinshawii*. Lactose may be

TABLE 20-9

Biochemical reactions of genus *Arizona*

Test	Reaction	Test	Reaction
Adonitol	−	Methyl red	+
Dulcitol	−	Voges-Proskauer	−
Glucose	+ with gas	Simmons citrate	+
Inositol	−	KCN	−
Lactose	+ or delayed	Phenylalanine deaminase	−
Mannitol	+	Sodium malonate	+
Salicin	−	Lysine decarboxylase	+
Sucrose	−	Arginine dihydrolase	+
Indole	−	Ornithine decarboxylase	+

fermented with acid and gas in 24 hours, but most strains ferment the carbohydrate after 7 to 10 days. The reaction on TSI agar slants closely resembles that of salmonellae, including hydrogen sulfide production. Gelatin is liquefied by these organisms in 7 to 30 days. They are sensitive to KCN[64] (negative) and do not produce urease.

These organisms[25,59] can be important in human infections. Many serotypes can cause disease in chickens, dogs, and cats. An antigenic scheme has been established that contains approximately 35 different O antigenic groups with a total of more than 350 serotypes.

The members of this genus show the biochemical reactions listed in Table 20-9.

Because of the similarity of arizonae to salmonellae, they are frequently mistaken for the latter in initial biochemical screening tests. However, fermentation of lactose, although usually delayed, failure to ferment dulcitol, growth in sodium malonate, and slow gelatin liquefaction help distinguish arizonae from salmonellae.

Genus Citrobacter

The genus *Citrobacter* includes the type species *C. freundii* and two other species, *C. diversus* and *C. amalonaticus*.[9,23] *C. diversus* comprises those strains of *Citrobacter* that are indole positive, KCN negative, and adonitol positive, whereas members of *C. amalonaticus* are indole positive, KCN positive, and adonitol negative. The members of this genus are gram-negative motile rods that can ferment lactose. Because of their biochemical reactions, particularly during preliminary screening, they are often confused with *Salmonella* and *Arizona*. They are not truly pathogenic and are considered opportunists. Nevertheless, *Citrobacter* is found in a variety of infections, particularly urinary tract infection and bacteremia, on occasion. Seventy-four cases of neonatal meningitis with a high rate of complicating brain abscess have been described (Graham and Band; J.A.M.A. **245**:1923-1925, 1981). A summary of the biochemical reactions for the genus is shown in Table 20-10.

Certain *C. freundii* strains possess the Vi antigen found in *S. typhi*. The KCN test is positive only for *C. freundii* and *C. amalonaticus* (the organisms grow in this medium), whereas *Salmonella* and *Arizona* are inhibited.

Considerable work has been done on the development of a serologic test scheme for members of this genus, but to date none has evolved for routine use.

TABLE 20-10

Biochemical reactions of genus *Citrobacter*

Test	Reaction			Test	Reaction		
	C. freundii	*C. diversus*	*C. amalonaticus*		*C. freundii*	*C. diversus*	*C. amalonaticus*
Adonitol	-	+	-	Voges-Proskauer	-	-	-
Dulcitol	+ or -	+ or -	-	Simmons citrate	+	+	+
Glucose	+ with gas	+ with gas	+ with gas	Gelatin	-	-	Variable
Inositol	- or delayed	-	-	Urease	(+) or -	Variable	Variable
Lactose	+ or delayed	Variable	Variable	KCN	+	-	+
Mannitol	+	+	+	Phenylalanine deaminase	-	-	-
Salicin	Variable	Variable	(+)	Sodium malonate	- or +	+ or -	-
Sucrose	Variable	- or +	Variable	Lysine decarboxylase	-	-	-
Indole	-	+	+	Arginine dihydrolase	+	+	+ +
Methyl red	+	+	+	Ornithine decarboxylase	Variable	+	+

+ or -, majority are positive; - or +, majority are negative.

Genus Shigella

As determined by DNA-relatedness analysis, members of *Shigella* should be included in the genus *Escherichia*. However, because of the confusion that would be generated in the medical community by grouping these two genera together, *Shigella* has been retained as a separate genus.

All members of the genus *Shigella* are **nonmotile;** they do not produce hydrogen sulfide; and with a few exceptions (biotypes of *Shigella flexneri* 6) they are anaerogenic. Although many shigellae produce catalase,[14] for example *S. flexneri*, this is an inconsistent property within the genus. *Shigella dysenteriae* 1, the type species of the genus, is invariably negative.[13] Aside from bacillary dysentery, *Shigella* may occasionally cause bacteremia, pneumonia, or other infection.

Colonies of shigellae are usually smaller than those of salmonellae, but on occasion mucoid variants may be found in subgroup C. Lactose-negative colonies that resemble shigellae are picked from isolation plates to TSI agar (or KIA) slants. If these show an acid butt, no hydrogen sulfide, and an alkaline slant and prove to be urease negative, they may be tested with *Shigella* polyvalent typing sera. This procedure is recommended only for presumptive identification; cultures should always be checked for purity and motility and then confirmed with additional biochemical tests. The tests listed in Table 20-11 are recommended for screening of *Shigella* cultures. The reaction tree shown in Fig. 20-6 will serve as a guide in biochemical identification.

Serologic identification

The current antigenic scheme for *Shigella* was proposed by Ewing in 1949 and modified and extended by the Shigella Commission of the Enterobacteriaceae Subcommittee.[23] The scheme is based in part on biochemical characteristics, on antigenic relationships, and on tradition (the names of Shiga, Boyd, Flexner, and Sonne are obvious in the nomenclature). **Four**

TABLE 20-11

Biochemical reactions of genus *Shigella* (see Plate 59)

Test	Reaction	Test	Reaction
Adonitol	−	Methyl red	+
Dulcitol	Variable	Voges-Proskauer	−
Glucose	+ no gas*	Simmons citrate	−
Inositol	−	KCN	−
Lactose	Variable	Phenylalanine deaminase	−
Mannitol	Variable	Sodium malonate	−
Salicin	−	Lysine decarboxylase	−
Sucrose†	−	Arginine dihydrolase	−‡
Indole	Variable	Ornithine decarboxylase	−‡

*Some biotypes of *S. flexneri* produce gas.
†Some strains of *S. sonnei* ferment lactose and sucrose slowly.
‡*S. sonnei* and *S. boydii* 13 are usually ornithine decarboxylase positive and some strains are arginine dihydrolase positive. The other shigellae are negative for all three amino acids.

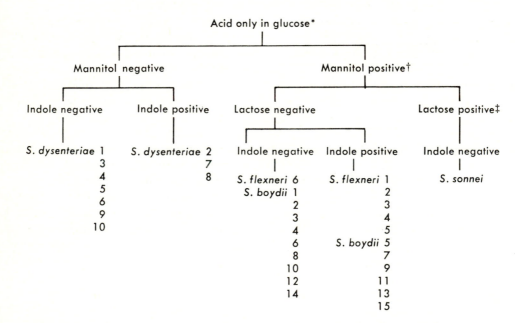

*S. flexneri 6 varieties may be aerogenic (Newcastle and Manchester).
†Certain cultures of *S. flexneri* 4, *S. flexneri* 6, and *S. boydii* 6 may not produce acid from mannitol.
‡Lactose fermentation is delayed with *S. sonnei* (usually 4 to 7 days). Closure of the fermentation tube with a tightly fitting stopper will hasten the reaction.

FIG. 20-6
Biochemical differentiation of genus *Shigella*. (Adapted from Edwards, P. R., and Ewing, W. H.:
Manual for enteric bacteriology, Atlanta, 1951, Center for Disease Control.)

subgroups (species) are presently identified: subgroup A—*S. dysenteriae* types 1 to 10; subgroup B—*S. flexneri* types 1 to 6, also X and Y variants; subgroup C—*S. boydii* types 1 to 15; subgroup D—*S. sonnei*.

Subgroup A consists of those types that are nonfermenters of mannitol. Each type exhibits a type-specific antigen not related to other shigellae.

The types that make up **subgroup B** are usually fermenters of mannitol (mannitol-negative variants of *S. flexneri* 6 do exist) and in addition are interrelated through group or subsidiary antigens. Each type, however, possesses a type-specific antigen that differentiates it from other shigellae. Serotypes 1, 2, 3, and 4 also possess subtypes based on group antigen differences. The X and Y variants represent those forms that have lost the type-specific antigen.

In **subgroup C** all types are fermenters of mannitol and possess individual type-specific antigens not related significantly to other shigellae.

Subgroup D comprises only one type, *S. sonnei*, and this organism possesses a type-specific antigen that bears no significant relationship to other shigellae. There exist different "forms" of *S. sonnei* that differ antigenically.

In view of the number of serotypes, it is recommended that preliminary serologic screening be carried out with **polyvalent** typing antisera. Groups A, B, C, and D antisera for slide agglutination tests are available commercially.* The overall technique is quite similar to that used for the *Salmonella* O antigens. Since K antigens are present also in some shigellae, live bacteria **may fail to agglutinate** in any of the groups mentioned. Thus, one is advised to heat the test suspension in 0.5% NaCl at 100 C for 30 to 60 minutes, cool, and retest with the same antisera.

---

*Lederle Laboratories, Pearl River, N.Y.; Difco Laboratories, Detroit; Baltimore Biological Laboratory, Cockeysville, Md.; Lee Laboratories, Grayson, Ga.

Type determination of shigellae can be carried out with monovalent antisera against the specific antigens. These are prepared from known types and are absorbed with suspensions of appropriate cultures to obtain type-specific diagnostic antisera. Agglutinin absorption is particularly necessary for most types in group B because of their group or minor antigens.

Colicin typing

In North America and in the United Kingdom, **S. sonnei** has become the most common etiologic agent in bacillary dysentery or shigellosis. In the United States, 85% of *Shigella* isolates are *S. sonnei* and 14% are *S. flexneri*.[81] Colicin typing of strains of *S. sonnei* is being performed in some reference laboratories. **Colicins**, which are produced by different gram-negative enteric bacteria, are antibiotic-like substances that may have a lethal effect on other bacteria from the same habitat. Colicin typing of shigellae is based on colicinogeny rather than colicin susceptibility.

Fifteen colicin types of *S. sonnei* are currently recognized,[1] and these appear to be sufficiently stable to use in epidemiologic investigations. Carpenter[13] reported that during 1964 to 1969 approximately one third of the strains isolated in England were noncolicinogenic (CTO), that of the typable strains one third were of type 7, and that the remainder comprised the other 14 types. The most prevalent of the latter in the United Kingdom were colicin types 1A, 2, 4, and 6.

In evaluating the colicin-typing method for differentiating epidemic strains of *S. sonnei* in the United States, Morris and Wells[66] reported that 40% of their strains were nontypable. The remaining 60% were distributed among all 15 established colicin types, with type 9 accounting for 22% of the total. These authors felt colicin typing offered a useful method of differentiating strains with reasonably good reproducibility, although it should not be interpreted with the same degree of confidence as some other characteristics, such as serotyping. They recommended that known type strains be included as controls in each run to ensure uniformity of results.

Genus Escherichia

The genus *Escherichia* includes the former *Alkalescens-Dispar* group, which although anaerogenic are biochemically and antigenically related to the escherichiae. The type species of the genus is *E. coli*.

Typical escherichiae are readily recognized and may be differentiated from other members of the Enterobacteriaceae by their rapid **fermentation of lactose** with acid and gas and their response to the classical **IMViC** tests (++−−). Some strains, however, either fail to ferment lactose or do so slowly. Both motile and nonmotile forms occur.

Most strains produce large, characteristic lactose-fermenting colonies on MacConkey agar and EMB agar. They are usually inhibited in enrichment broths and the more highly selective agar plating media, as stated earlier in this chapter. For direct isolation of *Escherichia*, the less inhibitory (differential) media, such as MacConkey agar and EMB agar, are recommended. Blood agar plates should also be used, because certain enteropathogenic strains may not grow on MacConkey agar but will grow well on blood plates. Most strains are nonhemolytic.

Pure cultures of typical *E. coli* will give the reactions shown in Table 20-12.

E. coli may be associated with a number of disease syndromes. Among these are (1) often severe and sometimes fatal infections, such as cystitis, pyelitis, pyelonephritis, appendicitis, peritonitis, gallbladder infection, septicemia, meningitis, and endocarditis; (2) epidemic diarrhea of adults and children; and (3) "traveler's" diarrhea.

The antigenic complexity of the genus is very similar to that of *Salmonella* and other genera within the Enterobacteriaceae. Approximately 162 O antigens are recognized. Many of these strains also possess K and H antigens, which now number 100 and 52, respectively. The K antigens may be of the L, A, or B type and thus exhibit various physical and immunologic properties. *E. coli* serotypes have been established on the basis of the O, K, and H antigens. K antigens are somatic antigens that occur as envelopes or capsules. This antigen masks or otherwise makes inaccessible the O complex. The O inagglutinability caused by K antigens is analogous to the O and Vi relationship in *S. typhi*.

TABLE 20-12

Biochemical reactions of genus *Escherichia*

Test	Reaction	Test	Reaction
Adonitol	−	Methyl red	+
Dulcitol	Variable	Voges-Proskauer	−
Glucose	+ with gas	Simmons citrate	−
Inositol	−	KCN	−
Lactose*	+	Phenylalanine deaminase	−
Mannitol	+	Sodium malonate	−
Salicin	Variable	Lysine decarboxylase	Variable
Sucrose	Variable	Arginine dihydrolase	Variable
Indole	+	Ornithine decarboxylase	Variable

*Some are late or nonlactose fermenting.

Enteropathogenic *Escherichia coli*

Based on mechanisms of pathogenicity, three principal types of enteropathogenic *E. coli* have been described: (1) enterotoxigenic *E. coli* (ETEC), toxin-producing strains; (2) enteroinvasive *E. coli*, associated with invasion of intestinal epithelium; and (3) enteropathogenic *E. coli* (EPEC), which may produce enterotoxins. The ETEC strains are associated with diarrhea in infants and adults.[87,89] At present the ETEC strains that have been described belong to one of eight O groups (i.e., 6, 8, 16, 25, 27, 78, 148, and 159).[69] The enteroinvasive strains also produce diarrheal disease in adults and infants, and they, too, are associated with a relatively small number of serotypes (see below). Although the enteropathogenic strains (O groups 26, 55, 86, 111, 114, 119, 125, 126, 127, 128, and 142) are primarily associated with infantile diarrhea, they may rarely cause enteric disease in adults.[44,90]

Toxigenicity. Recent studies of the pathogenesis of bacterial diarrhea have identified intestinal secretion of fluid and electrolytes in diseases associated with **enterotoxins.** The enterotoxins of both cholera and certain of the noninvasive (toxigenic) strains of *E. coli* cause diarrhea through a similar mechanism(s), that is, stimulation of adenylate cyclase in the small intestine (and in nonintestinal tissue), thereby giving rise to excessive secretion of fluid by the small intestine.[4,34] Enterotoxins have been identified in *Shigella* and *Salmonella*, but it is not known what role, if any, they play in enteritis.[86]

Much evidence has accumulated in recent years to implicate the **enterotoxigenic** strains of *E. coli* as a cause of severe diarrheal disease in human beings.*

Two distinct enterotoxins, one heat stable and nonantigenic (**ST**) and the other heat labile, antigenic (**LT**), and choleralike (see below), have been characterized from *E. coli*.[27,97] Production of both of these toxins is controlled by transfer-

able plasmids (Ent plasmid).[98] LT has been definitely shown to cause diarrheal disease in humans,[38,93] and recent evidence implicates ST as well.[65] A cytotoxin has also been described.

Although toxins are definitely involved in the disease process, other factors, such as the ability of the organism to adhere to the intestinal epithelium and colonize the bowel, are necessary for pathogenesis. A plasmid-mediated colonizing factor has been identified.[28] The colonizing factor is controlled by a transferable plasmid that is distinct from the Ent plasmid.

Several assay methods for detecting these enterotoxins are currently available. They vary in their ability to detect one or the other of the enterotoxins. When observed at 18 hours, the rabbit ileal loop test[108] detects primarily LT, a positive test being dilatation of the ligated segment with accumulated fluid. The infant rabbit examined at 6 hours presumably indicates the presence of both enterotoxins.[27] Two tissue culture assays have been developed that are highly sensitive assays for LT only. One is the adrenal cell technique,[18] and the other employs a Chinese hamster ovary tissue culture cell line as described by Guerrant and Dickens.[44] The infant mouse assay method detects ST.[17] Since these assays are not easily performed in clinical laboratories, efforts are being made to develop specific and sensitive polyvalent antisera against strains of ETEC (as well as EPEC and enteroinvasive *E. coli*).[62] If the use of such antisera proves to be efficacious, serotyping will provide clinical laboratories with a practical method for the routine identification of diarrhea-inducing *E. coli*.

In an attempt to determine the *E. coli* serotypes of the enterotoxigenic strains obtained from diarrhea in adults and children, Ørskov and co-workers[69] examined 106 strains submitted to them from many parts of the world for O and H antigens (K antigens were not studied because a reliable procedure to test for these antigens was not yet available). These researchers found some O:H types consistently from dif-

---

*See references 17, 21, 38, 39, 88, 91, 92, and 95.

ferent geographic locations (i.e., O6:H16, O8:H9, O15:H11, O25:H42, O78:H11 and O78:H12).

Certain strains of *E. coli* are capable of invading the bowel epithelium and producing an enteric disease resembling shigellosis. Serologic typing revealed that enteroinvasive strains were restricted to nine serogroups of *E. coli* (i.e., O groups 28, 112, 115, 124, 136, 143, 144, 147, and 152).[94] Although not routinely performed in the clinical laboratory, the Sereny test is used to identify these strains.[65] The development of keratoconjunctivitis in the guinea pig eye following inoculation with the test organism is indicative of enteroinvasive *E. coli*. Again, the development of a specific polyvalent antiserum against the enteroinvasive strains would provide a means for routinely identifying these strains in clinical laboratories.

Genus Edwardsiella

The type species of this genus is *Edwardsiella tarda*. Members of this genus are motile, and their biochemical pattern conforms to that of the family Enterobacteriaceae. The first isolates were reported in 1959 and examined under biotype 1483-59 by various workers between 1962 and 1964. The generic term was suggested by Ewing and co-workers[31] in 1965.

These organisms have been isolated from a variety of human sources, including diarrheal disease; from normal stools, blood, wounds, visceral abscesses, and urine; and also from warm- and cold-blooded animals. The biochemical reactions are shown in Table 20-6 (see Plate 66).

Genus Klebsiella

The establishment of *Klebsiella* and *Enterobacter* as separate genera was effected in 1962, following the recommendations of the ICSB Enterobacteriaceae Subcommittee.[26,50,52,63] The tribe Klebsielleae currently comprises the genera *Klebsiella*, *Enterobacter*, *Serratia*, and *Hafnia*.

Members of the genus *Klebsiella* are gram-negative, **nonmotile,** encapsulated, short rods that possess the characteristics shown in Table 20-13. The type species is *K. pneumoniae*. Approximately 95% of the clinical isolates of *Klebsiella* are *K. pneumoniae*. *K. oxytoca* (Plate 63) isolates make up the majority of the remaining 5%. *K. ozaenae* is occasionally isolated, and *K. rhinoscleromatis* is rarely isolated. The klebsiellae can cause severe enteritis in infants* and pneumonia (Plate 15), septicemia, meningitis, wound infection, peritonitis, and hospital-acquired urinary tract infections in adults. On blood agar, EMB agar, MacConkey agar, trypticase soy agar, and other routine plating media they generally give rise to large **mucoid** colonies (Plate 55) that have a tendency to coalesce and usually string out when touched with a needle. Growth in broth also can be very stringy and difficult to break up when making transfers.

Some 75 capsular types have been identified. Cross-reactions between types are known to occur; in the preparation of pooled typing sera related types are placed in the same pool. Epidemiologic significance of these bacteria, particularly in hospital-acquired infections, is perhaps best served by the methods of serotyping. It should be emphasized that greater accuracy in identification of the *Klebsiella* types is obtained by use of the quellung reaction rather than reliance on agglutinating antisera.

K. rhinoscleromatis is the cause of scleroma of the nose, pharynx, and other respiratory tract structures. This disease is endemic in Central and South America and northern Africa but is seen rarely in the United States.

Genus Enterobacter

According to current classification (Table 20-14), the genus *Enterobacter* contains five species—*E. cloacae*, *E. aerogenes*, *E. gergoviae*,[9] *E. sakazakii*,[9] and *E. agglomerans*,[29] which

---

*Enterotoxin-producing klebsiellae have been isolated from the small intestine of individuals with tropical sprue.

TABLE 20-13

Biochemical reactions of *Klebsiella* species

Test	Reaction			
	K. pneumoniae	*K. oxytoca*	*K. ozaenae*	*K. rhinoscleromatis*
Adonitol	+ or −	+ or −	+	+
Dulcitol	− or +	− or +	−	−
Gas from glucose	+	+	Variable	−
Inositol	+	+	Variable	+
Lactose	+	+	Variable	Variable
Mannitol	+	+	+	+
Salicin	+	+	+	+
Sucrose	+	+	Variable	+ or (+)
Indole	−	+	−	−
Methyl red	− or +	− or +	+	+
Voges-Proskauer	+	+	−	−
Simmons citrate	+	+	Variable	−
KCN	+	+	+ or −	
Urease	+ (slow)	+	Variable	−
Gelatin liquefaction	−	(+) or −	−	−
Phenylalanine deaminase	−	−	−	−
Sodium malonate	+	+	−	+ or −
Lysine decarboxylase	+	+	Variable	−
Arginine dihydrolase	−	−	−	−
Ornithine decarboxylase	−	−	−	−

+ or −, majority are positive; − or +, majority are negative; (+), delayed reaction.

includes the former Herbicola-Lathyri bacteria. The clinical significance of *E. agglomerans* is presently undetermined. However, in 1972 Pien and associates[80] examined 56 strains of *E. agglomerans* isolated from 51 patients during an 18-month period at the Mayo Clinic. Infections occurred primarily in accident victims during the summer and autumn months. *E. agglomerans* was considered to be directly pathogenic in only six wound infections and one urinary tract infection. No cases of septicemia were seen. Practically all strains isolated were sensitive to the antibiotics tested, except that some were relatively resistant to ampicillin and cephalothin. *E. gergoviae* and *E. sakazakii* are not frequently isolated from clinical specimens. How-

ever, they have been associated with a variety of infections, including meningitis, septicemia, and infections of the urinary tract.[68,85] *E. gergoviae* is distinguished from other members of *Enterobacter* by its ability to hydrolyze urea and its inability to grow in KCN, ferment D-sorbitol, or liquefy gelatin. *E. sakazakii* is characterized by production of a yellow pigment at 25 C and DNase activity (36 C, 3 to 6 days).

The species of *Enterobacter* are found in soil, water, dairy products, and the intestines of animals, including humans. Considered as opportunists, they are now being isolated more frequently in urinary tract infection, in septicemia, and from other clinical sites, particularly in hospitalized patients who are quite ill.

TABLE 20-14

Biochemical reactions of *Enterobacter* species and *Hafnia alvei*

Test	E. cloacae	E. aerogenes	E. agglomerans	E. gergoviae	E. sakazakii	Hafnia alvei 35 C	Hafnia alvei 22 C
Adonitol	– or +	+	–	–	–	–	–
Dulcitol	– or +	–	– or +	–	–	–	+
Glucose (+ gas)	+	+	– or +	+	+	+	+
Inositol (+ gas)	d	+	d	–	d	–	–
Lactose	+	+	d	– or (+)	+	– or (+)	– or (+)
Sorbitol	+	+	d	–	–	–	–
Raffinose	+	+	d	+	+	–	–
Mannitol	+	+	+	+	+	+	+
Salicin	+ or (+)	+	d	–	+	d	d
Sucrose	+	+	d	+	+	d	d
Indole	–	–	– or +	–	–	–	–
Methyl red	–	–	– or +	d	– or +	+ or –	+
Voges-Proskauer	+	+	+ or –	+	+	+ or –	+
Simmons citrate	+	+	d	+	+	+ or –	d
KCN	+	+	– or +	+	+	+	+
Urease	+ or –	–	d	+	–	–	–
Gelatin liquefaction	(+) or –	– or (+)	+	–	–	–	–
Phenylalanine deaminase	–	–	– or +	–	–	–	–
Sodium malonate	+ or –	+ or –	+ or –	+	– or +	+ or –	+ or –
Mucate	d	+	d	–	–	–	–
Arginine dihydrolase	+	–	–	–	+	–	–
Lysine decarboxylase	–	+	–	+ or (+)	–	+	+
Ornithine decarboxylase	+	+	–	+	+	+	+
DNase	–	–	d	–	d	–	–
Yellow pigment	–	–		–	+	–	–

d, different biochemical types; + or –, majority are positive; – or +, majority are negative; (+), delayed reaction.

Genus Serratia

Members of the genus *Serratia* are gram-negative motile rods; only a small percentage of strains are **chromogenic** (Plate 57). Six species currently exist: *S. marcescens, S. liquefaciens, S. rubidaea (marinoruba)*,[29] *S. plymuthica*,[41,42] *S. odorifera*,[42] and *S. fonticola*.[33] The majority of human isolates are *S. marcescens*, the most clinically significant of the *Serratia* species.[40] It is also the only species of *Serratia* that is involved in nosocomial infections. Although *S. liquefaciens* and *S. rubidaea* are isolated from human specimens, particularly sputum, their role in infection has not been determined. Clinical isolates of *S. odorifera* and *S. plymuthica* are very infrequent and at present are not believed to be clinically significant. No human isolates of *S. fonticola* have been reported. The strains of *S. marcescens* that are chromogenic produce a red, non-water-soluble pigment at room temperature but seldom at 35 C or above. Considered for many years as innocuous, these bacteria are primarily found in water and soil. Only in recent years have they been directly implicated in human infection, including pulmonary infection, urinary tract infection, and septicemia.[40,72] This again reflects the vulnerability of the compromised patient to opportunistic pathogens. The indiscriminate use of antibiotics also must be considered a contributory factor, especially since all Serratiae are quite resistant to cephalosporins and polymyxins. Nonpigmented biotypes of *S. marcescens* are frequently associated with multiresistance and R-plasmid–mediated resistance factors.

Fifteen somatic antigens for *Serratia* have

TABLE 20-15

Biochemical reactions of *Serratia* species

Test	S. marcescens	S. liquefaciens	S. rubidaea	S. odorifera	S. plymuthica	S. fonticola
Arabinose	−	+	+	+	+	+
Adonitol	d	d	+ or (+)		−	(+) or +
Dulcitol	−	−	−	−		−
Gas (glucose)	+ or −	+ or −	d	−	− or +	+
Inositol	d	+ or (+)	d	d	+	+
Lactose	−	d	+	(+) or +		+
Mannitol	+	+	+	+	+	+
Salicin	+	+	+ or (+)	+		+
Sucrose	+	+	+	+ or −		(+) or −
Indole	−	−	−	+	−	−
Methyl red	− or +	+ or −	− or +	+		+
Voges-Proskauer	+ or −	+ or −	+ or −	+ or −	+ or −	−
Simmons citrate	+ or −	+ or −	+ or −	(+) or −	+ or −	− or +
Gelatin (22 C)	+ or −	+ or −	+ or −	+	+	+
KCN	+	+	− or (+)	− or (+)		+
Phenylalanine deaminase	−	−	−		−	−
DNase	+	+ or −	+			+
Sodium malonate	−	−	+ or −	−		+
Lysine decarboxylase	+	+ or (+)	+ or (+)	+	−	+
Arginine dihydrolase	−	−	−	−	−	−
Ornithine decarboxylase	+	+	−	+ or −	−	+

d, differential biochemical types; + or −, majority are positive; − or +, majority are negative; (+), delayed reaction.

been previously identified serologically, and there is good evidence that serotyping can be of value in studying nosocomial infections. The biochemical pattern exhibited by the genus is shown in Table 20-15; the biochemical speciation is shown in Table 20-6.

Genus Proteus

The tribe Proteeae consists of three genera: *Proteus, Providencia,* and *Morganella.*

Proteus species are gram-negative, somewhat pleomorphic motile rods. The type species is *Proteus vulgaris.* They are typically **lactose negative** and often rapidly **urease positive.** The species are actively motile at 25 C but often weakly motile at 35 C. *P. vulgaris* and *P. mirabilis* tend to swarm (Plate 54) on moist agar or agar of 1.5% concentration (usual strength for plating media), producing a bluish-gray confluent surface growth at both 25 and 35 C. Swarming may be inhibited on MacConkey and EMB plates if the agar concentration is increased to 5%.

The appearance of the spreading growth varies from a rippled form that is easily recognized to one that is smooth and almost transparent. This growth may sometimes go unobserved in examining plates containing mixed cultures, but a loop drawn over a seemingly colony-free area readily reveals its presence. Because of careless technique, *Proteus* is often the contaminant in "pure" cultures obtained from selected colonies.

Because of their lactose-negative characteristic, discrete *Proteus* colonies are sometimes selected from differential or selective media as suspicious salmonellae, shigellae, or other gram-negative organisms. This is one of the reasons why screening on TSI agar (or KIA), followed by a rapid urease test, is highly recommended, as was previously discussed.

Proteus organisms can frequently be found in large numbers in the stools of individuals undergoing oral antibiotic therapy. They are frequently responsible for infections of the urinary tract and may be seen in bacteremia, intraab-

TABLE 20-16

Biochemical characteristics of *Proteus* species* (Plate 64)

Test	P. mirabilis	P. vulgaris
Adonitol	−	−
Dulcitol	−	−
Glucose	+ (gas)	+ (gas)
Inositol	−	−
Lactose	−	−
Mannitol	−	−
Salicin	Variable	+
Sucrose	+ (3-8 days)	+
Maltose	−	+
Xylose	+	+
Gelatin	+	+
H₂S (TSI)	+	+
Indole	−	+
Methyl red	+	+
Voges-Proskauer	− or +	−
Simmons citrate	+ (variable)	− (variable)
Phenylalanine deaminase	+	+
Ornithine decarboxylase	+	−

*All *Proteus* species are urease positive.

dominal infection, wound infection, and so forth. The association of *P. mirabilis* with nosocomial infections has led to the development of group O–specific antisera for both *P. mirabilis* and *P. vulgaris.* Although these antisera are not commercially available at this time, they may be useful in the future for following the epidemiology of hospital-acquired *Proteus* infections.[76]

The biochemical reactions of the *Proteus* species are given in Table 20-16. Species identification of Proteeae isolates is certainly to be encouraged, since *P. mirabilis* responds more readily to antimicrobial therapy (the other species are more resistant).[111]

Genus Providencia

Formerly known as the 29911 paracolon bacterium,[105,106] the genus *Providencia* currently consists of three species: *P. alcalifaciens, P. stu-*

TABLE 20-17

Biochemical reactions of *Providencia* species and *Morganella morganii* (Plates 62 and 65)

Test	P. alcalifaciens	P. stuartii	P. rettgeri	M. morganii
H₂S (TSI)	-	-	-	-
Gelatin	-	-	-	-
Indole	+	+	+	+
Methyl red	+	+	+	+
Voges-Proskauer	-	-	-	-
Urease	-	- or +	+	+
Simmons citrate	+	+	+	-
KCN	+	+	+	+
Phenylalanine deaminase	+	+	d	+
Lysine decarboxylase	-	-	-	-
Arginine dihydrolase	-	-	-	-
Ornithine decarboxylase	-	-	-	+
Adonitol	+	-	+	-
Arabinose	-	-	-	-
Arabitol	-	-	+	-
Dulcitol	-	-	-	-
Glucose (gas)	+ or -	-	+	+ (gas)
Inositol	-	+	+	-
Lactose	-	-	-	-
Sodium malonate	-	-	-	-
Mannitol	-	d	+ or -	-
Salicin	-	d	d	-
Sucrose	d	d	d	-
Rhamnose	-	-	+ or -	-

d, different biochemical types; + or -, majority are positive; - or +, majority are negative.

artii, and *P. rettgeri*. *P. alcalifaciens* is the type species. *P. rettgeri* was formerly *Proteus rettgeri* biogroups 1 to 4. *Proteus rettgeri* biogroup 5 is now a biogroup of *Providencia stuartii*, referred to as the urease-positive *P. stuartii*. Transferable urease activity in *P. stuartii* has been described recently by Grant and colleagues (J. Clin. Microbiol. **13**:561-565, 1981). These changes were made on the basis of results of DNA-DNA hybridization and serotyping.[9] The three *Providencia* species are gram-negative motile rods that are lactose negative and grow well on most enteric isolation media. Because they are hydrogen sulfide negative and may or may not produce gas in glucose, they often resemble shigellae on TSI agar (or KIA). If sucrose is fermented, the reaction is usually delayed, and thus fermentation of this carbohydrate will not be detected in 48 hours in the TSI slant. *Providencia* may be distinguished from *Shigella*, however, by its motility and utilization of citrate. *Providencia* may be distinguished from other genera within the Enterobacteriaceae by its biochemical characteristics, indicated in Table 20-17.

The organisms (particularly *P. stuartii*) have been incriminated in urinary tract infection, especially in patients with underlying urologic disorders[35,114] and in various infections of patients in a burn unit.[70] *P. stuartii*, in particular, is not uncommonly resistant to multiple antibiotics, like so many other nosocomial pathogens. *Providencia* (particularly *P. alcalifaciens* serotype O3) has been believed to cause diarrhea,[49,73] but this is not well established.

An antigenic scheme has been established for each species on the basis of O-specific antigens.[74,77,79] At this time 15 O serotypes of *P. stuartii*, 47 O serotypes of *P. alcalifaciens*, and 93 O serotypes of *P. rettgeri* have been defined.[74,79] Penner and associates[77] serotyped 829 isolates of *P. stuartii* collected primarily from urologic specimens at 12 hospitals. Although the serotype distribution varied from hospital to hospital, the urine isolates were associated with a relatively small number of O serotypes (i.e., O groups 63, 4, 17, 55, 25, 52, 56, 24, 15, 43, and 49). Serotyping of *P. stuartii*, at least in reference laboratories, is encouraged by Penner and co-workers, since these organisms are responsible for nosocomial infections and serotyping may be the only means of detecting strains involved in inapparent and insidious infections.

P. rettgeri is also a causative agent of nosocomial infections, particularly of the urinary tract. In contrast with isolates of *P. stuartii*, which fall into a narrow range of serotypes, a wide range of *P. rettgeri* O groups have been associated with human infection.[74]

Genus Morganella

The genus *Morganella* is composed of a single species, *M. morganii*. As shown in Tables 20-6 and 20-17, *M. morganii* is distinguished from *Providencia* species by its ability to decarboxylate ornithine and its inability to utilize citrate. The following characteristics differentiate *M. morganii* from *Proteus*: it is H_2S negative, gelatin (22 C) negative, and D-mannose positive. In addition to the biochemically typical strains, two separate biogroups have been identified.[47] One biogroup is ornithine decarboxylase positive, and the other is lysine decarboxylase negative. *M. morganii* has been associated with urinary tract and other infections.[75,102] O antigen typing of clinical isolates from two hospitals revealed that 48% belonged to a single O group, O1.

Genus Yersinia

Recently incorporated into the family Enterobacteriaceae, this genus consists of the species *Yersinia pestis*, *Y. enterocolitica*, *Y. pseudotuberculosis*, *Y. intermedia*, *Y. frederiksenii*, *Y. kristensii* and *Y. ruckeri*. Only the first three species are clinically significant, and the distinguishing properties of these species are shown in Table 20-18.[16]

Yersinia pestis

Y. pestis is the etiologic agent of **plague,** a disease with a high mortality in human beings and rats and is infectious for mice, guinea pigs, and rabbits. Three clinical forms of plague are recognized in humans: **bubonic, pneumonic,** and **septicemic.** The main vector for transmission is the rat flea. Humans are accidental hosts of this flea. Plague bacilli are short, plump, nonmotile, gram-negative rods, sometimes elongated and pleomorphic, usually appearing singly or in pairs and occasionally in short chains. Bipolar staining can be demonstrated with polychrome stains, such as the Giemsa and Wayson stains, but **not** the Gram stain. Coccoid, round, filamentous, elongated, and other forms commonly occur, especially in old cultures. A capsule can be demonstrated in animal tissue and in young cultures. The latter will give a positive fluorescent antibody reaction, by which a presumptive diagnosis may be made.

Y. pestis grows slowly on nutrient agar and fairly rapidly on blood agar, producing small, nonhemolytic, round, transparent, glistening, colorless colonies with an undulate margin.[103] Older colonies enlarge, becoming opaque with yellowish centers and whitish edges, which develop a soft, mucoid consistency because of capsular material. A characteristic type of growth occurs in old broth cultures overlaid with sterile oil, in which a pellicle forms with "stalactite" streamers. Biochemical properties are shown in Table 20-18. A rapid (20-minute) diagnostic test that uses isocitrate lyase activity for identification of *Y. pestis* has been described recently (Hillier and Charnetsky: J. Clin. Microbiol. **13:**661-665, 1981).

Y. pestis is pathogenic for rats and guinea pigs. After subcutaneous inoculation, the animals die within 2 to 5 days and show certain postmortem characteristics, including ulceration at the site of injection, regional adenopathy, congested spleen and liver, and pleural effusion. The bacilli may be demonstrated in

TABLE 20-18

Distinguishing properties of *Yersinia* species

Property	Y. pestis	Y. enterocolitica	Y. pseudotuberculosis
Colony forms	Two	Two	Two
Optimal growth temperature	25 to 30 C	25 to 30 C	25 to 30 C
Motility at 25 C	−	+	+
Serogroups	One	Two	Five
Catalase	+	+	+
Oxidase	−	−	−
Coagulase	+*		−
Fibrinolysin	+		−
Hemolysis on blood agar	−	alpha	−
Medium containing bile salts	+	+	+
H_2S	−	−	−
Indole	−	−	−
Methyl red	+	+	+
Voges-Proskauer	−	+	−
Urease	−	+	+
Nitrate	Variable	Reduced	Reduced
Cellobiose	−	+	−
Glucose	+	+	+
Glycerol	Variable	+	+
Lactose	−	−	−
Melibiose	−	−	+
Maltose	+	+	+
Mannitol	+	+	+
Rhamnose	−	−†	+
Salicin	+	−	+
Sucrose	−	+	−

*Using rabbit plasma.
†Occasional strains are rhamnose positive.

splenic smears; they may also be recovered by culture. Cultures may be identified by specific bacteriophage typing, by the fluorescent antibody test, or by agglutination with specific antisera.

Great care must be taken by the laboratory worker when handling suspect cultures or pathologic materials. A biologic safety hood should be used. The worker should be masked and wearing rubber gloves. The creation of aerosols should be avoided, and all contaminated materials must be autoclaved.

Yersinia enterocolitica

This organism appears to be closely related to *Y. pseudotuberculosis*. *Y. enterocolitica* has been implicated in human disease with a variety of clinical syndromes; these include gastroenteritis, bacteremia, peritonitis, cholecystitis, visceral abscesses, and mesenteric lymphadenitis.*[104] Septicemia, with a 50% mortality, has been reported in the compromised host.[82]

*Outbreaks of illness caused by *Y. enterocolitica* have been traced to milk (Morbid. Mortal. Weekly Rep. **26**:53-54, 1977).

Y. enterocolitica is not easily isolated and identified in the microbiology laboratory.[103] The organism grows slowly at 35 C. Biochemical reactions for the most part resemble those of many members of the family Enterobacteriaceae; thus, these organisms may be frequently overlooked. The organism is a gram-negative coccobacillus occasionally showing bipolar staining. Table 20-18 shows biochemical and other properties of this microorganism.

The serologic and biochemical characteristics of 24 human isolates of *Y. enterocolitica* submitted to the California Department of Health from 1968 through 1975 were reported by Bissett.[5] Nine different serotypes were represented, with the majority of strains being serotype O:8 (6 strains) and O:5 (5 strains). Sources of the isolates included feces (12 cases), blood (3), sputum or throat (3), bile or bowel drainage (2), wounds (2), breast abscess (1), and skin abscess (1). Underlying medical conditions existed in 13 patients.

Y. enterocolitica is frequently resistant to penicillins and cephalosporins. Aminoglycosides, cotrimoxazole, chloramphenicol, and tetracycline are the drugs most active against this organism.[7]

Yersinia pseudotuberculosis

Y. pseudotuberculosis causes disease primarily in rodents, particularly guinea pigs, but it also causes two recognized forms of disease in human beings. Of these the most serious is a **fulminating septicemia,** which is usually fatal, while the more common form is a **mesenteric lymphadenitis,** which may simulate appendicitis. The organism has been responsible for many infections in Europe.[58] In recent years cases have been reported in the United States by Weber and co-workers.[117]

The bacterium is a small gram-negative coccobacillus, exhibiting pleomorphism, found singly, in short chains, and in small clusters. It grows well on blood agar and media containing bile salts, such as MacConkey agar.[103] **Two** colo-

nial forms may be observed: a smooth grayish-yellow translucent colony in 24 hours at 25 to 30 C, and a raised colony, with an opaque center and a lighter margin with serrations, that develops with continued incubation. A rough variant with an irregular outline may also develop. The characteristics of the species are shown in Table 20-18.

Tribe Erwinieae

Although a certain amount of confusion still exists with regard to the taxonomy of these organisms, it is reasonably well established that these bacteria, noted primarily as plant pathogens, are members of the family Enterobacteriaceae, hence their inclusion here. At this writing, there is very little else to add other than to point out that Ewing's current classification consists of the tribe Erwinieae and the two genera *Erwinia* and *Pectobacterium* (see Table 20-1). Biochemical reactions of a representative species for each genus are shown in Table 20-6. Readers interested in this group of organisms should consult Chapter 15 in Edwards and Ewing's text.[23]

IDENTIFICATION OF ENTEROBACTERIACEAE BY TEST KITS AND RAPID METHODS

Rapid procedures and test kits designed to reduce the amount of time for identifying members of the Enterobacteriaceae have been developed commercially and have been compared with conventional methods used in the identification of gram-negative bacterial isolates from clinical material. The results have been evaluated and reported by various investigators. In the performance of each, however, emphasis is placed on the competence and technical skill of the person or persons carrying out the tests, and it should be recognized that the **results will only be as good as the laboratory expertise shown.** Complete information on the use of any of these test systems can be obtained from the manufacturer. All systems have been rated as good, with an accuracy correlation ranging from 87% to 96% or higher, depending on the number and variety of cultures tested. In addition, many of these systems are in their third or fourth generation, which should increase their accuracy even more.

API 20 Enterobacteriaceae (API 20E) System* (Plate 72)

The API 20 enteric system utilizes 22 biochemical tests that can produce results from a single bacterial colony in 18 to 24 hours. Some identifications can be made within 5 hours if a dense suspension of organisms is used. The colony is emulsified in about 5 ml of distilled water to supply the inoculum, and inoculation is carried out with a Pasteur pipet. Viable cells are introduced into the small plastic cupules and tubes arranged on a plastic-covered strip that is incubated in a plastic tray, to which water has been added to provide humidity, for 18 hours. This system has been evaluated by several investigators, and correlation with conventional tests as high as 96.4%[45,101,113,115] has been reported. Washington noted that this kit was complete and accurate.

Enterotube II System†

The new, improved tube permits simultaneous inoculation and performance of 15 biochemical tests from a single colony. A well-isolated colony is usually selected from MacConkey, EMB, or Hektoen agar plates that have been inoculated with a clinical specimen. The multitest tube is inoculated by touching the needle to a single colony and drawing it through all media in the tube. It has been reported that the citrate and urease reactions tend to present the greatest problems in the interpretation of the test. Reports by Morton and Monaco,[67] Douglas

and Washington,[19] and Smith[99] provided evidence of the practical use of this system. Washington[113] noted that this was a simple and convenient kit to use.

Entero-Set 20* (Plate 73)

This system consists of a card with 20 capillary units containing 20 different reagents designed to differentiate between the genera of the Enterobacteriaceae on a reduced time schedule and to differentiate the species of *Enterobacter* and *Proteus*. The reliability of this test system in regard to accuracy of results and laboratory safety has been noted.[84,116] This system was recently evaluated by Aldridge and Hodges.[2] They found it to be accurate and reproducible when compared with conventional tube media, and its performance was equal to that of the API 20E.

Inoculum is prepared from a single colony selected from a primary isolation plate, and from this suspension the battery of tests is set up. Readings can be recorded in 20 to 24 hours at 35 C.

Minitek System† (Plate 71)

This test system utilizes paper disks impregnated with individual substrates. These disks are placed in wells in a plastic plate and inoculated with a broth suspension of the isolate. Subsequent identification is based on color reactions occurring in the disks following overnight incubation. There are presently 35 different disks available, permitting the user to select the tests most appropriate for identification.

Several reports have attested to the reliability and accuracy of the Minitek system in the identification of the Enterobacteriaceae.[36,46,56] However, Washington's experience was less favorable.[113] He believed that the accuracy of identification with Minitek was not of the same order as that achievable with the AP1 20E and

---

*Analytab Products, Inc., Plainview, N.Y.
†Roche Diagnostics, Division of Hoffman-LaRoche, Inc., Nutley, N.J.

*Inolex Corp., Glenwood, Ill.
†Baltimore Biological Laboratory, Cockeysville, Md.

Enterotube II systems at the time of his study.

Micro-ID System* (Plates 69 and 70)

The Micro-ID system uses substrate- and reagent-impregnated paper disks to biochemically differentiate Enterobacteriaceae. The major component of the system, a molded plastic tray with a hinged lid, contains 15 test chambers, one for each biochemical test. The first 5 chambers contain separate substrate and detection reagent disks. The remaining 10 chambers each contain a single substrate/reagent disk. All test chambers are inoculated with a saline bacterial suspension prepared from a single isolated colony. After incubation at 35 C for only 4 hours, reagents are added to the appropriate chambers and the color reactions are read and recorded. Each set of reactions generates a five-digit octal code number corresponding to the identity of the organism. Buesching and colleagues[12] found that the Micro-ID system compared favorably with other systems for the identification of *Enterobacteriaceae*.

R/B System† (Plate 75)

The basic system contains eight biochemicals in two tubes: phenylalanine deaminase, hydrogen sulfide, indole, motility, lysine and ornithine decarboxylase, gas from glucose, and lactose. Two additional tubes have been introduced, namely Cit/Rham (citrate and rhamnose) and Soranase (sorbitol, DNase, raffinose, and arabinose), permitting an expansion to 14 biochemicals in four tubes. The addition of these tubes permits differentiation of *Enterobacter* species and a differentiation of other genera.[51, 61, 100] The tests are read after overnight incubation at 35 C.

This system has been evaluated favorably by several investigators.[51,61]

Micro-Media Enteric System (MMES)*

This system consists of various plastic plates containing from 24 to 104 wells per plate. Different plates are available for (1) identifying one gram-negative isolate (enteric or nonenteric), (2) identifying three different gram-negative isolates (Trident panel), (3) identifying a single isolate while checking its sensitivity to several antibiotics, and (4) determining the minimal inhibitory concentration of several antibiotics for an already identified isolate. Identifications are based on the results of 30 biochemical reactions (27 in the plate and 3 additional tests). All materials are supplied frozen in the test wells, and plates must be stored in a freezer until just before use. The procedure for use is as follows: an isolated colony from a primary plate is suspended in sterile distilled water, and the suspension is poured into a seed trough. The transfer lid is placed over the trough so that the prongs come into contact with the bacterial suspension and pick up a predetermined amount of suspension. The transfer lid is then removed from the trough and inserted into the plastic plate so that each well receives a standard inoculum. After 18 to 24 hours of incubation at 35 to 37 C, the reactions are read and recorded to obtain a biotype number. This number is listed along with the possible identities of the organism in the code book provided. This system was evaluated by Kelly and Washington[55] (as well as others) and was found to be an effective and practical method for identifying Enterobacteriaceae.

Other approaches (Plate 76)

A recent study indicates that the Repliscan system, at present, does not reliably identify Enterobacteriaceae, although the authors believed that it would be desirable to pursue its further development.[118]

Most systems employ mathematical analysis of data from biochemical reactions for rapid identification of Enterobacteriaceae. Thus, API

---

*General Diagnostics Division, Warner-Lambert Co., Morris Plains, N.J.
†Flow Laboratories, Inc., McLean, Va.

---

*Micro-Media Systems, Inc., Potomac, Md.

has a Profile Register for computer use. Encise II is a large data base for use with the Enterotube; it can be approached by a binomial computer system or a four-digit number reference.

Computer-assisted bacterial identification utilizing antimicrobial susceptibility patterns has also been done.[15,96]

Other approaches to rapid identification of the Enterobacteriaceae include the use of bile-esculin agar to detect esculin hydrolysis in 4 hours,[58] a 3-hour DNase test,[39] and direct identification of colonies of *Salmonella* and *Shigella* by coagglutination of protein A–containing staphylococci sensitized with specific antibody.[22] von Graevenitz[110] found that use of a DNase-indole medium for non-lactose-fermenting gram-negative rods often led to rapid identification of a variety of Enterobacteriaceae and other gram-negative bacilli. An interesting simplified approach to prompt lactose-fermenting Enterobacteriaceae strains has been presented by Hicks and Ryan.[48] Flat, spot indole-positive colonies were identified as *E. coli*. Spot indole-negative organisms forming mucoid colonies were identified as *Klebsiella* or *Enterobacter* species on the basis of semisolid agar motility and ornithine decarboxylase tests. This very simple scheme yielded 97.4% accuracy as compared with conventional and API identifications.

Use of automated systems for rapid identification of Enterobacteriaceae is considered in Chapter 40.

ANTIMICROBIAL SUSCEPTIBILITY

Antimicrobial susceptibility patterns may vary widely in different institutions. It is helpful to the clinician to receive periodic summaries of specific susceptibility patterns to guide decisions regarding therapy until studies have been done on isolates from patients. In general, the organisms most commonly encountered that are frequently resistant are *Pseudomonas*, *Klebsiella*, *Enterobacter*, and *Serratia*. Resistance to cephalosporins and aminoglycosides is not un-

common in many institutions. Amikacin and some of the newer cephalosporins and penicillins are presently the most active of all antimicrobials against the Enterobacteriaceae.

REFERENCES

1. Abbott, J.D., and Shannon, R.: A method for typing *Shigella sonnei* using colicin production as a marker, J. Clin. Pathol. **11**:71-75, 1958.
2. Aldridge, K.E., and Hodges, R.L.: Correlation studies of Entero-Set 20, API 20E, and conventional media systems for enterobacteriaceae identification, J. Clin. Microbiol. **13**:120-125, 1981.
3. Bailey, W.R.: Studies on the transduction phenomenon. I. Practical applications in the laboratory, Can. J. Microbiol. **2**:549-553, 1956.
4. Banwell, J.G., and Sherr, H.: Effect of bacterial enterotoxins on the gastrointestinal tract, Gastroenterol. **65**:467-497, 1973.
5. Bissett, M.L.: *Yersinia enterocolitica* isolates from humans in California, 1968-1975, J. Clin. Microbiol. **4**:137-144, 1976.
6. Blachman, U., and Pickett, M.J.: Unusual aerobic bacilli in clinical bacteriology, Los Angeles, 1978, Scientific Developments Press.
7. Bottone, E.J.: *Yersinia enterocolitica:* a panoramic view of a charismatic organism, CRC Crit. Rev. Microbiol. **5**:211-214, 1977.
8. Brenner, D.J.: Taxonomy, classification, and nomenclature of bacteria. In Lennette, E.H., Balows, A., Hausler, W.J., Jr., and Truant, J.P., editors: Manual of clinical microbiology, ed. 3, Washington, D.C., 1980, American Society for Microbiology.
9. Brenner, D.J., Farmer, J.J., Hickman, F.W., Asbury, M.A., and Steigerwalt, A.G.: Taxonomic and nomenclature changes in Enterobacteriaceae, Atlanta, 1977, Center for Disease Control.
10. Brinton, C.C.: Non-flagellar appendages of bacteria, Nature **183**:782-786, 1959.
11. Buchanan, R.E., and Gibbons, N.E., editors: Bergey's manual of determinative bacteriology, ed. 8, Baltimore, 1974, The William & Wilkins Co.
12. Buesching, W.J., Rhoden, D.L., Esaias, A.O., Smith, P.B., and Washington, J.A., II: Evaluation of the modified Micro-ID system for identification of Enterobacteriaceae, J. Clin. Microbiol. **10**:454-458, 1979.
13. Carpenter, K.P.: Personal communication; 1969.
14. Carpenter, K.P., and Lachowicz, K.: The catalase activity of *Sh. flexneri*, J. Pathol. Bact. **77**:645-648, 1959.
15. Darland, G.: Discriminant analysis of antibiotic susceptibility as a means of bacterial identification, J. Clin. Microbiol. **2**:391-396, 1975.

16. Darland, G., Ewing, W.H., and Davis, B.R.: The biochemical characteristics of *Yersinia enterocolitica* and *Yersinia pseudotuberculosis*, DHEW Pub. No. (CDC) 75-8294, Washington, D.C., 1974, Department of Health, Education, and Welfare.

17. Dean, A.G., Ching, Y.C., Williams, G., and Barden, B.: Test for *Escherichia coli* enterotoxin using infant mice: application in a study of diarrhea in children in Honolulu, J. Infect. Dis. **125**:407-411, 1972.

18. Donta, S.T., Moon, H.W., and Whipp, S.C.: Detection of heat-labile *Escherichia coli* enterotoxin with the use of adrenal cells in tissue culture, Science **183**:334-336, 1974.

19. Douglas, G.W., and Washington, J.A., II: Identification of Enterobacteriaceae in the clinical laboratory, Atlanta, 1970, Center for Disease Control.

20. Duguid, J.P., Smith, I.W., Dempster, G., and Edmonds, P.N.: Non-flagellar filamentous appendages ("fimbriae") and haemagglutinating activity in *Bacterium coli*, J. Path. Bact. **70**:335-348, 1955.

21. DuPont, H.L., Formal, S.B., Hornick, R.B., Snyder, M.J., Libonati, J.P., Sheahan, D.G., LaBrec, E.H., and Kalas, J.P.: Pathogenesis of *Escherichia coli* diarrhea, N. Engl. J. Med. **258**:1-9, 1971.

22. Edwards, E.A., and Hilderbrand, R.L.: Method for identifying *Salmonella* and *Shigella* directly from the primary isolation plate by coagglutination of protein A–containing staphylococci sensitized with specific antibody, J. Clin. Microbiol. **3**:339-343, 1976.

23. Edwards, P.R., and Ewing, W.H.: Identification of Enterobacteriaceae, ed. 3, Minneapolis, 1972, Burgess Publishing Co.

24. Edwards, P.R., and Fife, M.A.: Lysine-iron agar in the detection of *Arizona* cultures, Appl. Microbiol. **9**:478-480, 1961.

25. Edwards, P.R., Kauffmann, F., and van Oye, E.: A new diphasic *Arizona* type, Acta Pathol. Microbiol. Scand. **31**:5-9, 1952.

26. Enterobacteriaceae Subcommittee: Third report, Int. Bull. Bact. Nomencl. Taxon. **8**:25-70, 1958.

27. Evans, D.G., Evans, D.J., Jr., and Pierce, N.F.: Differences in the response of rabbit small intestine to heat-labile and heat-stable enterotoxins of *Escherichia coli*, Infect. Immun. **7**:873-880, 1973.

28. Evans, D.G., Silver, R.P., Evans, D.J., Chase, D.G., and Gorbach, S.L.: Plasmid-controlled colonization factor associated with virulence in *Escherichia coli* enterotoxigenic for humans, Infect. Immun. **12**:656-667, 1975.

29. Ewing, W.H., Davis, B.R., Fife, M.A., and Lessel, E.F.: Biochemical characterization of *Serratia liquefaciens* (Grimes and Hennerty), Bascomb et al. (formerly *Enterobacter liquefaciens*) and *Serratia rubidaea* (Stapp) comb. nov. and designation of type and neotype strains, Int. J. Syst. Bacteriol. **23**:217-225, 1973.

30. Ewing, W.H., and Fife, M.A.: Biochemical characterization of *Enterobacter agglomerans*, DHEW Pub. No. (HSM) 73-8173, Washington, D.C., 1972, Department of Health, Education, and Welfare.

31. Ewing, W.H., McWhorter, A.C., Escobar, M.R., and Lubin, A.M.: *Edwardsiella*, a new genus of Enterobacteriaceae based on a new species *E. tarda*, Int. Bull. Bact. Nomencl. Taxon. **15**:33-38, 1965.

32. Ewing, W.H., McWhorter, A.C., and Montague, T.S.: Transport media in the detection of *Salmonella typhi* in carriers, J. Conf. State Prov. Public Health, Lab. Directors **24**:63-65, 1966.

33. Ferragut, F.G., Izard, C., Trinel, P.A., Leclerc, H., Lefebvre, B., and Mossel, D.A.A.: *Serratia fonticola*, a new species from water, Int. J. Syst. Bact. **29**:92-101, 1979.

34. Field, M.: Intestinal secretion, Gastroenterology **66**:1063-1084, 1974.

35. Fields, B.N., Uwaydah, M.M., Kunz, L.J., and Swartz, M.N.: The so-called "paracolon" bacteria: a bacteriologic and clinical reappraisal, Am. J. Med. **42**:89-106, 1967.

36. Finklea, P.J., Cole, M.S., and Sodeman, T.M.: Clinical evaluation of the Minitek differential system for identification of Enterobacteriaceae, J. Clin. Microbiol. **4**:400-404, 1976.

37. Gorbach, S.L., Kean, B.H., Evans, D.G., Evans, D.J., Jr., and Bessudo, D.: Travelers diarrhea and toxigenic *Escherichia coli*, N. Engl. J. Med. **292**:933-936, 1975.

38. Gorbach, S.L., and Khurana, C.N.: Toxigenic *Escherichia coli* as a cause of infantile diarrhea in Chicago, N. Engl. J. Med. **287**:791-795, 1972.

39. Greenwood, J.R., and Pickett, M.J.: Deoxyribonuclease: detection with a three-hour test, J. Clin. Microbiol. **4**:453-454, 1976.

40. Grimont, P.A.D., and Grimont, F.: The genus *Serratia*, Annu. Rev. Microbiol. **32**:221-248, 1978.

41. Grimont, P.A.D., Grimont, F., and Dulong de Rosnay, H.L.C., Taxonomy of the genus *Serratia*, J. Gen. Microbiol. **98**:39-66, 1977.

42. Grimont, P.A.D., Grimont, F., Richard, C., Davis, B.R., Steigerwalt, A.G., and Brenner, D.J.: Deoxyribonucleic acid relatedness between *Serratia plymuthica* and other *Serratia* species, with a description of *Serratia odorifera* sp. nov. (type strain: ICPB 3995), Int. J. Syst. Bacteriol. **28**:453-463, 1978.

43. Gross, R.J., Scotland, S.N., and Rowe, B.: Enterotoxin testing of *Escherichia coli* causing epidemic infantile enteritis in the U.K., Lancet **1**:629-631, 1976.

44. Guerrant, R.L., and Dickens, M.D.: Toxigenic bacterial diarrhea: a nursery outbreak involving multiple

strains, Fourteenth Interscience Conference on Antimicrobial Agents and Chemotherapy, Abstr. 130, 1974.

45. Guillermet, F.N., and Desbresles, A.M.B.: A propos de l'utilisation d'une micromethode d'identification des Enterbacties, Rev. Inst. Pasteur de Lyon **4**:71-78, 1971.

46. Hanson, S.L., Hardesty, D.R., and Myers, B.M.: Evaluation of the BBL Minitek system for the identification of Enterobacteriaceae, Appl. Microbiol. **28**:798-801, 1974.

47. Hickman, F.W., Farmer, J.J., III, Steigerwalt, A.G., and Brenner, D.J.: Unusual groups of *Morganella* *("Proteus") morganii* isolated from clinical specimens: lysine-positive and ornithine-negative biogroups, J. Clin. Microbiol. **12**:88-94, 1980.

48. Hicks, M.J., and Ryan, K.J.: Simplified scheme for identification of prompt lactose-fermenting members of the Enterobacteriaceae, J. Clin. Microbiol. **4**:511-514, 1976.

49. Hobbs, B.C., Thomas, M.E.M., and Taylor, J.: School outbreak of gastro-enteritis associated with a pathogenic paracolon bacillus, Lancet **257**:530-532, 1949.

50. Hormaeche, E., and Edwards, P.R.: A proposed genus *Enterobacter*, Int. Bull. Bact. Nomencl. Taxon. **10**:71-74, 1960.

51. Isenberg, H.D., and Painter, B.G.: Comparison of conventional methods, the R/B System, and modified R/B System as guides to major divisions of Enterobacteriaceae, Appl. Bact. **22**:1126-1134, 1971.

52. Julianelle, L.A.: A biological classification of *Encapsulatus pneumoniae* (Friedlander's bacillus), J. Exp. Med. **44**:113-128, 1926.

53. Kauffmann, F.: Ein kombiniertes Anreicherungsverfahren fur Typhus and Paratyphusbazillen, Zbl. Bakt. **119**:148-152, 1930.

54. Kauffmann, F.: Die Bakteriologie der Salmonella-Gruppe, Copenhagen, 1941, Einar Munksgaard.

55. Kelly, S.A., and Washington, J.A., II: Evaluation of Micro-Media quad panels for identification of the Enterobacteriaceae, J. Clin. Microbiol. **10**:515-518, 1979.

56. Kiehn, T.E., Brennan, K., and Ellner, P.D.: Evaluation of Minitek system for identification of Enterobacteriaceae, Appl. Microbiol. **28**:668-671, 1974.

57. Knapp, W., and Masshoff, W.: Zur Ätiologie der abszedierenden retikulozytären Lymphadenitis: einer praktisch wichtigen, vielfach unter dem Bilde einer aktuen Appendizitis verlaufenden Erkrankung, Deutsch Med. Wschr. **79**:1266-1271, 1954.

58. Lindell, S.S., and Quinn, P.: Use of bile-esculin agar for rapid differentiation of Enterobacteriaceae, J. Clin. Microbiol. **1**:440-443, 1975.

59. Martin, W.J., Fife, M.A., and Ewing, W.H.: The occurrence and distribution of the serotypes of *Arizona*, Atlanta, 1967, National Communicable Disease Center.

60. Martin, W.J., and Washington, J.A., II: Enterobacteriaceae. In Lennette, E.H., Balows, A., Hausler, W.J., Jr., and Truant, J.P., editors: Manual of clinical microbiology, ed. 3, Washington, D.C., 1980, American Society for Microbiology.

61. McIlroy, G.T., Yu, P.K.W., Martin, W.J., and Washington, J.A., II: Evaluation of modified R-B system for identification of members of the family Enterobacteriaceae, Appl. Microbiol. **24**:358-362, 1972.

62. Merson, M.H., Black, R.E., Gross, R.J., Rowe, B., Huq, I., and Eusof, A.: Use of antisera for identification of enterotoxigenic *Escherichia coli*, Lancet **2**:222-224, 1980.

63. Minutes of the Enterobacteriaceae Subcommittee meeting, Montreal, 1962; report of the Subcommittee on taxonomy of the Enterobacteriaceae, Int. Bull. Bact. Nomencl. Taxon. **13**:69-93, 139, 1963.

64. Moeller, V.: Diagnostic use of the Braun KCN test within Enterobacteriaceae, Acta Pathol. Microbiol. Scand. **34**:115-126, 1954.

65. Morris, G.K., Merson, M.H., Sack, D.A., Wells, J.G., Martin, W.T., DeWitt, W.E., Feeley, J.C., Sack, R.B., and Bessudo, D.M.: Laboratory investigation of diarrhea in travelers to Mexico: evaluation of methods for detecting enterotoxigenic *Escherichia coli*, J. Clin. Microbiol. **3**:486-495, 1976.

66. Morris, G.K., and Wells, J.G.: Colicin typing of *Shigella sonnei*, Appl. Microbiol. **27**:312-316, 1974.

67. Morton, H.E., and Monaco, M.A.J.: Comparison of Enterotubes and routine media for the identification of enteric bacteria, Am. J. Clin. Pathol. **56**:64-66, 1971.

68. Nissen, R., Nørholm, T., and Siboni, K.E.: A case of neonatal meningitis caused by a yellow *Enterobacter*, Danish Med. Bull. **12**:128-130, 1965.

69. Ørskov, F., Ørskov, I., Evans, D.J., Jr., Sack, R.B., Sack, D.A., and Wadström, T.: Special *Escherichia coli* serotypes among enteropathogenic strains from diarrhea in adults and children, Med. Microbiol. Immunol. **162**:73-80, 1976.

70. Overturf, G.D., Wilkins, J., and Ressler, R.: Emergence of resistance of *Providencia stuartii* to multiple antibiotics: speciation and biochemical characterization of *Providencia*, J. Infect. Dis. **129**:353-357, 1974.

71. Pai, C.H., Sorger, S., Lafleur, L., Lackman, L., and Marks, M.I.: Efficiency of cold enrichment techniques for recovery of *Yersinia enterocolitica* from human stools, J. Clin. Microbiol. **9**:712-715, 1979.

72. Patterson, R.H., Banister, G.B., and Knight, V.: Chromobacterial infection in man, Arch. Intern. Med. **90**:79-86, 1952.

73. Penner, J.L., Fleming, P.C., Whiteley, G.R., and Hennessy, J.N.: O-serotyping *Providencia alcalifaciens*, J. Clin. Microbiol. **10**:761-765, 1979.

74. Penner, J.L., and Hennessy, J.N.: Application of O-serotyping in a study of *Providencia rettgeri (Proteus rettgeri)* isolated from human and nonhuman sources, J. Clin. Microbiol. **10**:834-840, 1979.

75. Penner, J.L., and Hennessy, J.N.: O antigen grouping of *Morganella morganii (Proteus morganii)* by slide agglutination, J. Clin. Microbiol. **10**:8-13, 1979.

76. Penner, J.L., and Hennessy, J.N.: Separate O-grouping schemes for serotyping clinical isolates of *Proteus vulgaris* and *Proteus mirabilis*, J. Clin. Microbiol. **12**:304-309, 1980.

77. Penner, J.L., Hinton, N.A., Duncan, I.B.R., Hennessy, J.N., and Whiteley, G.R.: O serotyping of *Providencia stuartii* isolates collected from twelve hospitals, J. Clin. Microbiol. **9**:11-14, 1979.

78. Penner, J.L., Hinton, N.A., and Hennessy, J.N.: Biochemical differentiation of *Proteus rettgeri*, J. Clin. Microbiol. **1**:136-142, 1975.

79. Penner, J.L., Hinton, N.A., Hennessy, J.N., and Whiteley, G.R.: Reconstitution of the somatic (O)-antigenic schema for *Providencia* and preparation of O-typing antisera, J. Infect. Dis. **133**:283-292, 1976.

80. Pien, F.D., Martin, W.J., Hermans, P.E., and Washington, J.A., II: Clinical and bacteriologic observations on the proposed species, *Enterobacter agglomerans* (the Herbicola-Lathyri bacteria), Mayo Clin. Proc. **47**:739-745, 1972.

81. Pruneda, R.C., and Farmer, J.J., III: Bacteriophage typing of *Shigella sonnei*, J. Clin. Microbiol. **5**:66-74, 1977.

82. Rabson, A.R., Hallett, A.F. and Koornhof, H.J.: Generalized *Yersinia enterocolitica* infection, J. Infect. Dis. **131**:447-451, 1975.

83. Reller, L.B., and Mirrett, S.: Motility-indole-lysine medium for presumptive identification of enteric pathogens of Enterobacteriaceae, J. Clin. Microbiol. **2**:247-252, 1975.

84. Rhoden, D.L., Tomfohrde, K.M., Smith, P.B., and Balows, A.: Auxotab: a device for identifying enteric bacteria, Appl. Microbiol. **25**:284-286, 1973.

85. Richard, C., Joly, B., Sirot, J., Stoleru, G.H., and Popoff, M.: Étude de souches de *Enterobacter* appartenant à un group particulier proche de *E. aerogenes* Ann. Microbiol. (Inst. Pasteur) **127A**:545-548, 1976.

86. Roat, W.R., Formal, S.B., Dammin, G.J., and Giannella, R.A.: Pathophysiology of Salmonella diarrhea in the rhesus monkey: intestinal transport, morphological and bacteriological studies. Gastroenterol. **67**:59-70, 1974.

87. Rowe, B., Scotland, S.N., and Gross, R.J., Enterotoxigenic *Escherichia coli* causing infantile enteritis in Britain, Lancet **1**:90-91, 1977.

88. Rowe, B., Taylor, J., and Bettelheim, K.A.: An investigation of travellers diarrhea, Lancet **1**:1-5, 1970.

89. Sack, R.B.: Human diarrheal disease caused by enterotoxigenic *Escherichia coli*, Annu. Rev. Microbiol. **29**:333-353, 1975.

90. Sack, R.B.: Serotyping of *E. coli*, Lancet **1**:1132, 1976.

91. Sack, R.B., Gorbach, S.L., Banwell, J.G., Jacobs, B., Chatterjee, B.D., and Mitra, R.C.: Enterotoxigenic *Escherichia coli* isolated from patients with severe cholera like disease, J. Infect. Dis. **123**:378-385, 1971.

92. Sack, R.B., Hirschhorn, N., Brownlee, I., Cash, R.A., Woodward, W.E., and Sack, D.A.: Enterotoxigenic *Escherichia coli*-associated diarrheal disease in Apache children, N. Engl. J. Med. **292**:1041-1045, 1975.

93. Sack, R.B., Jacobs, B., and Mitra, R.: Antitoxin responses to infections with enterotoxigenic *Escherichia coli*, J. Infect. Dis. **129**:330-335, 1974.

94. Sakazaki, R., Tamura, K., and Saito, M.: Enteropathogenic *Escherichia coli*: associated with diarrhea in children and adults, Jpn. J. Med. Sci. Biol. **20**:387-399, 1967.

95. Shore, E.G., Dean, A.G., Holik, K.J., and Davis, B.R.: Enterotoxin producing *Escherichia coli* and diarrheal disease in adult travellers: a prospective study, J. Infect. Dis. **129**:577-582, 1974.

96. Sielaff, B.H., Johnson, E.A., and Matsen, J.M.: Computer-assisted bacterial identification utilizing antimicrobial susceptibility profiles generated by Autobac 1, J. Clin. Microbiol. **3**:105-109, 1976.

97. Smith, H.W., and Gyles, C.L.: The relationship between two apparently different enterotoxins produced by enteropathogenic strains of *Escherichia coli* of porcine origin, J. Med. Microbiol. **3**:387-401, 1970.

98. Smith, H.W., and Halls, S.: The transmissible nature of the genetic factor in *Escherichia coli* that controls enterotoxin production, J. Gen. Microbiol. **52**:319-334, 1968.

99. Smith, P.B.: Roundtable on Enterobacteriaceae, American Society for Microbiology Meeting, Miami Beach, May 1973.

100. Smith, P.B., Tomfohrde, K.M., Rhoden, D.L., and Balows, A.: Evaluation of the modified R/B system for identification of Enterobacteriaceae, Appl. Microbiol. **22**:928-929, 1971.

101. Smith, P.B., Tomfohrde, K.M., Rhoden, D.L., and Balows, A.: API system: a multitube micromethod for identification of Enterobacteriaceae, Appl. Microbiol. **24**:449-452, 1972.

102. Søgaard, H., Zimmerman-Nielsen, C., and Siboni, K.: Antibiotic resistant gram-negative bacilli in a urological ward for male patients during a nine-year period: relationship to antibiotic consumption, J. Infect. Dis. **130**:646-650, 1974.

103. Sonnenwirth, A.C.: *Yersinia*. In Lennette, E.H., Spaulding, E.H., and Truant, J.P., editors: Manual of clinical microbiology, ed. 2, Washington, D.C., 1974, American Society for Microbiology.

104. Sonnenwirth, A.C., and Weaver, R.E.: *Yersinia enterocolitica*, N. Engl. J. Med. **283**:1468, 1970.

105. Stuart, C.A., Wheeler, K.M., and McGann, V.: Further studies of one anaerogenic paracolon organism, type 29911, J. Bacteriol. **52**:431-438, 1946.

106. Stuart, C.A., Wheeler, K.M., Rustigian, R., and Zimmerman, A.: Biochemical and antigenic relationships of the paracolon bacteria, J. Bacteriol. **45**:101-119, 1943.

107. Stuart, R.D.: Transport medium for specimens in public health bacteriology, Public Health Rep. **74**:431-438, 1959.

108. Taylor, J., Maltby, M.P., and Payne, J.M.: Factors influencing the response of ligated rabbit-gut segments to injected *Escherichia coli*, J. Pathol. Bacteriol. **76**:491-499, 1958.

109. Thomas, M.E.M.: Disadvantages of rectal swabs in diagnosis of diarrhea, Br. Med. J. **2**:394-396, 1954.

110. von Graevenitz, A.: Detection of unusual strains of gram-negative rods through the routine use of a deoxyribonuclease-indole medium, Mt. Sinai J. Med. **43**:727-735, 1976.

111. Waisbren, B.A., and Carr, C.: Penicillin and chloramphenicol in the treatment of infections due to *Proteus* organisms, Am. J. Med. Sci. **223**:418-421, 1952.

112. Washington, J.A., II, editor: Laboratory procedures in clinical microbiology, Boston, 1974, Little, Brown and Co.

113. Washington, J.A., II: Laboratory approaches to the identification of Enterobacteriaceae, Human Pathol. **7**:151-159, 1976.

114. Washington, J.A., II, Senjem, D.H., Haldorson, A., Schutt, A.H., and Martin, W.J.: Nosocomially acquired bacteriuria due to *Proteus rettgeri* and *Providencia stuartii*, Am. J. Clin. Pathol. **60**:836-838, 1973.

115. Washington, J.A., II, Yu, P.K., and Martin, W.J.: Evaluation of accuracy of multitest micromethod system for identification of Enterobacteriaceae, Appl. Microbiol. **22**:267-269, 1971.

116. Washington, J.A., II, Yu, P.K., and Martin, W.J.: Evaluation of the Auxotab Enteric 1 System for identification of Enterobacteriaceae, Appl. Microbiol. **23**:298-300, 1972.

117. Weber, J., Finlayson, N.B., and Mark, J.B.D.: Mesenteric lymphadenitis and terminal ileitis due to *Yersinia pseudotuberculosis*, N. Engl. J. Med. **283**:172-174, 1970.

118. Woolfrey, B.F., Quall, C.O., and Fox, J.M.: Evaluation of the Repliscan system for Enterobacteriaceae identification, J. Clin. Microbiol. **13**:58-61, 1981.

21 VIBRIONACEAE

Vibrio

Aeromonas

Plesiomonas

GENUS VIBRIO

Vibrio has been assigned to the family *Vibrionaceae* in the eighth edition of *Bergey's Manual*. The species of medical importance are *V. cholerae*, *V. parahaemolyticus*, *V. vulnificus*, and *V. alginolyticus*. The El Tor vibrio is not considered a separate species but a biotype of *V. cholerae* (this assignment was adopted by the International Subcommittee on Cholera). Both the El Tor and *V. cholerae* biotypes produce **cholera,** but because of their biochemical and other differences, it is of epidemiologic significance to distinguish between them. *V. parahaemolyticus* is perhaps the most important member of this genus because of its pathogenic potential in this hemisphere.

As noted in Chapter 9, cholera has been found in the United States in recent years, and *V. cholerae* has been found in the environment in the United States.[27] *V. cholerae* non–O group 1 may produce a disease similar to cholera or may produce bloody diarrhea and may also be involved in extraintestinal disease. *V. parahaemolyticus* produces a gastroenteritis that is usually mild or moderate in severity. It may occur in outbreaks. On rare occasions *V. parahaemolyticus* may be isolated from extraintestinal infection. *V. vulnificus* may produce either infection in a preexisting wound or ulcer or primary sepsis that may be accompanied by shock and may be fatal. *V. alginolyticus* is recovered from infected wounds or cutaneous ulcers and from otitis media and external otitis. Bacteremia occurs occasionally.

Table 21-1 shows characteristics that differentiate between *Vibrio* and certain similar genera.

Vibrio cholerae (O group 1)

This species and its biotype El Tor are gram-negative, actively motile rods possessing a single polar flagellum (Plate 77). With careful preparation of stained smears one may observe the slightly curved rods. Most investigators believe the El Tor biotype is less susceptible to environmental changes than is the *V. cholerae* type, and for this reason it is more readily recovered from clinical specimens (usually stool) submitted to the laboratory. *V. cholerae* non–O group 1 (noncholera vibrios, nonagglutinating vibrios) does

not agglutinate in *V. cholerae* polyvalent O1 antiserum. At present there are 72 serotypes of non-O1 *V. cholerae*.[37] A recent report by Morris and associates (Ann. Intern. Med. **94:**656-658, 1981) described 14 sporadic cases of non–O group 1 *V. cholerae* gastroenteritis identified in 1979. All had diarrhea (bloody in 4 cases), and 10 had fever. All 9 domestically acquired cases were in patients who had eaten raw oysters within 72 hours of onset of illness. Only one isolate produced heat-labile toxin in a Y-1 adrenal cell assay.

As has been pointed out by Balows and co-workers,[1] the most effective and rapid bacteriologic diagnosis of cholera is accomplished only by **proper communication** between the clinician and the laboratory. As advocated by these investigators, a liquid stool is best collected by rectal catheter, and formed stools should be collected in disinfectant-free containers. Rectal swabs are most effective when inserted beyond the anal sphincter. In all cases specimens should be taken prior to any antimicrobial therapy and inoculated to appropriate media immediately at the laboratory. Thiosulfate citrate bile salts sucrose

TABLE 21-1

Differentiation of vibrios from other organisms

Test	Vibrio	Aeromonas	Plesiomonas	Pseudomonas	Enterobacteriaceae
Indophenol oxidase	+	+*	+	+	−
Gelatinase	+	+	−	+	V
O-F test, glucose	F	F	F	O	F
Glucose, gas	−	±	−	−	+
Inositol	−	−	+	NC	V
Mannitol	+	+	−	NC	V
Lysine decarboxylase	+	−	+	NC	V
Arginine dihydrolase	−	+	+	+	V
Ornithine decarboxylase	+	−	+	NC	V
O/129 inhibition†	+	−	±	−	−
String test	+‡	−	−	−	−
Polar monotrichous flagella	+	+	+	+§	−
Loss of motility in distilled water[7]	+	−	−	−	−

Modified from Wachsmuth and others.[37]

+, 90% or more positive within 1 to 2 days; −, 90% or more no reaction; V, different reactions within genus; F, fermentative; O, oxidative; NC, no change.

*Test only from nonselective media.[25]

†2,4-diamino-6,7-diisopropyl pteridine phosphate.

‡Data on *V. parahaemolyticus* and *V. alginolyticus* are contradictory; most are negative or weakly positive.

§May have more than one flagellum per pole.

(TCBS) agar at pH 8.6, tellurite taurocholate gelatin agar (TTGA), and taurocholate gelatin agar (TGA) give good results. The selective TCBS and TTGA media may be inoculated quite heavily. The TGA medium should be inoculated lightly.[37] A MacConkey agar plate should be inoculated moderately. An enrichment broth should also be used.

On TCBS at 35 C after 18 to 24 hours *V. cholerae* appears as medium-sized, smooth, **yellow colonies** with opaque centers and transparent periphery. A few strains of *V. cholerae* may appear green or colorless on TCBS because of delayed sucrose fermentation. On TTGA colonies develop dark centers because of tellurite reduction and are surrounded by cloudy zones of gelatinase activity.[37] On TGA the colonies are somewhat flattened and transparent and are surrounded by a cloudy halo. Refrigeration tends to accentuate this characteristic, which demonstrates gelatin liquefaction.

Enrichment broth media are sodium-gelatin-phosphate broth and alkaline peptone water. Culturing in these media should not be extended beyond 18 to 20 hours, because suppressed forms may begin to develop. Agar media may be inoculated from the enrichment broth after 6 to 8 hours of incubation.

Suspicious colonies are selected and inoculated to appropriate media or tested with O1 typing serum by slide test. The young enrichment broth culture also may be examined for the characteristic darting motility by darkfield microscopy. The motility test, if positive, can be extended by carrying out the immobilization test with *V. cholerae* polyvalent O1 antiserum.

TABLE 21-2

Distinguishing characteristics of *Vibrio* species

Test	*V. cholerae*	*V. cholerae* El Tor biotype	*V. parahaemolyticus*
String test after 45 to 60 seconds	+	+	−
Hemagglutination test	−	+	−
Polymyxin B susceptibility test	+	−	
Phage IV susceptibility test	+	−	
VP	−	+	−
Hemolysis of sheep RBC	−	+*	−
Sucrose	+	+	−
Salt-free broth	+	+	−
Broth containing 7% to 10% NaCl	−	−	+
Cholera red test	+	+	−
Agglutination in polyvalent O1 serum	+	+	−

+, susceptibility.

*Considerable variability in hemolytic activity has been reported.

If this is positive, it may be used as presumptive evidence of identity.

Several tests will help to distinguish *V. cholerae* from the noncholera vibrios and also differentiate between *V. cholerae* and its biotype El Tor. Among these are the "string test,"[22,32] the hemagglutination test,[10] the polymyxin B susceptibility test,[11] the phage IV susceptibility test,[21] the VP test, and the hemolysis test.[16]

The **string test** consists of testing for the viscid character of a cholera culture in 0.5% sodium desoxycholate on a slide. The "string" is detected by lifting a loop of the mixture from the slide. The **hemagglutination test** is performed by mixing a loopful of washed chicken red blood cells with a heavy suspension of a pure culture of the organism on a slide. Visible clumping of the red blood cells is a positive test. The **polymyxin B susceptibility test** determines the inhibitory effect of the antimicrobic on the organism by the appearance of a zone of inhibition around polymyxin B disks on a seeded plate. The **phage IV susceptibility test** aids in differentiating *V. cholerae* from El Tor. The **hemolysis test,** performed with washed sheep red blood cells, is claimed by

some investigators also to be effective in differentiating these biotypes (Table 21-2).

Characteristics that differentiate various *Vibrio* species are given in Table 21-3. Several of the tests noted in Table 21-3 are very useful for separating these organisms and are recommended for use in rapid presumptive identification.[37] These include the NaCl requirement, the decarboxylase reactions, the fermentation of sucrose and lactose, the oxidase test, and agglutination in *V. cholerae* O1 antiserum.

Although the primary treatment of cholera consists of adequate intravenous or oral fluid and electrolyte replacement, tetracycline has been a valuable adjunct in that it shortens the duration of the disease and the duration of excretion of vibrios and lessens the amount of fluid and electrolyte replacement required. Accordingly, it is disturbing to find evidence of antimicrobial resistance in *V. cholerae*. There have been a number of sporadic isolations of drug-resistant organisms and, more recently, two outbreaks involving plasmid-mediated multiple antibiotic resistance.[33] The organisms from the Bangladesh outbreak were resistant to tetracycline,

TABLE 21-3

Differentiation of various vibrios

Test	V. cholerae	V. parahaemolyticus	V. alginolyticus	V. vulnificus	V. fluvialis (group F; EF-6)	V. metchnikovii
Indole	+	+	+	+	−	V
Voges-Proskauer	V	−	+	−	−	+
Lysine	+	+	+	+	−	V
Arginine	−	−	−	−	+	V
Ornithine	+	+	V	V	−	−
Lactose	+	−	−	+*	−	V
Sucrose	+	−	+	−	+	+
Arabinose	−	V	−	−	+	−
Salicin	−	−	−	+	−	−
Nitrate to nitrite	+	+	+	+	+	−
Oxidase	+	+	+	+	+	−
Agglutination in O1 serum	V	−	−	−	−	−
Growth in						
0% NaCl	+	−	−	−	−	−
8% NaCl	−	+	+	−	V	V
10% NaCl	−	−	+	−	−	−

Modified from Wachsmuth and associates.[37]

+, 90% or more positive; −, 90% or more no reaction; V, variable.

*Reaction sometimes delayed.

sulfonamides, ampicillin, kanamycin, strepto-mycin, and trimethoprim.[33]

Vibrio parahaemolyticus

This species is perhaps more important in the United States, since *V. cholerae* and the El Tor biotype are rarely encountered. *V. parahaemolyticus* can cause gastroenteritis or food poisoning, associated with the consumption of contaminated seafood, and (rarely) more serious infection such as septicemia with shock, hemolytic anemia, disseminated intravascular coagulation, and other manifestations.[28,39] Infection with this organism is most prevalent in the Orient but has been reported from other countries, and the organism is present in most, if not all, of the coastal marine environment of the United States.[8] The organism is resistant to penicillin, colistin, and polymyxin; variable in sensitivity to ampicillin, erythromycin, and kanamycin; and sensitive to chloramphenicol and gentami-cin.[6,35] It is relatively sensitive to tetracycline (maximum minimal inhibitory concentration 6 μg/ml) and borderline in susceptibility to streptomycin.

The organism is **halophilic** and grows well in peptone water medium containing 7% to 8% NaCl, but it does not normally utilize citrate. For the characteristics of this species see Tables 21-2 and 21-3. Bottone and Robin[4] described a strain of *V. parahaemolyticus* that was selected from a TCBS plate but that gave aberrant biochemical and morphologic reactions on subculture until the media to which it was subcultured were supplemented with sodium chloride.

Strains of *V. parahaemolyticus* associated with gastrointestinal illness cause hemolysis of human or rabbit red blood cells. This is known as the Kanagawa phenomenon. Details of the test are provided by Wachsmuth and colleagues.[37] Immunologic methods have been described for detection of the Kanagawa phenomenon. These include a modified Elek test and an immunohalo test.[15] The modified Elek test correlates well with the standard test for the Kanagawa phenomenon and gets around the problem of false-positive results that may result from instability of the blood used in the medium.

Other vibrios

A newly described *Vibrio* species, *V. vulnificus,* produces noteworthy disease. There are two different types of clinical presentations.[2,5] In one the illness begins with septicemia, often within 24 hours after raw oysters are eaten. In a report by Blake and associates,[2] 18 of 24 patients with this form of the disease had preexisting hepatic disease, and 11 of the 24 died. Three fourths of the patients with bacteremia had secondary cutaneous lesions, some of which showed a marked necrotizing vasculitis in the skin and muscles with extensive inflammatory changes. Despite the fact that this unusual lactose-positive *Vibrio* appears to cross the gut mucosa rapidly to invade the bloodstream, it only causes gastrointestinal symptoms in a small percentage of patients. The second type of clinical presentation is a wound infection after exposure to sea water or an injury incurred during the handling of crabs. Of 15 such patients in the series by Blake and others, none had preexisting hepatic disease and only one died. The wound infections tend to progress rapidly. Mertens and co-workers[20] described a case of fatal bacteremia with enteritis caused by this organism, and Kelly and Avery[17] described a case of pneumonia and septicemia in an individual who was resuscitated after almost drowning in the sea. These investigators sampled seawater from 21 sites around Galveston Island over a period of 4 weeks and found that one third of the samples yielded *V. vulnificus.* Disk susceptibility studies on strains studied by Kelly and Avery showed the organism to be sensitive to ampicillin, chloramphenicol, tetracycline, cotrimoxazole, and aminoglycosides and resistant to colistin.

V. alginolyticus is differentiated from *V. parahaemolyticus* by growth in 10% NaCl, positive VP test, acid from sucrose, and negative methyl red. *V. alginolyticus* has been isolated from extraintestinal sources such as blood, otitis media, otitis externa, conjunctivitis, and infected wounds.[9,14,29,30]

There are two other vibrios that are possibly pathogenic for humans. One is designated group F by workers in England and EF-6 by the CDC.[3] This organism is widely distributed in the aquatic environment around Britain. It was isolated from more than 500 patients with diarrhea in Bangladesh between October 1976 and June 1977. It was rarely isolated before and has rarely been isolated since that time. Family members of infected patients showed the organism in fewer than 1% of stool specimens. The clinical symptoms were similar to those of cholera, except that some patients had blood and mucus in their stools and some had abdominal pain and fever. It is not certain that the organism is a pathogen in humans, although it does kill mice when injected intraperitoneally and produces a heat-labile toxin that causes fluid accumulation in ligated rabbit ileal loops. This organism is now called *V. fluvialis* (Lee et al.: J. Appl. Bacteriol. **50:**73-94, 1981). *Vibrio metchnikovii* (also known as enteric group EG-16) is also widely distributed in rivers, estuaries, and sewage and has been isolated from the intestines of humans and animals.[3] There is no real evidence that it causes disease in humans or animals, but it has been isolated from the blood of an elderly woman with gallbladder disease.

GENUS AEROMONAS

Members of the genus *Aeromonas* are gram-negative motile rods with a single polar flagellum. They utilize carbohydrates **fermentatively,** with the production of acid or acid and gas, and are oxidase positive. Their normal habitat appears to be natural bodies of water, nonfecal sewage, marine life, and foods; they have also been isolated from fecal specimens of asymptomatic persons. *Aeromonas hydrophila* has been suggested as the type species of the genus.

An increasing incidence of human infections

caused by *A. hydrophila* has been reported* and includes infected traumatic wounds (some with a history of exposure to soil or water), septicemia, meningitis, gastroenteritis, osteomyelitis, and postoperative wound infections (usually in mixed culture). A rapidly progressive pneumonia and bacteremia that proved fatal within 15 hours of onset in a previously healthy 29-year-old man was described by Scott and colleagues.[31] A unique presentation is a relatively benign or slow-moving myonecrosis, which may cause significant liquefaction of muscle. Patients with hematologic and other malignancies appear to be particularly susceptible to infection with this organism.

A. hydrophila grows well on routine laboratory media, producing on blood agar small (1 to 3 mm), smooth, convex **beta-hemolytic** colonies that become dark green after 3 to 5 days.[13] Good growth also can occur on enteric isolation media, including EMB, MacConkey, and Salmonella-Shigella agar, both at 25 and 35 C. Key differential reactions are shown in Table 21-1. An alkaline slant over an acid and gas butt is observed on TSI medium; indole is usually produced from tryptophan, which helps to separate the aeromonads from pseudomonads, *Alcaligenes,* flavobacteria, and others. Demonstration of a **positive oxidase reaction** (Kovacs' method) and **polar flagellation** are most useful in distinguishing these organisms from other facultative gram-negative bacilli of clinical importance. The usefulness of these two test procedures in the identification of members of the genus *Aeromonas* cannot be overemphasized, since these organisms may be misidentified as members of the Enterobacteriaceae. They show similarity to *Escherichia coli, Enterobacter species*, and *Providencia*, particularly on conventional biochemical test media used in the early stages of the identification process. At the Mayo Clinic isolates of *A. hydrophila* were most often confused with *Enterobacter*.[38]

---

*See references 12, 13, 18, 23, 26, 36, and 38.

It should be noted that some strains of *A. hydrophila* are oxidase negative when tested from differential media because they ferment lactose in the medium, lowering the pH below 5.2. This problem of false-negative oxidase reactions can be avoided by using a rapid, same-day oxidase test on colonies from differential media, as described by Hunt and others (J. Clin. Microbiol. **13**:1117-1118, 1981).

A. hydrophila is highly susceptible to the aminoglycosides gentamicin and kanamycin, to cotrimoxazole, and to chloramphenicol and is variably susceptible to tetracycline; little activity is demonstrated by penicillin, carbenicillin, ampicillin, or cephalothin.[24,38] Antibiotic-resistant strains of *A. hydrophila* have been isolated from aquatic environments in Chesapeake Bay and Bangladesh.[19] The Bangladesh strains carried resistance to chloramphenicol, streptomycin, and tetracycline with a plasmid coding for resistance to streptomycin and tetracycline.

A recent report indicated that *A. sobria* was more commonly associated with human infection than *A. hydrophila*.

GENUS PLESIOMONAS

The one species in this genus, *Plesiomonas shigelloides*, previously was in the genus *Aeromonas*. The organism has been isolated from fresh water sources as well as various animals. It is **oxidase positive** and produces acid without gas from carbohydrates. The organism is not beta hemolytic on blood agar and generally does not ferment lactose on enteric agars. It gives a positive arginine dihydrolase reaction, is usually lysine decarboxylase positive, and may be ornithine decarboxylase positive. It is lipase negative. Also, in contrast with *A. hydrophila*, it ferments inositol and does not ferment mannitol or sucrose. It does not break down gelatin. Most strains are sensitive to the vibriostatic agent, 2,4-diamino-6,7-diisopropyl pteridine. Like *Aeromonas*, it may grow on a number of enteric media. Motility is generally observed with polar, generally lophotrichous flagella, although young cultures may show lateral flagella, and monotrichous cells as well as nonmotile strains occur.[34]

P. shigelloides has been isolated from feces of humans and from blood and spinal fluid cultures. It has been thought to be a cause of acute gastroenteritis. *Plesiomonas* frequently is resistant to ampicillin and carbenicillin but is usually susceptible to cephalosporins, tetracycline, aminoglycosides, chloramphenicol, and cotrimoxazole.[34]

REFERENCES

1. Balows, A., Hermann, G.J., and DeWitt, W.E.: The isolation and identification of *Vibrio cholerae:* a review, Health Lab. Sci. **8**:167-175, 1971.
2. Blake, P.A., Merson, M.H., Weaver, R.E., Hollis, D.G., and Heublein, P.C.: Disease caused by a marine vibrio, N. Engl. J. Med. **300**:1-5, 1979.
3. Blake, P.A., Weaver, R.E., and Hollis, D.G.: Diseases of humans (other than cholera) caused by vibrios, Annu. Rev. Microbiol. **34**:341-367, 1980.
4. Bottone, E.J., and Robin, T.: *Vibrio parahaemolyticus:* suspicion of presence based on aberrant biochemical and morphological features, J. Clin. Microbiol. **8**:760-763, 1978.
5. Carpenter, C.C.J.: More pathogenic vibrios, N. Engl. J. Med. **300**:39-41, 1979.
6. Chatterjee, B.D., Neogy, K.N., and Chowdhury, B.R.R.: Drug-sensitivity of *Vibrio parahaemolyticus* isolated in Calcutta during 1969, Bull. WHO **42**:640-641, 1970.
7. Chester, B., and Poulos, E.G.: Rapid presumptive identification of vibrios by immobilization in distilled water, J. Clin. Microbiol. **11**:537-539, 1980.
8. Dadisman, T.A., Jr., Nelson, R., Molenda, J.R., and Garber, H.J.: *Vibrio parahaemolyticus* gastroenteritis in Maryland, Am. J. Epidemiol. **96**:414-426, 1973.
9. Fernandez, C.R., and Pankey, G.A.: Tissue invasion by unnamed marine vibrios, J.A.M.A. **233**:1173-1176, 1975.
10. Finkelstein, R.A., and Mukerjee, S.: Hemagglutination: a rapid method for differentiating *Vibrio cholerae* and El Tor vibrios, Proc. Soc. Exp. Biol. Med. **112**:355-359, 1963.
11. Gangarosa, E.S., Bennett, J.V., and Boring, J.R., III: Differentiation between *Vibrio cholerae* and *Vibrio* biotype El Tor by the polymyxin B disc test: comparative results with TCBS, Monsur's, Meuller-Hinton, and nutrient agar media, Bull. WHO **35**:987-990, 1967.

12. Gifford, R.R.M., Lambe, D.W., Jr., McElreath, S.D., and Vogler, W.R.: Septicemia due to *Aeromonas hydrophila* and *Mima polymorpha* in a patient with acute myelogenous leukemia, Am. J. Med. Sci. **263**:157-161, 1972.

13. Gilardi, G.L., Bottone, E., and Birnbaum, M.: Unusual fermentative gram-negative bacilli isolated from clinical specimens. II. Characteristics of *Aeromonas* species, Appl. Microbiol. **20**:156-159, 1970.

14. Hollis, L.G., Weaver, R.E., Baker, C.N., and Thornsberry, C.: Halophilic *Vibrio* species isolated from blood cultures, J. Clin. Microbiol. **3**:425-431, 1976.

15. Honda, T., Chearskul, S., Takeda, Y., and Miwatani, T.: Immunological methods for detection of Kanagawa phenomenon of *Vibrio parahaemolyticus*, J. Clin. Microbiol. **11**:600-603, 1980.

16. Hugh, R.: A comparison of *Vibrio cholerae*, Pacini and *Vibrio* El Tor, Int. Bull. Bact. Nomencl. Taxon. **15**:61-68, 1965.

17. Kelly, M.T., and Avery, D.M.: Lactose-positive *Vibrio* in seawater: a cause of pneumonia and septicemia in a drowning victim, J. Clin. Microbiol. **11**:278-280, 1980.

18. Ketover, B.P., Young, L.S., and Armstrong, D.: Septicemia due to *Aeromonas hydrophila*: clinical and immunologic aspects, J. Infect. Dis. **127**:284-290, 1973.

19. McNicol, L.A., Aziz, K.M.S., Huq, I., Kaper, J.B., Lockman, H.A., Remmers, E.F., Spira, W.M., Voll, M.J., and Colwell, R.R.: Isolation of drug-resistant *Aeromonas hydrophila* from aquatic environments, Antimicrob. Agents Chemother. **17**:477-483, 1980.

20. Mertens, A., Nagler, J., Hansen, W., and Gepts-Friedenreich, E.: Halophilic, lactose-positive *Vibrio* in a case of fatal septicemia, J. Clin. Microbiol. **9**:233-235, 1979.

21. Mukerjee, S.: The bacteriophage susceptibility test in differentiating *Vibrio cholerae* and *Vibrio* El Tor, Bull. WHO **28**:333-336, 1963.

22. Neogy, K.N., and Mukherji, A.C.: A study of the string test in *Vibrio* identification, Bull. WHO **42**:638-641, 1970.

23. Nygaard, B.S., Bissett, M.L., and Wood, R.M.: Laboratory identification of aeromonads from men and other animals, Appl. Microbiol. **19**:618-620, 1970.

24. Overman, T.L.: Antimicrobial susceptibility of *Aeromonas hydrophila*, Antimicrob. Agents Chemother. **17**:612-614, 1980.

25. Overman, T.L., D'Amato, R.F., and Tomfohrde, K.M.: Incidence of "oxidase-variable" strains of *Aeromonas hydrophila*, J. Clin. Microbiol. **9**:244-247, 1979.

26. Qadri, S.M.H., Gordon, L.P., Wende, R.D., and Williams, R.P.: Meningitis due to *Aeromonas hydrophila*, J. Clin. Microbiol. **3**:102-104, 1976.

27. Rennels, M.B., Levine, M.M., Daya, V., Angle, P., and Young, C.: Selective vs. nonselective media and direct plating vs. enrichment technique in isolation of *Vibrio cholerae*: recommendations for clinical laboratories, J. Infect. Dis. **142**:328-331, 1980.

28. Roland, F.P.: Leg gangrene and endotoxin shock due to *Vibrio parahaemolyticus*: an infection acquired in New England coastal waters, N. Engl. J. Med. **282**:1306, 1970.

29. Rubin, S.J., and Tilton, R.C.: Isolation of *Vibrio alginolyticus* from wound infections, J. Clin. Microbiol. **2**:556-558, 1975.

30. Schmidt, U., Chmel, H., and Cobbs, C.: *Vibrio alginolyticus* infections in humans, J. Clin. Microbiol. **10**:666-668, 1979.

31. Scott, E.G., Russell, C.M., Noell, K.T., and Sproul, A.E.: *Aeromonas hydrophila* sepsis in a previously healthy man, J.A.M.A. **239**:1742, 1978.

32. Smith, H.L.: A presumptive test for vibrios: the "string" test, Bull. WHO **42**:817-818, 1970.

33. Threlfall, E.J., Rowe, B., and Huq, I.: Plasmid-encoded multiple antibiotic resistance in *Vibrio cholerae* El Tor from Bangladesh, Lancet **1**:1247-1248, 1980.

34. von Graevenitz, A.: *Aeromonas* and *Plesiomonas*. In Lennette, E.H., Balows, A., Hausler, W.J., Jr., and Truant, J.P., editors: Manual of clinical microbiology, ed. 3, Washington, D.C., 1980, American Society for Microbiology.

35. von Graevenitz, A., and Carrington, G.O.: Halophilic vibrios from extraintestinal lesions in man, Infection **1**:54-58, 1973.

36. von Graevenitz, A., and Mensch, A.H.: The genus *Aeromonas* in human bacteriology, N. Engl. J. Med. **278**:245-249, 1968.

37. Wachsmuth, I.K., Morris, G.K., and Feeley, J.C.: *Vibrio*. In Lennette, E.H., Balows, A., Hausler, W.J., Jr., and Truant, J.P., editors: Manual of clinical microbiology, ed. 3, Washington, D.C., 1980, American Society for Microbiology.

38. Washington, J.A., II: *Aeromonas hydrophila* in clinical bacteriological specimens, Ann. Intern. Med. **76**:611-614, 1972.

39. Zide, N., Davis, J., and Ehrenkranz, N.J.: Fulminating *Vibrio parahaemolyticus* septicemia, Arch. Intern. Med. **133**:479-481, 1974.

22 NONFERMENTATIVE GRAM-NEGATIVE BACILLI

Pseudomonas

Alcaligenes

Achromobacter

Acinetobacter

Moraxella

Kingella

Flavobacterium

Eikenella

Agrobacterium

Predominantly opportunistic in nature, this group of organisms owes its invasiveness or infectivity to an altered or already debilitated host, who has been compromised by potent medications, varied instrumentation, or the dramatic and prolonged surgical procedures recently developed.

In the past several years major advances have been made in the characterization and taxonomy of these nonfermentative bacteria; excellent descriptions of this group can be found in several sources.[2,10,25,42,46] No doubt one of the most important tests in this area was introduced by Hugh and Leifson[26] in their fermentation (O-F) medium (Plates 86 to 88), enabling the bacteriologist to determine whether an isolate was oxidative, fermentative, or inactive with respect to carbohydrate metabolism. These workers recognized that conventional fermentation media contained a high content of peptone (1%) and, when attacked, gave rise to alkaline amines capable of neutralizing any acidity formed during the fermentation. This is not a problem when large amounts of acid are produced by active "fermenters," but the oxidative bacteria produce **low levels** of acidity, which can be masked because of the accumulation of the alkaline amines. With a carbohydrate medium low in peptone (0.2%) the oxidative, fermentative, or inactive properties of gram-negative bacilli can be determined.

The base medium* with bromthymol blue indicator is sterilized by autoclaving (see Chapter 42 for preparation); after it is cooled, a filter-sterilized solution of the desired carbohydrate is added to give a final concentration of 1%. The recommended carbohydrates include glucose, lactose, sucrose, maltose, mannitol, and xylose.

*Baltimore Biological Laboratory, Cockeysville, Md.; Difco Laboratories, Detroit.

For each isolate **two** tubes of glucose O-F medium are inoculated with a light stab from a young culture, and one of the tubes is overlaid with at least ¼ inch of sterile, stiff petrolatum or vaspar. Sterile mineral oil is not recommended for this purpose. The tubes are then incubated at 35 C for several days and examined daily. An acid reaction is indicated by a change from the uninoculated blue-green color to a **yellow** color. A key to the identification of nonfermenting bacteria is given on pp. 250-251.

Key media required for initial grouping of glucose-nonfermenting gram-negative bacteria are listed in Table 22-1. The characteristics of the organisms that can be determined from inocula-

---

KEY TO THE IDENTIFICATION OF NONFERMENTING BACTERIA

Glucose nonoxidizers
  MacConkey positive
    Oxidase negative
      Motile: *Pseudomonas maltophilia* (w Glu)
      Nonmotile: *Acinetobacter calcoaceticus* biotype lwoffii, *Acinetobacter calcoaceticus* biotype alcaligenes
    Oxidase positive
      Motile: *Pseudomonas acidovorans* (v Glu), *Pseudomonas pseudoalcaligenes* (v Glu), *Pseudomonas vesicularis* (v Glu, r Mac), *Pseudomonas testosteroni* (v Mac), *Pseudomonas alcaligenes*, *Pseudomonas diminuta*, *Alcaligenes faecalis*, *Alcaligenes odorans*, *Alcaligenes denitrificans*, *Bordetella bronchiseptica*, group IVc-2 (v Mac), group IVe (v Mac)
      Nonmotile: *Flavobacterium breve* (v Glu, v Mac), *Flavobacterium* sp. (v Mac), *Flavobacterium odoratum*, *Moraxella nonliquefaciens* (r Mac), *Moraxella osloensis* (v Mac), *Moraxella phenylpyruvica*, *Moraxella atlantae*, *Moraxella urethralis*, group M-5 (v Mac)
  MacConkey negative
    Oxidase negative
      Nonmotile: *Eikenella corrodens*
    Oxidase positive
      Motile: *Pseudomonas vesicularis* (v Glu, r Mac), *Pseudomonas extorquens*, *Pseudomonas testosteroni* (v Mac), group IVe (v Mac), group IVc-2 (v Mac)
      Nonmotile: *Flavobacterium breve* (v Glu, v Mac), *Flavobacterium* sp. (v Mac), *Moraxella lacunata*, *Moraxella nonliquefaciens* (r Mac), Moraxella osloensis (v Mac), group M-5 (v Mac), group M-6, group IIf, group IIj

---

From Rubin and associates.[46]
w, weakly positive; r, 10% to 25% positive; v, 26% to 80% positive; Mac, growth on MacConkey agar; Ox, oxidase; Mot, motility; Glu, glucose oxidizer.

KEY TO THE IDENTIFICATION OF NONFERMENTING BACTERIA—cont'd

Glucose oxidizers
  MacConkey positive
    Oxidase negative
      Motile: *Pseudomonas maltophilia,* group Ve-1, group Ve-2, group IIK (r Mac, v Mot)
      Nonmotile: *Acinetobacter calcoaceticus* biotype anitratus, *Acinetobacter calcoaceticus* biotype haemolyticus
    Oxidase positive
      Motile: *Pseudomonas aeruginosa, Pseudomonas fluorescens, Pseudomonas putida, Pseudomonas pseudomallei, Pseudomonas cepacia, Pseudomonas pickettii,* group Va-1, group Va-2, *Pseudomonas stutzeri, Pseudomonas mendocina, Pseudomonas putrefaciens,* group IIk-2 (r Mac, v Mot), *Pseudomonas acidovorans* (v Glu), *Pseudomonas pseudoalcaligenes* (v Glu), *Pseudomonas vesicularis* (v Glu, r Mac), *Achromobacter* sp. (biotype Vd-1, biotype Vd-2), *Achromobacter xylosoxidans, Agrobacterium radiobacter* (group Vd-3)
      Nonmotile: Group IIk-2 (r Mac, v Mot), *Flavobacterium meningosepticum* (v Mac), *Flavobacterium breve* (v Glu, v Mac)
  MacConkey negative
    Oxidase positive
      Motile: *Pseudomonas paucimobilis* (r Mac), group IIk-2 (r Mac, v Mot), *Pseudomonas vesicularis* (v Glu, r Mac)
      Nonmotile: Group IIk-1 (r Mac, v Mot), *Flavobacterium* IIB, *Flavobacterium meningosepticum* (v Mac), *Flavobacterium breve* (v Glu, v Mac)

Glucose weak oxidizers
  MacConkey positive
    Oxidase positive
      Motile: *Achromobacter xylosoxidans*
    Oxidase negative
      Motile: *Pseudomonas maltophilia*

Questionable or weak fermenters
  MacConkey positive
    Oxidase positive
      Nonmotile: *Flavobacterium meningosepticum* (v Mac)
  MacConkey negative
    Oxidase positive
      Nonmotile: *Kingella kingae, Kingella denitrificans, Kingella indologenes, Flavobacterium meningosepticum* (v Mac)

TABLE 22-1

Media for initial grouping of glucose-nonfermenting gram-negative bacteria

Medium	Inoculation procedure	Characteristic determined
Heart infusion broth		Motility, Gram reaction; inoculum for other tests (one drop/tube)
Blood agar plate	Streak and stab; examine growth with a hand lens	Colonial morphology, odor, pigment, hemolytic action on blood, indophenol oxidase
MacConkey agar (Plate 83)	Streak	Growth/no growth
TSI/Kligler iron agar slant	Stab butt and streak entire slant	Hydrogen sulfide production, fermentation of glucose
O-F glucose, O-F maltose, and O-F lactose	Stab four times to about 1.3 cm below the surface	Oxidation of glucose, lactose, and maltose

From Rubin and colleagues.[46]

tion of the media in Table 22-1 permit initial grouping of isolates by following the key. Other characteristics can subsequently be determined as necessary to correctly determine the genus and species. In the clinical laboratory usually only five to seven additional tests are required for identification beyond those indicated in the key. Of course, reference laboratories may use a large battery of tests to cover all unusual organisms. Test systems similar to those used in the identification of the Enterobacteriaceae are available for identification of nonfermentative gram-negative bacilli.* None of these systems presently are adequate for identification of nonfermentative bacteria other than *P. aeruginosa* and *Acinetobacter*. However, they are quick and convenient and can be very helpful when a few supplemental tests are used with them. The utility of these kits is illustrated by the fact that Otto and Blachman[39] found that the API (Plate 84) and Oxi/Ferm (Plate 74) systems accurately identified nonfermentative bacilli constituting

*API, Plainview, N.Y.; Flow Laboratories, McLean, Va.; Baltimore Biological Laboratory, Cockeysville, Md.; and Roche Diagnostics, Nutley, N.J.

92% of the total number of such organisms isolated at their medical center. They found that the oxidative attack system (not commercially available) was 100% accurate. Similarly, Chester and Cleary[5] found that the Minitek system correctly identified all strains of *Acinetobacter anitratus, Pseudomonas maltophilia, Pseudomonas fluorescens,* and *Pseudomonas putida* and all but one strain of *P. aeruginosa*. Less commonly encountered nonfermentative organisms were misidentified with some frequency, and supplemental tests were required for complete identification of strains.

There are several different conventional methodologies in use. One cannot mix these but must adhere rigidly to a particular scheme. Otto and Pickett[40] have described a practical scheme employing modified substrate tablets that permit some growth in addition to detecting preformed enzymes. Incubation is at 30 C; almost all reactions are positive in 48 hours. The system should lend itself to automation.

Generally, the nonfermentative bacteria are gram-negative, nonsporulating, obligately aerobic bacilli that produce no change on TSI (or Kligler's iron) agar (occasionally an alkaline slant) and are indole (except the flavobacteria) and ornithine decarboxylase negative.

Oberhofer and associates[37] have described a medium for rapid detection of lysine and ornithine decarboxylase and arginine dihydrolase, which gave results in 4 to 24 hours and generally agreed with results on the Moeller medium, which often requires 3 to 7 days' incubation.

Pickett[42] provided important perspective regarding the incidence of nonfermentative gram-negative rods in clinical laboratory practice. Among 1,032 strains of aerobic or facultatively anaerobic gram-negative bacilli recovered from clinical specimens in the UCLA Clinical Laboratories in June 1976, 705 (68%) were enteric bacilli and 169 (16%) were nonfermenters. Among 486 strains of nonfermentative bacilli recovered from clinical specimens in a 7-month period in 1968, 322 (66%) were *P. aeruginosa*. Other *Pseudomonas* species and *Pseudomonas*-like organisms accounted for 77 strains (16%). *Acinetobacter* strains totaled 45 (9%); *Flavobacterium* strains, 22 (4%); *Moraxella* strains, 11 (2%); and *Alcaligenes* strains, 6 (1%). There were two isolates of *Bordetella bronchiseptica* (see Chapter 23).

Only those organisms of proved clinical significance will be discussed in detail; the interested reader is referred to authors already cited for further information.

GENUS PSEUDOMONAS
Pseudomonas aeruginosa

Pseudomonas aeruginosa is the most frequently implicated member of the genus in human infections; it may infect burn sites, wounds, the urinary tract, and the lower respiratory tract, particularly in patients whose defenses have been compromised. Infection also may result in a serious septicemia (Plate 78). Although *P. aeruginosa* may be isolated from the skin and feces of normal humans, most of the infections are exogenous in origin. Since the organism is part of the hospital environment—it can survive and even multiply in moist environ-

ments with minimal amounts of organic matter—it has been incriminated in from 5% to 15% of all hospital-acquired infections.[9]

P. aeruginosa is a polar, **monotrichous,** gram-negative rod occurring singly, in pairs, or in short chains. On blood agar the organism grows as a large, flat colony (Plate 79) with a ground-glass appearance and produces a zone of hemolysis. **Mucoid** strains are frequently isolated from the sputum of patients with cystic fibrosis. The colonies tend to spread and give off a characteristic **grapelike odor.** Most strains excrete pyocyanin and fluorescein (pyoverdin), giving the colony a characteristic **blue-green** color; approximately 4% are apyocyanogenic. Reyes and colleagues (J. Clin. Microbiol. 13:456-458, 1981) used Tech agar* to help identify *P. aeruginosa* rapidly.

P. aeruginosa is **oxidase positive** (rare strains are oxidase negative[23]) by Kovacs' method[30] (described in Chapter 44) and utilizes glucose **oxidatively** in O-F medium; gluconate is oxidized to ketogluconate† (but not by other pseudomonads). *P. aeruginosa* is lysine and ornithine decarboxylase negative and arginine dihydrolase positive. Most strains grow at 42 C on trypticase agar slants; they also grow on a selective agar medium containing cetyltrimethylamine bromide (Cetrimide).‡ Most other members of the genus are generally inhibited on the latter medium.

The characteristic grapelike odor of *P. aeruginosa* in culture and infected wounds is now known to be caused by 2-aminoacetophenone. Gas chromatographic, fluorometric, and colorimetric methods can be used to assay this compound in a variety of media.[6] Its synthesis occurs relatively early in the growth cycle, so that one

---

*BBL Microbiology Systems, Cockeysville, Md.
†Gluconate tablets, from Key Scientific Products Co., Los Angeles.
‡Available as Pseudosel agar, Baltimore Biological Laboratory, Cockeysville, Md.; Cetrimide agar, Difco Laboratories, Detroit.

TABLE 22-2

Some characteristics of species of *Pseudomonas*

Organism	Pyocyanin CHCl₃ soluble	Oxidase (Kovacs')	Growth at 42 C	NO₃ reduction	Growth on SS	Maltose oxidation	Lysine decarboxylase	Ornithine decarboxylase	Arginine dihydrolase
P. aeruginosa	+(−)	+	+	+*	+	−	−	−	+
P. fluorescens	−	+	−	−*	+	var	−	−	+
P. putida	−	+	−	−	+	var	−	−	+
P. cepacia	−	var	−	+/−	−	+	+	−(+)	−
P. stutzeri	−	+	+	+*	−(+)	+	−	−	−
P. maltophilia	−	−	+	−(+)	−	+	−(+)	−	−
P. pseudomallei	−	+	+	+*	−	+	−	−	+

+, positive reaction; −, negative reaction; ( ), occasional strain; var, variable.
*Some strains reduce NO₃ to gas.

TABLE 22-3

Minimal characters for identification of *Pseudomonas aeruginosa* strains

Character	Sign	% Positive
Polar monotrichous, fewer than three flagella per pole	+	96
Motility	+	96
O-F glucose medium open, acid	+	97
O-F maltose medium, acid	−	4
Indophenol oxidase	+	100
L-Lysine decarboxylase	−	0
L-Arginine dihydrolase	+	99
L-Ornithine decarboxylase	−	0
Hydrogen sulfide, black butt in Kligler iron agar	−	0
Growth at 42 C	+	100

From Hugh and Gilardi.[25]

can routinely detect it after 24 hours of incubation on blood agar plates.

Because *P. aeruginosa* grows on EMB or MacConkey agar as a non-lactose-fermenting organism, it is frequently selected and transferred to TSI (or Kligler's) agar as a suspicious colony from stool cultures and may be incorrectly identified because of the alkaline slant and butt reaction, which is characteristic for this organism. One other pseudomonad, *P. putrefaciens*, also can be misidentified as an enteric organism because it produces an appreciable amount of H₂S in these media.[49]

Some characteristics of various *Pseudomonas* species are given in Table 22-2. The minimal characters for identification of strains of *P. aeruginosa* are noted in Table 22-3.

An identification system that uses a standardized technique of bacteriophage typing has been recommended for tracing *Pseudomonas* strains during an epidemiologic investigation. In addition, a system of typing by pyocin production and a serologic typing system have been used as markers to trace the sources of infections caused by this organism.

TABLE 22-4

Minimal characters for identification of
Pseudomonas maltophilia strains

Character	Sign	% Positive
Polar tuft of three or more flagella	+	100
Motility	+	100
O-F glucose medium open, acid	+	100
O-F maltose medium, acid	+	100
O-F maltose medium sealed, acid	−	0
Deoxyribonuclease, extracellular	+	100

From Hugh and Gilardi.[25]

P. aeruginosa is resistant to kanamycin but susceptible to the aminoglycosides gentamicin, tobramycin, and amikacin, the drugs of choice in the treatment of serious *Pseudomonas* infections. Unfortunately, in several centers significant resistance to the first two agents listed has been noted. Many strains are also sensitive to carbenicillin and ticarcillin, semisynthetic penicillins that are recommended for therapy primarily as an adjunct to aminoglycosides in serious infections. Certain of the so-called third generation cephalosporins are active against *P. aeruginosa*.

Pseudomonas maltophilia

P. maltophilia is ubiquitous in nature. Like *P. aeruginosa*, it is being increasingly isolated from blood, CSF, other body fluids, sputum, urine, and abscesses. It is the second most commonly isolated *Pseudomonas*, the first being *P. aeruginosa*.

P. maltophilia is multitrichous, with tufts of two or more flagella per pole. It produces a yellow to tan pigment on trypticase soy agar and an ammonia odor. Colonies of *P. maltophilia* show a characteristic lavender-green color on blood agar. There is also a greenish discoloration around areas of confluent growth. On glucose O-F medium it produces an early (overnight) alkaline reaction, becoming weakly acid on fur-

ther incubation; on **maltose** O-F medium acidity is promptly produced oxidatively.

P. maltophilia is **oxidase negative** and ONPG and DNase positive; it does not reduce nitrate to nitrogen gas. It is lysine decarboxylase positive and arginine dihydrolase negative. Minimal characters for identification of *Pseudomonas maltophilia* are noted in Table 22-4. Most strains are susceptible to polymyxin and colistin, chloramphenicol, cotrimoxazole,[35] minocycline, and moxalactam. Varying results occur with other antimicrobial agents. Combinations of cotrimoxazole and carbenicillin, of the latter two compounds and rifampin, and of gentamicin, carbenicillin, and rifampin often show synergistic activity.[14,51]

Other opportunistic pseudomonads

P. fluorescens (Table 22-5) and *P. putida* (Table 22-6) are occasionally isolated from humans; sources have included respiratory tract and urinary tract infections, wounds, septic arthritis, bacteremia, and contaminated blood bank blood. They fail to grow at 42 C (25 C optimal). *P. fluorescens* will grow at refrigerator temperatures. *P. fluorescens* can be differentiated from *P. putida* by the former's ability to liquefy gelatin and produce lecithinase. Both produce fluorescein but not pyocyanin or pyorubrin. They are generally resistant to carbenicillin and sensitive to kanamycin,[41] gentamicin, piperacillin, cefoperazone, polymyxin, and often tetracycline.[33]

P. stutzeri (Table 22-7) is a polar, monotrichous, nonfluorescent pseudomonad that produces a buff to light brown, leathery, wrinkled colony resembling that of *P. pseudomallei*. Oxidative in glucose O-F medium, it reduces nitrate to nitrogen gas and grows in 6.5% NaCl broth, which aids in differentiating it from other pseudomonads. It is lysine and ornithine decarboxylase negative and arginine dihydrolase negative. It is usually susceptible to aminoglycosides, carbenicillin, ampicillin, tetracycline, cefoperazone, moxalactam, and cefotaxime.

TABLE 22-5

Minimal characters for identification of *Pseudomonas fluorescens* strains

Character	Sign	% Positive
Polar tuft of three or more flagella	+	99
Motility	+	99
OF glucose medium open, acid	+	100
OF maltose medium, acid	− or +	41
Indophenol oxidase	+	100
Pyocyanin	−	0
Pyoverdin	+	94
L-Arginine dihydrolase	+	99
Gelatin hydrolysis	+	100
Growth at 42° C	−	0

From Hugh and Gilardi.[25]

TABLE 22-6

Minimal characters for identification of *Pseudomonas putida* strains

Character	Sign	% Positive
Polar tuft of three or more flagella	+	100
Motility	+	100
OF glucose medium open, acid	+	100
OF maltose medium, acid	− or +	24
Indophenol oxidase	+	100
Pyocyanin	−	0
Pyoverdin	+ or −	79
L-Arginine dihydrolase	+	98
Gelatin hydrolysis	−	0
Growth at 42° C	−	0

From Hugh and Gilardi.[25]

TABLE 22-7

Minimal characters for identification of *Pseudomonas stutzeri* strains

Character	Sign	% Positive
Polar monotrichous, fewer than three flagella per pole	+	100
Motility	+	100
OF glucose medium open, acid	+	100
OF lactose medium, acid	−	0
OF maltose medium, acid	+	100
Indophenol oxidase	+	100
Nitrate to gas	+	100
L-Arginine dihydrolase	−	2

Adapted from Hugh and Gilardi.[25]

TABLE 22-8

Minimal characters for identification of *Pseudomonas cepacia* strains

Character	Sign	% Positive
Polar tuft of three or more flagella	+	99
Motility	+	99
O-F glucose medium open, acid	+	100
O-F lactose medium, acid	+	98
O-F maltose medium, acid	+	96
O-F mannitol medium, acid	+	100
Nitrate to gas	−	0
L-Lysine decarboxylase	+	90
L-Arginine dihydrolase	−	0

From Hugh and Gilardi.[25]

P. cepacia (Table 22-8) (synonyms: *P. multivorans, P. kingii,* EO-1) has occasionally been recovered from clinical material, including blood cultures, particularly as a nosocomial pathogen, in drug addicts, and in cystic fibrosis patients. It has been isolated from contaminated detergent solutions in urinary catheter kits as well as from hospital water supplies and has been implicated in several outbreaks of infections in hospitals. The organism is motile with a tuft of 3 to 8 polar flagella. Included in its characteristics are a variable oxidase reaction, lack of growth on Salmonella-Shigella agar, presence of lysine decarboxylase, and resistance to polymyxin and colistin. Chloramphenicol is the drug most consistently active against it, with two thirds of strains susceptible to kanamycin. Piperacillin and cefoperazone are quite active. Many strains are susceptible to trimethoprim alone and to cotrimoxazole.[35] *P. cepacia* produces a diffusible pigment that fluoresces violet under ultraviolet light. Many strains produce a nonfluorescent yellow pigment (particularly on TSI) that diffuses into the agar medium.

P. alcaligenes, P. putrefaciens, P. diminuta, P. vesicularis, P. acidovorans, P. testosteroni, and *P. paucimobilis* are rarely isolated but occasionally pathogenic pseudomonads. A description of these and related pseudomonads may be found in references 25 and 45. Two additional homogeneous groups of pseudomonads, tentatively called *Pseudomonas* species 1 and *Pseudomonas* species 2, have recently been recovered from clinical specimens.[36] Pseudomonas IIk-2 has been shown to be much more closely related to *Flavobacterium* and will be discussed with that organism. The first reported infection caused by *P. denitrificans* was a fatal case of bacteremia and meningitis (Fischer et al.: J. Clin. Microbiol. **13**:1004-1006, 1981); the organism was resistant to aminoglycosides and susceptible to cotrimoxazole.

Pseudomonas pickettii, previously identified as VA-2, has been isolated from such clinical specimens as blood, urine, wounds and abscesses, and spinal fluid. It is oxidase and catalase positive and urea positive, produces acid oxidatively from glucose but not mannitol, produces gas during nitrate reduction, and is arginine dihydrolase negative. It does not grow on Salmonella-Shigella or cetrimide agar. It is motile by means of one to two polar flagella. A related organism, VA-1, is rarely pathogenic.

CDC groups VE-1 and VE-2[17] have occasionally been isolated from clinical material, particularly wounds and abscesses. They are oxidase negative and catalase positive and produce yellow pigment. The ends of the cells are slightly tapered. Colonies may be smooth, wrinkled, or semirough on blood agar, and the medium is discolored green or lavender-green. The organisms are motile by means of either one polar flagellum or a tuft of more than three polar flagella. The slant of TSI (Kligler's) is alkalinized, and no H_2S is produced. The organisms are oxidative and produce acid from a number of sugars. The VE group has a unique pattern of antimicrobial agent susceptibility; they are sensitive to aminoglycosides (including kanamycin), carbenicillin, ampicillin, piperacillin, moxalactam, cefotaxime, polymyxin, and tetracycline and sometimes chloramphenicol and erythromycin.

Pseudomonas pseudomallei

P. pseudomallei is the causative agent of **melioidosis** in humans. This disease presents a varying clinical picture, ranging from unsuspected asymptomatic infection to acute, severe pneumonia or overwhelming and highly fatal septicemia. The organism has been isolated frequently from moist soil, market fruits and vegetables, and well and surface waters in southeast Asia and other tropical areas. Although apparently rare in natives, the disease was an important and sometimes fatal infection in the U.S. Armed Forces in Vietnam. The disease may be activated years after exposure to an endemic area.[32] A closely related organism was recovered from an infection in the United States.[34] *P. pseudomallei* is multitrichous, with a tuft of three or more flagella per pole and morphology similar to *P. aeruginosa,* but the colonies frequently are **wrinkled** (Plate 82) and on prolonged incubation become umbonate in character, particularly on blood agar. An oxidative acidity is produced in O-F media containing glucose, maltose, and cellobiose. The oxidase reaction is positive, and growth occurs at 42 C, but pyocyanin or fluorescent pigment is not produced. The organism is arginine dihydrolase positive and lysine decarboxylase negative (see Table 22-9).

TABLE 22-9

Characters for identification of *Pseudomonas pseudomallei* and *Pseudomonas mallei* strains

Character	P. pseudo-mallei Sign	P. pseudo-mallei % Positive	P. mallei Sign	P. mallei % Positive
Polar tuft of three or more flagella	+	100	−	0
Motility	+	100	−	0
O-F glucose medium open, acid	+	100	+	100
O-F cellobiose medium, acid	+	100	(+) or +	100
O-F maltose medium, acid	+	100	(+)	100
Citrate, Simmons	+	96	−	0
Nitrate to gas	+	100	−	0
L-Lysine decarboxylase	−	0	−	0
L-Arginine dihydrolase	+	100	+ or (+)	100
Growth at 42° C	+	100	−	0

From Hugh and Gilardi.[25]

These pseudomonads may be cultivated on most laboratory media, growing well on trypticase soy agar, blood agar, and MacConkey agar but not Salmonella-Shigella or cetrimide agar. A selective medium for isolating *P. pseudomallei* from contaminated clinical material has been described.[11]

P. pseudomallei is generally resistant to most antimicrobials, with chloramphenicol and tetracycline being the drugs of choice and kanamycin showing good activity. Cotrimoxazole also offers promise.[29]

Thomason and associates[48] have reported that identification of *P. pseudomallei* in mixed culture may be made by the fluorescent antibody technique.

Pseudomonas mallei

Formerly classified as *Actinobacillus mallei*, this organism is the causative agent of **glanders,** an infectious disease of horses that has occasionally been transmitted to humans by direct contact through trauma or inhalation. *P. mallei* is a **nonmotile,** coccoid- to rod-shaped organism, sometimes occurring in filaments or, under special conditions, with branching involution forms. Colonies on infusion agar (especially when glycerol is added) appear in 48 hours as grayish-white and translucent, later becoming yellowish and opaque. *P. mallei* oxidizes glucose, fails to grow at 42 C, and may be weakly oxidase positive. It is lysine decarboxylase negative. See Table 22-9 for biochemical reactions. Male guinea pigs injected intraperitoneally with culture material containing *P. mallei* develop a tender and swollen scrotum 2 to 4 days later (Straus test).

GENERA ALCALIGENES AND ACHROMOBACTER

In the eighth edition of *Bergey's Manual* the genus *Alcaligenes* is listed under genera of uncertain affiliation, and *Achromobacter* is not listed as a genus. These groups have long been poorly defined and, accordingly, are difficult to identify.

Alcaligenes is best defined as rods that are gram-negative, motile with **peritrichous flagella, oxidase positive, nonsaccharolytic,** and **urease negative.** Growth occurs on MacConkey agar but is inhibited on Salmonella-Shigella agar. The three most important species of *Alcaligenes* are *A. faecalis, A. odorans,* and *A. denitrificans.* The three species are basically inert in tests that are commonly employed and can be differentiated from each other by only a few characteristics. *A. faecalis* does not grow in

6.5% NaCl broth, and approximately half the strains reduce nitrate to nitrite. Nitrogen gas is not produced. *A. odorans* grows in the presence of 6.5% NaCl. It does not reduce nitrate but does reduce nitrite to nitrogen gas. *A. denitrificans* also grows in 6.5% NaCl broth but reduces nitrate and nitrite to nitrogen gas. *A. odorans* produces a pronounced dark green color on blood agar, whereas the other species vary from indeterminate lysis to greenish-brown. *A. odorans* produces a **sweet odor** similar to that of strawberries or peeled apples. The most frequent clinical sources of these organisms are the ear, urine, blood, spinal fluid, pleural fluid, wounds and abscesses, and feces. Susceptibility patterns vary considerably. With *A. faecalis*, the most active drugs are amikacin, tetracycline, and polymyxin. With *A. odorans*, polymyxin, carbenicillin, cefotaxime, and amikacin are most active. Tetracyline and carbenicillin are most active against *A. denitrificans*. Moxalactam is very active against strains of all three species, and cefoperazone is also quite active. Group IVe closely resembles *Alcaligenes*. It has been recovered only from the urinary tract and blood so far. Further description has been given by Rubin and co-workers.[46]

Achromobacter is also **peritrichously flagellated** and **oxidase positive** but **attacks carbohydrates oxidatively.** This genus is strictly **aerobic** and **fails to produce 3-ketolactonate.** There are two biotypes of *Achromobacter* species (CDC group Vd) and one additional species, *A. xylosoxidans*. All grow on MacConkey and Salmonella-Shigella agars, and *A. xylosoxidans* usually grows on cetrimide agar. *Achromobacter* species is urease positive (Christensen agar); *A. xylosoxidans* is not.

Achromobacter is most often isolated from blood, the ear, spinal fluid, urine, the respiratory tract, wounds, and feces. Only cotrimoxazole, piperacillin, cefoperazone, polymyxin, and carbenicillin show significant activity against this group, with chloramphenicol active against two thirds of strains.

GENUS ACINETOBACTER

There is a single species, *Acinetobacter calcoaceticus*. Four biotypes are recognized, based on hemolysis, growth on Salmonella-Shigella agar, production of gelatinase, and acid production from glucose. They are known as *anitratus*, *haemolyticus*, *alcaligenes*, and *lwoffii* (Plate 80). Biotype *anitratus* is the third most frequently isolated nonfermenter, after *P. aeruginosa* and *P. maltophilia*.[2]

These organisms are **oxidase-negative, catalase-positive, nonmotile** diplococcoid to coccobacillary forms that **do not reduce nitrate** (some may show activity). They grow well on MacConkey agar. Biotypes *anitratus* and *haemolyticus* produce acidity in the open tube of glucose, 10% lactose, and other carbohydrate O-F media. Biotypes *alcaligenes* and *lwoffii* are negative in glucose and lactose. Biotypes *anitratus* and *lwoffii* give strongly positive tests for catalase. All biotypes fail to demonstrate decarboxylase, dihydrolase, or deaminase; none grow on cetrimide agar. A characteristic reaction on Sellers medium (blue slant, yellow band, green butt) is produced by biotype *anitratus*, which readily differentiates it from other nonfermentative bacilli.

A. calcoaceticus is part of the indigenous flora of the skin and respiratory, gastrointestinal, and genitourinary tracts of humans and many animals and is found frequently in various sites in the hospital environment.

A. calcoaceticus has been recovered from a wide variety of clinical sources, including the central nervous system, the upper and lower respiratory tracts, urinary tract, wounds, nosocomial infections, and bacteremia secondary to intravenous catheterization. Its role has been primarily one of an opportunistic pathogen, generally occurring in mixed cultures from low-grade infections, although occasional cases of septicemia or pneumonia have been reported in debilitated hospital patients.[15] Many of the patients who develop infections with this organism have undergone various manipulations involving respiratory therapy equipment, endotracheal intubation, peritoneal dialysis, or bladder or central venous catheterization. Community-acquired pneumonia has also been reported. Biotype *anitratus* has been recovered from infection much more commonly than is true for biotype *lwoffii*. There is very little information about the other biotypes. For that matter, the majority of isolates of *A. calcoaceticus* are not clinically significant. In the review by Glew and others[18] only 58 of the 3,382 isolates of this organism in a 2-year-period represented clinically significant infection.

All biotypes are susceptible in vitro to the aminoglycosides as well as carbenicillin. Cotrimoxazole, colistin, and polymyxin B have variable activity. Biotype *lwoffii* appears to be susceptible to a wider variety of antimicrobial agents. Cefotaxime and ceftizoxime are very active in vitro (Appelbaum et al.: Lancet **2**:472, 1981).

GENUS MORAXELLA

Moraxellae are **nonmotile** bacilli or coccobacilli that are **oxidase positive** and **penicillin sensitive**; most strains grow on MacConkey agar and are **biochemically inactive** with respect to carbohydrate oxidation, denitrification, and the production of deaminase, decarboxylase, and dihydrolase. Some strains are fastidious, requiring enriched media or increased humidity for growth. Six species are generally recognized by medical microbiologists: *M. lacunata* (incorporates *M. liquefaciens*), *M. osloensis*, *M. nonliquefaciens*, *M. phenylpyruvica*, *M. atlantae*, and *M. urethralis*. *M. lacunata* (Morax-Axenfeld bacillus) was originally described as the etiologic agent in chronic conjunctivitis. It is infrequently isolated; characteristically, it causes **pitting**, or lacunae, on the surface of Loeffler slants, with subsequent digestion of the medium. Serum is required for its growth, preferably under increased CO_2. This species does not grow on MacConkey agar. Most isolates have been from infections of the eye or from the respiratory tract.

M. osloensis is easily confused with *N. gonorrhoeae* from genitourinary sources, since it is also **oxidase positive** and appears as gram-negative coccobacillary forms resembling gonococci. *M. osloensis* **does not ferment** CTA glucose medium and grows on nutrient agar, whereas *N. gonorrhoeae* ferments CTA glucose and does not grow on nutrient agar. *M. osloensis* may be isolated (rarely) from blood and spinal fluid, among other sources, and therefore may also be confused with the meningococcus; differentiation should not be difficult.

M. nonliquefaciens resembles *M. osloensis* but is somewhat more fastidious. Some strains are very mucoid. *M. nonliquefaciens* reduces nitrate to nitrite, but only about one fourth of *M. osloensis* strains do this. *M. nonliquefaciens* occurs more frequently in the respiratory tract than any other *Moraxella* species. This species has been isolated most often from respiratory tract infections, including pneumonia and lung abscess. Bacteremia has also been reported.

M. phenylpyruvica is characterized chiefly by hydrolysis of urea and deamination of phenylalanine or tryptophan. Major clinical sources of this species have been urine, blood, spinal fluid, and the urethra and vagina.

M. atlantae resembles *M. phenylpyruvica* but lacks urease and phenylalanine and tryptophan deaminase activities. The organism has been recovered primarily from blood and spinal fluid cultures.

M. urethralis resembles both *M. osloensis* and *M. phenylpyruvica*, but it reduces nitrites, possesses phenylalanine deaminase, utilizes citrate, and is urease negative. It has been recovered primarily from urine and from female genital samples.

Moraxella species are uniformly susceptible to penicillin, ampicillin, tetracycline, chloramphenicol, aminoglycosides, and erythromycin in vitro.[16]

Two additional groups of organisms named M-5 and M-6 are gram-negative, oxidase-positive, nonmotile rods resembling certain species of *Moraxella*. Most M-5 strains have been recovered from infections following dog bites, and M-6 isolates have been primarily from respiratory tract infections.

GENUS KINGELLA

The relatively new genus *Kingella* accommodates the organism originally known as *Moraxella kingii* and subsequently as *M. kingae;* this organism is thus *K. kingae*. The genus was created primarily because the organism in question differed strikingly from other moraxellae in several respects: production of acid from certain supplemented sugars (glucose and maltose especially) and lack of catalase activity, in particular. The organism is oxidase positive. Growth on blood agar spreads and corrodes the agar and produces beta hemolysis; there is a tendency to pellicle formation in fluid media. The cells show polar fimbriation and twitching motility. Poor growth is obtained on nonenriched media. The organism has been isolated from the blood, nose, throat, joints, and bone lesions. It is very sensitive to penicillin, streptomycin, chloramphenicol, tetracycline, and erythromycin.

There are two additional species in this genus: *K. indologenes* (isolated from eye infections) and *K. denitrificans* (isolated from bacterial endocarditis).[19,47]

GENUS FLAVOBACTERIUM

Members of the genus *Flavobacterium* (Plate 81) are gram-negative, nonmotile, proteolytic bacilli that can weakly ferment carbohydrates. Presently four species are recognized: *F. meningosepticum*, *F. odoratum*, *F. breve*, and another unnamed *Flavobacterium* called group IIb. Biochemical tests and other characteristics readily permit differentiation of these species.[46] They grow on MacConkey agar (usually) or blood agar, usually producing a **lavender-green** color

on the latter as a result of extensive proteolytic enzymatic activity. Although these organisms are fermentative, they are often inactive during the first 24 to 48 hours of incubation. If they are inoculated into sealed glucose O-F medium, acid production is slight and often delayed. If inoculated in a liquid peptone medium with carbohydrates, reactions may not be recognized for 14 to 21 days. For this reason the flavobacteria are best treated like oxidizers of carbohydrates, using unsealed O-F media for carbohydrate reactions.

Pigment production by *F. meningosepticum* can be either **beige** or a **light yellow.**[46] Group IIb, however, is markedly yellow to orange. TSI (or Kligler's) reaction is alkaline over alkaline or alkaline over neutral for both organisms. They are oxidase positive and catalase positive, and all form indole except *F. odoratum*. Strains of *F. meningosepticum* are mostly positive in gelatin; most IIb strains are also positive, but the reaction is delayed. On O-F media the reactions generally are as follows for *F. meningosepticum*: glucose, mannitol, and maltose positive and xylose, lactose, and sucrose negative. Except for glucose, the O-F reactions are all negative for the IIb organism. The O-F reactions are negative for *F. odoratum*, whereas glucose and maltose are mostly positive for *F. breve*. On Gram stain the flavobacteria are long, thin, gram-negative bacilli that usually appear with slightly swollen ends.

Flavobacterium is widely distributed in nature, particularly in water, soil, and any moist area. It does not readily colonize in adult patients with intact host defenses. In hospitals the organisms have been isolated from water fountains, faucets, sinks, water baths, air conditioners, humidifiers, ice machines, and so forth.[38] The organism grows best in a cool environment and does not remain viable at 35 C when stored for 5 to 7 days. Organisms isolated from patients during an outbreak of postoperative fever did not survive at 38 C.[38] However,

Flavobacterium will survive at O C. Group IIb flavobacteria are only rarely pathogenic in infants or adults.[46] *F. meningosepticum,* however, may cause a variety of nosocomial infections. Most important is the organism's ability to produce outbreaks of **neonatal meningitis.**[4,46] In these outbreaks many infants had positive nasal and throat cultures for this organism but remained healthy. In those who developed meningitis, mortality was in excess of 50%. Epidemiologic investigation failed to delineate a definite source or mode of transmission in the outbreaks. Only infrequently is *F. meningosepticum* pathogenic in adult patients. Sporadic cases of bacteremia, subacute bacterial endocarditis, pneumonia, and meningitis have been described. The mode of transmission in such sporadic infections is not well understood. There are six serotypes of *F. meningosepticum,* A through F, and although serotyping may be of assistance during epidemiologic investigations, it is not widely employed or available. No typing system exists for Group IIb. Very little is known about the disease-causing potential of *F. odoratum* and *F. breve. Flavobacterium* species are frequently resistant to many antimicrobial agents. Among the more active compounds are rifampin, minocycline, clindamycin, cefoxitin, and cotrimoxazole. It should be noted that disk diffusion susceptibility studies do not reliably predict antimicrobial susceptibility patterns of flavobacteria.[1] Accordingly, one should use a more direct measure of minimal inhibitory concentration. It appears that erythromycin is not really as active against flavobacteria as had been considered earlier.

There are additional organisms that are closely related to flavobacteria. Groups IIf and IIj resemble flavobacteria in their colonial, physiologic, and biochemical characteristics. These organisms include oxidase-positive, nonmotile, gram-negative rods that are nonsaccharolytic and fail to grow on MacConkey agar. Growth on blood agar media produces a green discoloration of erythrocytes. Colonies are usually pigmented, producing a diffusible tan or amber to brown pigment. Group IIf strains have been recovered from a variety of clinical specimens including spinal fluid, blood, urine, the female genital tract, the umbilical stump, and the ear. Group IIj strains have most often been from infections following bites or scratches by cats or dogs. In addition, they have been recovered from spinal fluid, blood, and sputum. Additional data on these organisms are presented by Rubin and associates.[46]

Group IIk-2 has previously been classified with *Pseudomonas,* but studies of chromosomal DNA, DNA-DNA hybridization and cellular fatty acid composition[7] indicate that it is much more closely related to *Flavobacterium.* Organisms of this group have been isolated from blood, spinal fluid, urine, wounds, and abscesses as well as environmental sources. These organisms are weakly pigmented (yellow); they hydrolyze urea and usually produce acid from starch. This group is now (Holmes et al.: Int. J. Syst. Bacteriol. **31:**21-34, 1981) a new species, *Flavobacterium multivorum.*[31] A recent report records spontaneous bacterial peritonitis caused by a group IIk-2 strain.[8] Group IIk-2 strains are typically resistant to aminoglycosides, most penicillins, cephalosporins, and erythromycin. They are sensitive to carbenicillin, moxalactam, cefotaxime, minocycline, clindamycin, and cotrimoxazole and are moderately sensitive to chloramphenicol.

GENUS EIKENELLA

Eikenella corrodens, originally known as *Bacteroides corrodens*[27] and clearly distinct from that obligately anaerobic organism, is a well-documented pathogen that is not at all uncommon. It has also been known as HB-1.[3,28] It is usually recovered in mixed culture, primarily along with aerobic gram-positive cocci. Many or most *Eikenella* infections originate from the oral cavity or the bowel. Sources of cultures positive for *E. corrodens,* include abscesses of the face and neck, pneumonia, lung abscess,[21] empy-

TABLE 22-10

Biochemical characteristics of *Eikenella corrodens* (595 cultures)

Test or substrate	Sign	Percent
Oxidase	+	100
Catalase	−	9 (w)*
Growth on		
MacConkey agar	−	0.8
SS agar	−	0
Cetrimide agar	−	0
Hydrogen sulfide		
TSI agar	−	0
Lead acetate papers	(+) or −	0 (64)†
Oxidation-fermentation	I	100
Urease	−	0
Indole	−	0
Methyl red/Voges-Proskauer	−	0
Citrate (Simmons), alkaline reaction	−	0
Motility	−	0
Gelatin	−	0
Glucose, xylose	−	0
Mannitol, lactose	−	0
Sucrose, maltose	−	0
Esculin	−	0
Nitrate to nitrite only	+	99.7
Pigment (pale yellow)	+	100

From Rubin and colleagues.[46]
+, 90% or more positive in 1 or 2 days; −, no reaction (90% or more); (+) or −, most strains positive after 3 days or longer but some cultures negative; I, inactive.
*Weakly positive reaction.
†Percentage of delayed reactions (3 days or longer).

ema, abdominal wounds, blood, spinal fluid, brain abscess, and bone. Infections with *Eikenella* are seen with high frequency in association with methylphenidate (Ritalin) abuse.

E. corrodens is a straight gram-negative rod that is **nonmotile** and **nonsaccharolytic, oxidase positive,** usually catalase negative, lysine and ornithine decarboxylase positive, and arginine dihydrolase negative and that reduces nitrate to nitrite only. Biochemical characteristics are shown in Table 22-10. Colonies are small to tiny and frequently are situated in shallow **craters in the agar.** Colonies of *Eikenella* produce a slight greening of the surrounding medium on prolonged incubation on blood agar. When observed under a stereoscopic microscope, three distinct zones of growth are evident: (1) a clear, moist, glistening central zone, (2) a highly refractile pearllike circle of growth resembling mercury droplets, and (3) an outer nonrefractile perimeter of spreading growth. A pale **yellow pigment** is produced. Optimal growth is obtained under increased CO_2 tension. Goldstein and associates (J. Clin. Microbiol. **13**:951-953, 1981) have shown that chocolate agar is the best medium for growth of *E. corrodens* in all atmospheres. An **odor** similar to hypochlorite bleach is produced. Growth in broth is usually granular, with the granules adhering to the side of the tube.

Disk susceptibility tests are not reliable, but the **resistance** of *E. corrodens* to clindamycin is so striking that the organism grows right to the disk margin (this may facilitate recovery of the organism from mixed culture). *Eikenella* organisms are susceptible to penicillin, ampicillin, carbenicillin, and tetracycline and usually chloramphenicol and colistin. They are resistant to methicillin and clindamycin, relatively resistant to aminoglycosides, and of variable susceptibility to cephalosporins. Cefoxitin and moxalactam are very active.[20,22]

GENUS AGROBACTERIUM

There are four species in the genus *Agrobacterium*. All are plant pathogens but one has been isolated on rare occasion from clinical specimens as well. That species is *Agrobacterium radiobacter*. It has been isolated from blood, urine, sputum and wounds, although the clinical significance of these isolates is uncertain. It has been isolated from endocarditis recently.[43] This organism can easily be confused with other oxidase-positive, nitrate-positive, motile glucose oxidizers. The key reaction that differentiates this organism is the production of 3-ketolactonate, which differentiates *Agrobacterium* from *Achromobacter*.

REFERENCES

1. Aber, R.C., Wennersten, C., and Moellering, R.C., Jr.: Antimicrobial susceptibility of flavobacteria, Antimicrob. Agents Chemother. **14**:483-487, 1978.

2. Blazevic, D.J.: Current taxonomy and identification of non-fermentative gram negative bacilli, Human Pathol. **7**:265-275, 1976.

3. Brooks, G.F., and White, A.: *Eikenella corrodens* comes of age, South. Med. J. **69**:533-534, 1976.

4. Cabrera, H.A., and Davis, G.H.: Epidemic meningitis of the newborn caused by flavobacteria. I. Epidemiology and bacteriology, Am. J. Dis. Child. **101**:289-295, 1961.

5. Chester, B., and Cleary, T.J.: Evaluation of the Minitek system for identification of nonfermentative and non-enteric fermentative gram-negative bacteria, J. Clin. Microbiol. **12**:509-516, 1980.

6. Cox, C.D., and Parker, J.: Use of 2-aminoacetophenone production in identification of *Pseudomonas aeruginosa*, J. Clin. Microbiol. **9**:479-484, 1979.

7. Dees, S.B., Moss, C.W., Weaver, R.E., and Hollis, D.: Cellular fatty acid composition of *Pseudomonas paucimobilis* and groups IIk-2, Ve-1, and Ve-2, J. Clin. Microbiol. **10**:206-209, 1979.

8. Dhawan, V.K., Rajashekaraiah, K.R., Metzger, W.I., Rice, T.W., and Kallick, C.A.: Spontaneous bacterial peritonitis due to a group IIk-2 strain, J. Clin. Microbiol. **11**:492-495, 1980.

9. Eickhoff, T.C.: Hospital infections, Disease-a-month, Chicago, September 1972, Year Book Medical Publishers, Inc.

10. Elliott, T.B., Gilardi, G., Hugh, R., and Weaver, R.E.: ASM Workshop on identification of glucose non-fermenting gram negative rods, Washington, D.C., 1975, American Society for Microbiology.

11. Farkas-Himsley, H.: Selection and rapid identification of *Pseudomonas pseudomallei* from other gram-negative bacteria, Am. J. Clin. Pathol. **49**:850-856, 1968.

12. Fass, R.J.: In vitro activity of cefoperazone against nonfermenters and *Aeromonas hydrophila*, Antimicrob. Agents Chemother. **18**:483-486, 1980.

13. Fass, R.J., and Barnishan, J.: In vitro susceptibilities of nonfermentative gram-negative bacilli other than *Pseudomonas aeruginosa* to 32 antimicrobial agents, Rev. Infect. Dis. **2**:841-853, 1980.

14. Felegie, T.P., Yu, V.L., Rumans, L.W., and Yee, R.B.: Susceptibility of *Pseudomonas maltophilia* to antimicrobial agents, singly and in combination, Antimicrob. Agents Chemother. **16**:833-837, 1979.

15. Gardner, P., Griffin, W.B., Swartz, M.N., and Kunz, L.J.: Nonfermentative gram-negative bacilli of nosocomial interest, Am. J. Med. **48**:735-749, 1970.

16. Gilardi, G.L.: Antimicrobial susceptibility as a diagnostic aid in the identification of nonfermenting gram-negative bacteria, Appl. Microbiol. **22**:821-823, 1971.

17. Gilardi, G.L., Hirschl, S., and Mandel, M.: Characteristics of yellow-pigmented nonfermentative bacilli (groups VE-1 and VE-2) encountered in clinical bacteriology, J. Clin. Microbiol. **1**:384-389, 1975.

18. Glew, R.H., Moellering, R.C., and Kunz, L.J.: Infections with *Acinetobacter calcoaceticus* (*Herrellea vaginicola*): clinical and laboratory studies, Medicine **56**:79-97, 1977.

19. Goldman, I.S., Ellner, P.D., Francke, E.L., Garvey, G.J., Neu, H.C., and Squilla, N.: Infective endocarditis due to *Kingella denitrificans*, Ann. Intern. Med. **93**:152-153, 1980.

20. Goldstein, E.J.C., Gombert, M.E., and Agyare, E.O.: Susceptibility of *Eikenella corrodens* to newer beta-lactam antibiotics, Antimicrob. Agents Chemother. **18**:832-833, 1980.

21. Goldstein, E.J.C., Kirby, B.D., and Finegold, S.M.: Isolation of *Eikenella corrodens* from pulmonary infections, Am. Rev. Respir. Dis. **119**:55-58, 1979.

22. Goldstein, E.J.C., Sutter, V.L., and Finegold, S.M.: Susceptibility of *Eikenella corrodens* to ten cephalosporins, Antimicrob. Agents Chemother. **14**:639-641, 1978.

23. Hampton, K.D., and Wasilauskas, B.L.: Isolation of oxidase-negative *Pseudomonas aeruginosa* from sputum culture, J. Clin. Microbiol. **9**:632-634, 1979.

24. Henriksen, S.D., and Bøvre, K.: Transfer of *Moraxella kingae* Henriksen and Bøvre to the genus *Kingella* gen. nov. in the family *Neisseriaceae*, Int. J. Syst. Bacteriol. **26**:447-450, 1976.

25. Hugh, R., and Gilardi, G.L.: *Pseudomonas*. In Lennette, E.H., Balows, A., Hausler, W.J., Jr., and Truant, J.P., editors: Manual of clinical microbiology, ed. 3, Washington, D.C., 1980, American Society for Microbiology.

26. Hugh, R., and Leifson, E.: The taxonomic significance of fermentative versus oxidative metabolism of carbohydrates by various gram-negative bacteria, J. Bacteriol. **66**:24-26, 1953.

27. Jackson, F.L., and Goodman, Y.E.: Transfer of the facultatively anaerobic organism *Bacteroides corrodens* Eiken to a new genus, *Eikenella*, Int. J. Syst. Bacteriol. **22**:73-77, 1972.

28. Jackson, F.L., Goodman, Y.E., Bel, F.R., Wong, P.C., and Whitehouse, R.L.S.: Taxonomic status of facultative and strictly anaerobic "corroding bacilli" that have been classified as *Bacteroides corrodens*, J. Med. Microbiol. **4**:171-184, 1971.

29. John, J.F., Jr.: Trimethoprim-sulfamethoxazole therapy of pulmonary melioidosis, Am. Rev. Respir. Dis. **114**:1021-1025, 1976.

30. Kovacs, N.: Identification of *Pseudomonas pyocyanea* by the oxidase reaction, Nature **178**:703, 1956.

31. Levine, M.G., Pickett, M.J., and Mandel, M.: Taxonomy of nonfermentative bacilli: the IIk-2 group, Current Microbiol. **4**:41-44, 1980.

32. Mackowiak, P.A., and Smith, J.W.: Septicemic melioidosis: occurrence following acute influenza A six years after exposure in Vietnam, J.A.M.A. **240**:764-766, 1978.

33. Martin, W.J., Maker, M.D., and Washington, J.A., II: Bacteriology and *in vitro* antimicrobial susceptibility of the *Pseudomonas fluorescens* group isolated from clinical specimens, Am. J. Clin. Pathol. **60**:831-835, 1973.

34. McCormick, J.B., Wenser, R.E., Hayes, P.S., Boyce, J.M., and Feldman, R.A.: Wound infection by an indigenous *Pseudomonas pseudomallei*-like organism isolated from the soil: case report and epidemiologic study, J. Infect. Dis. **135**:103-107, 1977.

35. Moody, M.R., and Young, V.M.: In vitro susceptibility of *Pseudomonas cepacia* and *Pseudomonas maltophilia* to trimethoprim and trimethoprim-sulfamethoxazole, Antimicrob. Agents Chemother. **7**:836-839, 1975.

36. Oberhofer, T.R.: Cultural and biochemical characteristics of clinical isolates of unusual colistin-resistant pseudomonads, J. Clin. Microbiol. **12**:156-160, 1980.

37. Oberhofer, T.R., Rowen, J.W., Higbee, J.W., and Johns, R.W.: Evaluation of the rapid decarboxylase test for the differentiation of nonfermentative bacteria, J. Clin. Microbiol. **3**:137-142, 1976.

38. Olsen, H.: *Flavobacterium meningosepticum* isolated from outside hospital surroundings and during routine examination of patient specimens, Acta Pathol. Microbiol. Scand. **75**:313-322, 1969.

39. Otto, L.A., and Blachman, U.: Nonfermentative bacilli: evaluation of three systems for identification, J. Clin. Microbiol. **10**:147-154, 1979.

40. Otto, L.A., and Pickett, M.J.: Rapid method for identification of gram-negative nonfermentative bacilli, J. Clin. Microbiol. **3**:566-575, 1976.

41. Pedersen, M.M., Marso, M.A., and Pickett, M.J.: Nonfermentative bacilli associated with man. III. Pathogenicity and antibiotic susceptibility, Am. J. Clin. Pathol. **54**:178-192, 1970.

42. Pickett, M.J.: Nonfermentative gram-negative bacilli, Current Concepts in Clinical Microbiology Course, UCLA Extension Division, August 1976, 10 pp.

43. Plotkin, G.R.: *Agrobacterium radiobacter* prosthetic valve endocarditis, Ann. Intern. Med. **93**:839-840, 1980.

44. Riley, P.S., Hollis, D.G., and Weaver, R.E.: Characterization and differentiation of 59 strains of *Moraxella urethralis* from clinical specimens, Appl. Microbiol. **28**:355-358, 1974.

45. Riley, P.S., Tatum, H.W., and Weaver, R.E.: *Pseudomonas putrefaciens* isolates from clinical specimens, Appl. Microbiol. **24**:798-800, 1972.

46. Rubin, S.J., Granato, P.A., and Wasilauskas, B.L.: Glucose-nonfermenting gram-negative bacteria. In Lennette, E.H., Balows, A., Hausler, W.J., Jr., and Truant, J.P., editors: Manual of clinical microbiology, ed. 3, Washington, D.C., 1980, American Society for Microbiology.

47. Snell, J.J.S., and Lapage, S.P.: Transfer of some saccharolytic *Moraxella* species to *Kingella* Henriksen and Bøvre 1976, with descriptions of *Kingella indologenes* sp. nov. and *Kingella denitrificans* sp. nov., Int. J. Syst. Bacteriol. **26**:451-458, 1976.

48. Thomason, B.M., Moody, M.D., and Goldman, M.: Staining bacterial smears with antibody. II. Rapid detection of varying numbers of *Malleomyces pseudomallei* in contaminated materials and infected animals, J. Bacteriol. **72**:362-367, 1956.

49. von Graevenitz, A., and Simon, G.: Potentially pathogenic, nonfermentative, H_2S-producing gram-negative rod (1 b), Appl. Microbiol. **19**:176, 1970.

50. Washington, J.A., II: Antimicrobial susceptibility of enterobacteriaceae and nonfermenting gram-negative bacilli, Mayo Clin. Proc. **44**:811-824, 1969.

51. Yu, V.L., Felegie, T.P., Yee, R.B., Pasculle, A.W., and Taylor, F.H.: Synergistic interaction in vitro with use of three antibiotics simultaneously against *Pseudomonas maltophilia*, J. Infect. Dis. **142**:602-607, 1980.

23 GRAM-NEGATIVE COCCOBACILLARY FACULTATIVE BACTERIA

Pasteurella

Francisella

Bordetella

Brucella

Haemophilus

The bacteria that constitute the genera discussed in this chapter are, for the most part, small gram-negative rods, occurring singly, in pairs, in short chains, and in other arrangements. Encapsulation may occur, and some may show bipolar staining. Others exhibit pleomorphism. The organisms are aerobic to facultatively anaerobic. CO_2 in excess of normal atmospheric concentration may favor the growth of some species, whereas serum or blood as culture medium enrichment enhances the growth of others. X and V factors (p. 273) are required for the cultivation of certain fastidious species.

Some species have the capacity to invade living tissue, gaining entrance through the mucous membranes or the skin. Several zoonotic species are transmissible to humans, producing diseases such as brucellosis, tularemia, respiratory illness and meningitis. Many species are obligate animal parasites.

GENUS PASTEURELLA

Organisms of the genus *Pasteurella* are oxidase positive and include *Pasteurella haemolytica*, *P. multocida*, *P. pneumotropica*, *P. ureae*, *P. aerogenes*, and *Pasteurella* new species 1. The commercial oxidase tests are not suitable for *Pasteurella*. One should use fresh aqueous 1% tetramethyl-*p*-phenylenediamine dihydrochloride (TPD) without alpha-naphthol.[14] There should be incubation at 37 C for 24 hours on 5% sheep blood agar. This eliminates problems of false-negative reactions with *Pasteurella* and false-positive oxidase reactions with other organisms. The organism formerly known as *P. tularensis* is currently the type species of the genus *Francisella*.[37] In the genus *Pasteurella* the only species of clinical significance are *P. multocida* (*P. septica*) and *Pasteurella* new species 1. The other species may be isolated from human infection on occasion, but either they are of little importance or their role in disease is uncertain.

Pasteurella multocida

Primarily an animal pathogen, *Pasteurella multocida* causes a form of hemorrhagic septicemia in lower animals and cholera in chickens. Humans become infected through a **bite** (Plate 89) or **scratch** from a cat or dog[18] or (rarely) another animal or through contact with a diseased carcass, as may be the case with abattoir workers and veterinarians. Pulmonary infections also may occur, particularly in patients suffering from bronchiectasis.[4] Other infections described with this organism include bacteremia, meningitis, brain abscess, epiglottitis, renal infection, septic arthritis, osteomyelitis, appendiceal abscess, peritonitis, puerperal sepsis, and liver abscess.[24] An outbreak of *P. multocida* infection involving seven patients on two adjacent wards has been reported.[20] All patients were debilitated, had underlying chronic neuromuscular or pulmonary disease, and had tracheostomies. The isolates of *P. multocida* were of the same biotype and serotype and had an identical antibiogram. Clinical specimens include sputum, pus, blood, spinal fluid, and tissues.

P. multocida is a small, coccoid, nonmotile, gram-negative rod often showing bipolar staining (Plate 90). It grows well at 35 C on chocolate agar or blood agar, where it produces small, nonhemolytic, translucent colonies with a characteristic musty odor. Several colony forms are recognized. Many strains isolated from the respiratory tract or chronic infections produce mucoid, relatively avirulent colonies. This form is highly pathogenic for animals, however.

TABLE 23-1

Characteristics of *Pasteurella multocida*

Property	Observation	Property	Observation
Colony forms	Several	Voges-Proskauer	−
Optimal growth temperature	35 to 37 C	Urease	−
Motility at 25 C	−	Nitrates	Reduced
Serotypes	16	Glucose	+
Catalase	+	Glycerol	−
Oxidase	+	Lactose	− or +
Coagulase	−	Melibiose	−
Fibrinolysin	−	Maltose	− or +
Hemolysis on blood agar	−	Mannitol	+ or −
Medium containing bile salts	No growth	Rhamnose	−
H$_2$S	+	Salicin	−
Indole	+	Sucrose	+
Methyl red	−		

Highly virulent strains for humans produce smooth, fluorescent colonies. Nonfluorescent, smooth, transitional forms are weakly virulent, and the R form, which is granular and dry, is avirulent. Colonies may be blue, iridescent, or punctiform. *P. multocida* is inhibited on bile-containing media, such as Salmonella-Shigella, XLD, or HE agar. The biochemical properties and other characteristics are shown in Table 23-1.

In identifying *Pasteurella* (chiefly *P. multocida*), the reliability of commercial test systems was 81% for Oxi-Ferm,* 68% for API,† and 11% for Minitek,‡ according to Oberhofer (J. Clin. Microbiol. **13**:566-571, 1981).

Serologically, *P. multocida* has been found to have 16 serotypes.[15] Animal pathogenicity tests and serologic tests with specific typing sera are of value. The organism is **very susceptible to penicillin** in vitro. The zone of inhibition around a two-unit disk (Plate 91) can frequently lead one to suspect its presence on routine culture plates streaked with sputum or bronchoscopic secretions. Tetracycline and chloramphenicol are also effective therapeutic agents, but erythromycin, clindamycin, and aminoglycosides have relatively poor activity in vitro.[42]

Pasteurella new species 1

Pasteurella new species 1 is acquired by contact with animals, primarily by dog or cat bites. Most of the infections are wounds of the extremities that have been bitten, but pulmonary infection, bacteremia, and endocarditis have been described.

The organism is unique among the pasteurellae in producing gas from glucose and other carbohydrates. A relatively small volume of gas is produced, so that it most often is not detected in the usual fermentation vial. The major characteristics of the organism are fermentation of glucose, positive oxidase reaction, no growth on MacConkey agar, reduction of nitrate, formation of indole, hydrolysis of urea (usually), and a negative ornithine decarboxylase reaction.

---

*Roche Diagnostics, Nutley, N.J.
†Analytab Products, Plainview, N.Y.
‡BBL Microbiology Systems, Cockeysville, Md.

GENUS FRANCISELLA
Francisella tularensis

Francisella tularensis is the etiologic agent of **tularemia,** a disease of rodents (particularly rabbits) that is directly transmissible to humans through the handling of infected animals or indirectly transmissible by bloodsucking insects (chiefly ticks and deerflies in the United States). Tularemia may also be spread by water and by the aerosol route. In culture *F. tularensis* is a minute, highly pleomorphic, nonmotile, gram-negative rod with capsules occurring in vivo. The characteristic bipolar staining may be seen on Gram stain or, preferably, Giemsa stain.

The organism reproduces by different methods, including budding,[16] binary fission, and the production of filaments. The organism exhibits a filterable phase, and in this respect it resembles members of the pleuropneumonia mycoplasmas. Clinical specimens include blood (first week), sputum, tissue, pleural fluid, and conjunctival scrapings.

F. tularensis requires enriched media, such as blood-cystine-glucose agar (see Chapter 42). Minute, transparent, droplike, mucoid, readily emulsifiable colonies are formed on this medium after 2 to 5 days of incubation at 35 C. Colonies may take as long as 10 to 14 days to develop. The organism may also grow on chocolate agar and other media, including selective media, used for cultivating *Neisseria gonorrhoeae*.[46] The organism is an obligate aerobe and grows optimally at 35 C. Glucose, maltose, and mannose are fermented without gas; other carbohydrates are attacked irregularly.

Further identification procedures include cellular fatty acid composition,[21] the testing for susceptibility to specific bacteriophages, **agglutination by specific antisera,** direct or indirect fluorescent antibody staining (the best technique for rapid specific diagnosis from exudates or tissue impressions), and demonstration of virulence by intraperitoneal inoculation of guinea pigs. The danger of handling infected animals and virulent cultures of *F. tularensis* cannot be overemphasized. Work should be done in a vented hood. Personnel should wear gloves. Aerosols must be avoided. **Many laboratory workers have become infected, and some have died of tularemia.** It is advised that specimens be sent to a laboratory equipped for handling *F. tularensis,* such as a reference laboratory or state health laboratory. Streptomycin is the drug of choice therapeutically, with tetracycline or chloramphenicol as alternative drugs. *F. tularensis* is also quite susceptible to gentamicin, and gentamicin has proved effective in mouse tularemia and in 10 persons with tularemia.[32]

GENUS BORDETELLA

The genus *Bordetella* consists of three species that are minute, gram-negative, motile or nonmotile coccobacilli. It may be difficult to see the bacterial cells unless the safranin is left on for 2 full minutes. Some require complex media for primary isolation, and all three species have been implicated in whooping cough, or an infection clinically resembling it, in humans.

Recent DNA hybridization studies (Kloos et al.: Int. J. Syst. Bacteriol **31**:173-176, 1981) indicate that the various so-called species of *Bordetella* may be more appropriately considered subspecies of a single species, although this was not formally proposed.

Bordetella pertussis

Bordetella pertussis, the type species, is the etiologic agent of **whooping cough,** or **pertussis.** For initial isolation, it requires Bordet-Gengou agar (potato-blood-glycerol agar; see Chapter 42). The addition of 0.25 to 0.5 unit of penicillin per milliliter is recommended for reducing overgrowth of gram-positive organisms. Small, smooth, convex colonies with a pearllike luster (resembling **mercury droplets**) develop on this medium in 3 to 4 days. The colonies are mucoid and tenacious and are surrounded by a zone of hemolysis. The organism is **nonmotile** and may

TABLE 23-2

Characteristics of clinical isolates of *Bordetella species*

Characteristic	*B. pertussis*	*B. parapertussis*	*B. bronchiseptica*
Involvement in respiratory infections	Moderately common, humans only	Rare, humans only	Frequent in animals, uncommon in humans
Recovery from wounds, abcesses, etc.	−	−	+
Visible growth on Bordet-Gengou agar	In 3 to 4 days, occasionally longer	In 1 to 2 days	In 1 to 1.5 days
Growth on blood agar on primary isolation	−	+	+
Growth on heart infusion agar	−	+	+
Brown soluble pigment on heart infusion–tyrosine agar	−	+	−
Motility	−	−	+ (peritrichous flagella)
Urease (Christensen), heavy inoculum	−	+ (24 hours)	+ (4 hours)
Nitrate → nitrite	−	−	+
Carbohydrate utilization	−	−	−
Litmus milk	Alkaline, 12 to 14 days	Alkaline, 1 to 4 days	Alkaline, 1 to 2 days
Specific heat-labile antigen (for genus and species)	1, 7	7, 14	7, 12
Other heat-labile antigens	2, 3, 4, 5, 6	8, 9, 10	8, 9, 10, 11, 13

From Parker and Linnemann.[36]

occur singly, in pairs, and occasionally in short chains. The cells tend to show bipolar staining and may be encapsulated.

Indole is not produced by the organism, and citrate is not utilized. Nitrates are not reduced, nor is urea hydrolyzed. X and V factors (p. 273) are not required; catalase is produced.

When isolated from patients with pertussis (a nasopharyngeal swab is the specimen of choice and should be plated immediately), the organism gives rise to smooth, encapsulated phase-I colonies on Bordet-Gengou medium. The other phases of the organism (II, III, and IV) may be determined by antigenic analysis. Identification of *B. pertussis* is further confirmed by a slide agglutination test with a specific antiserum.*

*Difco Laboratories, Detroit, Mich.

Immunofluorescent procedures are preferable for identification and can also be used for direct demonstration of organisms in respiratory secretions. Differentiation of the three *Bordetella* species is outlined in Table 23-2.[26] *B. pertussis* is susceptible in vitro to several drugs, notably erythromycin, chloramphenicol, and tetracycline,[13] but results of treatment are remarkably disappointing. Perhaps very early institution of therapy might make a difference.

Bordetella parapertussis

Occasionally isolated from patients with an acute respiratory tract infection resembling mild whooping cough, *Bordetella parapertussis* is morphologically and colonially similar to *B. pertussis*. *B. parapertussis* develops a large colony on Bordet-Gengou agar and produces a **brown** pigment in the underlying medium. It is **non-motile** and does not require X or V factor for growth. Indole is not produced, and carbohydrates are not fermented. The organism is normally urease and catalase positive and utilizes citrate.

Although it is serologically homogeneous, *B. parapertussis* shares common somatic antigens with *B. pertussis* and *B. bronchiseptica* and may cross-agglutinate with these organisms. An absorbed high titer antiserum is available for the serologic identification of *B. parapertussis* (see Chapter 37).

Bordetella bronchiseptica

Bordetella bronchiseptica has been isolated occasionally from patients with a pertussislike disease or wound infection. It differs from *B. pertussis* in that it is **motile** and possesses peritrichous flagella. The organism grows readily on blood agar, producing smooth, raised, glistening colonies with hemolytic zones. Indole is not produced, and none of the carbohydrates are fermented. Urease is positive within **4 hours,** catalase is formed, nitrates are often reduced, and citrate is utilized as a source of carbon. Cross-agglutination occurs with *B. pertussis* and *B. parapertussis*. Once thought to cause canine distemper, *B. bronchiseptica* is a common cause of bronchopneumonia in guinea pigs and rabbits; it may also occur in these animals as normal flora of the respiratory tract.

GENUS BRUCELLA

The genus *Brucella* consists of four main species of nonmotile, gram-negative, rod- to coccoid-shaped cells; they are pathogenic for humans and a variety of domestic animals.

The brucellae are **obligate parasites,** characterized by their intracellular existence, and are capable of invading all animal tissue, where they cause various brucelloses, including contagious abortion in goats, cows, and hogs, as well as undulant fever in humans.[41] The disease is presently uncommon in the United States; only 172 cases were reported in the United States in 1978.[6]

A definitive diagnosis of brucellosis is established by the isolation and identification of the organism from clinical specimens. **Blood** is the material most frequently found to be positive on culture, particularly when drawn during the febrile period of illness. Brucellae may be recovered occasionally from cultures of bone marrow, from biopsied lymph nodes and other tissue, and also from urine and CSF. The use of the modified Castañeda bottle (see Chapter 42) is strongly recommended for culturing blood from multiple specimens. Incubation of these cultures in a candle jar or CO_2 (3% to 10%) incubator is imperative, along with high humidity; cultures should be retained for a minimum of 21 days before being discarded as negative. Blood cultures, as a rule, are negative after the acute symptoms have subsided, which generally coincides with the development of humoral antibodies in the patient.

The agglutination test (see Chapter 38), which uses a standardized, heat-killed, smooth *Brucella* antigen, is the most reliable of the serologic tests. The standard agglutination test does not detect antibodies to *B. canis*, but there is a specific serologic test for this agent.[34] A recent study (Brown et al.: J. Clin. Microbiol. **13:**398-400, 1981) found that a microagglutination procedure was quicker and used less antigen than the standard tube agglutination test. A new serologic test for human brucellosis has been described. It is identical to the standard tube *Brucella* agglutination test, except for the addition of 2-mercaptoethanol (2ME).[7] This test is valuable in determining the effectiveness of antibiotic therapy. A 2ME titer of 1:80 or less is strong evidence against the diagnosis of chronic or persistent brucellosis. Dithiothreitol (DTT) may be substituted for 2ME (Klein and Behan: J. Clin. Microbiol. **14:**24-25, 1981); DTT does not have the offensive odor or irritant properties of 2ME. A rose bengal plate agglutination test and CIE have been used on spinal fluid to diag-

TABLE 23-3

Differential characteristics of four species of the genus *Brucella*

Species	CO_2 requirement (5%)	Urease activity	H_2S production	Growth* Thionine A	Growth* Thionine B	Growth* Thionine C	Growth* Basic fuchsin B	Growth* Basic fuchsin C
B. melitensis	−	V	− to +/− (throughout 4 days)	−	+	+	+	+
B. abortus	+	1 to 2 hours	+ (first 2 days only)	−	+	+†	+†	+†
B. suis	−	0 to 30 minutes	+ (throughout 4 days)	+	+	+	−†	−†
B. canis	−	0 to 30 minutes	−	+	+	+	−	−

V, variable.
*Dye concentration: A, 1:25,000; B, 1:50,000; C, 1:10⁵.
†There is some strain variation; these reactions are the most typical.

nose brucella meningitis.[11] An indirect fluorescent antibody test has been reported successful for detecting antibody in human sera.[5] The opsonocytophagic test is of doubtful value.

The four important species may be readily differentiated by their susceptibility to certain bacteriostatic dyes (Plate 92), by their reaction in carbohydrates, by their requirements for additional concentrations of CO_2 for primary isolation on laboratory media, and by H_2S production (Table 23-3).

Guinea pigs are susceptible to all species and develop an infection within 30 days after injection of primary smooth isolates.

Brucellae are aerobic and grow best at 35 C. *Brucella abortus* requires increased CO_2 tension (3% to 10%) on primary isolation, although many strains lose this requirement on subculture. The nutrition of these organisms is complex. Best growth is obtained primarily on enriched media, such as liver infusion tryptose,*

trypticase,* or Brucella† agar at pH 7 to 7.2 (pH 7.5 to 7.8 in 3% CO_2). After 24 to 48 hours' incubation, small, convex, smooth, translucent colonies appear, which become brownish with age.

The three major species reduce nitrates, with *B. abortus* and *B. suis* carrying the reduction to nitrogen gas. **Urea** is rapidly hydrolyzed by *B. suis* but slowly, if at all, by *B. melitensis* and *B. abortus*. All strains are catalase positive, with *B. suis* the most active. *B. suis* strains isolated in the United States are active producers of hydrogen sulfide (lead acetate paper), whereas the other species produce only small amounts or none. Brucellae do not liquefy gelatin or produce indole and are MR and VP negative.

Species of *Brucella* show a **differential sensitivity** to a number of aniline dyes, such as thionine, basic fuchsin, crystal violet, pyronin, azure

*Baltimore Biological Laboratory, Cockeysville, Md.
†Pfizer Laboratories, Flushing, N.Y.; Difco Laboratories, Detroit, Mich.; Baltimore Biological Laboratory, Cockeysville, Md.

*Difco Laboratories, Detroit, Mich.

A, and so forth. These may be incorporated in the agar medium in concentrations of 1:25,000 to 1:100,000, depending on the dye content of each lot of dye and on the medium used (Table 23-3). Inhibition of growth may also be determined by the use of dye tablets* similar to antibiotic disks. An inhibition zone of 4 mm or more in diameter around the disks is interpreted as susceptibility.

B. melitensis also can be differentiated from *B. abortus* and *B. suis* by the use of the agglutination test, using absorbed monospecific antisera. The latter two species, however, cannot be so differentiated, since they share an equal concentration of two identical antigens. Phage typing is also available.[38] Antigenically rough strains of *B. suis* that cannot be differentiated from *B. canis* by conventional procedures can be distinguished by gas-liquid chromatographic determination of cellular fatty acids (Dees et al.: J. Clin. Microbiol. **14**:111-112, 1981).

B. canis has occasionally been implicated in human disease, usually a relatively mild illness.[34] Persons exposed to infected dogs have a low risk of disease, but infection has been transmitted to humans from the dog. Routine *Brucella* agglutinin tests do not detect antibody to *B. canis;* special serologic studies are available through CDC.

Tetracycline for 3 weeks is effective therapy for brucellosis. Some workers feel that the addition of streptomycin is desirable. Cotrimoxazole appears to be very effective.

GENUS HAEMOPHILUS

Haemophilus species are small, nonmotile, gram-negative rods that require hemoglobin in the culture medium or are stimulated by its presence. Whole blood contains the following two factors that are necessary for the growth of the type species *H. influenzae:*

X factor—a **heat-stable** substance, hemin, associated with hemoglobin.

V factor—a **heat-labile** substance, which is coenzyme I, nicotinamide adenine dinucleotide (NAD), supplied by yeast, potato extract, and certain bacteria, in addition to that found in blood.

Table 23-4 shows the characteristics of the pathogenic species. Table 23-5 differentiates the biotypes.

Trypticase soy agar or brain-heart infusion agar plates used with commercially available filter paper strips or disks* containing factors X and V are convenient means for testing the requirements of *Haemophilus* for these factors. To prevent carryover of X factor, which may be present in trace amounts in blood agar, it is recommended that colonies be inoculated into nutrient broth.[44] After thorough mixing, this broth suspension is inoculated to a trypticase soy agar plate by streaking with a sterile cotton swab. However, there is probably no complex medium that otherwise satisfies all growth requirements of *Haemophilus* and that is totally free from X factor. Therefore, even when care is being exercised to avoid carrying over X factor with the inoculum, this method leads to an erroneous result in about 18% of cases.[27] Unless the identity is confirmed by biochemical tests, *H. influenzae* strains may be misidentified as *H. parainfluenzae* and vice versa. The porphyrin test provides a more accurate and rapid means of determining the X factor requirement. This test is based on the observation that hemin-independent *Haemophilus* strains excrete porphobilinogen and porphyrins when supplied with delta-aminolevulinic acid. Strains of *Haemophilus* that require X factor do not excrete these compounds. The test has been described in detail by Kilian.[27] One should place paper strips (or disks) containing X factor, V factor, and both X and V factors (not too close together) on the inoculated plate and incubate at 35 C under an atmosphere of 3% to 10% CO_2. The presence or absence of

---

*Medical Research Specialties, Loma Linda, Calif.

*Difco Laboratories, Detroit, Mich.; Baltimore Biological Laboratory, Cockeysville, Md.

TABLE 23-4

Principal differential characteristics of *Haemophilus* species

| Species | Factor requirement | | Hemoly-sis | Fermentation of | | | Catalase | CO$_2$ en-hances growth |
	X*	V		Glucose	Sucrose	Lactose		
H. influenzae (H ae-gyptius)	+	+	−	+	−	−	+	−
H. haemolyticus	+	+	+	+	−	−	+	−
H. ducreyi	+	−	−	−	−	−	−	−
H. parainfluenzae (H. parahaemolyticus + H. segnis)	−	+	d	+†	+†	−	d	d
H. paraphrophilus	−	+	−	+	+	+	−	+
H. aphrophilus	−	−	−	+	+	+	−	+

From Kilian.[27]
d, difference encountered.
*As determined by the porphyrin test.
†Strains of *H. segnis* show weak fermentation reactions.

TABLE 23-5

Key to the differentiation of the biotypes of *H. influenzae* and *H. parainfluenzae*, *H. aegyptius* and *H. segnis*

Species and biotype	Indole	Urease	Ornithine decarbox-ylase
H. influenzae			
Biotype I	+	+	+
Biotype II	+	+	−
Biotype III	−	+	−
Biotype IV	−	+	+
Biotype V	+	−	+
Biotype VI	+	−	−
H. aegyptius	−	+	−
H. parainfluenzae			
Biotype I	−	−	+
Biotype II	−	+	+
Biotype III	−	+	−
H. segnis	−	−	−

From Kilian.[27]

growth around each strip determines the species of *Haemophilus* (Table 23-4).

The hemolytic properties of members of the genus *Haemophilus* are readily determined by streaking a loopful of the broth suspension to a rabbit blood agar plate and incubating it overnight.

Although all members of the genus are parasitic in nature and require growth factors, they may or may not be pathogenic for humans. Some are members of the normal flora of the respiratory tract; others are important human pathogens, capable of causing severe respiratory tract disease, meningitis, pyogenic arthritis, subacute bacterial endocarditis, chancroid, and other types of infection.

Haemophilus influenzae

H. influenzae is found primarily in the respiratory tract of humans. It plays an important etiologic role in acute respiratory tract infections and conjunctivitis and may also cause septicemia, subacute bacterial endocarditis,[17] septic arthritis, urinary tract infection,[1] and purulent meningitis (Plate 24) in children. This form of meningitis occurs only rarely in adults.[33] *H. influenzae* also can produce a characteristic obstructive epiglottitis or laryngotracheal infection that may prove fatal in children 2 to 5 years of age.

H. influenzae is a fastidious organism, requiring an infusion medium containing X and V factors (Plate 94). Luxuriant growth occurs on **chocolate agar** (see Chapter 42). Growth on this medium appears in 18 to 24 hours as small (1 to 2 mm), colorless, transparent, moist colonies with a distinct "mousy" odor. On transparent media with Fildes enrichment colonies are translucent and bluish; on richer media, such as Levinthal transparent agar, the colonies may be larger. On sheep blood agar the organism grows poorly, if at all, producing only tiny colonies. Colonies are large and characteristic on blood agar, however, when they are growing **near** colonies of staphylococci (Plate 93), neisseriae, pneumococci, and other organisms capable of synthesizing V factor. This factor diffuses into the surrounding medium and stimulates growth of *H. influenzae* in the vicinity of such colonies. This phenomenon is known as "**satellitism.**"

All strains of *H. influenzae* reduce nitrates to nitrites and are soluble in sodium desoxycholate.* Indole is produced by the encapsulated organisms. Fermentation reactions are variable. Glucose and other carbohydrates are utilized by some strains but not by others. Six serologic types—**a, b, c, d, e,** and **f**—are recognized by the quellung† method or by the precipitin reaction. Most meningeal infections are caused by **type b,** but the majority of respiratory strains are

not type specific and are apparently less virulent. Virulent *H. influenzae* strains appear to be immunologically related to the pneumococcus; cross-reactions occur between the capsular substances of these two organisms. For example, type b cross-reacts with pneumococcus types 6 and 29.

The importance of biotyping of strains is emphasized in two studies that showed that the majority of strains from meningitis were *H. influenzae*, biotype I[28] and that strains from bacteremia were biotype I with a somewhat lesser incidence of biotype II.[2] Among antibiotic-resistant isolates almost all were *H. influenzae* biotype I or II[28]. Biotyping of *Haemophilus* species may be done effectively by the Minitek system[3] and by the Micro-ID system.

H. influenzae strains have a unique cellular fatty acid pattern as studied by gas chromatography.[22]

Various methods for serotyping *H. influenzae* were evaluated.[19] Included were slide agglutination, quellung reaction, CIE, latex agglutination, and antiserum agar tests. Cross-reaction problems encountered with latex agglutination and the expense of CIE and the antiserum agar tests made these methods less practical than the slide agglutination test for identifying single strains that were already isolated. The quellung reaction and slide agglutination were the most rapid tests for typing an organism. The coagglutination test can also be used; there is a commercially available reagent (Phadebact*). In identifying *H. influenzae* type b organisms from clinical specimens (195 strains), the coagglutination test gave 100% correlation with the slide agglutination test but was 100 to 200 times more sensitive (Grasso et al.: J. Clin. Microbiol. **13:**1122-1124, 1981). A very sensitive enzyme-linked immunosorbent assay for detection of *H. influenzae* type b antigen in clinical specimens has been developed.[12] This test is considerably simpler than radioimmunoassay, and based on pre-

---

*To 0.8 ml of a young broth culture, add 0.2 ml of a 10% solution of sodium desoxycholate. Incubate for 2 hours at 35 C. The tube should become clear except for a slight opalescence.

†Polyvalent and type-specific antisera are available from Difco Laboratories, Detroit, Mich., and Burroughs Wellcome Co., Research Triangle Park, N.C.

---

*Pharmacia Diagnostics, Piscataway, N.J.

liminary results in comparison with CIE it appeared to be more sensitive.

Recently, ampicillin resistance caused by beta-lactamase production has been a problem.[25] A simple iodometric spot test for detecting beta-lactamase activity in *H. influenzae* was found to be comparable to the capillary procedure.[30] An ampicillin-resistant strain of *H. influenzae* that did not produce beta-lactamase has also been reported.[31] Spurious ampicillin resistance may be noted because of an ampicillin antagonist in certain lots of Difco Supplement C.[45] Resistance to tetracycline and chloramphenicol is also seen occasionally. Cotrimoxazole is active against this organism clinically.

Haemophilus aegyptius (Koch-Weeks bacillus)

Haemophilus aegyptius is associated with the highly communicable form of conjunctivitis known as **pinkeye.** It has also been recovered from patients with pneumonia. Resembling *H. influenzae* morphologically, it also requires both X and V factors for its growth, and it produces small, transparent, nonhemolytic colonies on blood agar. Satellitism occurs with neighboring *Staphylococcus* colonies. On transparent agar the colonies show a bluish sheen with transmitted light. Indole is not produced, and the reaction in carbohydrates is inconsistent. Nitrates are reduced to nitrites, and the organism is bile soluble. *H. aegyptius* is serologically related to and possibly identical with *H. influenzae.* It has the same biochemical characteristics as biotype III.

Haemophilus haemolyticus

Haemophilus haemolyticus is found normally in human upper respiratory tracts. It requires both X and V factors for growth. Colonies on blood agar resemble *H. influenzae* but are surrounded by a wide zone of **beta hemolysis.**

In examining throat cultures on blood agar*

*Rabbit and horse blood do not contain inhibitory substances against *Haemophilus* species; human and especially sheep blood greatly inhibit the growth of these organisms.

plates it is important that colonies of *H. haemolyticus* be differentiated from those of beta-hemolytic streptococci, since both are small colonies surrounded by a zone of clear hemolysis. Colonies of *H. haemolyticus* are generally soft, pearly, and translucent, in contrast with the firm, white, opaque colonies of group A streptococci. Gram stain of the colony readily differentiates the two.

Haemophilus parainfluenzae

H. parainfluenzae is found in the normal respiratory tract of humans and is seldom associated with infections. Several reports, however, implicate *H. parainfluenzae* in respiratory tract infections, septic arthritis, and endocarditis. It requires **only the V factor** for growth. *H. parainfluenzae* grows slowly in blood cultures and often does not show visible turbidity. There is a tendency for the organisms to cluster at the interface between the blood and the medium, occasionally forming puff balls.[23] Unless blood cultures are subcultured to chocolate agar and these plates are held for longer than 48 hours, some isolates may fail to be recovered. *H. parainfluenzae* resembles *H. influenzae* both morphologically and colonially; it may be hemolytic, and it exhibits satellitism around staphylococcal colonies. "*H. parahaemolyticus*" is just a hemolytic variant of *H. parainfluenzae;* it resembles *H. haemolyticus,* although it produces somewhat larger colonies on blood agar. These are surrounded by a zone of beta hemolysis. Ampicillin resistance may be noted in *H. parainfluenzae* also.[39]

H. paraphrophilus, an organism that is readily confused with *H. parainfluenzae,* has been reported as a cause of endocarditis.[10]

Haemophilus ducreyi

Haemophilus ducreyi is the causative agent of an ulcerative venereal disease known as **chancroid** (soft chancre) in humans. (This is one of the classic five venereal diseases.) This small gram-negative rod occurs in long strands in smears obtained from the genital ulcer, where it

TABLE 23-6

Differential tests for *Haemophilus aphrophilus*, *H. paraphrophilus*, and some related species

Species	V factor required	Indole	Urease	Ornithine decarboxylase	Lysine decarboxylase	Fermentation			Nitrate reduction	Catalase
						Glucose	Sucrose	Lactose		
H. aphrophilus	−	−	−	−	−	+	+	+	+	−
H. paraphrophilus	+	−	−	−	−	+	+	+	+	−
Actinobacillus actinomycetemcomitans	−	−	−	−	−	+	−	−	+	+
Eikenella corrodens	−	−	−	+	+	−	−	−	+	−
Cardiobacterium hominis	−	+	−	−	−	+	+	−	−	−

From Kilian.[27]

is usually associated with other pyogenic bacteria. *H. ducreyi* is grown with considerable difficulty and grows best in fresh clotted rabbit, sheep, or human blood heated to 55 C for 15 minutes. Smears made after 1 to 2 days of incubation will show the tangled chains of *H. ducreyi*, if present. As noted in Chapter 11, recovery rates of *H. ducreyi* have been quite good using either rabbit blood agar or chocolate agar containing vancomycin.

Patients infected with this microorganism can develop a hypersensitivity reaction, which can be detected by the intradermal injection of heat-killed cells. Since the test is positive 1 to 2 weeks after infection, this can be useful as a diagnostic aid.

Beta-lactamase production is apparently very common now among strains of *H. ducreyi*.[40]

Haemophilus aphrophilus

Haemophilus aphrophilus is a small, gram-negative coccobacillus that does not require V factor and is variable in X factor requirement. Fastidious in its growth requirements, this organism appears to grow best in humid air with 10% CO_2.[43] Colonies on blood agar plates are similar in appearance to other species of *Haemophilus* that grow on this medium, except that colonies of *H. aphrophilus* tend to be more

opaque (Plate 95). Easily confused with *Actinobacillus actinomycetemcomitans*, differentiation can be readily obtained by the catalase test; *H. aphrophilus* does not produce catalase. Other biochemical tests of value include fermentation by *H. aphrophilus* of lactose, sucrose, and trehalose but not mannitol and xylose. Conversely, *A. actinomycetemcomitans* does not ferment lactose, sucrose, or trehalose but does utilize mannitol and xylose. Table 23-6 shows tests used to differentiate *H. aphrophilus*, *H. paraphrophilus*, and some related species.

Infections caused by *H. aphrophilus* are infrequent but are often very severe and can occur in adults and children. They include endocarditis, septicemia, brain abscess, and meningitis.[29,35,43,47] Specimens include blood, spinal fluid, pus, and sputum.[35,43]

REFERENCES

1. Albritton, W.L., Hammond, G.W., and Ronald, A.R.: Bacteremic *Haemophilus influenzae* genitourinary tract infections in adults, Arch. Intern. Med. **138**:1819-1821, 1978.
2. Albritton, W.L., Penner, S., Slaney, L., and Brunton, J.: Biochemical characteristics of *Haemophilus influenzae* in relationship to source of isolation and antibiotic resistance, J. Clin. Microbiol. **7**:519-523, 1978.
3. Back, A.E., and Oberhofer, T.R.: Use of the Minitek system for biotyping *Haemophilus* species, J. Clin. Microbiol. **7**:312-313, 1978.

4. Beyt, B.E., Jr., Sondag, J., Roosevelt, T.S., and Bruce, R.: Human pulmonary pasteurellosis, J.A.M.A. **242:**1647-1648, 1979.

5. Biegeleisen, J.Z., Jr., Bradshaw, B.R., and Moody, M.D.: Demonstration of *Brucella* antibodies in human serum: a comparison of the fluorescent antibody and agglutination techniques, J. Immunol. **88:**109-112, 1962.

6. Brucellosis, United States, 1978, Morbid. Mortal. Weekly Rep. **28:**437-438, 1979.

7. Buchanan, T.M., and Faber, L.C.: The 2ME brucella agglutination test: its usefulness for predicting recovery from brucellosis, J. Clin. Microbiol. **11:**691-693, 1980.

8. Criswell, B.S., Marston, J.H., Stenback, W.A., Black, S.H., and Gardner, H.L.: *Haemophilus vaginalis* 594: a gram-negative organism? Can. J. Microbiol. **17:**865-869, 1971.

9. Criswell, B.S., Stenback, W.A., Black, S.H., and Gardner, H.L.: Fine structure of *Haemophilus vaginalis*, J. Bacteriol. **109:**930-932, 1972.

10. DeSilva, M., Rubin, S.J., Lyons, R.W., Liss, J.P., and Rotatori, E.S.: *Haemophilus paraphrophilus* endocarditis in a prolapsed mitral valve, Am. J. Clin. Pathol. **66:**922-926, 1976.

11. Diaz, R., Maravi-Poma, E., Delgado, G., and Rivero, A.: Rose bengal plate agglutination and counterimmunoelectrophoresis tests on spinal fluid in the diagnosis of *Brucella* meningitis, J. Clin. Microbiol. **7:**236-237, 1978.

12. Drow, D.L., Maki, D.G., and Manning, D.D.: Indirect sandwich enzyme-linked immunosorbent assay for rapid detection of *Haemophilus influenzae* type b infection, J. Clin. Microbiol. **10:**442-450, 1979.

13. Field, L.H., and Parker, C.D.: Antibiotic susceptibility testing of *Bordetella pertussis*, Am. J. Clin. Pathol. **74:**312-316, 1980.

14. Gadberry, J.L., Clemmons, K., and Drumm, K.: Evaluation of methods to detect oxidase activity in the genus *Pasteurella*, J. Clin. Microbiol. **12:**220-225, 1980.

15. Heddleston, K.L., and Wessman, G.: Characteristics of *Pasteurella multocida* of human origin, J. Clin. Microbiol. **1:**377-383, 1975.

16. Hesselbrook, W., and Foshay, L.: The morphology of *Bacterium tularense*, J. Bacteriol. **49:**209-231, 1945.

17. Hirschmann, J.V., and Everett, E.D.: *Haemophilus influenzae* infections in adults: report of nine cases and a review of the literature, Medicine **58:**80-94, 1979.

18. Holloway, W.J., Scott, E.G., and Adams, Y.B.: *Pasteurella multocida* infection in man, Am. J. Clin. Pathol. **51:**705-708, 1969.

19. Ingram, D.L., Collier, A.M., Pendergrass, E., and King, S.H.: Methods for serotyping nasopharyngeal isolates of *Haemophilus influenzae:* slide agglutination, quellung reaction, countercurrent immunoelectrophoresis, latex agglutination, and antiserum agar, J. Clin. Microbiol. **9:**570-574, 1979.

20. Itoh, M., Tierno, P.M., Milstoc, M., and Berger, A.R.: A unique outbreak of *Pasteurella multocida* in a chronic disease hospital, Am. J. Public Health **70:**1170-1173, 1980.

21. Jantzen, E., Berdal, B.P., and Omland, T.: Cellular fatty acid composition of *Francisella tularensis*, J. Clin. Microbiol. **10:**928-930, 1979.

22. Jantzen, E., Berdal, B.P., and Omland, T.: Cellular fatty acid composition of *Haemophilus* species, *Pasteurella multocida*, *Actinobacillus actinomycetemcomitans*, and *Haemophilus vaginalis* (*Corynebacterium vaginale*), Acta Pathol. Microbiol. Scand. **88**(B):89-93, 1980.

23. Jemsek, J.G., Greenberg, S.M., Gentry, L.O., Welton, D.E., and Mattox, K.L.: Haemophilus parainfluenzae endocarditis, Am. J. Med. **66:**51-56, 1979.

24. Johnson, R.H., and Rumans, L.W.: Unusual infections caused by *Pasteurella multocida*, J.A.M.A. **237:**146-147, 1977.

25. Kammer, R.B., Preston, D.A., Turner, J.R., and Hawley, L.C.: Rapid detection of ampicillin-resistant *Haemophilus influenzae* and their susceptibility to sixteen antibiotics, Antimicrobiol. Agents Chemother. **8:**91-94, 1975.

26. Kendrick, P.L., Eldering, G., and Eveland, W.C.: Application of fluorescent antibody techniques: methods for the identification of *Bordetella pertussis*, Am. J. Dis. Child. **101:**149-154, 1961.

27. Kilian, M.: *Haemophilus*. In Lennette, E.H., Balows, A., Hausler, W.J., Jr., and Truant, J.P., editors: Manual of clinical microbiology, ed. 3, Washington, D.C., 1980, American Society for Microbiology.

28. Kilian, M., Sørensen, I., and Frederiksen, W.: Biochemical characteristics of 130 recent isolates from *Haemophilus influenzae* meningitis, J. Clin. Microbiol. **9:**409-412, 1979.

29. King, E.O., and Tatum, H.W.: *Actinobacillus actinomycetemcomitans* and *Hemophilus aphrophilus*, J. Infect. Dis. **111:**85-94, 1962.

30. Lee, W-S., and Komarmy, L.: Iodometric spot test for detection of beta-lactamase in *Haemophilus influenzae*, J. Clin. Microbiol. **13:**224-225, 1981.

31. Markowitz, S.M.: Isolation of an ampicillin-resistant, non−β-lactamase-producing strain of *Haemophilus influenzae*, Antimicrob. Agents Chemother. **17:**80-83, 1980.

32. Mason, W.L., Eigelsbach, H.T., Little, S.F., and Bates, J.H.: Treatment of tularemia, including pulmonary tularemia, with gentamicin, Am. Rev. Respir. Dis. **121:**39-45, 1980.

33. Merselis, J.G., Sellers, T.F., Jr., Johnson, J.E., and Hook, E.W.: *Hemophilus influenzae* meningitis in adults, Arch. Intern. Med. **110:**837-846, 1962.

34. Munford, R.S., Weaver, R.E., Patton, C., Feeley, J.C., and Feldman, R.A.: Human disease caused by *Brucella canis*, J.A.M.A. **231:**1267-1269, 1975.

35. Page, M.I., and King, E.O.: Infection due to *Actinobacillus actinomycetemcomitans* and *Haemophilus aphrophilus*, N. Engl. J. Med. **275:**181-188, 1966.

36. Parker, C.D., and Linnemann, C.C., Jr.: *Bordetella*. In Lennette, E.H., Balows, A., Hausler, W.J., Jr., and Truant, J.P., editors: Manual of clinical microbiology, ed. 3, Washington, D.C., 1980, American Society for Microbiology.

37. Philip, C.B., and Owen, C.R.: Comments on the nomenclature of the causative agent of tularemia, Int. Bull. Bact. Nomencl. Taxon. **11:**67-72, 1961.

38. Renner, E.D., and Hausler, W.J., Jr.: *Brucella*. In Lennette, E.H., Balows, A., Hausler, W.J., Jr., and Truant, J.P., editors: Manual of clinical microbiology, ed. 3, Washington, D.C., 1980, American Society for Microbiology.

39. Smith, P.W., Chambers, W.A., and Walker, C.A.: Ampicillin resistant *Haemophilus parainfluenzae* endocarditis, Am. J. Med. Sci. **278:**173-176, 1979.

40. Sottnek, F.O., Biddle, J.W., Kraus, S.J., Weaver, R.E., and Stewart, J.A.: Isolation and identification of *Haemophilus ducreyi* in a clinical study, J. Clin. Microbiol. **12:**170-174, 1980.

41. Spink, W.W.: The nature of brucellosis, Minneapolis, 1956, University of Minnesota Press.

42. Stevens, D.L., Higbee, J.W., Oberhofer, T.R., and Everett, E.D.: Antibiotic susceptibilities of human isolates of *Pasteurella multocida*, Antimicrob. Agents Chemother. **16:**322-324, 1979.

43. Sutter, V.L., and Finegold, S.M.: *Haemophilus aphrophilus* infections: clinical and bacteriologic studies, Ann. N.Y. Acad. Sci. **174:**468-487, 1970.

44. Washington, J.A., II, editor: Laboratory procedures in clinical microbiology, Boston, 1974, Little, Brown and Co.

45. Washington, J.A., II, Snyder, R.J., and Kohner, P.C.: Spurious ampicillin resistance by testing *Haemophilus influenzae* with agar containing Supplement C, Antimicrob. Agents Chemother. **9:**199-200, 1976.

46. Weaver, R.E., and Hollis, D.G.: Gram-negative fermentative bacteria and *Francisella tularensis*. In Lennette, E.H., Balows, A., Hausler, W.J., Jr., and Truant, J.P., editors: Manual of clinical microbiology, ed. 3, Washington, D.C., 1980, American Society for Microbiology.

47. Witorsch, P., and Gorden P.: *Hemophilus aphrophilus* meningitis, Ann. Intern. Med. **60:**957-961, 1964.

24 SPIROCHETES AND CURVED RODS

Campylobacter

Spirillum

Borrelia

Treponema

Leptospira

Most of the curved bacteria encountered as pathogens in humans belong to two families, the Spirillaceae and the Spirochaetaceae.

Members of the Spirillaceae are rigid, **helically curved** rods with from less than one turn to many turns. They are motile with a corkscrew motion, by means of **polar flagella.** Pathogenic forms stain readily with aniline dyes (they are gram negative) and Giemsa or Wright stain. The two genera in this family are *Campylobacter* and *Spirillum*.

The Spirochaetaceae are **helically coiled** organisms. They consist of a protoplasmic cylinder intertwined with one or more **axial fibrils;** both of these are enclosed by an outer envelope. Although gram negative, only *Borrelia* stains well with aniline dyes; Giemsa or silver impregnation is best for staining. The three genera containing organisms pathogenic for humans are *Borrelia, Treponema,* and *Leptospira*.

GENUS CAMPYLOBACTER

One species, *Campylobacter fetus* (*Vibrio fetus*), contains organisms pathogenic for humans: two of the three subspecies, *C. fetus* ss. *intestinalis* and ss. *jejuni* (the latter had been called "related vibrio" by King).[15]

The manifestations of *Campylobacter* infection in humans are variable and include fever alone (which may be relapsing), thrombophlebitis, bacteremia, endocarditis, septic or reactive arthritis, meningoencephalitis (sometimes chronic and indolent and sometimes fulminant and lethal), pericarditis, pleuropulmonary infection, peritonitis, cholecystitis, diarrhea, fever, and septic abortion. Many patients have underlying disease, such as malignancy. Bacteremia and metastatic infection are uncommon in infections caused by ss. *jejuni*. The vast majority of the more serious infections are caused by ss. *intestinalis*. *C. fetus* ss. *jejuni* may be found occasionally in humans (in the intestinal tract) in the absence of disease; this has not been true for ss. *intestinalis*.

The organism is not uncommon in infections in cattle, sheep, and goats and may be found in poultry. There is evidence that both food and water are important vehicles of infection. One large waterborne outbreak in Vermont involved some 2,000 people in a township of 10,000.[25] Transmission to humans from infected puppies has been documented, and infected kittens and pet birds may be implicated.[4] Children with diarrhea have been implicated as the source of spread of infection, both within and outside affected households.[4,21] As with other enteric pathogens, proctitis caused by *Campylobacter* has been spread among homosexuals.

It is now clear that *Campylobacter* is a major cause of diarrhea in adults and children. Reports from a number of institutions throughout the world indicate that *C. fetus* ss. *jejuni* may be involved as a cause of diarrhea at least as frequently as are *Salmonella* and *Shigella*.[5,6,13,21] It has been isolated in from 3% to 11% of patients with diarrhea in various studies. Patients may have grossly bloody stools, and often stools contain large numbers of leukocytes. Patients may have severe abdominal pain.[5,21] The disease tends to be self limited; however, many patients do require treatment, and relapse may occur following treatment. On occasion the diarrhea may persist for longer than 2 weeks.

Information on transport of specimens and techniques for culture and isolation was presented in Chapter 9. A special Bio-Bag (type Cfj)* with a microaerophilic atmosphere generator is now available. This permits inspection of the plates at frequent intervals in the case of a seri-

---

*Marion Scientific Corp., Kansas City, Mo.

ously ill patient. Plates should be examined at 24 and 48 hours. The colonies of *C. fetus* ss. *jejuni* are nonhemolytic and can be flat and gray with an irregular edge or raised and round with a mucoid appearance.[13] Colonies are 1 to 2 mm in diameter and occasionally spread along the streak on the plate. Occasional strains may appear tan or slightly pink. Plates should be examined quickly and returned to the appropriate atmosphere to ensure viability for the more oxygen-sensitive strains.

Presumptive identification is based on the typical morphology of curved, S-shaped, or long spiral forms (Plate 96) and motility preparations showing the characteristic darting motility as well as positive oxidase and catalase reactions. Biochemical confirmation can be made by following the tests outlined in Table 24-1. Inability to grow at 25 C, sensitivity to a 30-μg nalidixic acid disk, and the detection of H_2S in an iron-containing medium only with the use of lead acetate strips are particularly useful indicators. *C. fetus* ss. *jejuni* can be rapidly differentiated from other *C. fetus* species by gas-liquid chromatography analysis of cellular fatty acids.[7]

The organism is an **obligate microaerophile,** growing under reduced oxygen tension but not aerobically or anaerobically. It is motile with a **single polar flagellum** at one or both ends of the cell. It is **nonfermentative** and reduces nitrate to nitrite. *C. fetus* ss. *jejuni* stains poorly with safranin as the counterstain in the Gram stain. Substituting 0.06% carbol fuchsin for safranin is much more effective.[24]

Significant antibody responses have been demonstrated by agglutination, complement fixation, serum bactericidal assay, indirect immunofluorescence, indirect hemagglutination, latex agglutination, and a rapid agglutination test.[13] These techniques are definitely useful in the course of an outbreak. Whether they can be depended upon for diagnosis of sporadic cases that are culture-negative remains to be determined.

C. fetus ss. *jejuni* is relatively susceptible to

TABLE 24-1

Differentiation of *Campylobacter* species

Test	*C. fetus* ss. *intestinalis*	*C. fetus* ss. *jejuni*
Oxidase	+	+
Catalase	+	+
Motility	+	+
H_2S lead acetate strips	+	+
H_2S in iron-containing media	−	−
Nalidixic acid (30-μg disk)	R	S
Cephalothin (30-μg disk)	S	R
Red growth in TTC medium	−	+
Growth at 25 C	+	−
Growth at 42 C	−+	+
Hippurate hydrolysis[12] (2 hour rapid test)	−	+−

TTC, 0.04% 2,3,5-triphenyltetrazolium chloride; R, resistant; S, sensitive.

antimicrobial agents. Representative minimal inhibitory concentrations are chloramphenicol, 4 μg/ml; tetracycline, 1 μg/ml; gentamicin, less than 1 μg/ml; streptomycin, 2 to 4 μg/ml, and erythromycin, 2 to 8 μg/ml. However, in one report 8% of strains were totally resistant to erythromycin,[23] and in another a similar percentage of strains were resistant to tetracycline.[22] Furazolidone and clindamycin have good activity.[22] The subspecies is resistant to penicillin, most cephalosporins, bacitracin, polymyxin, trimethoprim, and novobiocin. There is less information available on susceptibility patterns of *C. fetus* ss. *intestinalis*. It appears that tetracycline, erythromycin, gentamicin, chloramphenicol, and cephaloridine[14] are active.

In a recent report Spelhaug and associates (J. Infect. Dis. **143:**500, 1981) studied four strains of *C. fetus* ss. *intestinalis* and found all very sensitive to thienamycin, gentamicin, streptomycin, ampicillin, and moxalactam. Cefotaxime and cephalothin showed moderate activity, and cefoperazone was inactive.

SPIRILLUM MINOR

Spirillum minor (minus), already discussed in Chapter 7 on blood cultures, is one of the causes of **rat-bite fever** (sodoku), a disease characterized by an initially inflamed (occasionally ulcerating) wound associated with lymphadenopathy and an erythematous rash. The disease may also follow the bite of a mouse or a rodent-ingesting animal.[18] The organism may be visualized by darkfield examination of the blood or of material from the bite wound or affected lymph node. Blood films also should be stained by the Wright or Giemsa technique and examined microscopically. The organism has not been cultivated to date.

When the microscopic examination is unrevealing, one must resort to animal inoculation, using at least several mice and a guinea pig. Before laboratory animals are inoculated, their blood should be examined for naturally occurring organisms resembling *S. minor*. An equivalent number of control animals should be injected with a blood specimen previously heated to 52 C for 1 hour. These are injected intraperitoneally with 1 to 2 ml of the patient's blood, and the peritoneal fluid (mice) or defibrinated blood (guinea pig) is examined by darkfield microscopy or by Giemsa or Wright stain weekly for 4 weeks for the presence of short, thick (1.7 to 5 μm by 0.5 μm), actively motile spiral forms of two to three (up to six) spirals and **bipolar polytrichous tufts of flagella.** When organisms are scarce or not demonstrable in peritoneal fluid or blood of animals that have been inoculated with specimens from the patient, impression films of the heart muscle of these animals often reveal numerous organisms.[18] The heart of the animal is sliced in half, and a clean glass slide is passed with pressure across the cut surface. These are stained after fixation with a dilute Giemsa stain consisting of 1 drop of Giemsa spirochete stain added to 1 ml of distilled water.

One may also demonstrate organisms by silver impregnation stains of tissue sections of heart from the animals or by use of a Thedan blue solution T-5* stain of impression smears of crushed heart tissue.[18] Patients may manifest a false-positive complement fixation test for syphilis. Penicillin and streptomycin, and probably tetracycline, are effective therapeutically.

GENUS BORRELIA

These spirochetes normally are parasitic for several species of arthropods, including body lice and ticks; human beings or other animals acquire infection (**relapsing fever**) by the bite of the infected vector. *Borrelia recurrentis* is the only species transmitted by lice; this species is presently confined primarily to eastern Africa. There are nine species of *Borrelia* transmitted by ticks (various species of *Ornithodoros*); the principal species found in the United States are *B. hermsii*, *B. parkeri*, and *B. turicatae*.[8,10] The tick bite is usually painless, and the tick drops off the host after 30 to 60 minutes, so the subject may not be aware of tick contact.

Borreliae are best demonstrated in the blood of an infected individual early in the course of a febrile period by direct examination of stained blood films. Thick films should always be examined routinely, since the number of spirochetes in the blood may be few. A microhematocrit concentration technique has been described for detecting spirochetes in the blood of individuals who are mildly infected.[8] When this is inconclusive, a similar specimen of blood is inoculated intraperitoneally into suckling Swiss mice or rats, and the animals are examined daily for at least 14 days for *Borrelia* organisms in films of tail blood. The organisms are 10 to 20 μm long, with five to seven open spirals, and are actively motile in a corkscrew fashion; they stain relatively well with Giemsa or Wright stain, particularly with prolonged staining. Counterstaining of blood films, stained in the above manner,

---

*Allied Chemical Co., New York, N.Y.

with 1% crystal violet for 30 seconds, is effective. **Direct darkfield examination** of blood is recommended. A drop of blood is placed on a slide, a coverslip is placed over it, and the edges of the coverslip are sealed with lanolin. Under $400\times$ to $500\times$ magnification (high dry) movement of erythrocytes (occasioned by the movement of the spirochetes) is readily noted, and the organisms themselves may then be detected. They exhibit forward and backward motion, with bending and looping. One may also diagnose *Borrelia* infection by serologic techniques. The two tests most used are the borreliolysin and the *Borrelia* immobilization test.[8] Promising results have also been obtained with indirect immunofluorescence and the indirect immunoenzyme tests. The organism may also be cultured.[10]

The drug of choice in therapy is tetracycline. Erythromycin is also effective.

GENUS TREPONEMA

There are numerous species in the genus *Treponema*, and they comprise two major groups: the several pathogenic species and those normally present in the mouth, urogenital tract, and gastrointestinal tract of humans and other animals. In the latter group are found *T. macrodentium* and *T. orale* from the oral cavity (Plate 97), *T. refringens* from the genital area, and so forth. In the pathogenic group are *T. pallidum*, the causative agent of **syphilis**; *T. pertenue*, from the tropical disease **yaws**; and *T. carateum*, which causes a chronic skin disease, **pinta**, endemic in Central and South America.

All the treponemes are **obligate anaerobes.** They are actively motile and contain numerous tight, rigid coils. They are difficult to stain and are best observed by **darkfield microscopy** (see Chapter 2). This is an important laboratory procedure, since a diagnosis of syphilis in the early stages can be immediately confirmed by demonstrating *T. pallidum* in material from suspected lesions (usually anogenital) or affected regional lymph nodes. *T. pallidum* has not been cultivated in vitro.

Darkfield examination for T. pallidum

The following procedure is recommended for darkfield examination:

1. After donning rubber gloves, thoroughly cleanse the lesion with gauze sponge, removing crusts if present (after soaking in saline) and abrading it to produce serous fluid.
2. Pinch the lesion with gloved fingers so that a drop of fluid is expressed from its border or surface; if none is obtained (avoid blood), moisten with a drop of saline and after a minute or two, repeat the attempt to obtain fluid.
3. Touch a coverslip to the fluid, invert it over a microscope slide so as to eliminate air bubbles, seal the edges with lanolin, and **immediately examine** for characteristic forms of motile *T. pallidum*, using darkfield microscopy and an oil immersion objective.
4. Look for a thin, tightly wound, corkscrew-shaped organism of 8 to 14 uniform, rigid spirals, slightly longer than the size of an average red blood cell. Characteristic movement is slowly backward or forward or a corkscrew rotation about the long axis, sometimes with flexion, bending, and snapping.
5. Cautiously interpret a positive preparation from a lesion in the mouth—the commensal treponemes may be confused with *T. pallidum*.

Great care should be taken in performing the darkfield examination to avoid accidental infection. The examiner should always wear gloves. Slides containing darkfield samples, as well as materials used for obtaining these samples, should be placed directly into a disinfectant, such as 70% ethanol. Discarded materials should all be sterilized, preferably by autoclaving. After handling the specimens, one should wash the hands and swab the table tops with disinfectant.

A direct fluorescent antibody staining procedure for delayed examination of fluids to detect the presence of *T. pallidum* is of diagnostic value.[9]

It is beyond the scope of this text to discuss the clinical manifestations of primary, secondary, or tertiary syphilis. The serologic tests available for laboratory diagnosis of syphilis are discussed in Chapter 38. (See also references 2, 17, and 19.)

GENUS LEPTOSPIRA

The principal sources of leptospirae infecting humans are urine and tissues of **infected animals.** The disease is acquired by direct contact or indirectly through contact with contaminated water. The organisms enter through abrasions of the skin or through the mucosal surfaces of the body; occupational exposure is a prime factor for acquiring the infection. Clinical manifestations range from a mild illness to a severe infection with liver, kidney, and central nervous system involvement.

The species of *Leptospira* are also thin, flexible, tightly coiled spirals of approximately the same size as the species of *Treponema*. One or both ends of the spirochete, being more flexible than the center portion, may be bent to form a hook. Spinning takes place on the long axis of the cell. If one end only is hooked, forward movement is in the direction of the straight end. With both ends hooked, a lashing effect may be noticed as the cell spins.

The organism is **aerobic** and may be cultivated (from the blood during the first week of illness or from the urine subsequently) in a supplemented ascitic fluid medium or in the medium recommended by Fletcher (see Chapter 42), consisting of salts, amino acids, and rabbit albumin. A low-protein medium* has been described (Bey and Johnson: Infect. Immun. **19:**562-569, 1978). False-positive cultures have resulted from the use of water contaminated with *Leptospira biflexa* as a result of membrane filtration rather than heat sterilization.[20] Opti-

mal growth temperature is 30 C, and the incubation time for optimal growth ranges from a few days to longer than 4 weeks but is usually 6 to 14 days.[2]

All pathogenic leptospires are placed in one species, *Leptospira interrogans*, with many serovars. Serovars encountered in the United States include icterohemorrhagiae, canicola, ballum, grippotyphosa, bataviae, autumnalis, and pomona.[11] The manifestations of the disease and its severity are not related to the specific serovar involved.

The spirochetes can be observed in blood or spinal fluid drawn from a patient during the first week of the disease (see Chapter 7), when the symptoms are chills, fever, muscle pains, headache, and abdominal pain. During the second stage, manifested by jaundice and skin lesions, the spirochetes may be readily observed in the urine by the darkfield technique.[3] The concentration of leptospirae in the blood and spinal fluid of patients is low, so that it is difficult to demonstrate them by direct microscopy. Centrifugation techniques increase the likelihood of demonstrating the organisms but often result in misdiagnosis by mistaken identification of extrusions from red blood cells that simulate spirochetes.[2] Direct darkfield examination is of considerably greater value for examination of specimens in which there would be a high concentration of leptospirae. This would include blood, peritoneal fluid, and suspension made from the liver of hamsters or guinea pigs infected with clinical material.

The **serologic** detection of leptospiral antibodies in humans and animals is an invaluable adjunct in the diagnosis of leptospirosis. Various techniques have been used, including the microscopic agglutination test, the genus-specific hemolytic or indirect hemagglutination test, and the ELISA test.[1] Stable, formalized suspensions of *Leptospira* serotypes are available* and can be used in a rapid macroscopic slide agglu-

---

*Scientific Protein Laboratories, Inc., Waunakee, Wisc.

*Difco Laboratories, Detroit, Mich.; Fort Dodge Laboratories, Fort Dodge, Iowa.

tination test for serologic diagnosis of the infection.

The more serious symptoms of leptospirosis are related to the immune response to the organism. Antimicrobial therapy is generally believed to be of no value, unless initiated during the first 48 to 72 hours of illness. Penicillin is the drug of choice. Corticosteroids are contraindicated.

ANAEROBIC VIBRIOS

Certain obligately anaerobic vibrios cause disease in humans on rare occasion. These organisms are discussed in Chapter 27.

REFERENCES

1. Adler, B., Murphy, A.M., Locarnini, S.A., and Faine, S.: Detection of specific anti-leptospiral immunoglobulins M and G in human serum by solid-phase enzyme-linked immunosorbent assay, J. Clin. Microbiol. **11**:452-457, 1980.
2. Alexander, A.D.: Leptospira. In Lennette, E.H., Balows, A., Hausler, W.J., Jr., and Truant, J.P., editors: Manual of clinical microbiology, ed. 3, Washington, D.C., 1980, American Society for Microbiology.
3. Alston, J.M., and Broom, J.C.: Leptospirosis in man and animals, London, 1958, E. & S. Livingston, Ltd.
4. Blaser, M.J.: *Campylobacter fetus* subspecies *jejuni:* the need for surveillance, J. Infect. Dis. **141**:670-671, 1980.
5. Blaser, M.J., Berkowitz, I.D., LaForce, F.M., Cravens, J., Reller, L.B., and Wang, W.L.L.: *Campylobacter* enteritis: clinical and epidemiologic features, Ann. Intern. Med. **91**:179-185, 1979.
6. Blaser, M.J., LaForce, F.M., Wilson, N.A., and Wang, W.L.L.: Reservoirs for human campylobacteriosis, J. Infect. Dis. **141**:665-669, 1980.
7. Blaser, M.J., Moss, C.W., and Weaver, R.E.: Cellular fatty acid composition of *Campylobacter fetus*, J. Clin. Microbiol. **11**:448-451, 1980.
8. Burgdorfer, W.: *Borrelia*. In Lennette, E.H., Balows, A., Hausler, W.J., Jr., and Truant, J.P., editors: Manual of clinical microbiology, ed. 3, Washington, D.C., 1980, American Society for Microbiology.
9. Daniels, K.C., and Ferneyhough, H.S.: Specific direct fluorescent antibody detection of *Treponema pallidum,* Health Lab. Sci. **14**:164-171, 1977.
10. Felsenfeld, O.: *Borrelia:* Strains, vectors, human and animal borreliosis, St. Louis, 1971, Warren H. Green, Inc.
11. Finegold, S.M., and Meyer, R.D.: Leptospirosis. In Spittell's Clinical medicine, vol. 2, Hagerstown, Md., 1980, Harper & Row, Publishers.
12. Harvey, S.M.: Hippurate hydrolysis by *Campylobacter fetus*, J. Clin. Microbiol. **11**:435-437, 1980.
13. Kaplan, R.L.: *Campylobacter*. In Lennette, E.H., Balows, A., Hausler, W.J., Jr., and Truant, J.P., editors: Manual of clinical microbiology, ed. 3, Washington, D.C., 1980, American Society for Microbiology.
14. Karmali, M.A., DeGrandis, S., and Fleming, P.C.: Antimicrobial susceptibility of *Campylobacter jejuni* and *Campylobacter fetus* subsp. *fetus* to eight cephalosporins with special reference to species differentiation, Antimicrob. Agents Chemother. **18**:948-951, 1980.
15. King, E.O.: The laboratory recognition of *Vibrio fetus* and a closely related *Vibrio* isolated from cases of human vibriosis, Ann. N.Y. Acad. Sci. **98**:700-711, 1962.
16. The laboratory aspects of syphilis, Atlanta, 1971, Center for Disease Control.
17. Manual of tests for syphilis, Public Health Service Pub. No. 411, Washington, D.C., 1969, U.S. Government Printing Office.
18. Rogosa, M.: *Streptobacillus moniliformis* and *Spirillum minor*. In Lennette, E.H., Balows, A., Hausler, W.J., Jr., and Truant, J.P., editors: Manual of clinical microbiology, ed. 3, Washington, D.C., 1980, American Society for Microbiology.
19. Rohde, P., editor: BBL manual of product and laboratory procedures, Cockeysville, Md., 1969, Baltimore Biological Laboratory, Division of BioQuest, Becton, Dickinson and Co.
20. Rubin, S.J., Perlman, S., and Ellinghausen, H.C., Jr.: Isolation of *Leptospira biflexa* from commercially prepared deionized water labeled "Sterile for tissue culture," J. Clin. Microbiol. **12**:121-123, 1980.
21. Skirrow, M.B.: Campylobacter enteritis: a "new" disease, Br. Med. J. **2**:9-11, 1977.
22. Vanhoof, R., Gordts, B., Dierickx, R., Coignau, H., and Butzler, J.P.: Bacteriostatic and bactericidal activities of 24 antimicrobial agents against *Campylobacter fetus* subsp. *jejuni*, Antimicrob. Agents Chemother. **18**:118-121, 1980.
23. Walder, M.: Susceptibility of *Campylobacter fetus* subsp. *jejuni* to twenty antimicrobial agents, Antimicrob. Agents Chemother. **16**:37-39, 1979.
24. Wang, W.L., Blaser, M., and Cravens, J.: Isolation of campylobacter, Br. Med. J. **2**:57, 1978.
25. Waterborne *Campylobacter* gastroenteritis, Morbid., Mortal. Weekly Rep. **27**:207, 1978.

25 AEROBIC OR FACULTATIVE GRAM-POSITIVE SPORE-FORMING BACILLI

Bacillus

In this chapter discussion of the clinical significance of the gram-positive spore-forming bacilli is limited to certain species of *Bacillus*. The genus contains a large number of species that are aerobic or facultative, usually gram-positive, and spore forming. They are widely distributed in nature and are therefore frequent contaminants in laboratory cultures from clinical specimens. They may or may not grow on eosin–methylene blue (EMB) agar. Because they may vary in Gram stain and oxidase and other reactions and spores may not be evident, they may resemble nonfermentative gram-negative bacilli. Such organisms cannot be classified in any known gram-negative species or CDC taxon. Since some *Bacillus* strains are strict aerobes, they may appear as nonfermentative gram-negative rods on Kligler's or TSI agar.[4] Most do not grow on enteric agars, but some show a limited growth on these. However, several gram-negative nonfermenters also fail to grow on such media. The colonial morphology of the *Bacillus* strains that simulate gram-negative rods is not typical of the usual *Bacillus* species with large flat colonies and frequent beta hemolysis. Some of these strains even have minute colonies.

Spore formation often fails to occur within the time required to report a clinical isolate. Sporulation is often stimulated on esculin agar and may be facilitated on acidified media such as TSI agar. Two other tests may be helpful. One is susceptibility to vancomycin; with the exception of *Flavobacterium* species, no gram-negative nonfermenter is known to be susceptible to vancomycin by the Kirby-Bauer technique, whereas most *Bacillus* species are sensitive. However, there are strains of *Bacillus* species that are vancomycin resistant. Therefore, only vancomycin susceptibility can be used diagnostically. The second procedure that may be helpful is the KOH test described in Chapter 3, in which gram-negative organisms show a viscous thread. Some *Bacillus* strains, particularly from older cultures that have also lost their gram positivity, may give a "gram-negative" reaction by this test. Accordingly, the test is of value for identification of *Bacillus* species only if no viscous thread is formed.

Treatment of specimens or mixed cultures that may contain *Bacillus* species with ethanol (50% ethanol for 1 hour) is effective for selecting *Bacillus* species, just as it is for selecting spore-forming anaerobes.[12]

It should be noted that certain species of *Bacillus*, other than the well-recognized pathogen *Bacillus anthracis*, can be involved, though infrequently, in human disease processes. For example, *Bacillus cereus* has been implicated in food-borne illness both in Europe and in the United States and may be isolated from wounds. *B. cereus*, *B. subtilis*, *B. sphaericus*, *B. circulans*, and *B. pumilus* have also been incriminated in cases of meningitis, pneumonia, septicemia, endocarditis, and other serious infections, as reported by several authors.[1,5-7,13-15,17] Sepsis and peritonitis caused by *B. licheniformis* have also been described.[16] Eye and other closed-space infections may follow trauma. Studies on the antimicrobial susceptibility of *Bacillus* species note that they are generally susceptible to tetracycline, aminoglycosides, and chloramphenicol.[5,17] Susceptibility to penicillin G, ampicillin, methicillin, and cephalothin is species related, being high for *B. subtilis*, intermediate for *B. pumilus*, and low for *B. cereus*. The *B. licheniformis* strain was sensitive to penicillin and resistant to clindamycin.[16] Hypersensitivity pneumonitis related to exposure to wood dust contaminated with *B. subtilis* has been described.[11] The role of *B. cereus* in food poisoning was discussed in Chapter 9.

B. cereus colonies on laboratory media vary from small, shiny, and compact to the large, feathery, spreading type. A **lavender-colored** colony with beta hemolysis is seen on sheep blood agar. *B. subtilis* colonies are normally large, flat, and dull, with a ground glass appearance (Plate 98). Unlike *B. anthracis*, *B. cereus* is resistant to gamma phage, is usually resistant to penicillin, does not encapsulate on bicarbonate agar, and on fluorescent antibody–stained smears does not exhibit fluorescence of both cell wall and capsule.

BACILLUS ANTHRACIS

Bacillus anthracis is the primary human pathogen in the genus. However, it is seldom encountered in the average hospital or public health laboratory. Nevertheless, because of its importance in some areas, its identification and pathogenicity should be discussed. Cases in the United States are most often related to handling of imported wool or goat hair, animal hides, shaving brushes, and so forth (chiefly from Asia and Africa). The disease may also occur in persons exposed to cattle.[2,10] In 1978 there were six cases of anthrax in humans in the United States.[2] Four occurred in industrial settings (textile mills), and two were associated with anthrax in cattle.

The organism is a facultative, large, squared-ended, nonmotile rod, with an ellipsoidal to cylindrical centrally located spore. The sporangium is usually not swollen. The cells frequently occur in long chains, giving a **bamboo** appearance, especially on primary isolation from infected tissue or discharge. The chains of virulent forms are usually surrounded by a **capsule**.

Encapsulation occurs also in enriched media and when grown on sodium bicarbonate agar under 5% CO_2. Encapsulated strains may be used for fluorescent antibody staining, an important ancillary test. Smears may be sent to the CDC for the fluorescent antibody test. Both the cell wall and the capsule fluoresce simultaneously. Avirulent forms are usually nonencapsulated. Sporulation occurs in the soil and on inanimate media but not in living tissue.

The colonies of *B. anthracis* are normally large (4 to 5 mm), opaque, raised, and irregular, with a **curled margin.** When the margin of the colony is pushed inward and then lifted gently with an inoculating needle, the disturbed portion of the colony stands up like beaten egg whites. Comma-shaped colony outgrowths are common. On sheep blood agar the colonies are invariably **nonhemolytic.** Smooth and rough colony forms may be observed, and both of these may be virulent.

When working with suspected *B. anthracis*, one should use **extreme caution,** work in a bacteriologic safety hood, avoid creating aerosols, and decontaminate all areas thoroughly.

The optimal temperature for growth is 35 C, and when grown at 42 to 43 C, the organism becomes **attenuated** or avirulent. This was shown by Louis Pasteur years ago. The loss of virulence is attributed to loss of the capsule. In broth the bacillus produces a heavy pellicle with little if any subsurface growth. Biochemically the organism is characterized as follows:

Carbohydrate fermentation—Glucose, fructose, maltose, sucrose, and trehalose fermented with acid only; arabinose, xylose, galactose, lactose, mannose, raffinose, rhamnose, adonitol, dulcitol, inositol, inulin, mannitol, and sorbitol not fermented.

Gelatin—Inverted pine-tree growth; liquefaction (slow).

Nitrates—Reduced to nitrites.

Starch—Hydrolyzed.

Voges-Proskauer—Positive.

A simple presumptive test for identification of *B. anthracis* has been proposed.[3] It is a modification of the string of pearls test, which reflects the susceptibility of a strain to penicillin. Single streaks of the suspect organism, as well as positive and negative controls, are made on a Mueller-Hinton agar plate. Ten-unit penicillin disks are placed on each streak, and a coverslip is placed over the streak. After incubation for 3 to 6 hours at 37 C, growth from beneath the coverslip is examined microscopically for the presence of strings of spherical cellular forms of the organism. The presence of such cells resembling strings of pearls is considered a positive test.

Specific identification may be made by use of a gamma bacteriophage (at CDC or state health department laboratories). An indirect hemagglutination test for detecting antibodies to the organism is available through the CDC.

Pathogenicity of Bacillus anthracis

The organism is the cause of **anthrax,** which in humans may be manifested in three forms[9]:

1. **Cutaneous anthrax** (malignant pustule), the most common form in the United States. Infection is initiated by the entrance of bacilli through an abrasion of the skin. A pustule usually appears on the hands or forearms. The bacilli are readily recognized in the serosanguineous discharge.

2. **Pulmonary anthrax,** or woolsorters' disease. The bacilli may be found in large numbers in the sputum. Spores are inhaled during shearing or sorting of animal hair. If not properly treated, this form can readily progress to fatal septicemia.

3. **Gastrointestinal anthrax,** the most severe and rarest form. The bacilli or spores are swallowed, thus initiating an intestinal infection. The organisms may be isolated from the stools. This form is also usually fatal if not treated.

The pathogenicity of the organism is determined by injecting each of 10 white mice (2 to 3 weeks of age) subcutaneously with 0.2 ml of a saline suspension of the organism. Rabbits or guinea pigs may also be used. Details of the technique are given by Feeley and Patton.[8] Animals usually die 2 to 5 days after inoculation, but they may survive 10 days. Death is caused by **septicemia,** and the organism is readily recovered from the heart, blood, spleen, liver, and lungs of the animal.

REFERENCES

1. Allen, T.B., and Wilkinson, H.A.: A case of meningitis and generalized Shwartzman reaction caused by *Bacillus sphaericus*, Johns Hopkins Med. J. **125:**8-13, 1969.
2. Anthrax in humans, United States, 1978, Morbid. Mortal. Weekly Rep. **28:**160-165, 1979.
3. Bailie, W.E., and Stowe, E.C.: A simplified test for identification of *Bacillus anthracis*, Abstract C80, Abstracts of the Annual Meeting of the American Society for Microbiology, 1977, p. 48.
4. Blachman, U., Gilardi, G.L., Pickett, M.J., Slotnick, I.J., and von Graevenitz, A.: *Bacillus* spp. strains posing as nonfermentative gram-negative rods, Clin. Microbiol. Newsletter **2:**8, 1980.
5. Coonrod, J.D., Leadley, P.J., and Eickhoff, T.C.: Antibiotic susceptibility of *Bacillus* species, J. Infect. Dis. **123:**102-105, 1971.
6. Curtis, J.R., Wing, A.J., and Coleman, J.C.: *Bacillus cereus* bacteremia: a complication of intermittent haemodialysis, Lancet **1:**136-138, 1967.
7. Farrar, W.E., Jr.: Serious infections due to "nonpathogenic" organisms of the genus *Bacillus:* review of their status as pathogens, Am. J. Med. **34:**134-141, 1963.
8. Feeley, J.C., and Patton, C.M.: *Bacillus anthracis*. In Lennette, E.H., Balows, A., Hausler, W.J., Jr., and Truant, J.P., editors: Manual of clinical microbiology, ed. 3, Washington, D.C., 1980, American Society for Microbiology.
9. Hospital of the University of Pennsylvania: A symposium on anthrax in man, Philadelphia, 1954, University of Pennsylvania Press.
10. Human anthrax, Colorado, Morbid. Mortal. Weekly Rep. **29:**469-470, 1980.
11. Johnson, C.L., Bernstein, I.L., Gallagher, J.S., Bonventre, P.F., and Brooks, S.M.: Familial hypersensitivity pneumonitis induced by *Bacillus subtilis*, Am. Rev. Respir. Dis. **122:**339-348, 1980.
12. Koransky, J.R., Allen, S.D., and Dowell, V.R., Jr.: Use of ethanol for selective isolation of sporeforming microorganisms, Appl. Environ. Microbiol. **35:**762-765, 1978.
13. Leff, A., Jacobs, R., Gooding, V., Hauch, J., Conte, J., and Stulberg, M.: *Bacillus cereus* pneumonia, Am. Rev. Respir. Dis. **115:**151-154, 1977.
14. Pennington, J.E., Gibbons, N.D., Strobeck, J.E., Simpson, G.L., and Myerowitz, R.L.: *Bacillus* species infection in patients with hematologic neoplasia, J.A.M.A. **235:**1473-1474, 1976.
15. Stopler, T.V., Cămuescu, V., and Voiculescu, M.: Bronchopneumonia with lethal evolution determined by a microorganism of the genus *Bacillus (B. cereus)*, Romanian Med. Rev. **19:**7-9, 1969.
16. Sugar, A.M., and McCloskey, R.V.: *Bacillus licheniformis* sepsis, J.A.M.A. **238:**1180-1181, 1977.
17. Tuazon, C.V., Murray, H.W., Levy, C., Solny, M.N., Curtin, J.A., and Sheagren, J.N.: Serious infections from *Bacillus* sp., J.A.M.A. **241:**1137-1140, 1979.

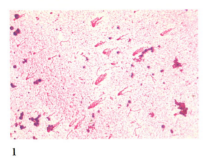
1

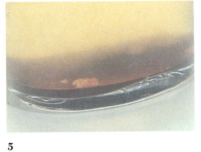
2

3

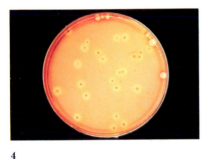
4

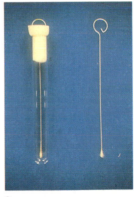
5

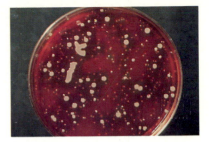
6

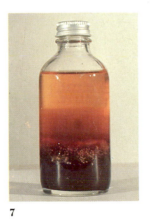
7

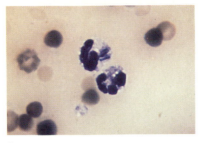
8

1. Flagella stain, *Proteus*.
2. Intracellular *Clostridium perfringens* in peripheral blood smear.
3. Pour plate blood culture, numerous colonies of *Staphylococcus aureus*.
4. Pour plate blood culture, positive for *Streptococcus pneumoniae*.
5. Positive blood culture. Note fluffy colonies at bottom of bottle (*Fusobacterium necrophorum*).
6. Gram stain from bottle shown in Plate 5.
7. Many colonies of *S. aureus* on layer of settled red blood cells in blood culture bottle.
8. Nasopharyngeal swab.

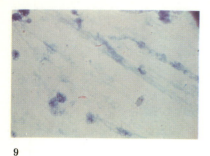

9

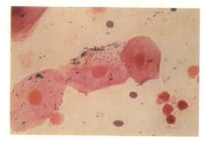

10

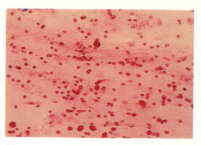

11

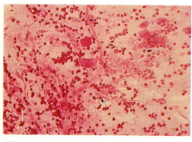

12

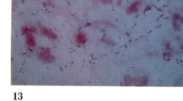

13

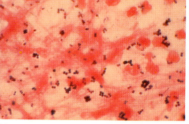

14

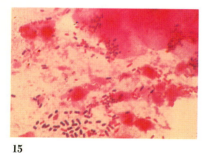

15

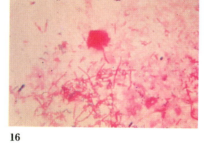

16

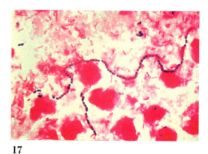

17

9. Positive acid-fast smear, sputum (*Mycobacterium tuberculosis*).

10. Sputum showing large squamous epithelial cells.

11. Sputum Gram stain (100×), numerous polymorphonuclear leukocytes (PMNs). Macrophages also present.

12. Sputum Gram stain (100×). Predominantly PMNs, but some squamous epithelial cells are also present.

13. Sputum Gram stain, numerous *Streptococcus pneumoniae*.

14. Sputum Gram stain, numerous *Staphylococcus aureus*.

15. Sputum Gram stain, *Klebsiella*. Note that some organisms are somewhat gram positive.

16. Transtracheal aspirate, *Fusobacterium necrophorum* predominant; *Bacteroides melaninogenicus* (small coccobacilli) and *Peptostreptococcus anaerobius* also present.

17. Transtracheal aspirate, *Peptostreptococcus* and *Bacteroides*.

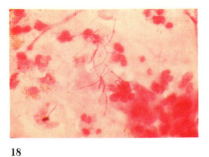
18

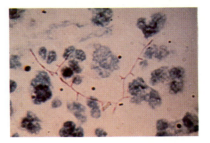
19

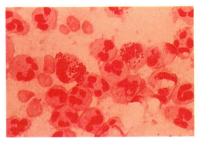
20

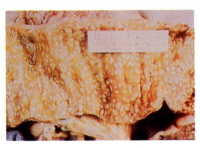
21

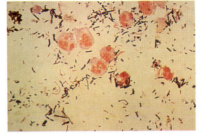
22

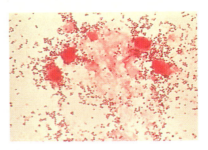
23

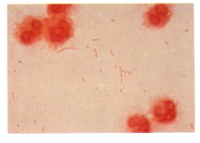
24

18. Sputum Gram stain, *Nocardia asteroides*.

19. Sputum acid-fast stain (1% sulfuric acid decolorization), *N. asteroides*.

20. Stool Gram stain, staphylococcal enterocolitis. Note PMNs.

21. Autopsy specimen of colon, pseudomembranous colitis. Note numerous yellow elevated plaques.

22. Stool Gram stain, *Clostridium difficile* pseudomembranous colitis. Note PMNs and predominance of large gram-positive rods with parallel sides.

23. Urethral smear, gonorrhea; gram-negative intracellular diplococci.

24. Spinal fluid Gram stain, *Haemophilus influenzae*.

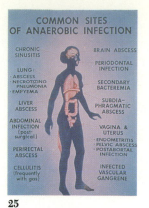

25

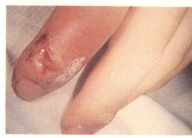

26

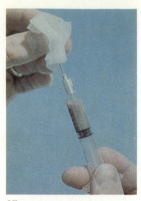

27

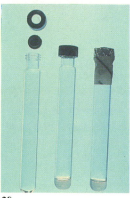

28

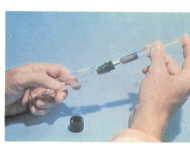

29

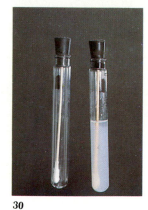

30

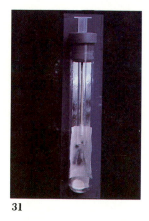

31

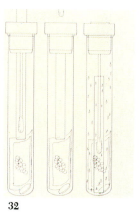

32

25. Common sites of anaerobic infection.

26. Human bite infection.

27. Eliminating air bubbles from syringe and needle to protect anaerobes in specimen from exposure to oxygen.

28. Transport tube with anaerobic atmosphere and nonnutritive fluid with resazurin indicator (pink indicates oxygen is present).

29. Injecting specimen into gassed-out tube.

30. Swab in anaerobic atmosphere. Companion tube (shown with specimen on swab in place) contains nonnutritive semisolid transport medium.

31. Vacutainer Anaerobic Transporter (B-D).

32. Vacutainer Anaerobic Transporter. *Left*, Remove tube from envelope. *Middle*, Remove plunger and attached swab. Collect sample. Insert swab into inner tube. *Right*, Press plunger through stopper.

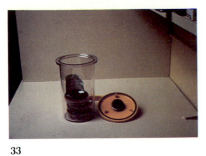

33

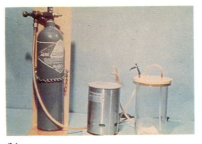

34

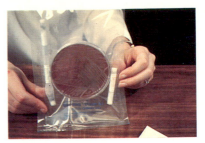

35

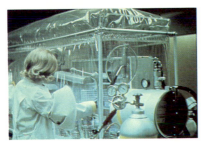

36

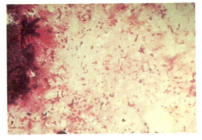

37

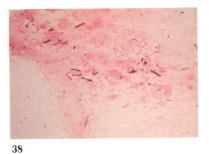

38

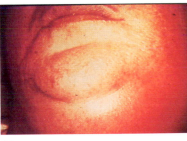

39

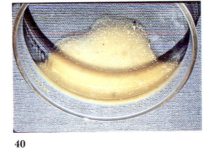

40

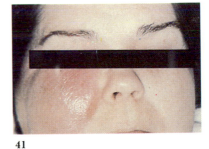

41

33. GasPak anaerobic jar; catalyst pellets in basket on lid.

34. Apparatus for continuous gassing of GasPak jar during holding period.

35. Anaerobic Bio-Bag for anaerobic incubation.

36. Anaerobic chamber.

37. Gram stain of intra-abdominal abscess. Irregularly staining gram-negative rods are *Bacteroides fragilis*.

38. Perineal gas gangrene, *Clostridium perfringens* (large, broad gram-positive rods), coliforms, and white blood cells badly distorted by toxin of *C. perfringens*.

39. Ludwig's angina.

40. Sulfur granules in thoracic empyema fluid, actinomycosis.

41. Erysipelas caused by *Streptococcus pyogenes*.

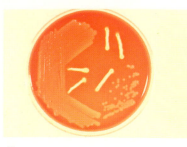
42

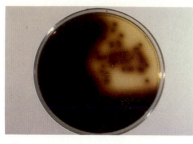
43

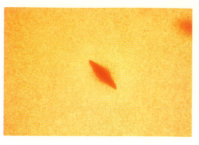
44

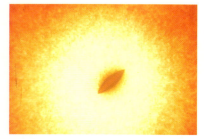
45

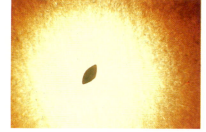
46

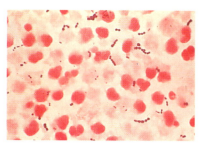
47

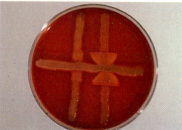
48

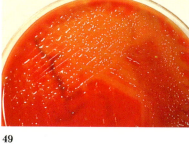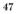
49

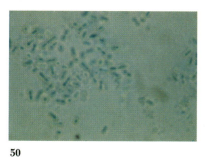
50

42. Group B streptococci with surface and subsurface inoculation.

43. Enterococcus colonies (esculin positive) on Pfizer selective streptococcus agar.

44. Alpha hemolysis, *Streptococcus*.

45. Alpha prime hemolysis, *Streptococcus*.

46. Beta hemolysis, *Streptococcus*.

47. Group A beta-hemolytic streptococci in pus.

48. CAMP test, groups A and B streptococci.

49. Mucoid colonies of type 3 pneumococci.

50. Quellung reaction with pneumococci from blood culture.

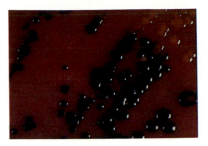

51

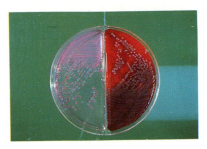

52

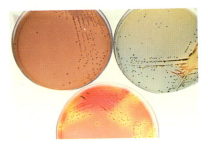

53

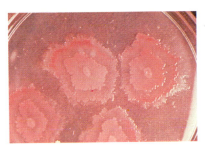

54

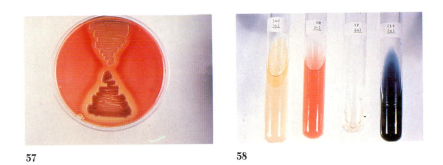

55

56

57

58

51. *Neisseria gonorrhoeae* colonies, positive oxidase test.
52. Mixture of *Escherichia coli* and *Salmonella* on MacConkey and blood agar.
53. *Shigella* in stool culture on EMB (colorless colonies), HE (not seen; would be colorless or blue-green), and XLD (red colonies) media.
54. Spreading *Proteus* colonies.
55. *Klebsiella pneumoniae* on Endo agar showing mucoid colonies.
56. *Salmonella typhi* on Wilson-Blair medium showing typical black sheen.
57. *Serratia marcescens*, nonpigmented and pigmented colonies.
58. IMViC reactions with *Salmonella*. *Left to right*, Indole negative, methyl red positive, V-P negative, and Simmon's citrate positive.

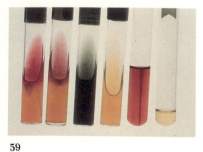

59

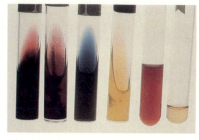

60

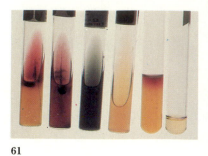

61

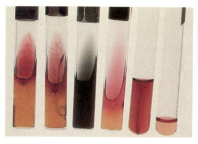

62

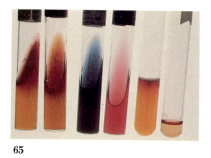

63

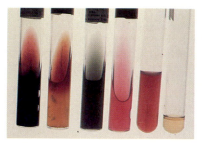

64

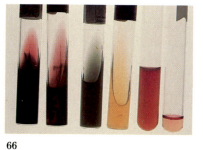

65

66

59 to 66. All have same six tubes, listed in same order (descending) below as they appear left to right.

	59 S. sonnei	60 S. infantis	61 S. typhi	62 Morganella	63 K. oxytoca	64 P. mirabilis	65 P. rettgeri	66 E. tarda
TSI	K/A⁻	K/Ag⁺⁺⁺⁺	K/A⁺	K/Ag	A/Ag	K/Ag⁺⁺⁺⁺	K/A⁻	K/A⁺⁺⁺⁺
LIA	K/A⁻	K/K⁺⁺	K/K⁺	R/Ag	K/Kg	R/Ag⁻	R/A	K/A⁺⁺⁺
Simmon's citrate	−	+	−	−	+	−	+	−
Christensen's urea	−	−	−	+	+ Delayed	+	+	−
Ornithine motility medium	Non-motile +	Motile +	Motile −	Motile +	Nonmotile −	Motile +	Motile −	Motile +
Peptone broth for indole	−	−	−	+	+	−	+	+

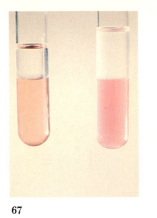

67

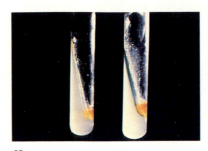

68

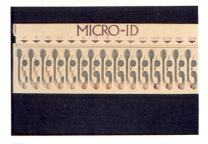

69

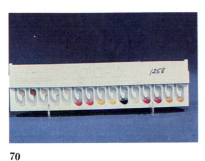

70

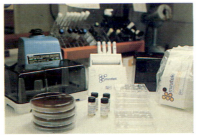

71

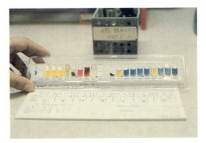

72

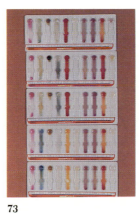

73

67. Arginine dihydrolase. *Left*, Control. *Right*, Positive.

68. Phenylalanine deaminase. *Left*, Negative. *Right*, Positive (blue-green slant after addition of ferric chloride).

69. Micro-ID kit, uninoculated.

70. Micro-ID kit with some positive reactions.

71. Minitek apparatus.

72. API-20E strip showing positive reactions, member of Enterobacteriaceae.

73. Entero-Set 20 (Auxotab system). *Top to bottom, Escherichia coli, Proteus mirabilis, Salmonella, Enterobacter, Klebsiella.*

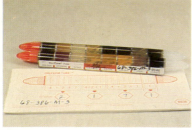

74

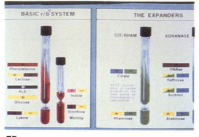
75

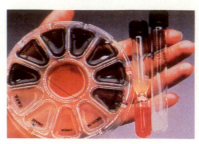
76

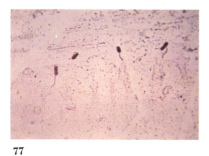
77

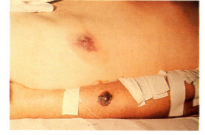
78

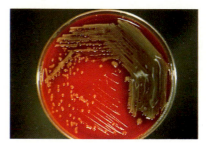
79

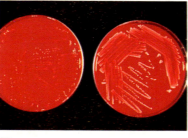
80

74. Oxi-Ferm tubes; back one uninoculated.
75. R/B system.
76. Flow system, uninoculated.
77. *Vibrio cholerae*, flagella stain.
78. Ecthyma gangrenosum caused by *P. aeruginosa*.
79. *Pseudomonas aeruginosa* colonies.
80. *Acinetobacter calcoaceticus* var. *lwoffi (left)*, var. *anitratus (right)*.

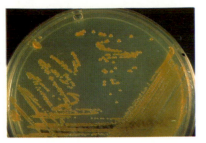

81

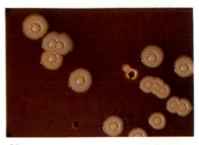

82

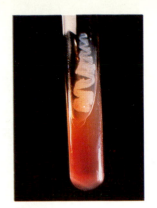

83

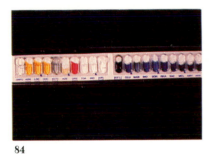

84

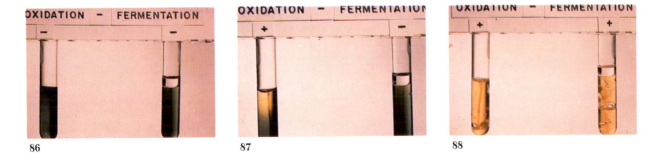

85

86

87

88

81. *Flavobacterium* colonies on Mueller-Hinton agar.
82. *Pseudomonas pseudomallei*, 96-hour growth on BAP.
83. MacConkey agar slant, nonfermenter.
84. API-20E, *Pseudomonas aeruginosa*.
85. Nitrate reduction test. *Left*, Uninoculated control. *Right*, Positive. itive.
86 to 88. O-F tests.

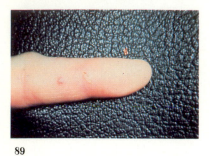

89

90

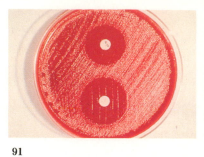

91

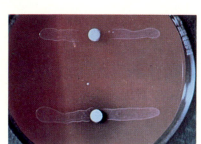

92

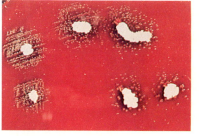

93

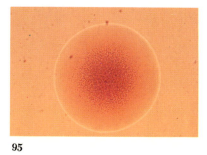

94

95

89. Animal bite infection caused by *Pasteurella multocida*.

90. *P. multocida*, bipolar staining (Wayson).

91. *P. multocida*, sensitivity to penicillin 2-unit disk.

92. *Brucella suis*. Growth inhibited by basic fuchsin *(above)* but not by thionin *(below)*.

93. *Haemophilus influenzae* satelliting about staphylococci.

94. *H. influenzae*, stimulation by XV disc but not V disc.

95. *Haemophilus aprophilus* colony.

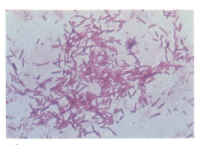

96

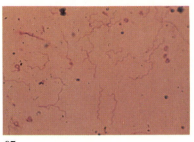

97

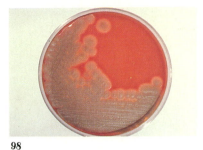

98

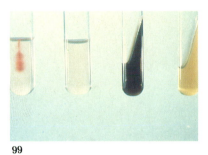

99

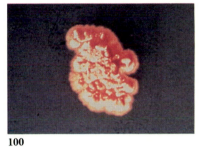

100

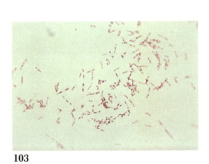

101

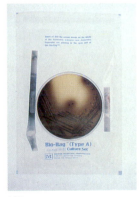

102

103

96. *Campylobacter fetus* in stool (plus few clostridia with spores).

97. *Treponema* from blood culture. Patient had oral lesion.

98. *Bacillus subtilis* on BAP.

99. *Listeria*. *Left*, Positive motility (inverted Christmas tree) with control tube (next to it). Right two tubes show positive reaction in bile esculin and control tube (*extreme right*).

100. *Nocardia asteroides* colony.

101. *Bacteroides fragilis* on BAP.

102. *B. fragilis* growing on *Bacteroides* bile esculin agar (positive esculin reaction) in Bio-Bag.

103. *B. fragilis*, irregular staining.

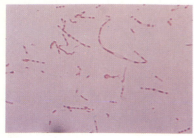

104

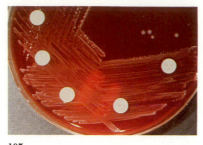

105

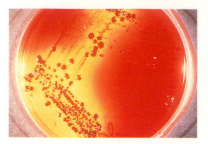

106

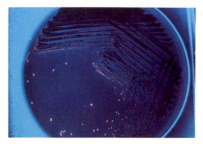

107

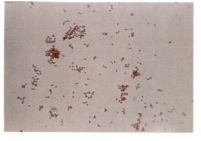

108

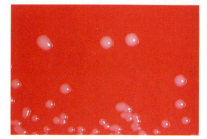

109

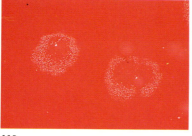

110

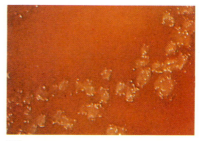

111

104. *Bacteroides fragilis*, irregular staining and pleomorphism.
105. *B. fragilis*, identification disks.
106. *Bacteroides melaninogenicus* on BAP.
107. *B. melaninogenicus*, red fluorescence under ultraviolet light.
108. *B. melaninogenicus*, microscopic.
109. *Bacteroides ruminicola* ss. *brevis* on BAP.
110. *Bacteriodes ureolyticus* on BAP. Note corroding of agar.
111. *Fusobacterium nucleatum* on BAP. Note greening.

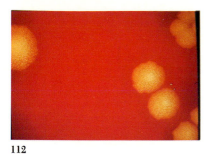
112

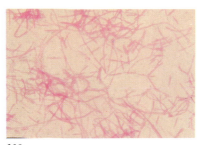

113

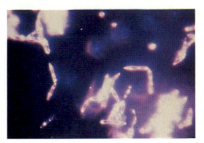
114

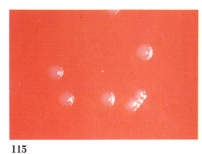
115

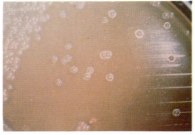
116

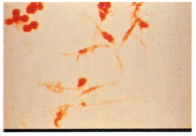
117

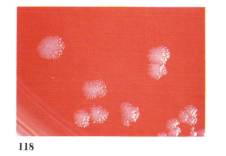
118

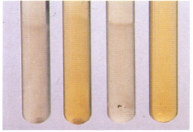
119

112. *Fusobacterium nucleatum.* Note internal speckling in colonies.

113. *F. nucleatum,* microscopic.

114. *F. nucleatum,* microscopic (darkfield).

115. *Fusobacterium necrophorum* on BAP.

116. *F. necrophorum* on Fusobacterium egg yolk agar, positive lipase reaction.

117. *Fusobacterium mortiferum.* Very pleomorphic.

118. *Leptotrichia buccalis* on BAP.

119. Bile test. *Left two tubes, Bacteroides fragilis* control and bile (no inhibition). *Right two tubes,* *F. nucleatum* control and bile (inhibition).

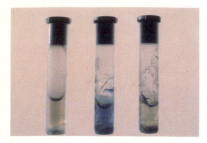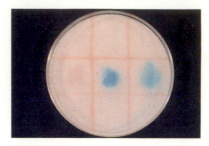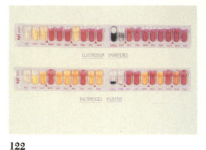

120   121   122

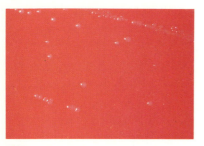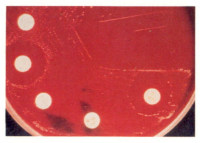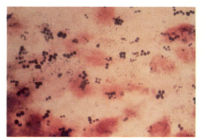

123   124   125

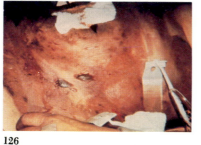

126   127

120. Glutamic acid decarboxylase test (Marion Scientific Corp.). *Left to right,* Uninoculated, positive, negative.

121. Spot indole test with paradimethylaminocinnamaldehyde. *Left,* negative. *Center and right,* Positive.

122. Reactions of *Clostridium sporogenes* and *Bacteroides vulgatus* on API test strips.

123. *Peptococcus asaccharolyticus* on BAP.

124. *Peptostreptococcus anaerobius,* disk identification tests.

125. *Peptococcus magnus* in pus (appearance identical to that of staphylococci).

126. Gas gangrene, abdominal wall. Note bronze discoloration and fluid-filled blisters (bullae).

127. *Clostridium perfringens,* double zone of hemolysis on BAP.

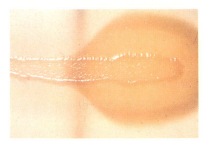
128

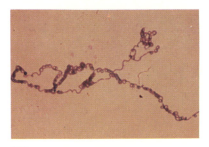
129

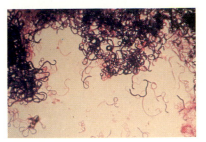
130

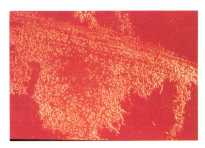
131

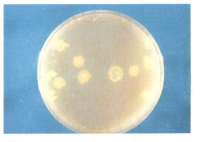
132

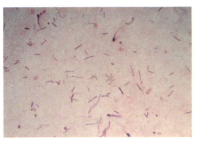
133

134

135

128. *Clostridium perfringens*, positive Nagler test on egg yolk agar. Inhibition of lecithinase reaction by antitoxin *(left)*.

129. *Clostridium ramosum*, microscopic.

130. *C. ramosum*, edge of colony.

131. *Clostridium septicum* on BAP.

132. *C. septicum*, edge of colony.

133. *C. septicum*, microscopic. Note spores.

134. *Clostridium difficile* on BAP.

135. *C. difficile* on cycloserine cefoxitin fructose agar.

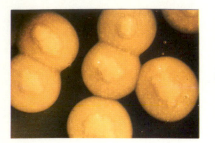

136

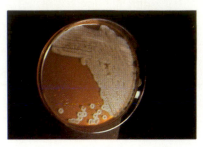

137

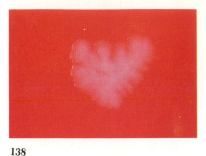

138

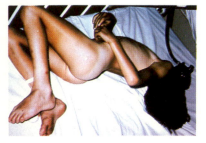

139

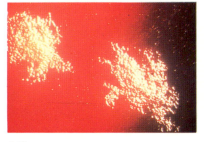

140

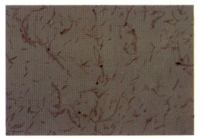

141

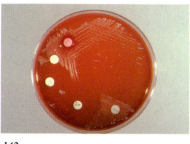

142

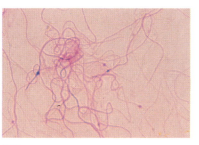

143

136. *Clostridium novyi* type A on egg yolk agar. Positive lecithinase and lipase reactions.
137. *Clostridium*, positive lipase reaction on egg yolk agar.
138. *Clostridium sordellii* on BAP.
139. Tetanus. Patient exhibits opisthotonos (head and legs bent backward toward each other).
140. *Clostridium tetani* on BAP.
141. *C. tetani*, microscopic.
142. *Propionibacterium acnes*, identification disks. Note positive nitrate test (*top*, red).
143. *Eubacterium lentum*, Gram stain.

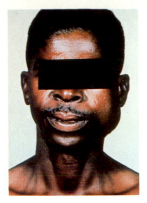

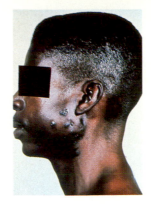

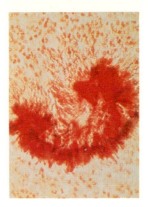

144   145   146

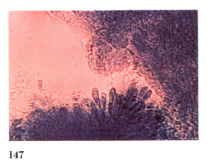

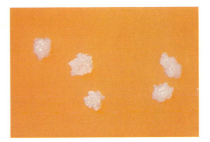

147   148   149

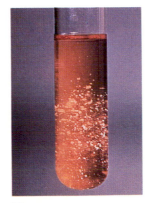

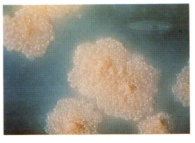

151

150

144. Actinomycosis. Note "lumpy" jaw.

145. Actinomycosis, side view. Note sinuses in skin of face and neck.

146. Sulfur granule, microscopic. Actinomycosis.

147. Edge of sulfur granule to show clubbing.

148. Sulfur granule, Gram stain.

149. *Actinomyces israelii,* "molar tooth" colonies.

150. *A. israelii* in thioglycollate broth (no growth near surface).

151. *Mycobacterium tuberculosis* colonies on L-J medium.

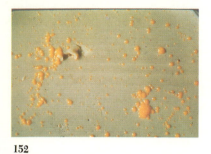

152

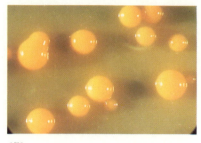

153

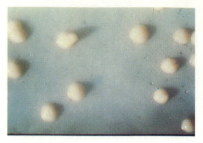

154

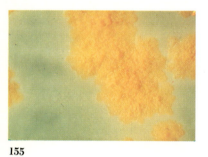

155

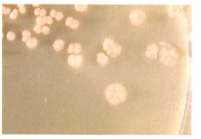

156

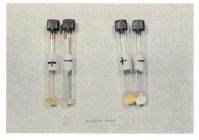

157

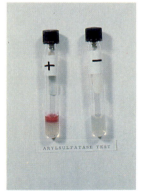

158

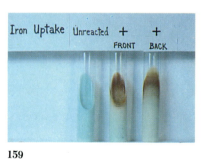

159

152. *Mycobacterium kansasii* colonies exposed to light.
153. Group II scotochromogen *Mycobacterium* with yellow colonies.
154. *Mycobacterium avium* complex, smooth colonies on L-J medium.
155. *Mycobacterium phlei* (rapid grower), rough colonies.
156. Smooth multilobate colonies of *Mycobacterium fortuitum* on L-J medium.
157. Niacin test for mycobacteria.
158. Arylsulfatase test for mycobacteria.
159. Iron uptake test for mycobacteria.

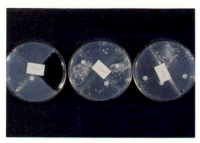

160

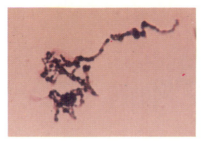

161

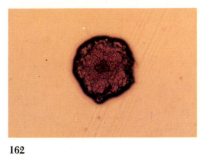

162

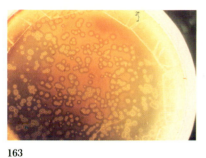

163

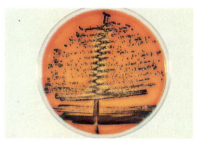

164

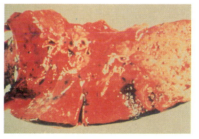

165

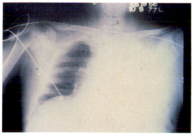

166

167

160. *Mycobacterium tuberculosis* susceptibility test (organism is INH resistant).

161. *Streptobacillus moniliformis*, Giemsa stain.

162. *Actinobacillus actinomycetemcomitans* colony. Note central star-shaped structure.

163. *Mycoplasma pneumoniae* colonies with sheep red blood cell overlay.

164. T strains of *Mycoplasma*, manganese chloride test.

165. *Chromobacterium violaceum* on BAP.

166. Chest radiograph, Legionnaires' disease. Severe pneumonia involving entire left lung.

167. Autopsy specimen, lung. Legionnaires' disease. Extensive consolidation.

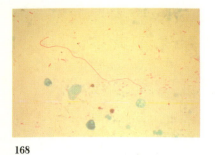

168

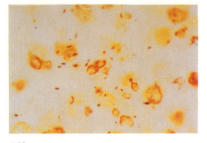

169

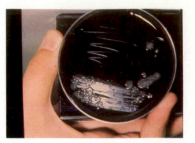

170

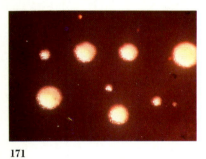

171

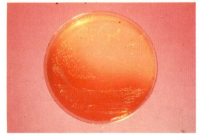

172

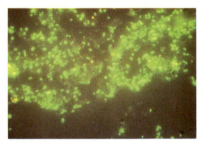

173

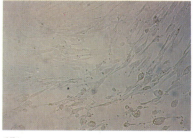

174

175

168. *Legionella pneumophila*, Giménez stain.
169. *L. pneumophila* in lung, Dieterle stain.
170. *L. pneumophila* on buffered charcoal yeast extract agar.
171. *L. pneumophila* colonies. Note internal flecking.
172. *L. pneumophila* on supplemented Mueller-Hinton agar. Note diffusible pigment (melanin).
173. Indirect FA test, Legionnaires' disease.
174. Herpes simplex infected human lung fibroblasts (100×).
175. Varicella-zoster infected human lung fibroblasts (100×).

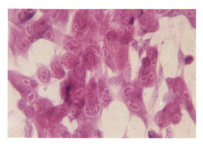

176

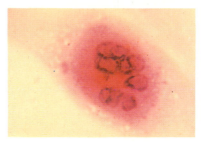

177

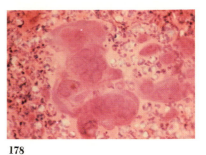

178

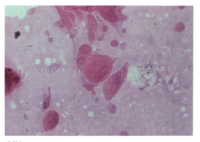

179

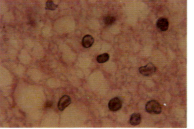

180

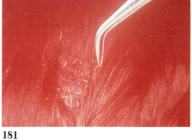

181

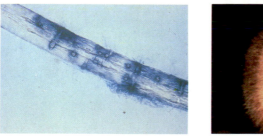

182

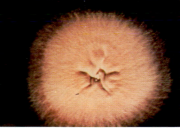

183

176. Cytomegalovirus infected human lung fibroblasts (HE stain; 1,000×).

177. Tzanck cell, HE stain (1,000×). Note multinucleated giant cell with intranuclear inclusions. Vesicle scraping. Varicella-zoster virus recovered on culture.

178. Vesicle scraping, HE stain (400×). Note multinucleated balloon cells.

179. Similar to Plate 178, but different patient.

180. Brain biopsy showing herpes simplex virus inclusions, PAS stain (400×).

181. Fluorescent hairs, Wood's lamp (mycotic infection).

182. *Trichophyton mentagrophytes*, in vitro hair perforation test.

183. *Trichophyton tonsurans* colony.

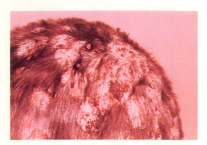

184

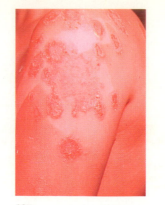

185

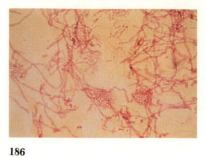

186

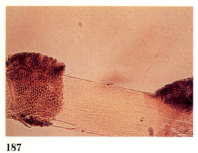

187

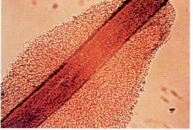

188

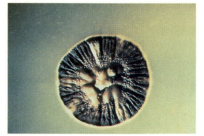

189

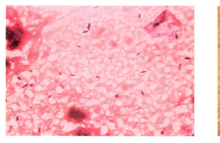

190

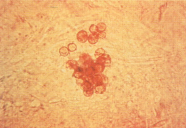

191

184. Scalp infection, *Trichophyton schoenleinii*.
185. *Trichophyton verrucosum* ringworm of skin.
186. *M. furfur*, microscopic (400×).
187. *Piedraia hortae*, hair (400×).
188. *T. beigelii*, hair (40×).
189. *S. schenkii* colony.
190. *S. schenkii* in mouse testes.
191. Chromomycosis cells in tissue (400×).

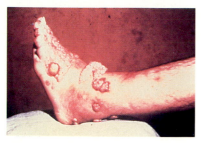

192

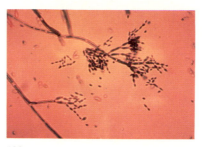

193

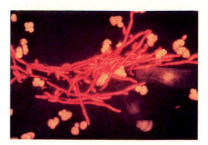

194

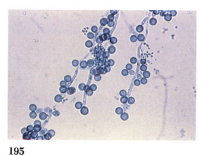

195

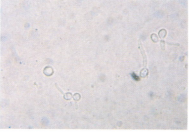

196

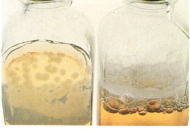

197

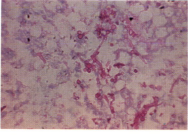

198

192. *Phialophora* infection, foot.
193. *Fonsecaea pedrosoi*.
194. *Candida albicans*, acridine orange stain.
195. *C. albicans*, blastospores and chlamydospores.
196. *C. albicans*, germ tubes.
197. *Candida tropicalis*, blood culture.
198. *Geotrichum* in tissues.

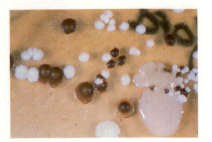

199

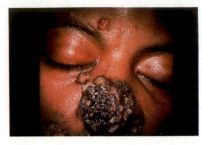

200

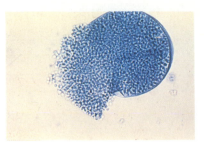

201

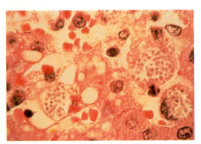

202

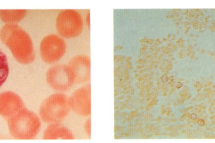

203

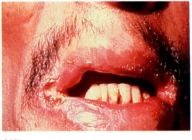

204

205

199. Birdseed agar, *Cryptococcus neoformans* and *Candida albicans*.
200. Disseminated coccidioidomycosis, coccidioidal granuloma.
201. *Coccidioides immitis*, ruptured spherule with endospores.
202. *Histoplasma capsulatum* in mononuclear cells of liver (1,000×).
203. *H. capsulatum* in neutrophil on peripheral blood smear (1,000×).
204. *Blastomyces dermatitidis* in tissue, Gridley stain (1,000×).
205. Lesions of South American blastomycosis about lips. Note purulent exudate at right edge of mouth.

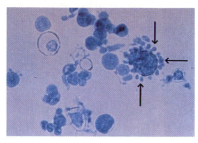

206

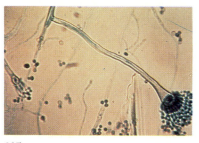

207

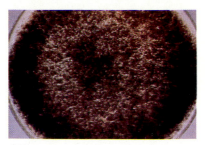

208

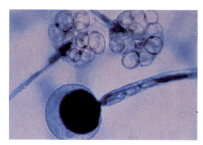

209

210

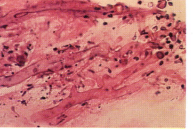

211

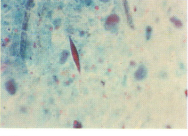

212

206. *Paracoccidioides brasiliensis*, numerous small buds.
207. *Aspergillus fumigatus* conidiophore and conidia (400×).
208. *Rhizopus* colony.
209. *Mucor*, spores inside sporangia.
210. Phycomycosis. Note large, nonseptate branched hyphae.
211. *Penicillium*. Spores borne in brushlike formation.
212. Charcot-Leyden crystals.

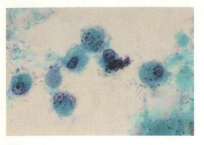

213

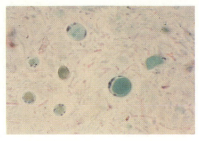
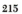

214

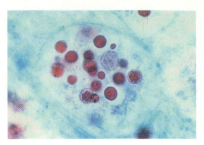

215

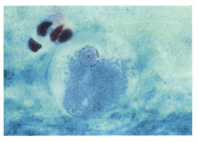

216

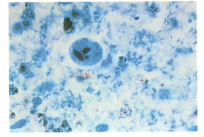

217

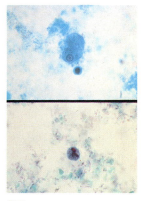
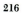

218

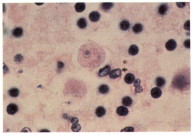

219

213. Polymorphonuclear leukocytes.
214. *Blastocystis hominis*.
215. *Entamoeba histolytica* trophozoite (contains ingested red blood cells).
216. *Entamoeba histolytica* trophozoite.
217. *E. histolytica* cyst.
218. *Top, Entamoeba hartmanni* trophozoite. *Bottom, E. hartmanni* cyst.
219. *Naegleria* in brain tissue, HE stain.

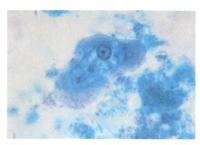

220

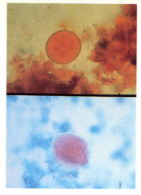

221

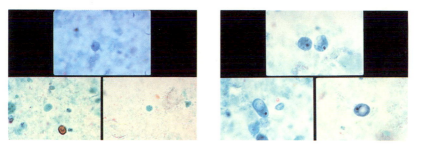

222   223

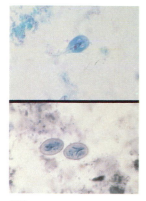

224

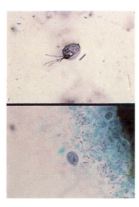

225

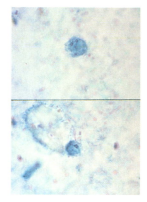

226

220. *Entamoeba coli* trophozoite.
221. *Top, E. coli* cyst, iodine stain. *Bottom, E. coli* cyst, trichrome stain (poor preservation).
222. *Top, Endolimax nana* trophozoite. *Bottom left, E. nana* cyst. *Bottom right, E. nana* cyst.
223. *Top, Iodamoeba hütschlii* trophozoites. *Bottom left, I. bütschlii* cyst. *Bottom right, I. bütschlii* cyst.
224. *Top, Giardia lamblia* trophozoite. *Bottom left, G. lamblia* cyst.
225. *Top, Chilomastix mesnili* trophozoite, silver stain. *Bottom left, C. mesnili* cyst.
226. *Top, Dientamoeba fragilis*, two nuclei. *Bottom left, D. fragilis*, one nucleus.

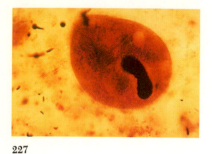
227

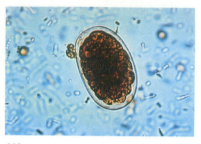
228

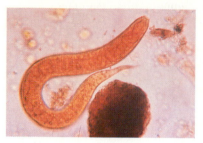
229

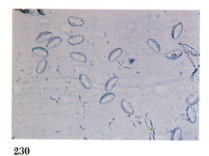
230

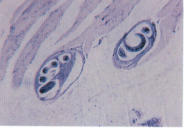
231

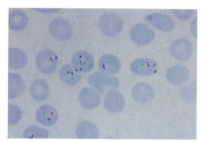
232

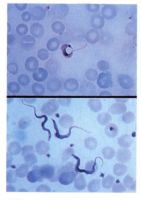
233

227. *Balantidium coli* trophozoite, iodine stain.
228. Hookworm egg, iodine stain.
229. *Strongyloides stercoralis* larva, iodine stain.
230. *Enterobius vermicularis* eggs (cellophane [Scotch] tape preparation).
231. *Trichinella spiralis* larvae (encysted in muscle).
232. *Plasmodium falciparum* early ring forms.
233. *Top, Trypanosoma cruzi* trypomastigote. *Bottom, Trypanosoma brucei gambiense* trypomastigotes.

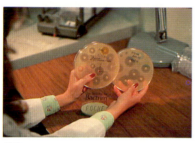

234

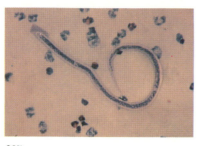

235

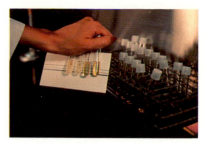

236

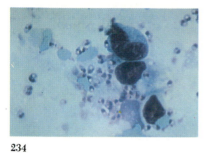

237

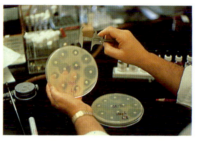

238

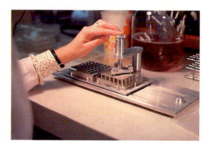

239

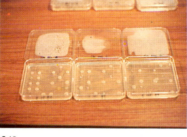

240

234. *Leishmania donovani* amastigotes.
235. *Wuchereria bancrofti* microfilaria.
236. McFarland nephelometer standards for turbidity measurement.
237. Kirby-Bauer disk susceptibility tests.
238. Disk susceptibility; measuring inhibition zones with calipers.
239. Steers replica inoculating apparatus for agar plate dilution susceptibility testing.
240. Plate dilution tests set up by Steers method.

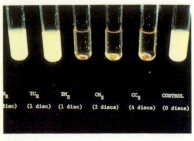

241

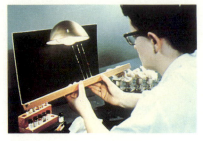

242

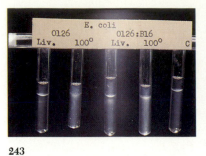

243

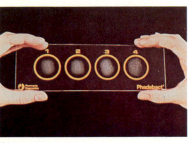

244

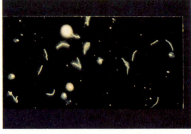

245

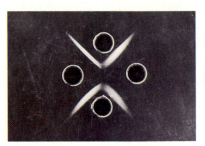

246

241. Broth disk technique for susceptibility testing of anaerobes.

242. Capillary precipitin test for identification of *Streptococcus* groups and types.

243. Quidin gel diffusion reaction. *Liv.*, Living cells; line of identity below meniscus. *C*, Control tube; it and heated tubes show no line.

244. Streptococcal coagglutination typing; positive reaction in circle 4, negative reactions in circles 1 to 3.

245. Positive FTA-ABS reaction with serum of syphilitic patient.

246. Ouchterlony gel diffusion reaction; antiserum in center well and antigens in other wells. Note line of identity.

26 GRAM-POSITIVE NON-SPORE-FORMING BACILLI

Corynebacterium

Kurthia

Listeria

Erysipelothrix

Nocardia

Actinomycetales, other

Rhodococcus

Rothia

Gardnerella

Lactobacillus

GENUS CORYNEBACTERIUM

The corynebacteria (Greek *koryne*, a club) are gram-positive, nonsporulating, nonmotile (with occasional exceptions) rods. They are often club shaped and frequently banded or beaded with irregularly staining granules (Fig. 26-1). These bacteria frequently exhibit characteristic arrangements resembling Chinese letters and palisades. The corynebacteria are generally aerobic or facultative, but microaerophilic species do occur. Anaerobic organisms formerly in this genus are now placed in the genus *Propionibacterium* (see Chapter 30). They have a wide distribution in nature. Some species are parasites or pathogens of plants and domestic animals; others are part of the normal human respiratory flora. The type species, *Corynebacterium diphtheriae*, produces a powerful exotoxin that causes **diphtheria** in humans.

Corynebacterium diphtheriae

Corynebacterium diphtheriae (Klebs-Loeffler bacillus) is a facultative, nonmotile, slender, gram-positive rod that is highly pleomorphic. In addition to straight or slightly curved bacilli,

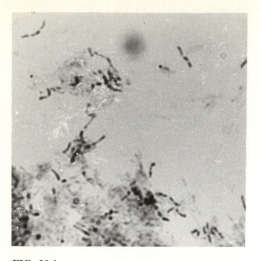

FIG. 26-1

Corynebacterium diphtheriae, granule stain
(1,000×).

club-shaped and branching forms are seen. The rods generally do not stain uniformly with methylene blue but show alternate bands of stained and unstained areas as well as deeply stained granules (metachromatic granules) that give the organism a beaded appearance. Individual cells tend to lie parallel or at acute angles to each other, resulting in V, L, or Y shapes. Although the appearance of *C. diphtheriae* in stained smears is highly characteristic, it **should not be identified by morphology alone;** many diphtheroids and actinomyces stain in the same irregular fashion and are also pleomorphic.

On primary isolation, *C. diphtheriae* should be cultivated on enriched media, such as infusion agar with added blood; the most characteristic morphologic forms, however, are found in smears made from a 12- to 18-hour culture on Loeffler serum medium (Chapter 42), which seems to enhance pleomorphism. The addition of potassium tellurite to blood or chocolate agar provides both a differential and selective medium. A cystine-tellurite agar plate is preferred by some workers. Bacterial contaminants are inhibited, and after 1 day *C. diphtheriae* appears as

gray or black colonies. This characteristic aids in distinguishing the organism in mixed culture and helps to differentiate the three types: *gravis*, *mitis*, and *intermedius*. Although the growth of *C. diphtheriae* is not distinctive on blood agar, specimens should be streaked on this medium (in addition to a tellurite plate), because a few strains are very sensitive to potassium tellurite.[16] Furthermore, the use of a blood agar plate permits isolation of group A beta-hemolytic streptococci, which may be responsible for the throat lesion or which may be part of a dual infection. The streptococci do not grow in the presence of the concentration of tellurite used for isolation of *C. diphtheriae*. However, it should be noted that some strains of streptococci, staphylococci, and diphtheroids can reduce tellurite and produce black colonies on cystine-tellurite agar.[16] The characteristics of *C. diphtheriae* are summarized in Table 26-1. In general, when grown on tellurite media the diphtheria bacilli are shorter, staining is more uniform, and the granules are less readily seen than when grown on Loeffler medium. For these reasons most laboratories use both media.

In nature *C. diphtheriae* occurs in the nasopharyngeal area (rarely on the skin or in wounds) of infected persons or healthy carriers. *C. diphtheriae* endocarditis has been described.[35] Cutaneous diphtheria is common in tropical areas and has accounted for a significant number of isolates of *C. diphtheriae* isolates from the northwestern United States and western provinces of Canada.[33] Most of the skin infections in North America are secondarily infected abrasions or insect bites, and staphylococci and streptococci may also be found. Diphtheritic lesions also occur in the nose, mouth, eye, middle ear, and, rarely, the vagina. The organisms are spread to susceptible individuals by droplets or direct contact. The **primary focus** of growth is on the mucous membrane of the respiratory tract, where the exotoxin is produced. Absorption of the toxin leads to the pathologic syndrome that characterizes the disease.

TABLE 26-1

Characteristics of *Corynebacterium diphtheriae* types

Organism	Morphology	Colonies on blood-tellurite agar	Hemo-lysis	Starch and gly-cogen	Glucose	Sucrose	Toxi-genic
C. diphtheriae type *gravis***	Short, evenly stain-ing	Large, dark gray centrally, matt, striated ("daisy-head"), irregular; brittle	–	+	+	–	+
C. diphtheriae type *mitis*	Long, curved, with many metachro-matic granules	Small, black, shiny, convex, entire, soft	+	–	+	–	+
C. diphtheriae type *inter-medius*	Long, barred forms with clubbed ends, few granules	Very small, flat, dry, gray, or black	–	–	+	–	+

*There is apparently no correlation between type and severity of disease in the United States.

Corynebacterium ulcerans also produces diphtheria toxin but usually causes mild disease. On occasion, however, it may cause severe classical diphtheria.[40] This disease may be related to drinking unpasteurized cow's milk. It appears that the organism is rarely spread from person to person.

Virulence test

Not all strains of *C. diphtheriae* elaborate exotoxin; however, it is now well established that infection of this bacterium by phage β or a closely related lysogenic bacteriophage is responsible for the production of diphtheria toxin. In this regard the one reliable criterion for identifying this organism is its **ability to produce exotoxin.** There are two primary methods for determining the toxigenicity of a suspect strain of *C. diphtheriae*—one in vivo and the other in vitro.

The **in vivo test** that yields satisfactory results for most workers is the one described by Fraser and Weld.[23] This is outlined below and may be applied to either a guinea pig or a white rabbit. The latter permits a greater number of tests.

1. Inoculate a Loeffler slant and a tube of sugar-free infusion broth from a suspect colony of each culture to be tested. Incubate both at 35 C. Check the slant culture for purity by staining after 24 hours. Use the broth culture after 48 hours of incubation for the test.
2. Prepare the test animal by clipping the back and sides closely. Disinfect the clipped area with alcohol or some suitable disinfectant. Make a line over the backbone with an indelible pen or pencil and mark off a series of 2-cm-square areas on both sides of the line.
3. Using a 2-ml syringe graduated in tenths of a milliliter and fitted with a 24-gauge needle, draw up 1 to 2 ml of each 48-hour culture and inject 0.2 ml intracutaneously into the marked squares, leaving in each case the square immediately adjacent (below) for the control. Refrigerate the syringe and contents for later use. **Inject a similar amount of a known toxigenic strain into one square as a positive control.**

4. After 5 hours, inject 500 units of diphtheria antitoxin intravenously into the rabbit's ear and wait 30 minutes. If a guinea pig is used, inject the antitoxin intraperitoneally.

5. Using the refrigerated syringe cultures, inject 0.2 ml of each culture into the corresponding square immediately adjacent (below) the original test site. This provides the **postantitoxin control.**

6. Read at 24 and 48 hours because the lesions are usually fully developed after the longer interval. A **toxigenic strain** produces a **central necrotic area,** about 5 to 10 mm in diameter, surrounded by a somewhat larger erythematous zone. The corresponding **control** should show only a **pinkish, swollen area** of 5 to 10 mm in diameter without any necrosis.

7. If both test sites show necrosis, toxigenicity of the test culture cannot be confirmed. This may be because the culture was not toxigenic or impure, because the antitoxin was inadequate or mislabeled, or because the test culture was some species other than *C. diphtheriae*. Some strains of *C. ulcerans*, a closely related organism, produce diphtheria toxin as well as an unrelated toxin that is not neutralized by diphtheria antitoxin.[16]

The **in vitro test,** first reported by Elek,[19] has been modified by a number of workers. The procedure recommended here is similar to the one described by Coyle and Tompkins.[16] To an autoclaved and cooled basal medium of proteose peptone agar* is added an enrichment of Tween 80, glycerol, and casamino acids* plus potassium tellurite. This is then thoroughly mixed in a Petri dish. Before the agar hardens, a 1- by 8-cm sterile paper strip saturated with diphtheria antitoxin* is placed on the agar surface and gently pressed below the surface with sterile forceps. The plate is dried at 35 C to ensure a moisture-

---

*Difco Laboratories, Detroit, Mich.

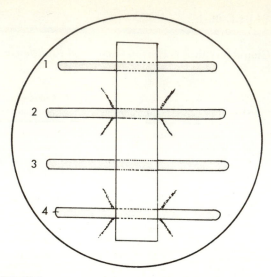

FIG. 26-2
Elek method for in vitro demonstration of toxigenicity of *Corynebacterium diphtheriae*. Filter paper strip impregnated with antitoxin (from top to bottom): *1,* known nontoxigenic strain (negative control); *2,* known toxigenic strain (positive control); *3,* unknown culture that is nontoxigenic; *4,* unknown culture that is toxigenic.

free surface. A loopful of the culture of suspected *C. diphtheriae* is then streaked across the plate perpendicular to the paper strip in a single line, as shown in Fig. 26-2. Four to five cultures may be tested on a single plate. The plate is incubated at 35 C and examined at 24, 48, and 72 hours. The antitoxin from the paper strip and any toxin produced by the growing diphtheria cultures diffuse through the agar medium and react in optimal proportions to produce thin lines of precipitate, as shown. These lines arise at angles of approximately 45° from those strains that are toxigenic. The test should include known **positive** and **negative** controls.

Two other types of tests for toxin production in *C. diphtheriae* have been described. One of these utilizes CIE,[61] which shows precipitin lines in 30 minutes. The second is a colorimetric tissue culture assay, using Chinese hamster ovary cell cultures in microtiter wells.[45] In the absence of toxin the cell culture produces sufficient acidic metabolites to change the phenol red indicator from pink to yellow within 56 hours. Growth inhibition can be observed within 24 hours in the presence of toxin.

It is important to recognize that several different strains or variants may be recovered on culture of a patient.[14] Some of these may be toxigenic and others nontoxigenic. The use of the Elek in vitro test for toxigenicity is helpful in this situation in that the plate is inoculated with a mass of growth, and therefore many colonies are screened simultaneously for toxin production with the one inoculum.[33]

The fluorescent antibody test has been considered useful in the rapid **presumptive** diagnosis of diphtheria when properly titered reagents are employed but should be used in conjunction with conventional cultural procedures.[15]

Antimicrobial therapy has little or no effect on the clinical course of diphtheria, but the use of antibiotics in patients may prevent additional toxin production, and the treatment of carriers may help limit an outbreak. Since erythromycin resistance has been noted in nontoxigenic strains, it is probably desirable to do susceptibility testing of all isolates of *C. diphtheriae*. In general, this organism is susceptible to penicillin, erythromycin, and most other drugs useful against gram-positive organisms.

Diphtheroid bacilli

As their collective name implies, diphtheroids are morphologically similar and sometimes indistinguishable from the diphtheria bacilli. *Corynebacterium pseudodiphtheriticum* occurs in the normal throat and is not pathogenic for human beings or laboratory animals. *C. xerosis* also occurs on mucous membranes of humans; it is basically nonpathogenic but has been recovered from patients with endocarditis, as have a number of other types of diphtheroids, and also from patients with other infections.[52] Other types of infection involving diphtheroids include meningitis, brain abscess, pneumonia and em-

pyema, osteomyelitis, and soft-tissue and wound infection.[31,47] Animal strains, such as *Corynebacterium bovis*,[64] have also been isolated from infection in humans.[10] This organism may be resistant to ampicillin, but it is sensitive to erythromycin. *Corynebacterium haemolyticum* has occasionally been isolated from infections, some of which are serious. *C. haemolyticum* may cause an infectious mononucleosis–like illness with sore throat, rash, and lymphadenopathy[21] (Green and LaPeter: J.A.M.A. **245**:2330-2331, 1981). *Corynebacterium pseudotuberculosis* produced pneumonia with eosinophilic pulmonary infiltrate and peripheral blood eosinophilia in a student of veterinary medicine.[34] *Corynebacterium pyogenes* or related diphtheroids have been involved in wound infections, empyema, pneumonitis, suppurative lymphadenitis, endocarditis, osteomyelitis, meningitis, brain abscess, and septic arthritis.[48] As noted in Chapter 11, *Corynebacterium genitalium* has been felt by some to be a cause of nonspecific urethritis; this requires further documentation.[20,22] Group E coryneform organisms, as identified by CDC, are now considered to be aerotolerant *Bifidobacterium adolescentis*.

In general, diphtheroids are relatively nonpathogenic and are primarily opportunistic pathogens, causing disease in persons with underlying valvular heart disease or with implanted foreign bodies or persons who are immunosuppressed.

Two poorly described species of *Corynebacterium*—*C. minutissimum* and *C. tenuis*—are said to be responsible for minor superficial infections, erythrasma, and trichomycosis axillaris, respectively.

Group JK diphtheroid bacilli

In 1964 Davis and associates[17] reported on four cases of bacterial endocarditis following surgery for repair of heart valve defects. An unusual fastidious diphtheroid was isolated repeatedly from the blood cultures of these patients. The

TABLE 26-2

Reactions obtained with some *Corynebacterium* species isolated from clinical specimens

Cultures	Catalase	Motility	Nitrate reduction	Urease	Carbohydrate fermentation	Acid from glucose	Acid from maltose	Acid from sucrose	Major acids produced[54]	ONPG	Pyrazin-amidase[60]
Group JK	+	–	–	–	+	+	–(+)	–		–	–
C. diphtheriae	+	–	+(–)	–	+	+	+	–	AFP (L)	NT	–
C. ulcerans	+	–	+	+	+	+	+	+(–)		NT	+
C. xerosis	+	–	–	–	+	+	+	+		NT	+
C. bovis	+	–	–	–	+	+	–	–	AL	+	+
C. minutissimum	+	–	–	–	+	+	+	–(+)		NT	+
C. pyogenes	+	–	–	–	+	+	+	±	AL	NT	
C. haemolyticum	–	–	–	+	+	+	+	+		NT	+
C. renale	+	–	–	+	+	+	–	+	L	NT	
C. striatum	+	–	+	–	+	+	–	+		NT	
C. pseudotuber-culosis	+	–	+(–)	+	+	+	+	–(+)	AFP	NT	+
C. kutscheri	+	–	+	+	+	+	+	+	PL	NT	+
C. pseudodiph-theriticum	+	–	+	+	–	–	–	–		NT	+
C. aquaticum	+	+	–(+)	–	–	+*	+*	+*		NT	

Modified from Riley and colleagues.[56]

ONPG, O-nitrophenyl-beta-D-galactopyranoside; A, acetic; F, formic; L, lactic; P, propionic; NT, not tested.

*Oxidative reaction.

( ), These reactions are recorded by a minority of cultures.

organism was very resistant to antimicrobial agents, and the infectious process was very destructive. Subsequently, there have been other reports of bacterial endocarditis and sepsis caused by this diphtheroid, often in immuno-suppressed patients. CDC has assigned the designation "group JK" to these diphtheroids and has presented data on 95 strains isolated from clinical specimens.[56] The majority have been isolated from blood cultures, with smaller numbers from genitourinary tract specimens, spinal fluid, wounds, pulmonary disease, and miscellaneous sources.[46,51,56,59,65] The organisms were uniformly susceptible to vancomycin but resistant to most of the other 17 antimicrobial agents tested.[17,31,56] Reactions of these organisms, in comparison with other *Corynebacterium* species isolated from clinical specimens, are presented in Table 26-2. The table includes data from two other studies—one concerned with acid metabolic products of corynebacteria and the other with pyrazine carboxylamidase activity in *Corynebacterium*.

GENUS KURTHIA

Kurthia is the only catalase-negative organism in the coryneform group of bacteria, although individual species of *Corynebacterium*, such as *C. haemolyticum*, are catalase negative. *Kurthia* is also motile, whereas most *Corynebacterium* species are not. *Kurthia* is motile at 35 C but not at 21 C, in contrast with *Listeria*. *Kurthia* does not attack carbohydrates. *Kurthia* was recently recovered from a patient with bacterial endocarditis.[49] The patient's heart valve was destroyed, and a cusp abscess was noted. This was the first definite report of infection involving *Kurthia*.

GENUS LISTERIA

The genus *Listeria* contains the clinically significant species *Listeria monocytogenes* plus the species *L. grayi*, *L. murrayi*, and *L. denitrificans*. *L. monocytogenes* is a small, nonsporulating, nonencapsulated, gram-positive rod, 0.5 μm by 1 to 2 μm in size, which exhibits distinctive **tumbling motility**. Isolated originally from

rabbits with a disease characterized by a great increase in circulating mononuclear leukocytes, it usually does not cause monocytosis in humans. *Listeria* has been isolated from blood, CSF, meconium, and various visceral and cutaneous lesions of humans. *L. monocytogenes* is responsible for an acute meningoencephalitis in infants and adults. It also is implicated in brain abscess, abortion and stillbirth, bacteremia, endocarditis, disseminated abscesses or granulomata in infants, spontaneous peritonitis in patients with cirrhosis, oculoglandular infection, and cutaneous infection. It is an important opportunistic pathogen in patients with hematologic and other malignancies and patients receiving immunosuppressive therapy. Special **cold enrichment** may be needed to effect recovery of the organism from sources with a heavily mixed flora.[4] A number of selective media for *L. monocytogenes* are available, but these are primarily for epidemiologic studies rather than clinical laboratory use.

L. monocytogenes is a facultative organism that grows well on infusion media, tryptose agar with or without added glucose and blood, or modified McBride medium (Chapter 42). It is not always isolated from tissue or other clinical material on the first attempt. The bacterium grows well at 25 and 35 C but poorly at 42 C and slowly (4 to 7 days) at 4 C. On sheep blood agar incubated at 35 C for 24 hours it produces small (1 to 2 mm), translucent, gray to white, **beta-hemolytic** colonies; hemolysis is slow to appear on sheep or rabbit blood agar. Most strains of *Listeria* show a narrow zone of beta hemolysis on blood agar plates. When cultivated on a clear medium, such as McBride agar, for 18 to 24 hours and examined by unfiltered, oblique illumination with a scanning microscope,* colonies appear characteristically **blue-green.** They are 0.2 to 0.8 mm in diameter, translucent, round, slightly raised, and watery in consistency.

Indole and hydrogen sulfide are not produced

---

*The plate may also be placed on a laboratory tripod and examined with a hand lens, with 45° oblique illumination.

by this organism; nitrate is not reduced; citrate is not utilized; urease is not formed; gelatin and coagulated serum are not liquefied. It is catalase positive and oxidase negative. The methyl red test is positive; the Voges-Proskauer reaction is negative with the O'Meara test but positive with Coblentz and other methods using alpha-naphthol, potassium hydroxide, and creatine. The organism hydrolyzes esculin, as demonstrated by the **blackening** of bile esculin agar after overnight incubation.

The **motility** of *L. monocytogenes* is best demonstrated by stab inoculating two tubes containing semisolid motility medium (see Chapter 42) and incubating one at room temperature (20 to 25 C) and the other at 35 C. Motility is more pronounced at room temperature than at the higher temperature, and a motile culture shows spread of growth from the line of the stab and the development of an "umbrella" 3 to 5 mm below the surface (Plate 99).

In meat extract broth with carbohydrates and bromcresol purple indicator (see Chapter 42) cultures of *Listeria* grown at 35 C for 1 week produce acid in glucose, levulose, rhamnose, maltose, and salicin; show irregular acidity in lactose, sucrose, xylose, arabinose, and dextrin; and rarely, if ever, produce acid in mannitol, inositol, sorbitol, dulcitol, or raffinose.

Test for pathogenicity

The **ocular** test (Anton) is reliable for pathogenicity. It is carried out by introducing two to three drops of an overnight tryptose agar slant culture, suspended in 5 ml of distilled water, into the conjunctival sac of a rabbit. A purulent conjunctivitis develops within several days and eventually heals completely. Keratitis may also occur.

Pathogenic strains of *L. monocytogenes* may be separated from nonpathogenic strains by three in vitro reactions. In a study by Groves and Welshimer[30] all CAMP-negative strains were nonpathogenic, and all but one CAMP-positive strain were pathogenic. All strains that produced acid in xylose were nonpathogenic, but not all nonpathogenic strains produced acid in xylose. All pathogenic strains but one showed an acid reaction in rhamnose, although not all strains showing acid in rhamnose were pathogenic.

Increasing evidence indicates the important role *L. monocytogenes* plays in both human and animal infections. The medical microbiologist should be fully aware that small, gram-positive, diphtheroidlike organisms isolated from CSF, blood, vaginal swabs, and so forth are not always contaminants. Because *Listeria* may appear coccoid and because it grows in 40% bile and 6.5% sodium chloride, hydrolyzes esculin and hippurate, and elicits the CAMP reaction, *L. monocytogenes* is confused not only with diphtheroids but also with group B streptococci and enterococci.[4]

Ampicillin and tetracycline are effective therapeutically in listeriosis. Penicillin appears to be less effective than ampicillin. Chloramphenicol is not effective therapeutically. The combination of penicillin and gentamicin worked effectively in synergistic fashion in experimental infection in mice.[18] Penicillin and streptomycin may be effective synergistically in human endocarditis involving *Listeria*.

GENUS ERYSIPELOTHRIX

Erysipelothrix rhusiopathiae (E. insidiosa) is the single member of the genus *Erysipelothrix*. It is a nonsporulating, nonencapsulated, nonmotile, gram-positive rod with a tendency to form long filaments. It decolorizes readily and may appear gram negative. It causes swine erysipelas and septicemia in mice. In humans it usually causes a self-limited infection of the fingers or hand (**erysipeloid**) but may cause bacteremia with arthritis or endocarditis. An erythematous, elevated, spreading lesion develops at the point of entrance of the organism; the disease generally can be traced to contact with animals or animal products. On blood agar medium smooth colonies are clear and very small (0.1 mm) and contain small slender rods. Rough colonies are 0.2 to 0.4 mm in diameter and contain long filamentous forms, showing beading and swelling; these colonies can spread out to simulate miniature anthrax-type colonies. Both forms stain evenly and may show deeply stained granules.

The organism is microaerophilic and facultatively anaerobic and grows best at 30 to 35 C. Hemolysis on blood agar occurs when 10% horse blood is used. A "test tube brush" type of growth (lateral, radiating projections) characteristically occurs in gelatin stab cultures at room temperature after 48 hours. Carbohydrate reactions are variable; most strains produce acid from glucose and lactose but not from sucrose and other carbohydrates. Hydrogen sulfide is produced; nitrate is not reduced; indole is not formed; and catalase is negative. *E. rhusiopathiae* is susceptible to penicillin, cephalosporins, and erythromycin, among other drugs. It is resistant to aminoglycosides.

The diagnosis rests on the isolation of the organism from a skin biopsy, tissue aspirate, or blood culture. Biopsy specimens or tissue aspirates should be placed into an infusion broth containing 1% glucose, which is then incubated at 35 C.[68] Subcultures should be made from this to a blood agar plate at 24-hour intervals. The catalase-negative *Corynebacterium* species, such as *C. haemolyticum,* can be differentiated from *E. rhusiopathiae,* because the former produce a beta-like hemolysis on blood agar and do not produce H_2S in the butt of TSI slants. *Listeria* can be differentiated from *Erysipelothrix* by catalase formation, motility, hemolysis, and H_2S production. Inoculation of white mice may be used to confirm the identification.[68]

GENUS NOCARDIA

Nocardiosis is a bacterial infection caused by species of *Nocardia* in humans and lower animals. It may result in chronic suppuration and draining sinuses of the subcutaneous tissue (mycetoma) or in a primary pulmonary infection resembling tuberculosis, which may spread to the pleural space and chest wall or metastasize to other organs, especially the brain and meninges.

Nocardia asteroides is an important opportunistic pathogen in patients with malignancy or those receiving immunosuppressive therapy and is usually responsible for a pulmonary infection. *Nocardia brasiliensis,* on the other hand, is the primary pathogen in mycetoma but may occasionally be found in pulmonary or disseminated disease, particularly in patients with poor host defense mechanisms.[13] *N. brasiliensis* also may cause a lymphocutaneous infection resembling sporotrichosis, as may *N. asteroides.*[42] *Nocardia caviae* may also cause pulmonary or disseminated infection. In a survey study carried out by Beaman and co-workers[8] involving 347 isolates of *Nocardia* strains recovered from disseminated pulmonary or primary central nervous system infection, only 83% were *N. asteroides;* the others were *N. brasiliensis, N. caviae,* or unspeciated strains. Bacterial endocarditis and other infections have been produced by a nocardioform organism, *Oerskovia turbata.*[55] This organism's taxonomic status is uncertain. *Nocardia farcinica* is also of uncertain taxonomic status.[43]

N. asteroides is a **partially acid-fast** aerobic to microaerophilic or capnophilic (CO_2-requiring) bacterium composed of branched filaments (**Fig. 26-3** and **Plate 19**) that fragment readily into bacillary and coccoid forms. The organism grows as a saprophyte in the soil, and systemic infection follows inhalation (**exogenous**) or introduction through skin abrasions, especially on the feet. *N. asteroides* may be demonstrated in direct smears of pus (opaque or pigmented sulfur granules are present occasionally) or sputum and in the sediment of centrifuged CSF. Gram-stained smears reveal thin, gram-positive, branching filaments (**Plate 18**) or coccoid and diphtheroid forms. An acid-fast stain* will show that some filaments retain the carbolfuchsin; young cultures are usually more strongly acid fast, whereas older cultures or subcultures are less so.

---

*The Kinyoun stain is recommended, followed by light decolorization with acid alcohol or, preferably, 0.5% to 1% aqueous sulfuric acid.

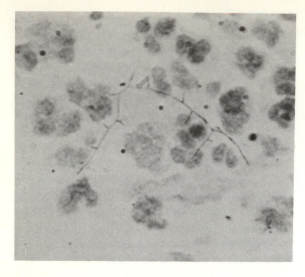

FIG. 26-3
Nocardia in Gram stain of sputum. Note thin, branching filamentous organism with irregular staining (1,000×).

All infected material in which delicate, branching, gram-positive filaments have been demonstrated should be inoculated heavily on two plates or tubes each of infusion blood agar and Sabouraud agar **without antibiotics***; both media should be incubated under 10% CO_2 at room temperature and at 35 C.† Enrichment media such as beef infusion broth or thioglycollate broth, to be incubated at 37 C, may be inoculated. Initial incubation at 45 C may help to recover *N. asteroides* from mixed culture, since *Nocardia* grows well at 45 C.[26] Cultures should also be set up for *Actinomyces* and *Arachnia* (see Chapter 30).

It should be pointed out that *N. asteroides* frequently survives the sodium hydroxide and other decontamination procedures used in pre-

paring sputum specimens for the isolation of *Mycobacterium tuberculosis* and grows well on the usual isolation media.[2] *N. asteroides* appears as a moist glabrous colony on the tuberculosis media and grows out within 1 to 2 weeks. The colonies resemble those of the saprophytic or other mycobacterial species; slide cultures reveal the branching acid-fast mycelium characteristic of *N. asteroides*.

On Sabouraud agar and blood agar growth may appear as early as 3 days as **small yellow colonies** resembling those of *M. tuberculosis*. After 5 to 10 days the colonies become waxy, cerebriform, irregularly folded, and yellow to deep orange (Plate 100). Microscopically, the colony is composed of delicate **branching** filaments that break up into bacillary forms. These are gram positive and acid fast.* Cultures should be held for 30 days before discarding.

Because of the similarity between some species of *Nocardia* and species of *Streptomyces* and other *Actinomycetales*, a variety of biochemical tests have been devised to differentiate them (Table 26-3).

1. **Demonstration of branching.** Demonstration of branching is best done in slide culture. *N. asteroides*, *N. brasiliensis*, and *Streptomyces* species branch, filamentous bacteria do not.
2. **Acid fastness.** As shown by the Kinyoun stain with 1% sulfuric acid decolorization, *N. asteroides* and *N. brasiliensis* are partially acid fast; spores of *Streptomyces* may be acid fast.
3. **Hydrolysis of casein.** See Chapter 44. *N. asteroides* does not hydrolyze casein, but casein is readily hydrolyzed by *N. brasiliensis* and *Streptomyces* species.
4. **Growth in gelatin.** See Chapter 44. *N. asteroides* either fails to grow or grows poorly, with a small, thin, flaky, white growth. *N. brasiliensis* grows well, form-

---

**N. asteroides* does not grow on media containing chloramphenicol.
†Growth on primary culture is much more rapid in an atmosphere of 10% CO_2.[11]

---

*Pure cultures grown in litmus milk for several weeks show a strong acid fastness when stained as described above.

TABLE 26-3

Cell wall and biochemical characteristics of pathogenic *Nocardia*, *Nocardiopsis*, *Actinomadura*, and *Streptomyces* species

Species	Cell wall type*	Decomposition† of							Acid from		Resistance to lyso-zyme
		Casein	Tyrosine	Xan-thine	Starch	Gela-tin	BCP milk	Urea	Lactose	Xylose	
Nocardia aster-oides	IV	−	−	−	−‡	−§	−‖	+	−	−	+
N. brasiliensis	IV	+	+	−	−‡	+	+	+	−	−	+
N. caviae	IV	−	−	+	−‡	−	−‖	+	−	−	+
Nocardiopsis das-sonvillei	IIIC	+	+	+	+	+	+ (rapid)	± (35%+)	−	+	−
Actinomadura madurae	IIIB	+	+ (14%−)		+	+	±	−	± (55%+)	+	−
A. pelletieri	IIIB	+	+	−	− (13%+)	+	±	−	−	−	−
Streptomyces so-maliensis	I	+	+	−	±	+	+	−	−	−	−
S. paraguayensis	I	+	+	+	−	+	+	+	−	−	
Streptomyces spp. (nonpathogenic)	I	+	+	−	(+)¶	(+)¶	(+)¶	± 50%+	+	+	(+)**
		+	+	+							
		−	+	+							

From Gordon.[26]

BCP, bromcresol purple.

*Cell walls of all actinomycetes contain glucosamine, muramic acid, glutamic acid, and alanine. In addition, major amounts of the following components are found in the respective groups: (I) L-diaminopimelic acid (DAP) and glycine; (III) *meso*-DAP; (IV) *meso*-DAP, arabinose, and galactose. Whole-cell hydrolysates of subgroup IIIB contain 3-*O*-methyl-D-galactose (madurose), absent in IIIC. *Nocardia* may be differentiated from *Actinomadura* and *Mycobacterium* by chromatographic lipid analysis and from the latter by the arylsulfatase test.

†Within 2 weeks at 27 C.

‡About 50% of strains positive by different method.

§Some strains reportedly liquefy certain gelatin media.

‖Usually turns alkaline.

¶Most species give positive results.

**Most species of *Streptomyces* are sensitive to lysozyme, as are *Mycobacterium phlei* and *M. smegmatis*; *M. fortuitum* and *M. marinum* are resistant.

ing discrete, compact, round colonies. *Streptomyces* species may grow well; growth is flaky or stringy.

5. **Animal pathogenicity.** Most isolates of *N. asteroides* are pathogenic for white mice and guinea pigs inoculated intraperitoneally; *N. brasiliensis* is usually not pathogenic. *Streptomyces* is not pathogenic, al-though some strains may cause a toxic death within 24 hours after inoculation.

As a test of pathogenicity for laboratory animals, a heavy suspension of the suspected culture should be prepared by grinding the growth from several slants of Sabouraud agar (incubated 1 to 2 weeks) with sterile saline, using a sterile mortar and pestle. This is combined with an equal amount of 5% hog gastric mucin, and 1 ml is injected intraperitoneally into a small (200-gm) guinea pig. The animal generally dies in 7 to 14 days, revealing a considerable amount of purulent peritoneal exudate at autopsy. Smears of this will reveal the characteristic gram-positive, acid-fast elements of *N. asteroides*. However, since there is considerable variation in strain virulence and guinea pig susceptibility to *N. asteroides*, animal injection is not reliable unless positive. *N. asteroides* is best identified by colonial and biochemical characteristics.

An early diagnosis of pulmonary nocardiosis, combined with vigorous treatment, is important to prevent metastasis to the brain. A microimmunodiffusion test for nocardiosis has been described.[9] Sera from 56 of 71 culturally proven cases of nocardiosis reacted positively. However, false-positive results are not infrequent, particularly in individuals who have tuberculosis or actinomycosis. The test has possibilities for improvement. In the meantime, it may serve as an adjunct in diagnosing nocardiosis. The majority of *Nocardia* strains produce beta-lactamase.[67] This beta-lactamase is most active against penicillin G and ampicillin, with lesser activity against carbenicillin. Sulfonamides appear to be the drugs of choice. It has been suggested that a sulfonamide combined with ampicillin or trimethoprim may be more effective.[1] Minocycline is very active in vitro, and limited clinical experience with cycloserine is encouraging. Amikacin is also very active in vitro, and one patient has been treated successfully with it.[70]

ACTINOMYCETALES, OTHER

The aerobic pathogenic actinomycetes are branched filamentous organisms related to the mycobacteria and include such major groups as *Nocardia* (already discussed), *Streptomyces*, *Actinomadura*, and *Nocardiopsis*.[26] Cell wall constituents and whole cell sugar patterns are very important in distinguishing between these various groups and related forms (Tables 26-3 to

26-6). (Further details concerning classification and differentiation of the various forms are given in the references cited.) Tisdall and Anhalt[62] described a liquid chromatographic method for analysis of isomers of diaminopimelic acid (DAP) in aerobic actinomycetes. It was possible to differentiate between *Streptomyces* and *Nocardia* by this means with a 1-hour liquid chromatographic procedure as compared with the 3 to 5 days required by thin-layer chromatography. A paper by Mishra and associates[41] provides a key for tentative identification of species of *Nocardia* and *Streptomyces*. This also includes members of *Actinomadura* and *Nocardiopsis*, although these are not labeled with those generic names in that key. The study of Mishra and others involves 658 isolates from laboratories of both human and veterinary medicine. Of the isolates received from clinical laboratories 35% were strains of *N. asteroides*. Strains of *Streptomyces* species accounted for 26% of the remaining isolates from medical laboratories. *Streptomyces somaliensis* is a recognized cause of mycetoma, but other *Streptomyces* have generally been considered saprophytic. These workers found that, after *N. asteroides* and *N. brasiliensis*, the third most common species from clinical isolates was *Streptomyces griseus*. They cited another report of a patient with cavernous sinus thrombosis and cerebellar abscess, from which *S. griseus* was isolated. Other organisms that may be found in mycetoma (madura foot) include *Actinomadura madurae*, *Actinomadura pelletieri*, *N. brasiliensis*, *N. asteroides*, and *N. caviae*. This form of mycetoma is sometimes called actinomycetoma to differentiate it from mycetoma caused by true fungi.

Some 50% to 75% of strains of *Streptomyces* produce beta-lactamase.[58] This beta-lactamase functions primarily as a penicillinase.

Dermatophilus congolensis is primarily pathogenic for animals. Occasionally, however, human infection may occur through contact with diseased animals.[26] In humans this results in pustules, furuncles, or similar lesions. The

TABLE 26-4

Major constituents of cell wall types of actinomycetes

Cell wall type	DAP		Glycine	Arabinose	Galactose
	Meso-	LL-			
I	−	+	+	−	−
II	+	−	+	−	−
III	+	−	−	−	−
IV	+	−	−	+	+

DAP, diaminopimelic acid.

TABLE 26-5

Whole cell sugar patterns of aerobic actinomycetes

Pattern	Arabinose	Galactose	Xylose	Madurose
A	+	+	−	−
B	−	−	−	+
C	−	−	−	−
D	+	−	+	−

TABLE 26-6

Distribution of cell wall types and whole cell sugar patterns in genera of *Actinomycetales* and certain other gram-positive rods

Streptomyces	I
Micromonospora	II
Actinomadura, Dermatophilus	IIIB
Nocardiopsis	IIIC
Cornybacterium, Nocardia, Rhodococcus	IV
Gardnerella, Kurthia, Lactobacillus, Rothia	No DAP
Listeria	DL-DAP
Erysipelothrix	No DL-DAP

organism grows readily on beef heart infusion blood agar plates, forming 0.5- to 1-mm colonies in 24 hours at 37 C. In 2 to 5 days these colonies develop orange pigment. Beta hemolysis may be noted. The organism is susceptible in vitro to many drugs, including penicillin, streptomycin, chloramphenicol, tetracyclines, erythromycin, kanamycin, and sulfonamides.

GENUS RHODOCOCCUS

Organisms of the so-called rhodochrous group that are taxonomically related to *Nocardia* and *Mycobacterium* have been assigned now to the genus *Rhodococcus*. Infections with these organisms are rare. A report by Broughton and co-workers[12] describing a young girl with osteomyelitis of fingers and a toe and septic arthritis of a knee caused by *Rhodococcus* also surveyed the literature and noted only nine cases of infection caused by *Rhodococcus* previously. These included pneumonia with septicemia, skin lesions, pericarditis, meningoencephalitis, and a ventriculoperitoneal shunt infection. Most of the infected patients have been immunocompromised or debilitated.

The organism forms orange or red colonies at 28 and 37 C when grown on Sabouraud dextrose agar. Growth usually takes 3 to 4 days. On microscopic examination one sees pleomorphic branching filaments without true mycelia or spores. The organism may be partially acid fast, but this property may be lost soon after isolation. *Rhodococcus* may be differentiated from the rapidly growing mycobacteria by its only slight acid fastness, its ability to utilize sucrose as a sole carbon source, and its inability to use trimethylene diamine as a simultaneous nitrogen and carbon source in the absence of arylsulfatase activity at 2 weeks. *Rhodococcus* may be distinguished from *Nocardia* by its ability to form acid from mannose, its usual ability to reduce nitrate, and its ability to utilize sucrose as a sole carbon source.

Antimicrobial agents showing activity against the *Rhodococcus* group include penicillin, tetracyclines (especially minocycline), erythromycin, and aminoglycosides.[12] Prolonged treatment is ordinarily necessary.

Corynebacterium equi has been reclassified into the genus *Rhodococcus* as *R. equi*. This organism is primarily an animal pathogen, but occasional cases of infection have been reported in humans. Gardner and colleagues[25] have reported a case of pneumonia caused by this organism. There are few reports of susceptibility studies with human isolates of this organism, and in most cases the disk diffusion method was used. These studies indicate that the organism is susceptible to erythromycin and aminoglycosides but resistant to penicillin. A study of susceptibility of 100 strains of nonhuman origin to 26 antimicrobial agents revealed the most active drugs to be penicillin G, doxycycline, erythromycin, lincomycin, and aminoglycosides.[69]

GENUS ROTHIA

Rothia dentocariosa is part of the normal oral flora of humans. It is also involved in dental caries and in periodontal disease.[5] However, it has rarely been recognized as a human pathogen. It has been described from a case of periappendiceal abscess, a case of pilonidal abscess[36] (along with a group F streptococcus), and two cases of endocarditis.[50,57] In the cases of endocarditis

the organism was not detected by gross visualization of the blood culture bottles. In one case it was seen on smear of the blood culture broth, and in the other case it was detected by blind subculture. It can be mistaken for *Streptococcus* or *Corynebacterium*, because it may appear either coccoid or diphtheroidal.

The organism forms off-white, smooth and creamy to rough and wrinkled colonies.[5] It grows best with CO_2 in the atmosphere. It is catalase positive in the absence of a source of hemin, which helps distinguish it from *Bifidobacterium* or *Lactobacillus*. It can be distinguished from *Actinomyces viscosus* and *Arachnia propionica* by lactose and mannitol fermentation (*Rothia* does not ferment either of these sugars). It can be distinguished from *Bacterionema* because the latter has characteristic whip-handle cells microscopically and produces metachromatic granules. Some strains of serotype 2 of *R. dentocariosa* produce an extracellular levan, a polymer of fructose. These strains can be detected as mucoid colonies on sucrose agar plates. The organism reduces nitrate and hydrolyzes esculin. Indole and urease are not produced.

R. dentocariosa is exquisitely sensitive to many antibiotics, including penicillin, aminoglycosides, erythromycin, tetracycline, and cephalosporins.[50,57]

GARDNERELLA VAGINALIS

The organism known as *Gardnerella vaginalis* is frequently recovered from genital tract specimens of women with clinically diagnosed vaginitis. Its role in vaginitis has been questioned, however. *G. vaginalis* has also been reported to be etiologically significant in cases of neonatal sepsis, postpartum bacteremia,[66] and bladder bacteriuria.[39]

Gardner and Dukes[24] originally placed the organism in the genus *Haemophilus*. Later work showed that neither X nor V factor is required for growth. Zinneman and Turner[71] recom-

TABLE 26-7

Characteristics of *Gardnerella vaginalis*

Property	Observation
Motility	−
Oxidase	−
Catalase	−
Indole	−
Gelatinase	−
Urease	−
Hemolysis on human blood agar	+
Hemolysis on sheep blood agar	−
Hippurate hydrolysis	+
Anaerobic growth	+
Nitrate to nitrite	−
Voges-Proskauer	−
Beta-galactosidase (ONPG)	Majority +
Glucose	+
Maltose	+
Dextrin	+
Starch	+
Sorbitol	−
Inulin	−
Salicin	−

mended placing *H. vaginalis* in the genus *Corynebacterium* because it stained gram positive. However, cell wall analysis, guanine plus cytosine ratios, and electron microscopy have shown *H. vaginalis* to be distinct from *Corynebacterium* and to have the cellular morphology and biochemical composition of a true gram-negative rod. It has recently been placed in a new genus, *Gardnerella*.[28]

Although several methods have been described for isolation of *G. vaginalis*, the medium described by Greenwood and others[29] seems to provide efficient isolation, rapid screening of plates, and quantification of this organism from clinical material. Colonies on this vaginalis agar (V agar) are used as inoculum for buffered single substrates (glucose, maltose, and starch).[29] *G. vaginalis* is glucose, maltose, and starch posi-

tive. Biochemical characteristics and other properties are shown in Table 26-7.

The finding of so-called clue cells (vaginal epithelial cells covered with bacteria) in wet mounts has been frequently stated to be diagnostic for the presence of *G. vaginalis*. Recent evidence, however, has questioned this method of identification because it lacks both sensitivity and specificity.[3]

As indicated in Chapter 11, there is question about the role of *G. vaginalis* in nonspecific vaginitis. It is likely that this infection is a mixed or synergistic infection involving one or more anaerobes in addition to *Gardnerella*. The disease is characterized by a malodorous vaginal discharge. When 10% KOH is added to such vaginal discharge, a fishy aminelike odor may be noted.[44] McCarthy and associates[38] have reported on the in vitro susceptibility of 56 strains of *G. vaginalis* to 21 antibiotics. Drugs that were very active included penicillin, ampicillin, vancomycin, cefazolin, erythromycin, clindamycin, chloramphenicol, and streptomycin. Other aminoglycosides and other cephalosporins were considerably less active. Tetracycline was variable in its activity, and cotrimoxazole was relatively inactive.

GENUS LACTOBACILLUS

Lactobacilli are gram-positive, pleomorphic, non-spore-forming, usually nonmotile rods. They are microaerophilic and catalase negative and produce lactic acid as the primary metabolic end product of glucose metabolism. They tolerate and produce acid well, giving a pH as low as 3 to 4 in well growing cultures. Some cultures may produce pigment. Microscopically, the organisms vary in shape from short plump rods, singly in chains or palisade arrangements, to long slender rods, singly or in chains. Surface colonies are variable in appearance from smooth to rough, "fried egg," and ground glass. Some are flat, grayish, and almost translucent. There is much variation in size. Some strains produce turbidity in liquid media, whereas others do not.

For the most part lactobacilli are not pathogenic, but there are a few reports of infection, including pneumonia,[37] bacteremia,[6] endocarditis,[63] and urinary tract infection.[53]

Concerning antimicrobial activity, penicillin, ampicillin, clindamycin, and cephalothin are all very active in terms of inhibitory activity but not in terms of minimal bactericidal concentration.[7] Cefoxitin and metronidazole have poor activity against these organisms.

REFERENCES

1. Adams, A.R., Jackson, J.M., Scopa, J., Lane, G.K., and Wilson, R.: Nocardiosis, Med. J. Aust. **1**:669-674, 1971.
2. Ajello, L., Grant, V.Q., and Gutzke, M.A.: The effect of tubercle bacillus concentration procedures on fungi causing pulmonary mycoses, J. Lab. Clin. Med. **38**:486-491, 1951.
3. Akerlund, M., and Mårdh, P.-A.: Isolation and identification of *Corynebacterium vaginale (Haemophilus vaginalis)* in women with infections of the lower genital tract, Acta. Obstet. Gynecol. Scand. **53**:85-90, 1974.
4. Albritton, W.L., Wiggins, G.L., DeWitt, W.E., and Feeley, J.C.: *Listeria monocytogenes.* In Lennette, E.H., Balows, A., Hausler, W.J., Jr., and Truant, J.P., editors: Manual of clinical microbiology, ed. 3, Washington, D.C., 1980, American Society for Microbiology.
5. Barksdale, L.: Identifying *Rothia dentocariosa*, Ann. Intern. Med. **91**:786-788, 1979.
6. Bayer, A.S., Chow, A.W., Betts, D., and Guze, L.B.: Lactobacillemia: report of nine cases, Am. J. Med. **64**:808-813, 1978.
7. Bayer, A.S., Chow, A.W., Concepcion, N., and Guze, L.B.: Susceptibility of 40 lactobacilli to six antimicrobial agents with broad gram-positive anaerobic spectra, Antimicrob. Agents Chemother. **14**:720-722, 1978.
8. Beaman, B.L., Burnside, J., Edwards, B., and Causey, W.: Nocardial infections in the United States, 1972-1974, J. Infect. Dis. **134**:286-289, 1976.
9. Blumer, S.O., and Kaufman, L.: Microimmunodiffusion test for nocardiosis, J. Clin. Microbiol. **10**:308-312, 1979.
10. Bolton, W.K., Sande, M.A., Normansell, D.E., Sturgill, B.C., and Westervelt, F.B., Jr.: Ventriculojugular shunt nephritis with *Corynebacterium bovis*, Am. J. Med. **59**:417-423, 1975.
11. Boncyk, L.H., Millstein, C.H., and Kalter, S.S.: Use of CO_2 for more rapid growth of the *Nocardia* species, J. Clin. Microbiol. **3**:463-464, 1976.
12. Broughton, R.A., Wilson, H.D., Goodman, N.L., and Hedrick, J.A.: Septic arthritis and osteomyelitis caused by an organism of the genus *Rhodococcus*, J. Clin. Microbiol. **13**:209-213, 1981.
13. Causey, W.A., and Sieger, B.: Systemic nocardiosis caused by Nocardia brasiliensis, Am. Rev. Respir. Dis. **109**:134-137, 1974.
14. Chang, D.N., Laughren, G.S., and Chalvardjian, N.E.: Three variants of *Corynebacterium diphtheriae* subsp. *mitis* (belfanti) isolated from a throat specimen, J. Clin. Microbiol. **8**:767-768, 1978.
15. Cherry, W.B., and Moody, M.D.: Fluorescent-antibody techniques in diagnostic bacteriology, Bacteriol. Rev. **29**:222-250, 1965.
16. Coyle M.B., and Tompkins, L.S.: Corynebacteria. In Lennette, E.H., Balows, A., Hausler, W.J., Jr., and Truant, J.P., editors: Manual of clinical microbiology, ed. 3, Washington, D.C., 1980, American Society for Microbiology.
17. Davis, A., Binder, M.J., Burroughs, J.T., Miller, A.B., and Finegold, S.M.: Diphtheroid endocarditis after cardiopulmonary bypass surgery for the repair of cardiac valvular defects: antimicrobial agents and chemotherapy, 1963, Ann Arbor, Mich., 1964, American Society for Microbiology, pp. 643-656.
18. Edmiston, C.E., Jr., and Gordon, R.C.: Evaluation of gentamicin and penicillin as a synergistic combination in experimental murine listeriosis, Antimicrob. Agents Chemother. **16**:862-863, 1979.
19. Elek, S.D.: The plate virulence test for diphtheria, J. Clin. Pathol. **2**:250-258, 1949.
20. Evangelista, A.T., Saha, A., Lechevalier, M.P., and Furness, G.: Analysis of the cell wall constituents of *Corynebacterium genitalium*, Int. J. Syst. Bacteriol. **28**:344-348, 1978.
21. Fell, H.W.K., Nagington, J., and Naylor, G.R.E.: *Corynebacterium haemolyticum* infections in Cambridgeshire, J. Hyg. Camb. **79**:269-274, 1977.
22. Felman, Y.M., and Nikitas, J.A.: Nongonococcal urethritis, J.A.M.A. **245**:381-386, 1981.
23. Fraser, D.T., and Weld, C.B.: The intracutaneous virulence test for *C. diphtheriae*, Trans. R. Soc. Can. Sect. **20**:343-345, 1926.
24. Gardner, H.L., and Dukes, C.D.: *Haemophilus vaginalis* vaginitis, Am. J. Obstet. Gynecol. **69**:962-976, 1955.
25. Gardner, S.E., Pearson, T., and Hughes, W.T.: Pneumonitis due to *Corynebacterium equi*, Chest **70**:92-94, 1976.

26. Gordon, M.A.: Aerobic pathogenic *Actinomycetaceae*, In Lennette, E.H., Balows, A., Hausler, W.J., Jr., and Truant, J.P., editors: Manual of clinical microbiology, ed. 3, Washington, D.C., 1980, American Society for Microbiology.

27. Gray, M.L., and Killinger, A.H.: *Listeria monocytogenes* and *Listeria* infections, Bacteriol. Rev. **30:**309-382, 1966.

28. Greenwood, J.R., and Pickett, M.J.: Transfer of *Haemophilus vaginalis* Gardner and Dukes to a new genus, *Gardnerella: G. vaginalis* (Gardner and Dukes) comb. nov., Int. J. Syst. Bacteriol. **30:**170-178, 1980.

29. Greenwood, J.R., Pickett, M.J., Martin, W.J., and Mack, E.G.: *Haemophilus vaginalis (Corynebacterium vaginale):* method for isolation and rapid biochemical identification, Health Lab. Sci. **14:**102-106, 1977.

30. Groves, R.D., and Welshimer, H.J.: Separation of pathogenic from apathogenic *Listeria monocytogenes* by three in vitro reactions, J. Clin. Microbiol. **5:**559-563, 1977.

31. Hande, K.R., Witebsky, F.G., Brown, M.S., Schulman, C.B., Anderson, S.E., Jr., Levine, A.S., Mac Lowry, J.D., and Chabner, B.A.: Sepsis with a new species of *Corynebacterium*, Ann. Intern. Med. **85:**423-426, 1976.

32. Hermann, G.J., Moore, M.S., and Parsons, E.I.: A substitute for serum in the diphtheria in vitro test, Am. J. Clin. Pathol. **29:**181-183, 1958.

33. Jellard, C.H.: Toxigenic and non-toxigenic *Corynebacterium diphtheriae*, Lancet **1:**650, 1980.

34. Keslin, M.H., McCoy, E.L., McCusker, J.J., and Lutch, J.S.: *Corynebacterium pseudotuberculosis*, Am. J. Med. **67:**228-231, 1979.

35. Love, J.W., Medina, D., Anderson, S., and Braniff, B.: Infective endocarditis due to *Corynebacterium diphtheriae:* report of a case and review of the literature, Johns Hopkins Med. J. **148:**41-42, 1981.

36. Lutwick, L.I., and Rockhill, R.C.: Abscess associated with *Rothia dentocariosa*, J. Clin. Microbiol. **8:**612-613, 1978.

37. Masure, O., Clavier, J., Gasser, F., Colloc, M.L., Kerbrat, G., and Chastel, C.: Pneumopathie aigue imputable à *Lactobacillus lactis*, Presse Méd. **9:**540, 1980.

38. McCarthy, L.R., Michelsen, P.A., and Smith, E.G.: Antibiotic susceptibility of *Haemophilus vaginalis (Corynebacterium vaginale)* to 21 antibiotics, Antimicrob. Agents Chemother. **16:**186-189, 1979.

39. McFadyen, I.R., and Eykyn, S.J.: Suprapubic aspiration of urine in pregnancy, Lancet **1:**1112-1114, 1968.

40. Meers, P.D.: A case of classical diphtheria, and other infections due to *Corynebacterium ulcerans*, J. Infect. **1:**139-142, 1979.

41. Mishra, S.K., Gordon, R.E., and Barnett, D.A.: Identification of nocardiae and streptomycetes of medical importance, J. Clin. Microbiol. **11:**728-736, 1980.

42. Mitchell, G., Wells, G.M., and Goodman, J.S.: Sporotrichoid *Nocardia brasiliensis* infection, Am. Rev. Respir. Dis. **112:**721-723, 1975.

43. Mordarski, M., Schaal, K.P., Szyba, K., Pulverer, G., and Tkacz, A.: Interrelation of *Nocardia asteroides* and related taxa as indicated by deoxyribonucleic acid reassociation, Int. J. Syst. Bacteriol. **27:**66-70, 1977.

44. Morse, S.A.: Sexually transmitted diseases. In Lennette, E.H., Balows, A., Hausler, W.J., Jr., and Truant, J.P., editors: Manual of clinical microbiology, ed. 3, Washington, D.C., 1980, American Society for Microbiology.

45. Murphy, J.R., Bacha, P., and Teng, M.: Determination of *Corynebacterium diphtheriae* toxigenicity by a colorimetric tissue culture assay, J. Clin. Microbiol. **7:**91-96, 1978.

46. Murray, B.E., Karchmer, A.W., and Moellering, R.C., Jr.: Diphtheroid prosthetic valve endocarditis, Am. J. Med. **69:**838-848, 1980.

47. Nazemi, M.M., and Musher, D.M.: Empyema due to aerobic diphtheroids following dental extraction, Am. Rev. Respir. Dis. **108:**1221-1223, 1973.

48. Norenberg, D.D., Bigley, D.V., Virata, R.L., and Liang, G.C.: *Corynebacterium pyogenes* septic arthritis with plasma cell synovial infiltrate and monoclonal gammopathy, Arch. Intern. Med. **138:**810-811, 1978.

49. Pancoast, S.J., Ellner, P.D., Jahre, J.A., and Neu, H.C.: Endocarditis due to *Kurthia bessonii*, Ann. Intern. Med. **90:**936-937, 1979.

50. Pape, J., Singer, C., Kiehn, T.E., Lee, B.J., and Armstrong, D.: Infective endocarditis caused by *Rothia dentocariosa*, Ann. Intern. Med. **91:**746-747, 1979.

51. Pearson, T.A., Braine, H.G., and Rathbun, H.K.: *Corynebacterium* sepsis in oncology patients, J.A.M.A. **238:**1737-1740, 1977.

52. Porschen, R.K., Goodman, Z., and Rafai, B.: Isolation of *Corynebacterium xerosis* from clinical specimens, Am. J. Clin. Pathol. **68:**290-293, 1977.

53. Poty, F.C., and Poty, J.A.: Infections urinaire à *Lactobacillus*, Presse Méd. **8:**3755, 1979.

54. Reddy, C.A., and Kao, M.: Value of acid metabolic products in identification of certain corynebacteria, J. Clin. Microbiol. **7:**428-433, 1978.

55. Reller, L.B., Maddoux, G.L., Eckman, M.R., and Pappas, G.: Bacterial endocarditis caused by *Oerskovia turbata*, Ann. Intern. Med. **83:**664-666, 1975.

56. Riley, P.S., Hollis, D.G., Utter, G.B., Weaver, R.E., and Baker, C.N.: Characterization and identification of 95 diphtheroid (group JK) cultures isolated from clinical specimens, J. Clin. Microbiol. **9:**418-424, 1979.

57. Schafer, F.J., Wing, E.J., and Norden, C.W.: Infectious endocarditis caused by *Rothia dentocariosa*, Ann. Intern. Med. **91**:747-748, 1979.

58. Schwartz, J.L., and Schwartz, S.P.: Production of β-lactamase by non-*Streptomyces Actinomycetales*, Antimicrob. Agents Chemother. **5**:123-125, 1979.

59. Stamm, W.E., Tompkins, L.S., Wagner, K.F., Counts, G.W., Thomas, E.D., and Meyers, J.D.: Infection due to *Corynebacterium* species in marrow transplant patients, Ann. Intern. Med. **91**:167-173, 1979.

60. Sulea, I.T., Pollice, M.C., and Barksdale, L.: Pyrazine carboxylamidase activity in *Corynebacterium*, Int. J. Syst. Bacteriol. **30**:466-472, 1980.

61. Thompson, N.L., and Ellner, P.D.: Rapid determination of *Corynebacterium diphtheriae* toxigenicity by counterimmunoelectrophoresis, J. Clin. Microbiol. **7**:493-494, 1978.

62. Tisdall, P.A., and Anhalt, J.P.: Rapid differentiation of *Streptomyces* from *Nocardia* by liquid chromatography, J. Clin. Microbiol. **10**:503-505, 1979.

63. Tornos, M.P., Perez-Soler, R., and Fernandez-Perez, R.: *Lactobacillus casei* endocarditis in tricuspid atresia, Chest **77**:713, 1980.

64. Vale, J.A., and Scott, G.W.: *Corynebacterium bovis* as a cause of human disease, Lancet **2**:682-684, 1977.

65. Van Scoy, R.E., Cohen, S.N., Geraci, J.E., and Washington, J.A., II: Coryneform bacterial endocarditis, Mayo Clin. Proc. **52**:216-219, 1977.

66. Venkataramani, T.K., and Rathbun, H.K.: *Corynebacterium vaginale (Hemophilus vaginalis)* bacteremia: clinical study of 29 cases, Johns Hopkins Med. J. **139**:93-97, 1976.

67. Wallace, R.J., Jr., Vance, P., Weissfeld, A., and Martin, R.R.: Beta-lactamase production and resistance to beta-lactam antibiotics in *Nocardia*, Antimicrob. Agents Chemother. **14**:704-709, 1978.

68. Weaver, R.E.: *Erysipelothrix*. In Lennette, E.H., Balows, A., Hausler, W.J., Jr., and Truant, J.P., editors: Manual of clinical microbiology, ed. 3, Washington D.C., 1980, American Society for Microbiology.

69. Woolcock, J.B., and Mutimer, M.D.: *Corynebacterium equi*: in vitro susceptibility to twenty-six antimicrobial agents, Antimicrob. Agents Chemother. **18**:976-977, 1980.

70. Yogev, R., Greenslade, T., Firlit, C.F., and Lewy, P.: Successful treatment of *Nocardia asteroides* infection with amikacin, J. Pediatr. **96**:771-773, 1980.

71. Zinneman, K., and Turner, G.C.: The taxonomic position of "*Haemophilus vaginalis*" (*Corynebacterium vaginale*), J. Pathol. Bacteriol. **85**:213-219, 1963.

27 ANAEROBIC GRAM-NEGATIVE NON-SPORE-FORMING BACILLI; IDENTIFICATION OF ANAEROBES

Bacteroides

Fusobacterium

Leptotrichia

Anaerobic vibrios

Five organisms or groups of organisms account for about two thirds of clinically significant anaerobic infections.[7] These are the *Bacteroides fragilis* group, the *Bacteroides melaninogenicus* group, *Fusobacterium nucleatum*, *Clostridium perfringens*, and the anaerobic cocci. Thus, the anaerobic gram-negative rods are very important. They are the most commonly encountered anaerobes in infections.

The identification of the anaerobic species of *Bacteroides* and *Fusobacterium* is based on a number of morphologic, physiologic, and genetic characteristics much too detailed to be considered satisfactorily in a text of this type. The interested reader is strongly advised to consult the excellent anaerobic bacteriology manuals currently available for full descriptions of technical procedures and methods of identification, including gas-liquid chromatography.[5,15,30]

Most of the anaerobes commonly encountered in clinically significant infections can be identified definitively, or with reasonable accuracy, by means of a relatively small number of tests that are easy to carry out in the clinical laboratory setting. It is not essential for all laboratories to do gas chromatography, but this procedure can be extremely helpful; more and more laboratories are using it. It is not a difficult procedure. These tests, noted in Tables 27-1 to 27-3, are described in Chapter 44.

Preliminary **grouping procedures** utilizing observations on colonial (Plate 102) and cellular morphology, susceptibility to antibiotic disks, and the results of a few simple biochemical tests are described in Chapter 13. These data may provide early and useful information to the clinician awaiting more definitive identification. Each "preliminary group" is studied by means of additional tests appropriate to definitive identification or further breakdown of identification within the group.

Definitive identification involves the use of additional tests beyond those used in the preliminary grouping procedures. Most laboratories should be able to perform these additional tests, which are not very complicated. As a minimum, however, every laboratory should be capable of isolating and maintaining an anaerobe in pure culture so that it can be sent to a reference laboratory for complete identification and susceptibility testing when necessary.

An acceptable standard system used by the CDC utilizes a thioglycollate base medium with added carbohydrates and other substrates.[28] The indicator is bromthymol blue, which turns yellow at pH 6. Various microtechniques have been developed, two of which are in common use. The API-20A* strip[11,12,23] (Plate 122) contains 16 carbohydrates as well as tests for indole, urea, gelatin, esculin, and catalase. The indicator is bromcresol purple, which turns yellow at pH 5.2. Unfortunately, a significant percentage of clinical isolates do not give clear-cut color reactions. Shades of brown that are difficult to interpret may be seen, especially with weakly saccharolytic organisms. This system is not helpful for identifying asaccharolytic organisms. A data base is available for identification after 24 hours as well as 48 hours. The tests may be easier to read at 24 hours. The Minitek*[11,12,29] system offers a wide choice of biochemical tests using microplates and disks saturated with various substrates. The indicator is phenol red, which turns yellow at pH 6.8. Only a true yellow color indicates a positive reaction. This system is also not helpful for identifying asaccharolytic organisms. The API Lactobacillus-50 strip can be used for additional substrates if desired. The API-ZYM system is not particularly helpful with gram-negative anaerobic rods.[14] A number of laboratories prefer to use prereduced anaerobically sterilized (PRAS) biochemicals.† PRAS biochemicals can be inoculated by open technique, using a special apparatus that provides gassing with oxygen-free gas during various manipulations. Scott Laboratories has recently introduced the PRAS II system, which employs small tubes of prereduced media and special systems for transferring inocula from plates to broth and then for inoculating biochemicals and reading the pH of these following incubation. Further details on these various systems are provided in laboratory manuals and elsewhere.[5,9,15,30]

Additional tests of value in differentiating gram-negative, anaerobic, non-spore-forming bacilli include the rapid glutamic acid decarboxylase test[22] (Plate 120) and gas chromatographic detection of phenylacetic acid.[18,21,33]

Various methods of **rapid processing** of cultures of anaerobes are outlined in Chapter 13. The fluorescent antibody technique is useful for rapid detection and identification of various gram-negative anaerobic rods.[1,19,25,34] Commercial fluorescent antibody reagents are available for the *B. fragilis* and *B. melaninogenicus* groups.‡ The *B. melaninogenicus* group reagent

---

*Analytab Products, Inc., Plainview, N.Y.

---

*Baltimore Biological Laboratory, Cockeysville, Md.
†Carr-Scarborough Microbiologicals Inc., Stone Mountain, Ga.; Nolan Biological Laboratories Inc., Tucker, Ga.; Scott Laboratories Inc., Fiskeville, R.I.
‡General Diagnostics Division, Warner-Lambert Co., Morris Plains, N.J.

(Fluoretec-M) also reacts with *Bacteroides biv-ius* and *B. disiens*.[34] Early studies with an immunoperoxidase method for identification of *B. fragilis* suggest that this technique might eventually replace fluorescent antibody techniques for identification of the organism directly in clinical specimens, as well as for identification of cultures.[17] The technique can be read macroscopically or rapidly with a light microscope at low power rather than a fluorescent microscope, and there are fewer nonspecific reactions. In the study just mentioned 91% of 44 strains of *B. fragilis* were identified. Other members of the *B. fragilis* group and other *Bacteroides* did not react with this antiserum. Other studies suggest that radioimmunoassay methods or other techniques will be useful ultimately in the clinical laboratory for detection of antibodies developed during the course of infection with *B. fragilis*.[16]

GENUS BACTEROIDES
Bacteroides fragilis group

Bacteroides fragilis group strains are the anaerobes **most frequently isolated from clinical infections**[7]; they are also the predominant organisms of the normal human intestinal tract. The importance of the group is further underlined by the fact that the organisms are more resistant to antimicrobial agents than are any other anaerobes. The group has been further divided into six species—*B. fragilis, B. distasonis, B. ovatus, B. thetaiotaomicron, B. uniformis,* and *B. vulgatus. B. fragilis* and *B. thetaiotaomicron* are the species most commonly found in infections. The *B. fragilis* group is important in infections related to disease, trauma, or surgery involving the bowel (Plate 37). However, these organisms may also be found in female genital tract infections and infections above the diaphragm, including pleuropulmonary infection, otitis media, mastoiditis, and intracranial infection.

On blood agar *B. fragilis* group strains grow as 1- to 3-mm, smooth, white to gray, nonhemolytic, translucent, glistening colonies (Plate 101). Gram stain shows a pale-staining, gram-negative bacillus with rounded ends; some are pleomorphic, with filaments and irregular staining (Plates 103 and 104). Bile is not inhibitory (it may be stimulatory) (Plate 119); catalase production is usually positive. *B. fragilis* group strains are uniformly resistant to colistin, kanamycin, and vancomycin (Plate 105) by the grouping technique described in Chapter 13. Speciation of *B. fragilis* and differentiation from the uncommonly encountered *Bacteroides eggerthii* and *Bacteroides splanchnicus*, which are also bile-resistant and saccharolytic, are done as noted in Table 27-1.

Bacteroides melaninogenicus group

This group was divided into two subspecies: *B. melaninogenicus* ss. *melaninogenicus* and *intermedius* and *Bacteroides asaccharolyticus*.[8] Subsequent studies show that the group is still heterogeneous. Two new species within the *B. melaninogenicus* group have been described. One of these is *Bacteroides gingivalis*, which has been split from *B. asaccharolyticus. B. gingivalis* can be distinguished from *B. asaccharolyticus* serologically (it does not react with Fluoretec-M) and by the fact that *B. gingivalis* produces phenylacetic acid.[4,18] Furthermore, *B. gingivalis* strains strongly agglutinate sheep red blood cells, whereas *B. asaccharolyticus* does not.[27] The second new species in this group is *Bacteroides macacae*, which is distinguished from *B. melaninogenicus* by the fact that it is catalase positive.[4] It is the only bile-sensitive pigmented *Bacteroides* that is catalase positive. There is still evidence of heterogeneity within the *B. melaninogenicus* group. Normally part of the microflora of the oropharynx and upper respiratory tract, gastrointestinal tract, and genitourinary tract, this group is less frequently isolated from human infections than is *B. fragilis*, but it is an important pathogen nonetheless. Charac-

TABLE 27-1

Characteristics of bile-resistant saccharolytic *Bacteroides* species

Species	Glutamic decarboxylase	Growth in 20% bile	Esculin hydrolysis	Catalase	Indole	Fermentation of — Glucose	Maltose	Rhamnose	Salicin	Sucrose	Trehalose	Fatty acids from PYG (or other fermentable carbohydrate)	Phenylacetic acid produced
B. fragilis group													
B. distasonis	+	+	+	$+^-$	−	+		V	+	+	+	A P IB IV S	+
B. fragilis	+	+	+	+	−	+		−	−	+	−	A P IB IV S	+
B. ovatus	+	+	+	−	+	+		+	+	+	+	A P IV S	+
B. thetaiotaomicron	+	+	+	$+^-$	+	+		+	$-^+$	+	+	A P IB IV S F	+
B. uniformis		+	+	$-^+$	+	+		$-^+$	$+^-$	+	−	A P IB IV S	
B. vulgatus	$-^+$	+	$-^+$	−	−	+		+	$-^+$	+		A P IV IB S F	−
Non-*B. fragilis* group													
B. eggerthii		+	+	$-^+$	+	+	+	$+^-$	−	−	−	A P IB IV S	
B. splanchnicus		+	+	−	+	+	−	−	−	−	−	A P IB B IV S	

Modified from Sutter and associates.[30]

−, negative reaction; +, positive reaction for majority of strains, includes weak as well as strong acid production from carbohydrates; V, variable reaction; $+^-$, most strains positive, reaction helpful if positive; $-^+$, most strains negative, some strains positive. Fatty acids: A, acetic; P, propionic; IB, isobutyric; B, butyric; IV, isovaleric; F, formic; S, succinic.

TABLE 27-2

Characteristics of nonpigmented and pigmented bile-sensitive *Bacteroides* species

Species	Glutamic acid decarboxylase	Growth in 20% bile	Pigment	Indole	Lipase	Urease	Arabinose	Glucose	Lactose	Salicin	Sucrose	Xylose	Esculin hydrolysis	Gelatin liquefaction	Fatty acids from PYG (or other fermentable carbohydrate)	Phenylacetic acid produced
											Fermentation of					
B. bivius	−	−	−	−	−	−	−	+	+	−	−	−	−	+	A IV S	
B. capillosus	−	−	−	−	−	−	−	+	−	−	−	−	+	−	A F S	
B. disiens	−	−	−	−	−	−	−	+	−	−	−	−	−	+	A P IV S	
B. oralis	−	−	−	−	−	−	−	+	+	−	+	−	+	+	A IB IV S	
B. praeacutus	−	−	−	−	−	−	−	−	−	−	−	−	−	+	A P IB B IV F	
B. putredinis	−	−	−	+	−	−	−	−	−	−	−	−	+	+	A P IB B IV F	
B. ruminicola ss. *brevis*	−	−	−	−	−	−	+	+	+	+	+	+	+	+	A P IB IV S F	
B. ruminicola ss. *ruminicola*	−	−	−	−	−	−	+	+	−	−	+	V	+	+	A S F	
*B. ureolyticus**	−	−	−	−	−	+	−	−	−	−	−	−	−	+	A S (F)	
B. asaccharolyticus	−	−	+	+	−	−	−	−	−	−	−	−	−	+	A P IB B IV	−
B. gingivalis	−	−	+	+	+⁻	−	−	−	−	−	−	−	−	+	A P IB B IV (S)	+
B. melaninogenicus ss. *intermedius*	−	−	+	+	−	−	−	+	−⁺	−	V	−	−	+	A P IB IV S F	−
B. macacae	−	−	+	+	−	−	−	+	−	−	−	−	−		A P IB B IV S	
B. melaninogenicus ss. *melaninogenicus*	−	−	+	−	−	−	−	+	+	−	+	−	+⁻	+	A IB IV S	−

Modified from Sutter and associates.[30]

−, negative reaction; +, positive reaction for majority of strains, includes weak as well as strong acid production from carbohydrates; V, variable reaction; +⁻, most strains positive, reaction helpful if positive; −⁺, most strains negative, some strains positive. Fatty acids: A, acetic; P, propionic; IB, isobutyric; B, butyric; IV, isovaleric; F, formic; S, succinic; ( ), sometimes detected.

*Formate-fumarate additive should be incorporated in all test media for this organism.

teristically it produces a **brown to black colony** on blood agar (Plate 106) after 5 to 7 days; it grows more rapidly and pigments much earlier on media containing **laked** blood. Young colonies on blood agar (prior to pigmentation) show a **brick red fluorescence** when examined under ultraviolet light (Plate 107).* By Gram stain the organism appears coccobacillary (Plate 108) and slightly pleomorphic in broth media. Bile inhibits its growth; catalase production is negative, except for *B. macacae;* indole is variable. The organism is resistant to kanamycin and variable to vancomycin and colistin by the disk identification technique described in Chapter 13. Further biochemical tests are required for identification within the group.[13] These are described in Chapter 44. Table 27-2 shows the characteristics of the members of the group.

Other Bacteroides species

Bacteroides oralis is of somewhat uncertain taxonomic status at this time. The organism formerly known as *Bacteroides ochraceus* is capable of growing in 5% to 10% CO_2 in air. It is now known to be *Capnocytophaga*.

Other less well-known *Bacteroides* are undoubtedly more important than has been appreciated. During a 6-year period at the Wadsworth Veterans Administration Medical Center, 22% of 679 specimens from infections caused by anaerobic bacteria yielded one or more *Bacteroides* species aside from those already considered.[20] The most commonly isolated were *Bacteroides ruminicola* ss. *brevis* (Plate 109), *Bacteroides ureolyticus* (formerly *B. corrodens*) (Plate 110), *B. bivius*, and *B. disiens*. It is important to note that some of these other *Bacteroides* species showed appreciable resistance to the beta-lactam antibiotics, erythromycin, and the tetracyclines. All strains were inhibited by chloramphenicol and metronidazole and almost all by clindamycin. These various lesser-known *Bacte-*

roides species were isolated from infections throughout the body, but there was a particular prevalence of infections involving them in the head and neck area, the pleuropulmonary region, bone and soft tissue infections, and, less commonly, intraabdominal and female genital tract infections. Bacteremia and central nervous system infections were very uncommon. Characteristics of these organisms are shown in Table 27-2. All these species are inhibited by bile; catalase is not produced.

GENUS FUSOBACTERIUM

A number of species belong to the genus *Fusobacterium;* included among those isolated from clinical specimens are *Fusobacterium necrophorum* (Plates 5, 6, and 115) (formerly *Sphaerophorus necrophorus*) and *Fusobacterium nucleatum* (formerly *F. fusiforme*). The study of 679 specimens from anaerobic infections at the Wadsworth Veterans Administration Medical Center revealed that 6% yielded less well-known species of *Fusobacterium*, as well as certain other uncommonly encountered genera of gram-negative anaerobic bacilli.[10] This group included *F. naviforme, F. gonidiaformans, F. varium, F. mortiferum* (Plate 117), and *F. russii*. Normally present in the upper respiratory tract, gastrointestinal tract, and genitourinary tract, the fusobacteria are responsible for serious pleuropulmonary, bloodstream, or metastatic suppurative infections (e.g., brain abscess, lung abscess, septic arthritis, and so forth). These organisms may also be found in intraabdominal infection and infection at other sites throughout the body.

Morphologically, members of this genus characteristically appear as long, slender, spear-shaped, pale-staining, gram-negative bacilli with **tapered ends** (Fig. 27-1 and Plates 113 and 114). Some species, such as *F. mortiferum*, show a bizarre pleomorphism, with spheroid swellings along irregularly stained filaments and free round bodies. Colonies on blood agar are generally nonhemolytic (some are alpha or

---

*"Blak-Ray" ultraviolet lamp and viewbox, Ultra-Violet Products, San Gabriel, Calif.

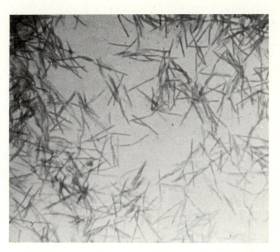

FIG. 27-1
Fusobacterium nucleatum. Note pointed ends (1,000×).

TABLE 27-3

Characteristics of *Fusobacterium* species

Species	Glutamic acid decarboxylase	Growth in 20% bile	Indole	Glucose	Fructose	Mannose	Hydrolysis of esculin	Propionate from lactate	Propionate from threonine	Fatty acids from PYG (or other fermentable carbohydrate)
				Fermentation of						
F. gonidiaformans	−	+	+	−	−	−	−	−	+	A P B F
F. naviforme	−	−	+	−	−	−	−	−	−	A P B L F
F. necrophorum	−	−	+	−	−	−	−	+	+	A P B F
F. nucleatum	−	−	+	−	+	−	−	−	+	A P B L F
F. russii	−	−	−	−	−	−	−	−	−	A P B F
F. mortiferum	−	+	−	+	+	+	+	−	+	A P B F (L)
F. varium	−	+	+⁻	+	+	+	−	−	+	A B L F

Modified from Sutter and associates.[30]

−, negative reaction; +, positive reaction for majority of strains, includes weak as well as strong acid production from carbohydrates; +⁻, most strains positive, reaction helpful if positive. Fatty acids: A, acetic; P, propionic; B, butyric; F, formic; L, lactic; ( ), sometimes detected.

slightly beta hemolytic) and vary from flat to convex, with opaque centers and translucent irregular margins (e.g., the "fried-egg" appearance of *F. mortiferum*). Convex, glistening alpha-hemolytic colonies (Plate 111) with a flecked internal structure (Plate 112), or bread crumb colonies, are characteristic of *F. nucleatum*. An excellent selective medium for *Fusobacterium* species is available (Plate 116) (Morgenstein et al.: J. Clin. Microbiol. **13:**666-669, 1981).

Bile is generally inhibitory (Plate 119), and indole is produced (*F. mortiferum* and *F. russii* are indole negative, and neither *F. mortiferum* nor *F. varium* is affected by bile); *F. necrophorum* often produces lipase on egg yolk agar (Plate 116). The fusobacteria are usually sensitive to colistin and kanamycin and are resistant to vancomycin on the disk identification test. Other biochemical tests are required for precise identification. Certain key characteristics are shown in Table 27-3.

LEPTOTRICHIA BUCCALIS

Leptotrichia buccalis is part of the normal flora of the oral cavity of humans and also has been found, on occasion, in the intestine and in the vagina. Human infections with this organism are uncommon. It has been recovered from dental infections, osteomyelitis of the mandible, bite wounds, infections of the head and neck, and the blood of a patient with lung abscess.[24] It has also been recovered from the blood of several asymptomatic patients following dental manipulation.

L. buccalis is a long, plump, straight or slightly curved, gram-negative bacillus that grows end to end in pairs or chains. The ends of cells that abut are flattened, whereas the other ends are often pointed. Colonies are 2 to 3 mm in diameter and have a characteristic convoluted appearance after 24 hours of incubation (Plate 118). The organism is saccharolytic, nonproteolytic, and nonmotile. Unlike other gram-negative anaerobic bacilli, *L. buccalis* produces lactic

acid as the sole organic acid end product of metabolism. *L. buccalis* is very sensitive to virtually all antimicrobial agents that are active against any of the anaerobes.

ANAEROBIC VIBRIOS

Anaerobic vibrios, usually not further identified, have been recovered, rarely, from central nervous system infection, bacteremia, pulmonary infection, abdominal infection, and soft-tissue infections.[7] *Butyrivibrio fibrisolvens* has been recovered from a patient with endophthalmitis and *Succinivibrio* from a patient with bacteremia.[7] *Desulfovibrio* and *Vibrio succinogenes* have also been isolated (rarely) from human infections. *Anaerobiospirillum succiniciproducens* was recovered from a patient with bacteremia (Rifkin and Opdyke: J. Clin. Microbiol. **13:**811-813, 1981).

CLINICAL EFFECTIVENESS OF ANTIMICROBIAL AGENTS

The in vitro testing of sensitivity of bacteroides and fusobacteria and other anaerobes to various antimicrobial agents is discussed in Chapter 36. Typical patterns of susceptibility to 23 antimicrobial agents are given elsewhere[31] (see Table 36-8).

Penicillin G is the drug of choice for infections caused by many of the gram-negative anaerobic rods other than the *B. fragilis* group, which is typically resistant. Resistance to penicillin G is also seen in some strains of the *B. melaninogenicus* group, *B. disiens*, *B. ureolyticus*, *B. putredinis*, *B. capillosus*, *B. bivius*, *B. ruminicola* ss. *brevis*, *F. mortiferum*, *F. naviforme*, and *F. varium*. Chloramphenicol is consistently active against all anaerobes and penetrates the central nervous system well. Clindamycin is also very effective,[3] but it does not cross the blood-brain barrier well, and a few strains of *B. fragilis*, 10% to 15% of strains of *B. ureolyticus* and *B. capillosus*, and many strains of *F. varium* are resistant. Metronidazole is consistently active against all gram-negative anaerobic rods[32]; it gets into the central nervous system well. It is the only agent consistently bactericidal against all susceptible anaerobes, including *B. fragilis*.[26] It should therefore be excellent for endocarditis. Surgical drainage and debridement are essential in the therapy of most anaerobic infections.

REFERENCES

1. Abshire, R.L., Lombard, G.L., and Dowell, V.R., Jr.: Fluorescent-antibody studies on selected strains of *Bacteroides fragilis* subspecies *fragilis*, J. Clin. Microbiol. **6**:425-432, 1977.
2. Bartlett, J.G., and Finegold, S.M.: Anaerobic pleuropulmonary infections, Medicine **51**:413-450, 1972.
3. Bartlett, J.G., Sutter, V.L., and Finegold, S. M.: Treatment of anaerobic infections with lincomycin and clindamycin, N. Engl. J. Med. **287**:1006-1010, 1972.
4. Coykendall, A., Kaczmarek, F.S., and Slots, J.: Genetic heterogeneity in *Bacteroides asaccharolyticus* (Holdeman and Moore, 1970) Finegold and Barnes 1977 (approved lists, 1980) and proposal of *Bacteroides gingivalis* sp. nov. and *Bacteroides macacae* (Slots and Genco) comb. nov., Int. J. Syst. Bacteriol. **30**:559-564, 1980.
5. Dowell, V.R., Jr., and Hawkins, T.M.: Laboratory methods in anaerobic bacteriology, CDC laboratory manual, DHEW Pub. No. (CDC) 74-8272, Washington, D.C., 1974, U.S. Government Printing Office.
6. Felner, J.M., and Dowell, V.R., Jr.: "Bacteroides" bacteremia, Am. J. Med. **50**:787-796, 1971.
7. Finegold, S.M.: Anaerobic bacteria in human disease, New York, 1977, Academic Press, Inc.
8. Finegold, S.M., and Barnes, E.M.: Report of the ICSB Taxonomic Subcommittee on gram-negative anaerobic rods: proposal that the saccharolytic and asaccharolytic strains at present classified in the species *Bacteroides melaninogenicus* (Oliver and Wherry) be reclassified in two species as *Bacteroides melaninogenicus* and *Bacteroides asaccharolyticus*, Int. J. Syst. Bacteriol. **27**:388-391, 1977.
9. Finegold, S.M., Shepherd, W.E., and Spaulding, E.H. In Shepherd, W.E., editor: Practical anaerobic bacteriology, Cumitech 5, Washington, D.C., 1977, American Society for Microbiology.
10. George, W.L., Kirby, B.D., Sutter, V.L., Citron, D.M., and Finegold, S.M.: Gram-negative anaerobic bacilli: their role in infection and patterns of susceptibility to antimicrobial agents. II. Little-known *Fusobacterium* species and miscellaneous genera, Rev. Infect. Dis. **3**:599-626, 1981.
11. Hansen, S.L., and Stewart, B.J.: Comparison of API and Minitek to Center for Disease Control methods for the biochemical characterization of anaerobes, J. Clin. Microbiol. **4**:227-231, 1976.
12. Hanson, C.W., Cassorla, R., and Martin, W.J.: API and Minitek systems in identification of clinical isolates of anaerobic gram-negative bacilli and *Clostridium* species, J. Clin. Microbiol. **10**:14-18, 1979.
13. Harding, G.K.M., Sutter, V.L., Finegold, S.M., and Bricknell, K.S.: Characterization of *Bacteroides melaninogenicus*, J. Clin. Microbiol. **4**:354-359, 1976.
14. Hofstad, T.: Evaluation of the API ZYM system for identification of *Bacteroides* and *Fusobacterium* species, Med. Microbiol. Immunol. **168**:173-177, 1980.
15. Holdeman, L.V., Cato, E.P., and Moore, W.E.C., editors: Anaerobe laboratory manual, ed. 4, Blacksburg, Va., 1977, Staff of the Anaerobe Laboratory, Virginia Polytechnic Institute and State University.
16. Hoppes, W.L., Rissing, J.P., Smith, J.W., and White, A.C.: Radioimmunoassay for *Bacteroides fragilis* infections, J. Clin. Microbiol. **12**:205-207, 1980.
17. Hsu, P.C., Minshew, B.H., Williams, B.L., and Lennard, E.S.: Use of an immunoperoxidase method for identification of *Bacteroides fragilis*, J. Clin. Microbiol. **10**:285-289, 1979.
18. Kaczmarek, F.S., and Coykendall, A.L.: Production of phenylacetic acid by strains of *Bacteroides asaccharolyticus* and *Bacteroides gingivalis* (sp. nov.), J. Clin. Microbiol. **12**:288-290, 1980.
19. Kasper, D.L., Fiddian, A.P., and Tabaqchali, S.: Rapid diagnosis of *Bacteroides* infections by indirect immunofluorescence assay of clinical specimens, Lancet **1**:239-242, 1979.
20. Kirby, B.D., George, W.L., Sutter, V.L., Citron, D.M., and Finegold, S.M.: Gram-negative anaerobic bacilli: their role in infection and patterns of susceptibility to antimicrobial agents. I. Little-known *Bacteroides* species, Rev. Infect. Dis. **2**:914-951, 1980.
21. Mayrand, D.: Identification of clinical isolates of selected species of *Bacteroides:* production of phenylacetic acid, Can. J. Microbiol. **25**:927-928, 1979.
22. Miranda, C.J., Edelstein, M.A., and Citron, D.M.: Evaluation of a Marion Scientific Corporation prototype rapid glutamic acid decarboxylase test for anaerobic bacteria, Abstract C36, Abstracts of the Annual Meeting of the American Society for Microbiology, 1980, p. 280.
23. Moore, H.B., Sutter, V.L., and Finegold, S.M.: Comparison of three procedures for biochemical testing of anaerobic bacteria, J. Clin. Microbiol. **1**:15-24, 1975.
24. Morgenstein, A.A., Citron, D.M., Orisek, B., and Finegold, S.M.: Serious infection with *Leptotrichia buccalis*, Am. J. Med. **69**:782-785, 1980.

25. Mouton, C., Hammond, P., Slots, J., and Genco, R.J.: Evaluation of Fluoretec-M for detection of oral strains of *Bacteroides asaccharolyticus* and *Bacteroides melaninogenicus*, J. Clin. Microbiol. **11**:682-686, 1980.

26. Nastro, L.J., and Finegold, S.M.: Bactericidal activity of five antimicrobial agents against *Bacteroides fragilis*, J. Infect. Dis. **126**:104-107, 1972.

27. Slots, J., and Genco, R.J.: Direct hemagglutination technique for differentiating *Bacteroides asaccharolyticus* oral strains from nonoral strains, J. Clin. Microbiol. **10**:371-373, 1979.

28. Stargel, M.D., Lombard, G.L., and Dowell, V.R., Jr.: Alternative procedures for identification of anaerobic bacteria, Am. J. Med. Technol. **44**:709-722, 1978.

29. Stargel, M.D., Thompson, F.J., Phillips, J.E., Lombard, G.L., and Dowell, V.R., Jr.: Modification of the Minitek miniaturized differentiation system for characterization of anaerobic bacteria, J. Clin. Microbiol. **3**:291-301, 1976.

30. Sutter, V.L., Citron, D.M., and Finegold, S.M.: Wadsworth anaerobic bacteriology manual, ed. 3, St. Louis, 1980, The C.V. Mosby Co.

31. Sutter, V.L., and Finegold, S.M.: Susceptibility of anaerobic bacteria to 23 antimicrobial agents, Antimicrob. Agents Chemother. **10**:736-752, 1976.

32. Tally, F.P., Sutter, V.L., and Finegold, S.M.: Treatment of anaerobic infections with metronidazole, Antimicrob. Agents Chemother. **7**:672-675, 1975.

33. Van Assche, P.F.D.: Differentiation of *Bacteroides fragilis* species by gas chromatographic detection of phenylacetic acid, J. Clin. Microbiol. **8**:614-615, 1978.

34. Weissfeld, A.S., and Sonnenwirth, A.C.: Rapid detection and identification of *Bacteroides fragilis* and *Bacteroides melaninogenicus* by immunofluorescence, J. Clin. Microbiol. **13**:798-800, 1981.

28 ANAEROBIC COCCI

Peptostreptococcus

Peptococcus

Veillonella

Acidaminococcus

Megasphaera

Next to the anaerobic gram-negative bacilli, the anaerobic gram-positive cocci are the anaerobes most commonly encountered in clinically significant infections.[10] Reflecting differences in their presence as normal flora, the **gram-positive** anaerobic cocci are relatively more prevalent in respiratory tract and related infections. They are seen in female genital tract infections and are less commonly encountered in intraabdominal processes than are the gram-negative anaerobic bacilli.[10,22] As with the gram-negative anaerobic rods, however, they may be found in virtually all types of infection. At the Mayo Clinic anaerobic cocci have been isolated from 31% of anaerobic cultures that yielded growth.[18] The most common isolate of the anaerobic cocci was *Peptococcus magnus* (Plate 125), which accounted for 32% of anaerobic gram-positive cocci recovered. Next most commonly encountered, in order, were *Peptococcus asaccharolyticus* (Plate 123) (16.5% of anaerobic gram-positive cocci isolated), *Peptococcus prevotii* (13.2%), *Peptostreptococcus micros* (12.7%), and *Peptostreptococcus anaerobius* (9.0%). At the Mayo Clinic the anaerobic cocci were involved in 6% to 12% of anaerobic bacteremias, with *P. magnus* being the predominant isolate from blood cultures. When *Peptococcus magnus* was isolated, it was usually recovered from septic arthritis, osteomyelitis, or soft tissue infections and was usually part of a polymicrobial infection, but in about 15% of cases it was present in pure culture. The **gram-negative** anaerobic cocci are not significant pathogens, as a rule, but may be found in mixed infections and, rarely, even in pure culture.[3]

Unfortunately, classification and characterization of the anaerobic cocci are somewhat complicated. For example, organisms formerly classified as *Peptococcus morbillorum*, *Peptococcus constellatus*, and *Peptostreptococcus intermedius* actually belong to the genus *Streptococcus*, since they produce lactic acid as a metabolic end product without significant amounts of other products. These organisms become aerotolerant after one or more subcultures. On the other hand, some strains of *Streptococcus* are obligately anaerobic. On the basis of DNA-DNA homology values, *Peptococcus saccharolyticus* was found to have relatedness to a number of staphylococcal species at the genus level and no significant genetic relatedness to other members of the genus *Peptococcus*.[13] This organism is relatively aerotolerant. The so-called **microaerophilic** streptococci have occasioned the greatest confusion. These organisms have often been included with the anaerobic cocci because they are readily overlooked if one does not use good anaerobic transport and culture techniques. Thus, workers interested in anaerobes have recovered these organisms much more commonly than have other investigators. However, the microaerophilic streptococci are actually members of the genus *Streptococcus* on the basis of metabolic end product analysis (Harder and associates, unpublished data). They can often be speciated and include, for example, *S. mutans*, *S. mitis*, *S. anginosus*, *S. sanguis*, *S. MG*, and *S. salivarius*. Although "viridans streptococci" have been said to be nonpathogenic, except in subacute bacterial endocarditis, it is clear that these organisms are not infrequently involved (and not uncommonly in pure culture) in such serious infections as brain abscess, necrotizing pneumonia, liver abscess, postabortal sepsis, and so forth.[10] Anaerobic cocci, particularly *Peptococcus*, may also be found as (skin) contaminants in blood cultures. *P. saccharolyticus* was found to be a numerically important organism on the skin of the antecubital fossa of the arm of about 20% of subjects studied.[9]

Preliminary grouping of these organisms is discussed in Chapter 13. The tests noted in Table 28-1, for further characterization, are described in Chapter 44. Additional data are found in three reference manuals.[8,12,20]

Definitive identification of the anaerobic cocci depends on gas chromatographic analysis of end products; nevertheless, as shown in Table 28-1, the use of a number of simple tests permits speciation of many of these organisms. Certainly characterization adequate for guidance regarding immediate treatment of the infected patient is possible by these means. Reference laboratories may be used for definitive identification where this is of interest.

Additional tests have been described recently for characterization of anaerobic cocci. A new tyrosine medium permits ready differentiation of *P. anaerobius* from other anaerobic gram-positive cocci.[1] *P. anaerobius* degrades tyrosine crystals in the medium, leading to a clear zone around the colony. In the study 135 of 136 other anaerobic gram-positive cocci failed to degrade tyrosine. The single strain that did degrade it was 1 of 13 strains of *P. micros* studied. Moss and colleagues[14] described the cellular fatty acid patterns of *Peptococcus variabilis* and *P. anaerobius*. The patterns of these two organisms differed markedly from each other and from a number of other bacteria studied by those workers. Additional studies are required before it can be determined whether this technique would be useful for distinguishing various anaerobic cocci. Graham and Falkler[11] were able to extract an antigen from *P. anaerobius* that could be used to

TABLE 28-1

Characteristics of anaerobic cocci*

Organism	Catalase	Indole production	Nitrate reduction	Gelatin liquefaction	Fermentation of						Esculin hydrolysis	Propionate from threonine	Growth stimulation with Tween 80	Fatty acids from PYG (or other fermentable carbohydrate)
					Cellobiose	Glucose	Lactose	Fructose	Maltose	Sucrose				
Gram-negative cocci														
Acidaminococcus fermentans	−	−	−	−	−	−	−	−	−	−	−	+	−	A B (P L)
Megasphaera elsdenii	−	−	−	−	−	+	−	+	+	−	−	+	−	A IB B IV V H (P F)
V. parvula	V	−	+	−	−	−	−	−	−	−	−	−	−	A P
Gram-positive cocci														
Peptococcus asaccharolyticus	V	+	−	−	−	−	−	−	−	−	−	−	V	A B (F L)
P. magnus†	V	−	−	V	−	−	−	−	−	−	−	−	V	A (F)
P. prevotii‡	V	−	−	−	−	−	−	+	−	−	−	−	V	A B (P F L)
P. saccharolyticus§	+⁻	−	+⁻	+	−	+	−	+	+	−	−	−	V	A
Peptostreptococcus anaerobius	−	−	−⁺	+	−	+	−	+	−	−	−	+	V	A IV IC (P IB B L)
P. micros	−	−	−	−	−	−	−	−	−	−	−	−	+	A (F)
P. parvulus	−	−	−	+	−	+	+	−	−	−	−	−	V	A L
P. productus	−	−	−	−	+	+	+	+	+	+	+	−	+	A S

Sutter and associates.[20]

−, negative reaction; +, positive reaction for majority of strains, includes weak as well as strong acid production from carbohydrates; V, variable reaction; +⁻, most strains positive, reaction helpful if positive; −⁺, most strains negative, some strains positive. Fatty acids: A, acetic; P, propionic; IB, isobutyric; B, butyric; IV, isovaleric; V, valeric; IC, isocaproic; H, hexanoic (caproic); F, formic; L, lactic; S, succinic; ( ), sometimes detected.

*Peptococcus morbillorum and Peptostreptococcus intermedius are not included, since they become aerotolerant after one or more subcultures and produce lactic acid without significant amounts of other acids or gas. Therefore, they should be identified as Streptococcus species. These organisms are commonly designated "microaerophilic streptococci."

†P. magnus is probably the same as Peptococcus anaerobius.

‡P. prevotii is not recognized in Bergey's Manual,[6] ed. 8, and may be a variant of P. asaccharolyticus.

§P. saccharolyticus is more closely related genetically to the genus Staphylococcus than to Peptococcus.

readily and rapidly identify *P. anaerobius* in a capillary precipitin test. Subsequently, Wong and others[24] prepared antisera against antigens of all of the *Peptostreptococcus* species. Following absorption, it was found that the antisera were specific for each *Peptostreptococcus* species by Ouchterlony tests or by coagglutination reaction. The species of *Peptostreptococcus* were serologically distinct from members of the genus *Peptococcus* and the genus *Streptococcus*.

GENUS PEPTOSTREPTOCOCCUS

Material suspected of harboring anaerobic streptococci should be plated without delay on fresh blood agar and enriched thioglycollate medium, placed immediately into an **anaerobic** atmosphere (see Chapter 13 for anaerobic methods), and examined after 48 hours' incubation. Peptostreptococci appear as minute, shiny, smooth, convex gray to white opaque colonies. Hemolysis is variable; gas and a foul odor are generally apparent in thioglycollate medium. Subcultures incubated aerobically and anaerobically should reveal only anaerobic growth of a catalase-negative, gram-positive streptococcus; this may sometimes exhibit a sharp, pungent odor.[17] See Table 28-1 for characterization tests. In addition, it has been noted that DNase is produced by *P. anaerobius* and *P. intermedius* (the latter is a *Streptococcus*).[16] However, occasional strains of other anerobic gram-positive cocci also produce DNase. One of the anaerobic cocci most commonly encountered in infections in our experience, *P. anaerobius* (Fig. 28-1), is readily identified by the SPS disk test[23] (Plate 124) (see Chapter 13, and the tyrosine degradation test previously mentioned).

The drug of choice in the treatment of infections caused by *Peptostreptococcus* is generally benzyl penicillin (penicillin G), although occasional strains require as much as 32 units/ml for inhibition[21] and therefore are best treated with another agent. Clindamycin and chloramphenicol have also proved effective, especially in

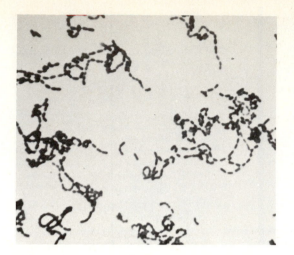

FIG. 28-1
Peptostreptococcus anaerobius (1,000×).

mixed anaerobic infections.[2] Metronidazole is active against 97% of strains.[21] There is evidence that the peptostreptococci may act synergistically with *Bacteroides* or *Staphylococcus aureus* to produce tissue necrosis in mixed infections.[15]

GENUS PEPTOCOCCUS

The species of this genus are **obligate anaerobes,** and although they are found normally in the respiratory and genital tracts and on the skin of humans, they have been isolated from a variety of infections, often in mixed culture. They occur in irregular masses, and some resemble *S. aureus* microscopically (Fig. 28-2). Such an appearance on direct Gram stain, with no staphylococci recovered on aerobic culture after 18 to 24 hours, should suggest the possibility of *Peptococcus*.

Peptococci are incriminated in anaerobic infections frequently. An excellent paper by Bourgault and co-workers[4] stresses the significance of *P. magnus* in infections. In a study covering a 3½-year period, this organism was the most common species of anaerobic gram-positive coccus isolated. Most of the infections were mixed, involving bones and joints, soft tissue,

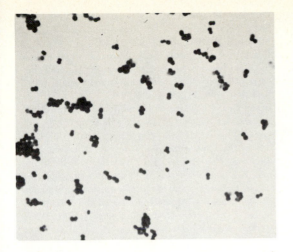

FIG. 28-2
Peptococcus prevotii (1,000×).

foot ulcers, the abdominal cavity, and miscellaneous types of infection. There were 18 patients with pure cultures of *P. magnus* isolated from their infections; 15 of these had foreign bodies present.

It may be possible to distinguish peptostreptococci from peptococci in that the latter are sometimes catalase positive. Peptococci do not produce a sharp, pungent odor. In general, however, there is no simple way to distinguish between *Peptococcus* and *Peptostreptococcus*. The tests noted in Table 28-1 often provide this differentiation and speciation.

Peptococci are usually very sensitive to penicillin G, and this drug would be the agent of choice in *Peptococcus* infections. Chloramphenicol is always effective. All but 2% of strains are susceptible to metronidazole. However, in the case of clindamycin significant resistance has become apparent recently; at present, 10% to 15% of strains are resistant.[21]

GRAM-NEGATIVE ANAEROBIC COCCI

Organisms in the genus *Veillonella* occur in pairs, short chains, and irregular clumps. They are gram negative and strictly **anaerobic.** The cells are smaller than neisseriae, and *Veillonella* is less fastidious in its nutritional requirements. It occurs normally in the respiratory tract, the intestinal tract, and the genitourinary tract of humans and animals. Normally *Veillonella* is not considered pathogenic, but it is found in mixed infection and, rarely, as a single infecting organism.[3] Chow and associates[7] reported that *Veillonella* strains fluoresce **red** under long-wave ultraviolet light. Unlike *B. melaninogenicus*, fluorescence does not depend on blood in the medium and is lost rapidly after exposure of colonies to air.

Acidaminococcus and *Megasphaera* differ from *Veillonella* in being nitrate negative. All three genera are distinct in terms of metabolic end products.[6] *Megasphaera* is fermentative, whereas *Acidaminococcus* is not (Table 28-1). *M. elsdenii* commonly stains gram positive, although it is really gram negative on the basis of cell wall composition. Both *Acidaminococcus* and *Megasphaera* are found normally in the lower intestinal tract of humans.[19] *M. elsdenii* presumably is indigenous to the oral cavity as well, since it has been recovered as part of the flora of a putrid lung abscess.[19] *A. fermentans* was found in a mixed aerobic-anaerobic intraabdominal abscess.[19] A case of endocarditis caused by *M. elsdenii* has been reported.[5]

REFERENCES

1. Babcock, J.B: Tyrosine degradation in presumptive identification of *Peptostreptococcus anaerobius*, J. Clin. Microbiol. **9:**358-361, 1979.
2. Bartlett, J.G., Sutter, V.L., and Finegold, S.M.: Treatment of anaerobic infections with lincomycin and clindamycin, N. Engl. J. Med. **287:**1006-1010, 1972.
3. Borchardt, K.A., Baker, M., and Gelber, R.: *Veillonella parvula* septicemia and osteomyelitis, Ann. Intern. Med. **86:**63-64, 1977.
4. Bourgault, A.-M., Rosenblatt, J.E., and Fitzgerald, R.H.: *Peptococcus magnus:* a significant human pathogen, Ann. Intern. Med. **93:**244-248, 1980.
5. Brancaccio, M., and Legendre, G.G.: *Megasphaera elsdenii* endocarditis, J. Clin. Microbiol. **10:**72-74, 1979.
6. Buchanan, R.E., and Gibbons, N.E., editors: Bergey's manual of determinative bacteriology, ed. 8, Baltimore, 1974, The Williams & Wilkins Co.

7. Chow, A.W., Patten, V., and Guze, L.B.: Rapid screening of *Veillonella* by ultraviolet fluorescence, J. Clin. Microbiol. **2:**546-548, 1975.

8. Dowell, V.R., Jr., and Hawkins, T.M.: Laboratory methods in anaerobic bacteriology, CDC laboratory manual, DHEW Pub. No. (CDC) 74-8272, Washington, D.C., 1974, U.S. Government Printing Office.

9. Evans, C.A., Mattern, K.L., and Hallam, S.L.: Isolation and identification of *Peptococcus saccharolyticus* from human skin, J. Clin. Microbiol. **7:**261-264, 1978.

10. Finegold, S.M.: Anaerobic bacteria in human disease, New York, 1977, Academic Press, Inc.

11. Graham, M.B., and Falkler, W.A., Jr.: Extractable antigen shared by *Peptostreptococcus anaerobius* strains, J. Clin. Microbiol. **9:**507-510, 1979.

12. Holdeman, L.V., Cato, E.P., and Moore, W.E.C., editors: Anaerobe laboratory manual, ed. 4, Blacksburg, Va., 1977, Staff of the Anaerobe Laboratory, Virginia Polytechnic Institute and State University.

13. Kilpper, R., Buhl, U., and Schleifer, K.H.: Nucleic acid homology studies between *Peptococcus saccharolyticus* and various anaerobic and facultative anaerobic gram-positive cocci, FEMS Microbiol. Lett. **8:**205-210, 1980.

14. Moss, C.W., Lambert, M.A., and Lombard, G.L.: Cellular fatty acids of *Peptococcus variabilis* and *Peptostreptococcus anaerobius*, J. Clin. Microbiol. **5:**665-667, 1977.

15. Pien, F.D., Thompson, R.L., and Martin, W.J.: Clinical and bacteriologic studies of anaerobic gram-positive cocci, Mayo Clinic. Proc. **47:**251-257, 1972.

16. Porschen, R.K., and Sonntag, S.: Extracellular deoxyribonuclease production by anaerobic bacteria, Appl. Microbiol. **27:**1031-1033, 1974.

17. Rogosa, M.: Peptococcaceae, a new family to include the gram-positive, anaerobic cocci of the genera *Peptococcus, Peptostreptococcus*, and *Ruminococcus,* Int. J. Syst. Bacteriol. **21:**234-237, 1971.

18. Rosenblatt, J.E.: Anaerobic cocci. In Lennette, E.H., Balows, A., Hausler, W.J., Jr., and Truant, J.P., editors: Manual of clinical microbiology, ed. 3, Washington, D.C., 1980, American Society for Microbiology.

19. Sugihara, P.T., Sutter, V.L., Attebery, H.R., Bricknell, K.S., and Finegold, S.M.: Isolation of *Acidaminococcus fermentans* and *Megasphaera elsdenii* from normal human feces, Appl. Microbiol. **27:**274-275, 1974.

20. Sutter, V.L., Citron, D.M., and Finegold, S.M.: Wadsworth anaerobic bacteriology manual, ed. 3, St. Louis, 1980, The C.V. Mosby Co.

21. Sutter, V.L., and Finegold, S.M.: Susceptibility of anaerobic bacteria to 23 antimicrobial agents, Antimicrob. Agents Chemother. **10:**736-752, 1976.

22. Thomas, C.G.A., and Hare, R.: The classification of anaerobic cocci and their isolation in normal human beings and pathological processes, J. Clin. Pathol. **7:**300-304, 1954.

23. Wideman, P.A., Vargo, V.L., Citronbaum, D.M., and Finegold, S.M.: Evaluation of the sodium polyanethol sulfonate disk test for the identification of *Peptostreptococcus anaerobius*, J. Clin. Microbiol. **4:**330-333, 1976.

24. Wong, M., Catena, A., and Hadley, W.K.: Antigenic relationships and rapid identification of *Peptostreptococcus* species, J. Clin. Microbiol. **11:**515-521, 1980.

29 ANAEROBIC GRAM-POSITIVE SPORE-FORMING BACILLI

Clostridium

The genus *Clostridium* contains the **anaerobic, spore-forming** bacteria. A large number of species are involved, and the majority are **obligate anaerobes.** Some species are aerotolerant, showing growth on enriched media on aerobic incubation. It is possible, then, to confuse these aerotolerant clostridia with certain facultative *Bacillus* species. Members of the genus *Clostridium* form spores under anaerobic conditions and usually do not produce catalase, whereas *Bacillus* species do not sporulate under anaerobic conditions and are usually catalase positive.[13] Also, aerotolerant clostridia form larger colonies under anaerobic conditions than under aerobic conditions, whereas the reverse is true for *Bacillus* species. The sporangia are often characteristically **swollen** (Fig. 29-1), showing spindle, drumstick, and "tennis-racket" forms and containing central, subterminal, and terminal spores. With rare exceptions in the aerotolerant forms, the enzymes catalase, cytochrome oxidase, and peroxidase are **not** produced. Many attack carbohydrates, and some are proteolytic.

True **exotoxins** are produced by many pathogenic clostridia, several species of which are important in medicine. The organisms are widely distributed in soil, dust, and water and are common inhabitants of the intestinal tract of animals, including humans. They are often found in unclean wounds and wound infections. Most clostridial infections are of endogenous origin, although clostridia from exogenous sources may be involved in certain conditions, such as botulism, tetanus, *Clostridium perfringens* food poisoning, and sometimes gas gangrene. The classical infections involving *C. perfringens* include myonecrosis (gas gangrene, Plate 126), gangrenous cholecystitis (with or without visceral gas gangrene), and postabortal sepsis with intravascular hemolysis. However, *C. perfringens* and a number of other species of clostridia are actually much more commonly involved in infections of diverse types throughout the body of the sort caused by non-spore-forming anaerobes. This would include such entities as brain abscess, aspiration pneumonia, empyema, intraabdominal infection, postoperative wound infection, infections related to gynecologic disease or surgery, and soft tissue infections.[3,7] Bacteremia is found in about 15% of patients with clostridial myonecrosis and may be seen on occasion in the course of other clostridial infections as well.

Tetanus (Plate 139) and botulism are classic toxin-related diseases. It is important to keep in mind that in botulism the disease may be related to wound infection as well as to ingestion of preformed toxin in contaminated food. It should also be appreciated that infant botulism, described relatively recently,[10] actually represents a different situation in that the organism colonizes the gastrointestinal tract of the infant (presumably because the infant's own flora is not yet fully developed) and produces toxin within the gastrointestinal tract, which is then absorbed to produce the disease.

Pseudomembranous colitis (Plate 21) related to antimicrobial therapy is now known to be

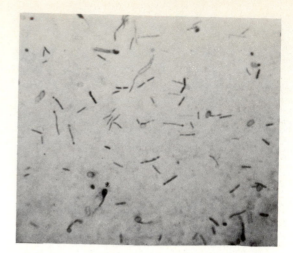

FIG. 29-1
Clostridium septicum. Note subterminal and free spores (1,000×).

caused primarily by *Clostridium difficile* (Plate 134).[1,4,5] This organism may also be involved in similar disease not related to the use of antimicrobial therapy, in disease following the use of methotrexate and other cytotoxic agents, in exacerbations of inflammatory bowel disease, and in complications of strangulation obstruction of the bowel. Most strains of *C. difficile* produce a toxin that is cytopathic for most tissue culture cell lines. CIE is useful in identifying toxigenic *C. difficile*.[16] Another toxin recently described is an enterotoxin. This toxin may prove to be more significant with regard to pathogenesis of the disease.

There is a definite association between *Clostridium septicum* (Plates 131 to 133) infection and malignancy, particularly in the colon.[3]

The spores of some pathogenic species (*Clostridium botulinum*) may appear in improperly home-canned produce, in which they can develop vegetatively under normal domestic conditions; in inefficiently sterilized surgical dressings and bandages; in plaster of Paris for casts; and on the clothing and skin of humans.

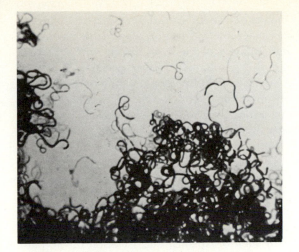

FIG. 29-2
Clostridium ramosum (1,000×).

RAPID PRESUMPTIVE IDENTIFICATION OF CLOSTRIDIA

The Gram stain may be very useful in helping the clinician or microbiologist to suspect the possibility of gas gangrene (clostridial myonecrosis). The two findings of note are absence or distortion of white blood cells and other host cells in the preparation and the presence of large, relatively short, fat, gram-positive rods

without evidence of spores (Plate 38). The changes in the host cells are related to toxin produced by *C. perfringens*.

Clostridium ramosum, the second most commonly encountered clostridium in clinical infections, is more slender and longer than *C. perfringens*, and the cells are often curved (Plates 129 and 130). With other clostridia spores may be apparent on Gram stain, but at times phase contrast microscopy reveals spores more readily.

Fluorescent antibody reagents are available commercially for *Clostridium septicum*, *C. novyi* (Plate 136), and *C. sordellii*.

C. perfringens colonies on blood agar plates are often surrounded by a double zone of hemolysis that is quite distinctive (Plate 127).[15] The inner zone shows complete hemolysis, and the outer zone shows discoloration and incomplete hemolysis. The Nagler plate, which may be used as a primary plate when *C. perfringens* is suspected, reveals a zone of precipitation around colonies on the control side of the plate and little or no precipitate around colonies on the side of the plate spread with antitoxin (Plate 128) (see below).[15] Three other clostridia are Nagler positive, as indicated in Table 29-1. One of these, *Clostridium paraperfringens*, is seldom encountered in clinical material. Another, *Clostridium*

TABLE 29-1

Characteristics of Nagler-positive *Clostridium* species

Species	Indole	Motility	Fermentation of lactose	Gelatin	Urease	Glutamic acid decarboxylase
C. perfringens	−	−	+	+		+
C. paraperfringens	−	−	+	−		−
C. bifermentans	+	+	−		−	−
C. sordellii	+	+	−		+⁻	+

Modified from Sutter and associates.[15]
−, negative reaction; +, positive reaction for majority of strains, includes weak as well as strong acid production from carbohydrates; +⁻, most strains positive, reaction helpful if positive.

sordellii (Plate 138), may be identified by the fluorescent antibody technique as previously noted. The third Nagler-positive strain is *Clostridium bifermentans*, which does not form a double zone of hemolysis and sporulates readily.

Gram stain of stool specimens from patients with *C. difficile* colitis often shows polymorphonuclear leukocytes and a predominance of relatively thin, long, gram-positive rods with perfectly parallel sides (Plate 22). There is an excellent selective and differential medium for *C. difficile* that permits early presumptive identification of the organism (Plate 135).[6] *C. difficile* is the one anaerobe of clinical significance that often does not grow by anaerobic jar technique. Accordingly, cultures for this organism should be set up in an anaerobic chamber. Plates may be placed in Bio-Bags* within the chamber after inoculation and then removed from the chamber for incubation in a standard incubator. In this manner plates can be examined at frequent intervals. Colonies of *C. difficile* are usually 2 mm or more in diameter after 24 hours of incubation. Relatively few organisms other than *C. difficile* grow on the cycloserine cefoxitin fructose agar (CCFA), and most of those that do form much smaller colonies. The colonies fluoresce yellow under ultraviolet light. Such colonies, which on Gram stain show typical gram-positive rods, constitute good presumptive evidence of the presence of *C. difficile*.

The presence of swarming growth on the surface of anaerobically incubated blood agar plates is suggestive of clostridia. Gram stain of such colonies should show gram-positive rods, and spores may be noted as well.

GENERAL METHODS OF ISOLATION AND CULTIVATION OF PATHOGENIC CLOSTRIDIA

The procedures for specimen collection and transport and for anaerobic culture discussed in Chapter 13 are applicable to the clostridia. It

---

*Marion Laboratories, Kansas City, Mo.

should be reemphasized here that any material for anaerobic cultivation should be inoculated **immediately,** using fresh media, without awaiting the results of aerobic culture. Egg yolk medium should be used, in addition to the others mentioned in Chapter 13, when clostridia are anticipated to be present. Media with 5% agar may also be useful to minimize swarming of colonies.

In most instances the clostridia occur in **mixed culture** with gram-negative bacteria, such as coliforms, *Proteus*, or *Pseudomonas*, and with various non-spore-forming anaerobes. The anaerobic plates, therefore, may be overgrown with such organisms, and isolation of the clostridia becomes difficult or impossible. Any or all of the following three methods may be used to combat this problem:

1. The original culture, shown to contain gram-positive sporulating rods, may be **heat shocked** at 80 C for 10 minutes and then streaked on blood agar and egg yolk agar plates for anaerobic cultivation. Alternatively, a fresh tube of enriched thioglycollate medium or starch broth may be inoculated from the original culture, heated immediately, and incubated for 24 to 48 hours. The plates may be streaked from this.
2. Treat mixed cultures with 50% ethanol for 1 hour to selectively isolate spore formers (see Chapter 13).
3. Incorporate 100 µg/ml of neomycin in blood agar plates or egg yolk agar plates. This compound can be autoclaved. Cycloserine, in a final concentration of 500 µg/ml, may also be useful; it should be added after autoclaving.

IDENTIFICATION OF THE PATHOGENIC CLOSTRIDIA

By virtue of the disease syndromes they produce, the pathogenic species may be placed in five categories or groups:

Group I—the **gas gangrene** group, includes

TABLE 29-2

Characteristics of Nagler-negative *Clostridium* species

Species	Glutamic acid decarboxylase	Spores	Aerobic growth	Motility	Lecithinase*	Lipase*	Indole production	Gelatin liquefaction	Meat digestion	Milk	Fermentation of — Fructose	Glucose	Lactose	Maltose	Mannitol	Esculin hydrolysis	Fatty acids from PY and PYG
C. butyricum		O S	−	$+^-$	−	−	−	−	−	C	+	+	+	+	−	+	A B F
C. cadaveris		O T	−	$+^-$	−	−	+	+	+	D	V	+	V	−	−	−	A P IB B IV
C. clostridiiforme	−	O S	−	V	−	−	$-^+$	−	−	C^-	+	+	+	+	+	+	A F
C. difficile		O S	−	$+^-$	−	−	−	+	+		+	+	−	−	+	+	A P IB B IV IC F
C. hastiforme		S	V	$+^-$	−	−	−	+	+	D	−	−	−	−	−	−	A P IB B IV IC
C. histolyticum	−	O S	V	$+^-$	−	−	−	+	+	D	−	−	−	−	−	−	A
C. innocuum	−	O T	−	−	+	−	−	−	−		+	+	−	−	+	+	A B L (F)
C. limosum		S	−	V	+	+	−	+	+	D	−	−	−	−	−	−	A F
C. novyi, type A	−	O S	−	$+^-$	+	+	−	+	−		+	+	−	V	−	+	A P B (V)
C. ramosum	−	R/O T	−	−	−	−	−	−	−	−	+	+	−	+	+	+	A L F
C. septicum	−	O S	−	$+^-$	−	−	−	+	−	C	+	+	+	+	−	+	A B F
C. sporogenes†	−	O S	−	$+^-$	$-^+$	+	−	+	+	C	−	V	−	−	−	−	A P IB B IV IC
C. subterminale	−	O S	−	$+^-$	$-^+$	−	−	+	+	D	−	−	−	−	−	−	A IB B IV
C. tertium	−	O T	+	$+^-$	−	−	−	−	−	C	+	+	+	+	+	+	A B L (F)
C. tetani	−	R T	−	$-^+$	−	−	$+^-$	+	+	−	−	−	−	−	−	−	A P B

Modified from Sutter and associates.[15]

O, oval; R, round; S, subterminal; T, terminal; C, clot; D, digested; −, negative reaction; +, positive reaction for majority of strains, includes weak as well as strong acid production from carbohydrates; V, variable reaction; $+^-$, most strains positive, reaction helpful if positive; $-^+$, most strains negative, some strains positive. Fatty acids: A, acetic; P, propionic; IB, isobutyric; B, butyric; IV, isovaleric; V, valeric; IC, isocaproic; F, formic; L, lactic; ( ), sometimes detected.

*See Plates 128, 136, and 137.

†*C. botulinum*, types A, B, and F, behave biochemically like *C. sporogenes* and can only be differentiated by toxin neutralization studies.

C. perfringens (type A), *C. novyi*, *C. septicum*, *C. bifermentans*, *C. histolyticum*, *C. sordellii*, *C. sporogenes* (Plate 122), and others. Of these, the three species first named are most important.

Group II—*C. tetani* (Plates 140 and 141).

Group III—the *C. botulinum* group.

Group IV—*C. difficile*, responsible for **pseudomembranous colitis.**

Group V—the miscellaneous infection group (wound infection, abscesses, bacteremia, and so forth). This group includes *C. perfringens*, *C. ramosum*, *C. bifermentans*, *C. sphenoides*, *C. sporogenes*, and a number of others.

C. perfringens and *C. ramosum* are by far the most commonly isolated clostridia. Group V infections are the most commonly encountered. However, clostridia are found in such infections only about one tenth as often as non-spore-forming anaerobes.

The **Nagler** reaction is recommended for the rapid identification of *C. perfringens* and other alpha-toxin producers. The medium for this reaction, 10% egg yolk in blood agar base (see Chapter 42, for preparation), is placed in a Petri dish, and one half of the surface is smeared with a few drops of *C. perfringens* type A antitoxin* (anti-alpha toxin). The culture is then streaked in a single line across the plate at a right angle to the antitoxin. The lecithinase toxin produces a precipitate (opalescence) about the growth in the line of streak in the absence of antitoxin, but it is inhibited on the half of the plate with antitoxin.† Gubash has proposed a synergistic hemolysis test in place of the Nagler test.[8] This test is based on synergistic hemolysis because of the interaction of the CAMP factor of group B streptococci and the lecithinase (phospholipase

C) of clostridia. The test requires the use of two human blood agar plates, one of which is supplemented with 0.066% calcium chloride. Details of the test are given in the publication by Gubash. This test avoids the need for the various tests listed in Table 29-1 for differentiating between Nagler-positive clostridia. It also uses a 1:6 dilution of type A *C. perfringens* antitoxin, thus saving this reagent.

Details on examination of specimens for *C. difficile* and its cytotoxin are presented in Chapter 9. Details on identification of various other species of clostridia are presented in Table 29-2. Further information on test procedures can be found in references 9, 11, 13, 15, and 16.

C. ramosum, although not as virulent as *C. perfringens*, takes on added importance by virtue of its **resistance** to antimicrobial agents. About 15% of strains are highly resistant to clindamycin, and many strains are resistant to tetracycline and erythromycin. Penicillin is the drug of choice against *C. ramosum* and clostridia in general, but minimal inhibitory concentrations of *C. ramosum* are as high as 8 units/ml. Occasional strains of *C. perfringens* and other clostridia are resistant to penicillin G. Some 20% to 30% of certain clostridial species other than *C. perfringens* are also resistant to clindamycin. One third of clostridia other than *C. perfringens* are resistant to cefoxitin. Chloramphenicol and metronidazole are universally active against clostridia. Oral vancomycin is the drug of choice for *C. difficile* colitis.

Most of the human pathogenic clostridia are pathogenic also for guinea pigs, mice, rabbits, and pigeons. To establish the toxigenicity of isolated strains, white mice, guinea pigs and hamsters are used in the laboratory. Susceptibility and rapidity of death may vary according to the virulence of the strain. This type of testing is beyond the scope of the clinical laboratory. Cultivation of *C. botulinum* should only be attempted by reference laboratories. Determination of toxigenicity, where indicated, should be done by reference laboratories.[2]

---

*No longer available commercially in the United States. It may be obtained from the Pasteur Institute, Paris.

†*C. bifermentans*, *C. sordellii*, and *C. paraperfringens* (*C. barati*) also produce alpha toxin and give a positive Nagler reaction. See Table 29-1 for means of differentiating these species.

For a further study of the clostridia, the reader is referred to some of the sources listed in this chapter.[2,7,12,17]

REFERENCES

1. Bartlett, J.G., Chang, T.W., Gurwith, M., Gorbach, S.L., and Onderdonk, A.B.: Antibiotic-associated pseudomembranous colitis due to toxin-producing clostridia, N. Engl. J. Med. **298**:531-534, 1978.
2. Dowell, V.R., Jr., and Hawkins, T.M.: Detection of clostridial toxins, toxin neutralization tests, and pathogenicity tests, Atlanta, 1968, Center for Disease Control.
3. Finegold, S.M.: Anaerobic bacteria in human disease, New York, 1977, Academic Press, Inc.
4. George, W.L.: Antimicrobial agent–associated colitis, Clin. Microbiol. Newslett. **2**:1-2, 1980.
5. George, W.L.: Antimicrobial agent–associated colitis and diarrhea, West. J. Med. **133**:115-123, 1980.
6. George, W.L., Sutter, V.L., Citron, D., and Finegold, S.M.: Selective and differential medium for isolation of *Clostridium difficile*, J. Clin. Microbiol. **9**:214-219, 1979.
7. Gorbach, S.L., and Thadepalli, H.: Isolation of *Clostridium* in human infections: evaluation of 114 cases, J. Infect. Dis. **131**: S 81-S 85, 1975.
8. Gubash, S.M.: Synergistic haemolysis test for presumptive identification and differentiation of *Clostridium perfringens*, *C. bifermentans*, *C. sordellii*, and *C. paraperfringens*, J. Clin. Pathol. **33**:395-399, 1980.
9. Holdeman, L.V., Cato, E.P., and Moore, W.E.C., editors: Anaerobe laboratory manual, ed. 4, Blacksburg, Va., 1977, Virginia Polytechnic Institute and State University.
10. Midura, T.F., and Arnon, S.S.: Infant botulism: identification of *C. botulinum* and its toxin in faeces, Lancet **2**:934-936, 1976.
11. Miranda, C.J., Edelstein, M.A., and Citron, D.M.: Evaluation of a Marion Scientific Corporation prototype rapid glutamic acid decarboxylase test for anaerobic bacteria, Abstract C36, Abstracts of the Annual Meeting of the American Society for Microbiology, 1980, p. 280.
12. Smith, L. DS.: The pathogenic anaerobic bacteria, ed. 2, Springfield, Ill., 1975, Charles C Thomas, Publisher.
13. Smith, L. DS., and Dowell, V.R., Jr. Revised by Allen, S.D.: *Clostridium*. In Lennette, E.H., Balows, A., Hausler, W.J., Jr., and Truant, J.P., editors: Manual of clinical microbiology, ed. 3, Washington, D.C., 1980, American Society for Microbiology.
14. Sterne, M., and van Heyningen, W.E.: The clostridia. In Dubos, R.J., and Hirsch, J.G.: Bacterial and mycotic infections of man, ed. 4, Philadelphia, 1965, J.B. Lippincott Co.
15. Sutter, V.L., Citron, D.M., and Finegold, S.M.: Wadsworth anaerobic bacteriology manual, ed. 3, St. Louis, 1980, The C.V. Mosby Co.
16. Welch, D.F., Menge, S.K., and Matsen, J.M.: Identification of toxigenic *Clostridium difficile* by counterimmunoelectrophoresis, J. Clin. Microbiol. **11**:470-473, 1980.
17. Willis, A.T.: Clostridia of wound infection, London, 1969, Butterworth & Co. (Publishers) Ltd.

30 ANAEROBIC GRAM-POSITIVE NON-SPORE-FORMING BACILLI

Bifidobacterium

Propionibacterium

Eubacterium

Lactobacillus

Actinomyces

Arachnia

The identification of this group of anaerobes requires the use of **gas chromatography** (or a substitute such as column chromatography), with rare exception. Comparative study of ultrastructure of *Actinomyces*, *Arachnia*, and certain nonanaerobic gram-positive rods indicates that ultrastructural features of the cell wall are probably reliable criteria for identification purposes.[8] This, of course, would be beyond the scope of the usual clinical laboratory. In general, morphologic features are not adequate for distinguishing between different gram-positive non-spore-forming anaerobic bacilli. Moreover, there may be problems distinguishing this group of organisms from others, since they may look coccoid at times, may destain and appear gram-negative, and may be confused with clostridia that do not demonstrate spores. The use of egg yolk agar can be helpful in differentiating clostridia from these organisms.[13] On this medium none of the non-spore-forming bacilli produce lecithinase and only a few produce lipase.

The catalase-positive forms, *Propionibacterium acnes*, *Propionibacterium granulosum,* and *Actinomyces viscosus*, may be recognized without gas chromatography. Fortunately, only *Acti-*

nomyces, Arachnia, and *Bifidobacterium eriksonii* are major pathogens, and none of these are encountered often. Laboratories not equipped for gas chromatography need to send selected cultures to reference laboratories.* In the case of actinomycosis, however, clinical and pathologic features may be very distinctive or diagnostic. The interested reader is referred to other sources for details of gas chromatographic and other identification procedures. Significant members of each genus are described on the following pages. Table 30-1 outlines identifying characteristics.

BIFIDOBACTERIUM ERIKSONII

Bifidobacterium eriksonii is part of the normal human oral and intestinal microflora and occurs principally in mixed pulmonary infections. It grows as a white, convex, shiny colony with an irregular edge. In thioglycollate medium growth is diffuse, and the Gram stain shows a diphtheroid to filamentous bacillus, branched or bifurcated. Catalase and indole are not produced; nitrate is not reduced; gelatin is not liquefied; but esculin is hydrolysed. Carbohydrate fermentation reactions and metabolic end products are characteristic.[6,14]

PROPIONIBACTERIUM ACNES

The anaerobe* *Propionibacterium acnes* produces propionic acid by fermentation of glucose and is part of the resident flora of **normal skin;** consequently, it is the most frequent contaminant of blood cultures and often contaminates other cultures as well. *Propionibacterium granulosum* is also a common contaminant from the skin. Accordingly, particular care must be exercised in the preparation of the skin before venipuncture, lumbar puncture, aspiration of pus from abscesses, and so on. One good procedure is to first cleanse the area carefully with soap solution and then remove the soap with 70% ethyl or isopropyl alcohol. Next 1% tincture of iodine is applied; finally, the iodine is removed with alcohol. *P. acnes* occasionally causes infection, especially endocarditis and

---

*For example, the Centers for Disease Control, Atlanta, through the referring state laboratory.

*Some strains are microaerophilic.

TABLE 30-1

Characteristics of gram-positive non-spore-forming bacilli*

Organism	Oxygen tolerance	Catalase	Indole production	Nitrate reduction	Gelatin liquefaction	Esculin hydrolysis	Starch hydrolysis	Urease	Fermentation of										Fatty acids from PYG
									Arabinose	Erythritol	Glucose	Inositol	Lactose	Mannitol	Raffinose	Ribose	Sorbitol	Trehalose	
Actinomyces israelii	A M	−	−	+	−	+	−	−	−	−	+	+	+	+	+	+	−	+	A L S F
A. meyerii	A	−	−	−	−	−	−	−	−	−	+	−	+	−	−	−	−	−	A S F
A. naeslundii	M F	−	−	+	−	+	−	+	−	−	+	V	+	−	+	V	−	+	A L S F
A. odontolyticus	A M	+	−	+	−	+	−	+	−	−	+	V	+	−	−	−	−	−	A S F
A. viscosus	A M	−	−	+	V	V	−	+	−	−	+	−	+	−	+	−	−	V	A L S F
Arachnia propionica	A M	−	−	+	+	−	−	−	−	−	+	−	V	V	V	+	−	V	A P S (L)
Propionibacterium acnes	A M	+	+⁻	+⁻	−	−	−	−	−	−	+	−	−	V	−	−	−	−	A P (IV L S F)
P. granulosum	A F	+⁻	−	−	V	−	−	−	−	−	+	−	−	−	−	−	−	−	A P (L)
Bifidobacterium eriksonii†	A	−	−	−	−	+	V	−	−	−	+	−	+	+	+	+	−	+	A L (F)
Lactobacillus catenaforme	A	−	−	−	−	+	+	−	−	−	+	−	+	−	−	−	−	−	L
Eubacterium alactolyticum	A	−	−	−	−	−	−	−	−	−	+	−	−	+	−	−	−	−	A B H (C F)
E. lentum	A	−⁺	−	+	−	−	−	+	−	−	−	−	−	−	−	−	−	−	(A)
E. limosum	A	−	−	−	−	+	−	−	+	+	+	−	−	+	−	+	−	−	A B L

Modified from Sutter and associates.[14]

A, anaerobic; M, microaerophilic; F, facultative; −, negative reaction; +, positive reaction for majority of strains, includes weak as well as strong acid production from carbohydrates; V, variable reaction; +⁻, most strains positive, reaction helpful if positive; −⁺, most strains negative, some strains positive. Fatty acids: A, acetic; P, propionic; B, butyric; IV, isovaleric; H, hexanoic (caproic); C, caprylic; F, formic; L, lactic; S, succinic; ( ), sometimes detected.

*Characteristics used to differentiate commonly encountered species after generic identification provided by fatty acid end product analysis. See VPI manual for other characteristics of these species and characteristics of other species.

†This organism is listed as *Actinomyces eriksonii*, species *incertae sedis* in *Bergey's Manual* ed. 8.

ventricular shunt infections. *P. acnes* character-istically grows as a small, white to pinkish, shiny to opaque colony with entire margins. A Gram stain of the colony shows slender, slightly curved rods, sometimes with false branching or a beaded appearance. Tests for catalase and indole production are usually positive; nitrates are usually reduced (Plate 142); gelatin is lique-fied; but esculin is not hydrolyzed. Characteris-tic patterns of carbohydrate fermentation and organic acid end products are obtained.[6,14] Flu-orescent antibody reagents are available for direct detection of *P. acnes*, *P. granulosum*, and other *Propionibacterium* species in direct smears of clinical materials and from cultures.[13] These are available from the CDC. *P. acnes* is very sensitive to penicillin G and most other antimicrobials, except aminoglycosides.[15]

GENUS EUBACTERIUM

Eubacterium species are isolated from wound and other infections and are almost always asso-ciated with other anaerobes or facultative bacte-ria; they are part of the normal fecal microflora. A coiled gram-positive anaerobic rod, which is undoubtedly a member of the genus *Eubacte-rium,* was isolated in pure culture from a gutter wall abscess.[12] *Eubacterium* is not particularly pathogenic but may cause endocarditis. Grow-ing as raised to convex, translucent to opaque colonies, they appear microscopically as pleomor-phic bacillary to coccobacillary forms, occurring in pairs and short chains. *Eubacterium lentum* (Plate 143) is relatively inactive biochemically; *Eubacterium limosum* hydrolyzes esculin and ferments several carbohydrates. Characteristic metabolic end products are observed.

GENUS LACTOBACILLUS

The anaerobic members of the genus *Lacto-bacillus* produce primarily lactic acid from the fermentation of glucose and are only occasional-ly involved in human infections, usually pleuro-pulmonary. One species, *Lactobacillus catena-forme*, was formerly classified as a member of the genus *Catenabacterium;* however, some strains of the latter were shown to produce spores, and therefore they belong to the clos-tridia.[6] *L. catenaforme* grows as a convex, trans-lucent colony; microscopic examination reveals pleomorphic gram-positive bacilli, sometimes in chains. Terminal swellings are also observed.

GENERA ACTINOMYCES AND ARACHNIA

The etiologic agents of **human actinomycosis** (Plates 144 and 145) include the most common and important organism, *Actinomyces israelii*, and several other species—*A. naeslundii*, *A. odontolyticus*, *A. viscosus*, and *Arachnia propi-onica*.[2,4] *A. meyerii* may also cause infection. These organisms are a part of the normal micro-biota of the mouth and female genital tract and produce infection primarily as endogenous opportunists. A large number of cases of actino-mycosis associated with the use of an intrauter-ine contraceptive device have been described. A procedure has been developed in which pepsin treatment and rhodamine conjugate of normal serum were used to reduce nonspecific staining so that satisfactory fluorescent antibody smears could be made of cervicovaginal material.[11] Studies by this technique indicated that *A. israelii* was found more commonly in women with intrauterine contraceptive devices, but this was not true for *A. naeslundii* or *Arachnia pro-pionica*. Although *A. israelii*, *A. odontolyticus*, and *Arachnia* grow best under anaerobic conditions (Plate 150), *A. naeslundii* and *A. vis-cosus* strains are either microaerophilic or facul-tative. *A. israelii* produces a characteristically heaped, rough, lobate colony resembling a **molar tooth** (Plate 149); microscopically it appears as long, filamentous, gram-positive bacilli, some of which may show branching. A Gram stain of "**sulfur granules**" (Fig. 30-1) from actinomycotic pus reveals a similar morphology (Plates 146 to 148), often with diphtheroid and coccal forms. Colonies of the other organisms generally are smooth, flat to convex, whitish,

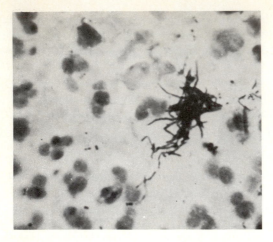

FIG. 30-1

Actinomyces israelii, crushed sulfur granule, showing bacterial forms and pus cells (Gram stain; 1,000×).

and transparent, with entire margins. *A. odontolyticus* colonies may develop a red color on blood agar after several days. Microscopically, the other causes of actinomycosis are gram-positive bacilli consisting of diphtheroidal forms and branched elements; some filaments may show clubbed ends (Plate 150).[3]

When the Putt acid-fast stain, which uses a weaker acid solution to decolorize, is used, *A. israelii* may be acid fast.[10] This could cause confusion with *Nocardia*, treatment for which would be typically distinctly different than that for *Actinomyces* infection. One may use the usual Ziehl-Neelsen stain, but the period of decolorization with acid alcohol should not exceed 5 to 10 seconds. The Kinyoun stain may also be employed, again with that same short period of decolorization. One may also use the Fite-Faraco method.

A. viscosus, being catalase positive, is often overlooked because it is assumed to be a *Propionibacterium* or diphtheroid and therefore not likely to be important. It differs from *P. acnes* by growing equally well aerobically and anaerobically, usually hydrolyzing esculin, not producing indole, not being proteolytic, not producing a pink sediment in thioglycollate broth, and fermenting melibiose, raffinose, sucrose, and salicin.[5]

A highly efficient selective medium for isolation of *A. viscosus* and *A. naeslundii* has been described.[7] This medium, containing metronidazole and cadmium sulphate, is designed for recovery of these organisms from dental plaque, but it should be suitable for clinical specimens as well. The selectivity of this medium and the characteristic cell morphology of the two organisms on it permit presumptive identification of the organisms.

Direct identification of *Actinomyces* and *Arachnia* by immunofluorescent techniques has proved successful (available from CDC, Atlanta).[9]

Penicillin G remains the drug of choice in the treatment of actinomycosis; tetracycline, clindamycin, and erythromycin also demonstrate activity against these organisms.[1]

REFERENCES

1. Bartlett, J.G., and Finegold, S.M.: Anaerobic pleuropulmonary infections, Medicine **51**:413-450, 1972.
2. Brock, D.W., Georg, L.K., Brown, J.M., and Hicklin, M.D.: Actinomycosis caused by *Arachnia propionica*: report of 11 cases, Am. J. Clin. Pathol. **59**:66-77, 1973.
3. Coleman, R.M., Georg, L.K., and Rozzell, A.R.: *Actinomyces naeslundii* as an agent of human actinomycosis, Appl. Microbiol. **18**:420-426, 1969.
4. Georg, L.K.: Diagnostic procedures for the isolation and identification of the etiologic agents of actinomycosis. In Proceedings of the International Symposium on Mycoses, Washington, D.C., 1970, Pan American Health Organization Scientific Pub. No. 205.
5. Gerencser, M.A., and Slack, J.M.: Identification of human strains of *Actinomyces viscosus*, Appl. Microbiol. **18**:80-87, 1969.
6. Holdeman, L.V., Cato, E.P., and Moore, W.E.C., editors: Anaerobe laboratory manual, ed. 4, Blacksburg, Va., 1977, Virginia Polytechnic Institute and State University.
7. Kornman, K.S., and Loesche, W.J.: New medium for isolation of *Actinomyces viscosus* and *Actinomyces naeslundii* from dental plaque, J. Clin. Microbiol. **7**:514-518, 1978.

8. Lai, C.-H., and Listgarten, M.A.: Comparative ultra-structure of certain *Actinomyces* species, *Arachnia*, *Bacterionema*, and *Rothia*, J. Periodontol. **51:**136-154, 1980.

9. Lambert, R.F., Jr., Brown, J.M., and Georg, L.K.: Identification of *Actinomyces israelii* and *Actinomyces naeslundii* by fluorescent antibody and agar-gel diffusion techniques, J. Bacteriol. **94:**1287-1295, 1967.

10. Lowe, R.N., Azimi, P.H., and McQuitty, J.: Acid-fast *Actinomyces* in a child with pulmonary actinomycosis, J. Clin. Microbiol. **12:**124-126, 1980.

11. Pine, L., Malcolm, G.B., Curtis, E.M., and Brown, J.M.: Demonstration of *Actinomyces* and *Arachnia* species in cervicovaginal smears by direct staining with species-specific fluorescent-antibody conjugate, J. Clin. Microbiol. **13:**15-21, 1981.

12. Pollock, H.M., and Rintala, L.: Unusual coiled gram-positive anaerobe isolated from a gutter wall abscess, J. Clin. Microbiol. **6:**642-644, 1977.

13. Sonnenwirth, A.C., and Dowell, V.R., Jr.: Gram-positive nonsporeforming anaerobic bacilli. In Lennette, E.H., Balows, A., Hausler, W.J., Jr., and Truant, J.P., editors: Manual of clinical microbiology, ed. 3, Washington, D.C., 1980, American Society for Microbiology.

14. Sutter, V.L., Citron, D.M., and Finegold, S.M.: Wadsworth anaerobic bacteriology manual, ed. 3, St. Louis, 1980, The C.V. Mosby Co.

15. Wang, W.L.L., Everett, E.D., Johnson, M., and Dean, E.: Susceptibility of *Propionibacterium acnes* to seventeen antibiotics, Antimicrob. Agents Chemother. **11:**171-173, 1977.

31 MYCOBACTERIA

The mycobacteria may vary morphologically from the coccobacillary form to long, narrow, rod-shaped cells ranging from 0.8 to 5 μm in length and about 0.2 to 0.6 μm in thickness. They do not stain readily, but once stained they resist decolorization with acid-alcohol and are therefore called **acid-fast bacilli.** Occurring as single bacilli or in small irregular clumps, mycobacteria are sometimes beaded, banded, or pleomorphic in stained smears. In addition to saphrophytic species the group includes numerous organisms pathogenic for humans, the most important of which is *Mycobacterium tuberculosis*.

LABORATORY DIAGNOSIS OF TUBERCULOSIS AND RELATED MYCOBACTERIOSES
General considerations

Tuberculosis is an infectious disease of a persistent and chronic nature that is usually caused by *Mycobacterium tuberculosis* but occasionally by other species, such as *Mycobacterium bovis* and *Mycobacterium kansasii*. Although capable of involving almost any organ of the body, tuberculosis is most commonly associated with the lungs, from which it spreads from person to person through coughing or expectoration. Tuberculosis is generally considered to be the most socioeconomically important specific communicable disease in the world today. Although it no longer ranks as the most common cause of death in nations with a high standard of living, it still remains a leading killer. Immunosuppressed patients are at increased risk of infection with various mycobacteria.

Only within the last two to three decades has it become generally accepted that mycobacteria other than *M. tuberculosis* can be the cause of human infections. Although *M. tuberculosis* is still the mycobacterium most frequently isolated from clinical specimens, *M. kansasii* and the *Mycobacterium avium* complex are also well-established human pathogens, and their recognition becomes equally important. Mycobacteria other than *M. tuberculosis* may account for as much as 10% of all human mycobacterial infections.[2]

Definitive proof of a tuberculous infection is provided only by the demonstration of *M. tuberculosis* (or *M. bovis*) in clinical specimens obtained from the patient. The laboratory procedures used include examination of a stained smear, isolation by cultural procedures, and identification.

Characteristics of the tubercle bacillus that differentiate it from other microorganisms are as follows:

1. The resistance of stained tubercle bacilli to decolorization with strong decolorizing agents. Acid-alcohol (3% hydrochloric acid in 95% ethanol) is the usual agent.

2. The resistance of acid-fast bacilli to digesting agents, such as strong acids and alkalis. The use of these agents on material that may contain contaminating bacteria destroys most contaminants without decreasing greatly the viability of any tubercle bacilli that may be present.

In 1967 Kubica and Dye proposed a "Levels of Laboratory Service" program for identification of mycobacterial disease. This approach, which we consider a very important concept that might well be applied to other areas of the microbiology laboratory, such as mycology and anaerobic bacteriology, is detailed further in two publications,[19,44] each with a slightly different approach. According to this concept, a laboratory decides how far it can reasonably go **reliably** and then depends on reference or regional laboratories for more sophisticated or complex procedures that may be beyond the scope of a small facility. Of course, a laboratory can always extend its level of service if conditions permit or warrant this. In the case of mycobacterial infection, Wayne and associates[44] suggested four levels of service (or areas of proficiency):

1. Collection and transport of specimens; preparation and examination of smears for acid-fast bacilli
2. Detection, isolation, and identification of *M. tuberculosis*
3. Determination of drug susceptibility of mycobacteria
4. Identification of mycobacteria other than *M. tuberculosis*

Collection of clinical specimens

In suspected mycobacterial infection, as in all other diseases of microbial origin, the **diagnostic procedure begins not in the laboratory but at the bedside of the patient.** In the collection of clinical specimens there should be the same careful attention to detail on the part of the attending physician, nurse, and ward personnel as is required of the bacteriologist in carrying out the cultural procedures.

Secretions from the **lung** may be obtained by any one of the following methods: spontaneous or induced expectoration of sputum, aspiration of secretions during bronchoscopy, transtracheal aspiration, aspiration of gastric contents that contain swallowed sputum, or swabbing of the larynx.

Sputum

Since it may not be practical to provide constant supervision during the collection of a sputum specimen, it is necessary to elicit the intelligent cooperation of patients by giving them detailed instructions for the collection and explaining the purpose and importance of the test. The importance of sputum expectoration "from deep down in the lungs" should be emphasized as opposed to the expectoration of saliva or nasopharyngeal secretions. The specimen should not be collected immediately after the patient has used a mouthwash.

A clean, sterile container must be provided for collection; the Falcon sputum collection kit* appears to be ideally suited for this purpose. It consists of a plastic disposable 50-ml graduated conical centrifuge tube with an aerosol-free screw cap, which is fitted inside a funnellike disposable plastic outer container in such a manner that the risk of accidental contamination by handling is almost eliminated. Not more than 5 to 10 ml of sputum is collected in this container, which is then labeled with the patient's name, date, and other data.

A 4- to 6-ounce, clean, sterile widemouthed glass jar with a screw cap and rubber or Teflon liner or a disposable sterile plastic cup with a tightly fitted lid may also be used. However, specimens in these containers must be transferred to an appropriate aerosol-free centrifuge tube in the laboratory, a procedure both unpleasant and hazardous to the laboratory worker.

For optimal recovery of mycobacteria a series of three to five single, fresh, **early morning** sputum specimens, not exceeding one fifth (10 ml) of the volume of the centrifuge tube, should be collected on successive days. If the amount of this specimen is insufficient, sputum may be collected over a 24-hour period. Extending the collection of a single specimen over a longer period or the pooling of several days' accumulation is **not** recommended, since a reduced number of positive isolations may result, along with an increased rate of contaminated cultures.

Nebulized and heated hypertonic saline may be used to induce sputum production in patients unable to raise a satisfactory coughed specimen. The specimen is obtained (preferably by a mem-

---

*Falcon Plastics, No. 9002, Division of Becton, Dickinson, and Co., Cockeysville, Md., and Los Angeles, Calif.

ber of the respiratory therapy service) 10 to 15 minutes after inhalation of aerosolized, warmed (45 C) 10% sodium chloride solution. Ultrasonic nebulizers are preferable to hypertonic saline inhalation for induction of sputum. Sputum induction gives a higher yield of positive cultures than does gastric lavage and is generally more acceptable to both patients and personnel. These specimens appear watery. They should be labeled "Induced sputum" so that the laboratory does not mistake them for saliva. The combination of sputum induction and gastric lavage yields more positive results than does either procedure alone. The optimal time for sputum induction and gastric lavage is early in the morning before meals.

Sputum, and other specimens, should be delivered to the laboratory with minimal delay; specimens that cannot be delivered or processed immediately should be refrigerated. Despite this, one study showed 90% agreement between fresh specimens and those examined after a delay of 1 to 8 days in the mail.

Gastric contents

If a patient is unable to raise a sufficient amount of sputum, is uncooperative, or cannot expectorate, a specimen of gastric contents is needed. Gastric lavage is frequently required with young children from whom it is difficult to obtain a sputum sample. A minimum of three specimens should be submitted.

The gastric lavage should be performed before the patient gets out of bed in the morning, after having fasted for at least 8 hours prior to the collection. A disposable plastic gastric tube* is used. It is first moistened with sterile water and then inserted into a nostril or into the mouth. As the tube is gently advanced, the patient is instructed to swallow small sips of sterile water to assist in swallowing the tube. After the gastric tube is properly in the stomach, gastric contents may be aspirated with a sterile 50-

ml syringe and transferred to a sterile flask. The patient should then be given 20 to 30 ml of sterile water (commercially distilled water for parenteral administration), either by mouth or by injection through the gastric tube.* The gastric washings are again aspirated and added to the first collection. The specimen is then delivered **immediately** to the laboratory, where prompt processing (within 4 hours) must be performed to neutralize the adverse effects of gastric acid on the tubercle bacillus. If this is not practical, some means of neutralizing the gastric acid must be used, such as the addition of 10% sodium carbonate until a pH of 7 is achieved, using phenol red as an indicator.

Urine

A minimum of three early morning midstream voided ("clean catch") or catheterized urine specimens is recommended; the entire volume of voided urine is collected in a sterile container. A 24-hour pooled specimen is sometimes used, although it is not recommended because it is likely to be contaminated and to contain fewer viable tubercle bacilli than a first-voided specimen. The specimen should be refrigerated prior to processing and processed as soon as possible.

Other materials

Since tuberculosis may occur in almost any site of the body, types of clinical material other than those previously mentioned may occasionally be examined. Specimens of CSF, pleural and pericardial fluid, pus, joint fluid, bronchial secretions, feces, resected lung tissue,† and autopsy material may be submitted for study. Anticoagulants may be used if indicated. Collection of these specimens does not generally require supervision by the bacteriologist; an

---

*Falcon Plastics, Los Angeles, Calif.

*Water should not be injected until one is certain that the tube is in the stomach and not the trachea.
†Tissue specimens may be frozen when a delay in processing is necessary.

adequate supply of sterile specimen containers must be available, however.

Processing of clinical specimens
Examination of stained smears

Although the demonstration of acid-fast bacilli in stained smears of sputum or other clinical material is only **presumptive** evidence of tuberculosis, the speed and ease of performance make the **stained smear** an important diagnostic aid, since it may be the first indication of a mycobacterial infection.

Because mycobacteria stain poorly by the Gram method, the conventional Ziehl-Neelsen carbolfuchsin stain or the fluorochrome staining technique, using auramine and rhodamine, is a required procedure. In the latter method, smears may be screened at 25 to 100 × magnification, permitting a larger area of the slide to be examined in the same time as compared with 1,000 × magnification using the conventional technique. By use of the fluorochrome stain (Truant technique described in Chapter 43) and a properly adjusted fluorescence optical system, the mycobacteria and acid-fast nocardias are readily discerned as bright, **yellow fluorescent bacilli** against a dark background. It should be noted that an antigen-antibody reaction is **not** involved in the fluorochrome procedure. It should not be considered, therefore, as a fluorescent antibody or immunofluorescence test. Some laboratories confirm all positive fluorescent smears by the more specific Ziehl-Neelsen or Kinyoun technique.

Preparation of the smear

Sputum specimen—direct smear
1. In a hood or biologic safety cabinet, transfer a portion of the sputum to a disposable Petri dish, and with a wooden applicator stick broken in half, tease out a small portion of caseous, purulent, or bloody material and transfer it to a clean **new** slide.
2. Press another slide on top of it, squeeze the slides together, then pull them apart.

This should result in two preparations of the proper thinness for staining and microscopy.
3. Label both slides and air dry and flame them immediately two or three times.
4. Stain the slides according to the Ziehl-Neelsen or Kinyoun acid-fast or Truant fluorochrome method (see Chapter 43). Do not use staining dishes, as they permit transfer of mycobacteria between slides.
5. Dry the slides in air or under an infrared lamp; do not blot them.
6. Examine the slides under oil immersion lens.

Sputum specimen—concentration. With the concentration method the specimen is digested by sodium hypochlorite, and any mycobacteria present are concentrated in the sediment by centrifugation. This procedure generally increases the number of positive smears and is best carried out on 24-hour specimens. Since sodium hypochlorite is actively tuberculocidal as well as an excellent digestant, the resulting sediments are considered nonviable and are useful **only for stained smears** and not for subsequent cultural procedures or animal inoculation.
1. Mix an equal volume (5 to 10 ml) of sputum and 5% sodium hypochlorite (Clorox household bleach is recommended) in a collection container of ample size; stir with a wooden applicator stick to ensure complete mixing. This should be done in an appropriately vented work area.
2. Shake the container for 2 to 3 minutes and keep it at room temperature for 10 minutes or until complete digestion has taken place.
3. Transfer a portion to a 15-ml centrifuge tube and centrifuge it for 10 minutes at 3,000 rpm.
4. Decant the supernatant fluid and allow the centrifuge tube to stand inverted on a paper towel to drain the sediment; no neutralization is necessary.

5. Transfer the creamy white sediment to a slide with a cotton-tipped applicator stick. Air dry (no fixing is required) and stain it by the usual method.

Concentration by polycarbonate membrane filtration was more effective than the standard centrifugation technique according to a recent report by Smithwick and Stratigos (J. Clin. Microbiol. **13:**1109-1113, 1981).

Spinal fluid specimen—direct smear

Prepare the smear in several layers in an area not more than 1 sq cm, so that much of the preparation can be examined within 30 minutes.

Reporting and interpreting the microscopic examination

One should examine all sputum smears stained by conventional methods by carefully scanning the long axis of the smear three times, right-left-right, before reporting as negative.[37] Typical acid-fast bacilli are **red stained,** slender, slightly curved, long or short rods (2 to 8 μm), sometimes beaded or granular (Plate 9). Atypical forms are unusually thick or diphtheroid, very long, and sometimes coccoid.*

Results of microscopic examination should be reported simply "**Positive for acid-fast bacilli**" or "**No acid-fast bacilli found**"; a positive finding should be based only on typical forms, but atypical rods should also be noted. When large numbers of typical acid-fast bacilli are found, it is reasonable to assume they are *M. tuberculosis;* when atypical rods are seen, they may represent other pathogenic or nonpathogenic mycobacteria or nocardias. It is desirable to report the number of acid-fast bacilli seen; the following criteria recommended by the American Lung Association may be used[2]:

Number of organisms seen	Report to read
1 to 2 in entire smear	Report number found and request another specimen
3 to 9 per slide	Rare (+)
10 or more per slide	Few (++)
1 or more per oil immersion field	Numerous (+++)

When only one or two acid-fast bacilli are seen in the **entire** smear, it is also recommended that they not be reported until confirmation is obtained by examining other smears from the same or another specimen. One study found that when **more than six** acid-fast organisms were present per high-power field, with either sputum or gastric contents, culture of the same material always yielded a pathogenic mycobacterium.[35]

In the case of CSF, if repeated specimens are examined, a high percentage of cases have acid-fast bacilli demonstrated by microscopy or culture. Microscopy is particularly important, of course, because of the need to treat patients as soon as possible when tuberculous meningitis is present. Smears were positive for 87% of 52 patients studied by Kennedy and Fallon,[16] but only 37% were positive on the first specimen (25% on the second, 19% on the third, and 6% on the fourth). Cultures were ultimately positive for 83% of the patients, 52% from the first specimen.

As previously noted, the demonstration of mycobacteria in sputum or other clinical material should be considered only as **presumptive** evidence of tuberculosis, since it does not specifically identify *M. tuberculosis.* The report form should indicate this in some manner. For example, *Mycobacterium gordonae*, a nonpathogenic scotochromogen commonly found in tap water, has been a particular problem when tap water or deionized water has been used in the preparation of smears or even when patients rinsed their mouths briefly with tap water prior

---

*It is important to wipe the objective thoroughly with lens paper **after every positive smear** to prevent the transfer of acid-fast organisms to the next slide by way of oil remaining on the objective. Use of a cover glass or Diaphane averts the problem.

to the use of aerosolized saline solution for inducing sputum.[10,11] The incidence of false-positive smears is very low when good quality control is maintained.[23]

The examination of stained smears is considered the least sensitive of the diagnostic methods for tuberculosis; **cultures** should be performed on all specimens examined microscopically.* Because of its simplicity and speed, however, the stained smear is an important and useful test, since smear-positive patients ("infectious reservoirs") are the greatest risk to others in their environment.

Digestion, concentration, and cultural methods
Culture of sputum and bronchial secretions by N-acetyl-L-cysteine-alkali method[29]

It has long been recognized that the conventional chemical methods of digestion and decontamination of sputum for the cultivation of tubercle bacilli result in the destruction of a large percentage of these organisms. For this reason, a milder decontamination and digestion procedure, using the mucolytic agent N-acetyl-L-cysteine (NALC), is advocated. (The preparation of the required reagents is described in Chapter 44.) The procedure is as follows:

1. Collect the sputum specimen as previously described and transfer approximately 10 ml to a 50-ml sterile, disposable, aerosol-free plastic centrifuge tube with a screw cap (Falcon Plastics, No. 2070).
2. Add an equal volume of NALC–sodium hydroxide solution.
3. Tighten the screw cap; mix the specimen well in a Vortex mixer† for 5 to 20 seconds or until digested. Violent agitation is not

recommended because denaturation of the NALC may take place.

4. Allow the tube to stand at room temperature for **15 minutes** to effect decontamination.*
5. Fill the tube within ½ inch of the top with either sterile M/15 phosphate buffer, pH 6.8 (preferred), or sterile distilled water. This dilution acts to minimize the action of the sodium hydroxide and reduce the specific gravity, thereby facilitating centrifugation.
6. Centrifuge the tube at or near 3,000 rpm (1,800 to 2,400 g) for **15 minutes** and carefully decant the supernatant fluid into a splash-proof can containing a phenolic disinfectant. Wipe the lip of the tube with a cotton ball soaked with 5% phenol. Retain the sediment.
7. If direct drug susceptibility tests are to be performed (see step 12), prepare a smear of the sediment by using a sterile applicator stick or 3-mm-diameter wire loop to spread one drop of the material over an area approximately 1 by 2 cm. Stain the material by the Ziehl-Neelsen or fluorochrome method and determine the approximate number of acid-fast bacilli (AFB) per oil immersion field.
8. Add 1 ml of 0.2% bovine albumin† to the sediment, using a sterile pipet. Shake the tube gently by hand to mix. No neutralization is required, since the dilution of the sodium hydroxide by the phosphate buffer wash in step 5 and the strong buffering capacity of the bovine albumin make this unnecessary. Refrigerate these albumin-suspended sediments overnight if inoculation to media is not practical at

---

*Authorities estimate that it requires from 10^4 to 10^5 organisms per milliliter of sputum to yield a positive direct smear, of which 10 to 100 organisms per milliliter are recoverable by culture.

†Vortex-type, Junior model, available from most laboratory supply houses.

---

*If contamination is expected to be heavy, the concentration of NaOH may be increased to 4%, but the exposure time must **not** be extended.

†Bovine albumin fraction V, adjusted to pH 6.8 with 4% NaOH; Pentex, Inc., Kankakee, Ill.

TABLE 31-1

Selective mycobacterial isolation media

Medium	Components	Inhibitory agents
Gruft modification of Löwenstein-Jensen	Fresh whole eggs, defined salts, glycerol, potato flour, ribonucleic acid (5 mg/100 ml)	Malachite green, 0.025 g/100 ml Penicillin, 50 U/ml Nalidixic acid, 35 μg/ml
Mycobactosel* Löwenstein-Jensen	Fresh whole eggs, defined salts, glycerol, potato flour	Malachite green, 0.025 g/100 ml Cycloheximide, 400 μg/ml Lincomycin, 2 μg/ml Nalidixic acid, 35 μg/ml
Middlebrook 7H10	Defined salts, vitamins, cofactors, oleic acid, albumin, catalase, glycerol, dextrose	Malachite green, 0.0025 g/100 ml Cycloheximide, 360 μg/ml Lincomycin, 2 μg/ml Nalidixic acid, 20 μg/ml
Selective 7H11 (Mitchison's medium)	Defined salts, vitamins, cofactors, oleic acid, albumin, catalase, glycerol, dextrose, casein hydrolysate	Carbenicillin, 50 μg/ml Amphotericin B, 10 μg/ml Polymyxin B, 200 U/ml Trimethoprim lactate, 20 μg/ml

From Sommers.[33]
*BBL Microbiology Systems, Cockeysville, Md.

TABLE 31-2

Dilution of concentrate for inocula

No. of acid-fast bacilli per oil immersion field	Control quadrant 1	Control quadrant 2	Drug quadrants
Less than 1	Undiluted	10^{-2}	Undiluted
1-10	10^{-1}	10^{-3}	10^{-1}
More than 10	10^{-2}	10^{-4}	10^{-2}

this time. It is recommended that bovine albumin be added **before** smears are made if the volume of sediment is small.

9. Make a 1:10 dilution of this sediment by adding 10 drops of it to 4.5 ml of sterile water.

10. Inoculate the following media, using 0.1 ml of the sediment for each tube or plate:

a. **Löwenstein-Jensen (L-J) slants**
One tube with undiluted sediment, one tube with 1:10 dilution

b. **7H10-Oleate-albumin-dextrose-catalase (OADC) (preferably) or 7H11 biplates**
One half of a plate with undiluted sediment, one half of a plate with 1:10 dilution
Spread with a glass spreader, using the 1:10 dilution first.

c. At least one of the selective media from Table 31-1

11. If the specimen shows a **positive** smear (step 7), dilute the concentrated sediment as shown in Table 31-2. Dilution is necessary to ensure an inoculum size that will yield at least 40 to 50 colonies on the control plate when performing drug susceptibility tests but not large enough to permit overgrowth of drug-resistant mutants, which can occur spontaneously in drug-susceptible populations.

12. **Direct** drug susceptibility testing* is encouraged for all specimens with **positive** smears. This may be carried out by inoculating the following media in Felsen quadrant 7H10 plates (Plate 160)† (see Chapter 42 for preparation), using sterile, disposable capillary pipets and adding to each quadrant 3 drops (0.15 ml) of the two dilutions selected in step 11:

Plate no.	Quad-rant no.	Drug	Amt (μg) per disk	Final drug concen-tration (μg/ml)
1	I	(Control no. 1)		0
	II	Isoniazid	1	0.2
	III	Isoniazid	5	1.0
	IV	Ethambutol	25	5.0
2	I	(Control no.2)		0
	II	Streptomycin	10	2.0
	III	Streptomycin	50	10.0
	IV	Rifampin	5	1.0
3	I	*p*-Aminosalicylic acid	10	2.0
	II	*p*-Aminosalicylic acid	50	10.0
	III			
	IV			

Tests involving the secondary antituberculous drugs, including kanamycin, viomycin, ethionamide, cycloserine, and others should be done only by reference laboratories.[44]

Paper disks impregnated with antituberculous drugs‡ are placed in sectors of quadrant plates that are then filled with 7H10 agar and incubated overnight to allow diffusion of the drug. They are then inoculated with the test strain as previously described.

13. Incubate L-J slants (steps 10 and 11) in a horizontal position for 1 to 2 days at 35 C in the dark. Examine weekly for 6 to 10 weeks. An atmosphere of CO_2 is beneficial for the growth of mycobacteria. Thus, L-J slants (loosen screw caps) should be incubated in a CO_2 incubator for the first 2 weeks. Incubation in a candle jar is not recommended, since an increase in contamination and a decrease in the amount of growth may occur, apparently as a result of oxygen depletion within the jar.

14. Incubate 7H10 or 7H11 plates (steps 10 and 12) right side up in permeable polyethylene bags,* closed by stapling, **in the dark** in a CO_2 (5% to 10%) incubator at 35 C for 3 weeks.

15. Examine 7H10 or 7H11 plates for growth both macroscopically and microscopically (a dissecting or other microscope with $100\times$ magnification is recommended) after 5 to 7 days' incubation and weekly thereafter.† The transparent 7H10 and 7H11 media permit good differentiation between corded and noncorded colonies under low-power magnification. **Group II scotochromogens** (see next section) are obvious by the presence of yellow, **noncorded** colonies on removal from the dark incubator; the development of **pigment** in colorless, noncorded colonies after exposure to light is characteristic of **Group I photochromogens.**

16. **Positive** cultures are reported as soon as growth is noted, and the final report is made after 6 to 8 weeks' or more incuba-

---

*These tests should be performed on all suspected isolates of *Mycobacterium tuberculosis;* if the tests are not available, the culture should be referred to a state laboratory or other specialized facility for susceptibility tests or speciation.
†Falcon Plastics, Los Angeles, Calif.
‡Antimicrobial drugs for use in culture media, Baltimore Biological Laboratory, Cockeysville, Md.

---

*Falcon Plastics, Los Angeles, Calif.; Baggies, Colgate-Palmolive Co., New York, N.Y.
†Runyon has written an excellent discussion of the identification of mycobacteria by microscopic examination of colonies.[28]

tion of 7H10 plates and L-J slants. All cultures, of any type, positive for mycobacteria should be saved at 5 C for 6 months in case special studies are required. Drug susceptibility tests are read as soon as possible, with the reservation that changes can occur in the final reading because of the slow growth of some initially susceptible strains in the presence of certain agents, particularly streptomycin.

In reporting results of the drug susceptibility tests, the report should include:
1. Type of test—direct or indirect
2. Number of colonies on control quadrant
3. Number of colonies on the drug quadrant
4. Concentration of the drug in each quadrant

From these data, a rough approximation of the percentage of organisms resistant to the drug may be calculated as follows:

$$\frac{\text{No. of colonies on drug quadrant}}{\text{No. of colonies on control quadrant}} \times 100 =$$

% resistance at that drug concentration

Refer to previously cited manual[37] and texts[29,39] for examples and photographs of these drug susceptibility tests.

Culture of sputum by other methods

In addition to the previously described NALC-alkali method for digestion and decontamination, two other methods, if properly performed, are acceptable.

Trisodium phosphate–benzalkonium chloride method.[45] The trisodium phosphate–benzalkonium chloride method requires digestion with trisodium phosphate for only 1 hour. Because of the low survival rate of mycobacteria, the 12- to 24-hour exposure of the original method is no longer an acceptable procedure. The preparation of the required reagents is described in Chapter 44. The technique is as follows:

1. Mix equal volumes of sputum and trisodium phosphate–benzalkonium chloride* in a 50-ml disposable, leakproof centrifuge tube†; shake it on a shaking machine‡ for 30 minutes.
2. Allow the tube to stand at room temperature for 20 to 30 minutes.
3. Centrifuge it at 3,000 rpm for 20 minutes.
4. Decant the supernatant fluid into a disinfectant, observing the necessary precautions.
5. Resuspend the sediment in 10 to 20 ml of M/15 sterile phosphate buffer, pH 6.6; recentrifuge it for 20 minutes.
6. Again decant the supernatant fluid and inoculate the sediment to egg media. If non-egg media, such as 7H10 agar, are used, residual benzalkonium chloride may inhibit the growth of mycobacteria. This inhibitory effect may be neutralized by adding 10 mg/100 ml of lecithin to the sterile buffer or by employing an additional wash with sterile buffer. This is not necessary when using egg-containing media, since neutralizing phospholipid compounds are already present.

Sodium hydroxide method
1. Mix equal volumes of sputum and 3% to 4% sodium hydroxide containing 0.004% phenol red in a disposable leakproof centrifuge tube; homogenize it on a shaking machine for 10 minutes.
2. Centrifuge the tube at 3,000 rpm for 20 minutes.
3. Decant the supernatant fluid into a disinfectant, observing bacteriologic precautions.
4. Using a sterile capillary pipet, add 2 N hydrochloric acid one drop at a time until a definite yellow endpoint is obtained.

*Zephiran, Winthrop Chemical Co., New York, N.Y.
†Falcon Plastics, No. 2070, Los Angeles, Calif.
‡Paint conditioner, laboratory model No. 34, Red Devil Tools, Union, N.J.

5. Back titrate with 4% sodium hydroxide to a **faint pink** endpoint (neutrality).
6. Inoculate the sediment to L-J medium and 7H10 or 7H11 agar. The use of one of the selective media from Table 31-1, along with digestion with 2% NaOH, has been found effective in the recovery of mycobacteria from heavily contaminated specimens.

When sputum specimens are consistently contaminated with *Pseudomonas* species and other similar organisms, the method of Corper and Uyei is recommended. It makes use of the decontaminating effect of oxalic acid as follows:

1. Mix equal volumes of sputum and 5% oxalic acid in a leakproof centrifuge tube; homogenize it in a Vortex mixer and allow it to stand at room temperature for 30 minutes, shaking it occasionally.
2. Add sterile physiologic saline to within 1 inch of the top of the tube; this lowers the specific gravity, permitting better concentration of bacilli in the sediment.
3. Centrifuge the tube at 3,000 rpm for 15 minutes.
4. Decant the supernatant fluid into a disinfectant, using bacteriologic precautions.
5. Neutralize the sediment with 4% sodium hydroxide containing phenol red indicator; inoculate the desired media.

Cetylpyridinium method. For specimens that will be in transport more than 24 hours, the CDC recommends mixing equal volumes of sputum and a solution of 1% cetylpyridinium chloride and 2% sodium chloride. This serves to decontaminate, liquefy, and concentrate the sputum. Tubercle bacilli remain viable for 8 days. This method is not suitable for fungi.

Culture of sputum without decontamination

Direct culture of sputum, without prior decontamination, onto selective 7H10 medium provided very good results.[27] Of 636 sputum specimens processed in this manner, 44 were positive and 2 were contaminated. By compari-son, specimens decontaminated with 1% sodium hydroxide–NALC and then cultured on nonselective 7H11 yielded 48 positive cultures and 18 contaminated cultures. Specimens decontaminated with 2% NaOH-NALC and then cultured on 7H11 yielded 48 positive cultures and 7 contaminated cultures.

Culture of gastric specimens

1. Add a pinch of NALC powder to about 25 ml of specimen in a 50-ml centrifuge tube.
2. Mix it in a Vortex mixer as with sputum.
3. Centrifuge the tuve at 3,000 rpm for 30 minutes.
4. Aseptically decant the supernatant fluid and resuspend the sediment in 2 to 5 ml sterile distilled water.
5. Add an equal volume of NACL-alkali reagent and proceed as with sputnum.
6. If the gastric specimen is quite fluid, centrifuge the tube directly and proceed with step 5.

Culture of urine

Clean-voided, early morning urine specimens are handled as follows:

1. Pour approximately 50-ml portions into one or more centrifuge tubes; centrifuge the tubes at 3,000 rpm for 30 minutes.
2. Aseptically decant the supernatant fluid, resuspend the sediment in 2 to 5 ml of sterile water, and handle as described under gastric specimens.

An alternate method described in the CDC manual[37] is as follows:

1. Centrifuge and combine the sediments as described above.
2. Add to the sediment an equal volume of 4% H_2SO_4.
3. Mix it in a Vortex mixer; let it stand for 15 minutes.
4. Fill the tube almost to the 50-ml mark with sterile distilled water, mix, and centrifuge as before.

5. After decanting the supernatant fluid, add 0.2% bovine albumin to the sediment and inoculate media as in sputum cultures.

Note: Since prolonged exposure to urine may be toxic to mycobacteria, urine should be decontaminated as soon as possible after receipt in the laboratory.

Culture of CSF and other body fluids

The isolation of *M. tuberculosis* from CSF and other body fluids is generally more difficult than that from sputum and gastric secretions. Since **very few** organisms may be present, success often depends on the amount of specimen available for culture—the larger the volume, the greater the chance of recovering the organism. At least 10 ml of fluid should be submitted.

The fluid specimen should be centrifuged for 30 minutes at 3,000 rpm and the supernatant fluid discarded. (CSF supernate may be saved for other examinations, such as serologic or chemical tests.) Half of the sediment is used for inoculating media and preparing a smear; the other half should be used for guinea pig injection.* Because these specimens generally contain no other bacteria, the decontaminating procedure is neither necessary nor desirable. It could result in the loss of the few organisms present. If the fluid specimen contains a clot, this is cut into small pieces with sterile scissors and subsequently accorded the same treatment as a sputum specimen. Purulent material is also handled in the manner used for sputum.

Kubica and Dye suggested that specimens that have been obtained aseptically—CSF, synovial fluid, pleural fluid, and small bits of biopsied tissue—be inoculated directly to a fluid medium, such as Middlebrook 7H9, Tween-Albumin medium, or Proskauer and Beck medium, in a volume ratio of 1:5. These media are incubated at 35 C in a CO_2 incubator, and acid-fast, stained smears are prepared and examined weekly. If mycobacteria are seen, the medium is inoculated to egg slants or 7H10 or 7H11 agar and incubated as previously described. If smears are negative after 4 weeks, the media are again subcultured at weekly intervals to L-J slants or 7H10 or 7H11 agar for 4 more weeks before discarding.

Specimens from superficial areas, such as skin lesions, should be set up in an additional culture to be incubated at **30 to 33 C** to permit detection of *M. marinum*.

Culture of feces

The examination of fecal material for *M. tuberculosis* is not very rewarding, and its use should be limited to special **unusual** circumstances. The presence of tubercle bacilli in the feces does not necessarily indicate intestinal tuberculosis; it more likely indicates sputum swallowed by a patient with pulmonary disease.

In the culture of fecal material, suspend about 5 g in 20 to 30 ml of distilled water and mix well. Add sufficient sodium chloride to make a saturated solution and allow it to stand for 30 minutes. With a sterile spoon skim off the film of bacteria that forms on the surface and transfer it to a sterile centrifuge tube. Add an equal volume of 4% sodium hydroxide, homogenize it with vigorous shaking, incubate it at 35 C for 3 hours, shaking at intervals, neutralize it with 2 N hydrochloric acid, and centrifuge it for 20 minutes at 3,000 rpm. Inoculate five tubes of media with the **top layer** of the supernatant fluid. Save a portion of the supernatant fluid, discarding the rest, and combine it with a portion of the sediment, to be later inoculated into a guinea pig if desired. Inoculate the remaining sediment to five additional tubes of media (**ten** tubes in all). This inoculation of ten tubes is advised because of the increased likelihood of subsequent loss from contamination in culturing fecal material.

---

*Wayne[39] has recommended the use of membrane filters for spinal fluid culture for mycobacteria.

Culture of tissue removed at operation or necropsy

Tissue removed surgically (lymph nodes, resected lung, and so forth) generally is not contaminated and does not require sodium hydroxide treatment. The specimen is finely minced with sterile scissors and transferred to a sterile tissue grinder,* where it is ground to a pasty consistency with sterile alundum and a small amount of sterile saline or 0.2% bovine albumin V. After settling, 0.2-ml portions of the supernatant fluid are removed and inoculated directly to egg media and 7H10 agar (liquid 7H9 medium also is desirable). Also, a smear is made.

Tissue that is obviously contaminated (such as tonsils and autopsy tissue) can be handled as just described, except that the supernatant fluid obtained after grinding is treated as is sputum (decontamination with NALC-alkali solution, homogenization, centrifugation, neutralization, and so forth) before inoculation to culture media.

ANIMAL INOCULATION TESTS

The inoculation of laboratory animals (generally guinea pigs) has been accepted in the past as definitive in determining the pathogenicity of an acid-fast bacillus. This is no longer true for human isolates, since some organisms, notably the mycobacteria other than tubercle bacilli and some isoniazid-resistant strains of *M. tuberculosis*, do not produce progressive disease in the injected animal.

Furthermore, the development of excellent cultural procedures and the more frequent use of **multiple specimens** from a suspected case of tuberculosis make it generally unnecessary for the hospital laboratory to inoculate laboratory animals.†

The procedure, however, is a useful diagnostic tool in the detection of **small numbers** of tubercle bacilli, as in CSF or specimens that are consistently contaminated on culture. For these reasons the technique has been included.

1. If clinical specimens are to be injected, they should be decontaminated and concentrated as described in previous sections under culture methods.
2. After a portion of the concentrated and neutralized sediment has been inoculated onto appropriate media, suspend the remainder in 1 ml of sterile physiologic saline and inject it either subcutaneously in the groin or intraperitoneally into a guinea pig.
3. If one is using pure cultures of mycobacteria, a dose consisting of approximately 0.1 mg (moist weight) is the usual inoculum. This is suspended in 1 ml of physiologic saline and injected subcutaneously into the right groin of each of **two** guinea pigs, the animals having been pretested and found negative to 0.1 ml of 5% old tuberculin (OT) or a satisfactory substitute injected intracutaneously. A subculture is also made of the suspension for control purposes.
4. Animals inoculated either with clinical material or with cultures should be examined weekly to detect the presence of enlarged lymph nodes draining the site of inoculation. Tubercle bacilli of human or bovine origin usually give rise to progressive disease in the guinea pig, with development of caseous nodes and involvement of the spleen and usually the liver and lungs. **Actual invasion of deep tissue** must be demonstrated—the microbiologist must not rely on the simple production of a local lesion alone.
5. If two guinea pigs have been injected, 0.5 ml of OT is administered to one at the end of 4 weeks. In most instances an animal eventually proved tuberculous is so sensitized to tuberculin by this time that it will

---

*Ten Broeck tissue grinder, small size, heavy-walled Pyrex glass, Bellco Glass, Inc., Vineland, N.J.
†Specimens for animal inoculation are best handled in a mycobacteriology reference laboratory.

die within 1 to 2 days of OT injection. If the tubrculin reaction is negative, the animals are held another 4 weeks before autopsy is performed.

6. Examine tissue showing gross pathology, using the acid-fast stain.

7. Involvement of only the regional nodes is considered a **doubtful** test, and the test should be repeated.

8. If only extensive lung tuberculosis is observed, **spontaneous** infection should be suspected and the test repeated; this also applies to animals that die in less than 4 weeks and show negative autopsy findings.

CULTURAL CHARACTERISTICS OF MYCOBACTERIA

It should be emphasized that the **acid-fast** nature of all colonies growing on culture media must be confirmed before they can be identified as mycobacteria. Cultures for the isolation of *M. tuberculosis* on L-J media should be incubated at 35 to 36 C for a total of 6 to 10 weeks and examined at weekly intervals; 7H10 media are held for at least 6 weeks. **Positive** cultures should be reported as soon as identification has been completed. Pathogenicity of the various species of *Mycobacterium* is noted in Table 31-3.

Mycobacterium tuberculosis

Colonies of human tubercle bacilli generally appear on egg media after 2 to 3 weeks at 35 C; no growth occurs at 25 or 45 C. Growth first appears as small (1 to 3 mm), dry, friable colonies that are rough, warty, granular, and buff colored. After several weeks these increase in size (up to 5 to 8 mm); typical colonies have a flat irregular margin and a "cauliflower" center (Plate 151). Because of their luxuriant growth, these mycobacteria are termed **eugonic.** Colonies are easily detached from the medium's surface but are difficult to emulsify. After some experience, one can recognize typical colonies of

human-type tubercle bacilli without great difficulty. However, final confirmation by biochemical tests must be carried out.

Virulent strains tend to orient themselves in tight, **serpentine cords,** best observed in smears from the condensation water or by direct observation of colonies on a cord medium. Catalase is produced in moderate amounts but not after heating at 68 C for 20 minutes in pH 7 phosphate buffer; human strains resistant to isoniazid (INH) are frequently catalase negative and yield smooth colonies on egg media. Nitrate reduction is positive. The niacin test (p. 358) is useful in that most **niacin-positive** strains encountered in the diagnostic laboratory prove to be *M. tuberculosis*. Susceptibility to antituberculous drugs is characteristically high.

Mycobacterium bovis

Bovine tubercle bacilli are rarely isolated in the United States but remain significant pathogens in other parts of the world. They require a longer incubation period—generally 3 to 6 weeks—and appear as tiny (less than 1 mm), translucent, smooth, pyramidal colonies when grown at 35 C. They adhere to the surface of the medium but are emulsified easily. On the basis of these characteristics, their growth is termed **dysgonic.** On 7H10 the colonies are rough and resemble those of *M. tuberculosis*.

M. bovis grows only at 35 C. It forms serpentine cords in smears from colonies on egg media; the niacin reaction and nitrate reduction tests are negative. *M. bovis* is also susceptible to thiophene-2-carboxylic acid hydrazide (TCH) (unless it is isoniazid resistant), a useful test to differentiate it from other mycobacteria.[43] Its susceptibility to the primary antituberculous drugs is similar to that of *M. tuberculosis*.

Mycobacterium ulcerans

M. ulcerans is associated with skin lesions and is considered the causative agent of Buruli ulceration, a necrotizing ulcer found in African natives.[5] The organism requires several weeks'

TABLE 31-3

Currently accepted species of *Mycobacterium*

Group	Strict or potential pathogen	Rarely or never a pathogen	
Slowly growing or "nonculturable" strict pathogens	*M. tuberculosis* *M. bovis* *M. africanum* *M. ulcerans* *M. leprae*		
Photochromogens	*M. kansasii* *M. marinum* *M. simiae* *M. asiaticum*		
Scotochromogens	*M. scrofulaceum* *M. szulgai* *M. xenopi*	*M. gordonae* *M. flavescens*	
Nonphotochromogens	*M. avium* *M. intracellulare* *M. malmoense* *M. haemophilum*	*M. terrae* *M. triviale* *M. nonchromogenicum*	
Rapidly growing	*M. fortuitum* *M. chelonei*	*M. vaccae* *M. smegmatis* *M. phlei* *M. parafortuitum* *M. neoaurum* *M. thermoresistible*	*M. chitae* *M. gadium* *M. gilvum* *M. duvalii* *M. aurum*
Animal pathogen	*M. lepraemurium* *M. microti* *M. paratuberculosis* *M. farcinogenes* *M. senegalense*		

From Good.[12]

incubation at 32 C. Unlike *M. marinum*, this organism is **nonphotochromogenic.** It is resistant to isoniazid, ethambutol, PAS, and ethionamide, but it is susceptible to rifampin, streptomycin, viomycin, kanamycin, and cycloserine.

Other mycobacteria

Although it has long been recognized that acid-fast bacilli other than *M. tuberculosis* are occasionally associated with both pulmonary and extrapulmonary disease, it has only been within the last two decades that these mycobacteria, variously called atypical, anonymous, unclassified, or nontuberculous acid-fast bacilli, have been associated with pulmonary and other disease clinically diagnosed as tuberculosis.[4] Evidence, obtained primarily from skin testing, suggests that many persons in the United States may become naturally infected with these myco-bacteria, although most of them do not show clinical evidence of disease.

In 1959 Runyon proposed a scheme for sepa-ration of the medically significant unclassified mycobacteria, dividing them into four large groups. This scheme served as an initial classifi-cation system until more precise speciation could be established for members within each group. For example, studies by individual work-ers and cooperative groups have demonstrated fundamental differences between various clini-cally significant and other mycobacteria through the use of easily performed metabolic and bio-chemical tests, many of which are described in a following section.

The non–*M. tuberculosis* strains account for a significant percentage of the total isolates of mycobacteria. In 1979 a survey of more than 24,000 isolates of mycobacteria revealed that *M. tuberculosis* accounted for 68% of the total, the *M. avium* complex 18%, *M. fortuitum* just less than 5%, *M. kansasii* 3%, *M. scrofulaceum* 3%, *M. chelonei* 1.5%, and several others less than 0.5% each.[12]

Group I photochromogens

Group I mycobacteria possess the outstanding characteristic of **photochromogenicity**—the ca-pacity to develop pigment when exposed to light. A young, actively growing culture on L-J slant medium that has been exposed to light for as little as 1 hour and reincubated in the dark will produce a bright lemon yellow pigment within 6 to 24 hours.

Three well-defined photochromogenic myco-bacteria constitute Runyon group I: *M. kansasii*, *M. marinum*, and *M. simiae*.

M. kansasii organisms are responsible for pul-monary disease in humans, often appearing in white, emphysematous men older than 45 years. The disease with its complications is indistin-guishable from that caused by *M. tuberculosis*, but it follows a more chronic and indolent

course. Other types of disease, including dis-seminated infection, may occur.[20] The disease is not communicable, in distinct contrast with that caused by the tubercle bacillus.

Optimal growth of *M. kansasii* occurs after 2 to 3 weeks at 35 C (slower at 25 C); growth does not occur at 45 C. Colonies are generally smooth, although there is a tendency to develop roughness. They are cream colored when grown in the dark and become a bright **lemon yellow** if exposed to light (Plate 152).

A practical procedure for photochromogenici-ty testing has been suggested by Kubica[18]:

1. Two slants of L-J medium are inoculated with a barely turbid suspension of the cul-ture; one tube is shielded from the light by wrapping with black x-ray paper or alumi-num foil.

2. Both tubes are incubated at 35 C (32 to 33 C is recommended for suspected cul-tures of *M. marinum*) until visible growth occurs on the uncovered slant.

3. The shield is removed from the covered tube and any pigment is noted; if none is observed, only **one half** of the tube is wrapped with the shield, while the other half is exposed either to a 60-watt bulb placed 8 to 10 inches from the tube or to bright daylight for 1 hour. The cap is loos-ened during exposure.

4. The shield is replaced, and both culture tubes are reincubated overnight with the caps loose. Pigments are compared in col-onies grown unshielded, shielded, and exposed to light for 1 hour. Three classes of pigments can then be established:
   a. **Scotochromogens**—pigmented in darkness
   b. **Photochromogens**—pigmented after exposure to light
   c. **Nonphotochromogens**—nonpig-mented either in darkness or light

If cultures are grown continuously under light (2 to 3 weeks), bright orange crystals of beta-carotene form on the surface of colonies, especially where growth is heavy. Nonphotochromogenic and scotochromogenic variants of *M. kansasii* occur very rarely.

Clinically significant strains of *M. kansasii* are strongly catalase positive, even after heating at 68 C at pH 7 (especially when using the semiquantitative test of Wayne, described on pp. 360-361). Low-catalase strains of *M. kansasii* have been described; these were not associated with human pathogenicity. Most strains do not produce niacin, although aberrant strains have been noted; nitrates are reduced; mature colonies show loose cords.

Stained preparations of *M. kansasii* show characteristically **long, banded, and beaded cells** that are strongly acid fast. There is variable susceptibility to INH and streptomycin, moderate susceptibility to rifampin, and resistance to para-aminosalicylic acid (PAS), but *M. kansasii* infections typically respond to conventional antituberculous therapy[3]; however, triple therapy, including rifampin, is desirable.[46]

Primarily associated with granulomatous lesions of the skin, particularly of the extremities, *M. marinum* infection usually follows exposure of the abraded skin to contaminated water. Known best for causing "swimming pool granuloma," this organism also has been implicated in infections related to home aquariums,[1] bay water, and industrial exposures involving water. It grows best at **25 to 32 C,** with sparse to no growth at 35 C (corresponding to the reduced skin temperature of the extremities), and is never isolated from sputum. It may be distinguished from *M. kansasii* by its source, its more rapid growth at 25 C, negative nitrate reduction, and weaker catalase production. The drugs most active against *M. marinum* are amikacin and kanamycin. Tetracyclines are inhibitory, chiefly at concentrations slightly below the expected blood levels.[31]

First isolated from monkeys, *M. simiae* has subsequently been recovered from humans with pulmonary disease. Pigmentation may be erratic. It has a positive niacin reaction, a high thermostable catalase activity, and a negative nitrate test; hydrolyzes Tween 80 slowly (more than 10 days); and is resistant to all first-line antituberculous drugs. It is sensitive to cycloserine and ethionamide.

Group II scotochromogens

The **scotochromogens** are **pigmented in the dark** (Greek *scotos*, dark), usually a deep yellow to orange, which darkens to an orange or dark red when the cultures are exposed to continuous light for 2 weeks (Plate 153). This pigmentation in the dark occurs on nearly all types of media at all stages of growth—characteristics that clearly aid in their identification.

The Group II scotochromogens include the potential pathogens *M. scrofulaceum*, *M. szulgai*, and *M. xenopi;* the so-called tap water scotochromogen, isolated from laboratory water stills, faucets, soil, and natural waters (now classified as *M. gordonae*); and *M. flavescens*.

Since the tap water scotochromogen is not associated with human disease, it is important to differentiate it from the potentially pathogenic mycobacteria. The former may contaminate equipment used in specimen collection, as in gastric lavage.

M. scrofulaceum is a slow-growing organism, producing smooth, domed to spreading, **yellow** colonies in both light and darkness. When exposed to continuous light, the colonies may increase in pigment to an **orange** or **brick red;** the paper shield should remain in place (see under photochromogens) until visible growth occurs in the unshielded tube; then colonies in the shielded tube should be exposed to continuous light. Initial growth may be inhibited by too much light.[37] The hydrolysis of Tween 80 (and urease activity) separates *M. scrofulaceum* from the tap water organisms in that the latter hydrolyze it within 5 days, whereas *M. scrofulaceum* remains negative up to 3 weeks. *M. scrofula-*

ceum is a cause of cervical adenitis and bone and other infections, particularly in children. It is often resistant to INH and PAS.

M. szulgai has been associated with pulmonary disease, cervical adenitis, cutaneous infection, tenosynovitis, and olecranon bursitis. It gives a positive nitrate reduction test. It is relatively susceptible to ethionamide, rifampin, ethambutol, and higher levels of INH.

M. xenopi has been isolated from the sputum of patients with pulmonary disease.[21] The optimal temperature for its growth is 42 C, and it fails to grow at 22 to 25 C. Four to five weeks' incubation is required to produce tiny dome-shaped colonies of a characteristic yellow color; branching **filamentous extensions** are seen around colonies on 7H10 agar, resembling a miniature bird's nest. Tween 80 hydrolysis and tellurite reduction tests are negative. Therapy with standard antituberculous drugs is generally successful.

Growth of *M. gordonae* appears late on L-J and 7H10 media, usually after 2 weeks and frequently after 3 to 6 weeks, as scattered small yellow-orange colonies in both light and darkness. Hydrolysis of Tween 80 characteristically occurs. *M. flavescens*, another nonpathogenic group II organism, also produces a yellow-pigmented colony in both light and darkness but is considerably more rapid in growth (usually within 1 week) and reduces nitrate as well as hydrolyzing Tween 80.

Group III nonphotochromogens

Runyon group III is made up of a heterogeneous variety of both pathogenic and nonpathogenic mycobacteria that do not develop pigment on exposure to light. The following species are among those recognized:

The *M. avium* complex (including *M. avium* and *M. intracellulare*) bacilli grow slowly at 35 C (10 to 21 days) and 25 C and produce characteristically thin, translucent, radially lobed to smooth, cream-colored colonies (Plate 154).

Rough variants* may show cording. These organisms are niacin negative (with rare exceptions[48]), do not reduce nitrate, and produce only a small amount of catalase. Tween 80 is not hydrolyzed in 10 days, but most of these organisms **reduce tellurite** within 3 days, a useful test to differentiate these potential pathogens from clinically insignificant members of group III.

The *M. avium* complex causes serious tuberculosislike disease that is most difficult to treat. However, these organisms may also occur in clinical specimens as nonpathogens. Multiple drug regimens (typically five drugs), usually including both isoniazid and rifampin, may be effective. Surgical resection of localized lesions may be necessary.

Mycobacterium gastri ("J" bacillus) has been described as occurring primarily as single colony isolates from gastric washings. However, it has not been associated with disease in humans. It is closely related to the low catalase-producing strains of *M. kansasii*, from which it may be readily differentiated by the photochromogenic ability of the latter. *M. gastri* may be differentiated from other members of Group III mycobacteria by its ability to hydrolyze Tween 80 rapidly, loss of catalase activity at 68 C, and nonreduction of nitrate.

M. malmoense was first described in 1977 in Sweden, where it was found associated with pulmonary disease.[32] Subsequently, it has been found in human pulmonary disease in Australia and Wales. The organism is nonphotochromogenic and grows slowly (2 to 3 weeks at 37 C and up to 6 weeks at 22 C). Colonies are colorless, smooth, glistening, grayish-white, opaque, domed, and circular, 0.5 to 1.5 mm in diameter. The organism does not produce niacin, is nitrate negative, hydrolyzes Tween-80 and pyrazinamide, and produces heat-labile catalase. It is resistant to isoniazid, streptomycin, PAS, and

---

*Most strains show a small proportion of rough colonies, which may resemble colonies of tubercle bacilli.

rifampin and is susceptible to ethambutol, cycloserine, kanamycin, and ethionamide.

M. haemophilum is a recently described organism isolated from skin lesions.[34] It requires hemin for growth and may be isolated on chocolate agar, 7H10 agar containing hemolyzed but not whole sheep red blood cells, or L-J medium containing 1% ferric ammonium citrate. Incubation should be at 32 C for a minimum of 2 to 4 weeks. The organism does not grow at 37 C. It should not be expected in specimens of sputum or gastric lavage. It is highly resistant to INH, streptomycin, and ethambutol but is susceptible to PAS.

M. terrae complex organisms have been called "radish" bacilli. A number of these mycobacteria have been isolated from soil and vegetables as well as from humans, where their pathogenicity remains questionable. The slow-growing (35 C) colonies may be circular or irregular in shape and smooth or granular in texture. They actively hydrolyze Tween 80, reduce nitrate, and are strong catalase producers, but they do not reduce tellurite in 3 days. *M. terrae* is resistant to INH.

M. triviale ("V" bacilli) occurs on egg media as rough colonies that may be confused with *M. tuberculosis* or rough variants of *M. kansasii*. These bacilli have been recovered from patients with previous tuberculous infections but are considered to be unrelated to human infections. There is one report of human infection with this organism. They are nonphotochromogenic, moderate to strong nitrate reducers, and maintain a high catalase activity at 68 C. They hydrolyze Tween 80 rapidly and do not reduce tellurite.

Group IV rapid growers

The Runyon group IV mycobacteria are characterized by their ability to **grow in 3 to 5 days** on a variety of culture media, incubated either at 25 or 35 C. Two members, *M. fortuitum* and *M. chelonei*, are associated with human pulmonary infection, although *M. fortuitum* is also a common soil organism and may frequently be recovered from sputum without necessarily being implicated in a pathologic process.

M. smegmatis, *M. phlei* (Plate 155), and *M. vaccae* are considered **saprophytes** and are nonpathogenic. *M. smegmatis* and *M. phlei* produce pigmented colonies and show filamentous extensions from colonies growing on cornmeal-glycerol agar. The ability of *M. phlei* ("hay bacillus") to produce large amounts of CO_2 has been utilized to stimulate primary growth of *M. tuberculosis* on 7H10 agar plates incubated in CO_2-impermeable (Mylar) bags.

M. fortuitum has been incriminated in progressive pulmonary disease, usually with a severe underlying complication, and has resulted in death. This potential pathogen also grows rapidly (2 to 4 days), is generally nonchromogenic, and may be readily separated from the rapidly growing saprophytes by its **positive 3-day arylsulfatase reaction** and by growing on MacConkey agar within 5 days, producing a change in the indicator. Both rough and smooth colonies are produced, with increased dye absorption (greening) on L-J medium (Plate 156). The niacin test is negative.

M. fortuitum is usually resistant to PAS, streptomycin, and INH but is susceptible to amikacin[8,46] and cefoxitin[7] and often the tetracyclines.[46]

M. chelonei (formerly *M. borstelense*) comprises two distinct subspecies: *M. chelonei*, which fails to grow on 5% NaCl medium, and *M. chelonei* ss. *abscessus*, which grows on the NaCl medium. *M. fortuitum* and *M. chelonei* are distinguished from each other by the combined use of five tests.[9] *M. fortuitum* is typically nitrate reductase positive, beta-glucosidase positive, penicillinase negative, and trehalose negative and produces acid from fructose. *M. chelonei* has the opposite reactions. A recent study indicates that a simple disk susceptibility test with pipemidic acid distinguishes between these two species readily (Casal and Rodriguez: J. Clin. Microbiol. **13**:989-990, 1981).

M. chelonei ss. *abscessus* is considered a significant but rarely isolated pulmonary pathogen, whereas *M. chelonei* is considered a saprophyte.[29,37] *M. chelonei*, along with unidentified mycobacteria, has been isolated from preimplantation cultures of porcine heart valve prostheses; there is evidence of infection subsequently in some patients receiving these implants. One report indicated susceptibility of this organism to erythromycin, streptomycin, and rifampin. Agents such as sulfonamides, trimethoprim, tetracyclines, and amikacin may be useful.

A recent report documents two outbreaks of sternal wound infection caused by *M. chelonei* in one case and *M. fortuitum* in the other (Hoffman et al.: J. Infect. Dis. **143**:533-542, 1981).

It should be noted that the majority of group IV mycobacteria are not stained by the fluorochrome (auramine-rhodamine) stain. All, however, are stained by the Ziehl-Neelsen technique.

Aids in identifying mycobacteria*

As soon as visible nonpigmented growth (5 to 6 days) is observed on any media, they should be exposed to light (previously described). After overnight incubation, *M. kansasii* strains become pigmented. All cultures of mycobacteria that are suspected of being members of Runyon's four groups (because of rapid growth, pigmentation, colonial characteristics, microscopic appearance, and so forth) should be subjected to the following procedures:

1. Subculture three L-J slants to obtain isolated colonies.
2. Incubate one at room temperature (20 to 25 C).

---

*The reader is referred to an excellent summary by Wayne and Doubek[41] of aids in the identification of most mycobacteria encountered in the clinical laboratory and to two publications by Wayne and colleagues.[42,43]

3. Incubate the second at 35 C in light, either continuously exposed to fluorescent light or frequently exposed to bright light at hourly intervals after growth appears.
4. Incubate the third at 35 C in the dark, wrapped in aluminum foil or black paper and placed next to the second tube.
5. When slant no. 2 shows good growth, remove the foil or paper from slant no. 3 and compare them.
6. Next, loosen the cap of slant no. 3 (grown in the dark), expose it to bright light, and observe for development of yellow pigment the next day.
7. Perform a niacin test on one of the original slants if growth is sufficient; subculture and reincubate if growth is scanty.
8. Other tests, such as cording, catalase, nitrate reduction, Tween 80 hydrolysis, arylsulfatase activity, and ability to grow at 45 C, may be required. See the following section for a description of these procedures.

Interpretation

M. tuberculosis and *M. bovis* do not grow at room temperature; rapid growers produce full-grown colonies in several days, even at room temperature. *M. kansasii* shows yellow colonies when grown in the light and white colonies when grown in the dark; the latter turn yellow overnight after exposure to light. Group II scotochromogens are yellow to orange in both the light and dark tubes, the pigment generally being deeper in the light tube. *M. avium* complex colonies are cream colored at first, becoming a deeper yellow with aging. Light exposure has no effect on pigment production. *M. tuberculosis* and a few others give a positive niacin test; a negative test does not preclude the possibility of *M. tuberculosis*, and it should be repeated at weekly intervals for a total of 6 weeks.

PROCEDURES USEFUL IN DIFFERENTIATING THE MYCOBACTERIA (INCLUDING CYTOCHEMICAL TESTS)

It should be emphasized that if facilities for carrying out these special procedures are lacking, the cultures should be **referred promptly** to a mycobacteriologic reference laboratory. In the meantime, an **interim report,** based on the available information (result of smear, growth on culture, and so forth) **should be sent to the clinician promptly.** Murray and Krogstad (J. Clin. Microbiol. **13:**468-471, 1981) preliminarily identified mycobacteria on the basis of colonial morphology, pigmentation, and growth rate and found this to be 92% accurate.

Table 31-4 summarizes control organisms, media, and duration of tests.

Niacin test

Strong niacin production by an acid-fast bacillus isolated from a clinical specimen is strong evidence of its possible identity as a **human tubercle bacillus.** Conversely, an accurately performed test resulting in a negative reaction generally indicates another species of *Mycobacterium*. *M. marinum* and *M. chelonei* may produce niacin and give doubtful or weakly positive results. *M. simiae* is also niacin positive.

The niacin test devised by Konno and modified by Runyon and co-workers depends on the formation of a complex color compound when a pyridine compound (niacin) from the organism reacts with cyanogen bromide (CNBr) and a primary or secondary amine (Plate 157).

If water of condensation is present on a culture slant of the organism to be tested (at least 3-week-old cultures **on egg media** should be used and have at least 100 colonies), it may be used for the niacin test. If not, the niacin may be extracted by adding a few drops of water or saline to the egg medium and placing the tube so that the liquid remains in contact with the colonies for 15 minutes. This serves to extract niacin if it is present. Puncturing the medium with the tip of a pipet aids in extracting niacin from the medium, especially if growth is confluent. One or two drops of the extract are then transferred to a white porcelain spot plate, and two drops of each of the following reagents are added: (1) 4% aniline in 95% ethanol, which should be nearly colorless, and (2) 10% aqueous CNBr. When not in use, both reagents are stored in the refrigerator in brown dropper bottles; they are made up fresh each month. A known positive strain of *M. tuberculosis* should always be included as a control.

Caution: The tests must be carried out in a chemical fume hood, since tear gas forms from CNBr. The production of an almost immediate **yellow color** indicates the presence of niacin. If a weak test is noted it should be repeated, using water in place of CNBr, and the results compared. On completion of the tests, several drops of 4% sodium hydroxide or 10% ammonia are added to the spot plate to destroy the residual CNBr and arrest tear gas formation. The plate may then be reconditioned by placing in boiling water for several minutes. Commercial niacin paper test strips are available and are strongly recommended.*

The only niacin-producing acid-fast organisms likely to be encountered in the clinical laboratory are those of *M. tuberculosis*. Most strains are niacin positive on L-J medium in 3 to 4 weeks; others may take up to 6 weeks. Some BCG strains (currently used in therapy of certain malignancies and sometimes causing disseminated infection in such patients) may give a weakly positive niacin test. Resistance to 1 μg/ml of thiophene-2-carboxylic acid[43] should also be tested in this situation. BCG strains are nitrate negative.

Nitrate reduction test

The test for reduction of nitrate (nitroreductase) is helpful in differentiating the slower-

---

*Bacto TB Niacin Test Strips, Difco Laboratories, Detroit, Mich.

TABLE 31-4

Controls and media used and duration of tests

No.	Biochemical test	Control organisms		Result		Medium used and amount	Duration of test	Remarks
		Positive	Negative	Positive	Negative			
1	Niacin	*M. tuberculosis*	*M. avium*	Yellow	No change of color	0.5 ml DH$_2$O	30 min	Room temp
2	Nitrate	*M. tuberculosis*	*M. avium*	Pink or red	No change of color	0.3 ml 7H9	2 hrs	37 C bath
3	Urease	*M. tuberculosis*	*M. avium*	Pink or red	No change of color	0.5 ml DH$_2$O	2 hrs	37 C bath
4	68 C Catalase	*M. avium*	*M. tuberculosis*	Bubbles	No bubbles	0.5 ml phosphate buffer [pH 7]	30 min	68 C bath
5	S.Q. Catalase	*M. fortuitum*	Medium	>50 mm	≤40 mm	Commercial medium	14 days	37 C incubator [with CO$_2$]
6	Tween	*M. kansasii*	*M. tuberculosis*	Pink or red	No change of color	1 ml DH$_2$O	5 days	37 C incubator [with CO$_2$]
7	Tellurite	*M. avium*	*M. tuberculosis*	Smooth fine black ppt. (smokelike) action	Gray clumps (no smokelike action)	Middlebrook 7H9 broth	10 days	37 C incubator [with CO$_2$]
8	Arylsulfatase	*M. fortuitum*	Medium	Pink or red	No change of color	Wayne's arylsulfatase medium	3 days	37 C incubator [with CO$_2$]
9	5% NaCl	*M. fortuitum*	*M. tuberculosis*	Substantial growth	Little or no growth	Commercial slant	28 days	37 C incubator [with CO$_2$]
10	T$_2$H, TCH	*M. bovis*	*M. tuberculosis*	No growth	Growth	T$_2$H flat and L-J	8 weeks	37 C incubator [with CO$_2$]

From Berlin and Martin: (Clin. Microbiol. Newsletter **2**:4-7, 1980).

growing organisms, *M. tuberculosis* and *M. kansasii*, from members of group II mycobacteria and the clinically significant *M. avium* complex organisms. The former are strong nitrate reducers, whereas the latter are generally negative. In group II, *M. szulgai* and *M. flavescens* are also positive. Other group III bacilli *(M. terrae, M. triviale)*, which are not considered clinically significant, are also strongly positive.

Nitrate broth,* in 2-ml amounts, is heavily inoculated (spadeful) from a 4-week slant culture and incubated in a 36 C water bath for 2 hours. The suspension is then acidified with one drop of a 1:2 dilution of hydrochloric acid, followed by two drops of sulfanilamide solution and two drops of the coupling reagent. (See Chapter 44 for preparation of these reagents.) Commercially available paper strips are equally satisfactory.

A **positive** test is indicated by the immediate formation of a **bright red** color (as compared with the reagent control). A **negative** test should always be confirmed by the addition of a small amount of zinc dust; a red color, caused by the reduction of nitrate by the zinc, confirms the negative test. An uninoculated reagent control and a negative and a positive control with a known strain of *M. tuberculosis* also should be included. Color standards (± to 5+) may be prepared from dilutions of sodium nitrate but are stable for only 10 to 15 minutes. (See Chapter 44 for preparation.)

Catalase activity

Acid-fast bacilli produce the enzyme **catalase,** which is detected by the breakdown of hydrogen peroxide and the subsequent active ebullition of gas (oxygen) bubbles. Detection of catalase activity, which should be tested routinely, has proved useful in several ways: (1) tubercle bacilli that become resistant to INH lose or show reduced catalase activity, (2) the catalase activity

of human or bovine strains may be selectively inhibited by heat, and (3) a group III mycobacterium *(M. gastri)* and isolates of clinically insignificant *M. kansasii* also lose their catalase activity at pH 7 and at 68 C.

Catalase activity may be determined in three ways:

1. At **room temperature,** add one drop of a 1:1 mixture of 10% Tween 80* and 30% hydrogen peroxide† directly to a slant culture of modified L-J medium or the control quadrant of a 7H10 agar plate. A **positive** catalase test is indicated by grossly visible gas bubbles (nascent O_2 from breakdown of H_2O_2 by catalase) within 2 minutes.

2. To determine the effect of pH and temperature on catalase activity, scrape several loopfuls or spadefuls of growth from a slant culture and suspend it in 0.5 ml of phosphate buffer pH 7 (M/15) in a screw-capped tube and place it in a **68 C** water bath for 20 minutes. After cooling the tube to room temperature, add 0.5 ml of the Tween 80–peroxide mixture and observe the reaction for 15 or 20 minutes for the formation of gas bubbles.

3. Perform a semiquantitative test, utilizing butt tubes (20 × 150 mm) of L-J medium‡ and a measurement of the height of the column of gas bubbles as follows. Inoculate the surface of the L-J medium with an actively growing egg slant or 7H9 broth culture and incubate the tube, with loosened cap, at 35 C for 2 weeks. Add 1 ml of the Tween 80–peroxide mixture, and after 5 minutes measure the height of the gas bubbles; record as follows:

Negative = no bubbles
≤ 45 = less than 45 mm bubbles (low)
≥ 45 = more than 45 mm bubbles (high)

---

*Cater, J.C., and Kubica, G.P. (unpublished data) have shown that Difco nitrate broth is a satisfactory substitute for the buffered nitrate substrate originally described.

*Atlas Chemicals Division, ICI America, Inc., Wilmington, Del.

†Must be refrigerated when not in use; Superoxol, Merck & Co., Rahway, N.J.

‡Lowenstein-Jensen Medium Deeps, Difco Laboratories, Detroit.

Interpretation

Except for *M. tuberculosis, M. gastri, M. malmoense, M. haemophilum,* and low-catalase *M. kansasii* strains, all other mycobacteria commonly isolated from human sources retain their ability to produce catalase after heating at 68 C at pH 7.

With the semiquantitative test most group II scotochromogens, group IV rapid growers (including *M. fortuitum*), and *M. kansasii* strains, as well as some group III nonphotochromogens (*M. terrae* and *M. triviale*), generally produce in excess of 45 mm of bubbles. *M. tuberculosis, M. bovis,* the *M. avium* complex, and clinically less significant strains of *M. kansasii* show less than 45 mm of foam; *M. marinum* and *M. xenopi* also produce less than 45 mm.

Tween 80 hydrolysis

Certain species of mycobacteria are capable of hydrolyzing Tween 80, a derivative of sorbitan monoleate, with the production of oleic acid. In the presence of the pH indicator neutral red, this acid is indicated by a change from amber to pink.

The test is performed by the method of Wayne and co-workers[42] (see Chapter 44 for reagents). One 3-mm loopful of an actively growing egg slant culture is suspended in a tube of substrate, which is incubated at 35 C. A control tube consisting of a known positive culture (*M. kansasii*) and an uninoculated (negative control) tube are also incubated. The tubes are examined after 5 days' and 10 days' incubation; a **positive** test is indicated by a change from amber to **pink** or **red.**

Generally, most strains of *M. kansasii* are positive within 5 days, whereas many strains of *M. tuberculosis* are positive in 10 to 20 days. Clinically significant group II and group III cultures usually remain negative for 3 weeks, whereas the clinically less significant strains are positive within 5 days.

A rapid Tween-80 hydrolysis test utilizing gas-liquid chromatography has been described.[6]

This test requires 1 hour of incubation, followed by simple extraction and chromatography of nonderivatized oleic acid.

Sodium chloride (NaCl) tolerance test

This procedure is useful for the general separation of the rapid-growing mycobacteria (positive) from the slow-growing strains (negative) and for aid in the identification of *M. triviale* (positive) and *M. flavescens* (sometimes positive).

The medium can be prepared by adding NaCl in a final concentration of 5% to either L-J or American Trudeau Society medium before inspissation. A light suspension (barely turbid) of growth from an L-J slant is prepared, and 0.1 ml is inoculated to the surfaces of the NaCl medium* and a control slant containing no NaCl. The tests are incubated at 35 C and examined for growth at weekly intervals for 4 weeks.

Arylsulfatase test

The enzyme arylsulfatase is present in varying concentration in many mycobacterial species, and its concentration in a controlled 3-day test is particularly useful in differentiating the potential pathogens *M. fortuitum* and *M. chelonei* from other group IV rapid growers.

This rapid test is performed by growing the suspected organism in Tween-albumin broth (available commercially) for 7 days and inoculating 0.1 ml of this into a substrate containing 0.001 M tripotassium phenolphthalein disulfate,† along with known negative, weakly positive, and positive control cultures. These are incubated at 35 C for 3 days,‡ and then 6 drops of 1 molar sodium carbonate are added to each tube. If appreciable amounts of arylsulfatase have been produced, phenolphthalein will be

---

*Difco Laboratories (No. 1423), Detroit, Mich.
†Nutritional Biochemical Corp., Cleveland, Ohio; L. Light & Co., Colinbrook, Bucks, England.
‡A 2-week test using a 0.003 M substrate also may be used.

TABLE 31-5

Distinctive properties of mycobacteria encountered in clinical specimens[a]

Runyon group	Complex name[b]	Species name	Incorrect or illegal synonym(s)	Clinical significance[c]	Growth rate[d] 45 C	37 C	31 C	24 C	Colony type — Usual colony morphology[e]	Colony type — Pigmentation[f]	Niacin
		M. leprae		1							
		M. ulcerans	buruli	1	−	−	S	−	R	N	−
	TB	M. tuberculosis		1	−	S	S	−	R	N	+
		M. bovis		1	−	S		−	Rt	N	−
I		M. marinum	balnei, platypoecilus	2		∓	M	M	S/SR	P	∓
		M. kansasii	luciflavum	2		S	S	S	SR/S	P	−
		M. simiae	habana	3-2	−	S			S	P	+
II	scrofulaceum	M. scrofulaceum	marianum, paraffinicum	3-2		S	S	S	S	S	−
		M. szulgai		1		S	S	S	S or R	S/P	−
		M. gordonae	aquae	4		S		S	S	S	−
		M. flavescens		4		M		M	S	S	−
		M. xenopi	littorale	3	S	S			Sf	S[k]	−
III	avium	M. avium		2	−/+	S		±	St/R	N	−
		M. intracellulare	brunense, Battey bacillus	2	−/+	S		±	St/R	N	−
		M. gastri		4		S		S	S/SR/R	N	−
		M. malmoense		1		S	S	S	S	N	−
		M. haemophilum		1	−	−	S[l]	S	R	N	−
		M. nonchromogenicum		4		S		S	SR	N	−
	terrae	M. terrae		4		S		S	SR	N	−
		M. triviale		4		M		S	R	N	−
IV		M. fortuitum	ranae, minetti, giae	4-3	−	R		R	Sf/Rf	N[m]	−
	fortuitum	M. chelonei	borstelense	4-3	−	R		R	S/R	N	V
		M. phlei	moelleri	4	R	R		R	R	S	
		M. smegmatis		4	R	R		R	R/S	N(V)	
		M. vaccae		4		R		R	S	S	

Modified from Runyon and colleagues.[29]

[a]Plus and minus signs indicate presence or absence of feature; blank spaces indicate either that information currently is not available or that the property is unimportant.

[b]For most clinical laboratories, designation to "complex" is usually sufficient.

[c]Potential clinical significance: 1, only as pathogens; 2, usually as pathogens; 3, commonly as nonpathogens; 4, usually as nonpathogens.

[d]S, Slow; M, moderate; R, rapid.

[e]R, Rough; S, smooth; SR, intermediate in roughness; t, thin or transparent; f, filamentous extensions.

Susceptibility to T2H[g] (5 µg/ml)	Nitrate reduction	Semi-quantitative catalase (>45 mm)	68 C catalase	Tween hydrolysis, 5 days	Tellurite reduction, 3 days	Tolerance to 5% NaCl	Iron uptake[h]	Arylsulfatase, 3 days	MacConkey agar	Urease	Pyrazinamidase, 4 days	Agglutination tests available
−	−		+	−		−					−	
−	+	−	−	−		−		−	+	+	+	
+	−	−	−	−		−		−		+	−	
−	−	−	+	+		−		∓[i]		+	+	+
−	+	+	+	+	−	−		−		+	−	+
−	⊣	+	+	−	−			−		+	−	+
−	−	+	+	−	−	−	−	−[i]		+	±	+
−	+	+		∓	−	−		±[i]		+	−	+
−		+	+	+	−	−	−	−		−	∓	+
−	+	+	+	+	−	+	−	−	−	+	+	
−	−	−	+	−	−		−	−[i]		−	+	+
−	−	−	+	−	+	−	−	−		−	+	+
−	−		+	−	+	−	−	−		−	+	+
−	−	−	−	+	−	−	−			+	−	
	−		−	+						−	+	
										+	+	
−	−	+	+	+	−	−	−			−		
−	+	+	+	+	−	−	−			−	∓	
−	+	+	+	+	−	+	−	±		−		
+	+	+	+	±	V	+	+	+	+	+		+
−		+	+	−	V	V[n]	−	+	+	+		+
+		+	+	+	+	+	+	−	−			
+		+	+	+	+	+	+	−	−			
+		+	+	+	+	V	+	−	−			

[f]P, Photochromogenic; S, scotochromogenic; N, nonphotochromogenic. Note: *M. szulgai* is scotochromogenic at 37 C and photochromogenic at 25 C.

[g]Thiophene-2-carboxylic acid hydrazide.

[h]Plate 159.

[i]Arylsulfatase, 14 days, is +.

[j]Tween hydrolysis, 10 days, is +.

[k]Young cultures may be nonchromogenic or possess only pale pigment which may intensify with age.

[l]Requires hemin as growth factor.

[m]May become green on media containing malachite green.

[n]*M. chelonei* subspecies *chelonei* is −, *M. chelonei* subspecies *abscessus* is +.

split from the sulfate and detected by alkaliniz-ing with sodium carbonate. The resulting color is then immediately compared with a set of stan-dards (see Chapter 44 for preparation), since the color is not stable. A **positive** test shows a range from a faint pink ($\pm$) to a **light red** (3+); a nega-tive test develops no color (Plate 158).

Growth on MacConkey agar

M. fortuitum and *M. chelonei* grow on Mac-Conkey agar in 5 days, thereby differentiating them from other group IV rapid growers, which are inhibited.

A Petri dish containing 15 ml of MacConkey agar* is inoculated on a turntable with a 3-mm loopful of a 7-day Tween-albumin broth culture of the organism in question by rotating the plate and slowly moving the loop along the surface of the medium. The plate is incubated at 35 C and observed at 5 days and 11 days for growth. A positive control of *M. fortuitum* and a negative control of *M. phlei* also should be included. Occasionally, other group IV organisms grow within 11 days.

Tellurite reduction

The tellurite reduction test appears to be most valuable in the separation of the potentially pathogenic *M. avium* complex strains from the saprophytic nonphotochromogens. Middle-brook 7H9 broth with ACD enrichment and Tween 80 is the base medium, to which is added a solution of tellurite. (See Chapter 42 for prep-aration.)

The medium is inoculated with the mycobac-terium and incubated at 35 C for 7 days. Two drops of a sterile 0.2% solution of potassium tel-lurite are then added to the medium, which is returned to the incubator and examined daily for reduction of the colorless tellurite salt to a black (or "dirty brown" in the case of highly pigmen-ted strains) metallic tellurium.

Most *M. avium* complex strains and the majority of group IV rapid growers reduce tellu-rite in 3 to 4 days; other mycobacteria, such as *M. terrae* and *M. xenopi*, react more slowly.

Other tests

Other tests are described in several sources in the references.

Commercially available urease test disks[22] are convenient and reliable. Additional tests that may be promising for identification of certain mycobacteria include the heat-stable acid phos-phatase test,[30] the amidase test[15] and a test for beta-glucosidase. Bacteriophage typing and se-rologic techniques for identification of mycobac-teria are not practical for clinical laboratory use.

Study of spinal fluid and serum from a patient with tuberculous meningitis using thin-layer polyacrylamide gel isoelectric focusing revealed five immunoglobulin zones in the spinal fluid without any in the serum.[17] This indicated local immunoglobulin production, and it was possible to show immunofixation with *M. tuberculosis* or BCG as antigens with autoradiography.

Table 31-5 summarizes results with most of the tests described and other tests. Fig. 31-1 is a flowchart for speciation of mycobacteria.

Gas-liquid chromatography

One of the more exciting developments with regard to identification of mycobacteria is the application of gas-liquid chromatography. Origi-nal work in this area was done by Ohashi and co-workers.[24] This work was extended by Tisdall and others.[36] The latter group identified 18 mycobacterial species by analysis of profiles obtained by the use of gas-liquid chromatogra-phy. By using gas-liquid chromatographic pro-files alone, approximately 60% of cultures were correctly identified to species level, and an addi-tional 39% were correctly identified to a group of two or three organisms. The method was eval-uated in a clinical laboratory over a 2-month period, during which chromatography proved to

---

*Plates, rather than slant cultures, should be used, since the latter medium supports growth of heavy inocula of *M. smeg-matis*.

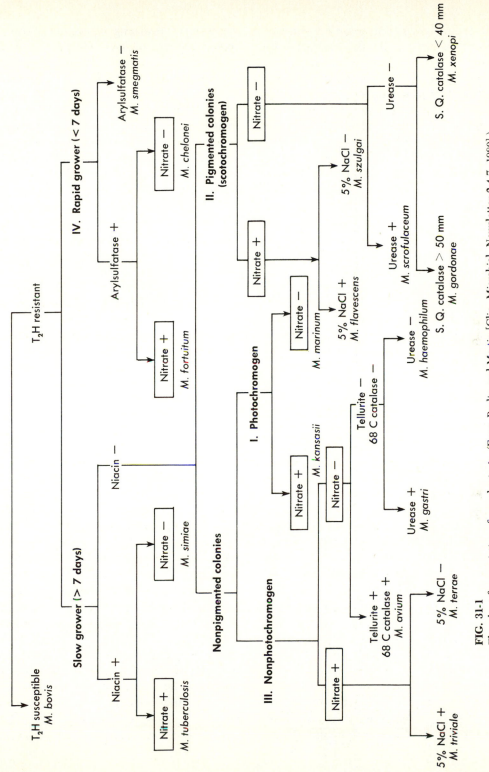

FIG. 31-1
Flowchart for speciation of mycobacteria. (From Berlin and Martin [Clin. Microbiol. Newsletter **2**:4-7, 1980].)

be as accurate as and more rapid than concurrent biochemical testing. In the case of chromatograms that differentiated to a group of two or three organisms, identification to species levels from these groups could usually be done by colonial morphology alone and could always be done by the addition of one selected biochemical test. Another procedure that appears promising has been described by Guerrant and colleagues (J. Clin. Microbiol. **13**:899-907, 1981).

Susceptibility testing

Direct susceptibility testing was discussed earlier in connection with culture technique. The procedure for conventional susceptibility testing is similar. Testing of second-line drugs or less commonly used drugs is best done in a reference laboratory. One may use disk diffusion testing to determine the susceptibility of *M. fortuitum* and *M. chelonei* to antibacterial agents, as outlined by Wallace and associates.[38]

Of particular interest is the radiometric (BACTEC) system for rapid susceptibility testing of mycobacteria.[26] This uses supplemented 7H9 broth plus ^{14}C-labeled substrate. Polymyxin B, carbenicillin, trimethoprim, and amphotericin are added to the broth to prevent growth of ordinary bacteria. Then the broth is inoculated directly with a concentrate for tubercle bacilli. The technique permits detection of the critical proportion of resistance—1% or greater of the bacterial population. Results are available in 4 to 6 days instead of the usual 2 to 3 weeks. There is excellent agreement with conventional susceptibility testing for *M. tuberculosis*. A recently published study also describes promising results (Snider et al.: Am. Rev. Respir. Dis. **123**:402-406, 1981).

MYCOBACTERIUM LEPRAE (LEPROSY BACILLUS OR HANSEN'S BACILLUS)

The leprosy bacillus was discovered by Hansen in 1872 in lepra cells (mononuclear epithelioid cells) of patients with leprosy. The conditions concerning communicability of the disease are still unclear. Humans are the only host; there is no known animal or soil reservoir.

Typical cells of *Mycobacterium leprae* are found predominantly in smears and scrapings obtained from the skin (not in the epidermis, but the corium) and mucous membrane (particularly of the nasal septum) of patients with nodular leprosy. When stained by the Ziehl-Neelsen method and decolorized and counterstained with 0.2% methylene blue in 4% sulfuric acid, large numbers of acid-fast bacilli are seen packed in lepra cells in parallel bundles, suggesting packets of cigars (globi). The bacilli are also found within endothelial cells of blood vessels, although they are rare or absent in tuberculoid lesions and undifferentiated lesions.

The organism has not been cultured on artificial media or human tissue culture cells. In 1960 Shephard was successful in producing infection in mouse foot pads with material obtained from cases of human leprosy. Other mycobacteria, such as *M. marinum* and *M. ulcerans*, also grow in foot pads of mice. Because of the prolonged generation time of these organisms, especially *M. leprae*, this procedure is not considered practical as a diagnostic test. The armadillo is susceptible to leprosy and has been used experimentally. However, an organism similar to *M. leprae* has been found in wild armadillos.

There are no serologic tests of value for diagnosis; serologic tests for syphilis in lepers frequently yield biologically false-positive results. Lepromin, a sterile extract of leprous tissue containing numerous *M. leprae* organisms, is used to determine relative resistance or susceptibility to the disease. Humans are relatively resistant to infection.

Although they are primarily bacteriostatic in their action, the sulfone drugs are the current therapy of choice in the treatment of human leprosy. Rifampin is an important adjunct in therapy.

REFERENCES

1. Adams, R.M., Remington, J.S., Steinberg, J., and Seibert, J.S.: Tropical fish aquariums: a source of *Mycobacterium marinum* infections resembling sporotrichosis, J.A.M.A. **211:**457-461, 1970.
2. American Lung Association: Diagnostic standards and classifications of tuberculosis and other mycobacterial diseases, New York, 1974, American Lung Association.
3. Bailey, W.C., Raleigh, J.W., and Turner, J.A.P.: Treatment of mycobacterial disease (official statement of American Thoracic Society), Am. Rev. Respir. Dis. **115:**185-187, 1977.
4. Chapman, J.S.: The atypical mycobacteria and human mycobacteriosis, New York, 1977, Plenum Medical Book Co.
5. Connor, D.H., and Lunn, H.F.: Buruli ulceration: a clinicopathologic study of 38 Ugandans with *Mycobacterium ulcerans* ulceration, Arch. Pathol. **81:**183-199, 1966.
6. Cox, F.R., Slack, C.E., Cox, M.E., Pruden, E.L., and Martin, J.R.: Rapid Tween 80 hydrolysis test for mycobacteria, J. Clin. Microbiol. **7:**104-105, 1978.
7. Cynamon, M.H., and Patapow, A.: In vitro susceptibility of *Mycobacterium fortuitum* to cefoxitin, Antimicrob. Agents Chemother. **19:**205-207, 1981.
8. Dalovisio, J.R., and Pankey, G.A.: In vitro susceptibility of *Mycobacterium fortuitum* and *Mycobacterium chelonei* to amikacin, J. Infect. Dis. **137:**318-321, 1978.
9. David, H.L., Traore, I., and Feuillet, A.: Differential identification of *Mycobacterium fortuitum* and *Mycobacterium chelonei*, J. Clin. Microbiol. **13:**6-9, 1981.
10. Dizon, D., Mihailescu, C., and Bae, H.C.: Simple procedure for detection of *Mycobacterium gordonae* in water causing false-positive acid-fast smears, J. Clin. Microbiol. **3:**211, 1976.
11. Gangadharam, P.R.J., Lockhart, J.A., Awe, R.J., and Jenkins, D.E.: Mycobacterial contamination through tap water, Am. Rev. Respir. Dis. **113:**894, 1976.
12. Good, R.C.: Nontuberculous mycobacteria, Clin. Microbiol. Newslett. **1:**1-3, 1979.
13. Good, R.C.: Isolation of nontuberculous mycobacteria in the United States, 1979, J. Infect. Dis. **142:**779-783, 1980.
14. Gruft, H.: Isolation of acid-fast bacilli from contaminated specimens, Health Lab. Sci. **8:**79-82, 1971.
15. Helbecque, D.M., Handzel, V., and Eidus, L.: Simple amidase test for identification of mycobacteria, J. Clin. Microbiol. **1:**50-53, 1975.
16. Kennedy, D.H., and Fallon, R.J.: Tuberculous meningitis, J.A.M.A. **241:**264-268, 1979.
17. Kinnman, J., Link, H., and Fryden, A.: Characterization of antibody activity in oligoclonal immunoglobulin G synthesized within the central nervous system in a patient with tuberculous meningitis, J. Clin. Microbiol. **13:**30-35, 1981.
18. Kubica, G.P.: Differential identification of mycobacteria, Am. Rev. Respir. Dis. **107:**9-21, 1973.
19. Kubica, G.P., Gross, W.M., Hawkins, J.E., Sommers, H.M., Vestal, A.L., and Wayne, L.G.: Laboratory services for mycobacterial diseases, Am. Rev. Respir. Dis. **112:**773-787, 1975.
20. Listwan, W.J., Roth, D.A., Tsung, S.H., and Rose, H.D.: Disseminated *Mycobacterium kansasii* infection with pancytopenia and interstitial nephritis, Ann. Intern. Med. **83:**70-73, 1975.
21. Marks, J., and Schwabacher, H.: Infection due to *Mycobacterium xenopei*, Br. Med. J. **1:**32-33, 1965.
22. Murphy, D.B., and Hawkins, J.E.: Use of urease test disks in the identification of mycobacteria, J. Clin. Microbiol. **1:**465-468, 1975.
23. Murray, P.R., Elmore, C., and Krogstad, D.J.: The acid-fast stain: a specific and predictive test for mycobacterial disease, Ann. Intern. Med. **92:**512-513, 1980.
24. Ohashi, D.K., Wade, T.J., and Mandle, R.J.: Characterization of ten species of mycobacteria by reaction-gas-liquid chromatography, J. Clin. Microbiol. **6:**469-473, 1977.
25. Roberts, G.D.: Mycobacteriology: laboratory procedure manual, Rochester, Minn., 1979, Mayo Foundation and Davies Printing Co.
26. Roberts, G.D.: Personal communication, 1981.
27. Rothlauf, M.V., Brown, G.L., and Blair, E.B.: Isolation of mycobacteria from undecontaminated specimens with selective 7H10 medium, J. Clin. Microbiol. **13:**76-79, 1981.
28. Runyon, E.H.: Identification of mycobacterial pathogens utilizing colony characteristics, Am. J. Clin. Pathol. **54:**578-586, 1970.
29. Runyon, E.H., Karlson, A.G., Kubica, G.P., and Wayne, L.G. Revised by Sommers, H.M., and McClatchy, J.K.: *Mycobacterium*. In Lennette, E.H., Balows, A., Hausler, W.J., Jr., and Truant, J.P., editors: Manual of clinical microbiology, ed. 3, Washington, D.C., 1980, American Society for Microbiology.
30. Saito, H., and Masai, H.: New heat-stable acid-phosphatase test for differentiation of mycobacteria, J. Clin. Microbiol. **11:**97-98, 1980.
31. Sanders, W.J., and Wolinsky, E.: In vitro susceptibility of *Mycobacterium marinum* to eight antimicrobial agents, Antimicrob. Agents Chemother. **18:**529-531, 1980.

32. Schröder, K.H., and Juhlin, I.: *Mycobacterium malmoense* sp. nov., Int. J. Syst. Bacteriol. **27**:241-246, 1977.

33. Sommers, H.M.: Mycobacterial diseases. In Henry, J.B., editor: Clinical diagnosis and management by laboratory methods, ed. 16, Philadelphia, 1979, W.B. Saunders Co.

34. Sompolinsky, D., Lagziel, A., Naveh, D., and Yankilevitz, T.: *Mycobacterium haemophilum* sp. nov.: a new pathogen of humans, Int. J. Syst. Bacteriol. **28**:67-75, 1978.

35. Strumpf, I.J., Tsang, A.Y., Schork, M.A., and Weg, J.G.: The reliability of gastric smears by auramine-rhodamine staining technique for the diagnosis of tuberculosis, Am. Rev. Respir. Dis. **114**:971-976, 1976.

36. Tisdall, P.A., Roberts, G.D., and Anhalt, J.P.: Identification of clinical isolates of mycobacteria with gas-liquid chromatography alone, J. Clin. Microbiol. **10**:506-514, 1979.

37. Vestal, A.L.: Procedures for the isolation and identification of mycobacteria, Public Health Service Pub. No. (CDC) 79-8230, Atlanta, 1978, Center for Disease Control.

38. Wallace, R.J., Jr., Dalovisio, J.R., and Pankey, G.A.: Disk diffusion testing of susceptibility of *Mycobacterium fortuitum* and *Mycobacterium chelonei* to antibacterial agents, Antimicrob. Agents Chemother. **16**:611-614, 1979.

39. Washington, J.A., II, editor: Laboratory procedures in clinical microbiology, Boston, 1974, Little, Brown & Co., pp. 100-117.

40. Wayne, L.G.: The use of Millipore filters in clinical laboratories, Am. J. Clin. Pathol. **28**:565-567, 1957.

41. Wayne, L.G., and Doubek, J.R.: Diagnostic key to mycobacteria encountered in clinical laboratories, Appl. Microbiol. **16**:925-931, 1968.

42. Wayne, L.G., Engbaek, H.C., Engel, H.W.B., et al.: Highly reproducible techniques for use in systematic bacteriology in the genus *Mycobacterium:* tests for pigment, urease, resistance to sodium chloride, hydrolysis of Tween 80, and beta-galactosidase, Int. J. Syst. Bacteriol. **24**:412-419, 1974.

43. Wayne, L.G., Engel, H.W.B., Grassi, C., et al.: Highly reproducible techniques for use in systematic bacteriology in the genus *Mycobacterium:* tests for niacin and catalase and for resistance to isoniazid, thiophene 2-carboxylic acid hydrazide, hydroxylamine, and *p*-nitrobenzoate, Int. J. Syst. Bacteriol. **26**:311-318, 1976.

44. Wayne, L.G., David, H., Hawkins, J.E., Kubica, G.P., Sommers, H.M., and Wolinsky, E.: Referral without guilt or how far should a good lab go? ATS News **2**:8-12, 1976.

45. Wayne, L.G., Krasnow, I., and Kidd, G.: Finding the "hidden positive" in tuberculosis eradication programs: the role of the sensitive trisodium phosphate–benzalkonium chloride (Zephiran) culture technique, Am. Rev. Respir. Dis. **86**:537-541, 1962.

46. Welch, D.F., and Kelly, M.T.: Antimicrobial susceptibility testing of *Mycobacterium fortuitum* complex, Antimicrob. Agents Chemother. **15**:754-757, 1979.

47. Wolinsky, E.: Nontuberculous mycobacteria and associated diseases, Am. Rev. Respir. Dis. **119**:107-159, 1979.

48. Zvetina, J.R., and Wichelhausen, R.H.: Pulmonary infection caused by niacin-positive *Mycobacterium avium*, Am. Rev. Respir. Dis. **113**:885-887, 1976.

32 MISCELLANEOUS AND UNCLASSIFIED PATHOGENS

GENUS STREPTOBACILLUS

Only one species, *Streptobacillus moniliformis*, constitutes the genus *Streptobacillus*. This is an **extremely pleomorphic, facultatively anaerobic,** gram-negative organism, which forms irregular chains of fairly uniform, small, slender rods 2 to 4 μm in length, to long, interwoven, looped or curved filaments up to 150 μm in length. These may be interspersed with fusiform enlargements and large, round, *Candida*-like swellings along the length of the filament (Latin *monile*, necklace), two to five times its width (Plate 161). These morphologic forms depend largely on the medium used, the conditions of incubation, and the age of the culture; the regular, rod-shaped cells predominate in clinical specimens and under favorable artificial conditions.

S. moniliformis is a normal inhabitant of the throat and nasopharynx of wild and laboratory rats and mice. It is extremely virulent for mice. Humans usually acquire infection with this organism by the **bite of a rat,** mouse, or other rodent, although ingestion of contaminated food, particularly milk, may also cause infection

369

(Haverhill fever). The infection is characterized by fever, rash, and polyarthritis. The organism may be recovered from the blood, joint fluid, skin lesions, or pus. Complications include endocarditis and pneumonia.

Streptobacillus moniliformis requires the presence of natural body fluid, such as ascitic fluid, blood, or serum, for its growth on artificial media. The addition of 10% to 30% ascitic fluid to thioglycolate medium makes an excellent recovery medium. The streptobacillus grows in the form of "fluff balls" or "breadcrumbs" near the bottom of the tube or on the surface of the sedimented red cells if blood is cultured (see Chapter 7). These colonies may be removed with a sterile Pasteur pipet and transferred to solid media or to slides for microscopic examination. (Giemsa or Wayson stain is preferable to the Gram stain.)

On slightly soft media, such as ascitic fluid agar or serum agar, incubated aerobically (some strains require increased CO_2, as in a candle jar) and with an excess of moisture, small discrete colonies develop in 2 to 3 days. These are smooth and glistening, irregularly round with sharp edges, and colorless or grayish. L-form colonies may develop beneath or adjacent to the colonies of *Streptobacillus;* the colonies measure 100 to 200 μm in diameter and show a dark center and lacy periphery ("fried-egg" appearance). This L form is a variant of *S. moniliformis*, arising spontaneously. Morphologically, L-form colonies consist of tiny, bipolar-staining, coccoid or coccobacillary elements. Biochemical characteristics of the organism are described by Rogosa.[36]

Agglutinins are formed in patients with *Streptobacillus* infections; titers of 1:80 or greater are considered indicative of infection. Penicillin is ordinarily effective in therapy. Penicillin-resistant infections respond to streptomycin, and some workers favor use of both drugs routinely. L-phase variant infections may respond to tetracyclines.

GENUS ACTINOBACILLUS

Actinobacillus actinomycetemcomitans is part of the normal human oral flora, and it is likely that most or all infections with this species are of endogenous origin. It is recovered from lesions of actinomycosis, along with members of the genus *Actinomyces* or *Arachnia* and often other organisms as well. Failure to eliminate the *Actinobacillus* may account for persistence of actinomycotic lesions, even when the *Actinomyces* or *Arachnia* are eliminated. *A. actinomycetemcomitans* is also recovered from bacteremia and endocarditis and occasionally from abscesses or pleural empyema. The other three species of *Actinobacillus*—*A. suis*, *A. equuli*, and *A. lignieresii*—are primarily animal pathogens but do cause infection in humans rarely. The types of infections from which these organisms are isolated include animal bite wounds, other wounds, bacteremia, pneumonia, meningitis, and endocarditis.[52]

Gram stain of these bacteria reveals a gram-negative, nomotile, non-spore-forming coccobacillus that can occur singly, in pairs, and in short chains. These bacteria also are pleomorphic, occurring as filaments, long rods, or coccal forms.

Considered primarily as a facultative organism, *Actinobacillus* grows best on blood agar or 10% serum agar at 35 C. Little or no growth occurs on MacConkey agar, and there is no growth on Salmonella-Shigella or eosin–methylene blue agar.[52] In broth media *A. actinomycetemcomitans* grows in granules that adhere to the walls of the tube, leaving the broth clear. After 24 hours of incubation on blood agar, colonies are punctate to 0.5 mm in diameter. Colonies are 2 to 3 mm in diameter by 7 days. Colony morphology may vary somewhat, but with prolonged incubation a 4- to 6-pointed star structure is often seen in the center of the colony growing into the agar (Plate 162) so as to leave an impression when the colony is scraped away. *A. actinomycetemcomitans* often does not grow on

TABLE 32-1

Characteristics of species of *Actinobacillus*

Characteristic	Actinobacillus equuli (n = 19) Sign	%+	Actinobacillus lignieresii (n = 30) Sign	%+	Actinobacillus suis (n = 33) Sign	%+	Actinobacillus actinomycetemcomitans (n = 120) Sign	%+
Hemolysis (clear zone)	−	0	−	4	V	76	−	0
Motility	−	0	−	0	−	0	−	0
Gas from glucose	−	0	−	0	−	0	V	28
Acid from								
Glucose	+	100	+	96(4)*	+	94(6)	+ or (+)	83(16)
Xylose	+	100	+ or (+)	87(13)	+	94(6)	V	33(9)
Mannitol	+	100	+ or (+)	91(9)	V	54	V	66(16)
Lactose	+	95	V	17(61)	+ or (+)	79(18)	−	0
Sucrose	+	100	+	96(4)	+	94(6)	−	0
Maltose	+	95	+ or (+)	83(17)	+	94(6)	+ or (+)	81(15)
Trehalose	+	100	−	0	+	96		
Melibiose	+ or (+)	79(21)	−	0	+	91		
Raffinose	+	100	V	25(46)	+	96		
Catalase	V	68(5)	V	89	V	85	+	99
Oxidase	+	100	+	100	+	100	V	19(2)
Growth on MacConkey	V	84(5)	V	67(8)	+ or (+)	82(12)	−	4(1)
Simmons citrate	−	0	−	0	−	0	−	0
Urease	+	100	+	100	+	97(3)	−	0
Nitrate reduction	+	100	+	100	+	100	+	100
Gas from nitrate	−	0	−	0	−	0	−	0
Indole	−	0	−	0	−	0	−	0
Gelatin hydrolysis	V	70	−	0		3	−	0
TSI slant, acid	+	100	+	100	+	100	+	100
TSI butt, acid	+	100	+	100	+	100	+	100
Esculin hydrolysis	−	0	−	0	+	100	−	0
Lysine decarboxylase	−	0	−	0	−	0		
Arginine dihydrolase	−	0	−	0	−	0		
Ornithine decarboxylase	−	0	−	0	−	0		

From Weaver and Hollis.[52]

+, 90% or more positive in 1 or 2 days; −, no reaction, 90% or more; + or (+), 90% or more positive, some strains positive after 3 or more days; V, more than 10% and less than 90% positive; TSI, triple sugar iron.

*Numbers in parentheses indicate percentage of delayed reactions (3 days or more).

TABLE 32-2

Key to identification of miscellaneous gram-negative fermentative bacteria

Growth on MacConkey agar

Oxidase negative
  Motile: *Chromobacterium violaceum*
  Nonmotile: HB-5

Oxidase positive
  Motile: *Chromobacterium violaceum*
  Nonmotile, urea positive
    Indole positive: *Pasteurella pneumotropica*
    Indole negative: *Actinobacillus equuli, Actinobacillus lignieresii, Actinobacillus suis, Pasteurella aerogenes*
  Nonmotile, urea negative
    Indole positive: HB-5
    Indole negative: *Kingella kingae, Pasteurella haemolytica*, EF-4

No growth on MacConkey agar

Oxidase negative
  Catalase positive: *Actinobacillus actinomycetemcomitans*
  Catalase negative, indole positive: HB-5
  Catalase negative, indole negative: *Capnocytophaga*

Oxidase positive
  Urea positive, indole positive: *Pasteurella pneumotropica; Pasteurella* new species 1
  Urea positive, indole negative: *Actinobacillus equuli, Actinobacillus lignieresii, Actinobacillus suis*
  Urea negative
    Indole positive, catalase positive: *Pasteurella multocida; Pasteurella* new species 1
    Indole positive, catalase negative: *Cardiobacterium hominis, Kingella indologenes*, HB-5
    Indole negative, catalase positive: *Actinobacillus actinomycetemcomitans, Pasteurella haemolytica,* DF-2, EF-4
    Indole negative, catalase negative: *Kingella denitrificans, Kingella kingae*

From Weaver and Hollis.[52]

solid media unless incubation is carried out in a candle jar or in a CO_2 incubator. In all cases growth is enhanced by increased CO_2 in the atmosphere. The biochemical characteristics of the four species of *Actinobacillus* are seen in Table 32-1. Table 32-2 differentiates a number of the organisms discussed in this chapter from each other and from certain similar forms.

A. actinomycetemcomitans is very sensitive to tetracyclines, chloramphenicol, and cotrimoxazole.[24,40] It is resistant to clindamycin and aminoglycosides. Some strains are highly resistant to penicillin G, ampicillin, erythromycin, cephalosporins, and metronidazole.

GENUS CAPNOCYTOPHAGA

Capnocytophaga is a genus of fastidious gram-negative gliding bacteria normally found in the oral cavity of humans. These organisms are involved in juvenile periodontosis and oral mucosal lesions and bacteremia in granulocytopenic and immunosuppressed patients.[32] There is evidence that infection with *Capnocytophaga* leads to changes in morphology and locomotion of neutrophils, which disappear when the infection is successfully managed. Organisms previously known as *Bacteroides ochraceus* and group DF-1 are now known to be identical to *Capnocytophaga*.[32] These organisms are fusiform shaped, have a fermentative metabolism, and grow under increased CO_2 tension, either anaerobically or aerobically. There are three species: *C. ochracea* (*B. ochraceus*), *C. gingivalis*, and *C. sputigena*. It appears that most of the strains isolated from pathologic processes are *C. ochracea*. However, *C. gingivalis* has been identified in at least one bacteremia. Strains have been isolated from spinal fluid, the eye, pleural fluid, amniotic fluid, the female genital tract, blood, and other respiratory tract sources. Colonial morphology is variable; colonies are typically very small after 18 to 24 hours' incubation and 2 to 3 mm in diameter by 2 to 4 days' incubation. Colonies are slightly convex, with a flat, spreading, fringelike edge; they may appear to pit the agar. Some strains have a smooth edge; others adhere firmly to the agar media. The color of colonies on blood agar may be gray to white, pink, or yellow. When scraped from the agar surface, the cell mass is usually yellow. Maximum spreading is noted on media

TABLE 32-3

Characteristics of *Capnocytophaga* species, *Cardiobacterium hominis,* and *Chromobacterium violaceum*

Characteristic	*Capnocytophaga* species (n = 155)		*Cardiobacterium hominis* (n = 32)		*Chromobacterium violaceum** (n = 36)	
	Sign	%+	Sign	%+	Sign	%+
Hemolysis (clear zone)	−	0	−	0	V	48
Motility	V	5(40)†	−	0	+	100
Gas from glucose	−	0	−	0	−	0
Acid from						
Glucose	+	90(10)	+ or (+)	78(22)	+	100
Xylose	−	0	−	0	−	0
Mannitol	−	0	+ or (+)	50(50)	−	0
Lactose	V	75(11)	−	0	−	0
Sucrose	+	90(9)	+ or (+)	61(39)	V	20(6)
Maltose	+ or (+)	86(14)	+ or (+)	72(28)	−	0(3)
Catalase	−	7	−	3	+	97
Oxidase	−	7	+	100	V	67
Growth on MacConkey	−	0	−	0	+	100
Simmons citrate	−	0	−	0	V	68(9)
Urease	−	0	−	0	V	5(14)
Nitrate reduction	V	63	−	0	+	97
Gas from nitrate	−	0	−	0	−	0
Indole	−	0	+	97	V	21
Gelatin hydrolysis	−	0	−	0	V	86
TSI slant, acid	V	73	+	96	−	8
TSI butt, acid	V	55	V	88	+	94
Esculin hydrolysis	V	81(2)	−	4	−	0
Lysine decarboxylase	−	0			−	0
Arginine dihydrolase	−	0			+	100
Ornithine decarboxylase	−	0			−	0

From Weaver and Hollis.[52]

+, 90% or more positive in 1 or 2 days; −, no reaction, 90% or more; + or (+), 90% or more positive, some strains positive after 3 or more days; V = more than 10% and less than 90% positive; TSI, triple sugar iron.

*92% produce a violet pigment.

†Numbers in parentheses indicate percentage of delayed reactions (3 days or more).

containing 3% agar. Gliding motility of log-phase cultures may be observed under darkfield microscopy. Motility is not ordinarily detectable in motility medium, but almost half of strains grow out slightly from the stab line in this medium after 3 to 7 days' incubation. An occasional cell is noted to have a single polar or lateral flagellum on special stain. Characteristics of the genus are noted in Table 32-3 and of the three species in Table 32-4. The organism grows on Thayer-Martin selective medium. Gas chromatographic end products of metabolism of glucose are acetic and succinic acids. All strains are highly susceptible to penicillin and most penicillin-type drugs, but they vary in susceptibility to cephalosporins[20] (see also Sutter et al.: Antimi-

TABLE 32-4

Differentiation of the species of *Capnocytophaga*

Characteristic	C. ochracea (n = 27)		C. sputigena (n = 6)		C. gingivalis (n = 5)	
	Sign	%+	Sign	%+	Sign	%+
Acid from						
Lactose	+	92	V	40	−	8
Galactose	V	83	−	0	−	0
Nitrate reduction	−	8	V	83	−	4

From Weaver and Hollis.[52]
Data from Socransky and colleagues (Arch. Microbiol. **122:**29-33, 1979).
+, 90% or more positive reactions; −, 90% or more negative reactions; V, 11 to 89% positive reactions.

crob. Agents Chemother. **20:**270-271, 1981). All strains are susceptible to tetracycline, chloramphenicol, and clindamycin. Most strains are susceptible to erythromycin. Aminoglycosides are generally inactive.

CALYMMATOBACTERIUM GRANULOMATIS

Calymmatobacterium granulomatis is the etiologic agent of **granuloma inguinale.** This venereal disease is characterized by an initial single or multiple swellings or "bubos" in the groin area, followed by involvement of the genitalia and sometimes the buttocks and abdomen with a hypertrophic, sclerotic granulomatous lesion. There may be ulceration or bleeding.

Calymmatobacterium is a nonmotile, gramnegative, pleomorphic rod with rounded ends and may occur singly or in clusters. "Safety-pin" forms may also occur as a result of bipolar condensation of chromatin. Wright stain of the encapsulated forms reveals a blue rod surrounded by a large, well-defined, pink capsule. The organisms may be found in the cytoplasm of large mononuclear cells in scrapings of lesions or biopsy of ulcers. Prominent polar granules are characteristically seen in addition to capsules.

Two factors are of importance in the cultivation of *C. granulomatis:* a low oxidation-reduction potential and growth factors found in egg yolk, phytone, and lactalbumin hydrolysate.[29] Inoculation of yolk sacs of 5-day-old chicken embryos and incubation for 72 hours at 35 C seem to be the method of choice, but growth has been obtained on coagulated egg yolk slants.

Therapy may be difficult. Active drugs include tetracycline, chloramphenicol, gentamicin, and streptomycin.

GENUS CARDIOBACTERIUM

Cardiobacterium hominis is the sole species in this genus. It is a **fermentative** gram-negative rod that is **oxidase positive, catalase negative,** and **nonmotile.** The organisms are pleomorphic with bulbous ends on media without yeast extract; they tend to retain some crystal violet stain. Cells may occur in clusters resembling rosettes. Colonies on blood agar are tiny after 24 hours' incubation and 1 mm in diameter after 48 hours. They are convex, circular, entire, smooth, and soft; no hemolysis is seen on rabbit blood. CO_2 and a moist atmosphere and yeast extract facilitate growth. Acid is produced throughout TSI (A/A), with no H_2S production, although lead acetate paper strips may give a positive reaction. The organism does not grow on enteric media. Urea is not hydrolyzed, and nitrate is not reduced. A small amount of indole is formed. Decarboxylase reactions are negative. Carbohydrate utilization may be determined in liquid peptone medium with added rabbit serum (2 drops). Acid is produced from glucose, mannitol, sucrose, and maltose in 2 to 7 days; xylose and lactose are not fermented. Reactions are shown in Table 32-3.

The organism is found in the human upper respiratory tract (nose and throat) and feces; it is not present in the genitourinary tract. Most isolates of this uncommon organism have been from cases of **endocarditis.**[16] Rarely, the organism has been recovered from sputum, pleural fluid, and spinal fluid.

C. hominis is quite susceptible to various penicillins, cephalothin, tetracycline, chloramphenicol, aminoglycosides, and colistin.

GENUS CHROMOBACTERIUM

One species of the genus *Chromobacterium* is encountered in humans, *Chromobacterium violaceum*. It is found primarily in soil and water but has been responsible for a small number of very serious infections in humans. Most of these infections have been fatal.

The genus is made up of gram-negative rods, sometimes slightly curved, motile by means of both one **polar flagellum** and one to four subpolar or lateral flagella. **Violet colonies** are produced (Plate 165), and in broth a **violet ring** is produced at the junction of the broth surface and the test tube wall. The pigment is soluble in ethanol but not in water or chloroform. Nonpigmented strains occur and are pathogenic.[39] The organism is usually **oxidase positive** (Kovacs method), but pigment may interfere with reading. It is **catalase positive** but **highly sensitive to hydrogen peroxide.** It is resistant to the vibriostatic agent 2,4-diamino-6,7-diisopropyl pteridine.

C. violaceum forms a fragile pellicle in broth. Nonpigmented variants occur. Gelatin is liquefied in 7 days. Carbohydrate attack is usually fermentative, sometimes oxidative. Acid is produced from glucose, fructose, and trehalose and often from maltose, mannose, sorbitol, and rhamnose. Rarely, strains produce gas. Chitin is usually digested. Casein is hydrolyzed. Nitrate is reduced, usually beyond nitrite but without gas. Arginine dihydrolase is positive. The organism produces HCN, and cultures smell of ammonium cyanide. Turbidity is produced on egg yolk medium. The organism is facultatively anaerobic with best growth at 30 to 35 C. It grows on MacConkey agar. Its characteristics are summarized in Table 32-3.

Infections in humans (only about 20 have been described) have usually involved abscess formation or bacteremia. Systemic infection with bacteremia has been almost uniformly fatal, at least partly resulting from delay in initiating appropriate therapy. One patient was cured recently with early institution of carbenicillin and gentamicin therapy.[51] Virtually all reported cases of human infection were from southeast Asia and the southeastern United States. Bacteremia is usually accompanied by necrotizing metastatic lesions. Although wounds not infrequently become infected with other soil and water organisms such as *Aeromonas* or *Edwardsiella*, this type of infection rarely occurs with *Chromobacterium*.

C. violaceum is resistant to penicillin and may produce beta-lactamase[17] at times. The strain studied by Victorica and co-workers was inhibited by 78 μg/ml of carbenicillin, an achievable level; by disk technique it was resistant to ampicillin, cephalothin, and colistin but sensitive to all aminoglycoside drugs, chloramphenicol, and tetracycline. The minimal inhibitory concentration of gentamicin was 5 μg/ml. All isolates have been uniformly susceptible to chloramphenicol and resistant to most penicillins and cephalosporins.[7] *C. violaceum* is relatively susceptible to ticarcillin, carbenicillin, and cefoxitin.

GROUP DF-2

As noted in Chapter 13, group DF-2 is an important cause of serious infection, chiefly in relation to dog bites.[6] The organism has been isolated from spinal fluid as well as blood. Usually the organisms are long thin rods, frequently curved and exhibiting variable degrees of pleomorphism. Growth is enhanced by blood or serum and usually by incubation in a candle jar.[52] Immunosuppressed individuals are at greater risk of infection and tend to get more severe infections. On occasion the organisms have been numerous enough to be observed directly in smears of peripheral blood. Endocarditis, meningitis, cellulitis, and arthritis occur in addition to bacteremia. There may be difficulty

TABLE 32-5

Characteristics of unclassified groups DF-2, EF-4, and HB-5

Characteristic	DF-2 (n = 27)		EF-4 (n = 97)		HB-5 (n = 44)	
	Sign	%+	Sign	%+	Sign	%+
Hemolysis (clear zone)	−	0	−	0	−	0
Motility	−	0	−	0	−	0
Gas from glucose	−	0	−	0	+	100
Acid from						
Glucose	V	85	+	100	+	100
Xylose	−	0	−	0	−	0
Mannitol	−	0	−	0	−	0
Lactose	+	100	−	0	−	0
Sucrose	−	0	−	0	−	0
Maltose	+	100	−	0	−	0
Catalase	+	100	+	100	−	2
Oxidase	+	96	+	100	V	54
Growth on MacConkey	−	0	V	42(8)*	V	34(23)
Simmons citrate	−	0	−	3(1)	−	0
Urease	−	0	−	0	−	0
Nitrate reduction	−	0	+	97	+	100
Gas from nitrate	−	0	V	62	−	0
Indole	−	0	−	0	+	100
Gelatin hydrolysis	−	0	V	79	−	0
TSI slant, acid	V	17	−	3	+	100
TSI butt, acid	V	15	V	73	+	95
Esculin hydrolysis	V	77	−	0	−	0
Lysine decarboxylase	−	0	−	0	−	0
Arginine dihydrolase	V	85	V	77(2)	−	0
Ornithine decarboxylase	−	0	−	0	−	0

From Weaver and Hollis.[52]

+, 90% or more positive in 1 or 2 days; −, no reaction, 90% or more; V, more than 10% and less than 90% positive; TSI, triple sugar iron.

*Numbers in parentheses indicate percentage of delayed reactions (3 days or more).

in subculturing the organism from blood cultures to agar media. Anaerobic incubation may help in this regard. Heart infusion agar with 5% rabbit blood in a candle jar seems to be very good. After 18 to 24 hours' incubation on heart infusion agar with rabbit blood, growth is smooth and has a purplish cast. The colonies are punctate. After an additional day of incubation, well-isolated colonies are 2 to 3 mm in diameter. Colonies are convex, smooth, and circular. To obtain consistent carbohydrate results one should supplement 3 ml of carbohydrate broth with 0.1 ml of rabbit serum and use a relatively heavy inoculum. Characteristics of the organism are outlined in Table 32-5.

Group DF-2 is susceptible to several antimicrobial drugs, including penicillin, tetracycline, chloramphenicol, erythromycin, and clindamycin. It is resistant to aminoglycosides and colistin.

GROUP EF-4

Group EF-4 is generally isolated from wounds, many of which are related to dog bites and some to cat bites. The organisms are gram-negative, short, rod-shaped bacteria, but coccoid forms, long rods, and chains of several cells may also be observed. After 24 hours of incubation, colonies average 1 mm in diameter and are convex, entire, circular, semiopaque, and smooth. A popcornlike odor is usually present. There may be slight yellow to orange pigmentation. They are unable to ferment any carbohydrates other than glucose. Other characteristics are listed in Table 32-5.

GROUP HB-5

HB-5 isolates have been primarily from the genitourinary tract, but there have been isolations from blood and from miscellaneous soft tissue infections. The organisms are gram-negative, coccoid, rod-shaped bacteria of medium length. They grow best under increased CO_2 tension. Under these conditions, colonies on blood agar plates average 0.5 to 1 mm in diameter after 18 to 24 hours' incubation. Colonies are smooth, entire, and convex. Sometimes they are mottled. Other characteristics of the organisms are shown in Table 32-5.

GENUS LEGIONELLA

Legionnaires' disease is manifested primarily as a severe pneumonia (Plates 166 and 167) with a mortality of 15% to 25%. The organism is rarely found outside of the lung at autopsy, but it may be found on occasion in other tissues, and pyelonephritis has been documented. There is involvement of many other organ systems in terms of the clinical picture. Included are the gastrointestinal, musculoskeletal, and central nervous systems and the kidneys. Bacteremia occurs probably not uncommonly in the sicker patients.

The causative agent of Legionnaires' disease is an unusual and fastidious gram-negative bacillus. The initial isolate has been designated as

TABLE 32-6

Proposed species of *Legionella*

Species	Other designations
L. pneumophila (6 serogroups)	OLDA
L. bozemanii	WIGA, GA-PH, ALLO-1 and 2, MI-15, *Fluoribacter bozemanae*
L. micdadei	HEBA, Tatlock, PPA, *Tatlockia micdadei*, L. pittsburghensis
L. dumoffii	TEX-KL, NY-23, ALLO-4, *Fluoribacter dumoffii*
L. gormanii	LS-13, *Fluoribacter gormanii*
L. longbeachae	Long Bch 4

Legionella pneumophila. There are now six species recognized, and *L. pneumophila* is now known to be composed of six serogroups (Table 32-6). Most of these species have been recovered from clinical material and the environment (Table 32-7). On electron microscopy, the cell wall structure of the organism is typical of gram-negative bacilli. However, in general, this organism does not stain well by the usual Gram stain when first isolated. It stains better with the Gram stain if one does not proceed with the decolorization and counterstain (the so-called half-a-Gram stain). Carbol fuchsin stains the organism relatively well, as does 1% toluidine blue in 1% sodium borate solution. The Giménez stain is excellent (Plate 168) and is suitable for demonstrating the organism in unembedded tissue as well. Various silver stains may be used, the Dieterle modification (Plate 169) being the best and suitable for paraffin-embedded tissues.

There is a direct fluorescent antibody procedure that is extremely useful diagnostically, inasmuch as it provides information very rapidly.[15,53] The direct fluorescent antibody test is relatively specific (90% to 95%) and moderately sensitive (65% to 70%).[15] Reagents are available from the CDC. It is necessary to use separate

TABLE 32-7

Sources of *Legionella* species

Species	Reference strain	Environmental isolations	Clinical isolates
L. pneumophila	Philadelphia 1	Yes	Yes
L. bozemanii	WIGA	No	Yes
L. micdadei	Tatlock	Yes	Yes
L. dumoffii	TEX-KL	Yes	Yes
L. gormanii	LS-13	Yes	No
L. longbeachae	Long Bch 4	No	Yes

reagents for each of the six serogroups, since there is relatively little cross-reaction. There is a polyvalent reagent available for serogroups 1 through 4.[48] As with any fluorescent antibody procedure, careful attention to detail and good quality control are essential. Organisms that stain by the fluorescent antibody procedure but cannot be cultivated (presumably dead *Legionella*) may be found occasionally in various materials employed in the fluorescent antibody procedure. An immunoperoxidase stain has been developed for demonstration of the organism in respiratory tract secretions and in formalin-fixed, paraffin-embedded lung sections.[4] A modified glucose oxidase immunoenzyme technique has been shown to be highly sensitive and specific for detecting the organism in paraffin-embedded tissue sections.[46] The organisms are short, pleomorphic rods 1 μm in diameter and 1 to 4 μm long. They sometimes show bipolar staining. Staining with Sudan black B reveals blue-black or blue-gray fat droplets.

Excellent culture techniques are now available, so that every laboratory that possesses a biologic safety hood should be able to culture for *Legionella* effectively. The best medium by far at present is buffered charcoal yeast extract (CYE) agar (Plate 170).[18,35] This is available commercially.* When inoculating plates, one should use a heavy inoculum and place it on two areas, side by side. One of the areas should be left as is and the second streaked out for isolation in the usual fashion. Incubation should be in an environment with high moisture content. A blood culture medium employing biphasic bottles with a buffered charcoal yeast extract agar slant and a clear broth such as Mueller-Hinton may be utilized; this is also available commercially.* A semiselective medium that has permitted recovery of the organism from lung tissue and on occasion from sputum is available.[14] An improved version of this medium, recently reported, greatly enhances recovery of *Legionella* from "contaminated" clinical specimens such as sputum (Edelstein: J. Clin. Microbiol. **14**:298-303, 1981). Vickers and others[50] have described a dye-containing buffered CYE medium that permits differentiation between different members of the family *Legionellaceae*. On this medium *L. pneumophila* grows as relatively flat, pale green colonies, whereas *L. micdadei* produces blue-gray colonies and *L. bozemanii* develops glistening colonies that are brighter green than those of *L. pneumophila*. When culturing suspensions of lung tissue, it may be helpful to culture diluted specimens as well as undiluted, as the lung tissue may be inhibitory. All species of *Legionella* grow well on buffered

*Remel Laboratories, Lenexa, Kan.

*Remel Laboratories, Lenexa, Kan.

TABLE 32-8

Characteristics of *L. pneumophila* and related organisms

	L. pneumophila	*L. bozemanii*	*L. dumoffii*	*L. micdadei*	*L. gormanii*	*L. longbeachae*
Primary growth on CYE agar	+	+	+	±	+	+
Primary growth on F-G agar	+	+	+	−		
Growth on other agars	None	None	None	None	None	None
Fluorescence, CYE	Yellow-green	Blue-white	Blue-white	Yellow-green	Blue-white	Yellow-green
Browning, F-G agar	+	±	+	−	+	+
Beta-lactamase	+	+	+	−	+	+
Erythromycin MIC, µg/ml	<1	<1	<1	<1	<1	<1
Gelatinase	$+^{w,a}$	+	+	−	+	+
Oxidase	$+^{w}$	−	$+^{w}$	±	−	+
Catalase	+	+	+	+	$+^{w}$	+
Starch hydrolysis	+	+	−	−	−	−
Hippurate hydrolysis	+	−	−	−	−	−
Acid fast in tissues (modified Kinyoun)	(+)	(+)	−	(+)	−	
Flagella	+	+	+	+	+	+
Major cellular fatty acid	i-16:0	a-15:0	a-15:0	a-15:0	a-15:0	i-16:0
a-17:1 acid present?	No	No	No	Yes	No	No

w, weak reaction; a, environmental isolates may be negative.
Direct FA—no cross-reactivity among the species; DNA homology—15% or less relatedness among the species.

CYE medium. Growth is often apparent in 3 to 4 days, but cultures should be held for 2 weeks. It should be appreciated that direct fluorescent antibody stains and cultures may remain positive for some period of time after successful therapy has been instituted.

On clear media such as Feeley-Gorman (F-G) and modified Mueller-Hinton media, a brown soluble pigment (Plate 172) develops in 3 to 5 days.[19] Colonies show internal flecking (Plate 171). The organism is weakly catalase positive, oxidase positive (Kovacs reagent), gelatin positive, urease negative, and ONPG negative; it does not produce acid from carbohydrates, and it hydrolyzes starch. Yellow fluorescence may be noted under long-wave (366 nm) ultraviolet light. Beta-lactamase is produced by several species. Characteristics of *L. pneumophila* and three other species that have been studied in detail are presented in Table 32-8. The cellular fatty acid composition of *Legionella* species is unique, as noted in Table 32-8.[30] Specific identification of isolates may be done by slide agglutination or a slide coagglutination test (Wilkinson and Fikes: J. Clin. Microbiol. **14:**322-325, 1981).

The standard test for detecting antibodies to *L. pneumophila* is the indirect fluorescent antibody procedure (Plate 173).[25] Paired acute and convalescent sera should be collected early in the illness and after 3 to 6 weeks, respectively. A fourfold or greater rise in titer to 1:128 or more is considered diagnostic. One must use reagents for all of the serogroups in order to detect all cases. The sensitivity of the indirect fluorescent antibody procedure is about 80%. Other procedures that have been used less commonly are the microagglutination test and the microenzyme-linked immunosorbent assay test. Immune adherence hemagglutination and indirect hemagglutination tests have also been used. An enzyme-linked immunospecific assay has been used to detect antigen of *Legionella* in urine, as has a radioimmunoassay, a reversed passive hemagglutination test, and a slide coagglutination test.

Erythromycin is the most effective drug therapeutically. Tetracycline may also be effective. Penicillins, cephalosporins, and aminoglycosides are ineffective. Rifampin is very active in vitro and in the egg yolk sac and animal models. It may be useful in combination therapy with other agents, but this remains to be studied.

HEMOTROPIC ORGANISMS

Archer and associates[1] noted an infection caused by an unusual gram-positive, rod-shaped bacterium in a 49-year-old splenectomized man. The organisms were found to be adherent to the majority of the patient's peripheral blood erythrocytes. On transmission electron microscopy, the bacterium was seen to be extraerythrocytic and 0.2 μm wide by 1 to 1.7 μm long. The organism had a thick granular cell wall, a trilamellar membrane external to the cell wall, and prominent mesosomes. It was not possible to cultivate the organism in vitro or to reproduce the patient's disease in splenectomized animals. The patient's clinical response to chemotherapy suggested that the organism was susceptible to cell wall–active antibiotics and chloramphenicol but not tetracycline. The organism was clearly different from *Bartonella bacilliformis* and an unidentified "bacteriumlike organism" seen in some patients with the hemolytic-uremic syndrome. Dooley[13] provided an excellent review of literature reports of infection with hemotropic bacteria.

CHLAMYDIA

Chlamydiae are nonmotile, gram-negative, **obligately intracellular parasites** that form characteristic intracellular microcolonies (inclusions). They differ from viruses in containing both RNA and DNA and possessing bacterial-type cell walls, ribosomes, and some metabolically active enzymes. They multiply by binary fission and are susceptible to certain antimicrobial drugs. The organisms are large enough to be seen by light microscopy; they are best stained with the Giemsa, Macchiavello, or Giménez stain. Both group and specific antigens are found. Fluorescent antibody techniques are also useful for demonstrating the organisms in impression smears, and so forth.

Details regarding collection and storage of specimens and of techniques for direct examination, cultivation and identification of chlamydiae are given by Schachter.[37] Except for chlamydial pneumonia in infants (which can be diagnosed by presence of high titers of IgM antibodies), the method of choice for diagnosing *Chlamydia trachomatis* infection is direct isolation of the organism in tissue culture systems. The systems of choice are iododeoxyuridine or cyclohexi-mide-treated McCoy cells.[37] Clinical specimens must be centrifuged into these cells, which are then incubated for 48 to 72 hours and examined microscopically for inclusions after staining with iodine, Giemsa stain, or an immunofluorescent procedure. Unfortunately, the reagents are not available commercially, so that a tissue culture laboratory is required for culturing. In the case of *Chlamydia psittaci* infections, particularly psittacosis, serologic testing may be very useful. Complement fixation has been the most widely used test, but the microimmunofluorescence method is much more sensitive. These techniques may be used for lymphogranuloma venereum diagnosis as well, except that often the patient does not seek treatment during the acute part of the illness, so it may be difficult to demonstrate a fourfold rise in titer of antibodies. Other serodiagnostic tests that have been used include ELISA, radioimmunoassay, and hemolysis in gel.

Chlamydiae are the causative agents of **psittacosis-ornithosis, lymphogranuloma venereum** (LGV), and **trachoma** and **inclusion conjunctivitis** (blennorrhea) (TRIC) in humans. A distinctive pneumonia syndrome has been described in infants infected with *C. trachomatis;* and pneumonia has also been described in immunosuppressed and other adults. As noted in Chapter 11, the organisms are important causes of "nonspecific" urethritis. In the latter case the use of urethral swabs is superior to urine specimens for recovery of the organisms.[42] They also play a role in epididymitis, proctitis, the acute urethral syndrome in women,[43] perihepatitis, endometritis, and acute salpingitis[54] and may cause endocarditis and meningoencephalitis.

Tetracycline is active therapeutically in all chlamydial infections. Sulfonamides are also quite effective in lymphogranuloma venereum, trachoma, and inclusion blennorrhea. Besides tetracycline and chloramphenicol, penicillin in large doses and erythromycin have been successful in some cases for psittacosis. In a cell-culture system ampicillin and amoxicillin were distinctly more active than penicillin G against *C. trachomatis*.[2] Minocycline and doxycycline were more active than tetracycline. Rifampin was the most active compound, and erythromycin also had good activity. Another study by Mourad and co-workers[31] showed that rosaramicin was highly active and that clindamycin was not very active. This study noted relative resistance to erythromycin in some isolates.

GENUS MYCOPLASMA

Dienes and Edsall, in 1937, were the first to report pleuropneumonialike organisms (PPLO) from a pathologic process in humans. Since that time, the role of these small microorganisms, which can be grown on culture media, has been studied in infections of the urogenital and respiratory tracts, in wound infections, as tissue culture contaminants, and in animal hosts other than humans. Mycoplasmas are generally considered as physiologically intermediate between the bacteria and rickettsiae and may be either parasitic or saprophytic. Presently seven identified species of mycoplasmas are indigenous to humans. One species, *Mycoplasma pneumoniae*, is a recognized human pathogen—the etiologic agent of **primary atypical pneumonia** and bronchitis. Other manifestations of *M. pneumoniae* infection include various rashes (including Stevens-Johnson syndrome), bullous hemorrhagic myringitis, arthritis, myocarditis, pericarditis, hemolytic anemia, meningoencephalitis, aseptic meningitis, and Guillain-Barré syndrome. *Ureaplasma urealyticum* may be responsible for some cases of nongonococcal ure-thritis.[47] *Mycoplasma hominis* rarely may cause significant infection in humans—chiefly pelvic inflammatory disease, postpartum and postabor-tal fever, and urinary tract infection.

The parasitic mycoplasmas are best recog-nized by such characteristics as their growth requirements (enriched media with sterols, conditions of incubation, and so forth), colonial morphology, inhibition by specific antisera, and resistance to penicillin. Another clue to their identity is the anatomic site from which the specimen was obtained, for example, *M. pneu-moniae* from lower respiratory tract secretions and *U. urealyticum* from a genitourinary source.

Growth of the parasitic mycoplasmas is best encouraged on an enriched medium containing heart infusion agar,* horse serum, yeast extract, and penicillin G (see Chapter 42 for prepara-tion). Colonies are best observed microscopical-ly under 45× magnification and appear large (250 to 750 μm in diameter) to small (1 to 10 μm), raised, pitted, and lacy to coarsely peb-bled. The central portion of the colony grows into the agar medium,† appearing darker than the periphery when examined by transmitted light, thus giving it the characteristic "fried-egg" appearance (Plate 163). In broth culture there is very faint turbidity, but some species show the presence of spherules (floating colonies). Stained preparations are best studied by the Dienes method, in which an agar block bearing the selected colony is cut out with a sterile scal-pel and placed upright on a glass microscope slide. A coverslip previously coated with the Dienes stain‡ and dried is carefully lowered, stain side down, on the agar block, and the

edges are sealed with Vaspar. The preparation may then be examined under oil immersion. Colonies of mycoplasma and bacteria (if selected in error) stain blue in a short time; after 15 minutes, however, the bacterial colonies lose their color because of the reduction of methy-lene blue by metabolizing organisms, whereas the mycoplasmas retain their stain. The method of Clark and others[8] is also recommended for microscopic study of mycoplasmas.

Isolation of M. pneumoniae, U. urealyticum, and M. hominis from clinical material

Primary cultures of clinical specimens—usu-ally swabs obtained from the throat, genital tract, and so forth—are promptly placed in a tube of transport medium consisting of 2 ml of trypticase soy broth with 0.5% bovine albumin. Sputum and tissue specimens may be submitted directly to the laboratory without the use of transport medium. A 0.1-ml amount of transport medium in which the swab has been extracted should be inoculated both into diphasic broth and onto an E agar plate.[27] Sputum, body fluids, and disrupted tissue materials should be diluted 1:10 and 1:100 before inoculation to reduce the amount of inhibitory substances normally present. The agar plates that have been set up for recovery of *M. pneumoniae* are incubated at 37 C aerobically in a sealed container and are examined microscopically at 2, 5, 10, 15, 25, and 30 days for the presence of typical colonies. Diphasic broth cultures should be examined microscopically by looking at the broth through the side of the tube for the presence of spherules (colonies), which appear as early as 5 days. Diphasic cultures should also be observed for a decrease in pH as judged by the phenol red indi-cator. Diphasic broth cultures should be trans-ferred to E agar plates at 21 days, and these cul-tures are observed for an additional 21 days. Most specimens that are positive for *M. pneu-moniae* show typical small colonies on agar and spherule and acid production in fluid medium

---

*Mycoplasma agar base, Baltimore Biological Laboratory, Cockeysville, Md.; PPLO agar, Difco Laboratories, Detroit, Mich. Broth media are also available.

†Colonies cannot be transferred with conventional needles or loops; an agar block cut from the plate is used.

‡Dienes stain contains methylene blue, azure II, and other ingredients; see Chapter 42 for preparation.

by 10 to 12 days, although some specimens may take up to 30 days to turn positive.

These factors allow a tentative identification of *M. pneumoniae*. This can then be verified by a test for hemolysis done on the original isolation plate if sufficient colonies exist. The only other organisms that can be isolated from the respiratory tract under the conditions indicated are *M. hominis*, which grows rapidly and forms large colonies, and, rarely, *A. laidlawii*, which also hemolyzes guinea pig erythrocytes. The hemolysis test is carried out by overlaying the colonies with a thin layer of 8% guinea pig erythrocytes in saline agar. Incubation is carried out overnight at 37 C, after which a zone of hemolysis may be observed surrounding the colonies. At this point specimens may be reported as positive for an organism with cultural characteristics resembling those of *M. pneumoniae*. Absolute identification requires inhibition of colonial growth with specific antiserum (see below). Modified New York City medium is also suitable for growing *M. pneumoniae* (studies done only with stock strains) and may yield more rapid growth.[22] A paper by Tully and colleagues[49] indicates that diphasic SP-4 medium may be much superior to conventional diphasic mycoplasma medium. In retesting 200 throat washings that had previously been screened and presumed to be negative for *M. pneumoniae*, they found that 34% of these specimens yielded *M. pneumoniae* on the diphasic SP-4 medium, in contrast with 5% on conventional diphasic medium. Their procedure involved examining possible mycoplasma colonies on agar plates by an epifluorescent antibody technique. They felt that the enhanced recovery of *M. pneumoniae* resulted not only from a superior culture medium but also from a more efficient identification procedure.

Kenny's recommendations for culture of *U. urealyticum* (Plate 164) and *M. hominis* follow.[27] The broth medium for *U. urealyticum* has been revised to include 1 mM sulfite and an optimal urea concentration. Mes (2-[N-morpholino] eth-

ane sulfonic acid) buffer is another important addition. Specimen amounts of 0.1 ml in collection medium should be inoculated onto E agar and Mes agar and into the urea broth. Plates must be incubated in a microaerophilic or anaerobic atmosphere. Plates are observed at 1, 2, 3, and 4 days for the presence of small colonies under 60× magnification. The urea broth is observed twice daily (early morning and late evening) for an increase in pH. Broth cultures should be transferred immediately to a new urea broth and to an agar plate if a pH change is observed. Colonies of *U. urealyticum* can be differentiated from colonies of *M. hominis* by applying a solution containing 0.1 M $CaCl_2$ and 0.1 M urea or by the single reagent urease test of Shepard. The plate is observed immediately after adding one drop of reagent to the agar plate with colonies. Colonies of *U. urealyticum* turn brown in 1 to 3 minutes, whereas *M. hominis* colonies are not affected. Isolates may be tentatively identified as *M. hominis* if they utilize arginine and produce typical large colonies. Their identity can be verified by disk inhibition, as for *M. pneumoniae* (see below). Urogenital mycoplasmas also grow in New York City medium.[21]

Identification by growth inhibition test

Early reports by various workers indicated that species-specific antisera prepared in rabbits were inhibitory to the growth of mycoplasmas and that this could be used in their identification.[9] Filter paper disks are saturated with individual growth-inhibiting antisera (made against prototype strains*) and pressed onto an E agar plate that has been previously seeded with a pure culture of the unknown strain. After incubation at 35 C for 1 week (or until good growth occurs), the plate is examined microscopically (10× to 45× magnification). **A clear zone** around

---

*Hyperimmune rabbit antisera are available for the mycoplasma prototypes previously listed from Microbiological Associates, Inc., Bethesda, Md.

any disk greater than the clear zone around a control disk that contains normal rabbit serum identifies the species of mycoplasma being tested. Since inhibition zones have been shown to be a function of the size of the inoculum and may vary from 0.1 to 17 mm in diameter, the most frequent error of "no zones" around any disk indicates that too heavy an inoculum was used. This may be remedied by repeating the test with varying dilutions of the unknown strain or by cutting out an agar block of growth and pushing it across the surface of the test plate in **one direction only,** and placing two disks along the line of inoculation, 1 inch apart. Further details of the disk technique may be found in other sources.[41]

Other identification tests

Several other in vitro tests are available, directed primarily toward the identification of *M. pneumoniae*, and include the following:

1. *M. pneumoniae* colonies produce beta hemolysis when coated with a layer of blood agar prepared with sheep or guinea pig erythrocytes; other species produce alpha-hemolytic, alpha-prime-hemolytic, or nonhemolytic reactions, but *Acholeplasma laidlawii*, which rarely may be isolated from the respiratory tract, also produces hemolysis. The unique cellular morphology of *M. pneumoniae* growing on glass has also been proposed as a rapid means of identification.[3]

TABLE 32-9

Biochemical characteristics of mycoplasmas isolated from humans

Sero-logical group*	Organism	Glucose fermen-tation	Arginine hydrol-ysis	Urea hydrol-ysis	Atmospheric conditions for isolation†		
					Air	Microaerophilic‡	Hydrogen-CO_2§
2	*Acholeplasma laidlawii*	+	−	−	? (1-4)‖	?	?
5	*Mycoplasma pneumoniae*	+	−	−	++++ (5-10)	+	±
6	*M. fermentans*	+¶	+¶	−	(2-10?)‖	?	?
7	*M. hominis*	−	+	−	++ (1-3)	+++	++++
7	*M. salivarium*	−	+	−	+	++++ (2-4)	++++
7	*M. orale#*	−	+	−	+	++	++++ (2-4)
8	*Ureaplasma urealyticum*	−	−	+	+++** (1-3)	+++ (1-3)	+++

From Kenny.[27]
*Groups are divided serologically. Organisms in a group show common antigens, whereas organisms in different groups do not cross-react in double immunodiffusion tests using hyperimmune sera. Numbering is that of Kenny, in which *M. mycoides* strains (bovine organisms) were group 1.
†Growth ranges from no growth (−) to maximum (++++). Figures in parentheses indicate the usual time (in days) when colonies appear from wild-type isolates under the indicated conditions on the recommended media.
‡A 95% N_2–5% CO_2 atmosphere from which oxygen is removed by flushing.
§An H_2–CO_2 atmosphere from which oxygen is removed catalytically (GasPak method).
‖Ideal atmosphere for isolation of wild-type strains is unknown; prototype organisms grow well both aerobically and microaerophilically.
¶Utilization of both arginine and glucose may be slow.
#Properties of *M. faucium* and *M. buccale* are similar to those of *M. orale*.
**Organisms on poorly buffered agar media will grow better in the presence of increased CO_2.

2. Colonies of *M. pneumoniae* reduce a tetrazolium salt incorporated in agar under aerobic conditions; the area around the colony becomes pink. *M. pneumoniae*, *M. fermentans*, and *A. laidlawii* utilize dextrose with the production of acid but no gas, a useful presumptive test.[10]

3. Mycoplasma colonies stained with homologous fluorescent antibody conjugates also show a characteristic yellow-green fluorescence when examined by incident light fluorescence microscopy.[12]

Other tests are noted in Table 32-9. The **recommended identification technique** is use of specific antisera for detection of growth inhibition, as previously described.

A complement fixation test may be used to detect antibody response to *M. pneumoniae* infection. There is also an ELISA for detection of *M. pneumoniae* antibodies[5] and an immunoperoxidase technique for demonstration of mycoplasmas in tissue.[23]

Primary atypical pneumonia caused by *M. pneumoniae* has been most successfully treated with the tetracyclines and erythromycin; the penicillins have not proved effective, and clindamycin is less effective than tetracycline or erythromycin. *U. urealyticum* is usually sensitive to tetracyclines and to erythromycin; it is resistant to cotrimoxazole.[11,44]

GENUS PROTOTHECA

Prototheca species are algae without chlorophyll that are morphologically similar to the green algae of the genus *Chlorella*. They cause infection in humans and, rarely, animals.[33] Two species are thought to be involved in infection in humans—*Prototheca wickerhamii* and *Prototheca zopfii*. These organisms grow rapidly in routine laboratory media without cycloheximide, producing soft white to tan yeastlike colonies. Microscopically, one sees large sporangia and endospores. Conventional identification involves the demonstration of assimilation of carbohydrates and alcohols and requires 2 weeks of incubation. Fluorescent antibody

techniques are available for more rapid identification, but these reagents can be found only in very specialized laboratories. The API-20 C clinical yeast identification system, which is commercially available, permits definitive identification of *Prototheca* species within 4 days. It is interesting that *P. wickerhamii* is susceptible in vitro to three different classes of antimicrobial agents—the polyenes (e.g., amphotericin B), the polymyxins, and imidazoles (e.g., miconazole).[45]

REFERENCES

1. Archer, G.L., Coleman, P.H., Cole, R.M., Duma, R.J., and Johnston, C.L., Jr.: Human infection from an unidentified erythrocyte-associated bacterium, N. Engl. J. Med. **301**:897-900, 1979.

2. Bowie, W.R., Lee, C.K., and Alexander, E.R.: Prediction of efficacy of antimicrobial agents in treatment of infections due to *Chlamydia trachomatis*, J. Infect. Dis. **138**:655-659, 1978.

3. Bredt, W., Lam, W., and Berger, J.: Evaluation of a microscopy method for rapid detection and identification of *Mycoplasma pneumoniae*, J. Clin. Microbiol. **2**:541-545, 1975.

4. Buschbaum, P.A., Cleary, T., Saldana, M., and Castro, A.: Immunoperoxidase staining for the serotype-specific demonstration of *Legionella pneumophila*, N. Engl. J. Med. **304**:613, 1981.

5. Busolo, F., Tonin, E., and Conventi, L.: Enzyme-linked immunosorbent assay for detection of *Mycoplasma pneumoniae* antibodies, J. Clin. Microbiol. **12**:69-73, 1980.

6. Butler, T., Weaver, R.E., Ramani, T.K.V., Uyeda, C.T., Bobo, R.A., Ryu, J.S., and Kohler, R.B.: Unidentified gram-negative rod infection, Ann. Intern. Med. **86**:1-5, 1977.

7. Chromobacteriosis—Florida, Morbid. Mortal. Weekly Rep. **29**:613-615, 1981.

8. Clark, H.W., Fowler, R.C., and Brown, T.M.: Preparation of pleuropneumonia-like organisms for microscopic study, J. Bacteriol. **81**:500-502, 1961.

9. Clyde, W.A., Jr.: *Mycoplasma* species identification based upon growth inhibition by specific antisera, J. Immunol. **92**:958-965, 1964.

10. Crawford, Y.E.: A laboratory guide to the mycoplasmas of human origin, Great Lakes, Ill., 1972, Naval Medical Research Unit No. 4.

11. Davis, J.W., and Hanna, B.A.: Antimicrobial susceptibility of *Ureaplasma urealyticum*, J. Clin. Microbiol. **13**:320-325, 1981.

12. Del Guidice, R.A., Robillard, N.F., and Carski, T.R.: Immunofluorescence identification of *Mycoplasma* on agar by use of incident illumination, J. Bacteriol. **93**:1205-1209, 1967.

13. Dooley, J.R.: Haemotropic bacteria in man, Lancet **2**:1237-1239, 1980.

14. Edelstein, P.H., and Finegold, S.M.: Use of a semiselective medium to culture *Legionella pneumophila* from contaminated lung specimens, J. Clin. Microbiol. **10**:141-143, 1979.

15. Edelstein, P.H., Meyer, R.D., and Finegold, S.M.: Laboratory diagnosis of Legionnaires' disease, Am. Rev. Respir. Dis. **121**:317-327, 1980.

16. Ellner, J.J., Rosenthal, M.S., Lerner, P.I., and McHenry, M.C.: Infective endocarditis caused by slow-growing, fastidious, gram-negative bacteria, Medicine **58**:145-158, 1979.

17. Farrar, W.E., Jr., and O'Dell, N.M.: β-Lactamase activity in *Chromobacterium violaceum*, J. Infect. Dis. **134**:290-293, 1976.

18. Feeley, J.C., Gibson, R.J., Gorman, G.W., Langford, N.C., Rasheed, J.K., Mackel, D.C., and Baine, W.B.: Charcoal-yeast extract agar: primary isolation medium for *Legionella pneumophila*, J. Clin. Microbiol. **10**:437-441, 1979.

19. Feeley, J.C., and Gorman, G.W.: *Legionella*. In Lennette, E.H., Balows, A., Hausler, W.J., Jr., and Truant, J.P., editors: Manual of clinical microbiology, ed. 3, Washington, D.C., 1980, American Society for Microbiology.

20. Forlenza, S.W., Newman, M.G., Horikoshi, A.L., and Blachman, U.: Antimicrobial susceptibility of *Capnocytophaga*, Antimicrob. Agents Chemother. **19**:144-146, 1981.

21. Granato, P.A., Paepke, J.L., and Weiner, L.B.: Comparison of modified New York City medium with Martin-Lewis medium for recovery of *Neisseria gonorrhoeae* from clinical specimens, J. Clin. Microbiol. **12**:748-752, 1980.

22. Granato, P.A., Poe, L., and Weiner, L.B.: Use of modified New York City medium for growth of *Mycoplasma pneumoniae*, Am. J. Clin. Pathol. **73**:702-705, 1980.

23. Hill, A.C.: Demonstration of mycoplasmas in tissue by the immunoperoxidase technique, J. Infect. Dis. **137**:152-154, 1978.

24. Höffler, U., Niederau, W., and Pulverer, G.: Susceptibility of Bacterium actinomycetemcomitans to 45 antibiotics, Antimicrob. Agents Chemother. **17**:943-946, 1980.

25. Jones, G.L., and Hébert, G.A.: "Legionnaires' ": the disease, the bacterium and methodology, U.S. Department of Health, Education, and Welfare, Atlanta, 1978, Center for Disease Control.

26. Jones, G.L., and Hébert, G.A.: *Legionella* update, DHEW Pub. No. (CDC) 80-8387, Atlanta, 1980, Centers for Disease Control.

27. Kenny, G.E.: Mycoplasmata. In Lennette, E.H., Balows, A., Hausler, W.J., Jr., and Truant, J.P., editors: Manual of clinical microbiology, ed. 3, Washington, D.C., 1980, American Society for Microbiology.

28. King, E.O., and Tatum, H.W.: *Actinobacillus actinomycetemcomitans* and *Hemophilus aphrophilus*, J. Infect. Dis. **111**:85-94, 1962.

29. Morse, S.A.: Sexually transmitted disease. In Lennette, E.H., Balows, A., Hausler, W.J., Jr., and Truant, J.P., editors: Manual of clinical microbiology, ed. 3, Washington, D.C., 1980, American Society for Microbiology.

30. Moss, C.W., Weaver, R.E., Dees, S.B., and Cherry, W.B.: Cellular fatty acid composition of isolates from Legionnaires' disease, J. Clin. Microbiol. **6**:140-143, 1977.

31. Mourad, A., Sweet, R.L., Sugg, N., and Schachter, J.: Relative resistance to erythromycin in *Chlamydia trachomatis*, Antimicrob. Agents. Chemother. **18**:696-698, 1980.

32. Newman, M.G., Sutter, V.L., Pickett, M.J., Blachman, U., Greenwood, J.R., Grinenko, V., and Citron, D.: Detection, identification, and comparison of *Capnocytophaga, Bacteroides ochraceus*, and DF-1, J. Clin. Microbiol. **10**:557-562, 1979.

33. Padhye, A.A., Baker, J.G., and D'Amato, R.F.: Rapid identification of *Prototheca* species by the API 20C system, J. Clin. Microbiol. **10**:579-582, 1979.

34. Page, M.I., and King, E.O.: Infection due to *Actinobacillus actinomycetemcomitans* and *Haemophilus aprophilus*, N. Engl. J. Med. **275**:181-188, 1966.

35. Pasculle, A.W., Feeley, J.C., Gibson, R.J., Cordes, L.G., Myerowitz, R.L., Patton, C.M., Gorman, G.W., Carmack, C.L., Ezzell, J.W., and Dowling, J.N.: Pittsburgh pneumonia agent: direct isolation from human lung tissue, J. Infect. Dis. **141**:727-732, 1980.

36. Rogosa, M.: *Streptobacillus moniliformis* and *Spirillum minor*. In Lennette, E.H., Balows, A., Hausler, W.J., Jr., and Truant, J.P., editors: Manual of clinical microbiology, ed. 3, Washington, D.C., 1980, American Society for Microbiology.

37. Schachter, J.: Chlamydiae (psittacosis-lymphogranuloma venereum-trachoma group). In Lennette, E.H., Balows, A., Hausler, W.J., Jr., and Truant, J.P., editors: Manual of clinical microbiology, ed. 3, Washington, D.C., 1980, American Society for Microbiology.

38. Shepard, M.C., and Howard, D.R.: Identification of "T" mycoplasmas in primary agar cultures by means of a direct test for urease, Ann. N.Y. Acad. Sci. **174**:809-819, 1970.

39. Sivendra, R., and Tan, S.H.: Pathogenicity of non-pigmented cultures of *Chromobacterium violaceum*, J. Clin. Microbiol. **5:**514-516, 1977.

40. Slots, J., Evans, R.T., Lobbins, P.M., and Genco, R.J.: In vitro antimicrobial susceptibility of *Actinobacillus actinomycetemcomitans*, Antimicrob. Agents Chemother. **18:**9-12, 1980.

41. Smith, T.F.: Isolation, identification, and serology of *Mycoplasma pneumoniae*. In Washington, J.A., II, editor: Laboratory procedures in clinical microbiology, Boston, 1974, Little, Brown & Co.

42. Smith, T.F., and Weed, L.A.: Comparison of urethral swabs, urine, and urinary sediment for the isolation of *Chlamydia*, J. Clin. Microbiol. **2:**134-135, 1975.

43. Stamm, W.E., Wagner, K.F., Amsel, R., Alexander, E.R., Turck, M., Counts, G.W., and Holmes, K.K.: Causes of the acute urethral syndrome in women, N. Engl. J. Med. **303:**409-415, 1980.

44. Stimson, J.B., Hale, J., Bowie, W.R., and Holmes, K.K.: Tetracycline-resistant *Ureaplasma urealyticum*: a cause of persistent nongonococcal urethritis, Ann. Intern. Med. **94:**192-194, 1981.

45. Sud, I.J., and Feingold, D.S.: Lipid composition and sensitivity of *Prototheca wickerhamii* to membrane-active antimicrobial agents, Antimicrob. Agents Chemother. **16:**486-490, 1979.

46. Suffin, S.C., Kaufmann, A.F., Whitaker, B., Muck, K.B., Prince, G.A., and Porter, D.D.: *Legionella pneumophila*: identification in tissue sections by a new immunoenzymatic procedure, Arch. Pathol. Lab. Med. **104:**283-286, 1980.

47. Taylor-Robinson, D., and McCormack, W.M.: The genital mycoplasmas, N. Engl. J. Med. **302:**1003-1010 and 1063-1067, 1980.

48. Thomason, B.M., Harris, P.P., Lewallen, K.R., and McKinney, R.M.: Preparation and testing of a polyvalent conjugate for direct fluorescent-antibody detection of *Legionella pneumophila*, Curr. Microbiol. **2:**357-360, 1979.

49. Tully, J.G., Rose, D.L., Whitcomb, R.F., and Wenzel, R.P.: Enhanced isolation of *Mycoplasma pneumoniae* from throat washings with a newly modified culture medium, J. Infect. Dis. **139:**478-482, 1979.

50. Vickers, R.M., Brown, A., and Garrity, G.M.: Dye-containing buffered charcoal-yeast extract medium for differentiation of members of the family *Legionellaceae*, J. Clin. Microbiol. **13:**380-382, 1981.

51. Victorica, B., Baer, H., and Ayoub, E.M.: Successful treatment of systemic *Chromobacterium violaceum* infection, J.A.M.A. **230:**578-580, 1974.

52. Weaver, R.E., and Hollis, D.G.: Gram-negative fermentative bacteria and *Francisella tularensis*. In Lennette, E.H., Balows, A., Hausler, W.J., Jr., and Truant, J.P., editors: Manual of clinical microbiology, ed. 3, Washington, D.C., 1980, American Society for Microbiology.

53. Winn, W.C., Jr., Cherry, W.B., Frank, R.O., Casey, C.A., and Broome, C.V.: Direct immunofluorescent detection of *Legionella pneumophila* in respiratory specimens, J. Clin. Microbiol. **11:**59-64, 1980.

54. Wølner-Hanssen, P., Weström, L., and Mårdh, P-A.: Perihepatitis and chlamydial salpingitis, Lancet **1:**901-903, 1980.

33 LABORATORY DIAGNOSIS OF VIRAL AND RICKETTSIAL DISEASES

In a text of this type it would be virtually impossible to provide adequate detail on the diagnosis of rickettsial and viral diseases. Therefore, we have attempted to provide only some guidelines and instructions on the collection and handling of appropriate specimens. For further information on virus isolation and identification, the reader may consult references 3, 4, 5, 8-10, 11, 15, and 16.

Drew and Stevens[2] provided excellent perspective on the question as to whether laboratories should perform viral studies. They pointed out that viral diseases are the most common infections experienced by humans and that the usual procedure in the past of simply sending serum to the county or state laboratory and waiting weeks or months for their results is frustrating for everyone. The laboratory personnel must request patient information, as well as a second specimen of serum, and must log these in and transport them. The physician must obtain the required data, recall the patient for a convalescent specimen, and wait for an extended period of time for the test results.

Drew and Stevens[2] pointed out that the actual

procedures used in a virology laboratory working with clinical specimens are relatively simple and should be well within the capability of any microbiologist or laboratory technician. Just as many hospital laboratories no longer make their own media, it is not necessary to maintain tissue culture cell lines to do viral cultures, since there are reliable commercial sources of such tissue culture tubes. Inoculation and incubation of viral cultures are simpler than in many types of cultures for bacteria. Just as several different media may be used for a particular specimen in bacteriology, several different types of tissue cultures are inoculated with each viral specimen. One may then detect the presence of a virus in the culture by observing the cytopathic effect (CPE) (Plates 174 to 176). With experience, a technologist can distinguish the CPE characteristic of certain particular virus groups and thus be able to make a presumptive judgment as to which virus has been isolated. This judgment is aided by noting which of the several tissue culture lines that were inoculated exhibited CPE and how rapidly and extensively it developed. For many clinical situations this pre-

sumptive identification may be sufficient, just as in bacteriology it is not always necessary to do definitive identification.

There is another means of detecting growth of viruses in certain cultures where CPE may not be evident. This is hemadsorption. This type of reaction is noted with mumps and parainfluenza virus, for example. In this procedure a suspension of guinea pig erythrocytes is added to the tissue culture tubes, and subsequently the tissue culture monolayers are examined to see whether these red blood cells adhere. If adherance occurs, a hemadsorbing virus may be present. Viral cultures are incubated for 10 days, unless cytomegalovirus is suspected. It is not necessary to perform blind subculture of specimens that do not show CPE, as the yield is very slight and probably not meaningful in those cases.

It is true that certain viruses require inoculation of embryonated eggs or inoculation into suckling mice, but there are few viruses of this type, and it is not worth the great increase in effort required to detect them. This would include certain serotypes of coxsackievirus and togaviruses. If it is warranted, one might send specimens to reference laboratories for culture in these systems. Other common viruses not isolated by the standard methods previously described include rubella, measles, and rotaviruses. Rotaviruses can be detected by direct electron microscopy and the ELISA technique, using commercially available reagents. Hepatitis viruses also cannot be cultured in any tissue culture system. Infections with these agents are best diagnosed serologically.

The direct detection of viral antigens by immunologic procedures (fluorescent antibody, radioimmunoassay, ELISA, etc.) is ideal, since it is more rapid than culture. Electron microscopy also detects viruses directly. There are an increasing number of viruses that may be detected directly. With future availability of high-titer monoclonal antibody reagents, this will become a much more available and reliable approach.

It may not be realistic for small microbiology laboratories to form a separate unit for viral diagnostic work. However, at the minimum, a small laboratory should accept specimens for viral culture and inoculate them into tissue culture tubes. These should be available in the laboratory and replaced weekly with fresh tubes from a reference viral diagnostic laboratory with which the small laboratory should establish a working relationship. After inoculation, the tubes can be forwarded to the support laboratory for daily inspection, hemadsorption, and so forth.

It is no longer true that viral infections are best diagnosed by serologic tests. When practical means exist for detecting viral antigen rapidly, of course this is ideal. An example of this is the test for HBsAg for detection of hepatitis B infection. For certain viruses such as rubella, measles, and the equine encephalitis viruses that require very specialized cultural procedures, a rising titer of antibodies in paired sera may be the most convenient diagnostic test. However, the time delay involved in establishing a diagnosis in this manner makes it a relatively useless clinical exercise. In general, the

convalescent serum must be obtained at least 10 to 14 days after the acute serum, and in practice it turns out that about 90% of the time a convalescent serum is not obtained. On occasion, it may be desirable to test acute and convalescent sera even when a virus is isolated to determine whether the patient was infected or merely colonized by the virus. However, in general, the decision on infection versus colonization is best made on clinical grounds, just as is true for recovery of group A beta-hemolytic streptococci from throat culture. It must also be remembered that on occasion false-positive or false-negative serologic responses may be obtained or an antibody rise may not be detected if the acute specimen is obtained too late in the course of the illness.

It has been said that the results of viral culture arrive so late that they cannot be used in managing the patient. Again, this is no longer true. As noted in Table 33-1, in a study of 1,000 viral isolates over a 6-year period (restricted to commonly isolated viruses) the average detection time was 4.1 days. Herpes simplex virus was isolated on an average after 2.7 days and influenza A virus after 3.8 days. One can speed up the recovery of certain viruses by direct inoculation of material at the patient's bedside. Utilizing this technique for throat cultures, Drew and Stevens[3] found that they improved the recovery of cytomegalovirus from only 43% in 10 days to 80% in 8 days. By direct inoculation of urine into tissue culture, on occasion they have been able to detect cytomegalovirus CPE within 1 day. These direct inoculations are used as transport tubes and are subcultured to new tubes when they reach the laboratory. As mentioned earlier, detection of viral antigen directly offers promise for much more rapid diagnosis. Varicella-zoster virus, which grows slowly or not at all in tissue culture, can be directly detected in smears from skin lesions by a fluorescent antibody technique. Commercial conjugates are available for the detection of herpes simplex, respiratory syncytial, and influenza viruses, and others are under development. Direct electron microscopy can

TABLE 33-1

Frequency of occurrence and average detection time for commonly isolated viruses at Mount Zion hospital and Medical Center, 1972 to 1978

Virus	Isolates		Average detection time in days
	No.	%	
Herpes simplex	416	42	2.7
Influenza A	66	7	3.8
Enteroviruses (echo, coxsackie A, B)	79	8	4.2
Cytomegalovirus	213	21	5.8
Respiratory syncitial virus	35	3	6.1
Varicella zoster	41	4	6.1
Adenovirus	80	8	6.4
Parainfluenza 1, 3	29	3	6.4
Other	41	4	
TOTAL/OVERALL AVERAGE	1,000	100	4.1

From Drew and Stevens.[3]

be completed within 15 minutes. This has been used for detection and identification of herpes virus and rotaviruses. Radioimmunoassay has been used to detect hepatitis B antigen and herpes simplex antigen.

Another point that has been made in the past is that since there is no treatment for viral infections, it is to no avail to establish a specific diagnosis. Even if this were true, which it is not, it would still be useful to establish a specific diagnosis to avoid unnecessary expense and hazard associated with other types of therapy which would be useless, to establish the prognosis for the patient, and to determine the possible risk of exposure of contacts of the patient. Viral culture may enable the clinician to quickly distinguish between herpetic ulcers on the genitalia and syphilitic chancres, chancroid, and other types of genital lesions. On occasion the recovery of a virus may establish a specific diagnosis in a patient with fever of undetermined origin and thus may save the patient from an expensive and sometimes hazardous workup for other causes. It should be appreciated also that now there are several drugs that are quite effective in treating

viral infections, and there is promise of more and better drugs in the not too distant future. Amantadine has a certain effectiveness therapeutically, as well as prophylactically, against influenza A. Idoxuridine is effective in the treatment of herpes simplex keratitis. Adenine arabinoside is at least as effective as this compound for this disease and is better tolerated. Trifluorothymidine is useful for the treatment of herpetic epithelial keratitis in humans. Adenine arabinoside has an effect in herpes simplex encephalitis and may be useful in varicella-zoster infections. Acyclovir looks very promising as an effective, safe antiviral agent for herpes simplex viral infections; it also has some activity against the varicella-zoster virus. Interferon has shown activity clinically in patients with herpes zoster, chronic hepatitis B, and viral respiratory tract infections.

GENERAL CONSIDERATIONS

Viruses exist as obligate intracellular parasites and cannot be visualized by light microscopy. As an order they can be divided into two groups, depending on the type of nucleic acid they contain: ribonucleic acid (**RNA viruses**) or deoxyribonucleic acid (**DNA viruses**). On the basis of their host association, they may be placed taxonomically in suborders: plant, insect, bacterial, or animal viruses. The animal viruses are generally destroyed by temperatures sufficient to kill most pathogenic bacteria but are preserved by freezing at low temperatures (below −40 C).

Because of their unique metabolic and reproductive mechanisms, viruses and rickettsiae cannot be propagated on cell-free media; they require **living cells** for replication. With advances in cell culture and the increasing availability of selectively sensitive cell lines, genetically sensitive strains of mice, embryonated eggs, electron microscopy, fluorescent microscopy, and various serologic and immunologic techniques, diagnosis of viral infection and the identification of viruses can be made with greater facility and speed in laboratories equipped for such procedures.

AVAILABLE TYPES
OF LABORATORY
EXAMINATION

Several types of laboratory examinations are presently available for the diagnosis of viral and rickettsial infections:

1. Isolation and identification of the agent by inoculation of cell cultures, chick embryos, or susceptible animals
2. Detection and measurement of antibodies developing during the course of the disease (serologic tests)
3. Histologic examination of infected tissues (skin lesions, biopsies, postmortem specimens)
4. Detection of specific antigens, using fluorescent antibody techniques, radioimmunoassay, ELISA and other immunologic techniques
5. Detection of virus particles by electron microscopy or immune electron microscopy

COLLECTION OF SPECIMENS FOR
VIRAL AND RICKETTSIAL DISEASE
DIAGNOSIS

Success of any laboratory diagnostic procedure depends on appropriate and timely specimen collection and the way in which specimens are handled after collection. So that a judicious choice of test systems can be made, the laboratory should be given information in the form of a brief clinical history. The following information is pertinent:

1. Date of onset of infection
2. Date specimen was collected
3. Clinical signs and symptoms
4. Suspected or differential diagnosis
5. Area of residence or travel
6. Similar cases in family or vicinity
7. Exposure to animals
8. Antimicrobial therapy

Finally, clearly specified test requisitions should accompany the specimen (cryptic requests for "viral studies" are useless).

The following is a brief description and outline for collecting specimens.[7]

Nasal secretion. Nasal secretions should be collected with a Culturette.*

Throat swabs. Best results are obtained by using a Culturette as for bacteriologic studies.

Autopsy and biopsy tissues. The tissues obtained depend on the nature of the disease. Lung and trachea specimens are most important in cases of respiratory illness. Brain (Plate 180), spinal cord, and colon tissue should be collected for central nervous system infections. Heart muscle and pericardial fluid should be collected in cases of myocarditis and pericarditis. Some infections are associated with widespread dissemination of the agent, and such tissues as liver, spleen, and kidney may be valuable sources of virus. Tissues submitted for virus isolation should **never** be placed in formalin but should be placed in sterile well-sealed, screw-capped jars or plastic freezer bags.

---

*Marion Scientific Corp., Kansas City, Mo.

Vesicular fluid or skin scrapings. Vesicular lesions should be opened and the exudate absorbed on a Culturette. For histologic studies (Plates 177 to 179) cells should be scraped from the base of lesions, with as little blood as possible, and placed on clean microscope slides followed by immersion in ether-alcohol for a minimum of 5 minutes. Study by fluorescent microscopy requires an adequate specimen and fixation in cold acetone (−20 C).

Blood specimens. For serologic tests, at least 5 ml of blood should be collected aseptically, without preservative or anticoagulant. One must not freeze whole blood but only separated serum. Smaller volumes may be acceptable from small children and infants. **Paired** sera, acute (onset) and convalescent (10 to 21 days later), are necessary for serodiagnosis.

Isolation of viruses from blood samples optimally requires coculture of blood leukocytes in tissue culture; therefore, a heparinized blood specimen is best for this purpose.

Stool specimens or rectal swabs. A fresh stool specimen (prune size) should be collected in a clean carton or jar. Rectal swabs (Culturette) may be used by passing the swab, moistened with broth, into the anus so that the cotton tip is no longer visible.

SUMMARY OF PROCEDURES FOR OBTAINING AND TRANSPORTING SPECIMENS FOR VIRAL STUDIES

General
Obtain specimens as early in the patient's illness as possible. Inoculate tissue cultures at patient's bedside if possible.

Throat
Use Culturette swab as for bacteriologic culture.

Nasopharynx
Obtain a nasopharyngeal swab or a nasal wash specimen using a bulb syringe and buffered saline.

Stool
Obtain as for bacteriologic culture. If a specimen cannot be passed, a rectal swab of feces may be obtained with a Culturette.

Cerebrospinal fluid
Obtain 1 ml as for bacteriologic culture.

Urine
Obtain as for bacteriologic culture.

Skin or mucosal scraping
Obtain with Culturette.

Biopsy material
Use sterile technique and submit in a sterile container (e.g., urine culture container).

Blood for culture
Submit at least 3 ml of heparinized blood (green-top Vacutainer* tube).

Blood for serologic studies
Submit at least 5 ml of clotted whole blood (red-top Vacutainer tube). In certain viral syndromes (e.g., lower respiratory) an acute-phase specimen should be submitted. If a virus is not isolated, a convalescent specimen should be obtained at least seven days after the acute specimen. Certain viral illnesses (e.g., rubella, rubeola, hepatitis, and arbovirus encephalitis) are diagnosed most readily by serologic studies.

Transportation
Transport specimens as rapidly as possible, using a messenger service. Specimens should be stored and transported at refrigerator temperature (4 C). **Do not freeze.** If transportation of swabs will be delayed, place them in a tube of buffered bacteriologic broth medium (e.g., trypticase soy yeast broth) rather than in the Culturette.

From Drew and Stevens.[3]
*Becton-Dickinson Co., Rutherford, N.J.

TABLE 33-2

Specimens for virus isolation and types of serological tests employed for diagnosis

Clinical manifestations and common etiological agents	Source of specimen for virus isolation		Serological tests*	
	Clinical	Postmortem	Usual	(Special)†
Upper respiratory tract infections				
Rhinovirus	Throat swab or nasal secretions		NA	(Nt)
Mycoplasma			CF	
Parainfluenza			CF, HI	
Epstein-Barr virus				(FA)
Adenovirus	Throat swab and feces		CF, HI, Nt	(Nt, HI)
Enterovirus			NA	
Reovirus			HI, Nt	
Lower respiratory tract infections				
Influenza	Throat swab and sputum	Lung, bronchus, trachea	CF, HI	
Adenovirus			CF, HI, Nt	
Parainfluenza			CF	
Mycoplasma			CF	
Chlamydiae			CF	
Pleurodynia				
Coxsackievirus	Feces and throat swab		NA	(Nt)
Cutaneous and mucous membrane diseases				
Vesicular				
Smallpox and vaccinia	Vesicle fluid and scrapings	Lung, liver, spleen, brain	CF, HI	(FA)
Herpes simplex			CF, Nt	(FA)
Varicella zoster			CF	(FA)
Enterovirus	Vesicle fluid, feces, and throat swab		NA	(Nt, HI)
Exanthematous				
Measles	Throat swab		CF, HI	(Nt, FA)
Rubella			HI, CF	(Nt)
Enterovirus	Feces and throat swab		NA	(Nt, HI)

From Lennette and associates.[9]

NA, tests either not available or generally not feasible as routine diagnostic procedure; Nt, neutralization; CF, complement fixation; HI, hemagglutination inhibition; FA, fluorescent antibody; CIE, counterimmunoelectrophoresis; RIA, radioimmunoassay; IEM, immunoelectron microscopy; CSF, cerebrospinal fluid.

*Usual indicates types of serological tests commonly performed.

†Serological tests which may be used for special studies, not feasible for routine diagnosis.

‡Occasional isolations reported from seminal fluid.

Spinal fluid. At least 1 ml and preferably 3 to 5 ml of spinal fluid should be collected in a sterile screw-capped or leakproof tube.

Urine. Voided urine should be collected in a sterile leakproof container.

Conjunctival swabs. One should use a Culturette and swab the upper and lower palpebral conjunctivae or obtain exudate if it is present.

A brief summary of procedures for obtaining and transporting specimens for viral studies, as

TABLE 33-2

Specimens for virus isolation and types of serological tests employed for diagnosis—cont'd

Clinical manifestations and common etiological agents	Source of specimen for virus isolation		Serological tests	
	Clinical	Postmortem	Usual	(Special)
Central nervous system infections				
Enterovirus	Feces and CSF	Brain tissue, intestinal contents	NA	(Nt, HI)
Herpes simplex	Throat swab and CSF	Brain tissue	CF	(Nt, FA)
Mumps			CF, HI	(Nt)
Lymphocytic choriomeningitis	Blood and CSF	Brain tissue	CF	(FA)
Arbovirus				
Western equine encephalitis	Blood and CSF	Brain tissue	CF, HI	(Nt)
Eastern equine encephalitis			CF	(Nt)
Venezuelan equine encephalitis			CF	(Nt)
California encephalitis	Usually not possible to isolate virus from clinical specimens	Brain tissue	CF	(Nt)
St. Louis encephalitis			CF	(Nt)
Japanese B encephalitis			CF	(Nt)
Rabies	Saliva	Brain tissue	Nt, FA	
Parotitis				
Mumps	Throat swab and urine		CF, HI	
Severe undifferentiated febrile illnesses				
Colorado tick fever	Blood	Liver, spleen, lung, brain	CF	
Yellow fever			CF	
Dengue			CF	
Congenital anomalies				
Cytomegalovirus	Urine and throat swab	Kidney, lung, other tissues	CF	(FA)
Rubella	Throat swab, CSF, and urine	Lymph nodes, lung, spleen, other tissues	HI, CF	(Nt, FA)
Hepatitis				
Virus B (HB Ag)	Agent not recoverable	Agent not recoverable	CF, CIE, RIA	
Virus A (HAV)				
Enteritis				
Rotavirus	Agent not recoverable	Agent not recoverable	CIE, RIA	(IEM)
Norwalk agent				
Hemorrhagic fevers				
Lassa	Blood, urine, and throat swab	Liver	FA	
Machupo				(Nt, CF)
Junin				(Nt, CF)
Marburg‡				
Ebola‡				

outlined by Drew and Stevens[3], is given on p. 393, and a detailed list of appropriate specimens for viral isolation and types of serologic tests employed for diagnosis is given in Table 33-2.

HOW TO SHIP SPECIMENS TO THE LABORATORY

The shorter the interval between collection of a specimen and its delivery to the laboratory, the greater the potential for isolating an agent. When feasible, inoculate all specimens other than blood, feces, and tissue into tissue culture tubes at the patient's bedside. These are then transported to the laboratory promptly. The Culturette is convenient for short-term transport (up to 4 hours). Storing specimens at temperatures above −60 C and freezing and thawing are **not** optimal procedures. The nature of the agent suspected can influence handling of specimens, and when doubt exists as to the most expedient method, a competent virologist should be consulted. In general, the following statements hold, but there may be a few exceptions:

1. Never leave a specimen at room or incubator temperature.

2. When it is impossible to deliver a specimen immediately, it should be **refrigerated** and packed in shaved ice for delivery to the laboratory within 12 hours of collection.

3. When the interval between collection and delivery is greater than 12 hours, **freeze** the specimen below −40 C (preferably −70 C). If possible, split the specimen and freeze one portion and pack the other in ice.

If CO_2 (dry) ice is needed for shipping frozen specimens, it can usually be obtained at an ice cream parlor or an ice plant. Specimens packed in dry ice must be in well-sealed containers to prevent contact with the CO_2, which lowers the pH and inactivates many viruses.

Specimens for isolation of cytomegalovirus and varicella virus should **not** be frozen. Respiratory syncytial virus is extremely labile and, if not processed immediately, will usually be lost. Arbovirus specimens should be frozen immediately (at least −40 C) if they must be held for delivery to the laboratory.

When diagnostic specimens are shipped by public carrier, packaging must conform with the

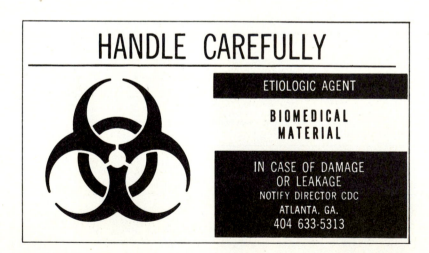

FIG. 33-1
Label for etiologic agents and biomedical material.

Department of Transportation and Interstate Quarantine regulations (49 CFR, Section 173.386.388, and 42 CFR, Section 72.25, Etiologic Agents). These regulations can be obtained from the Biohazards Control Officer, Centers for Disease Control, Atlanta, Georgia. In essence, regulations require that the specimen be wrapped in sufficient absorbent material to absorb the entire contents of the specimen in case of leakage or breakage. The wrapped specimen must then be enclosed in a durable watertight container, which is then enclosed in an outer shipping container. When dry ice is used, it should be placed between the outer shipping container and the watertight container, which must be secured with shock-absorbent material or tape so that it does not become loose as the dry ice sublimates.

The label for Etiologic Agents/Biomedical Material must appear on the outside of the shipping container (Fig. 33-1).

ISOLATION OF VIRUSES AND RICKETTSIAE FROM CLINICAL SPECIMENS

Table 33-3 provides a guideline for the types of specimens required for diagnosis of viral infections. Only generalizations relative to isolation and identification of viruses can be given. Additional information is provided in references cited at the end of this chapter.

Successful isolation of a viral agent depends on collection of the appropriate material from the patient, careful preservation while the specimen is being transported to the laboratory, and elimination of viable bacteria and fungi before inoculating the material into indicator hosts. The available indicator hosts are cell cultures of various derivations, embryonated eggs, and small animals. The choice of one or more of these systems is influenced by the clinical history submitted with the specimen. Presence of virus in cell cultures is recognized by cellular changes (or CPE) observed microscopically.[6] It must be remembered that bacterial toxins (e.g.,

the toxin of *C. difficile* in feces) may produce CPE. Characteristic lesions or new antigens may develop in embryonated eggs, and animals must be observed for signs of infection ranging from ruffled fur to paralysis or death. Final identification of a virus may require immunologic procedures such as are outlined in a following section.

Table 33-3 outlines procedures for processing of specimens submitted for viral culture and for inoculation of tissue culture cell lines. In Table 33-4 there is a brief description of the CPE and other requirements for identification of some of the more commonly encountered viruses.

Early diagnosis of Rocky Mountain spotted fever (as early as the fourth day of illness) may be made using a primary monocyte culture technique and demonstrating the organism in the monocytes by direct immunofluorescent or Giménez staining. The direct fluorescent antibody procedure can be used effectively for identification of rickettsiae in human skin biopsies as early as the fourth day of illness.[17] The indirect fluorescent antibody procedure is most useful for detection of antibody to rickettsiae but can also be employed for detection of antigen in infected tissue.

The difficulties and dangers of working with most rickettsiae are such that only class III containment facilities should attempt isolation in animals or embryonated eggs.[13]

SEROLOGIC AND OTHER DIAGNOSES OF VIRAL AND RICKETTSIAL INFECTIONS

Serologic tests provide the most easily accessible diagnostic aid for viral and rickettsial infections. They may be the only reliable diagnostic tests available and provide presumptive assessment of a disease etiology in the absence of an isolate. However, there are limitations to the usefulness of serologic tests, which depend on antibody formation: (1) early death, (2) the compromised host, (3) heterotypic serologic responses, (4) multiplicity of antigens in a virus

TABLE 33-3

Laboratory processing of viral specimens

Source	Specimen	Processing*	Tissue culture cell lines
Blood	Heparinized blood	Obtain buffy coat by centrifuging at 2,500 rpm for 10 to 15 minutes. Inoculate directly.	PMK, HFDL, Hep-2
CSF	1 ml CSF	Inoculate directly.	PMK, HFDL, Hep-2
Feces (preferred to rectal swab)	Pea-sized aliquot of feces	Place in 2 ml of antibiotic mixture.† Shake with mixer and hold at RT for 60 minutes. Centrifuge at 2,500 rpm for 15 minutes and use supernatant fluid for inoculum.	PMK, HFDL, Hep-2
Genital, skin	Culturette or swab in HFDL tube	Insert swab in HFDL tube for 30 minutes at RT. Use fluid from that tube to inoculate additional tubes.	PMK, Hep-2
Miscellaneous	Culturette, fluids	Swab: insert into PMK tube for 30 minutes at RT; use fluid from that tube to inoculate additional tubes. Fluid: inoculate directly.	PMK, HFDL, Hep-2
Respiratory	Culturette, nasopharyngeal or throat swab or washings	Insert swab directly into PMK tube for 30 minutes at RT. Use fluid from that tube to inoculate additional tubes. If infant specimen, inoculate Hep-2 first.	PMK, HFDL, Hep-2
Tissue	Tissue in sterile container	Mince with sterile scalpel and scissors. Prepare 20% suspension in antibiotic mixture and grind with sterile sand. Centrifuge at 2,500 rpm for 15 minutes and use supernatant fluid for inoculum.	PMK, HFDL
Urine	Fresh refrigerated urine or frozen volume with equal volume of sorbitol	Inoculate directly‡ into HFDL. Also, treat 5 to 10 ml urine with 0.3 ml antibiotic mixture for 60 minutes at RT. Centrifuge at 2,500 rpm for 15 minutes. Discard all but 1 ml of the supernate, resuspend the sediment in the remaining fluid, and use for inoculum.	HFDL, PMK (if mumps or adenovirus suspected)

From Drew and Stevens.[4]

RT, room temperature; CSF, cerebrospinal fluid; PMK, primary monkey kidney cells; HFDL, human fetal diploid lung cells.

*All inocula into tissue culture tubes are 0.25-ml volumes.

†Mixture consists of 100 ml of Eagle's minimal essential medium without bicarbonate in Earle's balanced salt solution plus 1.5 ml of gentamicin (10 mg/ml), 3 ml of amphotericin (250 µg/ml), and 3 ml of 7.5% $NaHCO_3$; dispense 5-ml aliquots into sterile tubes containing eight glass beads. For urine, antibiotic mixture contains 4 ml of gentamicin (50 mg/ml) and 10 ml of amphotericin (250 µg/ml); dispense 0.3-ml aliquots into test tubes and store at −20 C. Add 5 to 10 ml of urine to tube (thawed).

‡Treatment of urine with antibiotics is not necessary for direct inoculation of HFDL tube.

TABLE 33-4

Cultivation and identification of commonly isolated viruses

Virus	Tissue culture cell lines			CPE description	Rate of growth (days)	Identification and comments
	PMK	**Hep-2**	**HFDL**			
Influenza	++++	−	±	Destructive degeneration with swollen, vacuolated cells.	2-10	Detect by hemadsorption or hemagglutination with guinea pig RBCs. Identify by FA, HAD, or HI.
Parainfluenza	+++	−	−	CPE is often minimal or absent. PIV 3 produces fibroblastlike appearance at edges of cell sheet.	4-10	Detect by hemadsorption with guinea pig RBCs. Identify by FA or HAD.
Respiratory syncytial virus	+	+++	+	Syncytia in Hep-2, PMK. In HFDL, degeneration of cell sheet in definite foci.	3-10	Distinct CPE in Hep-2 is sufficient for presumptive identification. Confirm by FA.
Mumps	+++	±|	±	CPE usually absent. Occasionally syncytia are seen.	5-10	Detect by hemadsorption with guinea pig RBCs. Confirm by FA or HAD.
Enterovirus	++++	−	++	Characteristic refractile angular or tear-shaped CPE; progresses to involve entire monolayer.	2-8	Identify by cell culture neutralization test with intersecting pools of hyperimmune sera. Stable at pH 3.
Rhinovirus	±	−	+++	Characteristic refractile rounding of cells. In PMK, CPE is identical to that produced by enteroviruses.	4-10	Labile at pH 3.
Adenovirus	++++	++++	+	Rounding and aggregation of infected cells in grapelike clusters.	3-7	Stable to lipid solvents (ether, chloroform). Confirm by FA. Serotype by cell culture neutralization.
Herpes simplex virus	± (type 2)	++++	++++	Rounded, swollen refractile cells. Occasional syncytia, especially with type 2. Rapidly involves entire monolayer.	1-3 (may take up to 7)	Ether, chloroform labile. Distinct CPE. Confirmation usually unnecessary but may use FA.
Varicella-zoster virus	−	−	+++	Foci of enlarged cells.	5-10	Confirm by FA. Cell-associated virus; requires trypsin for passage.
Cytomegalovirus	−	−	++	Discrete small foci of rounded cells.	5-21	Distinct CPE sufficient to identify. Cell-associated virus; requires trypsin for passage.

From Drew and Stevens.[4]

FA, fluorescent antibody; HAD, hemadsorption; HI, hemagglutination inhibition.

group, or (5) viruses that are poor antigens. Antibody titer in a single specimen can rarely be considered significant; the titer merely indicates that infection has occurred at some nonspecified time. To be diagnostically significant the acute and convalescent specimens must be titrated at the same time, and **at least a fourfold rise** in antibody level should be demonstrated. Unfortunately, this provides the diagnosis rather late after onset of illness. It may be advantageous to study spinal fluid as well as blood.

Serologic tests in present use include complement fixation, neutralization, hemagglutination inhibition, passive hemagglutination, immune adherence hemagglutination, fluorescent antibody, immunoelectron microscopy, nonspecific agglutination tests, gel diffusion, CIE, radioimmunoassay, and ELISA. The choice of test depends on the nature of the infecting agent and the type of information required.[10] Immunoelectron microscopy, when it is feasible, may provide early diagnosis, since it does not depend on developing antibody.

Each one of the above tests can be adapted to demonstrate antibody response and to identify a particular agent.

Complement fixation is a highly satisfactory serologic test. Antibodies measured by this sytem generally develop slightly later in the course of an illness than those measured by other techniques; this lag provides a greater opportunity to demonstrate titer differences between acute and convalescent sera. Members of some virus groups, such as the adenoviruses, influenza A viruses, and influenza B viruses, possess common antigens demonstrable by complement fixation. Thus, antibody response to infection by any member of the particular group can be observed without resorting to a multiplicity of tests with individual antigens. A negative complement fixation titer does not necessarily indicate susceptibility to infection.

The **neutralization test** is essentially a protection test. When a virus is incubated with homologous type-specific antibody, the virus is rendered incapable of producing infection in an indicator host system. The test is technically more exacting than other serologic tests and is the principal method used for identifying virus isolates. A neutralizing-antibody response is virus type specific and develops with the onset of symptoms. Titers peak rapidly to a plateau and persist for long intervals, and measurable titers may be maintained indefinitely.

The **hemagglutination test** can be performed with a variety of viruses that have the capacity to agglutinate selectively red blood cells of various animal species (chicken, guinea pig, human O group, and others). The hemagglutinating capacity of a virus is inhibited by specific immune or convalescent serum. Hemagglutination-inhibiting antibody develops rapidly after the onset of symptoms, plateaus rapidly, declines slowly, and may last indefinitely at low levels.

In the **passive hemagglutination** procedure, certain viruses can be chemically coupled to the surface of erythrocytes, which then serve as indicators of the presence of homologous antibody in serum by the hemagglutination reaction.

For the **indirect fluorescent antibody test,** virus-infected cells are placed in prepared wells on microscope slides, then fixed in cold acetone and dried. Serum antibody is applied and, following incubation for antigen-antibody coupling, antihuman globulin-fluorescein conjugate is added to delineate, by fluorescence, the sites of antigen-antibody reaction. It is possible to identify specifically a virus in any adequately prepared specimen containing virus-infected cells, but the current lack of high-titer-specific antisera limits the usefulness of this method.

Immunoelectron microscopy has been used to visualize viruses and in very limited situations may provide the method of choice. Immunoelectron microscopy has not proved useful for the diagnosis of respiratory infections but has been applied to visualization of rotaviruses and the Norwalk agent associated with diarrhea of infancy and to detection of hepatitis A virus in feces.

The problem of obtaining sufficiently pure

antigen precludes the use of specific virus agglutination tests. However, **nonspecific agglutination** tests are used for the diagnosis of rickettsial infections (Weil-Felix), as is the heterophile agglutination test for diagnosis of infectious mononucleosis (see Chapter 38).

Other studies, such as gel diffusion, hemolysis in gel, CIE, reversed passive hemagglutination, latex agglutination, radioimmunoassay, and enzyme-linked immunoassay, have been used to test for antibodies against various viruses and rickettsiae. Some of these are discussed further in Chapters 37 and 38.

Even with careful attention to use of proper reagents and proper controls, the Weil-Felix test has limitations. Q fever and rickettsialpox do not give a positive Weil-Felix test. Immunofluorescence tests for the detection of specific rickettsial antibodies (as well as for detection of the organisms in tissues) represent a truly major advance in the serology of rickettsial diseases. These tests are relatively free from artifacts; they require very little antigen; they are sensitive, reproducible, and convenient; and they provide comprehensive detection of antibody. The microimmunofluorescent dot technique, the development of stable formalin-fixed standardized suspensions of rickettsial antigens, and the use of completely heavy-chain-specific antihuman IgG and antihuman IgM have permitted the indirect microimmunofluorescent test to become a routine, reliable, and sensitive procedure for measuring antibodies against rickettsiae.[13] It is possible to routinely test 10 dilutions of serum plus positive and negative serum controls against 9 different rickettsial antigens on a single microscope slide. In the case of Q fever endocarditis one must use specific phase 1 antigen, since the antibody response in rickettsial endocarditis is phase 1. One may distinguish between phase 1 and phase 2 antigen by the microimmunofluorescent test as well as other types of serologic tests.

The importance of attempting to detect viruses or rickettsiae directly rather than waiting for detection of antibodies developing against

TABLE 33-5

Techniques for rapid detection of human viruses

Technique	Detectable viruses
Electron microscopy* or immunoelectron microscopy	Smallpox, herpesvirus hominis, rotaviruses, Norwalk agent, hepatitis A, orf, CMV, herpes simplex, adenovirus, varicella-zoster
Fluorescent antibody techniques	Influenza A and B, parainfluenza viruses 1, 2, 3, 4a, and 4b, RSV, measles, adenovirus (group antigen), rubella, rabies, mumps (more difficult to detect), CMV (more difficult to detect), herpesvirus hominis, varicella-zoster
Immunoperoxidase	CMV, herpesvirus hominis, rabies
ELISA	Hepatitis A and B, influenza A, RSV, coxsackievirus A, CMV, parainfluenza, adenovirus, herpes simplex
Immunoelectroosmophoresis	Rotaviruses
Specific IgM detection	Rubella, measles, tick-borne encephalitis, influenza A
Gas chromatography	Picornaviruses
CIE	Adenovirus, coxsackieviruses A and B, ECHO, mumps
Radioimmunoassay	RSV, hepatitis B, adenovirus, rotavirus, parainfluenza
Fluorometric (4-methyl-umbelliferyl derivatives)	Neuraminidase of influenza A

CMV, cytomegalovirus; RSV, respiratory syncytial virus.
*Previous ultracentrifuge preparation increases the rate and yield of virus detection (Hammond et al.: J. Clin. Microbiol. **14:**210-221, 1981).

these organisms cannot be overemphasized. A significant amount of time can be saved by direct demonstration of the organisms, and this may have significant therapeutic implications. The value of the direct immunofluorescent procedure for detection of rickettsiae in tissues of patients has already been noted. Table 33-5 summarizes a number of techniques that have been utilized successfully for rapid detection of viruses in humans, along with a list of the various viruses that have been detected to date by each of these techniques. Gas chromatography of serum may reveal a typical profile in Rocky Mountain spotted fever as early as 1 day after onset (Brooks et al.: J. Clin. Microbiol. **14**:165-172, 1981).

A recent publication* provides a complete listing of sources of antigens, antisera, cell lines, and other reagents.

WHERE TO SEND SPECIMENS

If there is no local laboratory facility that can handle the desired viral or rickettsial studies, the following sources can be investigated:

1. Municipal, county, or state health department laboratories
2. The CDC (only through the local public health or state laboratory)
3. Local medical or research centers
4. Private laboratories engaged in virology
5. Military and Veterans Administration laboratories

In cases of suspected viral disease of obscure etiology or in instances of major outbreaks, **prompt consultation with a virologist is important.**

Linscott's Catalog of Immunological and Biological Reagents, 1980-1981, Linscott's Catalog, 40 Green Drive, Mill Valley, Calif. 94941.

REFERENCES

1. Acton, I.D., Kucera, L.S., Myrvik, Q.M., and Weiser, R.S.: Fundamentals of medical virology, Philadelphia, 1974, Lea & Febiger.
2. Drew, W.L., and Stevens, G.R.: Should your laboratory perform viral studies? Lab. Med. **10**:663-667, 1979.
3. Drew, W.L., and Stevens, G.R.: How your laboratory should perform viral studies: laboratory equipment, specimen types, cell culture techniques, Lab. Med. **10**:741-746, 1979.
4. Drew, W.L., and Stevens, G.R.: How your laboratory should perform viral studies (continued): isolation and identification of commonly encountered viruses, Lab. Med. **11**:14-23, 1980.
5. Fenner, F.J., and White, D.O.: Medical virology, ed. 2, New York, 1976, Academic Press, Inc.
6. Hsiung, G.D., Diagnostic virology, New Haven, Conn., 1973, Yale University Press.
7. Laboratory diagnosis of viral diseases, Course No. 8241-C, U.S. Department of Health, Education, and Welfare, Public Health Service, Atlanta, 1976, Center for Disease Control.
8. Lennette, E.H.: Laboratory diagnosis of virus infections: general principles, Am. J. Clin. Pathol. **57**:737-750, 1972.
9. Lennette, E.H., Balows, A., Hausler, W.J., Jr., and Truant, J.P., editors: Manual of clinical microbiology, ed. 3, Washington, D.C., 1980, American Society for Microbiology.
10. Lennette, E.H., and Schmidt, N.J.: Diagnostic procedures for viral, rickettsial, and chlamydial infections, ed. 5, Washington, D.C., 1979, American Public Health Association, Inc.
11. Lyerla, H.C., and Forrester, F.T.: Immunofluorescence methods in virology, Course No. 8231-C, U.S. Department of Health and Human Services, Atlanta, 1979, Center for Disease Control.
12. Madeley, C.R.: Guide to the collection and transport of virological specimens, Geneva, 1977, World Health Organization.
13. Ormsbee, R.A.: Rickettsiae. In Lennette, E.H., Balows, A., Hausler, W.J., Jr., and Truant, J.P., editors: Manual of clinical microbiology, ed. 3, Washington, D.C., 1980, American Society for Microbiology.
14. Pumper, R.W., and Yamashiroya, H.M.: Essentials of medical virology, Philadelphia, 1975, W.B. Saunders Co.
15. Smith, T.F. In Washington, J.A., II, editor: Laboratory procedures in clinical microbiology, Boston, 1974, Little, Brown & Co., pp. 217-277.
16. Smith, T.F.: Virology: laboratory procedure manual, Rochester, Minn., 1979, Mayo Foundation and Davies Printing Co.
17. Woodward, T.E., Pedersen, C.E., Oster, C.N., Bagley, L.R., Romberger, J., and Snyder, M.J.: Prompt confirmation of Rocky Mountain spotted fever: identification of rickettsiae in skin tissues, J. Infect. Dis. **134**:297-301, 1976.

34 LABORATORY DIAGNOSIS OF MYCOTIC INFECTIONS

Although the pathogenicity of certain fungi has been recognized since the first half of the nineteenth century, laboratory expertise in the handling of clinical specimens and in the subsequent isolation and identification of the causative agents of fungal disease has been developed only in comparatively recent years. It is recognized now that the **mycoses,** those diseases of fungal etiology, are more common than before; their incidence has increased through the widespread use of antibacterial agents and immunosuppressive drugs. It is incumbent on microbiologists, therefore, to become more knowledgeable about the pathogenic fungi and their identifying characteristics.

From basic microbiology one is reminded that fungi are multicellular heterotrophic members of the plant kingdom that lack roots and stems and are referred to as **thallophytes.** They are larger than the bacteria and more complex in their morphology. In addition, they are devoid of chlorophyll and fundamentally consist of a basic, branching, intertwining structure called a **mycelium,** composed of tubular filaments known as **hyphae** (sing. **hypha**). The latter may possess cross walls, or **septa,** in which case the mycelium is referred to as being **septate;** in the absence of septa, where the filaments are continuous, the mycelium is said to be **aseptate.** The mycelial cottony mass constitutes the **colony** of a **mold.** Colonies of **yeasts,** the other major form of fungi, are more like bacterial colonies. Certain fungi are **dimorphic;** these have both a mold phase and a yeast phase.

In septate hyphae only one nucleus is found per segment or cell, whereas aseptate hyphae exhibit a multinucleated condition in the continuous filament. The mycelium also has two parts: the **vegetative part** that grows in or on the substrate, absorbing nutrients, and the **reproductive or aerial part** that projects above the substrate, producing fruiting bodies bearing characteristic spores. Disseminated mature spores, when arriving on a suitable substrate, germinate by producing a **germ tube,** which finally leads to a new mature organism.

Fungi may reproduce sexually or asexually or by both means. **Sexual** reproduction is associated with the formation of specialized structures that facilitate fertilization and nuclear fusion, resulting in the production of specialized spores called **oospores, ascospores,** and **zygospores.** Fungi that exhibit a sexual phase are known as **perfect fungi. Imperfect fungi** are those in which no sexual phase has been demonstrated; the spores are produced directly by or from the mycelium. Most of the fungi of medical importance belong to the imperfect group, although the possibility of future recognition of a perfect phase must not be excluded.*

Since the form of sporulation and the type of spore are important criteria in the identification of the various fungi, the following morphologic data are provided to aid in the characterization of these microorganisms.

The simplest type of sporulation is the development of the spore directly from the vegetative mycelium. Three types of such spores are recog-

*The perfect state of some dermatophytes and other medically important fungi has been described.[5,18,26]

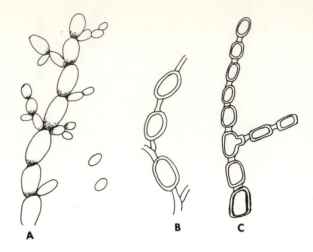

FIG. 34-1
Asexual spores produced from hyphae. **A,** Blastospores. **B,** Chlamydospores. **C,** Arthrospores.

nized: **blastospores or blastoconidia** (Fig. 34-1, A), simple budding forms in which the daughter cell is abstricted from a single mother cell or elongated budding cells that have not detached, called **pseudohyphae.** The resulting mycelium is called a pseudomycelium, as in *Candida* species; **chlamydospores** (Fig. 34-1, *B*), thick-walled, resistant, resting spores produced by the rounding up and enlargement of the terminal cells of the hyphae, as in *Candida albicans;* and **arthrospores or arthroconidia** (Fig. 34-1, *C*), resulting from simple fragmentation of the mycelium into cylindrical or cask-shaped, thick-walled spores, as in *Geotrichum candidum.*

Conidia are asexual spores produced singly or in groups by specialized vegetative hyphal stalks called **conidiophores** (Fig. 34-2, *B* and *C*). The conidia are freed from the point of attachment by pinching off, or abstriction. Some conidiophores become swollen at the end, and over their swollen surfaces are formed numerous small, flask-shaped stalks, from which conidia in chains (**catenate**) are pushed out. The swollen portion of the conidiophore is called a **vesicle;** the flask-shaped structures are **sterigmata** (Fig.

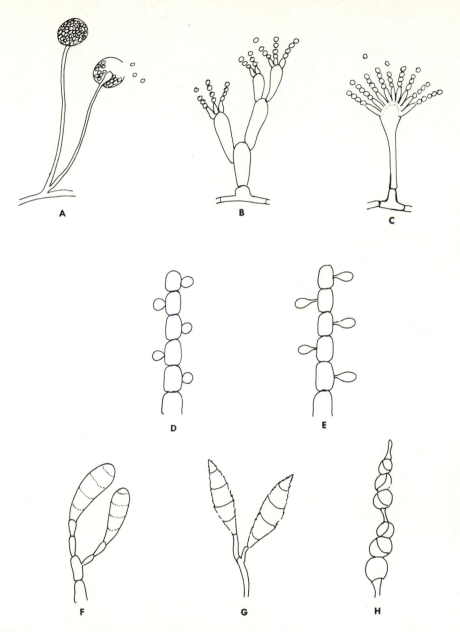

FIG. 34-2

Asexual spores produced on specialized hyphae. **A,** Sporangiospores in a sporangium. **B,** Conidia on branched conidiophore. **C,** Conidia on unbranched conidiophore. **D,** Sessile microconidia. **E,** Pedunculate microconidia. **F,** to **H,** Various macroconidia.

34-2, *C*). Many fungi produce conidia of two sizes: **microconidia** (Fig. 34-2, *D* and *E*) are small, unicellular, and round, elliptical, or pear shaped (pyriform); **macroconidia** (Fig. 34-2, *F* to *H*) are large, usually septate, and club shaped (clavate) or spindle shaped (fusiform). The microconidia may be borne directly on the hyphae (Fig. 34-2, *D*) and are said to be **sessile,** or they may develop directly from the end of a short conidiophore (Fig. 34-2, *E*) and are called **pedunculate.** If conidia have a rough or spiny surface, they are called **echinulate.**

Sporangiospores (Fig. 34-2, *A*) are asexual spores contained in **sporangia** produced terminally on **sporangiophores** (aseptate stalks). Sporulation takes place by a process called progressive cleavage. During maturation within the sporangium, the protospores divide into definitive uninucleate sporangiospores, which are released by irregular rupture of the sporangial wall (Fig. 34-2, *A*). This form of sporulation occurs in the zygomycetes, which exhibit an aseptate mycelium.

Other types of spores, produced sexually by the perfect fungi, have been referred to previously. Additional information may be gained from texts on general mycology.

Since the techniques commonly employed in medical bacteriology are not always practical for the identification of fungi, these microorganisms must often be recognized primarily by their **gross and microscopic characteristics.** This brings into focus certain questions. Is the colony rapid growing (2 to 5 days) or slow growing (2 to 3 weeks)? Is it flat, heaped up, or regularly or irregularly folded? Is its texture creamy and yeastlike or is it smooth and skinlike (glabrous)? Does it produce a mycelium that is powdery, granular, velvety, or cottony? Is a distinct surface pigment observed and is the pigment similar on the reverse side? These are the criteria that are important in the **gross characterization** of an unknown fungus.

A small portion of the colony and some of the medium may be removed with a 22-gauge ni-chrome needle or loop, and the mycelium teased apart in a drop of lactophenol cotton blue mounting fluid on a glass slide. This is covered with a thin coverglass heated *gently* over the pilot flame of a Bunsen burner and examined **microscopically,** using both low- and high-power objectives. One may also use cellophane tape, touching the sticky side to a colony and then mounting this on a slide in lactophenol blue. The size, shape, septation, and color of spores, if present, may be observed, and the morphology of the specialized structures bearing the spores is noted.

Frequently, it may be possible to identify a culture solely by this direct examination. Often, however, more sophisticated procedures may be required, and the preparation of a **slide culture** or hanging drop for the demonstration of the undisturbed relation of spores to specialized hyphae, such as conidiophores, is recommended. This technique is described in a later section.

Special culture media designed to suppress vegetative growth and stimulate **sporulation** of a fungus or to produce a special type of growth may also be required. Such media include potato dextrose agar, wort agar, brain-heart infusion agar, rice grain medium, chlamydospore agar, and others; their preparation and use are discussed in the section on culture media.

To identify a fungal culture properly, it may be necessary on occasion to carry out various **biochemical** studies, such as sugar assimilation tests and fermentations, nitrate assimilation tests, carbon and nitrogen utilization studies, and specific vitamin requirements. When indicated, these are described.

Finally, it may be necessary in certain instances to carry out **animal pathogenicity tests** to identify some species. These are discussed under the specific diseases.

Saprophytic fungi are frequently found as **contaminants** of clinical specimens as well as in the laboratory, where they readily contaminate cultures. It is essential, therefore, that the medical mycologist become well versed in differentiating these forms from recognized pathogens. Furthermore, some of these common saprophytes are important **opportunistic invaders** in debilitated patients who may have been treated with immunosuppressive drugs and the multiplicity of antimicrobial agents presently available to the clinician. Their recognition, therefore, is becoming important. The laboratorian should become familiar with about a dozen genera commonly considered as contaminants. Much help can be obtained from the excellent texts referred to at the end of this chapter.[18,26,86] Excellent training courses also are offered by the Mycology Branch of the CDC.*

In familiarizing oneself with the characteristics of the saprophytic genera, including *Penicillium, Aspergillus, Paecilomyces, Fusarium, Scopulariopsis, Rhizopus, Mucor,* and others, the student acquires experience in mycologic techniques and also gains an opportunity to recognize fungal morphology and its relation to the taxonomy of the group.

GENERAL LABORATORY METHODS

Mycologic examination of all clinical material should include a direct microscopic examination, culturing on appropriate media, and, if indicated, inoculation of susceptible laboratory animals. Although it is true that mycelial fragments, spores, and spore structures can sometimes be demonstrated in unstained preparations, it is essential that **all specimens be cultured** in an attempt to isolate the causative agent.

Collection of specimens

A prime requisite to good medical mycology is **a properly collected and properly handled specimen.** Procedural details are given under specific diseases; therefore, the following are general instructions only.

To obtain specimens of **skin** or **nails,** the affected site is carefully washed with 70% isopropanol and, after drying, the lesion is scraped with a sterile scalpel and the material obtained is placed in a sterile Petri dish or on a piece of white paper carefully folded in a packet to prevent loss of the specimen. **Hairs** from infected areas are clipped or plucked and sent to the laboratory in a similar manner.

In the **subcutaneous mycoses** (see later section in this chapter) a variety of materials may be submitted, including pus or exudate from draining lesions, material aspirated with syringe and needle from unopened abscesses or sinus tracts, and biopsied tissue.* These should be placed in sterile tubes or Petri dishes and submitted directly to the laboratory. If mailing of the specimen is necessary, the material first should be inoculated to a suitable culture medium. Under no circumstances should glass or plastic Petri dishes containing clinical specimens or fungus cultures be sent through the mails; they invariably break in transit. Neither should inoculated cotton swabs be mailed, as they are usually dried out on arrival. For best results **only pure cultures** on agar slants should be mailed. Scrapings of skin or nails and hair can be mailed in appropriate containers.

Material from suspected cases of **systemic mycoses** includes such varied specimens as blood, CSF, sputum, bronchial secretions, gastric washings, pus and exudates from abscesses and draining sinuses, bone marrow, and tissue. These specimens should be placed in sterile tubes or bottles and submitted promptly to the laboratory.

Sputum treated with cetylpyridinium chloride for shipment to a mycobacteriology laboratory is not satisfactory for culture for fungi, but the morphology and stainability of fungi are not

---

*Contact the Office of Training Activities, Bureau of Laboratories, Centers for Disease Control, Atlanta, Ga. 30333.

*Tissue for fungus culturing should not be ground in a tissue grinder; it fragments and may kill the larger fungal elements. Rather, the specimen should be minced with a sterile scalpel blade and pieces embedded directly into the culture medium.

affected.[63] To aid the laboratory in the proper examination of the specimen, some indication of the **suspected disease** should be noted on the laboratory request slip, along with the specimen source. This is necessary to guide laboratory personnel in the selection of the proper media and methods of incubation.

Direct microscopic examination

The following clinical specimens are preferably examined in the **unstained state:** sputum and bronchoscopic secretions, gastric washings, pus and exudates, sediments of CSF, pleural effusions, and urine. Several loopfuls of the material are placed on a clean glass slide, covered with a thin coverglass, and examined under both the low- and high-power objectives, using reduced light or phase contrast. If the material is opaque, 10% sodium hydroxide may be added and gentle heat applied. These preparations should be carefully searched for the following: broad mycelial fragments with septa (*Aspergillus* and *Penicillium* species) or without septa (*Mucor* species), arthrospores (*Geotrichum* species), thick-walled spherules (*Coccidioides immitis*), and budding cells (*Candida, Cryptococcus,* and *Blastomyces* species).

Dried and fixed films may be stained by the Gram method (mycelium and spores are gram positive), periodic acid–Schiff (PAS) stain, and Wright or Giemsa stain to reveal the presence of *Histoplasma capsulatum* in the macrophages or phagocytes of blood or bone marrow.* An India ink (use Pelikan brand) preparation of CSF may reveal encapsulated forms of *Cryptococcus neoformans.*

Cryptococcus neoformans may be difficult to recognize in Gram-stained smears because of the presence of the large capsule, which prevents good staining of the yeastlike cells. In this type of preparation *C. neoformans* may appear either as round cells with gram-positive granular

inclusions with a pale lavender cytoplasmic background or as gram-negative lipoid bodies.[14] When this type of appearance is noted, one should undertake other standard techniques, such as a mucicarmine stain, looking for cryptococci. India ink preparations, although excellent for CSF, are not useful for sputum, tissue homogenates, or other viscous material. In this type of specimen capsules can typically be detected readily in a wet preparation without India ink or stain, since small tissue particulates tend to adhere to the capsule, outlining it in much the same way as do India ink particles. Trumbull and Chesney[83] found that cytologic preparations of bronchial secretions stained by the Papanicolaou method were distinctly better than wet preparations for demonstrating *Blastomyces dermatitidis.* The cytologic technique yielded a positive diagnosis for 93% of patients (70% on the first specimen), in comparison with 61% by wet preparation (32% on the first specimen). Cytopathologic procedures are also very useful in diagnosing respiratory infections caused by other fungi.

Cultural procedures

Although the basic principles of microbiologic technique apply to the mycologist as well as the bacteriologist, certain differences should be noted. A 22-gauge nichrome needle, flattened at the end to a spade shape, is used to transfer mycelial growth. When the needle contains infectious material, care should be exercised to prevent spattering when flaming it; the needle should be gradually heated in the less intense part of the flame. Two stiff, sharp-pointed teasing needles in holders are useful in tearing apart the mycelial mat when immersed in mounting fluid on a glass slide.

Large (25- by 150-mm) borosilicate test tubes without lips are recommended for solid culture media rather than Petri dishes, to minimize the hazard of spore dissemination. Small, strong bottles with flat sides are also suitable for culture of fungi, such as *Coccidioides immitis,* to mini-

---

*Special histology stains for fungi are also extremely useful, including the Gridley and Gomori stains.[39]

mize the hazard to the laboratory worker. Screw-capped test tubes used for cultures are not recommended; they promote anaerobiosis and retain moisture, both of which prevent maximum sporulation. The large cotton-plugged test tubes afford ease of storage and handling, are less easily broken, and allow for a **thick butt** of agar that withstands drying during extended incubation. The disadvantage of culture tubes is that the surface area is too limited for satisfactory isolation of colonies. If a laboratory is equipped with an adequate biologic safety hood, one may utilize culture dishes in order to provide a large surface area on which mixed colonies can be more readily observed and to provide maximal aeration for colonies. The problem

TABLE 34-1

Fungal culture media: indications for use

Media	Indications for use
Primary isolation media	
Brain-heart infusion agar	Primary isolation of saprobic and pathogenic fungi
Brain-heart infusion agar with antibiotics	Primary isolation of pathogenic fungi exclusive of dermatophytes
Brain-heart infusion biphasic blood culture bottles	Recovery of fungi from blood
Dermatophyte test medium	Primary isolation of dermatophytes, recommended as screening medium only
Inhibitory mold agar	Primary isolation of pathogenic fungi exclusive of dermatophytes
Mycosel or mycobiotic agar	Primary isolation of dermatophytes
Sabouraud 2% dextrose agar	Primary isolation of saprobic and pathogenic fungi
SABHI agar	Primary isolation of saprobic and pathogenic fungi
Differential test media	
Ascospore agar	Detection of ascospores in ascosporogenous yeasts such as *Saccharomyces* species
Casein agar	Identification of *Nocardia* species and *Streptomyces* species
Cornmeal agar with Tween 80 and trypan blue	Identification of *Candida albicans* by chlamydospore production and speciation of *Candida* by colonial morphology
Cottonseed conversion agar	Conversion of dimorphic fungus *Blastomyces dermatiditis* from mold to yeast phase
Czapek's agar	Isolation and differential identification of aspergilli
Niger seed agar	Identification of *Cryptococcus neoformans*
Nitrate reduction medium	Detection of nitrate assimilation in confirmation of *Cryptococcus* species
Potato dextrose agar	Demonstration of pigment production by *Trichophyton rubrum* and preparation of microslide cultures
Rice medium	Identification of *Microsporum audouinii*
Trichophyton agars 1 to 7	Speciation of members of *Trichophyton* genus
Tyrosine agar	Identification of *Nocardia* species and *Streptomyces* species
Urea agar	Detection of *Cryptococcus* species, differentiation of *Trichophyton mentagrophytes* from *Trichophyton rubrum*, and detection of *Trichosporon* species.
Xanthine agar	Identification of *Nocardia* species and *Streptomyces* species
Yeast extract agar	Identification of *Histoplasma, Coccidioides,* and *Blastomyces*
Yeast fermentation broth	Speciation of yeasts by determining fermentations
Yeast nitrogen base agar	Speciation of yeasts by determining carbohydrate assimilations

Modified from Koneman and associates.[42]

of media in plates drying out during storage or prolonged incubation can be minimized by pouring at least 40 ml of agar into each plate and placing the plates into oxygen-permeable cellophane bags. Plates should be opened and examined only within an adequately vented safety hood. Pigment production is enhanced when there is free circulation of air, and a dry surface encourages the development of an aerial mycelium and spores.

Sabouraud 2% dextrose agar (SAB agar), brain-heart infusion (BHI) agar, with or without added blood, a combination of both (SABHI agar), inhibitory mold agar, and mycosel agar are the most useful media for primary isolation of most pathogens. (The preparation of these media is discussed in Chapter 42.) The addition of 0.5 mg/ml of cycloheximide and 0.016 mg/ml of chloramphenicol to these media effectively inhibits the growth of contaminating saprophytic molds and bacteria, especially when material likely to contain these contaminants in large numbers is cultured, such as skin and nail scrapings, sputum, pus, or autopsy material. One may also add gentamicin in a concentration of 0.005 mg/ml. On BHI agar with added antibiotics pathogenic fungi develop their typical colonial morphology, color, and microscopic appearance and can generally be identified without further subculturing. However, certain pathogens are partially or completely inhibited by these antibiotics. Included here are *Cryptococcus neoformans*, *Candida* species (including *C. parapsilosis* and *C. krusei*), and *Trichosporon beigelii (cutaneum)*. The yeast phases of *Histoplasma capsulatum* and *Blastomyces dermatitidis* are susceptible to cycloheximide when incubated at 35 C but not at 25 C; *Petriellidium boydii* and *Aspergillus fumigatus* are partially sensitive, but cycloheximide may inhibit sporulation. Table 34-1 lists various fungal culture media and their indications. Since the concentration procedure for mycobacteria is very detrimental to fungi, one must not rely on mycobacterial cultures to recover fungal pathogens.[7,70]

Some cultures neither sporulate nor produce pigment satisfactorily on SAB agar. To induce these, special media, including potato-dextrose agar, potato-carrot agar, cornmeal agar, rice grain agar, or SAB agar with added thiamine and inositol, have proved useful and can be recommended.

All isolation media should be held for a minimum of 4 weeks before discarding.

Slide culture

Microscopic observation of fungi in the natural state is often necessary for identification. The following method (Fig. 34-3) has proved successful for the culture of fungi on a glass slide:

1. With forceps dip a clean slide in alcohol and flame and burn it off. Repeat the procedure. Place the slide in a sterile Petri dish to cool.
2. Carefully apply aseptically quick-drying, tubed, plastic cement to the slide to form three sides of a square, equal in area to that of a coverglass or slightly less. The cement walls should be 1 to 2 mm high.
3. With a sterile dropping pipet place sufficient melted SAB agar at 45 C in the square to fill the space to the top of the walls. Place the slide in the Petri dish and allow the agar to set firmly.
4. Apply a minimal amount of inoculum (spores) to the center of the agar surface and then cover the surface squarely with a sterile coverglass (alcohol flamed and cooled).
5. Place a wide strip of filter paper in the Petri dish and moisten it with a few drops of water. Cover it with a lid, which assures a moist atmosphere.
6. Incubate the dish at the desired temperature and examine it after 48 hours or until sporulation occurs. This is determined by quick microscopic examination under the low-power objective.
7. Remove the damp filter paper at the desired stage and add a dry strip. Add sev-

eral drops of formalin to the strip and cover the dish.

8. Allow the dish to remain 30 minutes. Remove the slide, blot away excess moisture, and examine it under high-dry objective, with appropriate light adjustment.

9. Make a permanent mount by applying nail polish or asphalt tar varnish to all four sides of the square.

Hanging-drop culture

A hanging-drop culture preparation is recommended also for examining fungi in the natural state. Introduce a minute inoculum of the culture into a drop of Sabouraud broth on a coverglass, and invert it over a glass microslide ring* coated at both ends with petroleum jelly. Place this assembly on a 3- by 1-inch glass slide (with several drops of water for moisture), and incubate it at 25 C for 2 to 3 days until sporulation occurs.

Do not make slide cultures of *Histoplasma*, *Blastomyces*, or *Coccidioides*. This procedure is too hazardous.

---

*A.H. Thomas Co., Philadelphia, Penn.

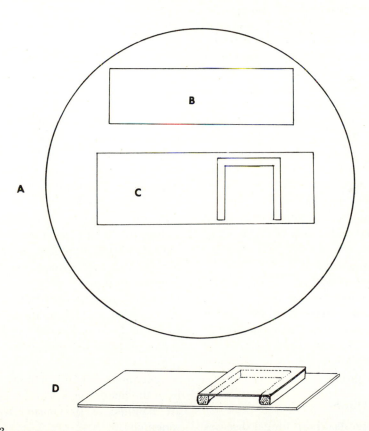

FIG. 34-3
Slide culture. **A,** Petri dish. **B,** Strip of filter paper. **C,** Slide with cement walls. **D,** Slide with agar medium and coverglass in place.

STUDY OF THE MYCOSES

Of the more than 50,000 valid species of fungi, only about 50 to 75 are generally recognized as being pathogenic for humans. A working taxonomic scheme is presented in Table 34-2. These organisms normally live a saprophytic existence in soil enriched by decaying nitrogenous matter, where they are capable of maintaining a separate existence, with a parasitic cycle in humans or animals. The systemic mycoses are not communicable in the usual sense of person-to-person or animal-to-person transfer; humans become **accidental hosts** by the inhalation of spores or by their introduction into tissues through trauma. Unusual circumstances, reflecting an **altered susceptibility** of the host, may also lead to infection by fungi that are normally considered saprophytes. Such conditions may occur in patients with debilitating diseases, diabetes mellitus, or impaired immunologic mechanisms resulting from steroid or antimetabolite therapy. Prolonged administration of antibiotic agents may also upset the host's normal microbiota, resulting in a **superinfection** by one of these fungi. The neophyte mycologist is cautioned, therefore, not to discard cultures as "contaminants" without first checking the clinical history of the patient and discussing findings with the patient's physician.

The **mycoses** may be conveniently considered in five groups, based on the tissues involved, as noted in Table 34-3.

1. The **dermatophytoses**
2. The **superficial mycoses**
3. Mycoses involving the **eye**
4. The **subcutaneous mycoses,** which involve the subcutaneous tissues and muscles
5. The **systemic mycoses,** which involve the deep tissues and organs; these are the most serious of the groups

DERMATOPHYTOSES

As the name suggests, these fungal diseases include infections that involve the superficial areas of the body, namely the **skin, hair,** and **nails.** The etiology for these diseases relates to the genera *Microsporum, Trichophyton,* and *Epidermophyton*. Such cutaneous mycoses are probably the most common fungal infections of humans and are usually referred to as **tinea** (Latin for gnawing worm or **ringworm**). The gross appearance is that of an outer ring of active, progressing infection with healing centrally within the ring. They may be characterized or qualified by another Latin noun in the genitive form to designate the area involved, for example, tinea corporis (body), tinea cruris (groin), tinea capitis (scalp and hair), tinea barbae (beard), and tinea unguium (nail). These fungi break down and use keratin (keratinolytic) as a source of nitrogen but are incapable of penetrating the subcutaneous layers.

Direct examination

The presence of the fungi can be readily demonstrated in direct slide preparations of digested skin scales, nail scrapings, or hair. The skin of the involved area is cleansed with 70% alcohol, and some epidermal scales at the active edge of the lesion are stripped off and placed on a microscope slide containing a drop of 10% potassium hydroxide. A coverglass is added, and the slide is gently warmed over a small flame to just short of boiling. The slide is then examined under low- and high-power magnification, using much-reduced light, for the presence of long branching threads of young hyphae or of older septate hyphae and barrel-shaped arthrospores. Occasionally, budding yeasts may be seen. Fungal elements must be differentiated from fibers of cotton, wool, and other fabrics as well as a mosaic of cholesterol crystals and other artifacts. Phase contrast microscopy can be useful in this regard.

Specimens of nail scrapings must be secured from the deeper layers of the infected nail; they are handled as previously described for skin scrapings.

Infected hairs are selected either by their characteristic appearance (broken-off hairs and

TABLE 34-2

Fungi of clinical laboratory importance: a practical working taxonomy

Molds				Yeasts
Hyphae aseptate	**Hyphae septate**			
Zygomycetes	Dematiaceous	Hyaline	Dimorphic molds	

Zygomycetes	Dematiaceous	Hyaline	Dimorphic molds	Yeasts
Commonly encountered *Rhizopus* *Mucor* *Absidia* **Rarely encountered** *Syncephalastrum* *Circinella* *Cunninghamella*	**Conidia multi-celled septa transverse and longitudinal** *Alternaria* *Stemphilium* *Epicoccum* **Conidia multicelled transverse septa only** *Curvularia* *Helminthosporium* *Heterosporium* **Conidia single-celled** *Cladosporium* *Nigrospora* *Aureobasidium* *(Pullularia)* **Slow-growing species** *Cladosporium carrionii* *Phialophora verrucosa* *Phialophora jeanselmei* *Fonsecaea pedrosi* *Fonsecaea compactum* **Others** *Drechstera* *Exophiala* *Phoma* *Wangiella*	**Conidiophores terminating in a swollen vesicle** *Aspergillus species* *A. fumigatus* *A. flavus* *A. niger* **Conidiophores branching into a "penicillus"** *Penicillium* *Paecilomyces* *Scopulariopsis* **Conidia in clusters** *Cephalosporium* *Trichoderma* *Gliocladium* *Fusarium* **Conidia borne singly** *Chrysosporium* *Sepedonium* *Petriellidium (Allescheria)*	**Dermatophytes** *Microsporum species* *M. audouinii* *M. canis* *M. gypseum* *Trichophyton species* *T. mentagrophytes* *T. rubrum* *T. tonsurans* *T. verrucosum* *T. schoenleinii* *T. violaceum* *Epidermophyton species* *E. floccosum* **Dimorphic molds** *Blastomyces dermatitidis* *Histoplasma capsulatum* *Coccidioides immitis* *Paracoccidioides brasiliensis* *Sporothrix schenckii*	**Hyphae formed on cornmeal Tween 80 agar** Pseudohyphae *Candida species* *C. albicans* *C. tropicalis* *C. parapsilosis* *C. pseudotropicalis* *C. krusei* Arthrospores *Geotrichum* *Trichosporon* **Hyphae not formed on cornmeal Tween 80 agar** *Cryptococcus* *Rhodotorula* *Torulopsis* *Saccharomyces**

Modified from Koneman and associates.[42]
*Rudimentary hyphae may be present.

TABLE 34-3

Disease-oriented taxonomy of pathogenic fungi

Cutaneous	Subcutaneous	Eye infections	Systemic
Superficial mycoses	Chromomycosis	Keratomycosis (corneal infection)	Aspergillosis
Tinea	*Phialophora*	*Fusarium solani*	Blastomycosis
Piedra	*Cladosporium*	*Candida albicans*	Candidiasis
Candidiasis	*Fonsecaea*	*Aspergillus fumigatus*	Coccidioidomycosis
		Many others	Histoplasmosis
Dermatophytosis	Sporotrichosis	Chorioretinal infection, endoph-	Cryptococcosis
Microsporum	Mycetoma (eumy-	thalmitis	Geotrichosis
Epidermophyton	cotic)	*Candida albicans*	Torulopsosis
Trichophyton	*Phialophora*	Other *Candida* species	South American
	Petriellidium	*Torulopsis glabrata*	blastomycosis
	(*Allescheria*)	*Petriellidium boydii*	Sporotrichosis
		Others	(rare)
			Zygomycosis
			(Phycomycosis)

Modified from Koneman and co-workers.[42]

twisted grayish stubs) or by their bright yellow-green fluorescence when examined under a Wood's lamp (Plate 181), using filtered ultraviolet light. Invasion of the inside of the hair (**endothrix**) or the outside of the hair shaft (**ectothrix**), as determined microscopically, can be helpful in identifying the fungus involved (see the Key to Direct Examination of Hair on p. 415).

Some workers find a stained preparation easier to examine than an unstained potassium hydroxide mount. The most convenient stain digestant is prepared from equal parts of Parker 51 blue-black ink and 10% sodium hydroxide and is used as previously described. One part of ink plus four parts of potassium hydroxide will give a lighter stain, and this method is preferred by some.

Cultural procedures

Specimens of skin and nail scrapings are obtained as described previously; hair stubs or scrapings of areas showing loss of hair (alopecia) are obtained without attempting to cleanse the scalp; however, a gentle wiping with 70% alcohol results in less contamination.

The specimen may be either inoculated directly to media in the clinic or submitted to the laboratory in sterile disposable Petri dishes or clean paper envelopes. The upper portion of the hairs should be clipped off with alcohol-flamed scissors; only the lower ends should be inoculated to media.

Primary isolation of the dermatophytes is readily accomplished by inoculating the hairs or scrapings on the surfaces of SAB agar slants; the specimen should be partially embedded in the agar. It is advisable to inoculate **duplicate sets** of media, one containing plain medium and one containing cycloheximide and chloramphenicol to inhibit the common bacterial and mold contaminants. These agents do not alter the cultural characteristics of dermatophytes and facilitate their isolation. Mycosel* and Mycobiotic† agars work well for isolation of dermatophytes.

---

*Baltimore Biological Laboratory, Cockeysville, Md.
†Difco Laboratories, Detroit, Mich.

KEY TO DIRECT EXAMINATION OF HAIR

Wood's lamp

1. Bright yellow-green fluorescence of hair shafts: *Microsporum audouinii*, *M. canis*, *M. distortum*, *M. ferrugineum*, rarely *Trichophyton schoenleinii*.
2. No fluorescence: all the other dermatophyte species.

KOH mounts

1. Ectothrix hairs
   a. Conidia 2 to 3 µm in diameter in mosaic, forming a sheath around the hair: *M. audouinii*, *M. canis*, *M. distortum*, *M. ferrugineum*.
   b. Conidia 3 to 5 µm in diameter, forming a sheath or in isolated chains on the surface of hairs: *T. mentagrophytes*.
   c. Conidia 5 to 8 µm in diameter, forming a sheath or in isolated chains on the surface of hair: *T. equinum*, rarely *T. rubrum*.
   d. Conidia 5 to 8 µm in diameter, in chains or in irregular masses of the hair surface: *M. fulvum*, *M. gypseum*, *M. nanum*.
   e. Conidia 8 to 10 µm in diameter, forming a sheath or in isolated chains on the surface of hair: *T. verrucosum*.
2. Endothrix hairs
   Short hair stubs, thick and usually twisted, filled with chains of large spores 4 to 8 µm in diameter: *T. soudanense*, *T. tonsurans*, *T. violaceum*, *T. yaoundii*.
3. Favic hairs
   Hairs invaded throughout their length by hyphal elements. Empty areas (tunnels) where hyphae have degenerated into fat droplets are commonly seen inside the hair: *T. schoenleinii*.

From Ajello and Padhye.[8]

Another medium, dermatophyte test medium (DTM), is valuable when trained personnel are not immediately available to identify cultures. This medium inhibits bacteria and saprophytic molds and becomes alkaline (red) when a dermatophyte has grown on it. The culture is then purified and maintained on media free of antibiotics. Various commercial DTM media have proved satisfactory.

All media should be incubated at room temperature (not over 30 C) and examined at 5-day intervals for at least 1 month before discarding. Sporulation of the dermatophytes generally occurs within 5 to 10 days of inoculation, and cultures should be examined during this period, because characteristic colonial appearance and microscopic morphology are more easily recognized before the cultures age.

Common species

Species of *Microsporum* attack the hair and skin (and nails very rarely) and include *M. audouinii*, *M. canis*, and *M. gypseum*. *Trichophyton* species are responsible for infection of the hair, skin, and nails and include principally *T. mentagrophytes*, *T. rubrum*, *T. tonsurans*, *T. schoenleinii*, *T. violaceum*, and *T. verrucosum*. *Epidermophyton* causes infection of the skin and nails but not the hair and includes a single species, *E. floccosum*.

Since these dermatophytes generally present an identical appearance on microscopic examination of infected skin or nails,[11] final identification can only be made by culture. Fig. 34-4 and Table 34-4 summarize colonial morphology and microscopic identification of these fungi.

Descriptions of the 10 principal species of fungi involved in dermatophytoses in the United States[4] follow; other geographically limited species are described in the references cited.

Genus Microsporum

The genus *Microsporum* is immediately identified by the presence of large (8 to 15 µm by 35 to 150 µm), spindle-shaped, rough or spiny mac-

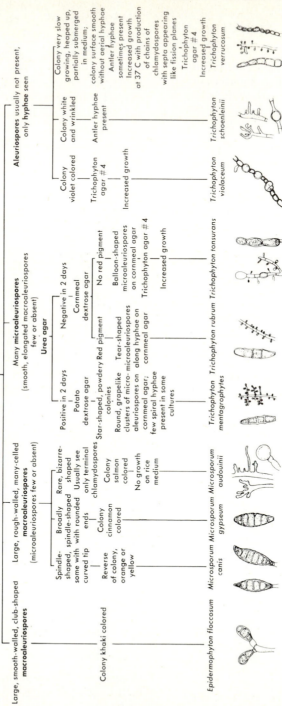
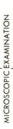

FIG. 34-4

Dermatophyte identification schema. Scheme used for dermatophytes commonly recovered by Mayo Clinic Mycology Laboratory. (From Koneman and associates.[42])

TABLE 34-4

Characteristics of more commonly isolated dermatophytes

Dermatophyte	Colonial morphology	Growth rate	Microscopic identification
Microsporum audouinii	Downy white to salmon pink colony. Reverse tan to salmon pink.	2 weeks	Sterile hyphae: terminal chlamydospores, favic chandeliers, and pectinate bodies. Macroaleuriospores rarely seen—bizarre shaped if seen. Microaleuriospores rare or absent.
Microsporum canis	Colony usually membranous with feathery periphery. Center of colony white to buff over orange-yellow. Lemon yellow or yellow-orange apron and reverse.	1 week	Thick walled, spindle-shaped, multi-septate, rough walled macroaleuriospores, some with a curved tip. Microaleuriospores rarely seen.
Microsporum gypseum	Cinnamon-colored, powdery colony. Reverse light tan.	1 week	Thick walled, rough, elliptical multi-septate macroaleuriospores, Microaleuriospores few or absent.
Epidermophyton floccosum	Center of colony tends to be folded and is khaki green; periphery is yellow. Reverse yellowish brown with observable folds.	1 week	Macroaleuriospores large, smooth walled, multi-septate, clavate and borne singly or in clusters of two or three. Microaleuriospores not formed by this species.
Trichophyton mentagrophytes	Different colonial types. White to pinkish, granular and fluffy varieties. Occasional light yellow periphery in younger cultures. Reverse buff to reddish brown.	7 to 10 days	Many round to globose microaleuriospores most commonly borne in grape-like clusters or laterally along the hyphae. Spiral hyphae in 30% of isolates. Macroaleuriospores are thin walled, smooth, club-shaped and multi-septate. Numerous or rare depending upon strain.
Trichophyton rubrum	Colonial types vary from white downy to pink granular. Rugal folds are common. Reverse yellow when colony is young; however, wine red color commonly develops with age.	2 weeks	Microaleuriospores usually teardrop, most commonly borne along sides of the hyphae. Macroaleuriospores usually absent, but when present are smooth, thin walled, and pencil-shaped.
Trichophyton tonsurans	White, tan to yellow or rust, suede-like to powdery. Wrinkled with heaped or sunken center. Reverse yellow to tan to rust red.	7 to 14 days	Microaleuriospores are teardrop or club-shaped with flat bottoms. Vary in size but usually larger than other dermatophytes. Macroaleuriospores rare and balloon forms found when present.
Trichophyton schoenleinii	Irregularly heaped, smooth white to cream colony with radiating grooves. Reverse white.	2 to 3 weeks	Hyphae usually sterile. Many antler-type hyphae seen (favic chandeliers).
Trichophyton violaceum	Port wine to deep violet colony, may be heaped or flat with waxy-glabrous surface. Pigment may be lost on subculture.	2 to 3 weeks	Branched, tortuous hyphae that are sterile. Chlamydospores commonly aligned in chains.
Trichophyton verrucosum	Glabrous to velvety white colonies. Rare strains produce yellow-brown color. Rugal folds with tendency to sink into agar surface.	2 to 3 weeks	Microaleuriospores rare. Large and teardrop when seen. Macroaleuriospores extremely rare, but form characteristic "rat-tail" types when seen. Many chlamydospores seen in chains, particularly when colony is incubated at 37 C.

From Koneman et al.[42]

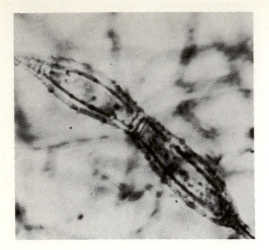

FIG. 34-5
Microsporum audouinii, showing macroconidium
(1,800×).

roconidia with thick (up to 4 μm) walls and containing 4 to 15 septa (Fig. 34-5). The microconidia are small (3 to 7 μm) and club shaped and are borne on the hyphae, either sessile or on short sterigmata. Cultures of *Microsporum* develop slowly or rapidly and produce an aerial mycelium that may be velvety, powdery, glabrous, or cottony, varying in color from whitish, buff, and bright yellow to a deep cinnamon brown, with varying shades on the reverse side of the colony.

M. audouinii has been the most important cause of epidemic tinea capitis among schoolchildren in the United States, but it rarely infects adults. *Trichophyton tonsurans* is now the major cause of tinea capitis in many parts of the country.[66,73] The fungus is known as an **anthropophilic,** or "man-loving" fungus and is spread directly by means of infected hairs on headwear, upholstery, combs, or barbers' clippers. The majority of infections are chronic; some heal spontaneously, whereas others may persist for several years. Infected hair shafts fluoresce yellow-green. A case of generalized infection with this organism has been described.[9]

On SAB agar *M. audouinii* grows slowly, producing a flat gray to tan colony with short aerial hyphae and a radially folded surface. The reverse of the colony is generally reddish-brown. *M. audouinii* sporulates poorly on SAB agar, and the characteristic macroconidia may be lacking in some cultures. The addition of yeast extract stimulates growth and production of both macroconidia and small club-shaped microconidia borne laterally along the hyphae. Abortive and bizarrely shaped macroconidia, hyphal cells with swollen ends (racquet hyphae), abortive branches (pectinate bodies), and chlamydospores are commonly observed.

*M. canis** is primarily a pathogen of animals (**zoophilic**); it is the most common cause of ringworm in dogs and cats in the United States. Children and adults acquire the disease through contact with infected animals, particularly puppies and kittens, although human-to-human transfer has been reported. Hairs infected with *M. canis* **fluoresce** a bright yellow-green under a Wood's lamp, which is a useful tool for screening pets as possible sources of human outbreaks. On direct examination in 10% potassium hydroxide small spores (2 to 3 μm) are found outside the hair (ectothrix), although cultural procedures must be carried out for specific identification.

On SAB agar *M. canis* grows rapidly as a flat, disklike colony with a bright yellow periphery and possesses a short aerial mycelium. On aging (2 to 4 weeks) the mycelium becomes dense and cottony, a deeper brownish-yellow or orange, and frequently shows an area of heavy growth in the center. The reverse side of the colony is **bright yellow,** becoming orange or reddish-brown with age. Rarely, strains are isolated that show no reverse-side pigment. Microscopically, *M. canis* shows an abundance of large (15 μm by 60 to 125 μm), spindle-shaped, multicelled (4 to 8) macroconidia (Fig. 34-6) with knoblike ends. These are thick walled and bear warty (echinulate) projections on their surfaces. Microconidia,

*Ascomycetous state: *Nannizzia otae*.

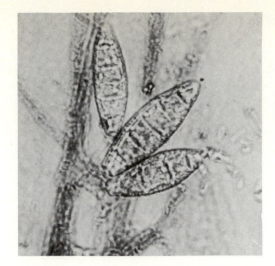

FIG. 34-6
Microsporum canis, showing several spindle-shaped, thick-walled, multicelled macroconidia (500×).

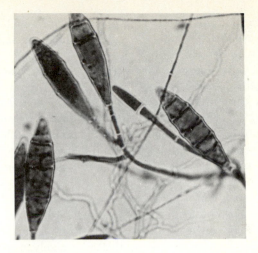

FIG. 34-7
Microsporum gypseum, showing ellipsoidal multicelled macroconidia (750×).

pectinate hyphae, racquet hyphae, and chlamydospores are found.

*M. gypseum** is a free-living saprophyte of the soil (**geophilic**) that only rarely causes human or animal infection. Infected hairs generally do not fluoresce under a Wood's lamp. However, microscopic examination of infected hairs shows them to be irregularly covered with clusters of spores (5 to 8 μm), some in chains. These arthrospores of the ectothrix type are considerably larger than those of other *Microsporum* species.

On SAB agar *M. gypseum* grows rapidly as a flat, irregularly fringed colony with a coarse powdery surface with a fawn to buff or **cinnamon brown** color. The underside of the colony is conspicuously orange to brownish. Macroconidia are seen in large numbers and are characteristically large, ellipsoidal, and multicelled (3 to 9) with echinulate surfaces (Fig. 34-7). Although spindle shaped, these macroconidia are not as pointed at the distal end as are those of *M. canis*. Microconidia are rare.

*Ascomycetous state: *Nannizzia gypsea*.

Genus Trichophyton

Species of this genus are widely distributed and are the most important causes of **ringworm** of the feet and nails; they may also be responsible for tinea corporis, tinea capitis, and tinea barbae. They are most commonly seen in adult infections, which vary considerably in their clinical manifestations. Most cosmopolitan species are anthropophilic; a few are zoophilic.

Generally, trichophyton-infected hairs **do not fluoresce** under a Wood's lamp; the demonstration of fungal elements inside the hair shaft (Plate 182), surrounding and penetrating the hair shaft, or within skin scrapings is needed to make a diagnosis of ringworm. Isolation and identification of the fungus are necessary for confirmation.

Microscopically, *Trichophyton* is characterized by club-shaped, **smooth,** thin-walled macroconidia with 8 to 10 septa ranging in size from 8 by 4 μm to 15 by 8 μm. The macroconidia are borne singly at the terminal ends of hyphae or on short branches; the microconidia are usually spherical or clavate and 2 to 4 μm in size. Although a large number of *Trichophyton* species have been described, many have proved to be colonial variants. Only the common species will be described.

*Trichophyton mentagrophytes** occurs in **two distinct colonial forms:** the so-called **downy** variety commonly isolated from human tinea pedis and the **granular** variety isolated from ringworm acquired from animals (zoophilic). It is possible to convert the downy form to the granular form by animal passage; the reverse may occur spontaneously in laboratory cultures.

Growth of *T. mentagrophytes* is rapid and abundant on SAB agar, appearing as white, cottony, or downy colonies to flat, cream-colored, or peach-colored colonies that are coarsely granular to powdery. The reverse side of the colony is rose-brown, occasionally orange to deep red. The white downy colonies produce only a few clavate microconidia; the granular colonies sporulate freely with numerous small, globose to club-shaped microconidia and thin-walled, slightly clavate, spindle- or pencil-shaped macroconidia measuring 6 by 20 μm to 8 by 50 μm in size, with 2 to 5 septa. (Fig. 34-8). Spiral hyphae and nodular bodies may be present. Macroconidia are demonstrated best in 5- to 10-day-old cultures.

Trichophyton rubrum is a slow-growing species, producing a flat or heaped-up colony with a white to reddish cottony or velvety surface. This characteristic **cherry red** color is best observed on the reverse side of the colony, commencing at the margin or spreading concentrically, but it may disappear on subculture. Occasional strains may lack the deep red pigmentation on first isolation.† Microconidia are rare in most of the fluffy strains and more common in the velvety or granular strains, occurring as globose to clavate spores, 2 to 5 μm in size, and growing in clusters

---

*Ascomycetous state: *Arthroderma benhamiae*.

†A useful method, utilizing in vitro hair cultures to differentiate aberrant forms of *T. mentagrophytes* from *T. rubrum*, has been described by Ajello and Georg.[5] This may be supplemented by cultivation on potato-carrot medium, which often induces sporulation.[79]

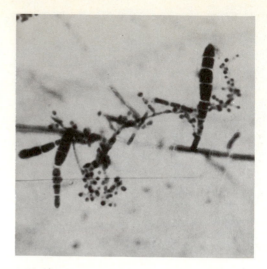

FIG. 34-8
Trichophyton mentagrophytes, showing numerous microconidia in grapelike clusters. Also shown are several thin-walled macroconidia (500×).

on the lateral sides of the mycelium. Macroconidia are rarely seen, although they are more common in the granular strains, where they appear as thin-walled, sausagelike cells with blunt ends, containing 3 to 8 septa (Fig. 34-9).

Trichophyton tonsurans, along with *M. audouinii*, is responsible for an **epidemic** form of tinea capitis occurring most commonly in children but occasionally in adults. As noted before, it has displaced *M. audouinii* as the primary cause of tinea capitis in much of the United States. The fungus causes a low-grade superficial lesion of varying chronicity and produces circular, scaly patches of alopecia. The stubs of hair remain in the epidermis of the scalp after the brittle hairs have broken off and may give the typical "black dot" ringworm appearance. Since the infected hairs do not fluoresce under a Wood's lamp, a careful search for the embedded stub should be carried out in a bright light, using a magnifying head loop.

The direct microscopic examination of infected stubs mounted in 10% potassium hydroxide reveals the hair shaft to be filled with masses

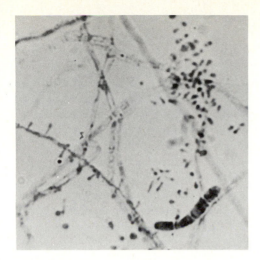

FIG. 34-9
Trichophyton rubrum, showing a sausage-shaped macroconidium and numerous pyriform microconidia borne singly on hyphae (750×).

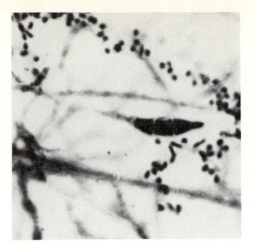
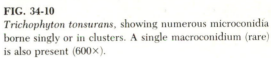

FIG. 34-10
Trichophyton tonsurans, showing numerous microconidia borne singly or in clusters. A single macroconidium (rare) is also present (600×).

of large (4 to 7 μm) arthrospores in chains, an endothrix type of invasion. Cultures of *T. tonsurans* develop slowly on SAB agar as flat, white, powdery colonies, later becoming velvety and varying in color from a gray through a sulfur yellow to tan (Plate 183). The colony surface shows radial folds, often developing a **craterlike** depression in the center with deep fissures. The reverse side of the colony is yellowish- to reddish-brown. Microscopically, numerous microconidia are observed, borne laterally on undifferentiated hyphae or in clusters. These vary greatly in size, from 2 by 3 μm to 5 by 7 μm. Macroconidia, although rarely encountered, are clavate or irregular in shape with thin walls (Fig. 34-10). Chlamydospores are abundant in old cultures; swollen and fragmented hyphal cells resembling arthrospores are also seen. The addition of thiamine to the isolation medium enhances the growth of *T. tonsurans*.

Favus is a severe type of ringworm of the scalp caused by *Trichophyton schoenleinii*. The infection is characterized by the formation of yellowish cup-shaped crusts, or scutulae, resulting in considerable scarring of the scalp and sometimes permanent baldness (Plate 184). A distinctive invasion of the infected hair, the favic type, is demonstrated by the presence of large inverted cones of hyphae and arthrospores at the mouths of the hair follicles along with a branching mycelium throughout the length of the hair (endothrix). Longitudinal tunnels or empty spaces appear in the hair shaft where the hyphae have disintegrated, which in potassium hydroxide preparations readily fill with fluid; air bubbles also can be seen in these tunnels.

On SAB agar *T. schoenleinii* grows slowly as a gray, glabrous, and waxy colony, somewhat hemispherical at first, but later spreading to resemble a sponge placed on the medium. The irregular border consists mostly of submerged mycelium, which tends to crack the agar. The surface of the colony is yellow to tan, furrowed, and irregularly folded. Old atypical strains show a powdery or downy surface with short aerial hyphae. The reverse side of the colony is usually tan or nonpigmented.

Microscopically, one sees only a few micro-

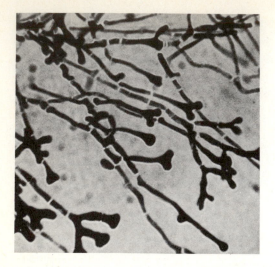

FIG. 34-11
Trichophyton schoenleinii, showing swollen hyphal tips, resembling antlers, with lateral and terminal branching (favic chandeliers). Microconidia and macroconidia are absent (500×).

conidia, which vary greatly in size and shape. Macroconidia are not produced; the mycelium is highly irregular. The hyphae tend to become knobby and club shaped at the terminal ends (pin heads), with the production of many short lateral and terminal branches (favic chandeliers) (Fig. 34-11). Chlamydospores are generally numerous. All strains of *T. schoenleinii* may be cultivated in a vitamin-free medium and grow equally well at both room temperature and 35 C.

Trichophyton violaceum causes ringworm of the scalp and body, mainly in the Mediterranean region, the Middle and Far East, and occasionally in the United States. Hair invasion is of the endothrix type; clinically, the typical black-dot ringworm is observed. Microscopically, direct examination of potassium hydroxide mounts of the short nonfluorescing hair stubs shows dark thick hairs filled with masses of arthrospores arranged in chains, similar to the appearance in *T. tonsurans* infections. On SAB agar the fungus is very slow growing, beginning

as a cream-colored, glabrous, cone-shaped colony, later becoming heaped up, verrucose (warty), and lavender to deep purple. The reverse side of the colony is purple or nonpigmented. Older cultures may develop a velvety aerial mycelium and sometimes lose their purple pigment. Microscopically, microconidia or macroconidia are generally absent; only sterile, thin, and irregular hyphae and chlamydospores are found. *T. violaceum* requires thiamine-enriched media to produce conidia.

Trichophyton verrucosum causes a variety of ringworm lesions in cattle (zoophilic) and humans (Plate 185); it is seen most often in farmers who are infected from cattle. The lesions are found chiefly on the beard, neck, wrist, and back of the hand; they are deep, boggy, and suppurating with sinus tracts. On pressure short stubs of hair can be recovered from the purulent lesion. On direct examination the outside of the hair shaft reveals sheaths of isolated chains of large (5 to 10 μm) spores and mycelium within the hair (ectothrix and endothrix type). Masses of these spores are also seen in the pus and germinate to form long thin filaments.

T. verrucosum grows very slowly (10 to 14 days) and poorly on SAB agar at room temperature but better at 35 C. Maximal growth is obtained on media enriched with thiamine and inositol or yeast extract; no growth occurs on vitamin-free media. Kane and Smitka[40] have described a new medium for the early detection and identification of *T. verrucosum.* The key ingredients of this medium are 4% casein and 0.5% yeast extract. The fungus is recognized by its early hydrolysis of casein and very slow growth. Chains of chlamydospores are formed regularly at 37 C. The early detection of hydrolysis, formation of characteristic chains of chlamydospores, and restrictive slow growth of *T. verrucosum* differentiate it from *T. schoenleinii.* The colony on SAB agar is small, heaped, and folded, occasionally flat and disk shaped. At first glabrous and waxy, the colony sometimes develops a short aerial mycelium on enriched media;

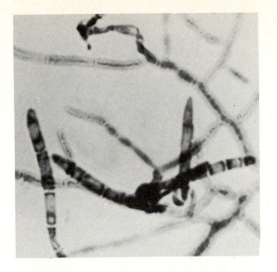

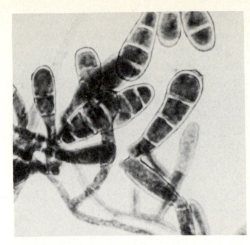

FIG. 34-12
Trichophyton verrucosum, showing multicelled, smooth, thin-walled macroconidia, which are rarely seen (500×).

FIG. 34-13
Epidermophyton floccosum, showing numerous smooth, multiseptate, thin-walled macroconidia with rounded ends (microconidia absent) (1,000×).

colonies vary from a gray, waxlike color to a bright ochre. The reverse of the colony is yellow but may be nonpigmented.

On SAB agar a thin, irregular mycelium is produced, with many terminal and intercalary (between two hyphal segments) chlamydospores; sometimes favic chandeliers are formed. Chlamydospores are more numerous on SAB agar incubated at 35 C. On enriched media *T. verrucosum* forms more regular mycelia and numerous small microconidia, borne singly along the hyphae. Macroconidia (Fig. 34-12) are rarely formed and vary considerably in size and shape.

Genus Epidermophyton

Epidermophytosis is caused by *Epidermophyton floccosum*, but a similar picture can be caused also by species of *Trichophyton* and *Microsporum*. The skin and nails are usually attacked, but not the hair. In the direct examination of scrapings mounted in potassium hydroxide, the fungus is seen as fine branching filaments in young lesions that form chains of arthrospores in older lesions.

E. floccosum grows slowly on SAB agar; primary growth appears as yellowish-white spots, developing into powdery or velvety colonies with centrally radiating furrows distinctively greenish-yellow. The reverse side of the colony is yellowish-tan. After several weeks, the colony develops a white aerial mycelium (pleomorphic), which completely overgrows the colony.

Microscopically, numerous smooth, thin-walled, multiseptate (2 to 4) macroconidia are seen, rounded at the tip and borne singly or in groups of two or three on the hyphae (Fig. 34-13). Microconidia are absent, spiral hyphae are rare, and chlamydospores are usually numerous.

SUPERFICIAL MYCOSES

Tinea versicolor (pityriasis versicolor)—a skin disease characterized by superficial brownish scaly areas on light-skinned persons and lighter areas on dark-skinned persons on the trunk, arms, shoulders, and face—is widely distributed throughout the world. It is caused by *Malassezia (Pityrosporum) furfur*, whose mycelial fragments and clusters of thickwalled, yeast-like spores may be observed microscopically in skin scrapings (Plate 186).

Cultivation of the fungus is not required to establish the diagnosis and is seldom employed. If one wishes to cultivate the organism, one must use SAB agar overlaid with olive oil. A Wood's lamp may be used to detect infected areas, which are difficult to spot otherwise. Most infected areas fluoresce dull reddish to orange.[8]

Tinea nigra is a disease manifested by blackish-brown macular patches on the smooth skin of the body. The palm of the hand is particularly susceptible. The causative agent is *Exophiala werneckii*, a dematiaceous fungus. Colonies of *E. werneckii* may be black and yeastlike or they may become woolly with age and gray to black. The annellids are hyphalike or consist of two-celled yeast cells that are clavate. One- to two-celled conidia are formed from the annellids.

Black piedra is a fungus infection of scalp hair and rarely of axillary and pubic hair. The causative agent is a dematiaceous fungus called *Piedraia hortae*. The dark-walled mycelium spreads over and around the hair shaft, forming a cemented mat of hyphae (Plate 187). Nodules are eventually formed that contain asci and ascospores and may attain a diameter of 0.1 cm. These nodules are hard and gritty. The disease occurs primarily in tropical areas of the world. Cases have been reported in Africa, Asia, and Latin America. Portions of hairs are examined in wet mounts of 2% KOH, which is gently heated. The mycelium is septate and 4 to 8 μm in diameter. The nodules themselves are composed of cemented mycelium. When mature nodules are crushed, oval asci, 44 to 50 μm by 24 to 30 μm, may be seen. These contain eight aseptate, curved, spindle-shaped ascospores that have a filament at each pole. The organism may be grown on SAB agar; it is important to use media

without cycloheximide, since *P. hortae* is inhibited by that compound. Chloramphenicol and other antibacterial drugs, however, are useful in the medium.

White piedra is an uncommon disease found in both tropical and temperate regions of the world. It is characterized by development of soft, yellow or pale brown accretions around hair shafts in the axillary, facial, genital, and scalp regions of the body. The responsible fungus is *Trichosporon beigelii*. It frequently invades the cortex of hair filaments and thus damages the hair (Plate 188). Nodules may be readily crushed by covering them with a coverslip and applying light pressure using a mount of 10% KOH. Hyaline mycelium 2 to 4 μm in width and arthroconidia are found in the preparation with a cement-like material binding the hyphae together. The organism is readily isolated on SAB agar that contains chloramphenicol, but cycloheximide must not be used in the medium, since it inhibits growth of *T. beigelii*. A cream-colored, yeast-like colony grows in a few days. It is composed of hyaline mycelium that produces blastoconidia and that fragments into arthroconidia. *T. beigelii* may be distinguished from the other seven species in the genus by its inability to ferment sugars and its ability to assimilate certain compounds. Rarely *T. beigelii* (incorrectly known as *Trichosporon cutaneum*) may produce systemic mycosis in immunosuppressed hosts.[27]

SUBCUTANEOUS MYCOSES

Subcutaneous mycoses are fungal infections that involve the skin and subcutaneous tissue, generally without dissemination to the internal organs of the body. This classification is artificial; for example, sporotrichosis on occasion involves the lungs, other viscera, the meninges, or joints or may disseminate. The other agents causing subcutaneous infection may also produce visceral infection occasionally. The agents are found in several unrelated fungal genera, all of which probably exist as saprophytes in nature. Humans and animals serve as **accidental hosts** through inoculation of the fungal spores into cutaneous and subcutaneous tissue after trauma. Three subcutaneous mycoses are considered here: **sporotrichosis, chromomycosis,** and **maduromycosis.**

Sporotrichosis

Sporotrichosis is a chronic infection of worldwide distribution caused by the **dimorphic** fungus *Sporothrix schenckii*, whose natural habitat is in the soil and on living or dead vegetation. Humans acquire the infection through wounds (thorns, splinters) of the hand, arm, or leg. The infection is characterized by the development of a nodular lesion of the skin or subcutaneous tissue at the point of contact and later involves the lymphatic vessels and nodes draining the area. The lesion then breaks down to form an indolent ulcer that later becomes chronic. Only rarely is the disease disseminated. The infection is an occupational hazard for farmers, nurserymen, gardeners, florists, and miners.*

The **tissue forms** of *S. schenckii* appear as small, oval, budding, yeastlike cells, which are not usually demonstrable in unstained or stained smears of material from suspected lesions, except by immunofluorescence procedures (see Chapter 39). However, the tissue form may be produced readily by inoculating (Plate 190) mice or rats (see p. 426). The organism can be demonstrated in tissue sections stained by the Gomori or Gridley procedure.

Pus from unopened subcutaneous nodules or from open draining lesions is inoculated to BHI agar incubated at 35 C and on SAB agar at room temperature. Chloramphenicol and cycloheximide should be added to the medium if contamination is anticipated. *S. schenckii* is not inhibited by these agents.

The tissue (yeast or parasitic) phase develops at 35 C, appearing in 3 to 5 days as smooth, tan, yeastlike colonies. Microscopically, such colo-

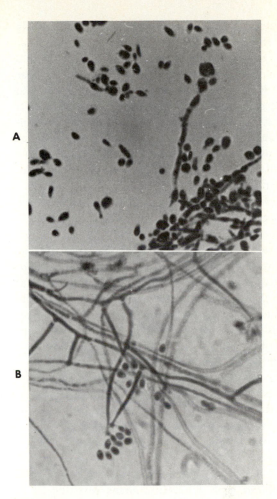

FIG. 34-14
Sporothrix schenckii. **A,** Yeast phase, showing cigar-shaped and oval-budding cells (500×). **B,** Mycelial phase, showing pyriform to ovoid microconidia borne bouquetlike at the tip of the conidiophore (750×).

nies show cigar-shaped (fusiform) cells, measuring 1 to 4 μm by 1 μm or less, and round or oval budding cells 2 to 3 μm in diameter (Fig. 34-14, *A*). Occasionally, a few large, pyriform cells, 3 to 5 μm in size, may be produced.

On SAB agar at room temperature growth appears in 3 to 5 days as small, moist, white to cream-colored colonies. On further incubation these become membranous, wrinkled, and

---

*An outbreak of sporotrichosis associated with sphagnum moss as the source of infection has been reported.[22]

coarsely tufted, the color becoming irregularly **dark brown or black** (Plate 189). Microscopically, the mycelium is made up of delicate (1 to 2 μm thick), branching, septate hyphae that bear pyriform or ovoid to spherical microconidia 2 to 5 μm in diameter. These are borne, bouquet-like, in clusters from the tips of the conidiophores or directly on the sides of hyphae as dense sleeves of conidia (Fig. 34-14, *B*). Older cultures may produce larger, thick-walled chlamydospores.

Because of their morphology, saprophytic species of the genus may be confused with *S. schenckii*, and it is necessary to distinguish between them by in vitro and in vivo culture. For the former moist slants of BHI agar containing 5% blood are inoculated and incubated at 35 C. It may require several transfers before the characteristic yeast form (tissue phase) develops. Animal inoculation may be employed if laboratory culture is nonproductive; to this end white rats are injected intratesticularly with pus, yeast cells, or mycelial fragments, using approximately 0.2 ml. In 3 weeks the animals are killed and examined for a purulent orchitis. Gram-stained pus reveals gram-positive cigar-shaped or oval budding forms of *S. schenckii* (Plate 190).

Comparison of clinical isolates of *S. schenckii* isolated from different sources revealed some interesting differences.[44] Strains isolated from cutaneous lesions without any involvement of the lymphatics or deeper tissues grew at 35 C but not 37 C and did not multiply in internal organs of mice injected by the intraperitoneal route, although they did grow well in the testes. In contrast, strains isolated from disease involving lymphatics or deeper tissues were able to grow both at 35 C and 37 C, and when injected into mice intraperitoneally, they multiplied well in the internal organs as well as the testes.

Chromomycosis

Chromomycosis is a chronic noncontagious skin disease characterized by the development of a papule at the site of infection that spreads to form warty or tumorlike lesions, later resembling a cauliflower. There may be secondary infection and ulceration. The lesions are usually confined to the feet and legs (Plate 192) but may involve the head, face, neck and other body surfaces. Brain abscess may also be caused by species in the genera *Phialophora* and *Cladosporium*.

The disease is widely distributed, but most cases occur in tropical and subtropical areas. Occasional cases are reported from temperate zones, including the United States. The infection is seen most often in areas where barefoot workers suffer thorn or splinter puncture wounds, through which the spores enter from the soil.

The etiologic agents of chromomycosis constitute a group of closely related fungi that produce a slow-growing, heaped-up, and slightly folded **dematiaceous** (dark-colored) colony with a grayish velvety mycelium. The reverse side of the colony is jet black. The different species are distinguished by the type of conidiophores they produce:

Cladosporium type (*Cladosporium carrionii*)—Conidia in branched chains are produced by conidiophores of various lengths.

Phialophora type (*Phialophora verrucosa*)—Conidia are produced endogenously in flasklike conidiophores or phialides (Fig. 34-15).

Acrotheca type (*Fonsecaea [Hormodendrum] pedrosoi, F. compacta*)—Conidia are formed along the sides of irregular club-shaped conidiophores (Fig. 34-16).

A laboratory diagnosis of chromomycosis is essential and is easily made. Scrapings or scales from encrusted areas mounted in 10% potassium hydroxide, xylol, or balsam show the presence of long, dark brown, thick-walled, branching septate hyphae 2 to 5 μm wide. In pus, tissue, or biopsy specimens thick-walled, rounded brown cells 4 to 12 μm in diameter may be observed (Plate 191). All of the fungi causing chromomycosis have the same appearance.

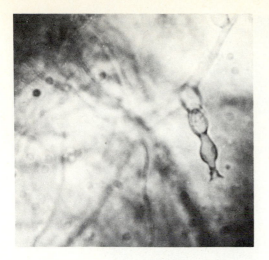

FIG. 34-15
Phialophora verrucosa, showing a single flasklike conidiophore (1,000×).

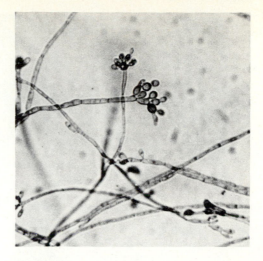

FIG. 34-16
Phialophora (Hormodendrum) pedrosoi, showing conidia produced terminally and in clusters on club-shaped conidiophores (cladosporium type) (400×).

Crusts, pus, and biopsy tissue are cultured on SAB agar with antibiotics (see Chapter 42) and incubated at room temperature. Identification of the dematiaceous isolates is based on the type of sporulation observed. *C. carrionii* exhibits only the *Cladosporium* type of sporulation, and the conidial chains are quite long. *F. compacta* and *F. pedrosoi* (Plate 193) may exhibit all three types of sporulation concurrently, although the cladosporium type predominates, with short chains of conidia. *P. verrucosa* exhibits only the *Phialophora* type of sporulation. A *Cladosporium* species, considered to be a saprophyte, also produces a cladosporium type of sporulation but, unlike *C. carrionii*, liquefies gelatin and hydrolyzes a Loeffler serum slant.

Mycetoma (maduromycosis)*

Mycetoma is a chronic granulomatous infection that usually involves the lower extremites but may occur on any part of the body. It was first described by Gill in 1842 while he was working in a dispensary near Madura, India. The term "Madura foot" probably originated from the natives' describing the deformed foot seen in infected patients. The disease is characterized by swelling, purplish discoloration and tumorlike deformities of the subcutaneous tissue, and multiple sinus tracts that drain pus containing yellow, red, or black granules. The infection gradually progresses to involve bone, muscle, or other contiguous tissue, ultimately requiring amputation. Occasionally there may be more significant invasion, with involvement of the brain or other internal organs.

Maduromycosis is common among the natives of the tropical and subtropical regions, whose outdoor occupations and shoeless habits often predispose them to trauma. These are significant factors in exposure to the fungus. More than 60 cases of mycetoma have been reported in the United States.[32]

There are two types of mycetoma: so-called actinomycotic mycetoma, or nocardiomycosis, caused by several species of *Nocardia*, *Actinomadura*, and *Streptomyces*; and fungal mycetoma or maduromycosis, caused by a heteroge-

*The interested reader is referred to Vanbreuseghem's excellent monograph on mycetoma.[85]

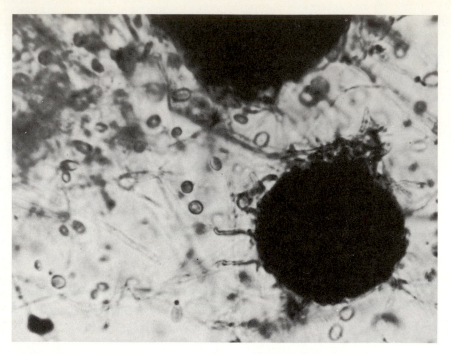

FIG. 34-17
Petriellidium boydii, showing perithecia and numerous ascospores (750×).

neous group of at least 17 species of septate true fungi with broad hyphae. The most common cause of maduromycosis in the United States is the perfect fungus *Petriellidium (Allescheria) boydii,** in the class Ascomycetes, since it produces sexual ascospores. The fungus is a common saprophyte in soil and sewage, and humans acquire the infection after such injuries as a scratch, bruise, or penetrating wound or by contaminating an open wound.

P. boydii is a **hyaline** (glassy, transparent) organism, producing white or yellow granules in pus. These are composed of tightly meshed, wide, septate mycelia and numerous large, hyaline chlamydospores. On SAB agar without antibiotics *P. boydii* grows rapidly at room temperature as a white fluffy colony that changes in sev-

eral weeks to a brownish-gray mycelium. The reverse of the colony is gray-black. Microscopic examination shows large, septate, hyaline hyphae and many conidia borne singly on conidiophores. The conidia are pyriform to oval in shape, are unicellular, and measure approximately 6 by 9 μm. Clusters of conidiophores (coremia) with conidia at the ends sometimes occur; these resemble ripened grains on sheaves of wheat.

Some strains of *P. boydii* produce **perithecia,** closed structures containing asci with ascospores. When the latter are fully developed, the large (50 to 200 μm), thin-walled perithecia rupture, liberating the asci and spores (Fig. 34-17). The ascospores are yellow, oval, and delicately pointed at each end and are somewhat smaller than the conidia.

P. boydii is also involved in a variety of infections elsewhere in the body. Included are

---

*Imperfect state: *Monosporium apiospermum.*

infections in and about the eye, sinusitis, brain abscess, meningitis, endocarditis, necrotizing pneumonia, and various bone and soft tissue infections. Most of these more serious infections occur primarily in immunosuppressed hosts.[87]

It should be noted that media containing antibiotics are not to be used alone in culturing clinical specimens from mycetomas or draining sinuses, since some of the agents of maduromycosis may be inhibited in their growth. This is particularly true with *P. boydii* and species of *Nocardia* and *Aspergillus*. Since "actinomycotic" lesions may respond to specific therapy, whereas maduromycoses may not, this etiologic differentiation must be made.

For information on other fungi involved in maduromycosis, one may refer to sources listed in the references.

EYE INFECTIONS

Keratomycosis (fungus infection of the cornea) is an uncommon but important fungal infection. Failure to recognize and treat it early and to avoid therapeutic use of corticosteroids may lead to deeper penetration of the infection and loss of the eye. Corneal involvement is typically in the form of an elevated ulcer with surrounding infiltrate and satellite lesions.

Except for *Candida albicans* infection, keratomycosis is **exogenous** in origin. Outdoor material, especially vegetable matter, is the primary source of the organism. Some 80 species of fungi in 35 genera may be causative agents. Most are saprophytes or plant pathogens; only a few are known as causes of other types of fungal infection. Accordingly, identification may often require the aid of mycologists with specialized knowledge. The most common causes of keratomycosis, in order of frequency, are *Fusarium solani*, *Candida albicans*, *Aspergillus fumigatus*, *Curvularia* species and other dematiaceous hyphomycetes, *Aspergillus flavus* and other *Aspergillus* species, *Penicillium*, *Paecilomyces*, *Fusarium episphaeria* and other *Fusarium* spe-

cies, *Cylindrocarpon*, *Acremonium* species and related genera, *Petriellidium boydii*, *Volutella* species, *Lasiodiplodia theobromae* and *Colletotrichum* species. Details on the fungi involved may be found in the chapter by Rebell and Forster.[67]

Other eye infections involving fungi include canaliculitis, dacryocystitis, orbital cellulitis, endophthalmitis following surgery or trauma, and the extension of cutaneous or systemic mycotic infection to the eye. Chorioretinitis is found relatively commonly in the course of systemic infection with *C. albicans*. These infections are embolic in origin and may spread from chorioretinal lesions to involve both the anterior and posterior chambers of the eye. Rarely other species of *Candida* may be involved,[80] as may *Torulopsis glabrata*.[28] Other fungi, including *Cryptococcus neoformans*,[82] *Petriellidium boydii*, and *Sporothrix schenckii*, may produce serious infections of the eye. Rarely, opportunistic fungi found only in keratomycosis may cause deep-seated infections elsewhere or even disseminated infection in immunosuppressed hosts.[88] There has been an outbreak of endophthalmitis associated with implantation of lenses; this was caused by contamination of the lens prostheses with *Paecilomyces lilacinus*.[17]

YEASTLIKE FUNGI

This group of imperfect fungi resembles the true yeasts both morphologically and culturally. They produce yeastlike, creamy colonies on solid media and are generally unicellular, although some produce a pseudomycelium or true mycelium. The genera discussed here include *Candida*, *Geotrichum*, *Torulopsis*, *Trichosporon*, *Saccharomyces*, *Rhodotorula*, and *Hansenula*.

Cryptococcus is also a yeast; this organism is discussed under **systemic mycoses**. Again, as with the subcutaneous mycoses, the division is arbitrary. The yeasts discussed here, except perhaps *Saccharomyces*, can all cause systemic disease. A practical approach to identification of yeasts is shown in Fig. 34-18.

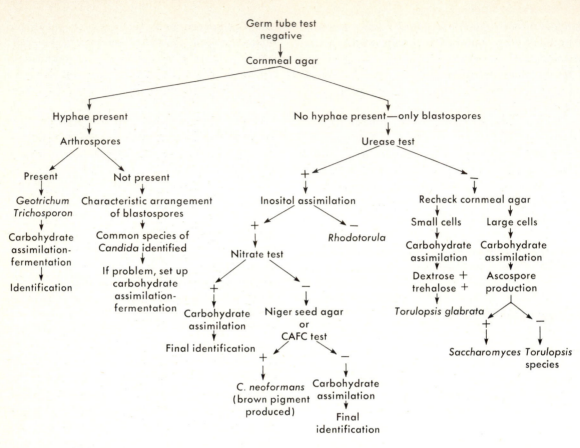

FIG. 34-18

Practical approach to the laboratory identification of yeasts. (From Koneman and associates.[42])

Candidiasis

Candidiasis is an acute or subacute infection caused by members of the genus *Candida*, chiefly *C. albicans*, although all species may be pathogenic.* The fungus may be isolated from the stools, genitourinary tract, throat, and skin of normal persons (**endogenous**), and it may produce lesions in the mouth, esophagus, genitourinary tract, skin, nails, bronchi, lungs, and other organs in patients whose normal defense mechanisms may have been altered by underlying disease, antimicrobial therapy, or immunosuppressive agents.[84] Bloodstream infection, endocarditis (primarily in drug addicts), and meningitis caused by *Candida* species have also been reported.

The isolation of *Candida* species from clinical materials is difficult to evaluate, since positive cultures may be obtained from various anatomic sites of a large percentage of normal persons. The organisms must be recovered repeatedly in significant numbers from **fresh specimens** and to

***Candida tropicalis* and *Candida parapsilosis*, although less commonly isolated from human infections, have been increasingly implicated in endocarditis and fungemia (Plate 197).

the exclusion of other known etiologic agents in patients with an appropriate clinical picture before a diagnosis of candidiasis can be entertained. Indeed, a Mayo Clinic group[55] concluded that *Candida* and other yeasts in respiratory secretions (aside from *C. neoformans*) probably represent normal flora and that their routine identification is not warranted.

Skin and nail scrapings should be examined directly; they are mounted in 10% potassium hydroxide with a coverglass and heated gently. Other material, such as exudate from the oropharynx or vagina or material from the intestinal tract, should be pressed under a coverglass and examined fresh, either unstained or Gram stained. *Candida* appears as small (2 to 4 μm), oval or budding, yeastlike cells, along with mycelial-like fragments of varying thickness and length (**tissue phase**). The yeastlike cells and pseudomycelial elements are strongly gram positive. It is advisable to report the approximate number of such forms seen, since the presence of large numbers in a fresh specimen may have diagnostic significance.

Since saprophytic yeasts are similar microscopically to the pathogenic species, all infected material should be **cultured** on duplicate sets of SAB agar with and without cycloheximide* and incubated at both room temperature and 35 C. Colonies of *Candida* species (and saprophytic yeasts) appear in 3 to 4 days as medium-sized, cream-colored, smooth, and pasty, with a characteristic yeastlike appearance. Most strains grow well at either temperature. On microscopic examination a slide mount shows budding cells along with elongated unattached cells (**pseudohyphae**) (Plate 194) with clusters of blastospores at constrictions (Fig. 34-19).

If the unknown culture is suspected of belonging to the genus *Candida*, subsequent proce-

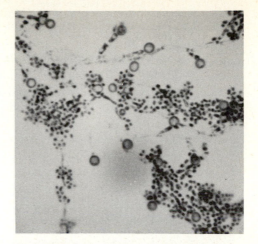

FIG. 34-19
Candida albicans, showing round, thick-walled chlamydospores, pseudomycelia, and numerous blastospores (750×).

dures must be carried out, including the demonstration of chlamydospore production (Plate 195), germ tube production (Plate 196), and sugar assimilation and fermentation tests. Although other species of *Candida* may be encountered in candidiasis, *C. albicans* is the most frequently isolated species and is the usual etiologic agent in oral or vaginal thrush, intertriginous or cutaneous monilial infection, paronychial infection, or bronchopulmonary candidiasis.

A simple test for production of germ tubes recommended by Ahearn[1] (modified) is as follows:

1. Cells from a young (not more than 96 hours) colony are transferred by means of the tip of a plastic straw* into about 0.5 ml of pooled **human** serum contained in a clean 12- by 75-mm test tube, leaving the straw immersed in the serum. The inoculum should be small.
2. The tube is incubated for 3 hours at 35 C; a

---

*A number of *Candida* species are inhibited by 0.5 mg/ml of cycloheximide; these include *C. parapsilosis*, *C. krusei*, and strains of *C. tropicalis*; most strains of *C. albicans* are resistant.

---

*Commercial cocktail straws cut into approximately 100-mm lengths, clean but not sterile.

drop of the suspension is placed on a glass slide, using the straw for transfer, and a coverslip is applied.

3. Microscopic examination of typical *C. albicans* reveals thin **germ tubes** 3 to 4 μm in diameter and up to 20 μm long; unlike pseudohyphae, they are **not constricted** at their point of origin.

4. Arthrospores of *Geotrichum* or *Trichosporon** species and structures produced by other organisms may be mistaken for germ tubes by the inexperienced. For this reason, a **known isolate** of *C. albicans* and *C. tropicalis* should be included as a control.

Another method of identification of *Candida* relates to morphology when grown on corn meal agar containing 1% Tween 80 and trypan blue at room temperature in a Petri dish for 24 to 48 hours. The inocula are cut into the agar at a 45° angle. The dish is inverted and examined microscopically under 100× magnification. All *Cryptococcus* and *Torulopsis* strains fail to produce hyphae or pseudohyphae, whereas *Candida*,† *Trichosporon*, and *Geotrichum* strains do show such structures.

Identification of Candida by assimilation tests

1. Prepare a sterile solution of yeast-nitrogen base‡ by weighing 6.7 g of the dehydrated medium. To this add 5.0 g of the appropriate carbohydrate§ and dissolve in 100 ml of distilled water.

2. Sterilize by membrane filtration and add to an agar solution (20 g in 900 ml of distilled water) that has been autoclaved and cooled to approximately 50 C.

3. Dispense into sterile, cotton-stoppered test tubes; solidify in the slanting position. The use of agar slants rather than plates facilitates handling and storage.

4. The inoculum is prepared from 24- to 36-hour cultures of the isolate in yeast-nitrogen broth plus 1 mg/liter of glucose, and one drop (approximately 0.01 ml) is added to each carbohydrate slant. The tests are read after 96 hours' incubation, and evidence of growth is noted on each of the carbohydrate slants when compared with a control slant of the basal medium.

A rapid technique using carbohydrate-impregnated disks was proposed by Huppert and colleagues[38] and supported by Segal and Ajello.[75] Correlation with reference techniques is 90% after incubation for 1 day, 97% after 2 days, and 98% after 3 days. Certain carbohydrates for assimilation studies, as well as certain other tests important in identification of yeasts, are available in commercial kits. These provide results rapidly and have received favorable evaluations.[15,16,21,34,46,72] The Autobac I instrument[57] and the AutoMicrobic system[58] have been shown to be satisfactory for studies of rapid assimilation testing and for rapid identification based on 26 biochemical reactions, respectively.

Identification of Candida by fermentation tests*

1. Obtain a pure culture by inoculating a tube of SAB dextrose broth and incubating it overnight at 35 C.

2. Shake the tube, and inoculate a loopful to a blood agar plate and incubate it overnight at 35 C.

3. Examine the plate and pick single colonies to SAB agar slants; incubate it overnight at 35 C.

4. Transfer the culture to sugar-free beef

---

*Trichosporon species produce pseudomycelia, true mycelia, blastospores, and arthrospores. This rapidly growing yeast may be part of the normal skin flora; it has also been isolated from infected fingernails.
†Occasional strains of *C. guilliermondii* and *C. parapsilosis* do not produce obvious hyphal structures.
‡Difco Laboratories, Detroit, Mich.
§Recommended: lactose, inositol, melibiose, cellobiose, erythritol, xylose, trehalose, and raffinose.

*A simple, rapid (24 hour) technique using tablets (available from Key Scientific Products, Los Angeles) and a Vaspar seal is described by Huppert and associates.[38]

extract agar slants for three successive transfers, incubating each transfer overnight at 35 C.

5. Inoculate growth from the third transfer to sugar media in the following manner:

    a. Make a suspension of the growth in 2 ml of sterile saline.

    b. Pipet 0.2 ml to each of five tubes containing 9.5 ml of beef extract broth with 0.04% bromthymol blue indicator.

    c. To each of these tubes add, respectively, 0.5 ml of a filter-sterilized 20% stock solution (Millipore or Seitz) of glucose, maltose, sucrose, lactose, and galactose.

    d. Overlay each tube with sterile melted petrolatum or paraffin and petrolatum, to form a plug about 1 cm thick.

    e. Hold five uninoculated tubes containing the sugars as sterility controls.

    f. Incubate all tubes at 35 C for 10 days and record the presence of acid or acid and gas.

Refer to Table 34-5 for test results.

Additional rapid tests have shown promise in identification of yeasts. One is a rapid technique for determining nitrate utilization by yeasts in which the reaction may be read after only 2 minutes of incubation.[37] A second is a rapid urea broth test in which 60% of urease-producing yeasts were positive within 30 minutes and the remainder within 4 hours.[69] Finally, preliminary studies with 17 4-methylumbelliferyl substrates for identifying yeast isolates looked promising.[13] The hydrolysis product of enzymatic action on these conjugates produces a light blue fluorescence when viewed with the long wavelength of a Wood's lamp. Three substrates in particular showed promise.

Geotrichosis

Geotrichosis is a rather rare infection caused by the yeastlike fungus *Geotrichum candidum* (not a true yeast), which reproduces by fragmentation of the hyphae into rectangular arthrospores. It may produce lesions in the mouth, bronchi, or lungs. Since *Geotrichum* has been isolated from the mouths and intestinal tracts of normal persons, it must be recovered repeatedly and in large numbers from freshly obtained clinical specimens in patients with an appropriate clinical picture and no other likely pathogens present to be considered of etiologic significance.

Sputum or pus is pressed in a thin layer on a slide under a coverglass and examined directly. *Geotrichum* appears as rectangular (4 by 8 μm) or large spherical (4 to 10 μm) arthrospores that stain heavily gram-positive; no budding forms are seen (Plate 198).

Since these cells may be confused with those of the saprophytic *Oospora* (which frequently occurs as a contaminant), with the filamentous *Coccidioides immitis* (the etiologic agent of coccidioidomycosis), or with *Blastomyces dermatitidis* (the etiologic agent of North American blastomycosis), all infected material should be **cultured.** The specimen is inoculated on duplicate sets of SAB agar and BHI blood agar slants with and without chloramphenicol and cycloheximide; one set is incubated at room temperature and one at 35 C for at least 3 weeks. At room temperature the fungus develops rather rapidly as a moist, creamy colony; as a colony with a dry, mealy surface and radial furrows; or as one with fluffy aerial mycelium. At 35 C the slowly growing fungus develops only a small waxlike surface growth with a distinct zone of mycelium penetrating the subsurface of the medium. Microscopically, the septate, branching hyphae are fragmented into chains of rectangular, barrel-shaped, or spherical arthrospores that break apart readily. The rectangular cells frequently germinate by germ tubes from **one corner,** which are at first rounded and later elongated, a characteristic of *Geotrichum* (Fig. 34-20). Blastospores are not produced. *G. candidum* does not ferment carbohydrates but assimilates glucose and xylose. Characteristics are shown in Table 34-5.

Animal inoculation and serologic testing procedures are of no value in diagnosis.

TABLE 34-5

Cultural and biochemical characteristics of yeasts frequently isolated from clinical specimens

	Growth at 37 C	Pellicle in broth	Pseudo/true hyphae	Chlamydospores	Germ tubes	Capsule, India ink	Assimilation												Fermentation						Urease	KNO₃ utilization	Phenol oxidase
							Glucose	Maltose	Sucrose	Lactose	Galactose	Melibiose	Cellobiose	Inositol	Xylose	Raffinose	Trehalose	Dulcitol	Glucose	Maltose	Sucrose	Lactose	Galactose	Trehalose			
Candida albicans	+	–	+	+	+	–	+	+	+	–	+	–	–	–	+	–	+	–	F	F	–	–	F	F	–	–	–
C. famata	+	–	–	–	–	–	+	+	+	+	+	+	+	–	+	+	+	+	W	F	W	–	–	W	–	–	–
C. glabrata	+	–	–	–	–	–	+	–	–	–	–	–	–	–	–	–	+	–	F	–	–	–	–	F	–	–	–
C. guilliermondii	+	–	+	–	–	–	+	+	+	–	+	+	+	–	+	+	+	+	F	–	F	–	F	F	–	–	–
C. krusei	+	–	+	–	–	–	+	–	–	–	–	–	–	–	–	–	–	–	F	–	–	–	–	–	+*	–	–
C. parapsilosis	+	–	+	–	–	–	+	+	+	–	+	–	–	–	+	–	+	–	F*	–	–	–	F*	–	–	–	–
C. pintolopesii	+†	–	–	–	–	–	+	–	–	–	–	–	–	–	–	–	–	–	F	–	–	–	–	–	–	–	–
C. pseudotropicalis	+	–	+	–	–	–	+	–	+	–	+	–	+	–	+	+	–	–	F	–	F	F	F	–	–	–	–
C. rugosa	+	–	+	–	–	–	+	–	–	–	+	–	–	–	+	–	–	–	–	–	–	–	–	–	–	–	–
C. stellatoidea	+	–	+	+	+	–	+	+	–	–	+	–	–*	–	+	–	*	–	F	F	–	–	F	–	–	–	–
C. tropicalis	+	–	+	‡	–	–	+	+	+	–	+	–	–	–	+	+	+	–	F	F	F	–	F	*	+	–	–
Cryptococcus neoformans	+	–	R	–	–	+*	+	+	+	–	+*	–	+	+	+	+*	+	+*	–	–	–	–	–	–	+	–	+
C. albidus var. albidus	–*	–	R	–	–	–	+	+	+	+	–*	+	+	+	+	+	+	+*	–	–	–	–	–	–	+	+	–
C. albidus var. diffluens	+*	–	–	–	–	–	+	+	+	+	–*	+	+	+	+	+	+	+	–	–	–	–	–	–	+	+	–
C. gastricus	+	–	–	–	–	–	+	+	+	–	+*	+*	+	–	+	+	+	+	–	–	–	–	–	–	+	+	–
C. laurentii	–*	–	–	–	–	–	+	+	+	+	+*	+	+	+	+	+*	+	+	–	–	–	–	–	–	+	–	–
C. luteolus	+	–	–	–	–	–	+	+	+	+	+	+	+*	–	+	+	+	–	–	–	–	–	–	–	+	–	–
C. terreus	–*	–	–	–	–	–	+	+*	+*	+*	+*	+*	+*	+	+	+*	+	+*	–	–	–	–	–	–	+	+	–
C. uniguttulatus	+	–	–	–	–	+*	+	+	+	–	+	+	+	+	+	+	+	+	–	–	–	–	–	–	+	–	–
Rhodotorula glutinis	+	–	–	–	–	–	+	+	+	–	+	+	+	+	+	+	+	+	–	–	–	–	–	–	+	+	–
R. rubra	+	–	–	–	–	–	+	+	+	–	+	+	+	–	+	+	+	–	–	–	–	–	–	–	+	–	–
Saccharomyces cerevisiae	+*	–	–*	–	–	–	+	+	+	–	+	–	–	–	–	+	+	–	F	F	F	–	F	–	–	–	–
Trichosporon beigelii	+*	+	+	–	–	–	+	+	+	+*	+	+*	+	+	+	+*	+*	+*	F	F	F	–	F	F*	+*	–	–
T. pullulans	+*	+	+	–	–	–	+	+	+	–	+	+	+	+	+	+	+	+	F	F	F	–	F	–	+	+	–
Geotrichum candidum	–*	+	+	–	–	–	+	–	–	–	+	–	–	–	+	–	–	–	–	–	–	–	–	–	–	–	–

From Silva-Hutner and Cooper.[78] Based on data from Ahearn and Schlitzer and Lodder.

R, rare; +, growth greater than that of the negative control; F, sugar is fermented (i.e., gas is produced); W, weak fermentation.

*Strain variation.

†*C. pintolopesii* is a thermophilic yeast capable of growth at 40 to 42 C.

‡Occasional strains of *C. tropicalis* produce teardrop-shaped chlamydospores.

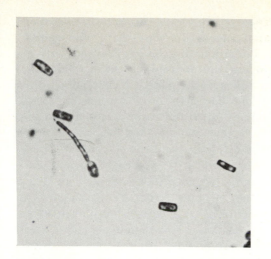

FIG. 34-20
Geotrichum candidum, showing barrel- to rectangular-shaped arthrospores, one with developing germ tube (500×).

Torulopsis glabrata

Torulopsis glabrata, closely related to *Cryptococcus* and *Candida* species, was once considered a nonpathogenic saprophyte from the soil, being widely distributed in nature. However, it is now clear that it is a potentially important opportunistic pathogen, particularly in the compromised host.[50] It has caused endocarditis.

On sheep blood agar *T. glabrata* appears as **tiny**, white, raised, nonhemolytic colonies after 1 to 3 days' incubation at 35 C. Gram stain of these colonies reveals round to oval budding yeasts, 2 to 4 µm in diameter; no hyphae or capsules are seen. Cultures on cornmeal-Tween agar are negative for mycelia or pseudohyphae; the germ tube test is also negative. *T. glabrata* ferments glucose and trehalose only and does not assimilate carbohydrates.[51] Characteristics are shown in Table 34-5.

Miscellaneous yeasts

Trichosporon has been discussed already as the cause of white piedra. This organism also causes occasional opportunistic invasion of mucous membranes or skin. *Saccharomyces* is responsible for occasional cases of thrush and vaginitis. Cells are oval to spherical, 3 by 5 µm; budding occurs, cells may form short chains and elongate as pseudohyphae. Ascospores are formed and are gram negative, in contrast with vegetative cells, which are gram positive. *Rhodotorula* resembles *Cryptococcus* closely, except for its distinctive pink pigment and general lack of pathogenicity. *Rhodotorula* may be involved in fungemia, but even here the pathogenic significance is uncertain.[64] *Hansenula*, not previously known to be pathogenic, was isolated from mediastinal lymph nodes of a child with chronic granulomatous disease.[53] This fungus develops globose asci containing 1 to 4 hemispherical ascospores with narrow brims. It ferments glucose but not several other carbohydrates and is able to assimilate several carbohydrates as well as potassium nitrate. Characteristics of *Trichosporon*, *Saccharomyces*, and *Rhodotorula* are given in Table 34-5.

SYSTEMIC MYCOSES

Systemic mycotic infections may involve any of the internal organs of the body, as well as lymph nodes, bone, subcutaneous tissue, and skin. **Asymptomatic infection** may go unrecognized clinically and may be detected only through skin sensitivity tests or serologic procedures; in some cases radiographic examination may reveal healed lesions. **Symptomatic infection** may present signs of only a mild or more severe but self-limited disease, with positive supportive evidence by culture or immunologic findings. **Disseminated or progressive infection** may reveal severe symptoms, with spread of the initial disease to visceral organs as well as the bone, skin, and subcutaneous tissues. This type of disease is frequently fatal. Some cases of disseminated infection may exhibit little in the way of signs or symptoms of the disease for long periods, only to exacerbate later.

Collection of specimens

The obtaining of a proper specimen for the laboratory diagnosis of systemic mycoses is of prime importance; success or failure in isolating the etiologic agent may well depend on it.

The most satisfactory **sputum** specimen is a single, early morning, coughed specimen, taken before the patient has eaten and after vigorous rinsing of the mouth with water after brushing the teeth. Twenty-four-hour specimens or those containing excessive amounts of postnasal discharge are not satisfactory. Sputum raised after inhalation of a heated 5% saline aerosol (prepared fresh and sterilized) and material obtained by bronchial aspiration are also satisfactory for mycologic examination. In all instances of suspected pulmonary infection, **at least six sputum specimens** should be obtained on successive days. It should also be emphasized that all of these types of specimens should be delivered promptly to the mycology laboratory and **cultured promptly,** since *Histoplasma capsulatum* dies rapidly in specimens held at room temperature; furthermore, saprophytic fungi, *C. albicans,* and commensal bacteria may multiply rapidly and prevent the isolation of significant pathogens.

Biopsy specimens, such as scalene lymph nodes, direct lung biopsies and so forth, are excellent specimens for the recovery of fungal pathogens; they should be submitted in sterile tubes or Petri dishes that are slightly moistened with sterile normal salt solution. Empyema fluid should be anticoagulated with heparin during aspiration to prevent clotting; gastric aspirates, CSF, synovial fluid, blood and bone marrow, urine, prostatic secretions (particularly in blastomycosis), and lesions of skin and mucous membranes afford significant sources for recovery of systemic fungal pathogens.

Introduction to systemic mycoses

The systemic mycoses to be considered in this section include **cryptococcosis, coccidioidomycosis, histoplasmosis, blastomycosis,** and **paracoccidioidomycosis.** The fungi responsible for these infections, although unrelated generically and dissimilar morphologically and culturally,

have (except for *Cryptococcus neoformans*) one characteristic in common—that of **dimorphism.** The dimorphic organisms involved exist in nature as the **saprophytic form,** sometimes called the **mycelial phase,** which is quite distinct from the **parasitic,** or tissue-invading form, sometimes called the **tissue phase.** The reader will note that reference has been made previously to this diphasic phenomenon in the fungal diseases candidiasis, sporotrichosis, and chromomycosis, where distinct morphologic differences may be observed both in vivo and in vitro. Temperature (35 C), certain nutritional factors, and stimulation of growth in tissue independent of temperature have been among the factors considered necessary to effect the transformation of mycelial forms to the parasitic phase.

Cryptococcosis

Cryptococcosis (torulosis) is a subacute or chronic mycotic infection involving primarily the brain and meninges and the lungs; at times the skin or other parts of the body may be involved. It is caused by a single species of yeastlike organism, *Cryptococcus neoformans.* Four serotypes of *C. neoformans* have been described—A, B, C, and D, with somewhat different geographic distribution. Serotypes B and C have been proposed as a separate species, *C. bacillisporus.*[45] However, there is no difference in disease produced or in response to therapy between these two species. On rare occasion other species of *Cryptococcus* have produced disease. Meningitis, pulmonary disease, and cutaneous infection have been produced by *Cryptococcus albidus* and *Cryptococcus laurentii.*[49] *C. neoformans* was first isolated by Sanfelice in 1894 from peach juice. Subsequently, the source of infection in humans and animals was erroneously assumed to be endogenous until Emmons, in 1950, reported the isolation of virulent strains of *C. neoformans* from barnyard soil. In 1955 he further reported a frequent association of virulent strains of *C. neoformans* with the excreta of pigeons and indicated that, until other sources are discovered, exposure to pigeon excreta was the most significant and important source of infection in humans and animals. This hypothesis has been substantiated by numerous reports that pigeon habitats serve as reservoirs for human infection; the pigeon manure apparently serves as an enrichment for *C. neoformans* because of its chemical makeup.[3] The organism is apparently the only pathogenic yeast not found in the normal human flora.

There is a strong association of cryptococcal infection with such debilitating diseases as leukemia and malignant lymphoma and the immunosuppressive therapy that may be required for these and other underlying diseases. The infection is probably more frequent than is commonly supposed; it is estimated that there are 2,000 undiagnosed cases for every proved case of infection caused by *C. neoformans*.

All clinical material, especially CSF,* should be mixed with a drop of Pelikan brand **India ink** (a cool loop must be used, since heat precipitates the ink particles) on a slide and examined under a coverglass using the oil immersion objective with reduced light. The India ink serves to delineate the large capsule, since the ink particles cannot penetrate the capsular material. *C. neoformans* appears as an oval to spherical, single-budding, thick-walled, yeastlike organism 5 to 15 μm in diameter, surrounded by a wide, **refractile, gelatinous capsule** (Fig. 34-21). This characteristic morphology occurs in India ink preparations of CSF, sputum, pus, urine, infected tissue, or gelatinous exudates. Frequently these capsules are more than twice the width of the individual cells. In CSF *C. neoformans* may be mistaken for a lymphocyte and is often observed first in the spinal fluid counting chamber.

Dried, heat-fixed, and stained preparations are not generally recommended; distortion of

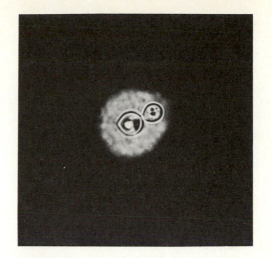

FIG. 34-21
Cryptococcus neoformans in spinal fluid, showing a large, encapsulated, single-budding, yeastlike cell (India ink; 1,000×).

the cryptococci may render them unrecognizable.

The infected material should be promptly cultured on infusion blood agar **without cycloheximide** (*C. neoformans* is inhibited) at 35 C and on SAB agar without cycloheximide at room temperature. Utz[84] recommended that when culturing CSF, the **uncentrifuged** fluid should be inoculated in generous amounts (15 to 20 ml) to a series of culture tubes, since the cryptococci may be present in very small numbers and the centrifugation may destroy the more fragile cells. After several days of incubation at either temperature, the organism produces a wrinkled, whitish colony, which on microscopic examination may show only budding cells without capsules. On further incubation the typical slimy (*Klebsiella*-like), mucoid, cream- to brown-colored colony develops. This colony has no mycelium and flows down to the bottom of the slant. At this time budding cells with large capsules can be readily demonstrated in India ink wet mounts, although some strains do not form large capsules (unless they are transferred

---

*The demonstration of encapsulated forms in the urine may precede their presence in CSF; urine may also be a good source for the isolation of *C. neoformans*.

several times) and generally produce a shiny, dry colony. Incubation in a candle jar may stimulate capsule production.

Of the yeastlike fungi, only members of the genus *Cryptococcus* (both saprophytic strains and *C. neoformans*) consistently produce **urease.** This can be detected by inoculating a urea agar slant (Christensen) with the suspected cryptococcus. If it is a *Cryptococcus* species, it will produce a positive reaction (red color) in the medium after 1 to 2 days of incubation at room temperature.* One may also use the rapid urease test described earlier. A still more impressive rapid urease test has been described by Zimmer and Roberts.[89] This detected urease activity of 99.6% of 286 isolates of *C. neoformans* within 15 minutes. *C. neoformans* characteristically does not assimilate nitrate or lactose but can assimilate glucose, maltose, and sucrose as carbon sources.

The incorporation of cycloheximide and chloramphenicol in SAB agar suffices in most instances for the isolation of pathogenic fungi from heavily contaminated material, **except** for *C. neoformans*, which is inhibited by cycloheximide. Staib[81] introduced a medium ("birdseed" or niger seed agar) containing creatinine and an extract of *Guizotia abyssinica* (a canary seed constituent) as a color marker for the selective isolation of *C. neoformans*, the growth of which produces a **brown** color (Plate 199). This medium, however, was rapidly overgrown with saprophytic fungi when inoculated with material from pigeon nests. The addition of diphenyl and chloramphenicol apparently increased the efficiency of the original preparation.[77] Caffeic acid, a constituent of *Guizotia* seeds, together with ferric citrate, has been used in a 6-hour paper disk test for brown pigment formation.[36] A simplified birdseed medium has been described,[62] as has a diagnostic medium containing inositol,

urea, and caffeic acid.[35] Growth and pigment production helped distinguish *C. neoformans* from other yeasts on this medium. Still another medium for isolation and identification of *C. neoformans* employs esculin as a substrate.[24] A portion of the esculin molecule is converted to a melaninlike pigment by *C. neoformans*. A commercially available medium known as the CN screen medium* is excellent for presumptive identification of *C. neoformans*. A positive test depends on phenol oxidase. A study of this medium by Cooper[19] revealed no false-positive results and a small number of false-negative results, which could be eliminated by using fresh isolates of *C. neoformans* preincubated at 25 C on SAB agar. Other methods for rapid identification of *C. neoformans*, as well as other yeasts, are described by Huppert and associates.[38]

Most saprophytic strains of cryptococci do not grow at 35 C.† The pathogenicity of suspected strains of *C. neoformans*, especially from the sputum or skin, should be demonstrated in mice. This is carried out by injecting two to four white mice with either 1 ml intraperitoneally or 0.02 ml intracerebrally (under light ether anesthesia) of a heavy saline suspension of a 4- or 5-day-old culture.

Mice injected **intraperitoneally** develop lesions in the brain in about **3 weeks,** whereas mice injected **intracerebrally** generally develop them in **less than 1 week.** Mice are killed at the end of 3 weeks if death has not occurred. At autopsy the animals show gelatinous masses in the abdominal viscera, lungs, and brain. India ink preparations reveal the typical budding and encapsulated *C. neoformans*, and the fungus may be cultivated from these lesions.

---

*Some strains of *Rhodotorula*, *Candida*, and *Trichosporon* occasionally hydrolyze urea.

*Flow Laboratories Inc., Roslyn, N.Y.
†*C. laurentii*, *C. albidus*, and *C. luteolus* sometimes grow at 35 C and may show a mild degree of mouse virulence. Therefore, when reporting to the clinician, microbiologists must make certain whether the cryptococcus isolated is or is not *C. neoformans*.

Coccidioidomycosis

Coccidioidomycosis is an infectious disease caused by a single species of fungus, *Coccidioides immitis*. Generally an acute, benign, and self-limiting respiratory tract infection, the disease less frequently becomes disseminated, with extension to other visceral organs, bone, lymphatic tissue, skin, and subcutaneous tissue (Plate 200).

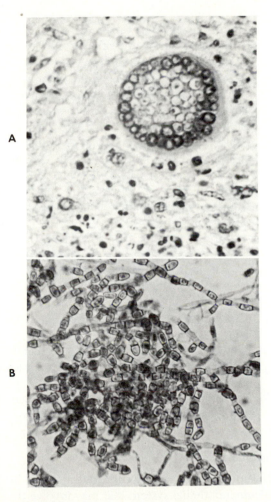

FIG. 34-22
Coccidioides immitis. **A,** Showing spherule containing many spherical endospores (1,000×). **B,** Showing thick-walled, rectangular- or barrel-shaped arthrospores in mycelial phase (500×).

C. immitis spores are found in the semiarid regions of the southwestern part of the United States and northern Mexico as well as in Central and South America; the disease, however, may be seen anywhere in the United States and can be traced to previous travel or residence in an endemic area.

Humans acquire the infection by inhaling **arthrospores** from contaminated soil, particularly during the dry and dusty season. Fewer than 0.5% of persons who acquire the infection ever become seriously ill; dissemination does, however, occur most frequently in dark-skinned races.

In **direct microscopic examination** (using wet, unstained preparations) of sputum, sediment from gastric washings or CSF, exudates, or pus, *C. immitis* appears as a nonbudding, thick-walled (up to 2 μm) **spherule** or sporangium 20 to 200 μm in diameter, containing either granular material or numerous small (2 to 5 μm in diameter) **endospores** (Fig. 34-22, A). These endospores are freed by rupture of the cell wall (Plate 201), and empty and collapsed "ghost" spherules may be present. Small, immature spherules measuring 10 to 20 μm may be confused with nonbudding forms of *Blastomyces dermatitidis*, since they are thick walled and endospores are not yet apparent. To check such structures, seal the edges of the coverglass with petrolatum and incubate overnight. If spherules are present, mycelial filaments will develop from the endospores.

The tissue phase cannot always be demonstrated by direct microscopic examination. Consequently, **all material** from suspected cases should be cultured on **duplicate** sets of SAB agar and BHI agar with and without chloramphenicol and cycloheximide,* one set incubated at room

---

*The mycelial growth of *C. immitis* is not appreciably affected by cycloheximide, whereas the white cottony growth of most saprophytes is inhibited. However, polymyxin B, which is incorporated in some media for fungi, is inhibitory to *C. immitis*.

temperature and one set at 35 C. Animal inoculation is also indicated on occasion.

Growth appears in 3 to 5 days at room temperature (more positive isolations at this temperature) as a moist, membranous colony growing close to the surface of the medium. This soon develops a white, cottony mycelium, turning from buff to brown with age. The central area of the colony frequently remains moist and glabrous. The slant should be **wetted down** before removing any of the mycelium (see following list of precautions). Microscopically, these cultures show a branching, septate mycelium, forming chains of thick-walled, rectangular or barrel-shaped **arthrospores,** 2 by 3 μm to 3 by 5 μm. In lactophenol cotton blue mounts, these chains show only **alternate** deeply stained arthrospores, with dried-out transparent cell tags on either side (Fig. 34-22, *B*). If such structures are observed, the identification should be confirmed by animal inoculation.

At 35 C only the saprophytic or mycelial phase develops, since spherule production generally cannot be induced on the usual artificial media. The tissue phase can be obtained, however, in embryonated eggs or by injecting ground-up mycelia intratesticularly into guinea pigs.* Mycelial suspension, 0.1 ml, is injected, and if orchitis does not develop (generally within 1 week), the animal is killed in 2 to 4 weeks. In either case the testicular tissue is examined for the presence of typical spherules, which verifies the identification of *C. immitis*. It is possible to get conversion to the spherule phase rapidly and consistently by means of slide culture on modified Converse liquid medium at 40 C in a candle jar. Slide culture, however, presents **significant**

hazards to laboratorians working with *C. immitis* unless specialized safety facilities are available.

Old (more than 10 days) cultures in the arthrospore stage are the **most dangerous** phase of the fungus, and dissemination of the highly infectious arthrospores in the air can lead to infection of laboratory personnel. Therefore, the following precautions must be taken in handling such cultures:

1. Never use Petri dishes—always employ cotton-plugged test tubes or bottles.
2. To prevent the escape of arthrospores, **as soon as a cottony mold grows out** (usually within 3 days), **wet down the slant with sterile saline before introducing an inoculating needle.** Carry out all procedures in a biologic safety hood.
3. Make mounts for microscopic examination in lactophenol cotton blue, which kills the spores; subculture to SAB slants if indicated.
4. Sterilize all contaminated equipment by autoclaving promptly.

In culture *C. immitis* must be differentiated from *Geotrichum* and *Oospora* (and other saprophytes), which produce arthrospores by mycelial fragmentation. The following features may be noted:

1. *Geotrichum* remains yeastlike on SAB agar.
2. *Oospora* does not produce alternately stained arthrospores and is not virulent for animals.
3. *C. immitis*, on animal injection, produces the characteristic endospore-filled spherules.

Histoplasmosis

Histoplasmosis is a mycotic infection of the reticuloendothelial system that may involve the lymphatic tissue, lungs, liver, spleen, kidneys, skin, central nervous system, and other organs. Endocarditis may also occur. It is caused by the **dimorphic** (saprophytic and tissue forms) fungus

---

*If guinea pigs are not available, white mice may be injected intraperitoneally with 1 ml of the spore suspension. After about 1 week they develop lesions containing the mature spherules of *C. immitis*. These methods may also be used with sputum or gastric washings by adding 0.05 mg/ml of chloramphenicol and incubating 1 hour with frequent shaking prior to injection.

*Histoplasma capsulatum,** which exists as a saprophyte in the soil. Humans and animals acquire the infection by the inhalation of spores from the environment; the severity of the disease is generally related directly to the intensity of the exposure. The growth of *H. capsulatum* in nature appears to be associated with decaying or composted manure of chickens, birds (especially starlings), and bats ("cave disease"). Humans may typically acquire the infection by cleaning a chicken house or silo that has not been disturbed for a long period or from working in soil under trees that have served as roosting places for starlings, grackles, or other birds. Although histoplasmosis may affect dogs and cats, there is no evidence of contagion between animals and humans or between persons. The domestic animals, as well as several species of wild animals, appear to be accidental hosts and play no role in distributing or encouraging growth of *H. capsulatum* in the soil.

Histoplasmosis, once considered a rare and generally fatal illness, is now recognized as a common and benign disease in endemic areas in the eastern and central United States, where it is estimated that 500,000 persons are infected annually. Further studies and proper utilization of laboratory facilities will probably reveal the disease to be global in distribution.

The most frequent site of **primary infection** in humans is the respiratory tract, usually resulting in an asymptomatic or mild pulmonary infection with cough, fever, and malaise. In some areas a positive histoplasmin skin test, indicating exposure to *H. capsulatum*, is elicited in 60% to 90% of the inhabitants, most of whom give no history of an unusual respiratory illness.

A chronic **cavitary form** of histoplasmosis also occurs in humans, with a productive cough, low-grade fever, and an x-ray picture of pulmonary cavitation that resembles tuberculosis. Undoubtedly, many such cases have been misdiag-

nosed, and patients have been hospitalized and given treatment for pulmonary tuberculosis.

In fewer than 1% of cases of histoplasmosis, a severe, **disseminated form** of the disease develops, with involvement of the reticuloendothelial system and many other sites.

Since *H. capsulatum* is primarily a parasite of the reticuloendothelial system, it is **rarely found extracellularly** in tissue. Therefore, direct and stained smears of clinical material are generally inadequate to demonstrate the fungus. Films of the buffy coat of the blood (white cell layer following sedimentation) (Plate 203), bone marrow, cut surfaces of lymph nodes, splenic and liver (Plate 202) biopsies, sputum, and scrapings should be stained with the Giemsa or Wright stain and carefully examined with the **oil immersion objective.** *H. capsulatum* occurs **intracellularly** as small, round or oval, yeastlike cells, 2 by 3 μm to 3 by 4 μm in size, with a large vacuole and a crescent or half-moon–shaped mass of red-stained protoplasm at the larger end of the cell. These may be found within the cytoplasm of macrophages and occasionally in the polymorphonuclear leukocytes or free in the tissue.

The following methods for the isolation of *H. capsulatum* from clinical material are those used by the Mycology Branch of the CDC[6] and are highly recommended. **Sputum** specimens should be requested in all cases in which pulmonary or disseminated disease is suspected. A series of **six** early morning specimens should be collected in sterile bottles; 1- to 10-ml quantities are adequate. If the specimen cannot be inoculated promptly to culture media (**immediate inoculation is recommended**), add 1 ml of a stock solution of chloramphenicol* to 1 to 10 ml of the specimen. It is advisable, however, to inoculate the specimen directly to duplicate sets of SAB agar and BHI blood agar, with and with-

---

*Perfect form: *Emmonsiella capsulata*.[43]

*To prepare a stock solution, suspend 20 mg of chloramphenicol in 10 ml of 95% ethanol and add 90 ml of distilled water. Heat gently to dissolve. The solution is stable. The concentration is approximately 0.2 mg/ml sputum.

out antibiotics; with antibiotics, pretreatment with chloramphenicol is unnecessary. **Never hold specimens at room temperature;** *Histoplasma* **will not survive.**

Another procedure that may be useful for recovery of *Histoplasma* as well as *Blastomyces* and *Coccidioides* from contaminated specimens involves placing one drop of concentrated NH$_4$OH on one side of an inoculated plate of yeast extract–phosphate medium (Smith and Goodman: Am. J. Clin. Pathol. **63:**276-280, 1975).

Gastric washings should be requested when sputum is unobtainable; a series of three to six specimens is adequate. These are centrifuged and the sediments inoculated to the media previously described. Induced sputum may also be useful. CSF is submitted only when cerebral or meningeal involvement is evident. It is also centrifuged, and the sediment is inoculated as described. Citrated blood and bone marrow are of value only in acute disseminated cases. The blood is centrifuged and the buffy coat used for inoculation of media or laboratory animals. Bone marrow is handled identically, without centrifugation.

Incubate the BHI blood agar without antibiotics at 35 C, and incubate the other media at room temperature. The yeast phase of *H. capsulatum* and other dimorphic fungi does not develop at 35 C on media containing the antibiotics.

The use of **mouse inoculation** is often helpful in the isolation of *H. capsulatum* from clinical specimens. Sputum and gastric washings are liquefied by agitation with glass beads and an equal part of physiologic saline; tissues are ground with alundum and physiologic saline in a tissue grinder. Chloramphenicol is added (0.05 mg/ml) for decontamination, and the specimen is incubated at 35 C for 1 hour. This is not necessary for buffy coat of blood or CSF. Two to four mice are inoculated intraperitoneally with 1-ml aliquots of the material. They are killed in 4 weeks, and cultures are made of portions of liver and spleen on cycloheximide media at room temperature

and on BHI agar without antibiotics at 35 C. These are examined at intervals for development of colonies of *H. capsulatum*.

On SAB agar at **room temperature** *H. capsulatum* grows slowly (10 to 14 days) as a raised, **white, fluffy mold,** becoming tan to brown with age.* Microscopically, these cultures show septate, branching hyphae bearing delicate, round to pyriform, smooth **microconidia** (2 to 4 μm in diameter), either on short lateral branches or attached directly by the base (sessile). Although at this stage the culture may be mistaken for *Blastomyces dermatitidis*, further incubation usually reveals the diagnostic **tuberculate macroconidia** (chlamydospores) (Fig. 34-23, *A*). These spores are large (7 to 25 μm in diameter), round, thick walled, and covered with knoblike or spikelike projections (tuberculate) that are sometimes difficult to see when focusing in only one plane.

On **moist** BHI blood agar incubated at 35 C† *H. capsulatum* grows slowly as a white to brown, membranous, convoluted (cerebriform), yeast-like colony, resembling that of *Staphylococcus aureus*, or a very mucoid colony. A mycelial or mixed type of growth also may be produced. Although these colonies do not produce typical spores, a higher percentage of isolations results on this medium.‡ Transfer of these colonies to SAB agar held at room temperature with ready access to air results in development of the typical macroconidia previously described, and this is recommended as a confirmatory procedure.

To convert the mycelial to the typical **yeast phase,** inoculate slants of moist BHI blood agar, seal with Parafilm, and incubate at 35 C for several weeks. Growth appears as dull, white,

---

*A white (albino) colony, showing only rare, smooth chlamydospores, may overgrow the typical colonies; the latter must be subcultured early to separate the two forms.

†**Note:** The yeast phase of the dimorphic fungi is suppressed by cycloheximide; media containing this agent must be incubated at **room temperature.**

‡Incubation under an increased CO$_2$ tension appears to improve the growth of *H. capsulatum*.

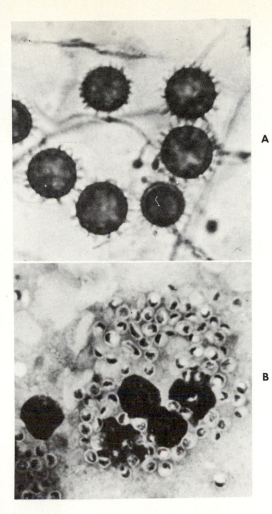

A

B

FIG. 34-23
Histoplasma capsulatum. **A,** Mycelial phase, showing characteristic tuberculate macroconidia (1,000×). **B,** Blood smear, showing intracellular oval- to pear-shaped yeastlike cells, deeply stained (2,000×).

yeastlike colonies, the contents of which appear microscopically as small (1 to 3 μm), oval, **budding cells** similar to those seen in tissues. Strains in the mycelial phase that cannot readily be converted to the yeast phase culturally may be converted by animal inoculation.

Confirmation of the identification of *H. cap-*

sulatum may also be made by **animal injection.** Inoculate several white mice intraperitoneally with a suspension of yeast phase cells harvested from several tubes of BHI blood agar in 5% hog gastric mucin* or a suspension of a 4- to 6-week mycelial growth ground in saline. One mouse is killed after 2 weeks and the others at weekly intervals thereafter; impression smears of the involved organs (generally liver and spleen) are made and stained with Giemsa (not hematoxylin-eosin) stain. Microscopic demonstration of the typical intracellular organisms confirms the identification (Fig. 34-23, *B*). Yeast phase cultures also may be obtained from these tissues by culturing on enriched media incubated at 35 C.

Sepedonium, a saprophytic fungus found on mushrooms, may be confused with *H. capsulatum,* since it produces tuberculate chlamydospores. However, it does not form a yeast phase and is not virulent for animals.

North American blastomycosis

North American blastomycosis is a chronic granulomatous and suppurative disease caused by the **dimorphic** fungus *Blastomyces dermatitidis.*† The disease is limited to the continent of North America, extending southward from Canada to the Mississippi Valley, Mexico, and Central America. Some isolated cases also have been reported from Africa.[3] The largest number of cases occurs in the Mississippi Valley region.

Blastomycosis, first described by Gilchrist in 1894, originates as a respiratory infection. Humans probably acquire the infection through inhalation of the spores from the dust of their environment. One case of blastomycosis was traced to a bag of pigeon manure used for fertilizer.[74] The infection may spread and involve the

---

*Intravenous injection of 0.2 ml of **chilled** (must be kept at 8 to 10 C until the moment of injection) cell suspension (without mucin) into the tail vein of white mice frequently gives better results.[6]
†The perfect stage, *Ajellomyces dermatitidis,* has been described.

lungs, bone, and soft tissue. It is not spread from person to person and generally occurs as sporadic cases. Small outbreaks appear to have been related to a common exposure; although blastomycosis is more common in men, there is no apparent association with occupational exposure.

Material from cutaneous lesions is collected by scraping bits of tissue or taking swabs of pus from the edge of the lesion. Pus from unopened subcutaneous abscesses should be aspirated with a sterile syringe and needle. Sputum, urine, and CSF also should be examined in suspected systemic blastomycosis.

Such material is prepared for direct microscopic examination by placing it on a slide and pressing it into a thin layer with a coverglass. If the material is opaque, it may be cleared in 10% potassium hydroxide with gentle heating. The specimen is examined under high power, using subdued light. *B. dermatitidis* appears as a large, spherical, **thick-walled** cell, 8 to 20 μm in diameter, usually with a single bud that is connected to the mother cell by a **wide base** (Plate 204). Some walls may be sufficiently thick to give a double-contoured effect.

The infected material should be cultured on BHI blood agar incubated at 35 C and on SAB agar incubated at room temperature. Material likely to be contaminated with bacteria should be inoculated on the aforementioned media with chloramphenicol and cycloheximide and incubated at room temperature. Growth of the yeast phase of *B. dermatitidis* may be suppressed when grown on these media incubated at 35 C. In suspected pulmonary disease fresh morning sputum specimens should be examined and cultured as previously described.

On SAB agar at **room temperature** *B. dermatitidis* generally forms a slowly growing, moist, grayish, mealy or prickly colony, which soon develops a **white, cottony,** aerial mycelium, becoming tan (rarely, dark brown to black) with age. Microscopically, these filamentous colonies are made up of septate hyphae bearing small,

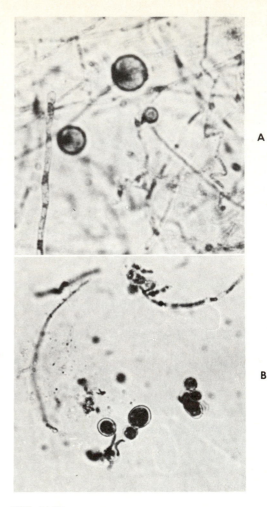

FIG. 34-24
Blastomyces dermatitidis. **A,** Mycelial phase, showing oval microconidia borne laterally on branching hyphae (1,000×). **B,** Yeast phase, showing thick-walled, oval to round, single-budding, yeastlike cells (500×).

oval (2 to 3 μm) or pyriform (4 to 5 μm) **conidia** (aleuriospores) laterally, near the point of septation (Fig. 34-24, *A*). Older cultures develop conidia 7 to 15 μm in diameter with thickened outer walls that suggest the appearance of chlamydospores.

At 35 C incubation on either SAB agar or BHI blood agar, *B. dermatitidis* grows as a **yeastlike** organism. The fungus develops slowly (1 week) as a creamy, wrinkled, waxy colony (similar to that of *Mycobacterium tuberculosis*) with a verrucose (warty) surface texture, cream to tan. Microscopic examination reveals thick-walled, budding, **yeastlike cells** 8 to 20 μm in diameter, resembling those seen in tissues or exudates (Fig. 34-24, *B*).

To identify an organism as *B. dermatitidis*, it is necessary to **convert** the mycelial phase at 25 C to the tissue phase at 35 C. This is done by subculturing to **fresh media** (BHI blood agar) and incubating at 35 C. Animal inoculation usually is unnecessary if the budding cells are demonstrated in direct smears of the infected material and the dimorphism is shown as described here.

If, however, the two phases are poorly defined, **animal injection** is required. A heavy suspension of either the mycelial or yeast phase is prepared, using physiologic saline, and 1 ml of this suspension is then injected intraperitoneally into several mice. These are killed in 3 weeks; microscopic examination of caseous material from the lesions or peritoneal fluid shows the thick-walled, budding, yeastlike tissue forms of *B. dermatitidis*. If these are not demonstrated, portions of the organs are cultured on BHI blood agar and incubated at 35 C. Yeast phase cultures are generally obtained.

Paracoccidioidomycosis (South American blastomycosis)

Paracoccidioidomycosis is a chronic progressive infection of the mucous membranes of the mouth (portal of entry) (Plate 205) and nose and the lymph nodes of the neck, which may give rise to metastatic lesions of the internal organs. It is caused by the **dimorphic** fungus *Paracoccidioides brasiliensis*. The disease is most common in Brazil, although it is seen in many areas, including Mexico, Central America, and Africa.

---

*Recommended as the most practical diagnostic method.[3]

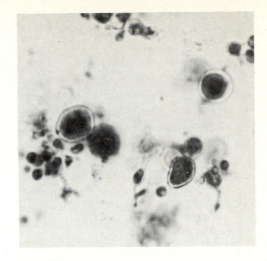

FIG. 34-25
Paracoccidioides brasiliensis, yeast phase, showing multiple budding (400×).

Materials for **direct examination*** are secured and prepared as described for North American blastomycosis. *P. brasiliensis* appears as large, round to oval, budding cells 8 to 40 μm in diameter, thick walled, refractile, and with characteristic **multiple** buds (Fig. 34-25 and Plate 206). Cells with single buds are indistinguishable from those of *B. dermatitidis;* therefore, a search should be made for the diagnostic multiple budding cells. The daughter buds, 1 to 2 μm in diameter, usually are attached to the thick-walled mother cell by narrow connections, giving the whole a **steering wheel** appearance.

Infected material should be cultured on BHI blood agar at 35 C and on SAB agar at room temperature, as in the study of North American blastomycosis. At room temperature the fungus develops as a very **slowly growing** (2 to 3 weeks), heaped-up folded colony with a short nap of white, velvety mycelium. Microscopically, small, delicate (3 to 4 μm), round or oval conidia may be seen, sessile or on very short sterigmata on septate hyphae. Usually, however, only a fine septate mycelium and chlamydospores are seen.

At 35 C *P. brasiliensis* grows slowly as a smooth, soft, yeastlike, cream to tan colony. These yeastlike colonies, which may appear either verrucous or smooth and shiny, are composed of single cells and multiple budding forms, identical with those seen in tissue and exudates. All cultures should be held at least 4 weeks before being discarded as negative.

As with *B. dermatitidis*, **conversion** of the mycelial to the yeast phase must be demonstrated by subculture and incubation at 35 C. If animal inoculation is required for further confirmation, guinea pigs injected intratesticularly (1 ml of a heavy saline suspension of yeast phase organisms) may be used. The guinea pigs are killed in 8 to 12 days and examined for the presence of the diagnostic multiple budding tissue forms of the fungus in pus from the draining sinuses.

LESS COMMON MYCOSES
Aspergillosis

Aspergilli are among the most common and troublesome contaminants in the laboratory; several are pathogenic and may produce either inflammatory or chronic granulomatous lesions in the bronchi or lungs, often with hematogenous spread to other organs. The external ear, cornea of the eye, nasal sinuses, and other tissues of humans or animals are frequently infected. Endocarditis may occur, as may allergic pulmonary disease. *Aspergillus fumigatus* is the species most frequently associated with pathologic processes. This may include pulmonary aspergillosis of a severe and invasive type or generalized infection, which is being observed with increasing frequency in debilitated patients receiving antibiotic or corticosteroid therapy and immunosuppressive or antimetabolite drugs.

Since aspergilli are found frequently in cultures of sputum, skin scrapings, and other specimens, it is essential that the fungus be **repeatedly demonstrated** in large numbers in direct smears of the fresh material and **repeatedly iso-**lated on culture in a patient with an appropriate clinical picture to be considered etiologically significant. Other factors that make the diagnosis of aspergillosis likely in a patient from whom *Aspergillus* has been isolated include known predisposition to invasive aspergillosis (malignancy, leukemia, granulocytopenia, corticosteroid therapy, etc.) and isolation of *Aspergillus fumigatus* and *Aspergillus flavus*, which do not usually represent laboratory contamination from respiratory secretions.[56] On the other hand, isolation of *Aspergillus niger* is only rarely associated with disease. Recovery of *A. fumigatus* or *A. flavus* from surveillance nose cultures is strongly correlated with subsequent invasive aspergillosis.[2] Absence of such a nasal culture does not preclude infection. Direct microscopic examination of sputum or other infected material may reveal fragments of branched, septate mycelium (3 to 6 μm wide) and, sometimes, conidial heads.

Suspected material should be inoculated on SAB agar without cycloheximide* and incubated at room temperature. *A. fumigatus* grows rapidly (2 to 5 days) and appears first as a flat, white filamentous growth, which rapidly becomes **blue-green and powdery** as a result of the production of spores.

Microscopically, *A. fumigatus*† is characterized by branching, septate hyphae, some of which terminally bear a conidiophore that expands into a large, inverted, flask-shaped vesicle (sac) covered with small sterigmata (Fig. 34-26 and Plate 207). These sterigmata occur only in a **single row** and around the **upper half** of the vesicle; from their tips are extruded parallel chains of small rough-surfaced, green conidia, giving the whole structure a flaglike appearance. A number of other species may cause serious infection, particularly in the compromised host.

A. fumigatus may be inhibited by cycloheximide.
†Although *A. fumigatus* is the most common agent in pulmonary aspergillosis, other species, including *A. flavus*, have been incriminated.

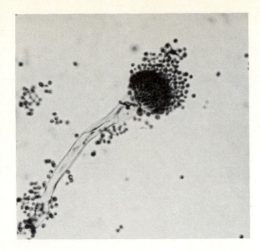

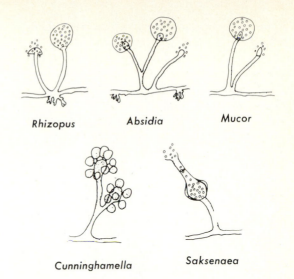

FIG. 34-26

Aspergillus fumigatus, showing conidia in chains, arising from a single row of sterigmata on the upper portion of the vesicle (500×).

FIG. 34-27

Diagrammatic representation of morphologic distinction between the genera *Rhizopus*, *Absidia*, *Mucor*, *Saksenaea*, and *Cunninghamella*. (From Greer.[33])

Animal inoculation is not necessary for the identification of *A. fumigatus*.

For differentiation of the various *Aspergillus* species, see the chapter by Austwick and Longbottom.[10]

Zygomycosis

Zygomycosis (mucormycosis, phycomycosis) is a rare but often fatal disease caused by fungi that produce aseptate mycelia and are ordinarily considered nonpathogenic laboratory contaminants. The genera involved include *Mucor*, *Rhizopus*, *Absidia*, *Saksenaea*, *Cunninghamella*, *Conidiobolus*, and *Basidiobolus*. Morphologic features of these genera are depicted in Fig. 34-27. The fungus most often enters the nose of susceptible patients, particularly uncontrolled diabetics and patients receiving prolonged antibiotic, corticosteroid, or cytotoxic therapy, and penetrates the arteries, producing thrombosis and death of the segment of tissue normally receiving its blood supply from the affected vessel. Later it invades the veins and lymphatics.

The disease assumes cerebral and pulmonary forms and, rarely, intestinal, ocular, bony, and disseminated forms. It is usually fatal. A number of cases of hospital-acquired zygomycosis involving the skin and subcutaneous tissue were related to the use of contaminated Elastoplast bandages.[30] The organism involved was *Rhizopus rhizopodiformis*.

The diagnosis of zygomycosis is usually made by examination of tissue specimens taken at biopsy or autopsy, in sections of which can be demonstrated broad (4 to 200 μm thick), branching, predominantly **nonseptate hyphae** (Plate 210). The culture of sputum, CSF, or exudate should be attempted in suspected cases.

On SAB agar incubated at room temperature *Rhizopus* species produce a rapidly growing (2 to 4 days), coarse, wooly colony, which soon fills the test tube with a loose, grayish mycelium dotted with brown or black sporangia (Plate 208). The fungus is characterized microscopically by a large, broad, **nonseptate**, hyaline mycelium that produces horizontal runners (stolons), which

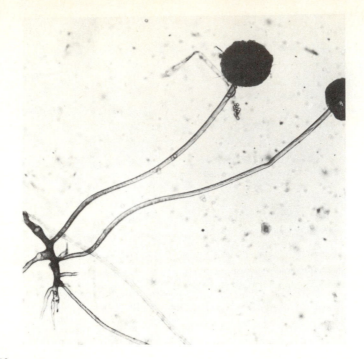

FIG. 34-28
Rhizopus species, showing sporangium on long sporangiophore arising from a nonseptate mycelium. Characteristic rhizoids are seen at the base of the sporangiophore (250×).

attach at contact points (medium or glass) by rootlike structures called **rhizoids** (Fig. 34-28). From these contact points arise clusters of long stalks, known as **sporangiophores,** the ends of which are terminated in large, round, dark-walled **sporangia** (spore sacs). When mature, these sporangia are filled with spherical hyaline spores. Since *Rhizopus* species are common contaminants, the recovery of this organism in culture is not in itself diagnostic.

On SAB agar at room temperature *Mucor* species produce a rapidly growing colony that fills the test tube with a white fluffy mycelium, becoming gray to brown with age. Microscopically, the fungus is characterized by a nonseptate, colorless mycelium without rhizoids; the sporangiophores arise singly from stolons and branch profusely, with sporangia containing many spores arising from the apex of each branch (Plate 209). The columellae (the persis-

tent dome-shaped apices of the sporangiophores) are usually well developed and of various shapes but **never hemispherical** as in *Rhizopus*. Empty sporangial sacs, still attached to the conidiophores after release of the spores, may be observed in both genera.

Organisms of the genus *Absidia* are similar to *Rhizopus* except that the sporangiophores arise on stolons at a **point between two nodes** from which rhizoids are formed. The sporangia are pear shaped (10 to 70 μm in diameter) rather than round.

Mycologic features of the other zygomycetes not described here can be found in the chapter by Greer.[33]

Miscellaneous systemic mycoses

Sporothrix schenckii may cause pulmonary or ther serious infection in addition to the less severe infections of the skin and subcutaneous tissue discussed under subcutaneous mycoses. The organism is described in that section.

Petriellidium boydii has been discussed under mycetoma. This organism can also produce necrotizing pneumonia, meningitis, eye and sinus infections, and disseminated infection. Infections occurring in immunosuppressed patients may be very severe and often are fatal. In infected organs *P. boydii* produces septate hyphae that are difficult to distinguish from *Aspergillus* species. The organism is seldom, if ever, a contaminant when isolated from sputum. Fungal infections have complicated dialysis. Peritonitis caused by *Drechslera spicifera* complicating continuous ambulatory peritoneal dialysis has been reported,[60] and there is a report of *Cephalosporium* infection of a dialysis access fistula in a patient receiving hemodialysis.[59] Many other fungi, such as *Alternaria, Paecilomyces, Penicillium* (Plate 211), and others that are ordinarily saprophytic may, on occasion, produce infection of one type or another.

TREATMENT OF SYSTEMIC MYCOSES

The agents available for treatment of systemic fungal infections include the polyene antibiotic amphotericin B, flucytosine, ketoconazole, miconazole, sulfonamides and iodides. Amphotericin B appears to be the drug of choice for blastomycosis, cryptococcal meningitis, systemic candidiasis, disseminated histoplasmosis, and coccidioidomycosis and is given parenterally. Flucytosine, given by mouth, has proved effective in candidemia and candidal urinary tract infections and is useful in combination with amphotericin for cryptococcosis. Iodides may be useful for selected cases of sporotrichosis. Sulfonamides and cotrimoxazole are useful for South American blastomycosis. Infections caused by *P. boydii* that typically do not respond well to any antifungal agents may be treated effectively with miconazole.[48] Ketoconazole is a very important new drug for management of mycoses.[31] This compound is an imidazole derivative. It has a broad spectrum of activity that includes *Candida* species, *Cryptococcus*

neoformans, Coccidioides immitis, Histoplasma capsulatum, Blastomyces dermatitidis, and various dermatophytes. Natamycin is a polyene antibiotic approved for topical treatment of fungal infections of the eye, including keratitis. Table 34-6 demonstrates the in vitro activity of four antifungal agents. It is disturbing to note that resistance may develop to polyene antibiotics such as amphotericin B and nystatin. Dick and co-workers[23] found that about 8% of fungi from oncology patients demonstrated resistance to these agents, whereas none of the isolates from nononcology services did. Resistant yeasts included *Candida albicans, Candida tropicalis*, and *Torulopsis glabrata*.

USE AND INTERPRETATION OF HYPERSENSITIVITY TESTS, SEROLOGIC REACTIONS, AND GAS CHROMATOGRAPHY FOR MYCOTIC INFECTIONS

Conclusive evidence of the presence of a fungal infection is best offered by the demonstration of the fungi, either by direct examination or by cultural procedures, in the exudate or in diseased tissue. However, **indirect evidence,** by the demonstration of a hypersensitive state or an increasing titer of specific antibody, may prove exceedingly helpful.

Intradermal skin tests have been widely used to aid in the diagnosis, treatment, and epidemiologic survey of the systemic mycoses, particularly blastomycosis, histoplasmosis, and coccidioidomycosis. In the hypersensitive patient the injection of mycelial or whole-cell extracts of these fungal agents (blastomycin, histoplasmin, coccidioidin, and spherulin*) elicits a **tuberculinlike response**—redness and induration—within 24 to 48 hours. The significance of this positive reaction is simply that a mycotic infection has occurred at some time during the patient's life. Since cross-reactions occur among

---

*Standardized skin test antigens may be obtained from Parke-Davis & Co., Eli Lilly & Co., Cutter Laboratories, and Michigan State Health Laboratories.

TABLE 34-6

In vitro antifungal activities of four antifungal agents against pathogenic fungi

Organism	Amphotericin B		Flucytosine (5-FC)		Miconazole		Clotrimazole	
	MIC (μg/ml)	MFC (μg/ml)	MIC (μg/ml)	MFC (μg/ml)	MIC (μg/ml)	MFC (μg/ml)	MIC (μg/ml)	MFC (μg/ml)
Pathogenic yeasts								
Cryptococcus neoformans	0.05-0.78*	0.1-12.5	0.10-100†	0.39->100	0.05-3.13	0.05-25	0.1-2	0.5-10
Candida albicans	0.2-0.78‡	0.39-0.78	0.05-12.5†	0.10->100	0.1-2.0‡	0.1-10	<0.1-10	0.1->10
Candida spp. not *C. albicans*	0.2-1.56‡	0.39-6.25	0.10-50†	0.20->100	<0.1-2.0	0.1->10	<0.1-10	<0.1->10
Torulopsis glabrata	0.1-0.4	0.2-0.78	0.05-1.56	0.4->100	0.5-10	2-10	1-10	2->10
Trichosporon sp.	0.78-3.13	1.56-3.13	25-100	>100	0.2-25	0.2->100		
Geotrichum sp.	0.4-1.56	0.78-3.13	1.56-12.5	25->100	0.1-2	0.5->10	<0.1-0.5	0.1-0.5
Filamentous fungi								
Petriellidium (Allescheria) boydii	1.56->100†	>100	Resistant		0.05§	0.05	0.5-2§	2-10
Aspergillus sp. including *A. fumigatus*	0.05-8	6.25->100	0.2-1.56†	>100	0.4->100	0.8->100	0.1-10	0.5-10
Blastomyces dermatitidis	0.05-0.2	0.1-0.4	Resistant		≤0.25	ND	0.8-3.13	0.8->100
Cladosporium trichoides	3.13->100	3.13->100	3.13-12.5†	12.5->100	0.5->64	ND	0.4δ	0.4-12.5
Coccidioides immitis	0.1-0.78	0.78-1.56	Resistant		0.25-1.0	ND	0.05-0.1	0.1-1.56
Histoplasma capsulatum	0.05-0.1	0.05-0.2	Resistant		≤0.25	ND	0.1-0.4	0.1-0.4
Phialophora spp. and other dematiaceous fungi	0.05->128	6.25->128	Variable susceptibility	Resistant	0.05-32	ND	0.5->128	ND
Sporothrix schenckii	1.56-12.5	3.13->100	Resistant		1-2	ND	0.5-10	2->10
Zygomycetes	0.78-1.56	1.56->100	Variable susceptibility	Resistant				
Dermatophytic fungi								
Epidermophyton floccosum					0.5-10	2-10	0.1-0.2	0.2-0.4
Microsporum spp.					0.5-10	0.5->10	0.1-0.8	0.1-0.8
Trichophyton spp.					0.5-10	0.5-10	<0.05-1.56	0.05-1.06

From Shadomy and Espinel-Ingroff.[76] Based both upon data obtained at the Medical College of Virginia, Virginia Commonwealth University, Richmond, Va., and a review of the literature. In vitro data for nystatin and pimaricin not included because of the narrow clinical spectra of these agents. Most isolates of *Candida* species and *Torulopsis* should be clinically susceptible (MIC, ≤ 10 μg/ml) to nystatin; many isolates of *Fusarium solani* and other *Fusarium* species as well as other etiological agents of mycotic keratitis will be inhibited by 1.8 to 10 μg of pimaricin per ml.

MFC, Minimal fungicidal concentration; MIC, results of agar dilution studies; ND, not determined.

*The expected ranges of MICs and MFCs.

†Resistance not uncommon.

‡Resistance reported but rare.

§Only a limited amount of data available.

these three antigens, some workers have applied all three **simultaneously,** using a separate needle and syringe uncontaminated by previous use with other skin test antigens. Skin testing is of questionable diagnostic value, however, in blastomycosis. Testing with histoplasmin may cause an antibody rise, which may prove confusing; immunodiffusion studies may avert the problem. In general, skin testing with histoplasmin also is of little diagnostic value. Results should be interpreted with caution; when negative, they may be valuable in ruling out the diagnosis of a systemic infection, particularly in histoplasmosis (patients who are very ill or who have serious underlying illness may be anergic). Skin tests have been used to demonstrate hypersensitivity to *Paracoccidioides brasiliensis, Sporothrix schenckii, Aspergillus fumigatus,* and other fungi, although standardized reagents are not yet commercially available.

Serum from patients infected with mycotic agents may contain **specific antibodies.** These may be demonstrated in the laboratory by utilizing complement fixation, precipitin, latex or colloidin particle agglutination, hemagglutination, agar gel immunodiffusion, and indirect immunofluorescence, radioimmunoassay, ELISA, and other procedures.* The need for standardized reference antigen-antibody systems has been stressed.[39] These serologic examinations are useful adjuncts in the diagnosis and prognosis of a mycotic infection. For example, in a case of a pulmonary infection in which no sputum can be obtained, or in a case where it is difficult or impossible to secure infected tissue or exudate, the diagnosis may well depend on the application of serologic tests and the interpretation of their results.

As is true of all serologic examinations, **a dependable diagnostic interpretation ordinarily cannot be made on a single serum specimen. A sharp rise** (fourfold or greater) or subsequent

fall in titer usually corroborates a clinical diagnosis. Because of cross-reactions, all three antigens should be used in the serologic tests performed.

The immunodiffusion test for blastomycosis is specific, and a positive reaction is an indication for treatment of the patient without the need for parallel tests with coccidioidin and histoplasmin.[41] The test has a sensitivity of approximately 70%. Negative tests do not exclude a diagnosis of blastomycosis. The complement fixation test is much less sensitive and specific.

In coccidiodomycosis the complement fixation and tube precipitin tests are valuable for diagnosis and prognosis. The tube precipitin test is most effective in detecting early primary infection or an exacerbation of illness. Complement-fixing antibodies persist for longer periods, and the complement fixation titer parallels the severity of the infection. Titers rise as the disease progresses and decline as the patient improves. As screening tests, one may use the latex particle agglutination and immunodiffusion tests, which yield results comparable with precipitin and complement fixation tests, respectively. Coccidioidin is more specific than spherulin in complement fixation tests for coccidioidomycosis.

Serologic testing is often the primary means available for a definitive diagnosis of histoplasmosis. The complement fixation test is most widely used. As many as 96% of culturally proved cases of histoplasmosis may be positive by the complement fixation test if the patient's illness is followed by testing sera collected at 2- to 3-week intervals. This test should be performed with the yeast phase antigen, and, where possible, this should be supplemented with either the immunodiffusion or CIE tests with histoplasmin. The latter two tests have greater than 90% agreement between them, and the results from them are very useful for examining sera that are anticomplementary. Because of their greater specificity, they provide a more accurate diagnosis with sera that cross-react in

---

*The reader is referred to an excellent summary of the serology of the systemic mycoses by Kaufman.[41]

complement fixation tests. Serial serologic studies on spinal fluid may be valuable for diagnosing culture-negative chronic *Histoplasma* meningitis.[65]

Latex agglutination, immunodiffusion, and CIE are valuable in the diagnosis of systemic *Candida* infections. On the other hand, the agglutination and complement fixation tests have proven to be unreliable. The latex agglutination, immunodiffusion, and CIE tests have a sensitivity of about 90% for proven cases of candidiasis. The CIE and immunodiffusion tests are the most specific and yield results that are comparable. The only cross-reaction with these two tests is with *Torulopsis*. On the other hand, the latex agglutination test shows more nonspecific reactions, including reactions with sera from patients with cryptococcosis and tuberculosis, in addition to *Torulopsis* infection. The latex agglutination test is quantitative and appears to have prognostic value. A fourfold rise in titer or a titer of 1:8 or more is considered highly suggestive of invasive candidiasis. Other tests that have been studied recently include passive hemagglutination, ELISA, and radioimmunoassay. Extracellular proteinase enzyme purified from culture filtrates of *Candida albicans* was a more specific antigen for the serologic diagnosis of candidiasis than were the traditional cytoplasmic extracts using a precipitin technique. Other tests used to diagnose candidiasis include ELISA and radioimmunoassay to detect cell wall mannan from *C. albicans* and mass spectrometry and gas liquid chromatography to measure concentrations of D-arabinitol in serum. This compound is a major metabolite of several *Candida* species. However, in patients both false-negative and false-positive (in renal failure) results occur (Eng et al.: J. Infect. Dis. **143:**677-683, 1981).

For the diagnosis of systemic sporotrichosis the latex agglutination and the tube agglutination tests are reliable and sensitive. The latex agglutination test is much more rapid. Both tests are performed at the CDC.

The latex slide agglutination test for detection of **cryptococcal antigen** in spinal fluid and serum is extremely useful diagnostically and prognostically. Antibody to *C. neoformans* may also be detected by a variety of tests, including indirect fluorescent antibody test, a charcoal particle agglutination test, and a tube agglutination test. The antibody tests are of value in detecting early or localized cryptococcal infection and in determining the prognosis. They are less specific than the latex particle agglutination test for cryptococcal antigen. One may rarely get false-positive cryptococcal antigen tests when using commercial kits that have not been evaluated adequately for the incidence of false positivity. False-negative cryptococcal antigen tests may occur rarely as the result of prozoning, as noted in Chapter 12.

The immunodiffusion test is effective for the diagnosis of aspergillosis and is specific. CIE is probably not as specific but might be useful for screening. The value of the complement fixation test is open to question. The greatest number of aspergillosis cases may be detected by the use of reagents for *A. fumigatus*, *A. flavus*, and *A. niger* in separate immunodiffusion tests performed at the same time. Precipitins can be found in more than 90% of cases of pulmonary mycetoma and in 70% of cases of allergic bronchopulmonary aspergillosis. They are found less frequently in patients with invasive disease. Other tests that are being evaluated for the diagnosis of aspergillosis are the passive hemagglutination assay, ELISA, and radioimmunoassay.

An immunodiffusion test employing antigens from four species of fungi involved in zygomycosis appears promising. Cross-reactions occur among the genera causing this problem, however.

The complement fixation test detects antibodies in 80% to 95% of patients with paracoccidioidomycosis. Complement-fixing antibodies are diagnostic. Cross-reactions are infrequent and occur mainly at levels of 1:8. The immunodiffusion test is also quite good and, when used with reference sera, is entirely specific. One can obtain an initial serodiagnosis of this disease in over 98% of cases with the concomitant use of the immunodiffusion and complement fixation tests.

Prognostic interpretation of the immunologic and serologic tests is based on the general observation that a patient reacting positively to an intradermal test and not showing a significant serologic titer has a better prognosis than does the patient with a negative skin test and a high titer of complement-fixing antibodies. This is particularly true in coccidioidomycosis. It should be noted that serum for histoplasmosis serologic testing should be drawn before, or not later than a few days after, an intradermal test is carried out, because the latter may induce the production of antibodies, as noted earlier.

Immunologic and other procedures may also be used for **identification of fungi.** Isolates of *Blastomyces dermatitidis, Coccidioides immitis, Histoplasma capsulatum, Petriellidium boydii,* and *Paracoccidioides brasiliensis* all produce cell-free antigens called exoantigens, which can be detected by immunodiffusion. *Cryptococcus neoformans* can be identified rapidly using an extract made from the yeast cells in phenolized saline and then tested by coagglutination or with a latex agglutination reagent.[54] *Candida* of eight medically important species may be identified rapidly (10 minutes to 5 hours) by a slide agglutination procedure (Shinoda et al.: J. Clin Microbiol. 13:513-518, 1981). Species of *Candida, Cryptococcus,* and *Torulopsis* have been identified by gas-liquid chromatography, using a fatty acid analysis of the whole cell hydrolysate.[29]

REFERENCES

1. Ahearn, D.G.: Identification and ecology of yeasts of medical importance. In Prier, J.E., and Friedman, H., editors: Opportunistic pathogens, Baltimore, 1973, University Park Press.
2. Aisner, J., Murillo, J., Schimpff, S.C., and Steere, A.C.: Invasive aspergillosis in acute leukemia: correlation with nose cultures and antibiotic use, Ann. Intern. Med. **90:**4-9, 1979.
3. Ajello, L.: Comparative ecology of respiratory mycotic disease agents, Bacteriol. Rev. **31:**6-24, 1967.
4. Ajello, L.: A taxonomic review of the dermatophytes and related species, Sabouraudia **6:**147-159, 1968.
5. Ajello, L., and Georg, L.K.: In vitro hair cultures for differentiating between atypical isolates of *Trichophyton mentagrophytes* and *Trichophyton rubrum,* Mycopathologia **8:**3-17, 1957.
6. Ajello, L., Georg, L.K., Kaplan, W., and Kaufman, L.: CDC manual for medical mycology, Public Health Service Pub. No. 994, Washington, D.C., 1963, U.S. Government Printing Office.
7. Ajello, L., Grant, V.Q., and Gutzke, M.A.: The effect of tubercle bacillus concentration procedures on fungi causing pulmonary mycoses, J. Lab. Clin. Med. **38:**486-491, 1951.
8. Ajello, L., and Padhye, A.: Dermatophytes and the agents of superficial mycoses. In Lennette, E.H., Balows, A., Hausler, W.J., Jr., and Truant, J.P., editors: Manual of clinical microbiology, ed. 3, Washington, D.C., 1980, American Society for Microbiology.
9. Allen, D.E., Snyderman, R., Meadows, L., and Pinnell, S.R.: Generalized *Microsporum audouinii* infection and depressed cellular immunity associated with a missing plasma factor required for lymphocyte blastogenesis, Am. J. Med. **63:**991-1000, 1977.
10. Austwick, P.K.C., and Longbottom, J.L.: Medically important *Aspergillus* species. In Lennette, E.H., Balows, A., Hausler, W.J., Jr., and Truant, J.P., editors: Manual of clinical microbiology, ed. 3, Washington, D.C., 1980, American Society for Microbiology.
11. Beneke, J.E. In Thomas, B.A., editor: Scope monograph on human mycoses, Kalamazoo, Mich., 1972, The Upjohn Co.
12. Bennett, J.E.: Chemotherapy of systemic mycoses, N. Engl. J. Med. **290:**30-32, 320-323, 1974.
13. Bobey, D.G., and Ederer, G.M.: Rapid detection of yeast enzymes by using 4-methylumbelliferyl substrates, J. Clin. Microbiol. **13:**393-394, 1981.
14. Bottone, E.J.: *Cryptococcus neoformans:* pitfalls in diagnosis through evaluation of gram-stained smears of purulent exudates, J. Clin. Microbiol. **12:**790-791, 1980.
15. Bowman, P.I., and Ahearn, D.G.: Evaluation of the Uni-Yeast-Tek kit for the identification of medically important yeasts, J. Clin. Microbiol. **2:**354-358, 1975.
16. Buesching, W.J., Kurek, K., and Roberts, G.D.: Evaluation of the modified API 20C system for identification of clinically important yeasts, J. Clin. Microbiol. **9:**565-569, 1979.
17. Center for Disease Control: Endophthalmitis associated with implantation of intraocular lens prosthesis—United States, Morbid. Mortal. Weekly Rep. **25:**369, 1976.

18. Conant, N.F., Smith, D.T., Baker, R.D., and Callaway, J.L.: Manual of clinical mycology, ed. 3, Philadelphia, 1971, W.B. Saunders Co.

19. Cooper, B.H.: Clinical laboratory evaluation of a screening medium (CN screen) for *Cryptococcus neoformans*, J. Clin. Microbiol. **11:**672-674, 1980.

20. Cooper, B.H.: Introduction to clinical mycology. In Lennette, E.H., Balows, A., Hausler, W.J., Jr., and Truant, J.P., editors: Manual of clinical microbiology, ed. 3, Washington, D.C., 1980, American Society for Microbiology.

21. Cooper, B.H., Johnson, J.B., and Thaxton, E.S.: Clinical evaluation of the Uni-Yeast-Tek system for rapid presumptive identification of medically important yeasts, J. Clin. Microbiol. **7:**349-355, 1978.

22. D'Alessio, D.J., Leavens, L.J., Strumpf, G.B., and Smith, C.D.: An outbreak of sporotrichosis in Vermont associated with sphagnum moss as the source of infection, N. Engl. J. Med. **272:**1054-1058, 1965.

23. Dick, J.D., Merz, W.G., and Saral, R.: Incidence of polyene-resistant yeasts recovered from clinical specimens, Antimicrob. Agents Chemother. **18:**158-163, 1980.

24. Edberg, S.C., Chaskes, S.J., Alture-Werber, E., and Singer, J.M.: Esculin-based medium for isolation and identification of *Cryptococcus neoformans*, J. Clin. Microbiol. **12:**332-335, 1980.

25. Edwards, J.E., Jr., Lehrer, R.I., Stiehm, E.R., Fischer, T.J., and Young, L.S.: Severe candidal infections: clinical perspective, immune defense mechanisms, and current concepts of therapy, Ann. Intern. Med. **89:**91-106, 1978.

26. Emmons, C.W., Binford, C.H., Utz, J.P. and Kwon-Chung, K.J.: Medical mycology, ed. 3, Philadelphia, 1977, Lea & Febiger.

27. Evans, H.L., Kletzel, M., Lawson, R.D., Frankel, L.S., and Hopfer, R.L.: Systemic mycosis due to *Trichosporon cutaneum*, Cancer **45:**367-371, 1980.

28. Fitzsimons, R.B., Nicholls, M.D., Billson, F.A., Robertson, T.I., and Hersey, P.: Fungal retinitis: a case of *Torulopsis glabrata* infection treated with miconazole, Br. J. Ophthalmol. **64:**672-675, 1980.

29. Gangopadhyay, P.K., Thadepalli, H., Roy, I., and Ansari, A.: Identification of species of *Candida, Cryptococcus*, and *Torulopsis* by gas-liquid chromatography, J. Infect. Dis. **140:**952-958, 1979.

30. Gartenberg, G., Bottone, E.J., Keusch, G.T., and Weitzman, I.: Hospital-acquired mucormycosis *(Rhizopus rhizopodiformis)* of skin and subcutaneous tissue, N. Engl. J. Med. **299:**1115-1118, 1978.

31. Graybill, J.R., and Drutz, D.J.: Ketoconazole: a major innovation for treatment of fungal disease, Ann. Intern. Med. **93:**921-923, 1980.

32. Green, W.O., Jr., and Adams, J.E.: Mycetoma in the United States, Am. J. Clin. Pathol. **42:**75-91, 1964.

33. Greer, D.L.: Agents of zygomycosis (phycomycosis). In Lennette, E.H., Balows, A., Hausler, W.J., Jr., and Truant, J.P., editors: Manual of clinical microbiology, ed. 3, Washington, D.C., 1980, American Society for Microbiology.

34. Haley, L.D., Trandel, J., and Coyle, M.B. In Sherris, J.C., editor: Practical methods for culture and identification of fungi in the clinical microbiology laboratory, Cumitech 11, Washington, D.C., 1980, American Society for Microbiology.

35. Healy, M.E., Dillavou, C.L., and Taylor, G.E.: Diagnostic medium containing inositol, urea, and caffeic acid for selective growth of *Cryptococcus neoformans*, J. Clin. Microbiol. **6:**387-391, 1977.

36. Hopfer, R.L., and Gröschel, D.: Six-hour pigmentation test for the identification of *Cryptococcus neoformans*, J. Clin. Microbiol. **2:**96-98, 1975.

37. Hopkins, J.M., and Land, G.A.: Rapid method for determining nitrate utilization by yeasts, J. Clin. Microbiol. **5:**497-500, 1977.

38. Huppert, M., Harper, G., Sun, S.H., and Delanerolle, V.: Rapid methods for identification of yeasts, J. Clin. Microbiol. **2:**21-34, 1975.

39. Huppert, M., Sun, S.H., and Vukovich, K.R.: Standardization of mycological reagents, Proceedings of the International Conference on Standardization of Diagnostic Materials, Atlanta, 1974, Center for Disease Control, pp. 187-194.

40. Kane, J., and Smitka, C.: Early detection and identification of *Trichophyton verrucosum*, J. Clin. Microbiol. **8:**740-747, 1978.

41. Kaufman, L.: Serodiagnosis of fungal diseases. In Lennette, E.H., Balows, A., Hausler, W.J., Jr., and Truant, J.P., editors: Manual of clinical microbiology, ed. 3, Washington, D.C., 1980, American Society for Microbiology.

42. Koneman, E.W., Roberts, G.D., and Wright, S.F.: Practical laboratory mycology, ed. 2, Baltimore, 1978, The Williams & Wilkins Co.

43. Kwon-Chung, K.J.: *Emmonsiella capsulata:* perfect state of *Histoplasma capsulatum*, Science **177:**368-369, 1972.

44. Kwon-Chung, K.J.: Comparison of isolates of *Sporothrix schenckii* obtained from fixed cutaneous lesions with isolates from other types of lesions, J. Infect. Dis. **139:**424-431, 1979.

45. Kwon-Chung, K.J., Bennett, J.E., and Theodore, T.S.: *Cryptococcus bacillisporus* sp. nov.: serotype B-C of *Cryptococcus neoformans*, Int. J. Syst. Bacteriol. **28:**616-620, 1978.

46. Land, G.A., Harrison, B.A., Hulme, K.L., Cooper, B.H., and Byrd, J.C.: Evaluation of the new API 20C strip for yeast identification against a conventional method, J. Clin. Microbiol. **10:**357-364, 1979.

47. Larsh, H.W. and Goodman, N.L.: Fungi of systemic mycoses. In Lennette, E.H., Balows, A., Hausler, W.J., Jr., and Truant, J.P., editors: Manual of clinical microbiology, ed. 3, Washington, D.C., 1980, American Society for Microbiology.

48. Lutwick, L.I., Rytel, M.W., Yãnez, J.P., Galgiani, J.N., and Stevens, D.A.: Deep infections from *Petriellidium boydii* treated with miconazole, J.A.M.A. **241:**272-273, 1979.

49. Lynch, J.P., III, Schaberg, D.R., Kissner, D.G., and Kauffman, C.A.: *Cryptococcus laurentii* lung abscess, Am. Rev. Respir. Dis. **123:**135-138, 1981.

50. Marks, M.I., Langston, C., and Eickhoff, T.C.: *Torulopsis glabrata:* an opportunistic pathogen in man, N. Engl. J. Med. **283:**1131-1135, 1970.

51. Marks, M.I., and O'Toole, E.: Laboratory identification of *Torulopsis glabrata:* typical appearance on routine bacteriological media, Appl. Microbiol. **19:**184-185, 1970.

52. McGinnis, M.R.: Dematiaceous fungi. In Lennette, E.H., Balows, A., Hausler, W.J., Jr., and Truant, J.P., editors: Manual of clinical microbiology, ed. 3, Washington, D.C., 1980, American Society for Microbiology.

53. McGinnis, M.R., Walker, D.H., and Folds, J.D.: *Hansenula polymorpha* infection in a child with chronic granulomatous disease, Arch. Pathol. Lab. Med. **104:**290-292, 1980.

54. Muchmore, H.G., Felton, F.G., and Scott, E.N.: Rapid presumptive identification of *Cryptococcus neoformans*, J. Clin. Microbiol. **8:**166-170, 1978.

55. Murray, P.R., Van Scoy, R.E., and Roberts, G.D.: Should yeasts in respiratory secretions be identified? Mayo Clin. Proc. **52:**42-45, 1977.

56. Nalesnik, M.A., Myerowitz, R.L., Jenkins, R., Lenkey, J., and Herbert, D.: Significance of *Aspergillus* species isolated from respiratory secretions in the diagnosis of invasive pulmonary aspergillosis, J. Clin. Microbiol. **11:**370-376, 1980.

57. Ngui Yen, J.H., and Smith, J.A.: Use of Autobac 1 for rapid assimilation testing of *Candida* and *Torulopsis* species, J. Clin. Microbiol. **7:**118-121, 1978.

58. Oblack, D.L., Rhodes, J.C., and Martin, W.J.: Clinical evaluation of the AutoMicrobic system yeast biochemical card for rapid identification of medically important yeasts, J. Clin. Microbiol. **13:**351-355, 1981.

59. Onorato, I.M., Axelrod, J.L., Lorch, J.A., Brensilver, J.M., and Bokkenheuser, V.: Fungal infections of dialysis fistulae, Ann. Intern. Med. **91:**50-52, 1979.

60. O'Sullivan, F.X., Steuwe, B.R., Lynch, J.M., Brandsberg, J.W., Wiegmann, T.B., Patak, R.V., Barnes, W.G., and Hodges, G.R.: Peritonitis due to *Drechslera spicifera* complicating continuous ambulatory peritoneal dialysis, Ann. Intern. Med. **94:**213-214, 1981.

61. Padhye, A., and Ajello, L.: Fungi causing eumycotic mycetomas. In Lennette, E.H., Balows, A., Hausler, W.J., Jr., and Truant, J.P., editors: Manual of clinical microbiology, ed. 3, Washington, D.C., 1980, American Society for Microbiology.

62. Paliwal, D.K., and Randhawa, H.S.: Evaluation of a simplified *Guizotia abyssinica* seed medium for differentiation of *Cryptococcus neoformans*, J. Clin. Microbiol. **7:**346-348, 1978.

63. Phillips, B.J., and Kaplan, W.: Effect of cetylpyridinium chloride on pathogenic fungi and *Nocardia asteroides* in sputum, J. Clin. Microbiol. **3:**272-276, 1976.

64. Pien, F.D., Thompson, R.L., Deye, D., and Roberts, G.D.: *Rhodotorula* septicemia, Mayo Clin. Proc. **55:**258-260, 1980.

65. Plouffe, J.F., and Fass, R.J.: Histoplasma meningitis: diagnostic value of cerebrospinal fluid serology, Ann. Intern. Med. **92**(Part 1):189-191, 1980.

66. Prevost, E.: Nonfluorescent tinea capitis in Charleston, S.C., J.A.M.A. **242:**1765-1767, 1979.

67. Rebell, G.C., and Forster, R.K.: Fungi of keratomycosis. In Lennette, E.H., Balows, A., Hausler, W.J., Jr., and Truant, J.P. editors: Manual of clinical microbiology, ed. 3, Washington, D.C., 1980, American Society for Microbiology.

68. Roberts, G.D.: Mycology: laboratory procedure manual, Rochester, Minn., 1979, Mayo Foundation and Davies Printing Co.

69. Roberts, G.D., Horstmeier, C.D., Land, G.A., and Foxworth, J.H.: Rapid urea broth test for yeasts, J. Clin. Microbiol. **7:**584-588, 1978.

70. Roberts, G.D., Karlson, A.G., and DeYoung, D.R.: Recovery of pathogenic fungi from clinical specimens submitted for mycobacteriological culture, J. Clin. Microbiol. **3:**47-48, 1976.

71. Roberts, G.D., Wang, H.S., and Hollick, G.E.: Evaluation of the API 20 C microtube system for the identification of clinically important yeasts, J. Clin. Microbiol. **3:**302-305, 1976.

72. Rogers, A.L.: Opportunistic and contaminating saprophytic fungi. In Lennette, E.H., Balows, A., Hausler, W.J., Jr., and Truant, J.P., editors: Manual of clinical microbiology, ed. 3, Washington, D.C., 1980, American Society for Microbiology.

73. Rudolph, A.H.: The clinical recognition of tinea capitis from *Trichophyton tonsurans*, J.A.M.A. **242:**1770, 1979.

74. Sarosi, G.A., and Serstock, D.S.: Isolation of *Blastomyces dermatitidis* from pigeon manure, Am. Rev. Respir. Dis. **114:**1179-1183, 1976.

75. Segal, E., and Ajello, L.: Evaluation of a new system for the rapid identification of clinically important yeasts, J. Clin. Microbiol. **4:**157-159, 1976.

76. Shadomy, S., and Espinel-Ingroff, A.: Susceptibility testing with antifungal drugs. In Lennette, E.H., Balows, A., Hausler, W.J., Jr., and Truant, J.P., editors: Manual of clinical microbiology, ed. 3, Washington, D.C., 1980, American Society for Microbiology.

77. Shields, A.B., and Ajello, L.: Medium for selective isolation of *C. neoformans*, Science **151**:208-209, 1966.

78. Silva-Hutner, M., and Cooper, B.H.: Yeasts of medical importance. In Lennette, E.H., Balows, A., Hausler, W.J., Jr., and Truant, J.P., editors: Manual of clinical microbiology, ed. 3, Washington, D.C., 1980, American Society for Microbiology.

79. Sinski, J.T., van Avermaete, D., and Kelley, L.M.: Analysis of tests used to differentiate *Trichophyton rubrum* from *Trichophyton mentagrophytes*, J. Clin. Microbiol. **13**:62-65, 1981.

80. Sixbey, J.W., and Caplan, E.S.: *Candida parapsilosis* endophthalmitis, Ann. Intern. Med. **89**:1010-1011, 1978.

81. Staib, F.: Membranfiltration und Negersaat (Guizotia abyssinica)—Nährboden für den *Cryptococcus neoformans*—Nachweis (Braunfarbeffekt), Z. Hyg. Infektionskr. **149**:329-336, 1963.

82. Staib, F., Mishra, S.K., Grosse, G., and Abel, T.: Ocular cryptococcosis: experimental and clinical observations, Zentralbl. Bakteriol. [Orig. A] **237**:378-394, 1977.

83. Trumbull, M.L., and Chesney, T.M.: The cytological diagnosis of pulmonary blastomycosis, J.A.M.A. **245**:836-838, 1981.

84. Utz, J.P.: Recognition and current management of the systemic mycoses, Med. Clin. North Am. **51**:519-527, 1967.

85. Vanbreuseghem, R.: Early diagnosis, treatment, and epidemiology of mycetoma, Rev. Med. Vet. Mycol. **6**:49-60, 1967.

86. Wilson, J.W., and Plunkett, D.A.: The fungous diseases of man, Berkeley, 1965, University of California Press.

87. Winston, D.J., Jordan, M.C., and Rhodes, J.: *Allescheria boydii* infections in the immunosuppressed host, Am. J. Med. **63**:830-835, 1977.

88. Young, N.A., Kwon-Chung, K.J., Kubota, T.T., Jennings, A.E., and Fisher, R.I.: Disseminated infection by *Fusarium moniliforme* during treatment for malignant lymphoma, J. Clin. Microbiol. **7**:589-594, 1978.

89. Zimmer, B.L., and Roberts, G.D.: Rapid selective urease test for presumptive identification of *Cryptococcus neoformans*, J. Clin. Microbiol. **10**:380-381, 1979.

35 LABORATORY DIAGNOSIS OF PARASITIC INFECTIONS

Lynne Shore Garcia

The field of parasitology is often associated with tropical areas; however, many parasitic organisms that infect humans are worldwide in distribution and occur with some frequency in the temperate zones. Many organisms endemic elsewhere are seen in the United States in persons who have lived or traveled in those areas. Consequently, laboratory personnel should be aware of the possibility that these organisms may be present and should be trained in the performance of appropriate procedures for their recovery and identification.

The identification of parasitic organisms is dependent on morphologic criteria; these criteria are in turn dependent on correct specimen collection and adequate fixation. Improperly submitted specimens may result in failure to find the organisms or in their misidentification. The information presented here should provide the reader with appropriate laboratory techniques and examples of morphologic criteria to permit the correct identification of the more common parasitic organisms.

FECAL SPECIMENS
Collection

The ability to detect and identify intestinal parasites (particularly protozoa) is directly related to the quality of the specimen submitted to the laboratory. Certain guidelines are recommended to ensure proper collection and accurate examination of specimens.[68]

Collection of fecal specimens for intestinal parasites should always be performed prior to radiologic studies involving barium sulfate. Because of the excess crystalline material in the stool specimen, the intestinal protozoa may be impossible to detect for at least 1 week after the use of barium. Certain medications may also prevent the detection of intestinal protozoa; these include mineral oil, bismuth, nonabsorbable antidiarrheal preparations, antimalarials, and some antibiotics (e.g., tetracyclines). The organisms may be difficult to detect for several weeks after the medication is discontinued.

Fecal specimens should be collected in clean, widemouthed containers; most laboratories use a waxed, cardboard half-pint container with a tight-fitting lid. The specimen should not be contaminated with water that may contain free-living organisms. Contamination with urine should also be avoided to prevent destruction of motile organisms in the specimen. All specimens should be identified with the patient's name, physician's name, hospital number if applicable, and the time and date collected. Every fecal specimen represents a potential source of infectious material (e.g., bacteria, viruses, and parasites) and should be handled accordingly.

The number of specimens required to demonstrate intestinal parasites will vary depending on the quality of the specimen submitted, the accuracy of the examination performed, and the severity of the infection. For a routine examination for parasites prior to treatment, **a minimum of three fecal specimens** is recommended—two specimens collected from normal movements and one specimen collected after a cathartic, such as magnesium sulfate or Fleet Phospho-Soda. A cathartic with an oil base should not be used, and all laxatives are contraindicated if the patient has diarrhea or significant abdominal pain. Stool softeners are inadequate for produc-

ing a purged specimen. The examination of at least six specimens ensures detection of 90% of infections[82]; six are usually recommended when amebiasis is suspected.

Many organisms do not appear in fecal specimens in consistent numbers on a daily basis[60]; thus, collection of specimens on **alternate days** tends to yield a higher percentage of positive findings. The series of three specimens should be collected within no more than 10 days, and a series of six within no more than 14 days.

The number of specimens to be examined after therapy will vary depending on the diagnosis; however, a series of three specimens collected as previously outlined is usually recommended. A patient who has received treatment for a protozoan infection should be checked 3 to 4 weeks after therapy. Patients treated for helminth infections may be checked 1 to 2 weeks after therapy, and those treated for *Taenia* infections, 5 to 6 weeks after therapy.

Since the age of the specimen directly influences the recovery of protozoan organisms, the **time the specimen was collected** should be recorded on the laboratory request form. Freshly passed specimens are mandatory for the detection of trophic amebae or flagellates. **Liquid specimens should be examined within 30 minutes of passage** (not 30 minutes from the time they reach the laboratory), or the specimen should be placed in polyvinyl alcohol fixative (PVA) or another suitable preservative (see following section on preservation of specimens). **Semiformed or soft specimens should be examined within 1 hour of passage;** if this is not possible, the stool material should be preserved. Although the time limits are not as critical for the examination of a formed specimen, it is recommended that the material be examined on the day of passage. If these time limits cannot be met, portions of the sample should be preserved. Stool specimens should not be held at room temperature but should be refrigerated at 3 to 5 C and stored in closed containers to prevent dessication. At this temperature eggs, larvae, and protozoan cysts remain viable for several days. Fecal specimens should never be incubated or frozen prior to examination. When the proper criteria for collection of fecal specimens are not met, the laboratory should request additional samples.

Collection kit for clinic use

A collection kit that can be used for outpatient laboratory services contains the following items:

1. One 5- to 7-dram brown glass, screwcapped vial containing approximately 10 ml of PVA. Some laboratories also request that some fecal material be placed in a separate vial containing 10 ml of 10% formalin, whereas others may also request a vial containing a portion of the unpreserved sample. Some workers recommend using a vial of Schaudinn's fixative in place of PVA.[84]

2. One half-pint cardboard carton with a tight-fitting lid.

3. Four 6-inch applicator sticks.

4. Instruction sheet containing information on proper collection procedures.

5. Small paper bag in which all supplies can be returned to the laboratory after specimen collection.

Since examination of three specimens is usually recommended, a kit can be prepared with 3 vials of preservatives, 3 cartons, and 10 or 12 applicator sticks. If the patient's clinical status permits, all preserved specimens in the requested series may be collected prior to delivery.

Caution: PVA solution contains a large amount of mercury; for safety reasons and protection of the patient, each vial containing PVA or any type of preservative should have a childproof cap and should be marked **Poison.** In some areas of the country it may be helpful to label the vials in more than one language, depending on the population using the medical facility.

Collection kit delivered by regular mail service

Specimens may be submitted to a referral laboratory through the regular postal service; how-ever, the following United States postal regulations must be followed: the final kit size may vary according to individual needs; there must be two separate containers—one screwcapped metal container, which is placed inside a screwcapped cardboard container. The inner mailing tube should contain one vial of PVA (individual laboratories may wish to include a vial of 10% formalin, one of schaudinn's fixative, or an empty vial) and several applicator sticks. The instruction sheet may be placed around the inner tube, which is then placed in the cardboard mailing container. This kit would be adequate for a single specimen; if three examinations were requested, the patient should submit three separate mailing kits.

The PVA-preserved portion of the specimen may be used for the complete examination,[31] although some laboratories may prefer to use the sample in 10% formalin for the concentration procedure. Other laboratories may prefer to use Schaudinn's fixative for collection. The unpreserved portion of the specimen (many laboratories do not request this sample unless an occult blood procedure is requested) may be examined to determine the specimen type (e.g., liquid, soft, or formed).

Preservation

Depending on specimen-to-laboratory transportation time, the laboratory work load, and the availability of trained personnel, it may often be impossible to examine the specimen within specified time limits. To maintain protozoan morphology and prevent further development of certain helminth eggs and larvae, the fecal specimen should be placed in an appropriate preservative for examination at a later time. A number of preservatives are available; four of these methods—PVA, formalin, merthiolate-iodine-formalin (MIF), and sodium acetate–formalin (SAF)—will be discussed. When selecting an appropriate fixative, it is important to realize the limitations of each. PVA and SAF are the only fixatives included here from which a permanent stained smear can be easily prepared.

The stained smear is extremely important in providing a complete and accurate examination for intestinal protozoa. The other fixatives mentioned permit the examination of the specimen as a wet mount only, a technique much less accurate than the stained smear for the identification of protozoa.[31,32,34]

There is presently a great deal of interest in developing a preservative without the use of mercury compounds; preliminary studies indicate that substitute compounds may provide the quality of preservation necessary for good protozoan morphology on the permanent stained smear. Another reason for investigation in this area is the problem of mercury disposal, a problem many laboratories are trying to solve.

PVA fixative

PVA fixative solution is highly recommended as a means of preserving protozoan cysts and trophozoites for examination at a later time. The use of PVA also permits specimens to be shipped by regular mail service to a laboratory for subsequent examination. PVA, which is a combination of modified Schaudinn's fixative and a water-soluble resin, should be used in the ratio of 3 parts PVA to 1 part fecal material. Perhaps the greatest advantage in the use of PVA is that permanent stained slides can be prepared from PVA-preserved material. This is not the case with many other preservatives that permit the specimen to be examined as a wet preparation only, a technique that may not be adequate for the correct identification of protozoan organisms. PVA can be prepared in the laboratory[31] or purchased commercially.* This fixative remains

stable for long periods (months to years) when kept in **sealed containers** at room temperature. However, when dispensed in small vials, PVA may become viscous and turn cloudy or white after 2 or 3 months; these vials should be discarded.

The following procedure for preparation of PVA fixative is modified from Brooke and Goldman.[9]

FORMULA

PVA, Elvanol 71-24	10 g
95% ethyl alcohol	62.5 ml
Mercuric chloride, saturated aqueous	125 ml
Glacial acetic acid	10 ml
Glycerin	3 ml

PREPARATION

1. Mix liquid ingredients in a 500-ml beaker.
2. Add PVA powder (stirring not recommended).
3. Cover beaker with a large Petri dish, heavy waxed paper, or foil and allow to soak overnight.
4. Heat solution slowly to 75 C. When this temperature is reached, remove beaker and swirl mixture until a homogeneous, slightly milky solution is obtained (30 seconds).

Formalin preservation (10% formalin)

FORMULA

Formaldehyde (USP)	100 ml
0.85% saline solution	900 ml

PREPARATION. Dilute 100 ml of formaldehyde with 900 ml of 0.85% saline solution (distilled water may be used instead of saline).

---

*Elvanol, grades 71-24, 71-30, and 90-25, can be obtained from E. I. du Pont de Nemours and Co., Electrochemical Department, Niagara Falls, N.Y. (or their local representatives), in a minimum of 50-pound bags. One could check with a local chemical supply house to see if small quantities might be available. When ordering PVA powder, be sure to specify the pretested powder for use in PVA fixative. The PVA powder should be water soluble and of medium viscosity. Prepared liquid PVA (ready for use) can be obtained from Medical Chemical Corporation, P.O. Box 445, Santa Monica, Calif. 90404; Meridian Diagnostics, Inc., P.O. Box 44216, Cincinnati, Ohio 45244; Marion Scientific Corporation, 9233 Ward Parkway, Kansas City, Mo. 64114; Regional Media Laboratories, 12076 Santa Fe Drive, Lenexa, Kan. 66215; Trend Scientific, Inc., 13895 Industrial Park Blvd., Suite 175, Minneapolis, Minn. 55441; Medical Media Lab, 15575 Southeast Amifigger Rd., Boring, Ore. 97009; and Bio Spec, Inc., 6499 Sierra Lane, Dublin, Calif. 94566.

Protozoan cysts, helminth eggs, and larvae are well preserved for long periods in 10% formalin. It is recommended that hot formalin (60 C) be used for helminth eggs to prevent further development of the eggs to the infective stage. Formalin should be used in the ratio of at least 3 parts formalin to 1 part fecal material; thorough mixing of the fresh specimen and fixative is necessary to ensure good preservation.

MIF solution

The Merthiolate (thimerosal)-iodine-formalin solution of Sapèro and Lawless[81] can be used as a stain-preservative for most kinds and stages of intestinal parasites and may be helpful in field surveys. Helminth eggs, larvae, and certain protozoa can be identified without further staining in wet mounts, which can be prepared immediately after fixation or several weeks later. This type of wet preparation may not be adequate for the diagnosis of all intestinal protozoa, and another fixative preparation may be necessary to provide a permanent stained smear. There are certain disadvantages with the MIF method, which may include the instability of the iodine component of the fixative. For a more thorough discussion of this technique, the reader may refer to Dunn.[21] This publication also contains a discussion of the concentration procedure that uses MIF-preserved material; this technique is referred to as the merthiolate-iodine-formalin concentration (MIFC) or thimerosal-iodine-formalin concentration (TIFC) method.

SAF fixative

SAF fixative contains formalin combined with sodium acetate, which acts as a buffer. This combination ensures good preservation and stability of morphology. It is a liquid fixative much like 10% aqueous formalin. When the sediment is used to prepare permanent stained smears, there may be some difficulty in getting material to adhere to the slide. Mayer's albumin has been recommended as an adhesive.[83] Although it has a long shelf life and is easy to prepare in the laboratory, this technique may be more difficult to use for less experienced laboratory personnel who are not familiar with fecal specimen differences in consistency related to adhesion to the slide.

Macroscopic examination

The consistency of the stool (formed, semiformed, soft, or liquid) may give an indication of the protozoan stages present. When the moisture content of the fecal material is decreased during **normal passage** through the intestinal tract, the trophozoite stages of the protozoa encyst to survive. **Trophozoites** (motile forms) of the intestinal protozoa are usually found in soft or liquid specimens and occasionally in a semiformed specimen; the **cyst stages** are normally found in formed or semiformed specimens, rarely in liquid stools.

Helminth eggs or larvae may be found in any type of specimen, although the chances of finding any parasitic organism in a liquid specimen will be reduced because of the dilution factor.

Occasionally adult helminths, such as *Ascaris lumbricoides* or *Enterobius vermicularis* (pinworm), may be seen in or on the surface of the stool. Tapeworm proglottids may also be seen on the surface, or they may actually crawl under the specimen and be found on the bottom of the container. Other adult helminths, such as *Trichuris trichiura* (whipworm), hookworms, or perhaps *Hymenolepis nana* (dwarf tapeworm), may be found in the stool, but usually this occurs only after medication.

The presence of blood in the specimen may indicate a number of things and should always be reported. Dark stools may indicate bleeding high in the gastrointestinal tract, whereas fresh (bright red) blood most often is the result of bleeding at a lower level. In certain parasitic infections blood and mucus may be present; a soft or liquid stool may be highly suggestive of an amebic infection. These areas of blood and mucus should be carefully examined for the presence of trophic amebae. Occult blood in the stool may or may not be related to a parasitic infection and can result from a number of different conditions. Ingestion of various compounds may give a distinctive color to the stool (iron, black; barium, light tan to white).

Microscopic examination

The identification of intestinal protozoa and helminth eggs is based on recognition of specific morphologic characteristics; these studies require a good binocular microscope, good light source, and the use of a calibrated ocular micrometer.

The microscope should have 5× and 10× oculars (widefield oculars are often recommended) and three objectives: low power (10×), high-dry (40× to 44×), and oil immersion (97× to 99×). The microscope should be kept covered when not in use, and all lenses should be carefully cleaned with lens paper. The light source should provide light of variable intensity in the blue-white range.

Calibration of microscope

Parasite identification depends on several parameters, one of which is size; any laboratory doing diagnostic work in parasitology should have a calibrated microscope available for precise measurements.

Measurements are made by means of a micrometer disk placed in the ocular of the microscope; the disk is usually calibrated as a line divided in 50 units. Since the divisions in the disk represent different measurements, depending on the objective magnification used, the ocular disk divisions must be compared with a known calibrated scale, usually a stage micrometer with a scale of 0.1- and 0.01-mm divisions. Specific directions may be found in the work of Garcia and Ash.[31]

Note: After each objective power has been calibrated on the microscope, **the oculars containing the disk or these objectives cannot be interchanged with corresponding objectives or oculars on another microscope.** Each microscope that will be used to measure organisms must be calibrated as a unit; **the original oculars and objectives that were used to calibrate the microscope must also be used when an organism is measured.**

Diagnostic procedures

A combination of techniques yields a greater number of positive specimens than does any one technique alone. Procedures recommended for a complete ova and parasite examination are discussed in the following section.

Direct smears

Normal mixing in the intestinal tract usually ensures even distribution of helminth eggs or larvae and protozoa. However, examination of the fecal material as a direct smear may or may not reveal organisms, depending on the parasite density. The direct smear is prepared by mixing a small amount of fecal material (approximately 2 mg) with a drop of physiologic saline; this mixture provides a uniform suspension under a 22- by 22-mm coverslip. Some workers prefer a 1½- by 3-inch glass slide for the wet preparations, rather than the standard 1- by 3-inch slide most often used for the permanent stained smear. A 2-mg sample of fecal material forms a low cone on the end of a wooden applicator stick. If more material is used for the direct mount, the suspension is usually too thick for an accurate examination; any less than 2 mg results in the examination of too thin a suspension, thus decreasing the chances of finding any organisms. If present, blood and mucus should always be examined as a direct mount. The entire 22- by 22-mm coverslip should be systematically examined using the low-power objective (10×) and low light intensity; any suspect objects may then be examined on high-dry power (43×). The use of the oil immersion objective on mounts of this kind is not recommended unless the coverslip (No. 1 thickness coverslip is recommended when the oil immersion objective is used) is sealed to the slide with a cotton-tipped applicator stick dipped in equal parts of heated paraffin and petroleum jelly. Many workers believe the use of oil immersion on this type of preparation is impractical, especially since morphologic detail is most easily seen and the diagnosis confirmed with oil immersion examination of the permanent stained smear.

The **direct wet mount** is used primarily to detect motile trophozoite stages of the protozoa. These organisms are very pale and transparent, two characteristics that require the use of low light intensity. Protozoan organisms in a saline preparation usually appear as refractile objects. If suspect objects are seen on high-dry power, one should allow at least 15 seconds to detect motility of slow-moving protozoa. Heat applied by placing a hot penny on the edge of a slide may enhance the motility of trophic protozoa.

Note: With few exceptions, protozoan organisms should not be identified on the basis of a wet mount alone. Permanent stained smears should be examined to confirm the specific identification of suspected organisms.

Helminth eggs or larvae and protozoan cysts may also be seen on the wet film, although these forms are more often detected after fecal concentration procedures.

After the wet preparation has been thoroughly checked for trophic amebae, a drop of iodine may be placed at the edge of the coverslip, or a new wet mount can be prepared with iodine alone. A weak iodine solution is recommended; too strong a solution may obscure the organisms. Several types of iodine are available: Dobell and O'Connor's, Lugol's, and D'Antoni's. Gram's iodine used in bacteriologic work is not recommended for staining parasitic organisms.

Modified D'Antoni's iodine[65]

FORMULA

Distilled water	100 ml
Potassium iodide (KI)	1 g
Powdered iodine crystals	1.5 g

PREPARATION. The potassium iodide solution should be saturated with iodine, with some excess remaining in the bottle. Store in brown, glass-stoppered bottles in the dark. The solution is ready for use immediately and should be decanted into a brown-glass dropping bottle; when the solution lightens, it should be discarded and replaced with fresh stock. The stock solution remains good as long as an excess of iodine remains on the bottom of the bottle. The iodine solutions eventually lighten in color and lose their staining strength; fresh solutions should be prepared every 2 to 3 weeks.

Protozoan cysts correctly stained with iodine contain yellow-gold cytoplasm, brown glycogen material, and paler refractile nuclei. The chromatoidal bodies may not be as clearly visible as they were in the saline mount.

Several staining solutions are available that may be used to reveal nuclear detail in the trophozoite stages. Nair's[71] buffered methylene blue stain is effective in showing nuclear detail when used at a low pH; a pH range of 3.6 to 4.8 allows more active penetration of the organism with the biologic dye. After 5 to 10 minutes, Nair's buffered methylene blue stain stains the cytoplasm a pale blue and the nuclei a darker blue. Methylene blue (0.06%) in an acetate buffer at pH 3.6 usually gives satisfactory results; the mount should be examined within 30 minutes.

ACETATE BUFFER SOLUTION. Stock solution A consists of 0.2 M solution of acetic acid (11.55 ml in 1,000 ml of distilled water). Stock solution B consists of 0.2 M solution of sodium acetate (16.4 g of $C_2H_3O_2Na$, or 27.2 g of $C_2H_3O_2Na \cdot 3H_2O$ in 1,000 ml of distilled water).

Proportions of A and B for specific pH are as follows: mix the indicated quantity of stock solutions A and B and dilute with distilled water to a total of 100 ml.

Desired pH	Stock solution A (ml)	Stock solution B (ml)
3.6	46.3	3.7
3.8	44.0	6.0
4.0	41.0	9.0
4.2	36.8	13.2
4.4	30.5	19.5
4.6	25.5	24.5

Concentration procedures

Often a direct mount of fecal material fails to reveal the presence of parasitic organisms in the gastrointestinal tract. Fecal concentration procedures should be included for a complete examination for parasites; these procedures allow the detection of small numbers of organisms that may be missed using only the direct mount.

A number of concentration procedures are available, which are either **flotation or sedimentation techniques** designed to separate the parasitic components from excess fecal debris through differences in specific gravity.[24] A flotation procedure permits the separation of protozoan cysts and certain helminth eggs through the use of a liquid with a high specific gravity. The parasitic elements are recovered in the surface film, while the debris will be found in the bottom of the tube. This technique yields a cleaner preparation than does the sedimentation procedure; however, some helminth eggs (operculated eggs or very dense eggs, such as unfertilized *Ascaris* eggs) and some protozoa do not concentrate well with the flotation method. The specific gravity may be increased, although this may produce more distortion in the eggs and protozoa. Any laboratory that uses a flotation procedure only may fail to recover all the parasites present; to ensure detection of all organisms in the sample, both the surface film and the sediment should be carefully examined.

Note: Directions for any flotation technique must be followed exactly to produce reliable results.

Sedimentation procedures (using gravity or centrifugation) allow the recovery of all protozoa, eggs, and larvae present; however, the sediment preparation contains more fecal debris. If a single technique is selected for routine use, the **sedimentation procedure is recommended** as the easiest to perform and least subject to technical error.

FORMALIN-ETHER[31,78] SEDIMENTATION TECHNIQUE

1. Transfer ¼ to ½ teaspoon of fresh stool into 10 ml of 10% formalin in a 15-ml shell vial, unwaxed paper cup, or 16- by 125-mm tube (container may vary depending on individual preferences) and comminute thoroughly. Let stand 30 minutes for adequate fixation.

2. Filter this material (funnel or pointed paper cup with end cut off) through two layers of gauze into a 15-ml centrifuge tube.

3. Add physiologic saline to within ½ inch of the top and centrifuge for 2 minutes at 1,500 rpm (or 1 minute at 2,000 to 2,500 rpm).

4. Decant, resuspend the sediment (should have 0.5 to 1 ml sediment) in saline to within ½ inch of the top, and centrifuge again for 2 minutes at 1,500 rpm (or 1 minute at 2,000 to 2,500 rpm). This second wash may be eliminated if the supernatant fluid after the first wash is light tan or clear.

5. Decant and resuspend the sediment in 10% formalin (fill the tube only half full). If the amount of sediment left in the bottom of the tube is very small, do not add ether in step 6; merely add the formalin, then spin, decant, and examine the remaining sediment.

6. Add approximately 3 ml of ether (**do not use near open flames**), stopper, and shake vigorously for 30 seconds. Hold the tube so that the stopper is directed away from your face; remove stopper carefully to prevent spraying of material caused by pressure within the tube.

7. Centrifuge for 2 to 3 minutes at 1,500 rpm. Four layers should result: a small amount of sediment in the bottom of the tube, containing the parasites; a layer of formalin; a plug of fecal debris on top of the formalin layer; and a layer of ether at the top.

8. Free the plug of debris by ringing with an applicator stick, and decant all the fluid. After proper decanting, a drop or two of fluid remaining on the side of the tube will drain down to the sediment. Mix the fluid

with the sediment and prepare a wet mount for examination.

The formalin-ether sedimentation procedure may be used on PVA-preserved material.[31] Steps 1 and 2 differ as follows:

1. Fixation time with PVA should be at least 30 minutes. Mix contents of PVA bottle (stool-PVA mixture: 1 part stool to 2 or 3 parts PVA) with applicator sticks. Immediately after mixing, pour approximately 2 to 5 ml (amount will vary depending on the viscosity and density of the mixture) of the stool-PVA mixture into a 15-ml shell vial, 16- by 125-mm tube, or such, and add approximately 10 ml physiologic saline.

2. Filter this material (funnel or paper cup with pointed end cut off) through two layers of gauze into a 15-ml centrifuge tube.

Steps 3 through 8 will be the same for both fresh and PVA-preserved material.

Note: Tap water may be substituted for physiologic saline throughout this procedure; however, saline is recommended. Some workers prefer to use 10% formalin for all the rinses (steps 3 and 4).

Note: The introduction of ethyl acetate as a substitute for diethyl ether (ether) in the formalin-ether sedimentation concentration procedure provides a much safer chemical for the clinical laboratory. Tests comparing the use of these two compounds on formalin-preserved and PVA-preserved material indicate that the differences in organism recovery and identification are minimal and probably do not reflect clinically relevant differences.[33,113]

When examining the sediment in the bottom of the tube:

1. Prepare a saline mount (1 drop of sediment and 1 drop of saline solution mixed together), and scan the whole 22- by 22-mm coverslip under low power for helminth eggs or larvae.

2. Iodine may then be added to aid in the detection of protozoan cysts and should be examined under high-dry power. If iodine is added prior to low-power scanning, be certain that the iodine is not too strong; otherwise, some of the helminth eggs will stain so darkly that they will be mistaken for debris.

3. Occasionally a precipitate is formed when iodine is added to the sediment obtained from a concentration procedure using PVA-preserved material. The precipitate is formed from the reaction between the iodine and excess mercuric chloride that has not been thoroughly rinsed from the PVA-preserved material. The sediment can be rinsed again to remove any remaining mercuric chloride, or the sediment can be examined as a saline mount without the addition of iodine.

ZINC SULFATE FLOTATION PROCEDURE (MODIFIED).[25] Protozoan cysts may be more distorted using this method, and the technique is unsuitable for stool specimens containing large amounts of fatty material. The specific gravity of the zinc sulfate should be 1.18 and should be checked frequently with a hydrometer. If this technique is used to concentrate formalin-preserved material, the specific gravity should be increased to 1.20.

Zinc sulfate solution ($ZnSO_4$, specific gravity 1.18; approximately 330 g of dry crystals in 670 ml of distilled water). A 33% solution usually approximates the correct specific gravity but may be adjusted to 1.18 by the addition of zinc sulfate or distilled water.

1. Prepare a fecal suspension of ¼ to ½ teaspoon of feces (more if the specimen is diarrheal) in 10 to 15 ml of tap water.

2. Filter this material through two layers of gauze into a small tube (Wassermann tube). Fill the tube with tap water to within 2 to 3 mm of the top, and centrifuge for 1 minute at 2,300 rpm.

3. Decant the supernatant fluid, fill the tube with water, and resuspend the sediment by stirring with an applicator stick. Centrifuge for 1 minute at 2,300 rpm.

4. Decant the water, add 2 to 3 ml zinc sulfate solution, resuspend the sediment, and

fill the tube with zinc sulfate solution to within 0.5 cm of the top.

5. Centrifuge for 1 to 2 minutes at 2,500 rpm. Do not "brake" the centrifuge; allow the tubes to come to a stop without interference or vibration.

6. Without removing the tubes from the centrifuge, touch the surface film of the suspension with a wire loop (diameter 5- to 7-mm; loop should be parallel with the surface of the fluid). **Do not go below the surface of the film with the loop.** Add the material in the loop to a slide containing a drop of dilute iodine or saline.

Note: Material recovered from the zinc sulfate flotation procedure must be examined within several minutes; prolonged contact with the high specific gravity solution leads to organism distortion.

Permanent stained smears

The detection and correct identification of **intestinal protozoa** are frequently dependent on the examination of the permanent stained smear. These slides not only provide the microscopist with a permanent record of the protozoan organisms identified but also may be used for consultations with specialists when unusual morphologic characteristics are found. In view of the number of morphologic variations possible, organisms may be found that are very difficult to identify and do not fit the pattern for any one species.

The smaller protozoan organisms are often seen on the stained smear and missed using only the direct smear and concentration methods. Although an experienced microscopist can occasionally identify certain organisms on a wet preparation, most identifications should be considered tentative until confirmed by the permanent stained slide. For these reasons, **the permanent stain is recommended for every stool sample submitted for a routine examination for parasites.**[13,34,74]

A number of staining techniques are available;

individual selection of a particular method may depend on the degree of difficulty and amount of time necessary for staining. The older classical method is the long Heidenhain's iron-hematoxylin method; however, for routine diagnostic work most laboratories select one of the shorter procedures, such as the **trichrome method** or one of several methods using iron-hematoxylin. Other procedures are available[35]; however, those included here generally tend to give the best and most reliable results with both fresh and PVA-preserved specimens.

Preparation of fresh material. When the specimen arrives, use an applicator stick or brush to smear a small amount of stool on two clean slides and immediately immerse them in Schaudinn's fixative. If the slides are prepared correctly, one should be able to read newsprint through the fecal smear. The smears should fix for a minimum of 30 minutes; fixation time may be decreased to 5 minutes if the Schaudinn's solution is heated to 60 C.

If a liquid specimen is received, mix three or four drops of PVA with one or two drops of fecal material on a slide, spread the mixture, and allow the slides to dry for several hours at 35 C or overnight at room temperature. The following fixative solutions may be used.

SATURATED MERCURIC CHLORIDE

Mercuric chloride ($HgCl_2$)	110 g
Distilled water	1,000 ml

Use a beaker as a water bath; boil (use a hood if available) until the $HgCl_2$ is dissolved; let stand until crystals form.

SCHAUDINN'S FIXATIVE (STOCK SOLUTION)

Saturated aqueous solution of $HgCl_2$	600 ml
95% ethyl alcohol	300 ml

Immediately prior to use add 5 ml of glacial acetic acid per 100 ml of stock solution.

Preparation of PVA-preserved material. Stool specimens preserved in PVA should be allowed to fix at least 30 minutes. After fixation, the sample should be thoroughly mixed and a

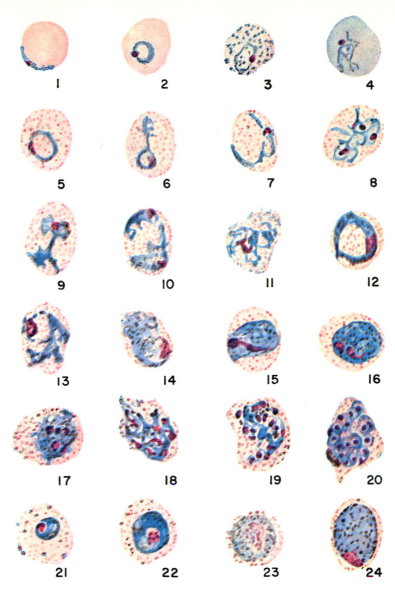

PLATE 247.

Plasmodium vivax. **1,** Normal-sized red cell with marginal ring form trophozoite. **2,** Young signet ring form trophozoite in macrocyte. **3,** Slightly older ring form trophozoite in red cell showing basophilic stippling. **4,** Polychromatophilic red cell containing young tertian parasite with pseudopodia. **5,** Ring form trophozoite showing pigment in cytoplasm, in enlarged cell containing Schüffner's stippling (dots). (Schüffner's stippling does not appear in all cells containing growing and older forms of *P. vivax,* as would be indicated by these pictures, but it can be found with any stage from fairly young ring form onward.) **6, 7,** Very tenuous medium trophozoite forms. **8,** Three ameboid trophozoites with fused cytoplasm. **9, 11-13,** Older ameboid trophozoites in process of development. **10,** Two ameboid trophozoites in one cell. **14,** Mature trophozoite. **15,** Mature trophozoite with chromatin apparently in process of division. **16-19,** Schizonts showing progressive steps in division (presegmenting schizonts). **20,** Mature schizont. **21, 22,** Developing gametocytes. **23,** Mature microgametocyte. **24,** Mature macrogametocyte. (From Wilcox.[111])

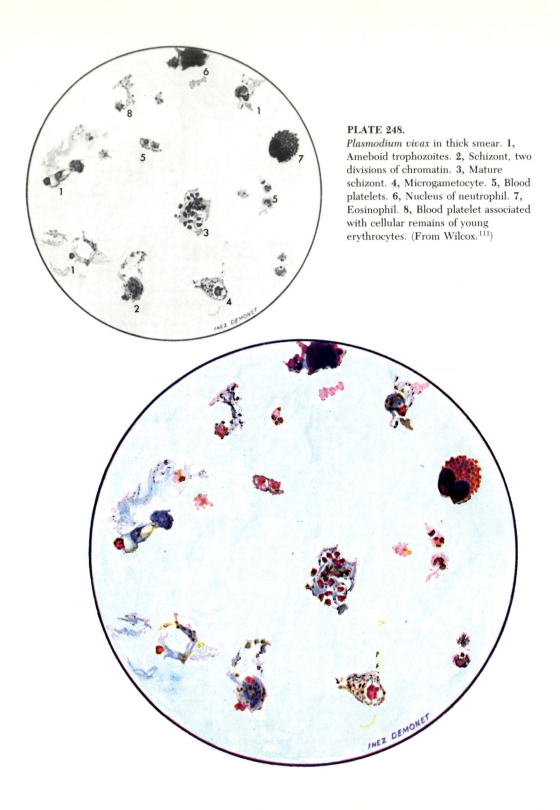

PLATE 248.

Plasmodium vivax in thick smear. **1,** Ameboid trophozoites. **2,** Schizont, two divisions of chromatin. **3,** Mature schizont. **4,** Microgametocyte. **5,** Blood platelets. **6,** Nucleus of neutrophil. **7,** Eosinophil. **8,** Blood platelet associated with cellular remains of young erythrocytes. (From Wilcox.[111])

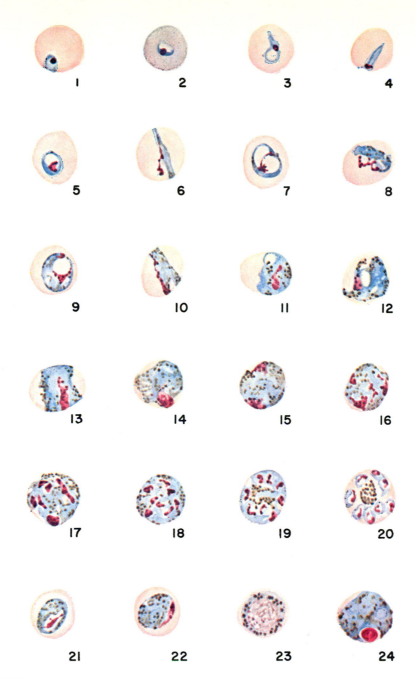

PLATE 249.

Plasmodium malariae. **1,** Young ring form trophozoite of quartan malaria. **2-4,** Young trophozoite forms of parasite showing gradual increase of chromatin and cytoplasm. **5,** Developing ring form trophozoite showing pigment granule. **6,** Early band form trophozoite, elongated chromatin, some pigment apparent. **7-12,** Some forms that developing trophozoite of quartan may take. **13, 14,** Mature trophozoites, one a band form. **15-19,** Phases in development of schizont (presegmenting schizonts). **20,** Mature schizont. **21,** Immature microgametocyte. **22,** Immature macrogametocyte. **23,** Mature microgametocyte. **24,** Mature macrogametocyte. (From Wilcox.[111])

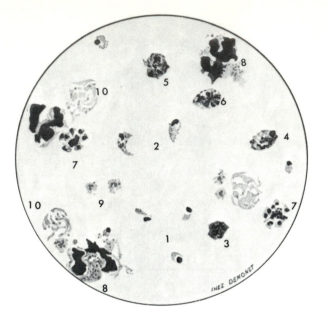

PLATE 250.

Plasmodium malariae in thick smear. **1,** Small trophozoites. **2,** Growing trophozoites. **3,** Mature trophozoites. **4-6,** Schizonts (presegmenting) with varying numbers of divisions of chromatin. **7,** Mature schizonts. **8,** Nucleus of leukocyte. **9,** Blood platelets. **10,** Cellular remains of young erythrocytes. (From Wilcox.[111])

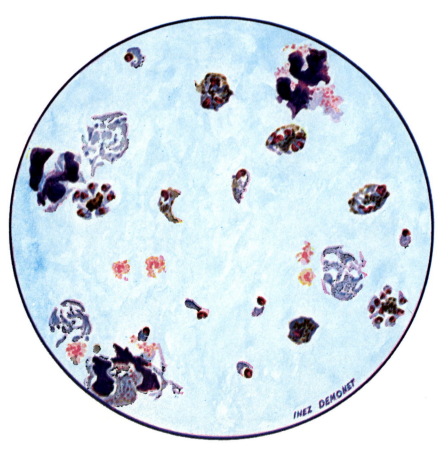

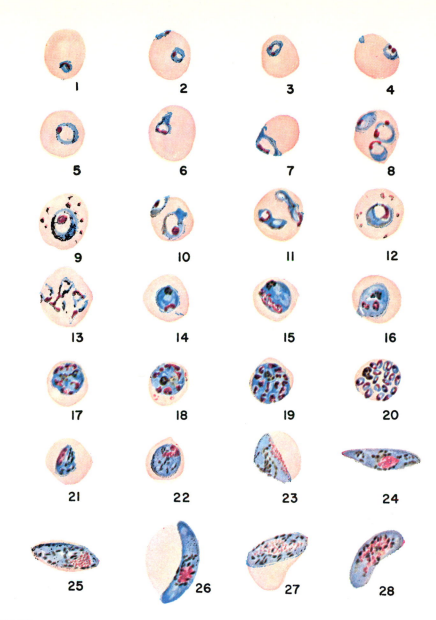

PLATE 251.

Plasmodium falciparum. **1,** Very young ring form trophozoite. **2,** Double infection of single cell with young trophozoites, one a marginal form, the other signet ring form. **3, 4,** Young trophozoites showing double chromatin dots. **5-7,** Developing trophozoite forms. **8,** Three medium trophozoites in one cell. **9,** Trophozoite showing pigment in cell containing Maurer's dots. **10, 11,** Two trophozoites in each of two cells, showing variations of forms that parasites may assume. **12,** Almost mature trophozoite showing haze of pigment throughout cytoplasm. Maurer's dots in cell. **13,** Estivoautumnal "slender forms." **14,** Mature trophozoite showing clumped pigment. **15,** Parasite in process of initial chromatin division. **16-19,** Various phases of development of schizont (presegmenting schizonts). **20,** Mature schizont. **21-24,** Successive forms in development of gametocyte, usually not found in peripheral circulation. **25,** Immature macrogametocyte. **26,** Mature macrogametocyte. **27,** Immature microgametocyte. **28,** Mature microgametocyte. (From Wilcox.[111])

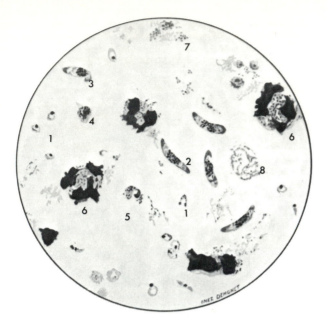

PLATE 252.
Plasmodium falciparum in thick film.
1, Small trophozoites. **2,** Normal gametocytes. **3,** Slightly distorted gametocyte. **4,** "Rounded-up" gametocyte. **5,** Disintegrated gametocyte. **6,** Nucleus of leukocyte. **7,** Blood platelets. **8,** Cellular remains of young erythrocyte. (From Wilcox.[111])

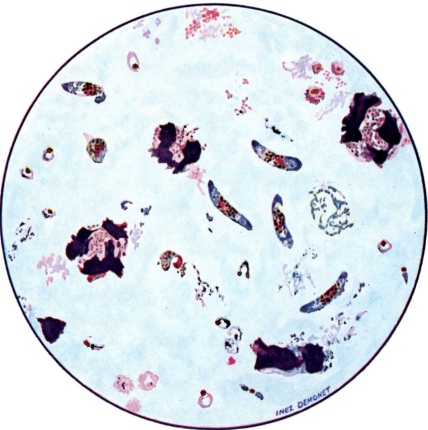

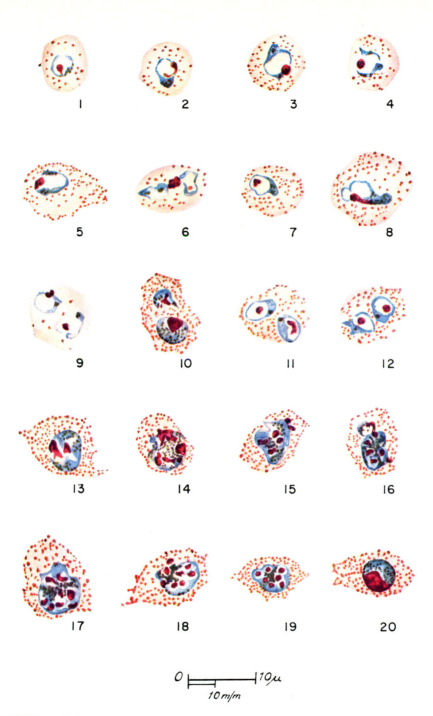

PLATE 253.

Plasmodium ovale. **1,** Young ring-shaped trophozoite. **2-5,** Older ring-shaped trophozoites. **6-8,** Older ameboid trophozoites. **9, 11, 12,** Doubly infected cells, trophozoites. **10,** Doubly infected cell, young gametocytes. **13,** First stage of the schizont. **14-19,** Schizonts, progressive stages. **20,** Mature gametocyte. (From Markell and Voge.[65])

small amount of the material poured onto a paper towel to absorb the excess PVA. This is an important step in the procedure; allow the PVA to soak into the paper towel for 2 to 3 minutes before preparing the slides. With an applicator stick apply some of the stool material from the paper towel to two slides and let them dry for several hours at 37 C or overnight at room temperature. The PVA-stool mixture should be spread to the edges of the glass slide; this causes the film to adhere to the slide during staining. It is also important to thoroughly dry the slides to prevent the material from washing off during staining.

Trichrome stain. This stain was originally developed by Gomori[36] for tissue differentiation and was adapted by Wheatley[110] for intestinal protozoa. It is an uncomplicated procedure that produces well-stained smears from both fresh and PVA-preserved material.

FORMULA

Chromotrope 2R	0.6 g
Light green SF	0.3 g
Phosphotungstic acid	0.7 g
Acetic acid (glacial)	1 ml
Distilled water	100 ml

PREPARATION. The stain is prepared by adding 1 ml of glacial acetic acid to the dry components. Allow the mixture to stand for 15 to 30 minutes to "ripen," then add 100 ml of distilled water. This preparation gives a highly uniform and reproducible stain; the stain should be purple.

PROCEDURE
1. Prepare fresh fecal smears or PVA smears as described.
2. Place in 70% ethyl alcohol for 5 minutes.* (Step 2 may be eliminated for PVA smears.)
3. Place in 70% ethyl alcohol plus D'Antoni's iodine (dark reddish-brown) for 2 to 5 minutes.

4. Place in two changes of 70% ethyl alcohol—one for 5 minutes* and one for 2 to 5 minutes.
5. Place in trichrome stain solution for 10 minutes.
6. Place in 90% ethyl alcohol, acidified (1% acetic acid) for up to 3 seconds (**do not leave the slides in this solution too long**).
7. Dip once in 100% ethyl alcohol.
8. Place in two changes of 100% ethyl alcohol for 2 to 5 minutes each.*
9. Place in two changes of xylene or toluene for 2 to 5 minutes each.*
10. Mount in Permount or some other mounting medium; use a No. 1 thickness coverglass.

The trichrome stain can be used repeatedly, and stock solution may be added to the dish when the volume is decreased. Periodically, the staining strength can be restored by removing the lid and allowing the 70% alcohol carried over from the preceding dish to evaporate. Each lot number or batch of stain (either purchased commercially or prepared in the laboratory) should be checked to determine the optimum staining time, which is usually a few minutes longer for PVA-preserved material.

The 90% acidified alcohol is used as a destaining agent that will provide good differentiation; however, prolonged destaining (more than 3 seconds) may result in a poor stain. To prevent continued destaining, the slides should be quickly rinsed in 100% alcohol and then dehydrated through two additional changes of 100% alcohol.

INTERPRETATION OF STAINED SMEARS. Many problems in interpretation may arise when poorly stained smears are examined; these smears are usually the result of inadequate fixation or incorrect specimen collection and submission. An old specimen or inadequate fixation may

---

*Slides can be held several hours or overnight.

*Slides can be held several hours or overnight.

result in organisms that fail to stain or that appear as pale pink or red objects with very little internal definition. This type of staining reaction may occur with *Entamoeba coli* cysts, which require a longer fixation time; mature cysts in general (need additional fixation time) may not be as well stained as immature cysts. Degenerate forms or those that have been understained or destained too much may stain pale green.

When the smear is well fixed and correctly stained, the background debris will be green, and the protozoa will have a blue-green to purple cytoplasm with red or purple-red nuclei and inclusions. The differences in colors between the background and organisms provide more contrast than in hematoxylin-stained smears.

Helminth eggs and larvae usually stain dark red or purple; they are often distorted and difficult to identify. White blood cells, macrophages, tissue cells, yeast cells, and other artifacts still present diagnostic problems, since their color range on the stained smear approximates that of the parasitic organisms (Plates 212 to 214).

Iron-hematoxylin stain. Although the original method produces excellent results[62] most laboratories that use an iron-hematoxylin stain select one of the shorter methods. A number of procedures are available; both of those presented here can be used with either fresh or PVA-preserved material. Both background debris and the organisms stain gray-blue to black, with the cellular inclusions and nuclei appearing darker than the cytoplasm.

The method described by Spencer and Monroe[93] is a bit longer than the trichrome procedure. Although the slides do not require destaining, decolorizing in 0.5% hydrochloric acid after a longer initial staining time may provide better differentiation.

SOLUTION I. Solution I is hematoxylin, 10 g in 1,000 ml of absolute ethyl alcohol. Keep the stain in a stoppered flask, and allow to ripen in sunlight for at least a week.

SOLUTION II

Ferrous ammonium sulfate	10 g
Ferric ammonium sulfate	10 g
HC1, concentrated	10 ml
Distilled water	1,000 ml

WORKING SOLUTION. Mix equal parts of solutions I and II; this working solution will last for about 7 days.

PROCEDURE

1. Prepare fresh fecal smears or PVA-preserved smears as previously described.
2. Place in 70% ethyl alcohol for 5 minutes.*
3. Place in 70% ethyl alcohol plus D'Antoni's iodine (dark reddish-brown) for 2 to 5 minutes.
4. Place in 70% ethyl alcohol for 5 minutes.*
5. Wash in running tap water for 10 minutes.
6. Place in working solution of iron-hematoxylin staining solution for 4 to 5 minutes.
7. Wash in running tap water for 10 minutes.
8. Place in 70% ethyl alcohol for 5 minutes.*
9. Place in 95% ethyl alcohol for 5 minutes.
10. Place in two changes of 100% ethyl alcohol for 5 minutes each.*
11. Place in two changes of xylene or toluene for 5 minutes each.*
12. Mount in Permount or some other mounting medium; use a No. 1 thickness coverglass.

Another iron-hematoxylin method, described by Tompkins and Miller, [104] includes the use of phosphotungstic acid as a destaining agent. This procedure also gives good, reproducible results.

---

*Slides can be held several hours or overnight.

PROCEDURE

1. Prepare fresh fecal smears or PVA-preserved smears as previously described.
2. Place in 70% ethyl alcohol D'Antoni's iodine (dark reddish-brown) for 2 to 5 minutes.
3. Place in 50% ethyl alcohol for 3 minutes.
4. Wash in running tap water for 3 minutes.
5. Place in 4% ferric ammonium sulfate mordant for 5 minutes.
6. Wash in tap water for 1 minute.
7. Place in 0.5% aqueous hematoxylin for 2 minutes.
8. Wash in tap water for 1 minute.
9. Place in 2% aqueous phosphotungstic acid for 2 to 5 minutes.
10. Wash in running tap water for 10 minutes.
11. Place in 70% ethyl alcohol (plus a few drops of saturated aqueous lithium carbonate) for 3 minutes.
12. Place in 95% ethyl alcohol for 5 minutes.
13. Place in two changes of 100% ethyl alcohol for 5 minutes each.*
14. Place in xylene or toluene for 5 minutes.*
15. Mount in Permount or some other mounting medium; use a No. 1 thickness coverglass.

General information

The most important step in preparing a well-stained fecal smear is adequate fixation of a specimen that has been submitted within specified time limits. To ensure best results, the acetic acid component of Schaudinn's fixative should be added just prior to use; fixation time (room temperature) may be extended overnight with no adverse effects on the smears.

---

*Slides can be held several hours or overnight.

After fixation it is very important to completely remove the mercuric chloride residue from the smears. The 70% alcohol-iodine mixture removes the mercury complex; the iodine solution should be changed often enough (at least once a week) to maintain a dark reddish-brown color. If the mercuric chloride is not completely removed, the stained smear may contain varying amounts of highly refractive granules, which may prevent finding or identifying any organisms present.

Good results in the final stages of dehydration (100% alcohol) and clearing (xylene) depend on the use of **fresh reagents.** It is recommended that solutions be changed at least weekly and more often if large numbers of slides (10 to 50 per day) are being stained. Stock containers and staining dishes should have well-fitting lids to prevent evaporation and absorption of moisture from the air. If the clearing agent turns cloudy on addition of the slides from 100% alcohol, there is water in the solution. When clouding occurs, immediately return the slides to 100% alcohol, replace all dehydrating and clearing agents with fresh stock, and continue with the dehydration process.

Additional procedures
Sigmoidoscopy material

When repeated fecal examinations fail to reveal the presence of *Entamoeba histolytica*, material obtained from sigmoidoscopy may be valuable in the diagnosis of amebiasis. However, this procedure does not take the place of routine fecal examinations; a series of at least three (six is preferable) fecal specimens should be submitted for each patient having a sigmoidoscopy examination. Material from the mucosal surface should be obtained by **aspiration or scraping,** not with a cotton-tipped swab. If swabs must be used, most of the cotton should be removed (leave just enough to safely cover the end) and should be tightly wound to prevent absorption of the material to be examined.

The specimen should be processed and examined immediately; the number of techniques used will depend on the amount of material obtained. If the specimen is sufficient for both wet preparations and permanent stained smears, proceed as follows. The direct mount should be examined immediately for the presence of moving trophozoites; it may take time for the organisms to become acclimated to this type of preparation, thus motility may not be obvious for several minutes. Care should be taken not to confuse protozoan organisms with macrophages or other tissue cells; any suspect cells should be confirmed with the use of the permanent stained slide. The smears for permanent staining should be prepared at the same time the direct mount is made by gently smearing some of the material onto several slides and immediately placing them into Schaudinn's fixative. The slides can then be stained by any of the techniques mentioned for routine fecal smears. If the material is bloody, contains a lot of mucus,

or is a "wet" specimen, one or two drops of the sample can be mixed with three or four drops of PVA right on the slide. Allow the smears to dry (overnight if possible) prior to staining.

Duodenal contents

In some instances repeated fecal examinations may fail to confirm a diagnosis of *Giardia lamblia* and *Strongyloides stercoralis* infections (Fig. 35-1). Since these two parasites are normally found in the duodenum, the physician may submit duodenal drainage fluid to the laboratory for examination. The specimen should be submitted without preservatives and should be received and examined within 1 hour after being taken. The amount of fluid may vary. It should be centrifuged and the sediment examined as wet mounts for the detection of motile organisms. Several mounts should be prepared and examined; because of the dilution factor, the organisms may be difficult to recover using this technique.

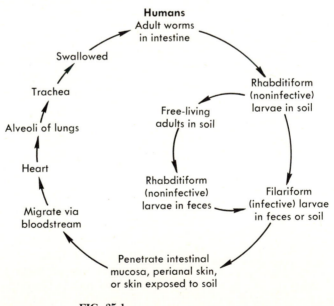

FIG. 35-1
Life cycle of *Strongyloides stercoralis*.

Another convenient method of sampling duodenal contents, which eliminates the necessity for intubation, is the use of the Entero-Test.[3] This device consists of a gelatin capsule containing a weighted, coiled length of nylon yarn. The end of the line protrudes through the top of the capsule and is taped to the side of the patient's face. The capsule is then swallowed, the gelatin dissolves, and the weighted string is carried by peristalsis into the duodenum. After approximately 4 hours, the string is recovered, and the bile-stained mucus attached to the string is examined as a wet mount for the presence of organisms. This type of specimen should also be examined immediately after the string is recovered. When the mucus is examined from either duodenal drainage or the Entero-Test capsule, typical "falling leaf" motility of *G. lamblia* trophozoites is usually not visible. The flagella usually are visible as a rapid "flutter," with the organism remaining trapped in the mucus.

Cellophane-covered thick smear

This procedure, which is commonly referred to as the Kato thick-smear technique, was originally developed in Japan by Kato and Miura.[52] It can be used for examination for **helminth eggs** but is not suitable for larvae or protozoa; it is not recommended for examination of stool containing large amounts of fiber or gas.

PROCEDURE
1. Cut wettable cellophane of medium thickness (30 to 50 μm) in 22- by 30-mm strips and soak for 24 hours or longer in a mixture of 100 parts glycerine, 100 parts water, and 1 part 3% aqueous malachite green.
2. Place 50 to 60 mg of feces on a clean slide and cover with a strip of cellophane prepared as above.
3. Turn the slide upside down on paper towels and press to spread the fecal material to the edges.
4. Reverse the slide and allow to dry at 40 C for 30 minutes or at room temperature for 1 hour.

5. Examine the slide under low power; higher magnification can be used if necessary.

As the film dries, the fecal debris clears more rapidly than the helminth eggs; however, with time the eggs also clear, making accurate identification impossible. Thus, the optimum drying time must be determined; overdrying causes distortion in many of the delicate eggs.

Martin and Beaver[66] modified the technique and concluded that egg counts made using their technique provided reliable results for the quantitative diagnosis of helminth infections.

Estimation of worm burdens

Circumstances may arise when it is helpful to know the degree of infection in a patient or perhaps to follow the effectiveness of therapy. In certain helminth infections that have little clinical significance, the patient may not be given treatment if the numbers of parasites are small. The **parasite burden** may be estimated by counting the number of eggs passed in the stool. In addition to the procedures presented here, the direct smear method of Beaver[4,5] has proved to be very helpful in estimating the parasite burden.

Stoll's dilution egg-count technique. This technique developed by Stoll and Hausheer[97] has been widely used to estimate the number of adult worms present in several helminth infections, specifically hookworm, *Ascaris*, and *Trichuris*. The value of this type of procedure is based on repeated egg counts to detect changes in the numbers present.

PROCEDURE
1. Save the entire 24-hour stool specimen, and determine the weight in grams.
2. Weigh out accurately 4 g of feces.
3. Place the feces in a calibrated bottle or large test tube, and add sufficient 0.1 N sodium hydroxide to bring the volume to 60 ml.
4. Add a few glass beads, and shake mixture vigorously to make a uniform suspension.

If the specimen is hard, the mixture may be placed in a refrigerator overnight, before shaking, to aid in its comminution.

5. With a pipet, quickly remove 0.15 ml of the suspension, and drain it onto a slide.
6. Do not use coverglass; place the slide on mechanical stage, and count all the eggs.
7. Multiply the egg count by 100 to obtain the number of eggs per gram of feces and by weight of 24-hour specimen to get total number of eggs per 24 hours.
8. The estimate (eggs per gram) obtained will vary depending on the consistency of the feces. The following correction factors should be used to convert the estimate to a formed-stool basis: mushy formed, ×1.5; mushy, ×2; mushy diarrheal, ×3; diarrheal, ×4; watery, ×5.

The following figures indicate the correlation between egg counts and need for therapy. *Trichuris trichiura* and hookworm are generally the only helminth infections where the egg count may determine whether the patient will receive therapy; low egg counts usually correlate with a lack of clinical symptoms in patients infected with these parasites. The effectiveness of therapy for any helminth infection may be checked by doing repeated egg counts.

Note: The presence of even one *Ascaris* is potentially dangerous; when irritated, the parasite tends to migrate while in the gastrointestinal tract, and this migratory habit may cause severe clinical symptoms in the patient.

With *Trichuris trichiura* approximately 30,000 eggs per gram indicate the presence of several hundred worms. This type of worm burden usually causes definite symptoms.

With hookworm approximately 2,500 to 5,000 eggs per gram usually indicate a clinically significant infection.

Recovery of larval-stage nematodes

Nematode infections that give rise to larval stages, which hatch either in the soil or in tissues, may be diagnosed by using culture techniques designed to concentrate the larvae. These procedures are used in hookworm, *Strongyloides*, and trichostrongyle infections. Some of these techniques, which permit the recovery of infective-stage larvae, may be helpful, since the eggs of many species are identical and specific identifications are based on larval morphology.

Harada-Mori filter paper strip culture. As a means of detecting light infections and providing specific identifications, the Harada-Mori filter paper strip culture technique is very useful. The method was originally introduced by Harada and Mori[38] in 1955 and has been modified by several workers.[43] Fecal specimens should not be refrigerated prior to culture; some of the nematodes are susceptible to cold and do not undergo further development. Since infective-stage larvae may be recovered from the culture system, gloves should be worn to handle the filter paper strip and other equipment.

PROCEDURE

1. To each 15-ml centrifuge tube add approximately 3 to 4 ml of distilled water.
2. In the center of each filter paper strip (3/8 inch by 5 inches) smear, in a relatively thin film, approximately 0.5 to 1 g of feces.
3. The identification of the specimen can be written in pencil on the piece of filter paper between the waterline and the fecal material.
4. Insert the strip in the tube so that the end of the filter paper strip, usually cut so that it is slightly tapered, is near the bottom of the tube. Caps are not required for the tubes.
5. Maintain the tube in a rack at 24 to 28 C, and add water to original level as it is needed. Usually there is rapid evaporation over the first day or two, and then the culture becomes stabilized.
6. The capillary flow of water up the filter paper strip keeps the feces moist. Soluable elements in the feces will be carried out of

the fecal mass and accumulate as a dark area at the top of the paper.

7. Tubes should be kept for approximately 10 days, but infective larvae may be found any time after the fifth day.

8. Using a glass pipet, one may withdraw a small amount of fluid from the bottom of the tube; larvae will generally be alive and very active. They may be heat killed within the tube or after removal to the slide; iodine may also be used to kill larvae.

9. Examination of the larvae for typical morphologic features reveals either hookworm, *Strongyloides*, or *Trichostrongylus*.

Baermann technique. When the stools from a patient suspected of having strongyloidiasis are repeatedly negative the Baermann technique may be helpful in recovering larvae. The apparatus is designed to allow the larvae to migrate from the fecal material through several layers of damp gauze into water, which is centrifuged, thus concentrating the larvae in the bottom of the tube (Fig. 35-2). Specimens for this technique should be collected after a mild saline cathartic, not a stool softener.

PROCEDURE

1. Attach rubber tubing with pinch clamp to the bottom of a 6-inch funnel. Fill the funnel with water. Place wire gauze, with one or two layers of gauze padding, in the funnel.

2. Place a large amount of fecal material on the gauze so that it is covered with water. If the fecal matter is too firm, it should be broken up slightly.

3. Allow the apparatus to stand for at least 2 hours. Draw off 10 ml of fluid by releasing the pinch clamp, spin down in a centrifuge, and examine the sediment for larvae.

Hatching procedure for schistosome eggs

When schistosome eggs are recovered from either urine or stool, they should be carefully

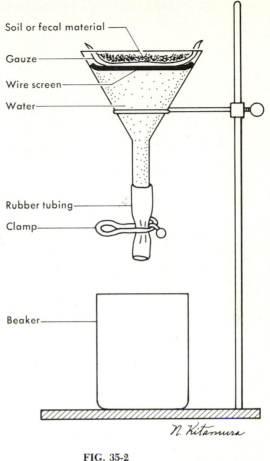

FIG. 35-2
Baermann apparatus.

examined to determine viability. The presence of living miracidia within the eggs indicates an active infection, which may require therapy. The viability of the miracidium larvae can be determined in two ways: (1) the cilia on the flame cells (primitive excretory cells) may be seen on high-dry power and are usually actively moving, and (2) the larvae may be released from the eggs with the use of a hatching procedure. The eggs usually hatch within several hours when placed in 10 volumes of dechlorinated or spring water. The eggs, which are recovered in the urine, are easily obtained from the sediment and can be examined under the microscope to determine viability.

PROCEDURE

1. Thoroughly mix a stool specimen in saline and strain through two layers of gauze.
2. Allow the material to settle, pour off the supernatant fluid, and repeat the process.
3. Decant the saline, add spring water, and pour the solution into a 500- or 1,000-ml Erlenmeyer flask or sidearm flask. Add enough fluid so that the level rises into the neck of the flask.
4. Cover the flask with foil or black paper, leaving 1 to 2 ml of fluid in the neck of the flask exposed to light.
5. Leave the flask at room temperature in subdued light for 2 to 3 hours.
6. Place a bright light at the side of the flask directly opposite and close to the surface of exposed water.
7. The miracidia will come to the illuminated portion of the fluid and can be identified with a hand lens.

Cellulose tape preparations.[10,37] *Enterobius vermicularis* is a roundworm that is worldwide in distribution. It is very common in children and is known as the **pinworm** or the seatworm. The adult female migrates from the anus during the night and deposits her eggs on the perianal area. Since the eggs are deposited outside the gastrointestinal tract, examination of a stool specimen may produce negative results. Although some laboratories use the anal swab technique, pinworm infections are most frequently diagnosed by using the cellulose tape method for egg recovery (Fig. 35-3). Occasionally the adult female may be found on the surface of a formed stool or on the cellulose tape. Specimens should be taken in the morning **before bathing** or going to the bathroom. A series of at least **four to six consecutive negative tapes** should be obtained before ruling out infection with pinworms.

PROCEDURE

1. Place a strip of cellulose tape on a microscope slide, starting ½ inch from one end and, running toward the same end, con-

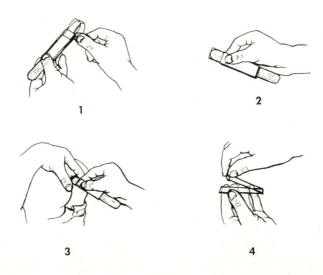

FIG. 35-3
Collection of *Enterobius vermicularis* eggs using cellulose tape method. (Illustration by Nobuko Kitamura.)

tinuing around this end across the slide; tear off the strip even with the other end. Place a strip of paper, ½ inch by 1 inch, between the slide and the tape at the end where the tape is torn flush.

2. To obtain the sample from the perianal area, peel back the tape by gripping the label, and with the tape looped adhesive side outward over a wooden tongue depressor held against the slide and extended about 1 inch beyond it, press the tape firmly against the right and left perianal folds.

3. Spread the tape back on the slide, adhesive side down.

4. Place name and date on the label. **Note:** Do not use Magic transparent tape, but regular clear cellulose tape.

5. Lift one side of the tape and apply one **small drop** of toluene or xylene; press the tape down onto the glass slide.

6. The tape is now cleared; examine under low power and low illumination. The eggs should be visible if present; they are described as football shaped with one slightly flattened side.

Identification of adult worms[31]

Most adult worms or portions of worms that are submitted to the laboratory for identification are *Acaris lumbricoides, Enterobius vermicu-* *laris,* or segments of tapeworms. The adult worms present no particular problems in identification; however, identification of the *Taenia* species tapeworms is dependent on the gravid proglottids, which contain the fully developed uterine branches. Identification as to species is based on the number of lateral uterine branches that arise from the main uterine stem in the gravid proglottids. Often the uterine branches are not clearly visible; one technique that can be used is the injection of the branches with India ink, which allows them to be easily seen and counted. With a 1-ml syringe and 25- to 26-gauge needle, India ink can be injected into the central stem or into the uterine pore, filling the uterine branches with ink. The proglottid can then be pressed between two slides and held up to the light, and the branches can be counted (see Fig. 35-38). Euparol is another mounting medium that can be used for tapeworm proglottids.[6]

Note: Caution should be used in handling proglottids of *Taenia* species, since the eggs of *T. solium* are infective for humans (Fig. 35-4).

UROGENITAL SPECIMENS

The identification of *Trichomonas vaginalis* is usually based on the examination of wet preparations of vaginal and urethral discharges and prostatic secretions. These specimens are diluted with a drop of saline and examined under low

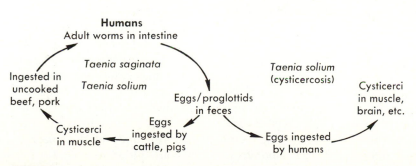

FIG. 35-4
Life cycle of *Taenia saginata* and *Taenia solium*.

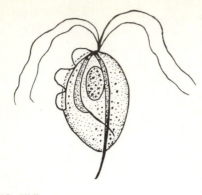

FIG. 35-5
Trichomonas vaginalis trophozoite. (Illustration by Nobuko Kitamura.)

power with reduced illumination for the presence of actively motile organisms; urine sediment can be examined in the same way. As the jerky motility of the organisms begins to diminish, it may be possible to observe the undulating membrane, particularly under high-dry power (Fig. 35-5). Stained smears are usually not necessary for the identification of this organism; often the number of false-positive and false-negative results reported on the basis of stained smears would strongly suggest the value of confirmation (i.e., observation of the motile organisms).[75]

Some studies indicate that the most sensitive method of detecting *T. vaginalis* is culture. This technique may not be the most practical, and expense may limit its availability.[90,92] Although commercial media are available, positive control strains should be used each time patient material is cultured.

SPUTUM

When sputum is submitted for examination, it should be "deep sputum" from the lower respiratory passages, not a specimen that is mainly saliva. The specimen should be collected early in the morning (before eating or brushing teeth) and immediately delivered to the laboratory. Sputum is usually examined as a saline or iodine wet mount under low and high-dry microscope power. If the quantity is sufficient, the formalin-ether sedimentation technique can be used. A very mucoid or thick sputum can be centrifuged after the addition of an equal volume of 3% sodium hydroxide. With any technique, the sediment should be carefully examined for the presence of brownish spots or "iron filings," which may be *Paragonimus* eggs.

Note: Care should be taken not to confuse *Entamoeba gingivalis,* which may be found in the mouth and might be seen in the sputum, with *E. histolytica* from a pulmonary abscess. *E. gingivalis* will contain ingested polymorphonuclear neutrophils (PMN); *E. histolytica* will not.

ASPIRATES

The diagnosis of certain parasitic infections may be based on procedures using aspirated material. These techniques include microscopic examination, animal inoculation, and culture.

Examination of aspirated material from lung or liver abscesses may reveal the presence of *Entamoeba histolytica;* however, the demonstration of these parasites is often extremely difficult for several reasons. Hepatic abscess material taken from the peripheral area, rather than the necrotic center, may reveal organisms, although they may be trapped in the thick pus and not exhibit any motility. The Amoebiasis Research Unit, Durban, South Africa, has recommended using proteolytic enzymes to free the organisms from the aspirate material.[58]

PROCEDURE
1. A minimum of two separate portions of exudate should be removed. The first portion, usually yellowish-white, seldom contains organisms. Later portions, which are reddish, are more likely to contain amebae. The best material to examine is the final portion from the wall of the abscess.
2. Ten units of the enzyme streptodornase are added to each 1 ml of thick pus; this mixture is incubated for 30 minutes at 37 C, with repeated shaking.

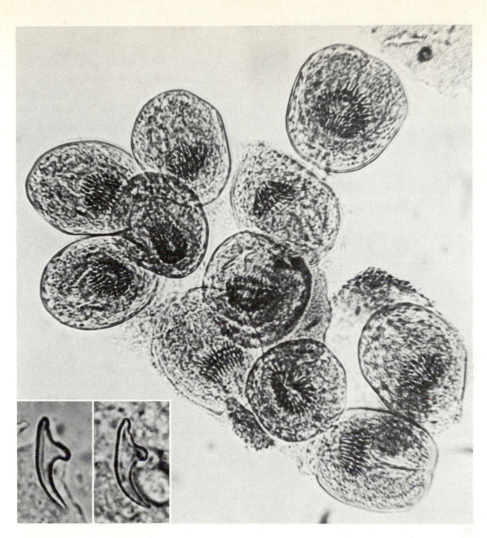

FIG. 35-6
Echinococcus granulosus, hydatid sand. *Inset*, two individual hooklets (300×; inset 1,000×).

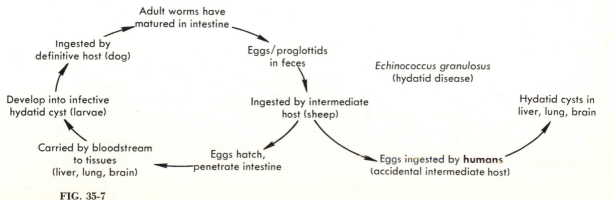

FIG. 35-7
Life cycle of *Echinococcus granulosus* (hydatid disease).

3. Centrifuge the mixture at 1,000 rpm for 5 minutes. The sediment may be examined microscopically as wet mounts or used to inoculate culture media. Some of the aspirate can be mixed directly with PVA on a slide and examined as a permanent stained smear.

Aspiration of cyst material (usually liver or lung) for the diagnosis of hydatid disease is usually performed when open surgical techniques are used for cyst removal. The aspirated fluid is submitted to the laboratory and examined for the presence of hydatid sand (scolices) or hooklets; the absence of this material does not rule out the possibility of hydatid disease, since some cysts are sterile (Figs. 35-6 and 35-7).

Material from lymph nodes, spleen, liver, bone marrow, or spinal fluid may be examined for the presence of trypanosomes or leishmanial forms. Part of the specimen should be examined as a wet preparation to demonstrate motile organisms. Impression smears can also be prepared and stained with Giemsa stain (see the section Detection of Blood Parasites). This type of material can also be cultured (specific details are presented in the section Culture Techniques).

Specimens obtained from cutaneous ulcers should be aspirated from below the ulcer bed rather than the surface; this type of sample will be more likely to contain the intracellular leishmanial organisms and will be free of bacterial contamination. A few drops of sterile saline may be introduced under the ulcer bed (through uninvolved tissue) through needle (25 gauge) and syringe (1 or 2 ml). The aspirated fluid should be examined as stained smears and should be inoculated into appropriate media (see the section Culture Techniques).

SPINAL FLUID

Cases of primary meningoencephalitis are infrequently seen, but the examination of spinal fluid may reveal the causative agent, *Naegleria fowleri* (Plate 219), if present. The spinal fluid may range from cloudy to purulent (with or without red blood cells). The cell count ranges from a few hundred to more than 20,000 white blood cells per milliliter, primarily neutrophils; the failure to find bacteria in this type of spinal fluid should alert one to the possibility of primary meningoencephalitis. Motile amebae may be found in unstained spinal fluid; however, one should be very careful not to confuse organisms with various blood and tissue cells that may also be motile. Isolation of these organisms from tissues or soil samples may be accomplished with the use of the *Acanthamoeba* medium developed by Culbertson and co-workers.[15]

The classification, transmission, virulence, and disease pathogenesis of the free-living amebic genera *Naegleria*, *Hartmannella*, and *Acanthamoeba* are receiving considerable attention at this time. The question of increasing infections has not been answered, although studies of thermally polluted or enriched waters indicate the presence of such amebae in these situations. Studies have also shown that these organisms have been recovered from asymptomatic human carriers (nasal passages, nasopharyngeal secretions) and have been implicated in chronic or subacute meningoencephalitis as well as acute primary amebic meningoencephalitis.[20,46,102]

BIOPSY MATERIAL

In some cases biopsy material may be used to confirm the diagnosis of certain parasitic infections. Most of these specimens are sent for routine tissue processing (fixation, embedding, sectioning, and staining).[86] However, fresh material may be sent directly to the laboratory for examination; it is imperative that these specimens be received immediately to prevent deterioration of any organisms present.

Pneumocystis carinii is usually classified with the sporozoa and is recognized as an important cause of pulmonary infection in patients who are immunosuppressed as a result of therapy or patients with congenital or acquired immuno-

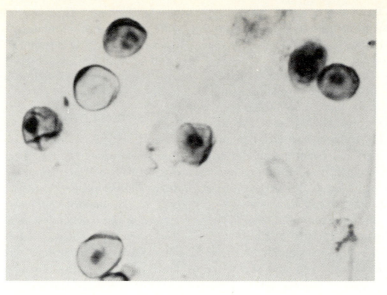

FIG. 35-8
Pneumocystis carinii from tracheobronchial aspirate; stained with methenamine silver (1,600×). (From Markell and Voge.[65])

logic disorders.[30] The organisms can be demonstrated in stained impression smears of lung material obtained by open or brush biopsy. *Pneumocystis* can be seen in stained smears of tracheobronchial aspirates, although preparations of lung tissue are more likely to reveal the organisms. Sputum specimens are generally considered unacceptable for the recovery of *Pneumocystis*. The recommended stain is Gomori's silver methenamine,[62] which clearly outlines *Pneumocystis* organisms (or various fungi) in dark brown or black (Fig. 35-8). The staining procedure is relatively complex, and positive control slides should be included with each specimen to ensure accurate interpretation of the smears.

The genus *Cryptosporidium* is a coccidial protozoan of the intestinal tract. Human cryptosporidiosis has been identified from intestinal biopsy material from patients whose immune responses were compromised, although it is uncommon in humans.[57,96,109] Cryptosporidia differ from other coccidia in that they are limited to the microvillus layer of gastrointestinal cells. Diagnosis has been based on electron microscopy studies and Giemsa-stained smears from jejunal biopsy material and routine tissue processing (paraffin embedding and sectioning). This may represent another organism that will become more widely recognized as a potential pathogen for the immunosuppressed host.

Skin biopsies for the diagnosis of cutaneous amebiasis or cutaneous leishmaniasis should be submitted for tissue processing. A portion of the tissue for the diagnosis of leishmaniasis can be teased apart with sterile needles and inoculated into appropriate culture media (see the section Culture Techniques.)

The diagnosis of onchocerciasis (*Onchocerca volvulus*) may be confirmed by the examination of "skin snips," very thin slices of skin, which are teased apart in saline to release the microfilariae.

Biopsy specimens taken from lymph nodes

are submitted for routine tissue processing; impression smears can also be prepared and stained with Giemsa stain (see the section Detection of Blood Parasites).

The diagnosis of trichinosis is usually based on clinical findings; however, confirmation may be obtained by the examination of a muscle biopsy (Plate 231). The encapsulated larvae can be seen in small pieces of fresh tissue, which are pressed between two slides and examined under low power of the microscope. At necropsy the larvae are most abundant in the diaphragm, masseter muscle, or tongue. Larvae can also be recovered from tissue that has undergone digestion in artificial digestive fluid at 37 C[31] (Fig. 35-9).

Tapeworm larvae may occasionally be recovered from a muscle specimen and should be carefully dissected from the capsules. They should then be pressed between two slides and examined under low power for the presence of a scolex with four suckers and a circle of hooks. If no hooks are present, it may be a species other than *Taenia solium*.

In some cases of schistomiasis the eggs may not be recovered in the stool or urine; however, examination of the rectal or bladder mucosa may reveal eggs of the appropriate species. The mucosal tissue should be compressed between two slides and examined under low power and decreased illumination. The eggs should be carefully examined to determine viability (see p. 473). Small pieces of tissue may also be digested with 4% sodium hydroxide for 2 to 3 hours at 60 to 80 C. The eggs, which are recovered by sedimentation or centrifugation, can be examined under the microscope.

CULTURE TECHNIQUES

Most clinical laboratories do not provide culture techniques for the diagnosis of parasitic organisms; however, the lack of culture procedures should not prevent the correct identification of the majority of parasites. Isolation of intestinal amebae yields a higher number of positive results, provided fresh specimens are received by the laboratory within specified time limits.[58] Most of the intestinal amebae do not culture as well as *Entamoeba histolytica;* however, once the organisms are established in culture, they must be speciated on the basis of morphology. Accurate identification of the organisms can be determined by the examination of permanent stained smears of culture sediment material, although the morphlogy may not appear typical from stained culture sediment.

Many different media have been developed for the culture of protozoan organisms (some of which are available commercially), and specific directions for their preparation are available in the literature. Types of media that have been

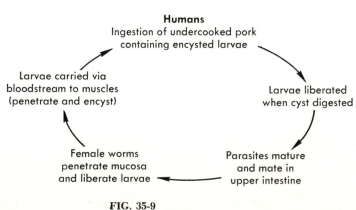

Humans
Ingestion of undercooked pork
containing encysted larvae

Larvae carried via
bloodstream to muscles
(penetrate and encyst)

Larvae liberated
when cyst digested

Female worms
penetrate mucosa
and liberate larvae

Parasites mature
and mate in
upper intestine

FIG. 35-9
Life cycle of *Trichinella spiralis*.

widely used include: amebae—Balamuth's aqueous egg yolk infusion[65] and Boeck and Drbohlav's Locke-egg-serum medium[65]; *Trichomonas vaginalis*—Lash's casein hydrolysate serum medium[31] and Feinberg medium[26]; leishmaniae and trypanosomes—Novy-Mac-Neal-Nicolle medium[31], diphasic blood agar medium (NIH method)[58] and Schneider's Drosophilia medium.[41] Techniques for the culture and isolation of other organisms (*Giardia lamblia, Plasmodium* species, and some of the helminths) are more difficult and are often reserved for research purposes.

ANIMAL INOCULATION

Most laboratories have neither the time nor facilities for animal care to provide animal inoculation procedures for the diagnosis of parasitic infections. Host specificity for many parasites also limits the kinds of laboratory animals available for these procedures. Occasionally animal studies may be requested; included here are several procedures [31]that can be used.

The hamster is the animal of choice for inoculation procedures designed to recover leishmanial organisms. After intraperitoneal or intratesticular inoculation, the infection may develop very slowly over a period of several months; in some cases a generalized infection develops more quickly, and the animal may die in several

days. Splenic and testicular aspirates should be examined for the presence of intracellular organisms; stained smears should be prepared and carefully examined with the oil immersion lens.

Mice are generally used for the isolation of *Toxoplasma gondii*, although most cases are diagnosed on clinical and serologic findings (Fig. 35-10). Mice that are inoculated through the peritoneum develop a fulminating infection that leads to death within a few days. Organisms can be easily recovered from the ascitic fluid and should be examined as stained smears. Giemsa stain is recommended for both types of inoculation studies listed above (specific staining techniques are found in the section Detection of Blood Parasites).

SERODIAGNOSIS

Although serologic procedures for the diagnosis of parasitic diseases have been available for many years, they are generally not performed by most clinical laboratories. The procedures vary both in sensitivity and specificity and at times may be difficult to interpret. The CDC offers a number of serologic procedures for diagnostic purposes, some of which are still in the experimental stages and not available elsewhere. For a detailed discussion of specific procedures, consult Kwapinski.[55] The procedures mentioned here have been found to give fairly reproducible results at CDC. Although commercial antigens and diagnostic kits are available, Kagan[58] emphasizes the variability of the results from different reagents. Diagnostic tests for 18 parasitic infections are presented in Table 35-1.

The ELISA procedure is presently being evaluated for a number of parasitic infections. A significant contribution of the ELISA method will be detection of antigen in the body fluids of patients with parasitic diseases. With purified antigens the usefulness of techniques such as radioimmunoassay, ELISA, FIAX, and defined antigen substrate spheres (DASS) will be greatly expanded.[47]

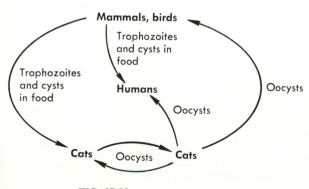

FIG. 35-10
Life cycle of *Toxoplasma gondii*.

TABLE 35-1

Immunodiagnostic tests for parasitic diseases

| Parasitic diseases | Complement fixation | Agglutination tests | | | Special tests | Indirect immunofluorescence | Immunodiffusion | Immunoelectrophoresis | Countercurrent electrophoresis | Enzyme linked immunoassay | Radioimmunoassay | Detection of circulating antigen |
		Bentonite flocculation	Indirect hemagglutination	Latex								
African Trypanosomiasis	▲		▲			■	■			■		
Amebiasis	■	■	■	■	○AC	■	■	■	■	▲		○
Ancylostomiasis	○		■	▲		○		○				
Ascariasis	■	■	■			▲	▲	○		■	○	
Chagas	■	■	■	■	■A	■	○	▲	■	▲		○
Clonorchiasis	■					○	○	○				○
Cysticercosis	▲	▲	■	▲		▲	▲	○	○	○		
Echinococcosis	■	■	■	■		■	■	■	■	○	○	
Fascioliasis	■	○	■	▲		■	■	■	■	○		
Filariasis	▲	■	■	○		■		▲	▲	▲		▲
Giardiasis						▲	○			▲		
Leishmaniasis	■		■	■	■A	■	○	○	○	▲	○	
Malaria	▲		■	▲		■	■	○	▲	■	○	▲
Paragonimiasis	■	○	○			▲	▲	○	○			○
Pneumocystosis	■			○		■						▲
Schistosomiasis	■	■	■	○	■BC	■	▲	■	▲	■	○	■
Strongyloidiasis			■			▲				○		
Toxocariasis	○	■	■			▲	■	○		■	○	○
Toxoplasmosis	■		■	■	■C	■	○			■	○	▲
Trichinellosis	■	■	■	■		■	■	▲	■	■		○

From Kagan, I.G.: personal communication.

○, reported in the literature; ■, evaluated test; ▲, experimental test; A, direct agglutination; B, circumoval precipitin test (COPT); C, FIAX automated fluoroimmunoassay.

At the present time immunodiagnostic procedures are most widely used for amebiasis, toxoplasmosis, leishmaniasis, Chagas' disease, trichinosis, schistosomiasis, cysticercosis, and hydatid disease.

Amebiasis

The sensitivity of the procedures for amebiasis depend on the type of disease present; a very low degree of sensitivity is found with sera from asymptomatic carriers, increased sensitivity from patients with amebic dysentery, and the greatest sensitivity with sera from those patients with extraintestinal disease. The complement fixation (CF) procedure has generally been replaced by the indirect hemagglutination (IHA), countercurrent electrophoresis (CEP), [105]and indirect flourescent antibody (IF) procedures; these three have approximately the same degree of sensitivity.

A new test that has been adapted to a routine diagnosis of amebiasis is the FIAX, a new flourescence technique in which the flourescence is measured in a flourometer. [47, 101]Techniques have also been developed for detection of antigen in feces. The sensitivity is reported to be quite good, although the only organism detected would be *E. histolytica*.[73,85]

Toxoplasmosis

The methylene blue dye test (MBD; Sabin-Feldman dye test) has been used for many years for the serologic diagnosis of toxoplasmosis.[57] However, this procedure is being replaced by the IHA and IF procedures, both of which are technically simple to perform and utilize a killed antigen rather than live organisms (used in the MBD test). Although all three procedures are approximately the same in terms of specificity and sensitivity, the IF procedure can be performed using specific conjugates of IgM, although interpretation of such results may be difficult and must be correlated with the patient's clinical status. Congenital infections are indicated when sera from newborns are positive with IgM conjugates.

Since two different types of antigens are used, the combination of the IF and IHA procedures allows more accurate interpretation, particularly if the titers are borderline in terms of clinical significance.

Pneumocystosis

The tests of choice for pneumocystosis are the CF and IF tests. Antigens from either infected rat or human lung tissue are used in both tests and can detect disease in approximately 85% of infected patients. A direct fluorescent antibody test has been developed for the detection of organisms in mucus and sputum smears and tissue biopsies.[59] The development of culture techniques for this organism should lead to more specific antigen production.

Leishmaniasis

The serologic procedures (IHA, IF, and CF) available for visceral leishmaniasis are quite helpful in making the diagnosis, and the IF test is now being used routinely with excellent results being reported using amastigote antigen for cutaneous leishmaniasis. The IF test is more specific that ELISA for the diagnosis of cutaneous leishmaniasis, but neither is as satisfactory as microscopic examinations.[22] Both methods were acceptable for the diagnosis of visceral leishmaniasis when promastigote forms of *L. donovani* were used as antigen.

Chagas' disease

Although both the IHA and CF procedures, are used for the diagnosis of Chagas' disease, the CF is more sensitive. A direct agglutination technique introduced by Vattuone and Yanovsky[106] in 1971 is very sensitive when used with sera from patients with acute disease; the procedure also provides good specificity in terms of cross-reactivity with leishmaniasis. The ELISA technique has been used with a reported sensitivity of 98%, and eluates of blood samples collected on filter papers can be used. The CEP and CF techniques have shown a 92% agreement; however, the sensitivity of the CEP test was less than that of the CF test. Studies also indicate that serum from patients with a positive CF for Chagas' disease contain immunoglobins that bind to cryostat sections of heart muscle (animals, including the mouse). The antibody binds to the endothelial lining of the blood vessels, the vascular musculature around the arteries, and the interstitium of striated musles; the fluorescence of the triad of tissues constitutes a positive test (essentially no false-positive tests with normal individuals or patients with other cardiovascular diseases).[14]

Trichinosis

A number of procedures are available for the diagnosis of trichinosis. The bentonite flocculation (BF) test has a high degree of specificity and is the standard procedure used at CDC; it is used to measure an increase or decrease in serum titers during the acute phase of the infection, yet it is not too sensitive and does not react with residual antibodies from past exposure to the parasite. It is important diagnostically when a series of serum samples from one patient show a rise in titers. When low titers are obtained, it is recommended that additional serologic tests (different types) may be valuable in confirming the diagnosis. The IF procedure is the most sensitive[51,56,98] and can be used to detect antibodies in pigs infected with less than one larva per gram of diaphragm muscle tissue.[51] The ELISA technique has also been found to be sensitive enough to detect low trichina infection in naturally infected pigs.[58]

Schistosomiasis

Several different tests (cholesterollecithin flocculation, BF, CF, and IF) are used for the diagnosis of schistosomiasis; however, they all share problems associated with both specificity and sensitivity. Although results with the CF procedure correlate closely with active clinical infections, Buck and Anderson[58] reported poor sensitivity with sera from infected children and from people with chronic schistosomiasis infections. There has been increased use of the IF procedure, which uses sections of adult worms for the antigen and which has proved to be the most sensitive technique (less cross-reactivity with trichina sera).

The circumoval precipitin test is used extensively in the Orient for the diagnosis of *Schistosoma japonicum*. There are also a number of studies using the ELISA technique; one study reports this test to be as sensitive as the IF and CF tests with adult worms used as antigen but indicates that the ELISA was more specific.[67]

Cysticercosis

Extensive evaluation of the diagnostic tests for cysticercosis has been difficult to achieve because of the low number of sera available from

proved human infections in the United States. Workers in south Africa reported the IHA procedure as providing 85% positive results with sera from proved cases of human infection.[76,77] Although the IHA was 100% reactive with sera from heavily infected animals, only 26% of those that were lightly infected were reactive. Biagi and associates[7] in Mexico reported the best results with the IHA. There are still difficulties with both specificity and sensitivity, and a higher positive titer with human sera may have to be selected as the standard to rule out false-positive reactions. The double-diffusion procedure, when evaluated by CDC, was found to be insensitive using both animal and human sera.[58] Cross-reactions with sera from patients infected with *Echinococcus* species, *Taenia saginata*, and *Coenurus* species have been reported.[57]

Echinococcosis

The IHA, IF, and immunoelectrophoresis (IE) procedures are considered to be the tests of choice for the diagnosis of echinococcosis. The IHA and BF procedures are routinely used at CDC, the IHA being the more sensitive test. High IHA titers usually indicate the presence of hydatid disease; however, low titers are difficult to interpret and have been found in sera from patients with collagen diseases or liver cirrhosis.[49] Hydatid cysts in the lung (sera, 33% to 50% sensitivity) are less likely to be diagnosed by serologic means than those found in the liver (sera, 82% to 86% sensitivity).[49] The IE test has been evaluated in a number of countries; however, a double-diffusion band 5 (DD5) test has been reported to be more sensitive and more specific than the IE test.[12] CEP tests have also been reported to be very specific and sensitive, and the ELISA has also been evaluated.[23]

DETECTION OF BLOOD PARASITES
Malaria

Malaria is caused by four species of the protozoan genus *Plasmodium: P. vivax, P. falciparum* (Plate 232), *P. malariae*, and *P. ovale*. Humans become infected when the sporozoites are introduced into the blood from the salivary secretion of the infected mosquito when the mosquito vector takes a blood meal. These sporozoites then leave the blood and enter the parenchymal cells of the liver, where they undergo asexual multiplication. This development in the liver prior to red cell invasion is called the preerythrocytic cycle; if further liver development takes place after red cell invasion, it is called the exoerythrocytic cycle. The length of time for the preerythrocytic cycle and the number of asexual generations vary depending on the species; however, the schizonts eventually rupture, releasing thousands of merozoites into the bloodstream, where they invade the erythrocytes.

The early forms in the red cells are called ring forms or young trophozoites. As the parasites continue to grow and feed, they become actively ameboid within the red cell. They feed on hemoglobin, which is incompletely metabolized; the residue left is called malarial pigment and is a compound of hematin and protein (hemozoin).

During the next phase of the cycle the chromatin (nuclear material) becomes fragmented throughout the organism, and the cytoplasm begins to divide, each portion being arranged with a fragment of nuclear material. These forms are called mature schizonts and are composed of individual merozoites. The infected red cell then ruptures, releasing the merozoites and also metabolic products into the bloodstream. If large numbers of red cells rupture simultaneously, a malarial paroxysm may result from the amount of toxic materials released into the bloodstream. In the early stages of infection or in a mixed infection with two species, rupture of the red cells is usually not synchronous; consequently, the fever may be continuous or daily rather than intermittent. After several days, a 48- or 72-hour periodicity is usually established.

After several generations of erythrocytic schizogony, the production of gametocytes begins. These forms are derived from merozoites, which do not undergo schizogony but continue to grow and form the male and female gametocytes, which circulate in the bloodstream. When the mature gametocytes are ingested by the appropriate mosquito vector, the sexual cycle is initiated within the mosquito, with the eventual production of the sporozoites, the infective stage for humans (Fig. 35-11).

The asexual and sexual forms just described circulate in the human bloodstream in three species of *Plasmodium*. However, in *P. falciparum* infections, as the parasite continues to grow the red cell membrane becomes sticky, and the cells tend to adhere to the endothelial lining of the capillaries of the internal organs; thus, only the ring forms and crescent-shaped gametocytes occur in the peripheral blood. Interference with normal blood flow in these vessels gives rise to additional problems, which are responsible for the different clinical manifestations of this type of malaria.

Laboratory diagnosis of malaria

Malaria is one of the few acute parasitic infections that can be life threatening. For this reason any laboratory that offers this type of diagnostic service must be willing to provide technical expertise on a 24-hour basis, 7 days per week.

The definitive diagnosis of malaria is based on the demonstration of the parasites in the blood. Two types of blood films are used. The **thick film** allows the examination of a larger amount of blood and is used as a screening procedure[28]; the **thin film** allows speciation of the parasite.

Blood films are usually prepared when the patient is admitted; samples should be taken at intervals of 6 to 18 hours for at least 3 successive days. Two-hundred miscroscopic fields should be examined before a film is signed out as negative. If possible, the smears should be prepared from blood obtained from the finger or earlobe; the blood should flow freely. If patient contact is not possible and the quality of the submitted

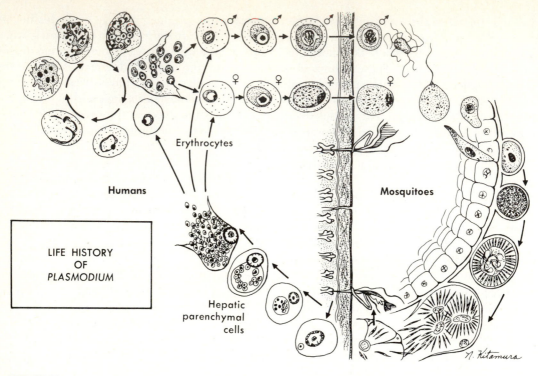

FIG. 35-11

Life cycle of *Plasmodium*. (Adapted from Wilcox.[114]) (Illustration by Nobuko Kitamura.)

slides may be poor, a tube of fresh blood should be requested (EDTA) anticoagulant is recommended) and smears prepared immediately after the blood is received.

To prepare the thick film place two or three small drops of fresh blood (no anticoagulant) on an alcohol-cleaned slide. With the corner of another slide, and using a circular motion, mix the drops and spread the blood over an area about 2 cm in diameter. Continue stirring for about 30 seconds to prevent formation of fibrin strands, which may obscure the parasites after staining. If the blood is too thick or any grease remains on the slide, the blood will flake off during staining. Allow the film to air dry (room temperature) in a dust-free area. Never apply heat to a thick film, since heat will fix the blood, causing the red blood cells to remain intact during staining; the result is stain retention and subse-

quent inability to identify any parasites present.

The thin blood film is used primarily for specific parasite identification, although the number of organisms per field is much reduced compared with the thick film (see Table 35-2 and Plates 248 to 254). The thin film is prepared exactly as one used for the differential blood count. After the film has air dried (do not apply heat), it may be stained. The necessity for fixation prior to staining depends on the stain selected.

Staining blood films.[88,89] For accurate identification of blood parasites, it is very important that a laboratory develop proficiency in the use of at least one good staining method. As a general rule, blood films should be stained as soon as possible, since prolonged storage results in stain retention.

TABLE 35-2

Microscopic identification of plasmodia of humans in Giemsa-stained thin blood smears[28,108,111]

	Plasmodium vivax	*Plasmodium malariae*	*Plasmodium falciparum*	*Plasmodium ovale*
Appearance of parasitized red blood cells: size and shape	1½ to 2 times larger than normal; oval to round	Normal shape; size may be normal or slightly smaller	Both normal	60% of cells larger than normal and oval; 20% have irregular, frayed edges
Schuffner's dots (eosinophilic stippling)	Usually present in all cells except early ring forms	None	None; occasionally commalike red dots are present (Maurer's dots)	Present in all stages including early ring forms, dots may be larger and darker than in *P. vivax*
Color of cytoplasm	Decolorized, pale	Normal	Normal, bluish tinge at times	Decolorized, pale
Multiple infections	Occasional	Rare	Common	Occasional
All developmental stages present in peripheral blood	All stages present	Ring forms few, as ring stage brief; mostly growing and mature trophozoites and schizonts	Young ring forms and no older stages; few gametocytes	All stages present
Appearance of parasite: young trophozoite (early ring form)	Ring is ⅓ diameter of cell; cytoplasmic circle around vacuole; heavy chromatin dot	Ring often smaller than in *P. vivax*, occupying ⅙ of cell; heavy chromatin dot; vacuole at times "filled in"; pigment forms early	Delicate, small ring with small chromatin dot (frequently 2); scanty cytoplasm around small vacuoles; sometimes at edge of red cell (appliqué form) or filamentous slender form; may have multiple rings per cell	Ring is larger and more ameboid than in *P. vivax*, otherwise similar to *P. vivax*
Growing trophozoite	Multishaped irregular ameboid parasite; streamers of cytoplasm close to large chromatin dot; vacuole retained until close to maturity; increasing amounts of brown pigment	Nonameboid rounded or band-shaped solid forms; chromatin may be hidden by coarse dark brown pigment	Heavy ring forms fine pigment grains	Ring shape maintained until late in development

Continued.

TABLE 35-2

Microscopic identification of plasmodia of humans in Giemsa-stained thin blood smears[28,108,111]—cont'd

	Plasmodium vivax	*Plasmodium malariae*	*Plasmodium falciparum*	*Plasmodium ovale*
Mature trophozoite	Irregular ameboid mass; 1 or more small vacuoles retained until schizont stage; fills almost entire cell; fine brown pigment	Vacuoles disappear early; cytoplasm compact, oval, band shaped, or nearly round, almost filling cell; chromatin may be hidden by peripheral coarse dark brown pigment	Not seen in peripheral blood (except in severe infections); development of all phases following ring form occurs in capillaries of viscera	Compact; vacuoles disappear; pigment dark brown, less than in *P. malariae*
Schizont (presegmenter)	Progressive chromatin division; cytoplasmic bands containing clumps of brown pigment	Similar to *P. vivax* except smaller, darker, larger pigment granules peripheral or central	Not seen in peripheral blood (see above)	Smaller and more compact than *P. vivax*
Mature schizont	16 (12 to 24) merozoites, each with chromatin and cytoplasm, filling entire red cell, which can hardly be seen	8 (6 to 12) merozoites in rosettes or irregular clusters filling normal-sized cells, which can hardly be seen; central arrangement of brown-green pigment	Not seen in peripheral blood (rare exceptions)	¾ of cells occupied by 8 (8 to 12) merozoites in rosettes or irregular clusters

Macrogametocyte	Rounded or oval homogeneous cytoplasm; diffuse delicate light brown pigment throughout parasite; eccentric compact chromatin	Similar to *P. vivax*, but fewer in number, pigment darker and more coarse	Sex differentiation difficult; "crescent" or "sausage" shapes characteristic; may appear in "showers"; black pigment near chromatin dot, which is often central	Smaller than *P. vivax*
Microgametocyte	Large pink to purple chromatin mass surrounded by pale or colorless halo; evenly distributed pigment	Similar to *P. vivax*, but fewer in number, pigment darker and more coarse	See above	Smaller than *P. vivax*
Main criteria	Large, pale red cell; trophozoite irregular; pigment usually present; Schuffner's dots not always present; several phases of growth seen in one smear; gametocytes appear early	Red cell normal in size and color; trophozoites compact, stain usually intense, band forms not always seen; coarse pigment; no stippling of red cells; gametocytes appear late	Development following ring stage takes place in blood vessels in internal organs; delicate ring forms and crescent-shaped gametocytes are only forms normally seen in peripheral blood	Red cell enlarged, oval, with fimbriated edges; Schuffner's dots seen in all stages

The stains that are generally used are of two types. One has the fixative in combination with the staining solution, so that both fixation and staining occur at the same time. Wright stain is an example of this type of staining solution. Giemsa stain represents the other type of staining solution, in which the fixative and stain are separate; thus, the thin film must be fixed prior to staining. There are also methods available for the identification of malarial parasites with the use of acridine orange and other DNA-binding dyes, the smears being examined using fluorescence microscopy.[43,87]

When slides are removed from either type of staining solution, they should be dried in a vertical position. After being air dried, they may be examined under oil immersion by placing the oil directly on the uncovered blood film.

Specimens may be submitted from patients with *Plasmodium falciparum* infections who do not yet have gametocytes in the blood. Consequently, a low-level parasitemia with delicate ring forms might be missed without extensive oil immersion examination of the blood films (at least 200 oil immersion fields).[13]

Giemsa stain. Giemsa stain is available commercially as a concentrated stock solution or as a powder for those who wish to make their own stain; there seems to be very little difference between the two preparations.

REAGENTS

1. Stock Giemsa stain:

Giemsa stain powder, certified	600 mg
Methanol, absolute and certified neutral, acetone free	50 ml
Glycerine, neutral, certified	50 ml

Grind well small portions of stain and glycerine in mortar and collect mixtures in a 500- or 1,000-ml flask until all measured material is mixed. Stopper flask with cotton plug, cover with heavy paper, place in 55 to 60 C water bath for 2 hours, making sure that the water reaches the level of the stain. Shake gently at ½-hour intervals. Allow to cool; add alcohol. Use a portion of the measured alcohol to wash out the mortar and add to the flask. Store in brown bottle. Allow to stand for 2 to 3 weeks. Filter before use.

2. 10% stock solution of Triton X-100:

Triton X-100	10 ml
Distilled water	100 ml

3. Stock buffers:

   a. Disodium phosphate buffer:

Na_2HPO_4 anhydrous	9.5 g
Distilled water	1,000 ml

   b. Sodium acid phosphate buffer:

$NaH_2PO_4H_2O$	9.2 g
Distilled water	1,000 ml

4. Buffered water: pH range 7.0 to 7.2; check with pH meter before use.

Disodium phosphate buffer	61 ml
Sodium acid phosphate buffer	39 ml
Distilled water	900 ml

5. Triton–buffered water solutions:
   a. 0.01% Triton–buffered water:

Stock 10% aqueous Triton X-100	1 ml
Buffered water	1,000 ml

   Use for thin blood films or combination of thin and thick blood films.

   b. 0.1% Triton–buffered water:

Stock 10% aqueous Triton X-100	10 ml
Buffered water	1,000 ml

   Use for thick blood films.

PROCEDURE FOR STAINING THIN FILMS

1. Fix blood films in absolute methyl alcohol (acetone free) for 30 seconds.
2. Allow slides to air dry.
3. Immerse slides in a solution of 1 part Giemsa stock (commercial liquid stain or stock prepared from powder) to 10 to 50 parts of Triton–buffered water (pH 7.0 to 7.2). Stain 10 to 60 minutes (see note below). Fresh working stain should be prepared from stock solution each day.

4. Dip slides briefly in Triton–buffered water.

5. Drain thoroughly in vertical position and allow to air dry.

Note: A good general rule for stain dilution versus staining time is that if dilution is 1:20, stain for 20 minutes; if 1:30, stain for 30 minutes; and so forth. However, a series of stain dilutions and staining times should be tried to determine the best dilution/time for each batch of stock stain.

PROCEDURE FOR STAINING THICK FILMS. The procedure to be followed for thick films is the same as for thin films, except that the first two steps are omitted. If the slide has a thick film at one end and a thin film at the other, fix only the thin portion, and then stain both parts of the film simultaneously.

RESULTS. Giemsa stain colors the components of blood as follows: erythrocytes, pale gray-blue; nuclei of white blood cells, purple and pale purple cytoplasm; eosinophilic granules, bright purple-red; neutrophilic granules, deep pink-purple.

There have been many studies using immunodiagnostic procedures for the diagnosis of malaria[44,54,64,91,103,107]; however, these procedures are not routinely performed in most laboratories. Sulzer and Wilson[99] have reported the use of thick-smear antigens prepared from washed parasitized blood cells. This type of antigen is used in the IF procedure, which has a 95% sensitivity and a false-positive rate of 1% at a titer of 1:16.[100] The IHA has also been used and evaluated by a number of workers.[18,68,78,94]

In some areas of the world where *P. falciparum* is endemic, there is also a high incidence of hemoglobin S (HbS), thalassemia, and glucose-6-phosphate dehydrogenase (G-6-PD) deficiency carriers. The young heterozygous carrier of HbS gains some protection against *P. falciparum*.[1] Apparently, G-6-PD deficiency[2] and thalassemia[11] are also associated with increased resistance.

Miller and co-workers[70] reported that Duffy-positive human erythrocytes are easily infected with *P. knowlesi;* however, Duffy-negative human erythrocytes are resistant to infection. They suggest that the resistance of many west Africans and approximately 70% of American blacks to *P. vivax* may be related to the high incidence of Duffy-negative erythrocytes in these groups. In east Africa, where there is a higher incidence of Duffy-positive red cells, *P. vivax* is more common.

Babesiosis

Babesia are tick-borne (can be transmitted via a blood transfusion) sporozoan parasites, which have generally been considered parasites of animals (Texas cattle fever) rather than humans.[45] However, there are now a number of documented human cases, some infections occurring

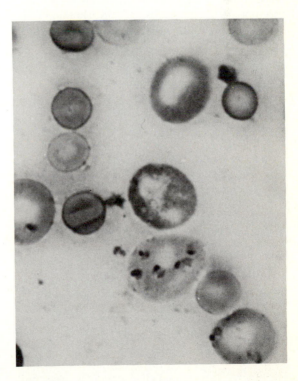

FIG. 35-12
Babesia in red blood cells. (Photomicrograph by Zane Price. From Markell and Voge.[65])

in splenectomized patients and others in patients with intact spleens.[29,65,80] *Babesia* organisms infect the red blood cells and appear as pleomorphic ringlike structures when stained with any of the recommended stains used for blood films (Fig. 35-12). They may be confused with the ring forms in *Plasmodium* infections; however, in a *Babesia* infection there are often many rings (four or five) per red cell, and the individual rings are quite small as compared with those found in malaria infections.[39,40]

Hemoflagellates

Hemoflagellates are blood and tissue flagellates, two genera of which are medically important for humans: *Leishmania* and *Trypanosoma*. Some species may circulate in the bloodstream or at times may be present in lymph nodes or muscle. Other species tend to parasitize the reticuloendothelial cells of the hemopoietic organs. The hemoflagellates of human beings

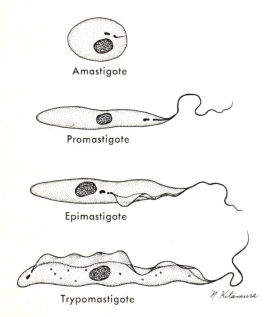

Amastigote

Promastigote

Epimastigote

Trypomastigote

N. Kitamura

FIG. 35-13
Characteristic stages of species of *Leishmania* and *Trypanosoma* in human and insect hosts. (Illustration by Nobuko Kitamura.)

have four morphologic types (Fig. 35-13): amastigote (leishmanial form, or Leishman-Donovan body), promastigote (leptomonal form), epimastigote (crithidial form), and trypomastigote (trypanosomal form).

The amastigote form is an intracellular parasite in the cells of the reticuloendothelial system and is oval, measuring approximately 1½ to 5µm, and contains a nucleus and kinetoplast. Species of the genus *Leishmania* usually exist as the amastigote form in humans and in the promastigote form in the insect host. The life cycle is essentially the same for all three species, and the clinical manifestations vary depending on the species involved. As the vector takes a blood meal, the promastigote form is introduced into a human, thus initiating the infection. Depending on the species, the parasites then move from the site of the bite to the organs of the reticuloendothelial system (liver, spleen, bone marrow) or to the macrophages of the skin.

Species based on clinical grounds are morphologically the same; however, there are differences in serologies and in growth requirements for culture. There is a great deal of biologic variation among the many strains that make up these groups. *Leishmania tropica* causes oriental sore or cutaneous leishmaniasis of the Old World; *L. braziliensis* causes mucocutaneous leishmaniasis of the New World; and *L. donovani* causes visceral leishmaniasis (Dumdum fever, or kala azar) (Fig. 35-14, *A*, and Plate 234). Additional species have been delineated based on buoyant density of kinetoplast DNA, isoenzyme patterns, and serologic testing.

In tissue impression smears or sections *Histoplasma capsulatum* must be differentiated from the Leishman-Donovan (L-D) bodies. *H. capsulatum* does not have a kinetoplast and stains with both periodic acid–Schiff (PAS) stain and Gomori methenamine silver stain, neither of which stains L-D bodies.

Diagnosis of leishmanial organisms is based on the demonstration of the L-D bodies or the recovery of the promastigote culture stages.

Three species of trypanosomes are pathogenic for humans: *Trypanosoma gambiense* causes west African sleeping sickness; *Trypanosoma rhodesiense* causes east African sleeping sickness; and *Trypanosoma cruzi* causes South American trypanosomiasis, or Chagas' disease (Plate 233). The first two species are morphologically similar and produce African sleeping sickness (Fig. 35-14, *B*), an illness characterized by both acute and chronic stages. In the acute stage of the disease the organisms can usually be found in the peripheral blood or lymph node aspirates. As the disease progresses to the chronic stage the organisms can be found in the CSF (comatose stage: "sleeping sickness"). *T. rhodesiense* produces a more severe infection, usually resulting in death within 1 year.

In the early stages of infection with *T. cruzi*, the trypomastigote forms appear in the blood but do not multiply (Fig. 35-15, *A*). They then

A
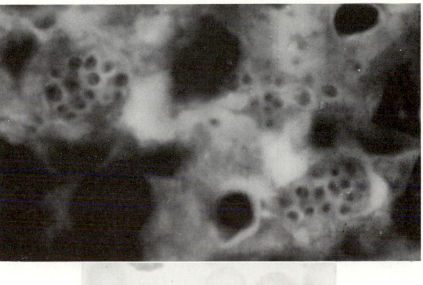

B
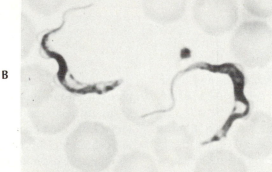

FIG. 35-14
A, *Leishmania donovani* parasites in Küpffer cells of liver (2,000×). **B,** *Trypanosoma gambiense* in blood film (1,600×).

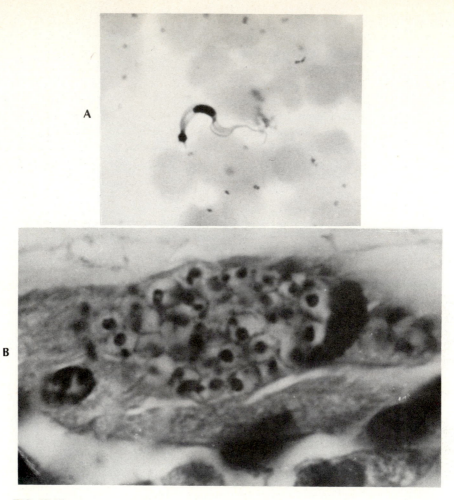

FIG. 35-15
A, *Trypanosoma cruzi* in blood film (1,600×). **B,** *Trypanosoma cruzi* parasites in cardiac muscle (2,500×). (From Markell and Voge.[65])

invade the endothelial or tissue cells and begin to divide, producing many L-D bodies, which are most often found in cardiac muscle (Fig. 35-15, *B*). When these forms are liberated into the blood, they transform into the trypomastigote forms, which are then carried to other sites, where tissue invasion again occurs.

Diagnosis of the organisms is based on demonstration of the parasites, most often on wet unstained or stained blood films. Both thick and thin films should be examined; these can be prepared from peripheral blood or buffy coat. The sediment recovered from CSF can also be examined for the presence of trypomastigotes. Specific techniques for culture, animal inoculation, handling of aspirate and biopsy material, and serologic procedures are presented in earlier sections of this chapter.

Another technique often used in endemic areas for the diagnosis of Chagas' disease is xeno-

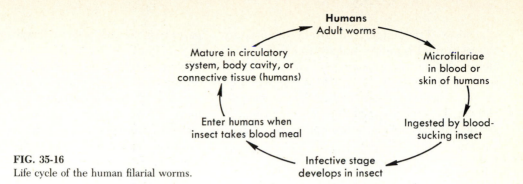

FIG. 35-16
Life cycle of the human filarial worms.

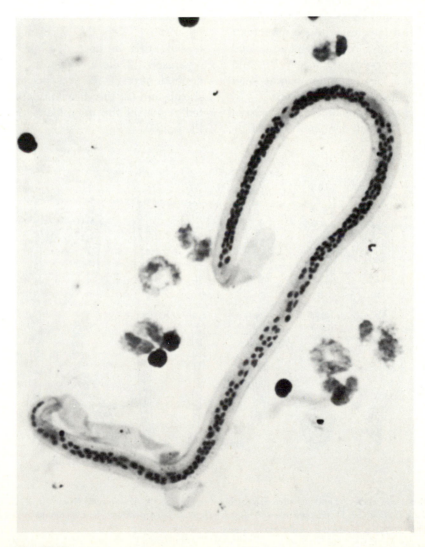

FIG. 35-17
Microfilaria of *Wuchereria bancrofti* in thick blood film. (From Markell and Voge.[65])

diagnosis. Triatomids, the insect vector, are raised in the laboratory and are free from infection with *T. cruzi*. These insects are allowed to feed on the blood of an individual suspected of having Chagas' disease, and after 2 weeks the intestinal contents are checked for the presence of the epimastigote forms. For additional information consult Maekelt.[63]

Filariae

The filarial worms are long, thin nematodes, that inhabit parts of the lymphatic system and the subcutaneous and deep connective tissues (Fig. 35-16). Most species produce microfilariae, which can be found in the peripheral blood; two species, *Onchocerca volvulus* and *Dipetalonema streptocerca,* produce microfilariae found in the subcutaneous tissues and dermis.

Diagnosis of filarial infections is often based on clinical grounds, but demonstration of the parasite is the only accurate means of confirming the diagnosis (Fig. 35-17). Fresh blood films may be prepared; actively moving microfilariae can be observed in a preparation of this type. If the patient has a light infection, thick blood films can be prepared and stained. The Knott concentration procedure[53] and the membrane filtration technique[16,17] may also be helpful in recovering the organisms. Microfilariae of some strains tend to exhibit nocturnal periodicity; thus, the time the blood is drawn may be critical in demonstrating the parasite. The microfilariae of *O. volvulus* and *D. streptocerca* are found in "skin snips," very thin slices of skin, which are teased apart in normal saline to release the organisms. Differentiation of the species is dependent on (1) the presence or absence of the sheath and (2) the distribution of nuclei in the tail region of the microfilaria (Fig. 35-18, and Plate 235).

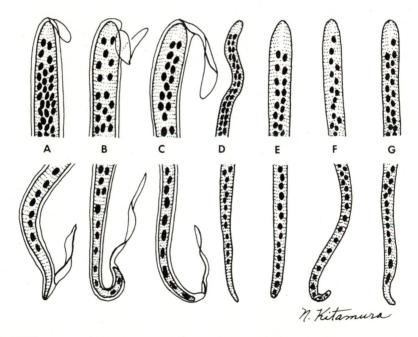

FIG. 35-18
Anterior and posterior ends of microfilariae found in humans. **A,** *Wuchereria bancrofti.* **B,** *Brugia malayi.* **C,** *Loa loa.* **D,** *Onchocerca volvulus.* **E,** *Dipetalonema perstans.* **F,** *Dipetalonema streptocerca.* **G,** *Mansonella ozzardi.*

IDENTIFICATION OF ANIMAL PARASITES

The animal parasites of humans are found in five major groups of phyla: the Protozoa; the Platyhelminthes, or flatworms; the Nematoda, or roundworms; the Acanthocephala, or thorny-headed worms; and the Arthropoda, which include ticks, mites, spiders, insects, and various other groups. The Protozoa, Platyhelmenthes, and Nematoda phyla are discussed here, since they contain the majority of organisms parasitic for humans. Within each phylum are various classes, which can be subdivided into orders and further subdivided into families with their own genera and species. These subdivisions are based on morphologic criteria; thus, identification of the organisms requires a certain knowledge of basic structures and their definitions.

Intestinal protozoa

The protozoa are unicellular organisms, most of which are microscopic. They possess a number of specialized organelles, which are responsible for life functions and which allow further division of the group into classes.

The class Sarcodina contains the organisms that move by means of cytoplasmic protrusions called pseudopodia. Included in this group are free-living organisms, as well as nonpathogenic and pathogenic organisms found in the intestinal tract and other areas of the body.

The Mastigophora, or flagellates, contain specialized locomotor organelles called flagella: long, thin cytoplasmic extensions that may vary in number and position depending on the species. Different genera may live in the intestinal tract, the bloodstream, or various tissues. The blood- and tissue-dwelling flagellates are discussed in the section Detection of Blood Parasites.

The class Ciliata contains a number of species that move by means of cilia, short extensions of cytoplasm that cover the surface of the organism. This group contains only one organism that infects humans: *Balantidium coli* infects the intestinal tract and may produce severe symptoms.

Members of the class Sporozoa are found in the blood and other tissues and have a complex life cycle that involves both sexual and asexual generations. The four species of *Plasmodium*, the cause of malaria, are found in this group and are discussed in the section Detection of Blood Parasites. Members of the genera *Isospora* and *Cryptosporidium* are found in the intestinal mucosa.

The majority of the intestinal protozoa live in the colon, with the exception of the flagellate *Giardia lamblia* and the coccidian parasites *Isospora belli* and *Cryptosporidium*, which are found in the small intestine. *I. belli* is the only protozoan that is an obligate tissue parasite in the intestinal tract and is passed in the stool as oocysts; the other members of the group, with the exception of *Cryptosporidium*, exist in the intestinal tract in the trophozoite or cyst stages. The important characteristics of the intestinal protozoa are found in Tables 35-3 to 35-7. The clinically important intestinal protozoa are generally considered to be *Entamoeba histolytica*, *Dientamoeba fragilis*, *Giardia lamblia*, *Isospora belli*, *Cryptosporidium*, and *Balantidium coli*. *E. histolytica* is the most important species and may invade other tissues of the body, resulting in severe symptoms and possible death. *D. fragilis* has been associated with diarrhea, nausea, vomiting, and other nonspecific abdominal compliants. *G. lamblia* is probably the most common protozoan organism found in persons in this country and is known to cause symptoms ranging from mild diarrhea, flatulence, and vague abdominal pains to steatorrhea and a typical malabsorption syndrome. There have been a number of documented waterborne/foodborne outbreaks during the past several years, and the beaver has been implicated as an animal reservoir host for *G. lamblia*. It is speculated that other animals may be involved as well. With present improved culture techniques and the

Text continued on p. 503.

TABLE 35-3

Morphologic criteria used to identify intestinal protozoa[10,31,65]: amebae, trophozoites

	Entamoeba histolytica	Entamoeba hartmanni	Entamoeba coli	Endolimax nana	Iodamoeba bütschlii
Size (diameter or length)*	12 to 60 μm; usual range, 15 to 20 μm; invasive forms may be over 20 μm	5 to 12 μm; usual range, 8 to 10 μm	15 to 50 μm; usual range, 20 to 25 μm	6 to 12 μm; usual range, 8 to 10 μm	8 to 20 μm; usual range, 12 to 15 μm
Motility	Progressive with hyaline, fingerlike pseudopods, motility may be rapid	Usually nonprogressive	Sluggish, nondirectional, with blunt pseudopods	Sluggish, usually nonprogressive	Sluggish, usually nonprogressive
Number of nuclei	Difficult to see in unstained preparations; usually not seen; 1	Usually not seen in unstained preparations; 1	Often visible in unstained preparations; 1	Occasionally visible in unstained preparations; 1	Usually not visible in unstained preparations; 1
Nucleus					
Peripheral chromatin (stained)	Fine granules, uniform in size, usually evenly distributed; may have beaded appearance	Nucleus may stain more darkly than E. histolytica, although morphology is similar; chromatin may appear as solid ring rather than beaded	May be clumped and unevenly arranged on membrane; may also appear as solid, dark ring with no beads or clumps	No peripheral chromatin	No peripheral chromatin
Karyosome (stained)	Small, usually compact; centrally located but may also be eccentric	Usually small and compact; may be centrally located or eccentric	Large, not compact; may or may not be eccentric; may be diffuse and darkly stained	Large, irregularly shaped; may appear "blotlike"; many nuclear variations common	Large, may be surrounded by refractile granules that are difficult to see
Cytoplasm					
Appearance (stained)	Finely granular, "ground-glass" appearance; clear differentiation of ectoplasm and endoplasm; if present, vacuoles usually small	Finely granular	Granular with little differentiation into ectoplasm and endoplasm; usually vacuolated	Granular, vacuolated	Coarsely granular; may be highly vacuolated
Inclusions (stained)	Noninvasive organsim may contain bacteria; presence of red blood cells diagnostic	May contain bacteria; no red blood cells	Bacteria, yeast, other debris	Bacteria	Bacteria, yeast, other debris

*These sizes refer to wet preparation measurements. Organisms on a permanent stained smear may be 1 to 1½ μm smaller because of artificial shrinkage

TABLE 35-4

Morphologic criteria used to identify intestinal protozoa[10,31,65]: amebae, cysts

	Entamoeba histolytica	*Entamoeba hartmanni*	*Entamoeba coli*	*Endolimax nana*	*Iodamoeba bütschlii*
Size*	10 to 20 µm; usual range, 12 to 15 µm	5 to 10 µm; usual range, 6 to 8 µm	10 to 35 µm; usual range, 15 to 25 µm	5 to 10 µm; usual range, 6 to 8 µm	5 to 20 µm; usual range, 10 to 12 µm
Shape	Usually spherical	Usually spherical	Usually spherical; occasionally oval, triangular, or other shapes; may be distorted on stained slide if fixation poor	Spherical, ovoidal, or ellipsoidal	Ovoidal, ellipsoidal, or other shapes
Number of nuclei	Mature cyst, 4; immature, 1 or 2 nuclei may be seen; nuclear characteristics difficult to see on wet preparation	Mature cyst, 4; immature, 1 or 2 nuclei may be seen; 2 nucleated cysts very common	Mature cyst, 8; occasionally 16 or more nuclei may be seen; immature cysts with 2 or more nuclei occasionally seen	Mature cyst, 4; immature cysts, 2 (very rarely seen and may resemble cysts of *Enteromonas hominis*)	Mature cyst, 1
Nucleus					
Peripheral chromatin (stained)	Peripheral chromatin present; fine, uniform granules, evenly distributed; nuclear characteristics may not be as clearly visible as in trophozoite	Fine granules evenly distributed on membrane; nuclear characteristics may be difficult to see	Coarsely granular and may be clumped and unevenly arranged on membrane; nuclear characteristics not as clearly defined as in trophozoite; may resemble *E. histolytica*	No peripheral chromatin	No peripheral chromatin
Karyosome (stained)	Small, compact, usually centrally located	Small, compact, usually centrally located	Large, may or may not be compact or eccentric; occasionally appears to be centrally located	Smaller than karyosome seen in trophozoite, but generally larger than those of genus *Entamoeba*	Large, usually eccentric refractile granules may be on one side of karyosome ("basket nucleus")

*See footnote to Table 35-3.

Continued.

TABLE 35-4

Morphologic criteria used to identify intestinal protozoa[10,31,65]: amebae, cysts—cont'd

	Entamoeba histolytica	Entamoeba hartmanni	Entamoeba coli	Endolimax nana	Iodamoeba bütschlii
Cytoplasm Chromatoidal bodies (stained)	May be present; bodies usually elongate with blunt, rounded, smooth edges	Often present; bodies elongate with blunt, rounded, smooth edges	May be present (less frequently than E. histolytica); splinter shaped with rough, pointed ends	No chromatoidal bodies present; occasionally small granules or inclusions seen; also, fine linear structures may be faintly visible on well-stained smears	No chromatoidal bodies present; occasionally small granules may be present
Glycogen (stained)	May be diffuse or absent in mature cyst; clumped chromatin mass may be present in early cysts (stains reddish-brown with iodine)	May or may not be present, as in E. histolytica	May be diffuse or absent in mature cysts; clumped mass occasionally seen in immature cysts (stains reddish-brown in iodine)	Usually diffuse if present (stains reddish-brown in iodine)	Large, compact, well-defined mass (stains reddish-brown in iodine)

TABLE 35-5

Morphologic criteria used to identify intestinal protozoa[10,31,65]: flagellates, trophozoites

	Dientamoeba fragilis	*Trichomonas hominis*	*Giardia lamblia*	*Chilomastix mesnili*	*Enteromonas hominis*	*Retortamonas intestinalis*
Shape and size	Shaped like amebae; 5 to 15 μm; usual range, 9 to 12 μm	Pear shaped; 8 to 20 μm; usual range, 11 to 12 μm	Pear shaped; 10 to 20 μm; usual range, 12 to 15 μm	Pear shaped; 6 to 24 μm; usual range, 10 to 15 μm	Oval; 4 to 10 μm; usual range, 8 to 9 μm	Pear shaped or oval; 4 to 9 μm; usual range, 6 to 7 μm
Motility	Usually nonprogressive; pseudopodia angular, serrated, or broad lobed and almost transparent	Jerky and rapid	"Falling leaf." Organisms may be trapped in mucus; only flagella flutter seen.	Stiff, rotary	Jerky	Jerky
Number of nuclei	Percentage may vary, but approximately 40% of organisms have 1 nucleus and 60% 2 nuclei; not visible in unstained preparations; no peripheral chromatin, karyosome composed of cluster of 4 to 8 granules	Not visible in unstained mounts; 1	Not visible in unstained mounts; 2	Not visible in unstained mounts; 1	Not visible in unstained mounts; 1	Not visible in unstained mounts; 1
Number of flagella (usually difficult to see)	No visible flagella	3 to 5 anterior, 1 posterior	4 lateral, 2 ventral, 2 caudal	3 anterior, 1 in cytostome	3 anterior, 1 posterior	1 anterior, 1 posterior
Other features	Cytoplasm finely granular and may be vacuolated with ingested bacteria, yeasts, and other debris	Axostyle (slender rod) protrudes beyond posterior end and may be visible; undulating membrane extends length of body	Sucking disk occupying ⅓ to ½ of ventral surface; pear-shaped front view, spoon-shaped side view	Prominent cytostome extending ⅓ to ½ length of body; spiral groove across ventral surface	One side of body flattened; posterior flagellum extends free posteriorly or laterally	Prominent cytostome extending approximately ½ length of body

TABLE 35-6

Morphologic criteria used to identify intestinal protozoa[10,31,65]: flagellates, cysts

	Dientamoeba fragilis	Trichomonas hominis	Giardia lamblia	Chilomastix mesnili	Enteromonas hominis	Retortamonas intestinalis
Shape	No cyst	No cyst	Oval, ellipsoidal, or may appear round	Lemon shaped with anterior hyaline knob	Elongate or oval	Pear shaped or slightly lemon shaped
Size*			8 to 9 µm; usual range, 11 to 12 µm	6 to 10 µm; usual range, 8 to 9 µm	6 to 8 µm; usual range, 4 to 10 µm	4 to 7 µm; usual range 4 to 9 µm
Number of nuclei			Not distinct in unstained preparations; usually located at one end; 4	Not visible in unstained preparations; 1	Usually 2 lying at opposite ends of cyst; not visible in unstained mounts; 1 to 4	Not visible in unstained mounts; 1
Other features			Longitudinal fibers in cyst may be visible in unstained preparations; deep-staining fibers usually lie across longitudinal fibers; there is often shrinkage, and cytoplasm pulls away from cyst wall; may also be "halo" effect around outside of cyst wall	Cytostome with supporting fibrils, usually visible in stained preparation; curved fibril along side of cytostome usually referred to as "shepherd's crook"	Resembles *E. nana* cyst; fibrils or flagella usually not seen	Resembles *Chilomastix* cyst; shadow outline of cytostome with supporting fibrils extending above nucleus

*See footnote to Table 35-3.

TABLE 35-7

Morphologic criteria used to identify intestinal protozoa[10,31,65]: ciliates and coccidia

	Balantidium coli		*Isospora belli*
	Trophozoite	**Cyst**	
Shape and size*	Ovoid with tapering anterior end; 50 to 100 μm in length, 40 to 70 μm wide, usual range, 40 to 50 μm	Spherical or oval; 50 to 70 μm; usual range, 50 to 55 μm	Ellipsoidal oocyst; usual range, 30 μm long, 12 μm wide; sporocysts rarely seen broken out of oocysts, but measure 9 by 11 μm
Motility	Rotary, boring, may be rapid		Nonmotile
Number of nuclei	1 large kidney-shaped macronucleus; 1 small round micronucleus, which is difficult to see even in stained smear; macronucleus may be visible in unstained preparation	1 large macronucleus visible in unstained preparation	
Other features	Body covered with cilia, which tend to be longer near cytosome; cytoplasm may be vacuolated	Macronucleus and contractile vacuole visible in young cysts; in older cysts, internal structure appears granular	Mature oocyst contains 2 sporocysts with 4 sporozoites each; usual diagnostic stage is immature oocyst containing spherical mass of protoplasm

*See footnote to Table 35-3.

ability to harvest material for antigen, serologic tests for giardiasis have been developed for both antibody and antigen.[8]

The identification of intestinal protozoan parasites is difficult, at best, and the importance of the permanent stained slide should be reemphasized. It is important to remember that many artifacts (vegetable material, debris, cells of human origin) may mimic protozoan organisms on a wet mount (Fig. 35-19). The important diagnostic characteristics will be visible on the stained smear, and the final identification of protozoan parasites should be confirmed with the permanent stain.

Amebae

Occasionally when fresh stool material is examined as a direct wet mount, motile tropho-zoites may be observed. *E. histolytica* is described as having directional and progressive motility, whereas the other amebae tend to move more slowly and at random. The cytoplasm usually appears finely granular, less frequently coarsely granular, or vacuolated. Bacteria, yeast cells, or debris may be present in the cytoplasm. The presence of red blood cells in the cytoplasm is usually considered to be diagnostic for *E. histolytica* (Plates 215 to 217).

Nuclear morphology is one of the most important criteria used for identification; nuclei of the genus *Entamoeba* contain a relatively small karyosome and have chromatin material arranged on the nuclear membrane (Figs. 35-20 to 35-22 and Plates 218, 220, and 221). The nuclei of the other two genera, *Endolimax* and *Ioda-*

Text continued on p. 508.

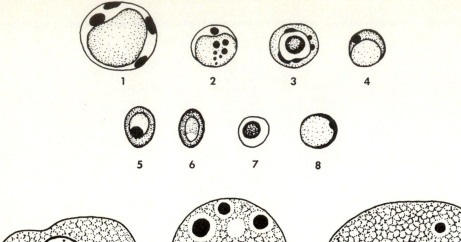

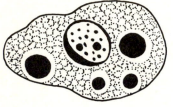

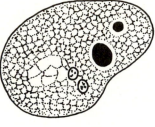

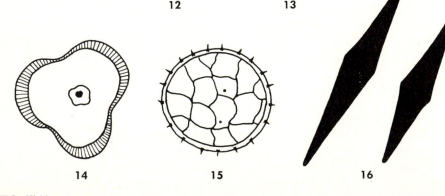

FIG. 35-19

Various structures that may be seen in stool preparations. **1, 2, 4,** *Blastocystis hominis*. **3, 5-8,** Various yeast cells. **9,** Macrophage with nucleus. **10, 11,** Deteriorated macrophage without nucleus. **12, 13,** Polymorphonuclear leukocytes. **14, 15,** Pollen grains. **16,** Charcot-Leyden crystals. (Adapted from Markell and Voge.[65] Illustration by Nobuko Kitamura.)

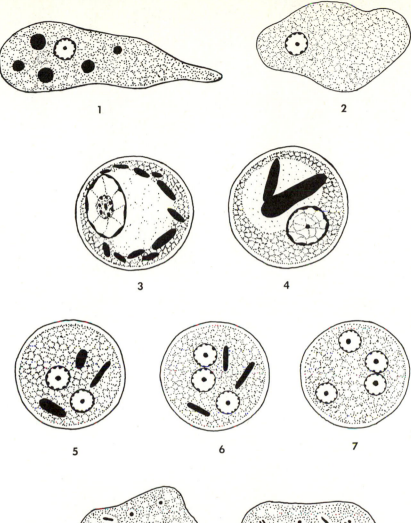

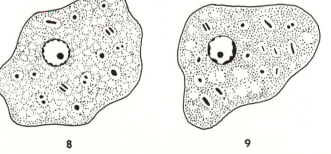

Continued.

FIG. 35-20

1, 2, Trophozoites of *Entamoeba histolytica*. 3, 4, Early cysts of *E. histolytica*. 5-7, Cysts of *E. histolytica*. 8, 9, Trophozoites of *Entamoeba coli*. 10, 11, Early cysts of *E. coli*. 12-14, Cysts of *E. coli*. 15, 16, Trophozoites of *Entamoeba hartmanni*. 17, 18, Cysts of *E. hartmanni*. (From Garcia and Ash.[31] Illustrations 4 and 11 by Nobuko Kitamura.)

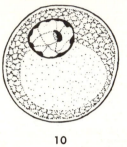

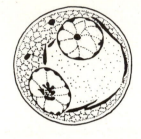

10   11

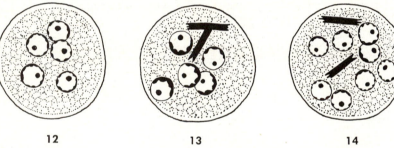

12   13   14

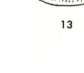

15   16   17   18

FIG. 35-20, cont'd
For legend see p. 505.

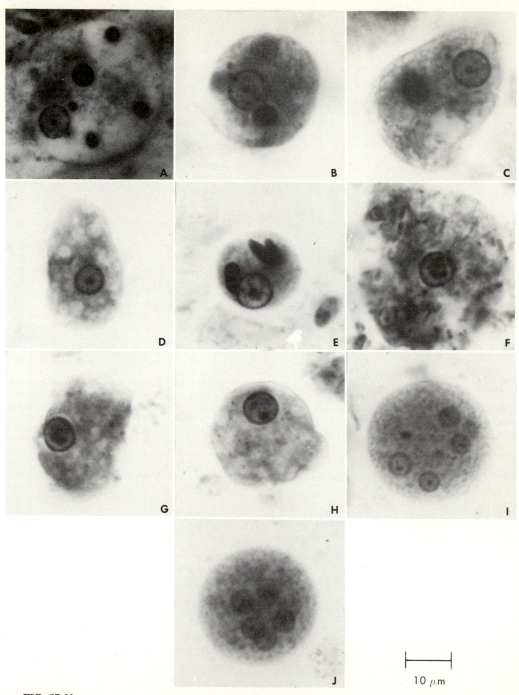

FIG. 35-21
A-D, Trophozoites of *Entamoeba histolytica*. **E,** Early cyst of *E. histolytica*. **F-H,** Trophozoites of
Entamoeba coli. **I, J,** Cysts of *E. coli*.

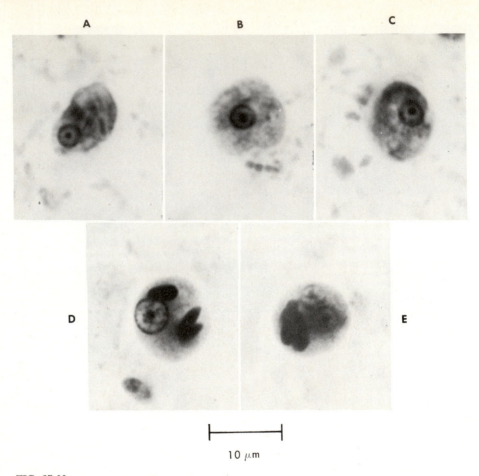

FIG. 35-22

A-C, Trophozoites of *Entamoeba hartmanni*. **D, E,** Cysts of *E. hartmanni*.

moeba, tend to have very large karyosomes with no peripheral chromatin on the nuclear membrane (Figs. 35-23 to 35-25 and Plates 222 and 223).

The trophozoite stages may often be pleomorphic and asymmetrical, whereas the cysts are usually less variable in shape, with more rigid cyst walls. The number of nuclei in the cysts may vary, but their general morphology is similar to that found in the trophozoite stage. There are various inclusions in the cysts, such as chromatoidal bars or glycogen material, which may be helpful in identification.

Flagellates

Four common species of flagellates are found in the intestinal tract: *Giardia lamblia, Chilomastix mesnili, Trichomonas hominis,* and *Dientamoeba fragilis* (Plates 224 to 226). Several other smaller flagellates, such as *Enteromonas hominis* and *Retortamonas intestinalis* (Fig. 35-26), are rarely seen, and none of the flagellates in the intestinal tract, with the exception of *G. lamblia* and *D. fragilis,* are considered pathogenic. *Trichomonas vaginalis* is pathogenic but occurs in the urogenital tract. *Trichomonas tenax* is occasionally found in

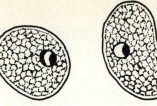

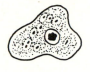
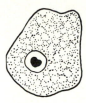
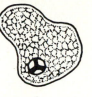

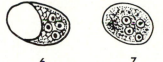
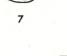

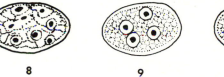
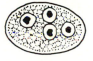
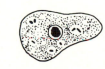
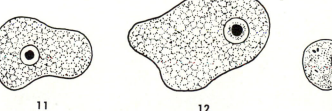
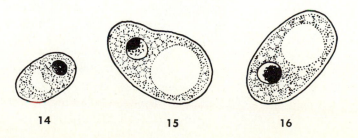
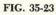

FIG. 35-23
1-5, Trophozoites of *Endolimax nana*. 6-10, Cysts of *E. nana*. 11-13, Trophozoites of *Iodamoeba bütschlii*. 14-16, Cysts of *I. bütschlii*. (From Garcia and Ash.[31])

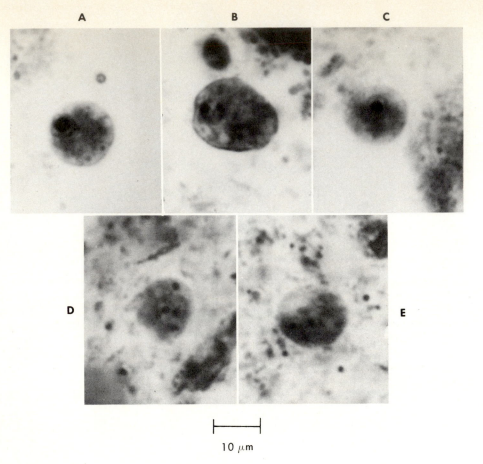

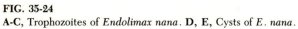

10 µm

FIG. 35-24
A-C, Trophozoites of *Endolimax nana*. **D, E,** Cysts of *E. nana*.

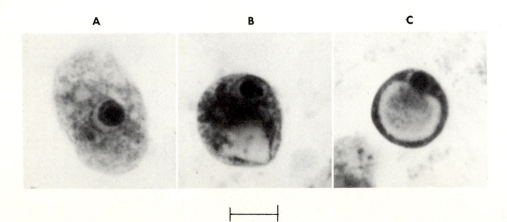

10 µm

FIG. 35-25
A, Trophozoite of *Iodamoeba bütschlii*. **B, C,** Cysts of *I. bütschlii*.

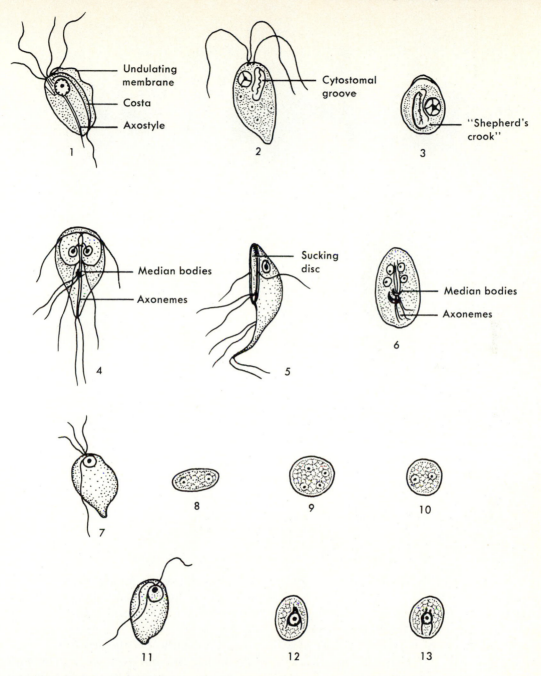

FIG. 35-26

1, Trophozoite of *Trichomonas hominis*. **2**, Trophozoite of *Chilomastix mesnili*. **3**, Cyst of *C. mesnili*. **4**, Trophozoite of *Giardia lamblia* (front view). **5**, Trophozoite of *G. lamblia* (side view). **6**, Cyst of *G. lamblia*. **7**, Trophozoite of *Enteromonas hominis*. **8-10**, Cysts of *E. hominis*. **11**, Trophozoite of *Retortamonas intestinalis*. **12**, **13**, Cysts of *R. intestinalis*. (From Garcia and Ash.[31] Illustration **5** by Nobuko Kitamura; illustrations **7** to **13** adapted from Markell and Voge.[65])

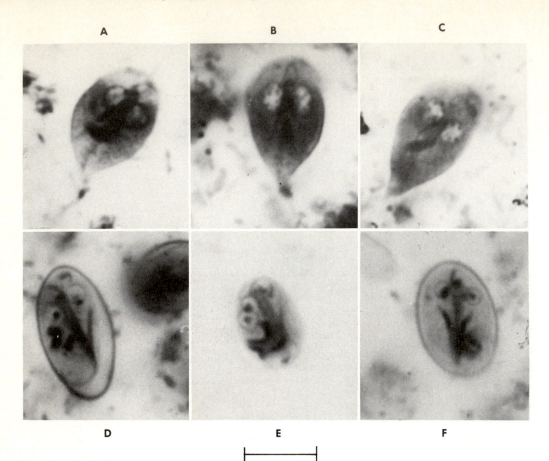

FIG. 35-27
A-C, Trophozoites of *Giardia lamblia.* **D-F,** Cysts of *G. lambia.*

the mouth and may be associated with poor oral hygiene.

With the exception of *Dientamoeba,* the flagellates are easily recognized by their characteristic rapid motility, which has been described as a "falling leaf" motion for *Giardia* and a jerky motion for the other species. Most of the flagellates have a characteristic pear shape and possess different numbers and arrangements of flagella, depending on the species. The sucking disk and axonemes of *Giardia,* the cytostome and spiral groove of *Chilomastix,* and the undulating membrane of *Trichomonas* are all distinctive criteria for identification (Figs. 35-26 to 35-28).

Until recently *Dientamoeba* was grouped with the amebae; however, electron microscopy studies have confirmed its correct classification with the flagellates, specifically the trichomonads.[65] *Dientamoeba* has no known cyst stage and is characterized by having one or two nuclei, which have no peripheral chromatin and

A   B   C

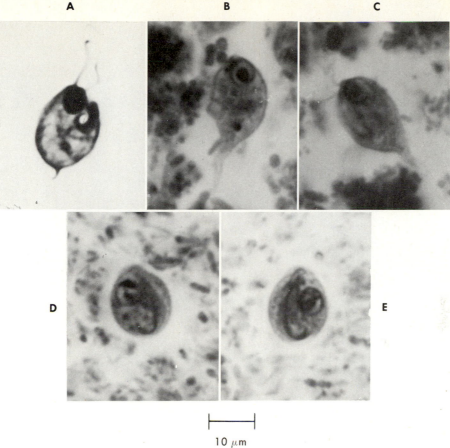

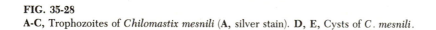

D   E

10 μm

FIG. 35-28
A-C, Trophozoites of *Chilomastix mesnili* (**A,** silver stain). **D, E,** Cysts of *C. mesnili*.

which have four to eight chromatin granules in a central mass. This organism is quite variable in size and shape and may contain large numbers of ingested bacteria and other debris. *Dientamoeba* is inconspicuous in the wet mount and is consistently overlooked without the use of the stained smear (Figs. 35-29 and 35-30).

Organisms can be recovered in fecal specimens from asymptomatic individuals, but reports in the literature describe a wide range of symptoms, which include intermittent diarrhea,

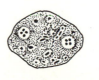 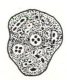

FIG. 35-29
Trophozoites of *Dientamoeba fragilis*. (From Garcia and Ash.[31])

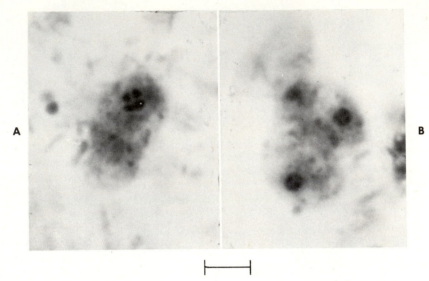

10 μm

FIG. 35-30
A, B, Trophozoites of *Dientamoeba fragilis*.

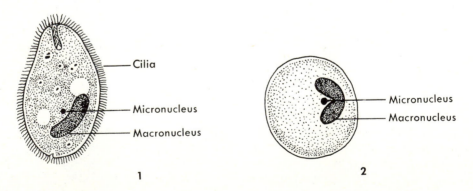

Cilia

Micronucleus

Macronucleus

Micronucleus

Macronucleus

1

2

FIG. 35-31
1, Trophozoite of *Balantidium coli*. 2, Cyst of *B. coli*. (From Garcia and Ash.[31])

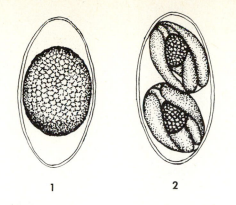

FIG. 35-32
1, Immature oocyst of *Isospora belli*. **2,** Mature oocyst of *I. belli*. (Illustration by Nobuko Kitamura.)

abdominal pain, nausea, anorexia, malaise, fatigue, poor weight gain, and unexplained eosinophilia.[19,94,112]

Ciliates

Balantidium coli is the largest protozoan and the only ciliate that infects humans (Plate 227). The living trophozoites have a rotatory, boring motion, which is usually rapid. The surface of the organism is covered by cilia, and the cytoplasm contains both a kidney-shaped macronucleus and a smaller, round micronucleus that is often difficult to see. The number of nuclei in the cyst remains the same as that in the trophozoite. *B. coli* infections are rarely seen in this country; however, the organisms are quite easily recognized (Fig. 35-31).

Sporozoa

Isospora belli is now considered to be the only valid species of the genus *Isospora* that infects humans. This organism is released from the intestinal wall as immature oocysts, so all stages from the immature oocyst containing a mass of undifferentiated protoplasm to those containing fully developed sporocysts and sporozoites are found in the stool (Fig. 35-32). If passed in the immature condition, they mature within 4 or 5 days to form sporozoites. This organism is rarely seen; however, it is not easily recognized in the stool and may be more common than statistics would indicate.

Intestinal helminths

The intestinal helminths that infect humans belong to two phyla: the Nematoda, or roundworms; and the Platyhelminthes, or flatworms. The Platyhelminthes, most of which are hermaphroditic, have a flat, bilaterally symmetrical body. The two classes, Trematoda and Cestoda, contain organisms that are parasitic for human beings (p. 517).

The trematodes (flukes) are leaf-shaped or elongate and slender organisms (blood flukes: *Schistosoma* species) that possess hooks or suckers for attachment. Members of this group, which parasitize humans, are found in the intestinal tract, liver, blood vessels, and lungs.

The cestodes (tapeworms) typically have a long, segmented, ribbonlike body, which has a special attachment portion, or scolex, at the anterior end. Adult forms inhabit the small intestine; however, humans may be host to either the adult or larval forms, depending on the species. The cestodes, as well as the trematodes, require (with few exceptions) one or more intermediate hosts for the completion of the life cycle.

The phylum Nematoda, or roundworms, are elongate, cylindrical worms containing a well-developed digestive tract. The sexes are separate, the male usually being smaller than the female. Intermediate hosts are required for larval development in certain species; a large number of species parasitize the intestinal tract and certain tissues of humans (Figs. 35-33 and 35-34).

Diagnosis of most intestinal helminth infections is based on the detection of the characteristic eggs and larvae in the stool; occasionally adult worms or portions of worms may also be found. No permanent stains are required, and

Key to helminth eggs

a. Egg nonoperculated, spherical or subspherical, containing a six-hooked embryo   b
Egg other than above   e

b. Eggs separate   c
Eggs in packets of twelve or more   *Dipylidium caninum*

c. Outer surface of egg consists of a thick, radially striated capsule or embryophore   *Taenia* sp.
Outer surface of egg consists of very thin shell, separated from inner embryophore by gelatinous matrix   d

d. Filamentous strands occupy space between embryophore and outer shell   *Hymenolepis nana*
No filamentous strands between embryophore and outer shell   *H. diminuta*

e. Egg operculated   f
Egg nonoperculated   j

f. Egg less than 35 μm long   *Clonorchis (Opisthorchis)* sp. or *Heterophyes heterophyes* or *Metagonimus yokogawai*
Egg 38 μm or over   g

g. Egg 38 to 45 μm in length   *Dicrocoelium dendriticum*
Egg over 60 μm in length   h

h. Egg with shoulders into which operculum fits   *Paragonimus westermani*
Egg without opercular shoulders   i

i. Egg more than 85 μm long   *Fasciolopsis buski* or *Fasciola hepatica* or *Echinostoma* sp.
Egg less than 75 μm long   *Diphyllobothrium latum*

j. Egg 75 μm or more in length, spined   k
Egg less than 75 μm long, not spined   m

k. Spine terminal   *Schistosoma haematobium*
Spine lateral   l

l. Lateral spine inconspicuous (perhaps absent)   *S. japonicum*
Lateral spine prominent   *S. mansoni*

m. Egg with thick tuberculated capsule   *Ascaris lumbricoides*
Egg without thick tuberculated capsule   n

n. Egg barrel shaped, with polar plugs   o
Egg not barrel shaped, without polar plugs   p

o. Shell nonstriated   *Trichuris trichiura*
Shell often striated   *Capillaria* spp.

p. Egg flattened on one side   *Enterobius vermicularis*
Egg symmetrical   q

q. Egg with large blue-green globules at poles   *Heterodera marioni*
Egg without polar globules   r

r. Egg bluntly rounded at ends, 56 to 76 μm long   hookworm
Egg pointed at one or both ends, 73 to 95 μm long   *Trichostrongylus* sp.

From Markell and Voge.[65]

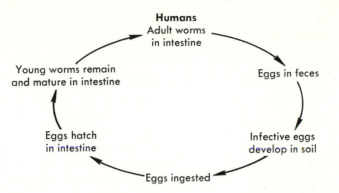

FIG. 35-33
Life cycle of *Enterobius vermicularis* and *Trichuris trichiura* (direct type of cycle).

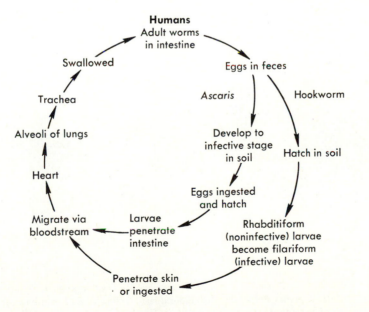

FIG. 35-34
Life cycle of *Ascaris lumbricoides* and hookworms (indirect type of cycle).

most diagnostic features can easily be seen on direct wet mounts or in mounts of the concentrated stool material.

Nematodes

The majority of nematodes are diagnosed by finding the characteristic eggs in the stool (Fig. 35-35). The eggs of *Ancylostoma duodenale* and *Necator americanus* are essentially identical, so an infection with either species is reported as "Hookworm eggs present" (Plate 228). *Trichostrongylus* eggs may easily be mistaken for those of hookworms; however, the eggs of *Trichostrongylus* are somewhat larger, and one end tends to be more pointed.

Strongyloides stercoralis is passed in the feces as the noninfective rhabditiform larva (Plate 229). Although hookworm eggs are normally passed in the stool, these eggs may continue to develop and hatch if the stool is left at room temperature for several days. These larvae may be mistaken for those of *Strongyloides*. Fig. 35-36 shows the morphologic differences between the rhabditiform larvae of hookworm and *Strongy-*

loides. Recovery of *Strongyloides* larvae in duodenal contents is mentioned in the section Duodenal Contents.

The appropriate techniques for recovery of *Enterobius vermicularis* (pinworm) eggs are given on pp. 474-475 (Plate 230). Eggs of the other nematodes are fairly easy to find and to differentiate from one another.

Cestodes

With the exception of *Diphyllobothrium latum*, tapeworm eggs are embryonated and contain a six-hooked oncosphere (Fig. 35-37 and Table 35-8).

Taenia saginata and *Taenia solium* cannot be speciated on the basis of egg morphology; gravid proglottids or the scolices must be examined (Fig. 35-38). *T. saginata* (beef tapeworm) proglottids have approximately 15 to 30 main lateral branches, and the scolex has no hooks; the proglottids of *T. solium* have 7 to 12 main lateral branches, and the scolex has a circle of hooks.

The eggs of *Hymenolepis nana* (more common) and *Hymenolepis diminuta* are very simi-

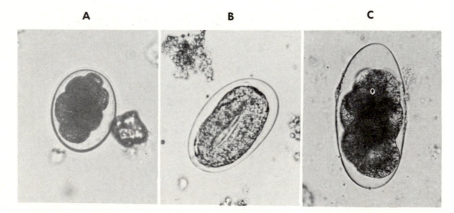

FIG. 35-35

A, Immature hookworm egg. **B,** Embryonated hookworm egg. **C,** *Trichostrongylus orientalis,* immature egg. **D,** *Strongyloides stercoralis,* rhabditiform larva (200 μm). **E,** *Enterobius vermicularis* egg. **F,** *Trichuris trichiura* egg. **G,** *Ascaris lumbricoides,* fertilized egg. **H,** *A. lumbricoides,* fertilized egg, decorticate. **I,** *A. lumbricoides,* unfertilized egg. **J,** *A. lumbricoides,* unfertilized egg, decorticate.

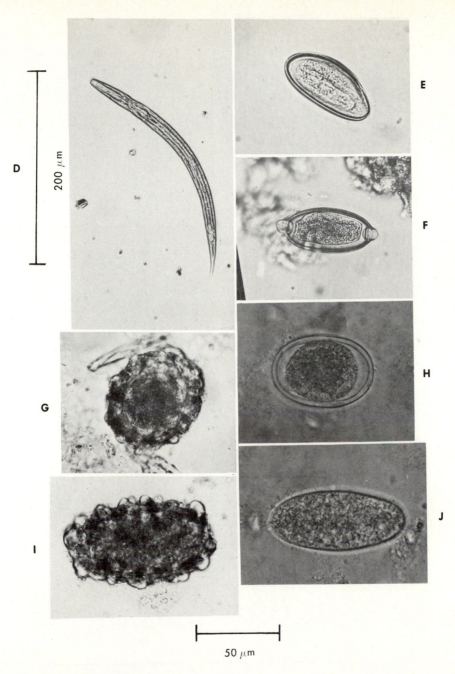

FIG. 35-35, cont'd
For legend see opposite page.

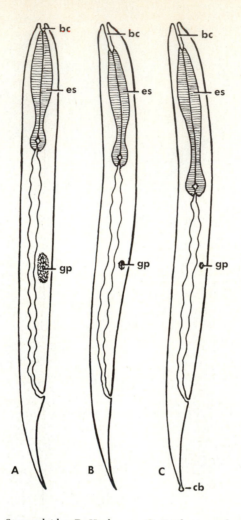

FIG. 35-36
Rhabditiform larvae. **A,** *Strongyloides.* **B,** Hookworm. **C,** *Trichostrongylus. bc,* Buccal cavity; *es,* esophagus; *gp,* genital primordia; *cb,* beadlike swelling of caudal tip. (Illustration by Nobuko Kitamura.)

FIG. 35-37
A, *Taenia* species egg. **B,** *Diphyllobothrium latum* egg. **C,** *Hymenolepis diminuta* egg. **D,** *Hymenolepis nana* egg. **E,** *Dipylidium caninum* egg packet.

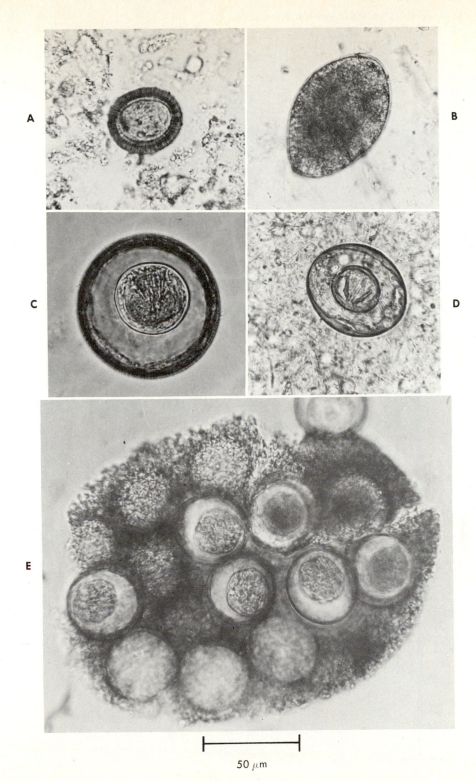

50 μm

Fig. 35-37
For legend see opposite page.

TABLE 35-8

Differential characteristics of some important tapeworms of humans[10,31,65]

	Taenia saginata	*Taenia solium*	*Hymenolepis nana*	*Diphyllobothrium latum*
Length	4 to 8 m	3 to 5 m	2.5 to 4 cm	4 to 10 m
Scolex				
Shape	Quadrilateral	Globular	Usually not seen	Almondlike
Size	1 by 1.5 mm	1 by 1 mm		3 by 1 mm
Rostellum and hooklets	No	Yes		No
Suckers	4	4		2 (grooves)
Terminal proglottids (gravid)				
Size	19 by 7 mm, longer than wide	11 by 5 mm	Usually not seen	3 by 11 mm, wider than long
Primary lateral uterine branches	15 to 30 on each side	6 to 12 on each side		Rosette shaped
Color	Milky white	Milky white		Ivory
Appearance in feces	Usually appear singly	5 or 6 segments		Varies from a few inches to a few feet in length
Ova				
Shape	Spheroid	Spheroid	Broadly oval	Oval
Size	35 μm	35 μm	30 by 47 μm	70 by 45 μm
Color	Rusty brown	Rusty brown	Pale	Yellow-brown
Embryo with hooklets	Yes	Yes	Yes	No
Operculum	No	No	No	Yes (difficult to see)

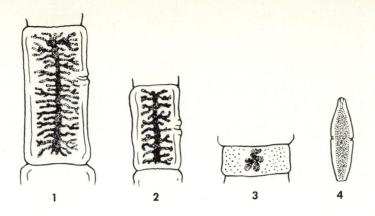

FIG. 35-38
Gravid proglottids. **1,** *Taenia saginata*. **2,** *Taenia solium*. **3,** *Diphyllobothrium latum*. **4,** *Dipylidium caninum*. (From Garcia and Ash.[31])

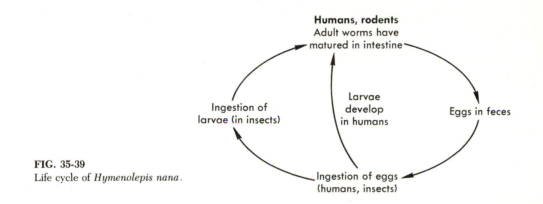

FIG. 35-39
Life cycle of *Hymenolepis nana*.

lar; however, *H. nana* eggs are smaller and have polar filaments, which are present in the space between the oncosphere and the egg shell (Fig. 35-39).

Eggs of *Dipylidium caninum* are occasionally found in humans (particularly children) and are passed in the feces in packets of 5 to 15 eggs each (Fig. 35-40). The proglottids may also be found; they may resemble cucumber seeds or, when dry, may look like rice grains (white).

The fish tapeworm, *Diphyllobothrium latum*, does not have embryonated eggs; these eggs have a somewhat thicker shell and are operculated, much like the trematode eggs (Fig. 35-41).

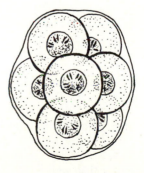

FIG. 35-40
Dipylidium caninum egg packet. (Illustration by Nobuko Kitamura.)

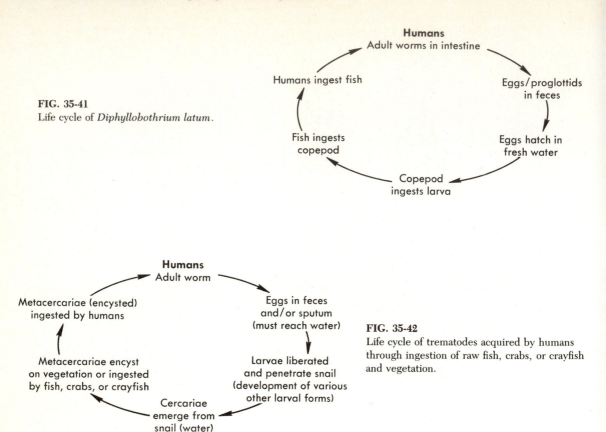

FIG. 35-41
Life cycle of *Diphyllobothrium latum*.

FIG. 35-42
Life cycle of trematodes acquired by humans through ingestion of raw fish, crabs, or crayfish and vegetation.

Key to gravid proglottids of the major human tapeworms

a. Uterus forms rosette in center of proglottid
   Diphyllobothrium latum
   Uterus otherwise disposed   b
b. Uterus with central stem running length of proglottid   c
   Uterus without central stem   d
c. Central stem with 7 to 13 main lateral branches
   Taenia solium
   Central stem with 15 to 20 main lateral branches   *T. saginata*
d. Proglottid wider than long   *Hymenolepis* sp.
   Proglottid longer than wide
   Dipylidium caninum

From Markell and Voge.[65]

Trematodes

Most of the trematodes have operculated eggs, which are best recovered by the sedimentation concentration technique rather than the flotation method (Fig. 35-42). Many of these eggs are very similar, both in size and morphology, and often careful measurements must be taken to speciate the eggs (Fig. 35-43). The eggs of *Clonorchis (Opisthorchis)*, *Heterophyes*, and *Metagonimus* are very similar and quite small; they are easily missed if the concentration sediment is examined with the 10× objective only. The eggs of *Fasciola hepatica* and *Fasciolopsis buski* are also very similar but much larger than those just mentioned.

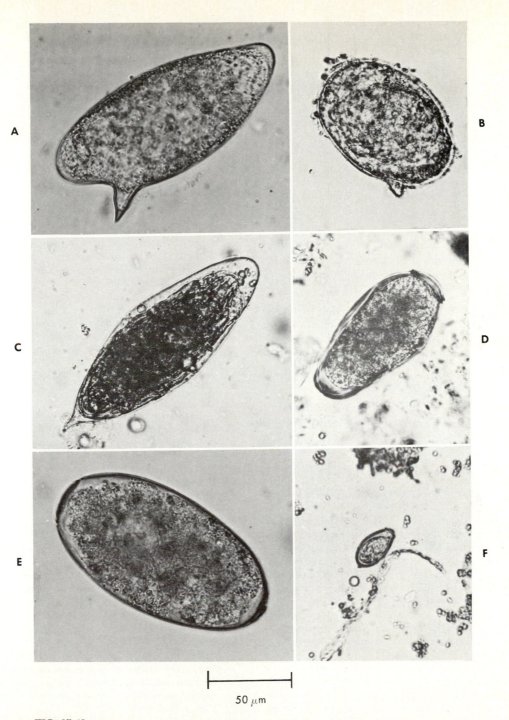

50 μm

FIG. 35-43

A, *Schistosoma mansoni* egg. B, *Schistosoma japonicum* egg. C, *Schistosoma haematobium* egg. D, *Paragonimus westermani* egg. E, *Fasciola hepatica* egg. F, *Clonorchis (Opisthorchis) sinensis* egg.

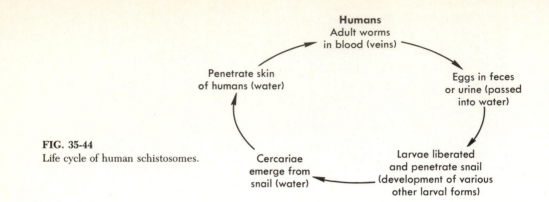

FIG. 35-44
Life cycle of human schistosomes.

Paragonimus westermani eggs are not only found in the stool but may be found in sputum. These eggs are very similar in size and shape to the egg of the fish tapeworm, *D. latum*.

Probably the easiest trematode eggs to identify are those of the schistosomes: *Schistosoma mansoni* eggs are characterized by having a very prominent lateral spine, *S. haematobium* a terminal spine, and *S. japonicum* a small lateral spine that may be difficult to see (Fig. 35-44). These eggs are nonoperculated. Specific procedures for their recovery and identification are found on p. 473.

REFERENCES

1. Allison, A.C.: Genetic factors in resistance to malaria, Ann. N.Y. Acad. Sci. **91**:710, 1961.
2. Allison, A.C., and Clyde, D.F.: Malaria in African children with deficient erythrocyte glucose-6-phosphate dehydrogenase, Br. Med. J. **1**:1346, 1961.
3. Beal, C.B., Viens, P., Grant, R.G.L., and Hughes, J.M.: A new technique for sampling duodenal contents: demonstration of upper small-bowel pathogens, Am. J. Trop. Med. Hyg. **19**:349-352, 1970.
4. Beaver, P.C.: A nephelometric method of calibrating the photoelectric meter for making egg-counts by direct fecal smear, J. Parasitol. **35**(Section 2):13, 1949.
5. Beaver, P.C.: The standardization of fecal smears for estimating egg production and worm burden, J. Parasitol. **36**:451-456, 1950.
6. Berlin, O.G.W., and Miller, M.J. Euparol as a permanent mounting medium for helminth eggs and proglottids, J. Clin. Microbiol. **12**:700-703, 1980.
7. Biagi, F., Navarrete, F., Piña, A., Santiago, A.M., and Tapia, L.: Estudio de tres reacciones serologicas en el diagnostico de la cisticercosis, Rev. Med. Hosp. Gen. Mexico City **24**:501-508, 1961.
8. Brandborg, L.L.: Giardiasis and traveler's diarrhea, Gastroenterology **78**:1602-1614, 1980.
9. Brooke, M.M., and Goldman, M.: Polyvinyl alcohol-fixative as a preservative and adhesive for Protozoa in dysenteric stools and other liquid material, J. Lab. Clin. Med. **34**:1554-1560, 1949.
10. Brooke, M.M., and Melvin, D.: Morphology of diagnostic stages of intestinal parasites of man, DHEW Pub. No. (HSM) 72-8116, Atlanta, 1969, U.S. Government Printing Office.
11. Chatterjea, J.B., Saha, T.K., Ray, R.N., and Chaudluri, R.N.: Response of tropical splenomegaly and thalassemia to induce malaria, Bull. Calcutta Sch. Trop. Med. **4**:105-106, 1956.
12. Coltorti, E.A., and Varela-Diaz, V.M.: Detection of antibodies against *Echinococcus granulosus* arc 5 antigens by double diffusion test, Trans. R. Soc. Trop. Med. Hyg. **72**:226-229, 1978.
13. Committee on Education, American Society of Parasitologists: Procedures suggested for use in examination of clinical specimens for parasitic infection, J. Parasitol. **63**:959-960, 1977.
14. Cossio, P.M., Diez, C., Szarfman, A., Kreutzer, E., Candiolo, B., and Arana, R.M. Chagasic cardiopathy: demonstration of a serum gamma globulin factor which reacts with endocardium and vascular structures, Circulation **49**:13-21, 1974.
15. Culbertson, C.G., Ensminger, P.W., and Overton, W.M.: The isolation of additional strains of pathogenic *Hartmanella* sp. (Acanthamoeba): proposed culture method for application to biological material, Am. J. Clin. Pathol. **43**:383-387, 1965.
16. Dennis, D.T., and Kean, B.H.: Isolation of microfilariae: report of a new method, J. Parasitol. **57**:1146-1147, 1971.

17. Desowitz, R.S., and Hitchcock, J.C.: Hyperendemic brancroftian filariasis in the Kingdom of Tonga: the application of the membrane filter concentration technique to an age-stratified blood survey, Am. J. Trop. Med. Hyg. **23**:877-879, 1974.

18. Desowitz, R.S., Saave, J.J., and Stein, B.: The application of the indirect haemagglutination test in recent studies on the immuno-epidemiology of human malaria and the immune response in experimental malaria, Milit. Med. **131**(Supp.):1157-1166, 1966.

19. Desser, S.S., and Yang, Y.J.: *Dientamoeba fragilis* in idiopathic gastro-intestinal disorders, Can. Med. Assoc. J. **114**:290-293, 1976.

20. Duma, R.J.: Free-living amebic meningoencephalitis, TINS 1980,

21. Dunn, F.L.: The TIF direct smear as an epidemiological tool, Bull. WHO **39**:439-449, 1968.

22. Edrissian, G.H., and Darabian, P. A comparison of enzyme-linked immunosorbent assay (ELISA) and indirect fluorescent antibody (IFA) in serodiagnosis of cutaneous and visceral leishmaniasis in Iran, Trans. R. Soc. Trop. Med. Hyg. **73**:289-292, 1979.

23. Farag, H., Bout, D., and Capron, A.: Specific immunodiagnosis of human hydatidosis by the enzyme-linked immunosorbent assay (ELISA), Biomedicine **23**:276-278, 1975.

24. Faust, E.C., D'Antoni, J.S., Odom, V., Miller, M.F., Peres, C., Sawitz, W., Thomen, L.F., Tobie, J., and Walker, J.H.: A critical study of clinical laboratory technics for the diagnosis of protozoan cysts and helminth eggs in feces, Am. J. Trop. Med. **18**:169-183, 1938.

25. Faust, E.C., Russell, P.F., and Jung, R.C.: Craig and Faust's clinical parasitology, ed. 8, Philadelphia, 1970, Lea & Febiger.

26. Feinberg, J.G., and Whittington, M.J.: A culture medium for *Trichomonas vaginalis* Donne and species of *Candida,* J. Clin. Pathol. **10**:327-329, 1957.

27. Field, J.W., Sandosham, A.A., and Fong, Y.L.: The microscopical diagnosis of human malaria. I. A morphological study of the erythrocytic parasites in thick blood films, ed. 2, Malaya, 1963, Institute of Medical Research.

28. Field, J.W., and Shute, P.G.: The microscopic diagnosis of human malaria. II. A morphological study of the erythrocytic parasites, Malaya, 1956, Institute of Medical Research.

29. Filstein, M.R., Benach, J.L., White, D.J., Brody, B.A., Goldman, W.D., Bakal, C.W., and Schwartz, R.S.: Serosurvey for human babesiosis in New York, J. Infect. Dis. **141**:518-521, 1980.

30. Fossieck, B.E., and Spagnolo, S.V.: *Pneumocystis carinii* pneumonitis in patients with lung cancer, Chest **78**:721-722, 1980.

31. Garcia, L.S., and Ash, L.R.: Diagnostic parasitology: clinical laboratory manual, ed. 2., St. Louis, 1979, The C.V. Mosby Co.

32. Garcia, L.S., Brewer, T.C., and Bruckner, D.A.: A comparison of the formalin-ether concentration and trichrome-stained smear methods for the recovery and identification of intestinal protozoa, Am. J. Med. Technol. **45**:932-935, 1979.

33. Garcia, L.S., and Shimizu, R.: Comparison of clinical results on the use of ethyl acetate and diethyl ether in the formalin-ether sedimentation technique performed on polyvinyl alcohol-preserved specimens, J. Clin. Microbiol. **13**:709-713, 1981.

34. Garcia, L.S., and Voge, M.: Diagnostic clinical parasitology. I. Proper specimen collection and processing, Am. J. Med. Technol. **46**:459-467, 1980.

35. Gleason, N.N., and Healy, G.R.: Modification and evaluation of Kohn's one-step staining technic for intestinal protozoa in feces or tissue, Am. J. Clin. Pathol. **43**:494-496, 1965.

36. Gomori, G.: A rapid one-step trichrome stain, Am. J. Clin. Pathol. **20**:661-663, 1950.

37. Graham, C.F.: A device for the diagnosis of *Enterobius* infection, Am. J. Trop. Med. **21**:159-161, 1941.

38. Harada, Y., and Mori, O.: A new method for culturing hookworm, Yonago Acta Med. **1**:177-179, 1955.

39. Healy, G.R.: *Babesia* infections in man, Hosp. Pract. June, 1979, pp. 107-116.

40. Healy, G.R., and Ruebush, T.K., II.: Morphology of *Babesia microti* in human blood smears, Am. J. Clin. Pathol. **73**:107-109, 1980.

41. Hendricks, L., and Wright, N.: Diagnosis of cutaneous leishmaniasis by in vitro cultivation of saline aspirates in Schneider's drosophila medium, Am. J. Trop. Med. Hyg. **28**(6):962-964, 1979.

42. Howard, R.J., and Battye, F.L.: *Plasmodium berghei:* infected red cells sorted according to DNA content, Parasitology **78**:263-270, 1979.

43. Hsieh, H.C.: A test-tube filter-paper method for the diagnosis of *Ancylostoma duodenale, Necator americanus,* and *Strongyloides stercoralis,* WHO Tech. Rep. Ser. **255**:27-30, 1962.

44. Ingram, R.L., Otken, Jr., L.B., and Jumper, J.R.: Staining of malarial parasites by the fluorescent antibody technic, Proc. Soc. Exp. Biol. Med. **106**:52-54, 1961.

45. Jacoby, G.A., Hunt, J.V., Kosinski, K.S., Demirjian, Z.N., Huggins, C., Etkind, P., Marcus, L.C., and Spielman, A.: Treatment of transfusion-transmitted babesiosis by exchange transfusion, N. Engl. J. Med. **303**:1098-1100, 1980.

46. Jonckheere, J.F.: Growth characteristics, cytopathic effect in cell culture, and virulence in mice of 36 type strains belonging to 19 different *Acanthamoeba* spp., Appl. Environ. Microbiol. **39**:(4)681-685, 1980.

47. Kagan, I.G.: Diagnostic epidemiologic and experimental parasitology: immunologic aspects, Am. J. Trop. Med. Hyg. **28**:429-439, 1979.

48. Kagan, I.G.: Serodiagnosis of parasitic diseases. In Lennette, E.H., Balows, A., Hausler, W.J., Jr., and Truant, J.P., editors: Manual of clinical Microbiology, ed. 3, Washington, D.C., 1980, American Society for Microbiology.

49. Kagan, I.G., Norman, L., Allain, D.S., and Goodchild, C.G.: Studies on echinococcosis: nonspecific serologic reactions of hydatid-fluid antigen with serum of patients ill with diseases other than echinococcosis, J. Immunol. **84**:635-640, 1960.

50. Kagan, I.G., Osimani, J.J., Varela, J.C., and Allain, D.S.: Evaluation of intradermal and serologic tests for the diagnosis of hydatid disease, Am. J. Trop. Med. Hyg. **15**:172-179, 1966.

51. Kagan, I.G., and Quist, K.D.: An evaluation of five serologic tests for the diagnosis of trichinosis in lightly infected swine. In Singh, K.S., and Tandan, B.K., editors: H.D. Srivastava Commemoration Volume, Iznatnagar, U.P. India, 1970, India Veterinary Research Institute.

52. Kato, K., and Miura, M.: Comparative examinations (Japanese text), Jpn. J. Parasitol. **3**:35, 1954.

53. Knott, J.I.: A method for making microfilarial surveys on day blood, Trans. R. Soc. Trop. Med. Hyg. **33**:191-196, 1939.

54. Kuvin, S.F., Tobie, J.E., Evans, C.B., Coatney, G.R., and Contacos, P.G.: Fluorescent antibody studies on the course of antibody production and serum gamma globulin levels in normal volunteers infected with human and simian malaria, Am. J. Trop. Med. Hyg. **11**:429-436, 1962.

55. Kwapinski, J.B.: Methods of serological research, New York, 1965, John Wiley & Sons, Inc.

56. Labzoffsky, N.A., Baratawidjaja, R.K., Kuitunen, E., Lewis F.N., Kavelman, D.A., and Morrissey, L.P.: Immunofluorescence as an aid in the early diagnosis of trichinosis, Can. Med. Assoc. J. **90**:920-921, 1964.

57. Lasser, K.H., Lewin, K.J., and Ryning, F.W.: Cryptosporidial enteritis in a patient with congenital hypogammaglobulinemia, Hum. Pathol. **10**(2):234-240, 1979.

58. Lennette, E.H., Balows, A., Hausler, W.J., Jr., and Truant, J.P., editors: Manual of clinical microbiology, ed. 3, Washington, D.C., 1980, American Society for Microbiology.

59. Lim, S.K., Eveland, W.C., and Porter, R.J.: Direct fluorescent-antibody for the diagnosis of *Pneumocystis carinii* pneumonia from sputa or tracheal aspirations from humans, Appl. Microbiol. **27**:144-149, 1974.

60. Lincicome, D.R.: Fluctuation in numbers of cysts of *Endamoeba histolytica* and *Endamoeba coli* in the stools of rhesus monkeys, Am. J. Hyg. **36**:321-337, 1942.

61. Lopez, C.E., Dykes, A.C., Juranek, D.D., Sinclair, S.P., Conn, J.M., Christie, R.W., Lippy, E.C., Schultz, M.G., and Mires, M.H.: Waterborne giardiasis: a community-wide outbreak of disease and a high rate of asymptomatic infection, Am. J. Epidemiol. **112**(4):495-507, 1980.

62. Luna, L.G.: Manual of histologic staining methods of the Armed Forces Institute of Pathology, ed. 3, New York, 1968, McGraw-Hill Book Co.

63. Maekelt, G.A.: A modified procedure of xenodiagnosis for Chagas' disease, Am. J. Trop. Med. Hyg. **13**:11-15, 1964.

64. Mahoney, D.F., Redington, B.C., and Schoenbechler, M.J.: Preparation and serologic activity of plasmodial fractions, Milit. Med. **131**(Supp.):1141-1151, 1966.

65. Markell, E.K., and Voge, M.: Medical parasitology, ed. 5, Philadelphia, 1981, W.B. Saunders Co.

66. Martin, L.K., and Beaver, P.C.: Evaluation of Kato thick-smear technique for quantitative diagnosis of helminth infections, Am. J. Trop. Med. Hyg. **17**:382-391, 1968.

67. McLaren, M., Draper, C.C., Roberts, J.M., Minter-Goedbloed, E., Ligthart, G.S., Teesdale, C.H., Amin, M.A., Omer, A.H.S., Bartlett, A., and Voller, A.: Studies on the enzyme linked immunosorbent assay (ELISA) test for *Schistosoma mansoni* infections, Ann. Trop. Med. Parasitol. **72**:243-253, 1978.

68. Melvin, D.M., and Brooke, M.M.: Laboratory procedures for the diagnosis of intestinal parasites, DHEW Pub. No. (CDC) 75-8282, Washington, D.C., 1974, U.S. Government Printing Office.

69. Meuwissen, J.H.E.T., and Leeuwenberg, A.D.E.M.: Indirect haemagglutination test for malaria with lyophilized cells, Trans. R. Soc. Trop. Med. Hyg. **66**:666-667, 1972.

70. Miller, L.H., Mason, S.J., Dvorak, J.A., McGinniss, M.H., and Rothman, I.K.: Erythrocyte receptors for (*Plasmodium knowlesi*) malaria: Duffy blood group determinants, Science, **189**:561-562, 1975.

71. Nair, C.P.: Rapid staining of intestinal amoebae on wet mounts, Nature **172**:1051, 1953.

72. Osterholm, M.T., Forfang, J.C., Ristinen, B.A., Dean, A.G., Washburn, J.W., Godes, J.R., Rude, R.A., and McCullough, J.G.: An outbreak of foodborne giardiasis, N. Engl. J. Med. **304**:24-28, 1981.

73. Palacios, B.O., de la Hoz, R., and Sosa, H.: Determinación del antígeno amibiano en heces por el metodo elisa (enzyme linked immunosorbent assay) para la identificación de *Entamoeba histolytica*, Arch. Invest. Med. **1**(Supp. 9)**1**:339-348, 1978.

74. Parasitology Subcommittee, Microbiology Section of Scientific Assembly, American Society for Medical Technology: Recommended procedures for the examination of clinical specimens submitted for the diagnosis of parasitic infections, Am. J. Med. Technol. **44**:1101-1106, 1978.

75. Perl, G.: Errors in the diagnosis of *Trichomonas vaginalis* infection, Obstet. Gynecol. **39**:7-9, 1972.

76. Proctor, E.M., and Elsdon-Dew, R.: Serological tests in porcine cysticercosis, S. Afr. J. Sci. **62**:264-267, 1966.

77. Proctor, E.M., Powell, S.J., and Elsdon-Dew, R.: The serological diagnosis of cysticercosis, Ann. Trop. Med. Parasitol. **60**:146-151, 1966.

78. Ritchie, L.S.: An ether sedimentation technique for routine stool examinations, Bull. U.S. Army Med. Dept. **8**:326, 1948.

79. Rogers, W.A., Jr., Fried, J.A., and Kagan, I.G.: A modified indirect microhemagglutination test for malaria, Am. J. Trop. Med. Hyg. **17**:804-809. 1968.

80. Ruebush, T.K., II: Human babesiosis in North America, Trans. R. Soc. Trop. Med. Hyg. **74**:149-152, 1980.

81. Sapero, J.J., and Lawless, D.K.: The MIF stain-preservation technique for the identification of intestinal protozoa, Am. J. Trop. Med. Hyg. **2**:613-619, 1953.

82. Sawitz, W.G., and Faust, E.C.: The probability of detecting intestinal protozoa by successive stool examinations, Am. J. Trop. Med. **22**:131-136, 1942.

83. Scholten, T.H.: An improved technique for the recovery of intestinal protozoa, J. Parasitol. **58**:633-634, 1972.

84. Scholten, T.H., and Yang, J.: Evaluation of unpreserved and preserved stools for the detection and identification of intestinal parasites, Am. J. Clin. Pathol. **62**:563-567, 1974.

85. Serafin-Anaya, F.J., Castañeda-Castañeira, E., Diaz, S., Palacios, O., Gutierrez-Trujillo, G.: Amebiasis intestinal en niños. II. Evaluación de diversas téchnicas diagnósticas y distintos esquemas terapéuticos, Arch. Invest. Med. **1**:(Supp. 9):371-374, 1978.

86. Sheehan, D.C., and Hrapchak, B.B.: Theory and practice of histotechnology, ed. 2, St. Louis, 1980, The C.V. Mosby Co.

87. Shute, G.T., and Sodeman, T.M. Identification of malaria parasites by fluorescence microscopy and acridine orange staining, Bull. WHO **48**:591, 1973.

88. Shute, P.G.: The staining of malaria parasites, Trans. R. Soc. Trop. Med. Hyg. **60**:412-416, 1966.

89. Shute, P.G., and Maryon, M.E.: Laboratory technique for the study of malaria, ed. 2, London, 1966, J & A Churchill, Ltd.

90. Smith, R.F., and Horen, P.: Inhibition of *Trichomonas*

vaginalis by fungi during associative growth, Sex. Transm. Dis. **7**:172-174, 1980.

91. Sodeman, W.A., Jr., and Jeffery, G.M.: Indirect fluorescent antibody test for malaria antibody, Public Health Rep. **81**:1037-1041, 1966.

92. Spence, M.R., Hollander, D.H., Smith, J., McCaig, L., Sewell, D., and Brockman, M.: The clinical and laboratory diagnosis of *Trichomonas vaginalis* infection, Sex. Transm. Dis. **7**:168-171, 1980.

93. Spencer, F.M., and Monroe, L.S.: The color atlas of intestinal parasites, ed. 2, Springfield, Ill., 1976, Charles C Thomas, Publisher.

94. Spencer, M.J., Garcia, L.S., and Chapin, M.R.: *Dientamoeba fragilis:* an intestinal pathogen in children? Am. J. Dis. Child. **133**:390-393, 1979.

95. Stein, B., and Desowitz, R.S.: The measurement of antibody in human malaria by a formalized sheep cell hemagglutination test, Bull. WHO **30**:45-49, 1964.

96. Stemmermann, G.N., Hayashi, T., Glober, G.A., Oishi, N., and Frankel, R.I. Cryptosporidiosis: report of a fatal case complicated by disseminated toxoplasmosis, Am. J. Med. **69**:637-642, 1980.

97. Stoll, N.R., and Hausheer, W.C.: Concerning two options in dilution egg counting: small drop and displacement, Am. J. Hyg. **6**:134-145, 1926.

98. Sulzer, A.J., and Chisholm, E.S.: Comparison of the IFA and other tests for *Trichinella spiralis* antibodies, Public Health Rep. **81**:729-734, 1966.

99. Sulzer, A.J., and Wilson, M.: The use of thick-smear antigen slides in the malaria indirect fluorescent antibody test, J. Parasitol. **53**:1110-1111, 1967.

100. Sulzer, A.J., Wilson, M., and Hall, E.C.: Indirect fluorescent antibody tests for parasitic diseases. V. An evaluation of a thick-smear antigen in the IFA for malaria antibodies, Am. J. Trop. Med. Hyg. **18**:199-205, 1969.

101. Taylor, R.G., and Perez, T.R. Serology of amebiasis using FIAX system. Arch. Invest. Med. **1**:(Supp. 9):363-366, 1978.

102. Thong, Y.H.: Primary amoebic meningoencephalitis fifteen years later, Med. J. Aust. **1**:352-354, 1980.

103. Tobie, J.E., and Coatney, G.R.: Fluorescent antibody staining of human malaria parasites, Exp. Parasitol. **11**:128-132, 1961.

104. Tompkins, V.N., and Miller, J.K.: Staining intestinal protozoa with iron-hematoxylin-phosphotungstic acid, Am. J. Clin. Pathol. **17**:755-758, 1947.

105. Tosswill, J.H.C., Ridley, D.S., and Warhurst, D.C.: Counterimmunoelectrophoresis as a rapid screening test for amoebic liver abscess, J. Clin. Pathol. **33**:33-35, 1980.

106. Vattuone, N.H., and Yanovsky, J.F.: *Trypanosoma cruzi:* agglutination activity of enzyme-treated epimastigotes. Exp. Parasitol. **30**:349-355, 1971.

107. Voller, A., and Bray, R.S.: Fluorescent antibody staining as a measure of malarial antibody, Proc. Soc. Exp. Biol. Med. **110**:907-910, 1962.

108. Walker, A.J.: Manual for the microscopic diagnosis of malaria, ed. 3, Science Pub. No. 161, Washington, D.C., 1968, Pan American Health Organization.

109. Weisburger, W.R., Hutcheon, D.F., Yardley, J.H., Roche, J.C., Hillis, W.D., and Charache, P. Cryptosporidiosis in an immunosuppressed renal transplant recipient with IgA deficiency, Am. J. Clin. Pathol. **72**(3):473-478, 1979.

110. Wheatley, W.B.: A rapid staining procedure for intestinal amoebae and flagellates, Am. J. Clin. Pathol. **21**:990-992, 1951.

111. Wilcox, A.: Manual for the microscopical diagnosis of malaria in man, Washington, D.C., 1960, U.S. Public Health Service.

112. Yang, J., and Scholten, T.H.: *Dientamoeba fragilis:* a review with notes on its epidemiology, pathogenicity, mode of transmission, and diagnosis, Am. J. Trop. Med. Hyg. **26**:16-22, 1977.

113. Young, K.H., Bullock, S.L., Melvin, D.M., and Spruill, C.L.: Ethyl acetate as a substitute for diethyl ether in the formalin-ether sedimentation technique, J. Clin. Microbiol. **10**:852, 1979.

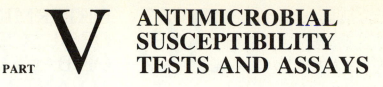

PART **V** **ANTIMICROBIAL SUSCEPTIBILITY TESTS AND ASSAYS**

36

DETERMINATION OF SUSCEPTIBILITY OF BACTERIA TO ANTIMICROBIAL AGENTS; ASSAY OF ANTIMICROBIAL AGENTS

According to Isenberg,[16] the value of the clinical laboratory can be measured only by the significance of the guidance it gives the physician in the treatment of his or her patients. In no other area of clinical microbiology does this statement become more pertinent than in the testing of clinical isolates for susceptibility to antimicrobial agents. With the increasing number of these agents at the physician's disposal and the changing pattern of resistance and susceptibility among bacteria—particularly the gram-negative enteric bacilli—the clinician must rely more and more on susceptibility testing to guide the selection of appropriate drugs or the altering of an already imposed regimen. Therefore, to a large extent, a laboratory report showing susceptibility or resistance to a particular antimicrobial agent becomes an endorsement of its usefulness or withdrawal.

Since the clinical microbiologist is in a position to advise the physician regarding proper antimicrobial therapy, it follows that he or she must maintain a high level of accuracy in testing procedures and a high degree of reproducibility of the results.[16] **Only through close cooperation and exchange of information between the labo-**

ratory staff and the clinician can the best possible management of an infectious process be achieved.

The principle methods used by the laboratory to determine susceptibility of a microorganism to an antimicrobial agent include the **dilution tests,** such as broth dilution (tube dilution and microdilution) and agar plate dilution procedures, and the **disk agar diffusion test,** utilizing antibiotic-impregnated disks. Each method has its advantages and its limitations, and these must be fully understood and appreciated to obtain maximum usefulness from the results.[32] Since all of these methods have a place in the clinical laboratory, the procedures and directions for the use of each will be described in detail.

In the interpretation of any in vitro susceptibility tests, one should remember that they are essentially **artificial measurements.** The data obtained from these tests give only the approximate range of effective inhibitory action against the microorganisms. The only absolute criterion of the efficacy of an antibiotic is the **clinical response** of the patient after an adequate dose of the appropriate drug is administered.

DILUTION METHODS FOR DETERMINING SUSCEPTIBILITY TO ANTIMICROBIAL AGENTS

In dilution methods for determining the susceptibility of an organism to antimicrobial agents, specific amounts of the antibiotic, prepared in decreasing concentration in broth or agar by serial dilution technique, are inoculated with a standardized suspension of the bacterium to be tested. The susceptibility of an organism is determined, after a suitable period of incubation, by macroscopic observation of the presence or absence of growth in the varying concentrations of the antimicrobial agent. The lowest concentration of drug demonstrating no observable growth is a measure of the bacteriostatic effect of the agent on the bacterium and is commonly referred to as the minimal inhibitory concentration (MIC). When using a broth medium, this technique can be further adapted to the determination of the bactericidal effects of an antibiotic, or the minimal bactericidal concentration (MBC).

A number of factors must be considered in establishing dilution procedures and in evaluating the results of these tests.[11] They include (1)

TABLE 36-1

"Breakpoints"* for activity of antimicrobial agents

Drug	Breakpoint†
Penicillin G	32
Ampicillin	16
Carbenicillin	128
Cephalexin	8
Cephalothin	16
Cefazolin	32
Cefaclor	8
Cefamandole	32
Cefoxitin	32
Cefoperazone (T-1551)	32
Moxalactam (LY-127935)	32
Chloramphenicol	24
Clindamycin	8
Erythromycin	4
Metronidazole	16
Tetracycline	4
Doxycycline	4
Amikacin	24
Gentamicin	8
Tobramycin	8
Kanamycin	24
Vancomycin	8 to 12

*The term "breakpoint" as used here means a concentration of an antimicrobial agent in blood that can be achieved with optimal therapy. Breakpoints for cefaclor, cefamandole, cefoperazone, and moxalactam were selected on the basis of information supplied by the manufacturers of these agents; some of these may change with additional clinical experience.

†Levels expressed as µg of drug/ml, except for penicillin G, which is expressed as units of drug/ml.

the medium in which the tests are performed, (2) the drug's stability, (3) the size of the inoculum, (4) the organism's rate of growth, and (5) the period of incubation of the tests. Any variation in one or more of these factors may influence the test results, and those obtained by one procedure may not agree with those determined by a slightly different method.[6] However, if a standard procedure using only pure cultures is adopted and strictly adhered to, reproducible results can usually be obtained, and the reports from a given laboratory can be interpreted readily by the clinical staff. Minimal inhibitory concentrations are interpreted in light of achievable blood and body fluid levels with various drugs (Table 36-1).

Preparation of stock solutions of antimicrobial agents for dilution testing

Stock solutions of drugs are prepared from concentrated, dehydrated sterile material of known potency that may be obtained directly from the pharmaceutical manufacturer. Generally, they are prepared in concentrations of 1,000 µg/ml or higher and dispensed in small volumes in sterile, tightly sealed vials.

When stored in the frozen state at −20 C, most antibiotics remain stable for at least 8 weeks; when refrigerated at 5 C, most show no appreciable loss of potency in 1 week. However, storage at −60 to −70 C is recommended, particularly for the more labile antibiotics, including the penicillins and cephalosporins. Any unused thawed solutions of drugs should be discarded; each aliquot should be sufficient for only 1 day of use and should not be refrozen.

When preparing stock solutions, one must take into consideration the assay potency of each drug. The activity of the drug may differ from the actual weight of the powder. For example, an antimicrobial agent with an assay potency stated as 900 µg/mg actually contains only 900 µg of active drug for each 1,000 µg (1 mg) weighed out. The following formulas may be applied when preparing stock solutions:

$$\text{Weight (mg)} = \frac{\text{Volume (ml)} \times \text{concentration (µg/ml)}}{\text{Assay potency (µg/mg)}}$$

$$\text{Volume (ml)} = \frac{\text{Weight (mg)} \times \text{assay potency (µg/mg)}}{\text{Concentration (µg/ml)}}$$

Only fine electronic balances should be used for accurate weighing of powders. The solvents and diluents used in preparation of the more common antimicrobial agents are listed in Table 36-2.

TABLE 36-2

Stock solution preparation

Antimicrobial agent	Manufacturer	Solvent	Diluent
Amikacin	Bristol Labs.	Water	Water
Amoxicillin	Bristol Labs.	7.5% NaHCO$_3$	pH 7.0, 0.1 M phosphate buffer
Amphotericin B	E.R. Squibb & Sons, Inc.	Dimethyl sulfoxide	Water
Ampicillin	Bristol Labs.	7.5% NaHCO$_3$	Water
Bacitracin	The Upjohn Co.	Water	Water
Carbenicillin	Pfizer, Inc.	Water	Water
Cefamandole	Eli Lilly & Co.	Water	Water
Cefoxitin	Merck, Sharp & Dohme	Water	Water
Cephalexin	Eli Lilly & Co.	pH 6.0, 0.1 M phosphate buffer	Water
Cephalothin	Eli Lilly & Co.	pH 6.0, 0.1 M phosphate buffer	Water
Cefazolin	Eli Lilly & Co.	Water	Water
Chloramphenicol	Parke-Davis & Co.	95% ethanol	Water
Clindamycin	The Upjohn Co.	Water	Water
Cloxacillin	Bristol Labs.	Water	Water
Colistin	Parke-Davis & Co.	Water	Water
Dicloxacillin	Bristol Labs.	Water	Water
Erythromycin	Eli Lilly & Co.	Water	Water
Flucytosine	Hoffman LaRoche	Water	Water
Gentamicin	Schering Corp.	Water	Water
Kanamycin	Bristol Labs.	Water	Water
Methicillin	Bristol Labs.	Water	Water
Nafcillin	Wyeth Labs.	Water	Water
Nalidixic acid	Sterling Winthrop Research Institute	NaOH	Water
Neomycin	The Upjohn Co.	Water	Water
Nitrofurantoin	Norwich-Eaton Pharmaceuticals	Dimethylsulfoxide	Water
Oxacillin	Bristol Labs.	Water	Water
Penicillin	Bristol Labs.	Water	Water
Polymyxin B	Pfizer, Inc.	Water	Water
Rifampin	Ciba Pharmaceutical Co.	Dimethylsulfoxide	pH 7.0, 0.1 M phosphate buffer
Spectinomycin	The Upjohn Co.	Water	Water
Streptomycin	Pfizer, Inc.	Water	Water
Sulfonamides	Burroughs Wellcome Co.	Warm 1 N NaOH	Water
Tetracycline	Bristol Labs.	Water	Water
Ticarcillin	Beecham Labs.	Water	Water
Tobramycin	Eli Lilly & Co.	Water	Water
Trimethoprim	Burroughs Wellcome Co.	Warm 0.05 N HCl	Water
Vancomycin	Eli Lilly & Co.	Water	Water

ROUTINE PROCEDURE FOR TUBE DILUTION TESTS

The tube dilution method is considered one of the most accurate for determination of susceptibility to measured amounts (either units or micrograms) of an antimicrobial agent. It is a time-consuming and expensive procedure, however, especially when the clinician wants to know the susceptibility of an organism to a number of drugs. For this reason its use may well be restricted to special cases when quantitative results, which may include minimal bactericidal concentration determinations, may be of value. In any event, it is strongly recommended that all clinical laboratories should be prepared to provide this service to the clinician, either directly or through a referral laboratory.

The tube dilution method may be recommended, as a minimum, for determining the susceptibility of organisms isolated in the following instances: (1) from blood cultures, (2) from patients who fail to respond to apparently adequate therapy, (3) from immunosuppressed patients, and (4) from patients who relapse while undergoing such therapy. The study of organisms isolated from patients who relapse while receiving therapy usually involves determination of any increase in resistance on subsequent isolations and may require special methods.

Selection of media

The broth media in which tube dilution susceptibility tests are carried out must be of a kind that supports optimal rapid growth of the test organism in pure culture. A medium that supports the growth of clinical isolates without the addition of serum or blood is preferable, since the addition of such enrichment adds another variable to the test and may influence the results. It has been found that the concentration of the divalent cations (Ca^{++} and Mg^{++}) in the medium may affect results obtained with the aminoglycosides, polymyxins, and tetracyclines, particularly when testing *Pseudomonas aeruginosa*.[30] It is recommended that Mueller-Hinton broth be supplemented with these ions to obtain approximate physiologic concentrations in order to obtain consistent results.[27] Mueller-Hinton broth* is recommended for routine susceptibility testing. A medium more enriched than Mueller-Hinton broth may be necessary for testing fastidious organisms. The growth requirements should be determined before susceptibility tests are performed, so that the broth medium supporting the most luxuriant and rapid growth may be selected for the procedure. Mueller-Hinton broth or Schaedler broth supplemented with 5% Fildes enrichment† is adequate for testing *Haemophilus* species. Todd-Hewitt broth (without dextrose)† may be used for testing fastidious *Streptococcus* species. Mueller-Hinton broth containing 2% Fildes extract is usually adequate for testing *Corynebacterium* species and other fastidious organisms. The supplements may be added to the broth before it is distributed into the test tubes, or it may be added with the inoculum.

Preparation of serial dilutions and determination of susceptibility

Dilute antimicrobial stock solutions to obtain a working solution to contain 200 μg (or units)/ml. Number 10 sterile, capped, 13- by 100-mm tubes. Using aseptic technique, pipet 1 ml of appropriate broth into tubes 2 through 10. Add 1 ml of the working solution (200 μg/ml) of the drug into tubes 1 and 2. Mix the contents of the second tube well, and transfer 1 ml to tube 3. Continue this procedure to tube 9, discarding 1 ml from tube 9. Separate pipets must be used for each transfer to avoid carryover. Tube 10 serves as a positive growth control (broth plus inoculum). An additional tube containing broth alone should be set up to serve as a negative control.

---

*This medium is low in tetracycline and sulfonamide inhibitors and shows good batch-to-batch consistency.
†Baltimore Biological Laboratory, Cockeysville, Md.

TABLE 36-3

Suggested setup for the tube dilution method

Tube	Diluent (medium) added (ml)	Antimicrobial agent added	Diluted culture added (ml)	Final drug concentration (units or μg/ml)
1	None	1 ml working solution	1	100
2	1	1 ml working solution	1	50
3	1	1 ml from tube 2	1	25
4	1	1 ml from tube 3	1	12.5
5	1	1 ml from tube 4	1	6.25
6	1	1 ml from tube 5	1	3.125
7	1	1 ml from tube 6	1	1.56
8	1	1 ml from tube 7	1	0.78
9	1	1 ml from tube 8*	1	0.39
10	1	None	1	0

*Discard 1 ml from tube 9.

Inoculation of tubes

Add 1 ml of an inoculum containing approximately 10^5 to 10^6 organisms per milliliter. This inoculum may be prepared by making a 1:1,000 dilution of an overnight (6 hour, if the organism is a rapid grower) broth culture of the organism to be tested. Alternatively, adjust a log phase suspension of the test organism to match the turbidity of a 0.5 McFarland standard (corresponding to 1.5×10^8 organisms per milliliter), and further dilute 1:200 in broth. With slow-growing organisms, such as the fastidious streptococci, it may be necessary to use cultures incubated as long as 48 hours, and increased CO_2 may be desirable.

The final volume in each tube should be 2 ml, and the concentration of drugs should be from 100 μg (or units) to 0.39 μg (or unit)/ml in two-fold steps (Table 36-3). For organisms considered highly susceptible to antimicrobial agents, such as streptoccocci, a lower range of dilutions may be employed by further diluting the working solution (200 μg [or units]/ml) to 1:10. Thus, the final concentrations in Table 36-3 would be 10, 5, 2.5, 1.25, 0.63, 0.3, 0.15, 0.08 and 0.04 μg (or units)/ml.

Incubation and reading of tubes

Incubate tubes at 35 C for 16 to 20 hours, and examine macroscopically for evidence of growth. As noted earlier, the lowest concentration of drug in the series showing no growth is taken as the minimal inhibitory concentration and is expressed as micrograms (or units) per milliliter. One should remember that in the serial dilution technique there is a possible error equivalent to one tube dilution. This, together with the fact that the "true" minimal inhibitory concentration may fall anywhere between two consecutive dilutions, emphasizes the fact that the results are not necessarily absolute values.

Minimal bactericidal concentration determinations

One method that can be used to determine the minimal bactericidal concentration is to pipet 0.5 ml from each tube that shows no visible turbidity into 12 ml of infusion agar, mix, and make a pour plate. In addition, a colony count of the **initial inoculum** is prepared by making a pour plate of the 1:1,000 (or 1:200) dilution as described previously. By comparing colony counts after an appropriate incubation period of 48 to 72 hours, one may calculate the lowest concentration of the antimicrobial that demonstrated bactericidal activity (defined as 99.9% decrease in inoculum). A quantitative loop or sterile-tipped automatic micropipet may be used in lieu of the more cumbersome pour plate technique.

It should be noted that tolerance (considerably higher minimal bactericidal concentration than minimal inhibitory concentration after 18 to 24 hours with bactericidal antimicrobial agents) has been described.[37] The significance of this phenomenon clinically is uncertain, as discussed in Chapter 16. The entire issue of in vitro testing for bactericidal activity is very complex and is currently under investigation.

MICRODILUTION SUSCEPTIBILITY TEST PROCEDURES

During the past few years the standard tube dilution or "macrobroth" dilution susceptibility test has been modified and miniaturized into a system known as the microdilution MIC or microdilution susceptibility test. The principle of the microdilution susceptibility test is identical to that of the tube dilution procedure; this miniaturized adaptation provides a practical approach for routine use of a broth dilution MIC system.

Microdilution MICs are performed in small plastic microtiter trays that were originally developed for serologic procedures. The final volume of organism–antimicrobial agent suspension is generally 0.1 ml. Microdilution trays may contain up to 96 wells, which allows the subsequent testing of as many as 94 different antimicrobial concentrations (generally 2 wells are reserved for positive and negative controls). The number of drugs to be tested governs how many different dilutions of each antimicrobial agent can be incorporated.

There are several automated or semiautomated devices available that allow a laboratory to prepare its own microdilution trays. One type of system dispenses antimicrobial solution into the first wells and broth into the remaining wells and then serially dilutes each of the antimicrobial solutions (Minidiluter,* Mini MIC). The other major type of system available utilizes multichannel dispensers (MIC 2000*). Large volumes of the desired antimicrobial dilutions are prepared, and the dispenser automatically fills each well simultaneously. One of the most important advantages of in-house preparation of trays is the versatility in selecting the antimicrobial solutions and the concentrations to be tested.

There are several commercial suppliers of prefilled microdilution MIC trays. Depending on the manufacturer, these are available frozen (Micro Media†), lyophilized (Sceptor‡), or dried (bonded to the tray wells [Sensititre§]). Since preparation of trays involves considerable effort, the commercial trays present a more practical approach to microdilution MICs for the smaller laboratory.

Preparation of microdilution trays

As mentioned above, the type of equipment available for preparation of microdilution trays varies considerably. Consequently, the preparation procedures vary also, and a complete discussion of this is beyond the scope of this text. For more information, one should consult reference 27.

Inoculation of microdilution trays

As in other susceptibility test procedures, an actively growing suspension of the test organisms is required. There are various means of inoculating the trays, that utilize plastic or metal replicator devices, generally delivering 1 to 5 μl. The system in use determines what adjustments or dilutions of the test suspension are

---

*Dynatech Laboratories, Alexandria, Va.
†Micro Media Systems, Inc., Potomac, Md.
‡Baltimore Biological Laboratory, Cockeysville, Md.
§Gibco, Grand Island, N.Y.

required, so that the final concentration of organisms in the test wells is approximately 10^5 organisms per milliliter.

Incubation and reading of trays

Since small volumes of broth are utilized in this procedure, the microdilution trays must be sealed prior to incubation in order to minimize evaporation. This may be accomplished by using sealing tape or by stacking trays (up to five) on top of one another, ending with an empty tray or sealing tape on the top tray. Incubation is generally at 35 C for 16 to 18 hours. Following incubation, the microdilution trays are examined from the bottom by using a mirrored viewer. The minimal inhibitory concentration is read as the lowest concentration showing no growth. Here growth may be defined as turbidity or a button of organisms. As in other dilution susceptibility tests, it is imperative to compare growth in the antimicrobial wells to the positive and negative control wells.

AGAR PLATE DILUTION METHOD FOR DETERMINING SUSCEPTIBILITY TO ANTIMICROBIAL AGENTS

The agar plate dilution method is similar in principle to the broth dilution methods, except that a solid medium is used. Mueller-Hinton agar is recommended and is commonly prepared in 100-ml amounts. Some workers incorporate 3% to 5% blood or chocolatized blood in the medium when using it for testing organisms that require enriched media, such as *Streptococcus* and *Haemophilus*. There appears to be no significant inactivation of the drugs by the addition of the blood.

Preparation of antimicrobial dilutions

Prepare dilutions of the stock solutions of antimicrobial agents, so that a convenient volume may be added to the 100-ml volumes of agar to obtain the desired final concentrations in the plates. For example, to obtain an 8-µg/ml plate, add 0.8 ml of 1,000-µg/ml stock solution to 100

TABLE 36-4

Concentrations of antimicrobials tested at UCLA Hospital and Clinics against bacterial isolates by the agar dilution method

Antimicrobial agent	Concentrations (µg/ml)															
	0.06	0.12	0.25	0.5	1	2	4	8	16	32	50	64	100	128	200	256
Amikacin						x	x	x	x	x						
Ampicillin						x		x	x							
Carbenicillin												x		x		x
Cephalothin			x			x		x	x							
Chloramphenicol						x		x	x							
Clindamycin		x			x		x									
Erythromycin				x		x		x								
Gentamicin			x		x		x	x								
Oxacillin			x		x		x									
Penicillin	x	x			x		x									
Tetracycline						x	x	x								
Tobramycin			x		x		x	x								
Vancomycin						x	x	x								
Trimethoprim/sulfa-methoxazole					1/20	2/90	4/80									

ml of melted and cooled agar, and then pour the plate.

In an effort to simplify the agar dilution procedure, some laboratories prefer to increase the size of the dilution steps tested or to use only a limited number of concentrations per drug. Table 36-4 shows the concentrations of antimicrobial solutions used at the UCLA Hospital and Clinics. Concentrations were selected on the basis of anticipated serum levels at both high and low doses of the drugs.

Preparation of plate dilutions

Melt and cool sufficient flasks (or bottles) of agar medium for the number of plates to be prepared (about 20 ml of medium is required per 90-mm diameter plate), and allow them to equilibrate in a water bath at 50 C before adding the drugs. Add the required amount of the various dilutions to each flask (or bottle), mix gently by inversion, and pour into plates.* Allow the agar to harden, and store the plates in the refrigerator at 5 C until ready for use. If the plates are kept in tightly sealed plastic bags, they may be stored up to 4 weeks.[27]

Inoculation of plates

The inoculum should be adjusted to contain about 1.5×10^8 organisms per milliliter (equivalent to a McFarland 0.5 standard) (Plate 236); this ensures dense, nearly confluent growth on a control plate containing no antibiotic.

Spot inoculation of the plates is made with a 1-mm loop (approximately 0.001 ml), a capillary pipet, or (preferably) the inocula-replicator of Steers and co-workers (Plates 239 and 240).[42] With this device each manipulation can release 36 different cultures from the prongs on a replicator head to the surface of a 100-mm square plastic plate (Falcon) containing agar to a depth of 3 mm. Each prong delivers about 0.001 ml;

36 inoculations can be made simultaneously.

In using the Steers replicating device, it is recommended that four spaces on each plate be allocated for control organisms, for example, *Escherichia coli* (American Type Culture Collection [ATCC] 25922), *Pseudomonas aeruginosa* (ATCC 27853), *Staphylococcus aureus* (ATCC 29213), and *Streptococcus faecalis* (ATCC 29212). Thus, 31 spaces are available per plate for the testing of clinical isolates.

Organisms that spread, such as *Proteus*, may be contained by the use of 12- by 12-mm Raschig rings.*[51]

Incubation and reading of plates

Incubate the plates at 35 C for 16 to 20 hours, and examine them for the presence of growth. The lowest concentration of drug producing complete inhibition of growth is taken as the end point. A very fine growth or one or two visible colonies may be disregarded in the reading of the test. Control cultures on drug-free media should always show confluent growth.

QUALITY CONTROL OF DILUTION SUSCEPTIBILITY TEST PROCEDURES

In addition to the control measures already mentioned, standard quality control strains should be tested to monitor accuracy and precision of dilution test procedures.

The National Committee for Clinical Laboratory Standards (NCCLS) has recommended that *E. coli* (ATCC 25922), *P. aeruginosa* (ATCC 27853), *S. aureus* (ATCC 29213), and *S. faecalis* (ATCC 29212) be used for this purpose.[27] The expected minimal inhibitory concentrations are shown in Table 36-5. Upon repeated testing, the concentrations should fall within ± 1 doubling dilution of the concentration shown in the table, and the majority of minimal inhibitory concentrations should be at the values listed. For maintenance of these quality control strains, the guidelines suggested in the section Disk Diffu-

---

*The drug dilutions and culture medium should not be mixed directly in the plates; this may produce uneven distribution of the antibiotic in the agar.

*Scientific Glass Apparatus Co., Bloomfield, N.J.

TABLE 36-5

MICs (µg/ml)* for standard reference strains

Antimicrobic	Reference strain			
	S. aureus ATCC 29213	*S. faecalis* ATCC 29212	*E. coli* ATCC 25922	*P. aeruginosa* ATCC 27853
Amoxicillin	0.5	1	8	
Ampicillin	0.5	1	4	
Carbenicillin	4	32	8	32
Methicillin	1-2	>16		
Nafcillin	0.25	4-8		
Oxacillin	0.25	8		
Penicillin	0.25	2		
Ticarcillin	4	32	2-4	16
Cefamandole	1	32	0.25-0.5	
Cefoxitin	4	>128	2	
Cephalothin	0.12-0.25	16	8	
Amikacin	2	128	1-2	4
Gentamicin	0.5-1.0	8	0.5	2-4
Kanamycin	≤1	32-64	2-4	>128
Tobramycin	1	16	0.5	1
Chloramphenicol	4	8	4	>32
Clindamycin	0.06-0.12	8-16		
Colistin	>4	>128	0.5-1	2-4
Erythromycin	0.12-0.25	1	32	
Tetracycline	0.5	32	2	16-32
Vancomycin	1	2		
Nalidixic acid	128		2	
Nitrofurantoin	16	8	8	
Sulfisoxazole	64	64	16	>256
Trimethoprim/sulfameth-oxazole (1-19)†	<0.5/9.5	<0.5/9.5	<0.5/9.5	16/304

From NCCLS Subcommittee on Antimicrobial Susceptibility Testing.[27] An updated version of this table is available in Standard Method for Dilution Antimicrobial Susceptibility Tests for Bacteria which Grow Anaerobically (MIC) (M7-P), Villanova, May 1981, NCCLS Publications. Since this material is constantly being updated, the reader should obtain the latest publication from National Committee for Clinical Laboratory Standards, 771 E. Lancaster Ave., Villanova, PA 19085.
*These MICs obtained in several reference laboratories by agar dilution or by broth microdilution with cation supplemented broth.
†Very medium dependent, especially with enterococci.

sion Quality Control may be followed. Results of MICs and MBCs of 44 antimicrobial agents against 3 control strains, with and without serum, are given by Reimer and associates (Antimicrob. Agents Chemother. **19:**1050-1055, 1981).

For additional information on dilution testing in general, the standards proposed by the NCCLS for dilution antimicrobial susceptibility tests for bacteria that grow aerobically are recommended.[27]

STANDARDIZED DISK–AGAR DIFFUSION METHOD FOR DETERMINING SUSCEPTIBILITY TO ANTIBIOTICS

One of the most useful and widely used laboratory tests for antimicrobial susceptibility is the antimicrobial disk–agar diffusion procedure, the so-called disk method (Plates 237 and 238). Its simplicity, speed of performance, economy, and reproducibility (under standardized conditions) make it convenient for the busy diagnostic laboratory when more laborious dilution methods may not be practical.

As originally described by Bondi and associates[5], filter paper disks are impregnated with various antimicrobial agents of specific concentrations and are carefully placed on an agar plate that has been inoculated with a culture of the bacterium to be tested. The plate is incubated overnight and observed the following morning for a **zone of growth inhibition** around the disk containing the antimicrobial agent. Organisms that grow up to the edge of the disk are resistant.

No attempt is made here to discuss the complex physicochemical reactions that take place during diffusion of the antibiotic into the agar gel or the dynamics of bacterial growth under these conditions. The reader is referred to publications by Ericsson[9,10] for details.

Over the years numerous attempts have been made to standardize the disk procedure, including the work of Bauer and co-workers,[4] Ericsson,[10] the World Health Organization (WHO), the Food and Drug Administration,[12] and most recently the NCCLS. The NCCLS performance standards for antimicrobial disk susceptibility tests[25] are presented herein.

Numerous proficiency testing surveys, including a nationwide laboratory evaluation by the CDC, of the disk procedure have revealed that the procedure as practiced is not standardized and that there are numerous variables that may contribute to these discrepancies. Among those that have been identified are:

1. Selection and concentration of antimicrobial disks
2. Selection, age of agar plating medium, and agar depth
3. Storage and handling of disks
4. Methodology of testing
5. Criteria used for interpreting results

Selection of plating medium

Although an ideal medium has not yet been perfected for the disk test, the NCCLS Subcommittee considers Mueller-Hinton agar the best compromise for routine susceptibility testing, since it shows good batch-to-batch uniformity and is low in tetracycline and sulfonamide inhibitors. With the addition of 5% defibrinated sheep, horse, or other animal blood, it supports the growth of more fastidious pathogens (i.e., those that do not grow on nonenriched medium). When required, the blood-containing medium may be "chocolatized" for testing *Haemophilus* species.

Mueller-Hinton agar* is prepared according to the manufacturer's directions and should be immediately cooled in a 50 C water bath after removal from the autoclave. The cooled medium is then poured into sterile Petri plates (on a level, horizontal surface) to a uniform depth of 4 mm; this is equivalent to approximately 60 ml in a 140-mm (internal diameter) plate, or approximately 25 ml in a 90-mm plate. After solidifying at room temperature, the plates may be used the same day or refrigerated at 2 to 8 C for **no longer than 7 days,** unless some method is used to minimize water loss from evaporation, such as storage in polystyrene plastic bags. As a sterility control, several plates from each batch of blood-containing Mueller-Hinton agar should be incubated at 35 C for 24 hours or longer. These plates should not be used subsequently.

Each batch of Mueller-Hinton agar should be checked for pH when prepared; the **pH should be 7.2 to 7.4** at room temperature. This may be

---

*Baltimore Biological Laboratory, Cockeysville, Md.; Difco Laboratories, Detroit, Mich.; and others.

tested by macerating a small amount of medium in a little distilled water or by allowing a little of the medium to gel around a pH meter electrode in a small beaker. If available, a surface electrode may be used.

Just prior to use of the medium, the plates should be placed in a 35 C incubator with lids partly ajar, until excess surface moisture has evaporated. This usually requires about 20 minutes.

Storage and handling of disks

Antimicrobial disks are generally supplied in separate containers with a desiccant* and should be kept under refrigeration (from 4 to 5 C). Disks containing the penicillins (including ampicillin and carbenicillin) and the cephalosporin family of drugs should always be kept **frozen** (at less than −14 C) to maintain their potency; a small working supply may be refrigerated for up to **1 week.** For long-term storage disks are best kept in the frozen state until needed.

The unopened containers are removed as needed from the refrigerator or freezer 1 or 2 hours before the disks are to be used and allowed to adjust to room temperature. This is done to minimize condensation resulting from warm air reaching the cold containers. If disk dispensers are utilized, they should be equipped with tight covers and supplied with a satisfactory desiccant; when not in use, they should also be refrigerated.

Manufacturer's expiration dates should be noted and listed; **disks must be discarded on their expiration date.**

Preparation of inoculum

Various workers have shown that when certified antimicrobial disks and a single standard culture medium are used, the greatest factor contributing to reproducibility of the disk test is control of the inoculum size.

The currently recommended method of preparing a standardized inoculum is as follows:

1. With a sterile wire loop, the tops of four or five isolated colonies of a similar morphologic type are transferred to a tube containing 4 to 5 ml of soybean-casein digest broth or other suitable broth medium.*

2. The broth is incubated at 35 C until its turbidity exceeds that of the standard (described in step 3). This usually requires 2 to 8 hours' incubation.

3. The turbidity is then adjusted to match a McFarland 0.5 **barium sulfate standard.** This is prepared by adding 0.5 ml of 1.175% w/v (0.048M) barium chloride hydrate ($BaCl_2 \cdot 2\ H_2O$) to 99.5 ml of 1% w/v (0.36N) sulfuric acid. The standard is distributed in screw-capped tubes of the same size as those used in growing the broth culture, which contain approximately 4 to 6 ml per tube. These are then tightly sealed and stored at room temperature in the dark. Fresh standards must be prepared at least once every 6 months, although these standards can remain stable for a much longer period when heat sealed and stored in the dark.[55]

4. The barium sulfate standard must be vigorously agitated on a Vortex shaker just before use. The turbidity of the broth culture is then adjusted visually by adding sterile saline or broth, using adequate light and comparing the tubes against a white background with a contrasting black line.

Inoculation of the test plates

Within 15 minutes of adjusting the density of the inoculum, a sterile cotton swab on a wooden applicator stick (plastic or wire sticks are not satisfactory) is dipped into the standardized bacterial suspension. The excess fluid is removed by rotating the swab with firm pressure against the

---

*Humidity—particularly high humidity—heat, and contamination are important deteriorating factors.[14]

*Trypticase soy broth, Baltimore Biological Laboratory, Cockeysville, Md.; tryptic soy broth, Difco Laboratories, Detroit, Mich.; and others.

inside of the tube above the fluid level. The swab is then used to streak the dried surface of a Mueller-Hinton plate in three different planes (by rotating the plate approximately 60° each time) to ensure an even distribution of the inoculum.

Replace the plate lids and allow the inoculated plates to remain on a flat and level surface undisturbed for 3 to 5 minutes (no longer than 15 minutes) to allow for absorption of excess moisture, then apply the disks, as described in the following section.

Placement of disks

With alcohol-flamed, fine-pointed forceps (cooled before using) or a disk dispenser,* the selected disks are placed on the inoculated plate and pressed firmly into the agar with sterile forceps or needle to ensure **complete contact** with the agar. The disks are distributed evenly in such a manner as to be **no closer than 15mm from the edge of the Petri dish** and so that no two disks are closer than 24 mm from center to center. Once a disk has been placed, it should not be moved, since some diffusion of the drug occurs almost instantaneously.

An alternative method, using an agar overlay, has been described by Barry and colleagues.[2] This method is useful only for rapidly growing organisms, such as *S. aureus*, the enteric bacilli, and *P. aeruginosa*. This method also must be standardized to correspond with results obtained by the cotton swab–streak method already described.

The plates are inverted and placed in the 35 C incubator within 15 minutes after application of the disks. Incubation under increased CO_2 tension should not be practiced, since the interpretative zone sizes were developed under aerobic conditions; CO_2 incubation may significantly alter the zone sizes.

Reading of results

After incubation, the relative susceptibility of the organism to the antimicrobic is demonstrated by a clear zone of growth inhibition around the disk. This is the result of two processes: diffusion of the drug and growth of the bacteria. As the antimicrobic diffuses through the agar medium from the edge of the disk, its concentration progressively diminishes to a point where it is no longer inhibitory for the organism. The size of this area of suppressed growth, the **zone of inhibition,** is determined by the concentration of antimicrobic present in the area and the susceptibility of the test isolate. Therefore, within the limitations of the test, the **diameter of the inhibition zone denotes the relative susceptibility** to a particular antimicrobic.

After 16 to 18 hours' incubation (rapid growers can be read in 6 to 8 hours[19]), each plate is examined, and the diameters of the complete inhibition zones are noted and measured, using reflected light and sliding calipers (Plate 238), a ruler, or a template prepared for this purpose and held on the bottom of the plate.* The **end point,** measured to the nearest millimeter, should be taken as the area showing no visible growth that can be detected with the unaided eye. Faint growth or tiny colonies near the edge of the inhibition zones are ignored, as is the swarming that may occur in the inhibition zones with some strains of *Proteus vulgaris* and *P. mirabilis*. With sulfonamides slight growth (with 80% or more inhibition) is disregarded, and the margin of heavy growth is measured to determine the zone diameter.

Large colonies growing within a zone of inhibition may actually be a different bacterial species (a mixed, rather than a pure, culture) and should be subcultured, reidentified, and retested.

---

*Dispensers for both the 90- and 140-mm Petri plates are available from Baltimore Biological Laboratory, Cockeysville, Md.; Difco Laboratories, Detroit, Mich.; and others.

*Microbial growth should be almost or just confluent; if only isolated colonies are present, the inoculum was too light and the test must be repeated.

Interpretation of zone sizes

The diameters of the zones of inhibition are interpreted by referring to Table 36-6, which represents the NCCLS subcommittee's recommendations.

The term "susceptible" implies that an infection caused by the strain tested may be expected to respond favorably to the indicated antimicrobial agent for that type of infection and pathogen. "Resistant" strains, on the other hand, are not inhibited completely by therapeutic concentrations. "Intermediate" implies that strains may respond to unusually high concentrations of the agent, resulting from either high dosage or high levels achieved, as in the urinary tract. In other circumstances, intermediate results might warrant further testing if alternative agents are not available.

Limitations of the test

The modified Bauer-Kirby procedure has been standardized for testing rapidly growing bacteria, particularly members of the Enterobacteriaceae, *S. aureus*, and *Pseudomonas* species. For testing *Haemophilus*, Mueller-Hinton agar plates supplemented with 1% hemoglobin and 1% IsoVitaleX* are recommended. Prepare the inoculum by suspending growth from a 24-hour chocolate agar plate in Mueller-Hinton broth to the density of a 0.5 McFarland standard. *Streptococcus pyogenes* is considered susceptible to penicillin G and is not routinely tested; however, in patients hypersensitive to penicillin, the isolate may be tested against erythromycin or clindamycin. The susceptibility of *Neisseria gonorrhoeae* to penicillin can be determined by testing these isolates on GC agar base supplemented with 1% IsoVitaleX. The inoculum is prepared as for *Haemophilus influenzae*. Strains that produce beta-lactamase and are consequently resistant to penicillin have zones of 19 mm or less, and susceptible strains have zones of 20 mm or more. The recent development of resistance of *S. pneumoniae* to penicillin G (and other antimicrobial agents) is noted in Chapter 18.

A screen for penicillin susceptibility can be performed by using a 1-μg oxacillin disk and a Mueller-Hinton agar plate supplemented with 5% sheep blood. The inoculum is prepared using 24-hour growth from a blood agar plate and standardized as for *H. influenzae*. Penicillin-susceptible strains have oxacillin zones of 20 mm or more (MIC $\leq$ 0.06 μg/ml). Penicillin-resistant strains have oxacillin zones 12 mm or less (MIC $\geq$ 2 μg/ml.). So-called penicillin-"relatively resistant" strains have zones of 13 to 19 mm (MIC 0.12-1 μg/ml). Further tests must be performed on the relatively resistant isolates to more definitively characterize the effect of penicillin on them.[48] (See Chapter 18.)

Hoo and Drew[15] pointed out that nitrofurantoin disks gave inconsistent results related to differences in pH of different batches of disks. They indicated that nonantibiotic chemotherapeutic agent disks are not regulated by the FDA. Accordingly, problems might be anticipated with other agents, such as cotrimoxazole (trimethoprim/sulfamethoxazole), sulfonamides, and nalidixic acid. Daily inclusion of standard test strains alerts laboratories to batches of disks that give erroneous results.

In general, fastidious organisms that require increased CO_2 tension (other than *H. influenzae*, *N. gonorrhoeae*, and *S. pneumoniae*) or an anaerobic atmosphere or whose growth rate is unusually slow do not lend themselves to susceptibility testing by the standardized disk–agar diffusion method; agar plate or broth dilution test procedures are recommended. Susceptibility testing of anaerobes is described in a subsequent section.

Quality control procedures

It is essential that some form of quality control procedure be carried out to ensure precision and accuracy of the test results. The NCCLS

---

*Baltimore Biological Laboratory, Cockeysville, Md.

Text continued on p. 550.

TABLE 36-6

Zone size interpretative standards

Antimicrobic or chemotherapeutic agent	Disk potency	Inhibition zone diameter to nearest mm		
		Resistant	**Intermediate**	**Sensitive**
Amikacin[a]	30 μg	14 or less	15-16	17 or more
Ampicillin[b]	10 μg			
Enterobacteriaceae and enterococci		11 or less	12-13	14 or more
Staphylococci[c]		20 or less	21-28	29 or more
Haemophilus[d]		19 or less		20 or more
Carbenicillin	100 μg			
Pseudomonas species		13 or less	14-16	17 or more
Proteus and *Escherichia coli*		17 or less	18-22	23 or more
Cefamandole[e]	30 μg	14 or less	15-17	18 or more
Cefoxitin[e]	30 μg	14 or less	15-17	18 or more
Cephalothin[f]	30 μg	14 or less	15-17	18 or more
Chloramphenicol	30 μg	12 or less	13-17	18 or more
Clindamycin[g]	2 μg	14 or less	15-16	17 or more
Colistin[h]	10 μg	8 or less	9-10	11 or more
Erythromycin	15 μg	13 or less	14-17	18 or more
Gentamicin[a]	10 μg	12 or less	13-14	15 or more
Kanamycin	30 μg	13 or less	14-17	18 or more
Methicillin[i]	5 μg	9 or less	10-13	14 or more
Nalidixic acid[j]	30 μg	13 or less	14-18	19 or more
Neomycin	30 μg	12 or less	13-16	17 or more
Nitrofurantoin	300 μg	14 or less	15-16	17 or more
Penicillin G	10 U			
Staphylococci[k]		20 or less	21-28	29 or more
Other organisms[l]		11 or less	12-21	22 or more
Polymyxin B[h]	300 U	8 or less	9-11	12 or more
Streptomycin	10 μg	11 or less	12-14	15 or more
Sulfonamides[j,m]	250 or 300 μg	12 or less	13-16	17 or more
Tetracycline[n]	30 μg	14 or less	15-18	19 or more
Tobramycin[a]	10 μg	12 or less	13-14	15 or more
Trimethoprim-sulfamethoxazole	1.25 μg/23.75 μg	10 or less	11-15	16 or more
Vancomycin	30 μg	9 or less	10-11	12 or more

See footnotes on opposite page.

TABLE 36-6 footnotes

Recent papers provide additional data. One recommends modifying the standard for sensitive with gentamicin to ≥16 mm (Barry: Am. J. Clin. Pathol. **75**:524-531, 1981). Another proposes standards for susceptibility of *Pseudomonas* and Enterobacteriaceae to mezlocillin (75-μg disk) (susceptible, ≥16 mm; indeterminate, 13 to 15 mm; resistant, ≤12 mm). For *S. aureus* the breakpoints for susceptible are ≥29 mm and for resistant ≤28 mm (Fuchs et al.: Antimicrob. Agents Chemother. **20**:197-203, 1981). With moxalactam 30-μg disks, the proposed intermediate category is a zone of 15 to 22 mm (Barry et al.: Antimicrob. Agents Chemother. **18**:716-721, 1980).

An updated, expanded version of this table is available in First Supplement, Performance Standards for Antimicrobic Disk Susceptibility Tests (M2-A2S1) (Table 2), Villanova, May 1981, NCCLS Publications. Since this material is constantly being updated, the reader should obtain the latest publication from National Committee for Clinical Laboratory Standards, 771 E. Lancaster Ave., Villanova, PA 19085.

[a]The zone sizes obtained with aminoglycosides, particularly when testing *Pseudomonas aeruginosa*, are very medium dependent because of variations in cation content. The zone size interpretive standards for amikacin, gentamicin, and tobramycin are tentative standards recently agreed upon by a subcommittee of the NCCLS. These interpretive standards are to be used only with Mueller-Hinton medium that has yielded zone sizes within the correct range when performance tests were done with *P. aeruginosa* (ATCC 27853). In addition, the amikacin disk must be 30 μg rather than the 10-μg disk used previously. Organisms in the intermediate category may be either susceptible or resistant when tested by dilution methods and should therefore more properly be classified as "indeterminate" in their susceptibility to aminoglycosides.

[b]Class disk for ampicillin, hetacillin, and amoxicillin.

[c]Resistant strains of *S. aureus* produce beta-lactamase.

[d]For testing *Haemophilus* use Mueller-Hinton agar supplemented with 1% hemoglobin and 1% IsoVitaleX (BBL), Supplement VX (Difco) or an equivalent synthetic supplement. Adjust pH to 7.2. Prepare the inoculum by suspending growth from a 24-hour chocolate agar plate in Mueller-Hinton broth to the density of a turbidity standard. The vast majority of ampicillin-resistant strains of *Haemophilus* produce beta-lactamase.

[e]Cefamandole and cefoxitin were recently approved. They have a wider spectrum of activity on gram-negative bacilli then do other approved cephalosporins. Therefore, the cephalothin disk cannot be used as the class disk for these two drugs.

[f]The cephalothin disk is used for testing susceptibility to cephalothin, cephaloridine, cephalexin, cefazolin, cephacetrile, cephradine, cefaclor, and cephapirin. Cefamandole and cefoxitin must be tested separately. *S. aureus* exhibiting resistance to methicillin disks should be reported as resistant to cephalosphorin-type class antibiotics, regardless of zone size because in most cases infections caused by these organisms are clinically resistant to cephalosporins. Methicillin-resistant *S. epidermidis* infection may not respond to cephalosporins.

[g]The clindamycin disk is used for testing susceptibility to both clindamycin and lincomycin.

[h]Colistin and polymyxin B diffuse poorly in agar, and the diffusion method is thus less accurate than with other antibiotics. Resistance is always significant, but when treatment of systemic infections caused by susceptible strains is being considered, results of a diffusion test should be confirmed with those of a dilution method. MIC correlates cannot be calculated reliably from regression analysis.

[i]Of the antistaphylococcal beta-lactamase-resistant penicillins, methicillin is the class disk, and results also apply to cloxacillin, dicloxacillin, oxacillin, and nafcillin. Oxacillin and nafcillin are, however, more resistant to degradation in storage. Cloxacillin disks should not be used, because they may not detect methicillin-resistant *S. aureus*.

[j]Susceptibility data for nalidixic acid, nitrofurantoin, and sulfonamides apply only to organisms isolated from urinary tract infections.

[k]Penicillin G is used to test the susceptibility of all penicillinase-sensitive penicillins, except ampicillin, amoxicillin, hetacillin, and carbenicillin. Results can be applied to phenoxymethyl penicillin or phenethicillin.

[l]Intermediate category includes some microorganisms, such as enterococci, and certain gram-negative bacilli that may cause systemic infections treatable with high dosages of benzyl penicillin but not of phenoxymethyl penicillin or phenethicillin. For pneumococci and gonococci refer to special interpretations applied in section 4.4 of reference 25.

[m]The 250- or 300-μg sulfisoxazole disks can be used for any of the commercially available sulfonamides. Blood-containing media, except media containing lysed horse blood, are not satisfactory for testing sulfonamides. The Mueller-Hinton agar should be as thymidine-free as possible for sulfonamide or trimethoprim testing. (See section 3.1.1 of reference 25).

[n]Tetracycline is the class disk for all tetracyclines, and the results can be applied to chlortetracycline, demeclocycline, doxycycline, methacycline, oxytetracycline, minocycline, and rolitetracycline for most commonly isolated organisms. However, some in vitro data show that certain organisms may be more susceptible to doxycycline and minocycline than to tetracycline.

TABLE 36-7

Control limits for monitoring precision and accuracy of inhibitory zone diameters (mm) obtained in groups of five separate observations

Antimicrobial agent	Disk content	Individual test control Zone diameter (mm)	Accuracy control Zone diameter (mm) Mean of 5 values	Precision control Range* of 5 values Maximum	Precision control Range* of 5 values Average†
E. coli (ATCC 25922)					
Amikacin	30 µg	19 to 26	20 to 25	4	2.1
Ampicillin	10 µg	15 to 20	15.8 to 19.2	6	2.9
Carbenicillin	100 µg	24 to 29	25.0 to 28.0	7	3.5
Cefamandole‡	30 µg	24 to 31			
Cefoxitin‡	30 µg	23 to 28	23.8 to 27.2	6	2.9
Cephalothin§	30 µg	18 to 23	18.8 to 22.2	6	2.9
Chloramphenicol	30 µg	21 to 27	22.0 to 26.0	7	3.5
Colistin	10 µg	11 to 15	11.7 to 14.3	4	2.3
Erythromycin	15 µg	8 to 14	9.0 to 13.0	7	3.5
Gentamicin	10 µg	19 to 26	20.2 to 24.8	8	4.1
Kanamycin	30 µg	17 to 25	18.3 to 23.7	9	4.7
Nalidixic acid‡	30 µg	23 to 28			
Neomycin	30 µg	17 to 23	18.0 to 22.0	6	3.5
Nitrofurantoin‡	300 µg	21 to 26			
Polymyxin B	300 units	12 to 16	12.7 to 15.3	4	2.3
Streptomycin	10 µg	12 to 20	13.3 to 18.7	9	4.7
Sulfisoxazole‡	250 µg or 300 µg	18 to 26			
Tetracycline§	30 µg	18 to 25	19.2 to 23.8	8	4.1
Tobramycin	10 µg	18 to 26			
Trimethoprim sulfamethoxazole‡	1.25 µg 23.75 µg	24 to 32	25.3 to 30.7	9	4.7
S. aureus (ATCC 25923)					
Amikacin	30 µg	20 to 26	21.9 to 23.9	5	2.4
Ampicillin	10 µg	24 to 35	25.8 to 33.2	13	6.4
Cefamandole‡	30 µg	28 to 34			

Cefoxitin‡	30 μg	23 to 28	23.8 to 27.2	6	2.9
Cephalothin§	30 μg	25 to 37	27.0 to 35.0	14	7
Chloramphenicol	30 μg	19 to 26	20.2 to 24.8	8	4.1
Clindamycin	2 μg	23 to 29	24.0 to 28.0	7	3.5
Erythromycin	15 μg	22 to 30	23.3 to 28.7	9	4.7
Gentamicin	10 μg	19 to 27	20.3 to 25.7	9	4.7
Kanamycin	30 μg	19 to 26	20.2 to 24.8	8	4.1
Methicillin	5 μg	17 to 22	17.8 to 21.2	6	2.9
Neomycin	30 μg	18 to 26	19.3 to 24.7	9	4.7
Nitrofurantoin‡	300 μg	20 to 24			
Penicillin G	10 units	26 to 37	27.8 to 35.2	13	6.4
Polymyxin B	300 units	7 to 13			
Streptomycin	10 μg	14 to 22	15.3 to 20.7	9	4.7
Sulfisoxazole‡	250 μg	24 to 34			
Tetracycline§	30 μg	19 to 28	20.5 to 26.5	11	5.2
Tobramycin	10 μg	19 to 29			
Vancomycin	30 μg	15 to 19	15.7 to 18.3	4	2.3
Trimethoprim	1.25 μg	24 to 32	25.0 to 31.0	7	3.5
sulfamethoxazole	23.75 μg				
P. aeruginosa (ATCC 27853)					
Amikacin	30 μg	18 to 26			
Carbenicillin	100 μg	20 to 24			
Gentamicin	10 μg	16 to 21			
Polymyxin B‡§	300 units	11 to 16			
Tobramycin	10 μg	19 to 25			

From NCCLS Subcommittee on Antimicrobial Susceptibility Testing.[25] An updated, expanded version of this table is available in Performance Standards for Antimicrobic Disc Susceptibility Tests (M2-A2S1), Villanova, May 1981, NCCLS Publications. Since this material is constantly being updated, the reader should obtain the latest publication from National Committee for Clinical Laboratory Standards, 771 E. Lancaster Ave., Villanova, PA 19085. Quality control limits for mezlocillin (*E. coli*, 23 to 29 mm; *S. aureus*, 27 to 35 mm; and *P. aeruginosa*, 19 to 25 mm) and for piperacillin (*E. coli*, 24 to 30 mm; *S. aureus*, 27 to 35 mm; and *P. aeruginosa*, 25 to 33 mm) have been proposed by Gavan and colleagues (J. Clin. Microbiol. 14:67-72, 1981).

*Maximum value minus minimum value obtained in a series of five consecutive tests should not exceed the listed maximum limits, and the mean should fall within the range listed under "accuracy control."

†In a continuing series of ranges from consecutive groups of five tests each, the average range should approximate the listed value.

‡To be considered tentative for twelve months from publication of reference 25.

§Many laboratories have reported difficulties with these quality control parameters; therefore, the parameters are currently being reevaluated.

recommends that tests be monitored daily with stock cultures of *S. aureus* (ATCC 25923), *E. coli* (ATCC 25922), and *P. aeruginosa* (ATCC 27853) using disks representative of those to be used in testing of clinical isolates.[25] These cultures may be grown on soy-casein digest agar slants and refrigerated (4 to 8 C) and should be subcultured to fresh slants every 2 weeks. For long-term storage these cultures may be lyophilized or frozen at −70 C in a suitable broth, such as Brucella broth with 15% glycerol.

For testing the cultures are inoculated to soy-casein digest broth tubes, which are incubated overnight and streaked to agar plates to obtain isolated colonies; these are then picked to broth and tested as described in the preceding sections.

The control strains may be used as long as there are no significant changes in the mean inhibition zone diameters that are not otherwise attributable to technical error. If such changes occur, fresh strains should be obtained from a reference laboratory or other reliable source. Individual values of zone diameters and permissible variation are indicated in Table 36-7, which represents a computation based on standard statistical methods.[25]

It should be emphasized that some lots of Mueller-Hinton agar may contain increased concentrations of Ca^{++} and Mg^{++}. Since *S. aureus* and *E. coli* do not appear to be affected by these ions, they will not demonstrate changes in zone sizes. However, as mentioned earlier, the Ca^{++} and Mg^{++} concentration is significant when testing *P. aeruginosa* and the aminoglycosides. An increase in the concentration of Ca^{++} and Mg^{++} results in increased resistance, hence smaller zones. Thus, the effect of increased concentrations of these cations would influence the interpretation of susceptibilty and should be predetermined. It should be noted that solid media (agar) usually contain significant concentrations of Ca^{++} and Mg^{++}, whereas broth media do not. For susceptibility testing the aim is to supplement the test media with these divalent cations to attain concentrations comparable

to physiologic concentrations so that reproducible and meaningful results can be obtained.

Several studies indicated that reading Kirby-Bauer disk susceptibilty tests at 8 hours, instead of at the usual 18 to 20 hours, gave accurate readings at least 85% of the time and that even earlier readings could often be made accurately.[19,23] This is not recommended as a routine but could be very useful on occasion in the management of seriously ill patients.

In selected instances, limited to sites normally sterile but from which a single organism is likely to be recovered in the event of an infection (as in a positive blood culture), it may be feasible to do direct disk susceptibility testing on the primary culture plate.[56] Again, this should be done only in the case of a seriously ill patient and should be repeated using a standard procedure.

BETA-LACTAMASE TESTING

The beta-lactamase test has become a very popular method for the rapid detection of ampicillin and penicillin resistance in beta-lactamase–producing strains of *H. influenzae*, *N. gonorrhoeae*, and *S. aureus*. Several methods have been described, including the rapid acidometric method,[47] the rapid iodometric method,[8] and the rapid chromogenic cephalosporin method.[28] These three methods depend on the beta-lactamase enzyme's ability to act on the substrate and either directly or indirectly produce a color change. This is detailed in Cumitech 6.[46]

Chloramphenicol resistance in *H. influenzae* is usually related to production of chloramphenicol acetyltransferase; a rapid screening procedure for this enzyme has been described (Azemun et al.: Antimicrob. Agents Chemother. **20:**168-170, 1981).

TESTING OF ANTIMICROBIAL COMBINATIONS

It is frequently necessary to treat serious infections with a combination of antimicrobial agents. Depending on the drugs and the infecting bacterium, the combination may be synergistic, additive, or antagonistic. A combination is considered synergistic when the effect of the two drugs together is greater than the sum of the effects with either drug alone. An additive effect occurs when the effect of the combination is equal to the sum of the effects of the two drugs tested separately or equal to that of the most active drug in the combination. Finally, antagonism occurs when the combination is less effective than the most active drug in the combination.

In vitro testing can be performed to assess the effects of two antimicrobial agents on a bacterium. The primary methods used to perform in vitro combination studies include "checkerboard" broth dilution testing and killing curves.

The checkerboard technique, which is basically a broth dilution MIC procedure, involves serially diluting and combining the two drugs to obtain as many combinations as possible within therapeutically achievable levels. In addition, each drug is tested alone, and the effect of the combination is compared to the individual results to see if there is a synergistic effect.

When determining killing curves, the rates of killing by a specified concentration of each drug singly and in combination are compared. If the two drugs together kill the test organism at a more rapid rate than either drug alone, the combination is considered to be synergistic. A tenfold or greater difference in the number of viable cells at a given time is considered significant. Synergy studies are very complex and time consuming and should not be performed on a routine basis.

SUSCEPTIBILITY TESTING OF ANAEROBES

It can no longer be said that most anaerobes have predictable patterns of susceptibility to antimicrobial drugs and that if the organism is well identified, one may usually predict its susceptibility pattern fairly accurately. Susceptibility testing certainly is required for patients with

serious infections, patients with infections failing to respond to what was thought to be appropriate therapy, and patients who relapse after an initial response to therapy, as a minimum. In most cases of anaerobic infection antimicrobial therapy must be started before the availability of definite bacteriologic data and susceptibility testing.

Although a number of specialized types of antimicrobial susceptibility tests have been devised specifically for anaerobic bacteria, the conventional tests used for other organisms may be used under anaerobic conditions.[24,25] It is extremely important, however, to realize that the Bauer-Kirby technique was not standardized for anaerobes and that reliable results cannot be obtained with anaerobes by this method.[49] Standardized disk tests designed specifically for anaerobes are available, but different techniques must be used for organisms with different growth rates.[21,44] For testing occasional isolates most laboratories probably find a broth test most convenient. An abbreviated test can be used, with three tubes covering the range of concentrations likely to be achieved with specific agents that might be employed therapeutically. A good alternative introduced by Wilkins and Thiel[57] utilizes antimicrobial agent–impregnated disks in broth. The drug is eluted from the disks to provide the desired concentration in broth quickly and conveniently. However, their original method required prereduced broth and a gassing apparatus. Kurzynski and associates[20] have modified the broth disk procedure by substituting aerobically incubated thioglycollate broth (Plate 241); this simple procedure seems ideally suited for the small laboratory doing small numbers of susceptibility tests on anaerobes. However, we would suggest the use of the following concentrations of drugs: 3 μg/ml for tetracycline, 100 μg/ml for carbenicillin, 3 μg/ml for erythromycin, 18 μg/ml for chloramphenicol, 2 units/ml for penicillin, and 6 μg/ml for clindamycin. Another simple approach would be to freeze tubes with double the desired concentration of drugs in broth; tubes could be tak-

TABLE 36-8

Susceptibility of anaerobes to antimicrobial agents

Bacterium	Chloram-phenicol	Clinda-mycin	Metroni-dazole	Penicillin G	Tetra-cycline	Erythro-mycin	Vanco-mycin
Microaerophilic and anaerobic cocci	+++	++ to +++	++	+++ to ++++	++	++ to +++	+++
Bacteroides fragilis	+++	+++†	+++	+	+ to ++	+ to ++	+
Other *Bacteroides*	+++	+++†	+++	++ to +++	++ to +++	+++	+
Fusobacterium varium	+++	+ to ++	+++	++ to +++	++	+	+
Other *Fusobacterium* species	+++	+++	+++	++ to +++	+++	+	+
Clostridium perfringens	+++	+++†	+++	++++‡	++ to +++	+++	+++
Other *Clostridium* species	+++	++	++ to +++	+++	++	++ to +++	++ to +++
Eubacterium and *Actinomyces*	+++	++ to +++	+ to ++	++++	++ to +++	+++	++ to +++

++++, drug of choice; +++, good activity; ++, moderate activity; +, poor or inconsistent activity. There is usually no difference in activity between drugs rated +++ and those rated ++++; the symbol ++++ indicates a drug with good activity, good pharmacologic characteristics, and low toxicity.

*Aminoglycosides, such as gentamicin and kanamycin, are generally quite inactive against the majority of anaerobes. The activity of erythromycin varies significantly according to the testing procedure. Erythromycin and vancomycin are not approved by the FDA for anaerobic infections. Penicillin G: Other penicillins and cephalosporins are frequently less active. Ampicillin, carbenicillin, and cephaloridine are roughly comparable to penicillin G on a weight basis, but the high blood levels safely achieved with carbenicillin make it effective against 95% of the strains of *Bacteroides fragilis*. Cefoxitin, a compound resistant to penicillinase (beta-lactamase I) and cephalosporinase (beta-lactamase II) is active against 90% to 95% of strains of the *B. fragilis* group and most other anaerobes, but one third of clostridia other than *C. perfringens* are resistant. Tetracycline: Doxycycline and minocycline are more active than other tetracyclines, but susceptibility testing is indicated to ensure activity.

†Rare strains are resistant.

‡A few strains are resistant.

en out of the freezer as needed and thawed and an equal amount of broth with inoculum added.

The agar dilution method as described by the NCCLS is the reference anaerobic method for susceptibility testing.[26] Further details on various techniques are given in reference 44.

Table 36-8 is presented as a guide to the microbiologist and clinician. It is based largely on correlations of in vitro findings[45] and evaluation of clinical effectiveness.

SUSCEPTIBILITY TESTING OF MYCOBACTERIA AND FUNGI

Susceptibility testing of mycobacteria is discussed in Chapter 31. Fungal susceptibility tests are best sent to a reference laboratory.

AUTOMATION IN ANTIMICROBIAL SUSCEPTIBILITY TESTING

Within the past few years, serious attention has been given to the development of automated and semiautomated antimicrobial susceptibility test systems. Semiautomated devices including the Steers replicator and the microdilution diluting and dispensing devices have already been mentioned.

The major approach to automated susceptibility testing involves photometric measurement of the effect an antimicrobial drug has on bacterial growth (in a liquid medium) as compared with growth of the same bacterium in the absence of antimicrobial agents. Systems currently available include the Autobac 1 and the Autobac-MIC,* the MS-2,† the AutoMicrobic System,‡ and the API-1§ (see Chapter 40). The first three systems not only automatically read and print out the susceptibility results but do so in less then 8 hours, thus qualifying them as rapid test systems.

OTHER USES FOR ANTIMICROBIAL SUSCEPTIBILITY TESTS

Antimicrobic disks may be used for selectively isolating various microorganisms. Following Vera's suggestions[50] one may employ disks containing penicillin (10 units), neomycin (30 µg), and bacitracin (10 units) on all primary plates inoculated with a potentially mixed flora. The zones of inhibition around the neomycin disks have been particularly useful in exposing colonies of group A beta-hemolytic streptococci, pneumococci, enterococci, and other streptococci. *H. influenzae* has been easily isolated from within the zones surrounding the 10-unit bacitracin disk on blood agar plates inoculated with sputum and from material obtained from the throat and nasopharynx. Penicillin disks (10

units) have been helpful in unmasking colonies of coliform bacilli, pseudomonads, and species of *Proteus*, *Candida albicans*, and others. A 10-unit penicillin disk also is useful for revealing colonies of *Bordetella pertussis* on Bordet-Gengou plates of nasopharyngeal cultures. Kanamycin disks (30 µg) have been reported to be helpful in separating *Bacteroides* and *Clostridium* species from other wound bacteria when the plates are incubated anaerobically.[50]

Unique susceptibility patterns may also be useful in identification of bacteria and may help "fingerprint" isolates for epidemiologic purposes.[7,41]

DETERMINATION OF BACTERICIDAL ACTIVITY OF SERUM DURING ANTIMICROBIAL THERAPY

A direct method for determining the antibacterial activity of serum of patients receiving antimicrobial drugs was first described by Schlichter and associates.[38,39] In the Schlichter test (also known as the serum bactericidal test) the dilution of a patient's serum that kills the infecting organism is determined. In selected cases of infection, particularly bacterial endocarditis, the Schlichter test may prove useful for assessing the adequacy of antimicrobial therapy.

Schlichter test procedure*

1. Subculture a recent isolate of the organism to an infusion agar or blood agar slant and store it in the refrigerator until the test is run, then subculture to a tube of broth early on the day of the test.
2. Obtain the first blood specimen **before therapy,** if possible; this serves as a control. Then take blood samples at any desired interval, although it is recommended that the low point of the blood concentration curve be included if the patient is on intermittent dosage. Collect 10 ml of the patient's blood in a sterile tube. On receipt in the laboratory, the

*Pfizer, Inc., New York, N.Y.
†Abbot Laboratories, North Chicago, Ill.
‡Vitek Systems, Inc., St. Louis, Mo.
§Analytab Products, Plainview, N.Y.

*As modified by Washington.[51]

clot is separated and the serum is obtained by centrifugation. The serum is then transferred to a sterile, rubber-stopped tube; it may be tested at that time (or within 2 to 3 hours if refrigerated) or frozen at −20 C, a temperature at which it remains stable for several days.

3. Prepare serial twofold dilutions of serum in 1-ml amounts in Mueller-Hinton broth, using eight sterile, gauze-stoppered Kahn tubes (**use a separate pipet for each dilution**). Soy-casein digest broth or others, such as brain-heart infusion or Levinthal broth, can be used for organisms that do not grow in Mueller-Hinton medium. The first tube contains only **undiluted serum,** and a ninth tube contains only broth and serves as a culture **control.** The serum dilutions range from undiluted through 1:128. Very sensitive organisms, such as alpha-hemolytic streptococci, may require dilutions up to 1:2,048.

4. To each tube of the series add 0.05 ml of a 1:1,000 dilution of a 6-hour broth culture of the organism isolated from the patient. Also prepare a colony count pour plate using 1 ml of the inoculum.

5. Incubate the tubes at 35 C for 18 to 24 hours and examine. The **bacteriostatic end point** is taken as the highest dilution in which no visible growth occurs. Because of the inherent turbidity of some sera, it is recommended that subcultures be made from each tube to a sector of a blood agar plate. To determine **bactericidal end points,** transfer 0.05 ml from each tube showing no growth to a tube of thioglycolate medium. Mix and incubate at 35 C for 72 hours. The tube in the series that shows no growth in thioglycolate is taken as the end point. Good growth should be evident in the control tube.

6. In cases where the organism grows slowly, a loopful of an overnight broth culture may be used as the inoculum. With microaerophilic or anaerobic bacteria, the tubes should be incubated anaerobically.

7. Schlichter indicated that an optimal antimicrobial dosage (either single or combined drugs) had been achieved when a bactericidal level of 1:2 (complete inhibition in the first two tubes) had been demonstrated; others, however, believe that a bactericidal level of 1:4 or 1:8 is desirable.

Since the serum bactericidal test was first described by Schlichter in 1947, it has undergone numerous modifications.[31] A survey performed in 1973 demonstrated that there was considerable variation in the way the test was being performed in diagnostic laboratories.[29] This variation included such factors as inoculum size, test medium, and the method for determining the bactericidal end point. It is apparent that in order for the serum bactericidal test to be a meaningful test, a standardized procedure, such as that provided by the NCCLS for testing of bacterial isolates, needs to be established. This is currently being investigated.

ASSAY OF ANTIMICROBIAL AGENTS

In recent years much interest has been focused on the development of techniques for the assay of antimicrobial agents.[22,35,40,43,59] These permit a laboratory to rapidly and accurately determine the concentrations of these agents in various body fluids (serum, spinal fluid, urine, and so forth). Assays are useful in the following situations: (1) with drugs such as gentamicin, which do not give predictable levels; (2) when relatively toxic drugs are used, particularly in patients with impaired kidney or liver function; (3) when inactivation of drugs may occur; (4) when it is uncertain how well a drug will penetrate the blood-brain barrier; and (5) with new agents whose pharmacology is not yet well known. For example, the aminoglycoside gentamicin is widely used to treat serious and life-threatening infections. However, the therapeutic-toxic ratio is relatively low with this agent. Because of its potential for nephrotoxicity and ototoxicity, patients may receive suboptimal doses of gentamicin, and therefore inadequate blood levels are achieved.[17,18,58]

A number of methods are in use for assaying

antimicrobial agents in the body fluids. Included are microbiologic assay, radioimmunoassay, enzymatic radio assay and enzymatic immunoassay, turbidimetric assay, inhibition of pH or redox change, fluorescent immunoassay, chemical, and high-pressure liquid chromatography. It is not within the scope of this text to discuss these procedures in detail. Interested readers should consult references 13, 33, 36, 53, and 54.

REFERENCES

1. Anderson, T.G.: Testing of susceptibility to antimicrobial agents and assay of antimicrobial agents in body fluids. In Lennette, E.H., Blair, J.E., and Truant, J.P., editors: Manual of clinical microbiology, Washington, D.C., 1970, American Society for Microbiology.
2. Barry, A.L., Garcia, F., and Thrupp, L.D.: An improved single-disk method for testing the antibiotic susceptibility of rapidly-growing pathogens, Am. J. Clin. Pathol. 53:149-158, 1970.
3. Barry, A.L., and Lasner, R.A.: In vitro methods for determining minimal lethal concentrations of antimicrobial agents, Am. J. Clin. Pathol. 71:88-92, 1979.
4. Bauer, A.W., Kirby, W.M.M., Sherris, J.C., and Turck, M.: Antibiotic susceptibility testing by a standardized single disc method, Am. J. Clin. Pathol. 45:493-496, 1966.
5. Bondi, A., Spaulding, E.H., Smith, E.D., and Dietz, C.C.: A routine method for the rapid determination of susceptibility to penicillin and other antibiotics, Am. J. Med. Sci. 214:221-225, 1947.
6. Branch, A., Starkey, D.H., and Power, E.E.: Diversifications in the tube dilution test for antibiotic sensitivity of microorganisms, Appl. Microbiol. 13:469-472, 1965.
7. Buck, G.E., Sielaff, B.H., Boshard, R., and Matsen, J.: Automated rapid identification of bacteria by pattern analysis of growth inhibition profiles obtained with Autobac 1, J. Clin. Microbiol. 6:46-49, 1977.
8. Catlin, B.W.: Iodometric detection of *Haemophilus influenzae* beta-lactamase: rapid, presumptive test for ampicillin resistance, Antimicrob. Agents Chemother. 7:265-270, 1975.
9. Ericsson, H.: Rational use of antibiotics in hospitals, Scand. J. Clin. Lab. Invest. 12:1-59, 1960.
10. Ericsson, H.: The paper disc method in quantitative determination of bacterial sensitivity to antibiotics, Stockholm, 1961, Karolinska Sjukhuset.
11. Fink, F.C.: Special features of the tube dilution method of antibiotic susceptibility testing, Presented at the Interscience Conference on Antimicrobial Agents and

Chemotherapy, American Society for Microbiology, Chicago, 1962.
12. Food and Drug Administration: Standardized disc susceptibility test, Federal Register 37(191):20527-20529, September 30, 1972.
13. Gerson, B., and Anhalt, J.P.: High-pressure liquid chromatography and therapeutic drug monitoring, Chicago, 1980, American Society of Clinical Pathologists.
14. Griffith, L.J., and Mullins, C.G.: Drug resistance as influenced by inactivated sensitivity discs, Appl. Microbiol. 16:656-658, 1968.
15. Hoo, R., and Drew, W.L.: Potential unreliability of nitrofurantoin disks in susceptibility testing, Antimicrob. Agents Chemother. 5:607-610, 1974.
16. Isenberg, H.D.: A comparison of nationwide microbial susceptibility testing using standardized discs, Health Lab. Sci. 1:185-256, 1964.
17. Jackson, G., and Riff, L.J.: *Pseudomonas* bacteremia: pharmacologic and other bases for failure of treatment with gentamicin, J. Infect. Dis. 124 (Supp.): S185-S191, 1971.
18. Kaye, D., Levison, M.E., and Labovitz, E.D.: The unpredictability of serum concentrations of gentamicin: pharmacokinetics of gentamicin in patients with normal and abnormal renal function, J. Infect. Dis. 130:150-154, 1974.
19. Kluge, R.M.: Accuracy of Kirby-Bauer susceptibility tests read at 4, 8, and 12 hours of incubation: comparison with readings at 18 to 20 hours, Antimicrob. Agents Chemother. 8:139-145, 1975.
20. Kurzynski, T.A., Yrios, J.W., Helstad, A.G., and Field, C.R.: Aerobically incubated thioglycolate broth disk method for antibiotic susceptibility testing of anaerobes, Antimicrob. Agents Chemother. 10:727-732, 1976.
21. Kwok, Y-Y, Tally, F.P., Sutter, V.L., and Finegold, S.M.: Disk susceptibility testing of slow growing anaerobic bacteria, Antimicrob. Agents Chemother. 7:1-7, 1975.
22. Lewis, J.E., Nelson, J.C., and Elder, H.A.: Radioimmunoassay of an antibiotic: gentamicin, Nature (London) New Biol. 239:214-216, 1972.
23. Liberman, D.F., and Robertson, R.G.: Evaluation of a rapid Bauer-Kirby antibiotic susceptibility determination, Antimicrob. Agents Chemother. 7:250-255, 1975.
24. Martin, W.J., Gardner, M., and Washington, J.A., II: In vitro antimicrobial susceptibility of anaerobic bacteria isolated from clinical specimens, Antimicrob. Agents Chemother. 1:148-158, 1972.
25. NCCLS Subcommittee on Antimicrobial Susceptibility Testing: Performance standards for antimicrobial disc susceptibility tests. Approved Standard: ASM-2, October 1979, The National Committee for Clinical Laboratory Standards.

26. NCCLS Subcommittee on Antimicrobial Susceptibility Testing: Proposed reference dilution procedure for antimicrobic susceptibility testing of anaerobic bacteria. Proposed Standard: PSM-11, November 1979.

27. NCCLS Subcommittee on Antimicrobial Susceptibility Testing: Standard methods for dilution antimicrobial susceptibility tests for bacteria which grow aerobically. Proposed Standard: PSM-7, July 1980.

28. O'Callaghan, C.H., Morris, A., Kirby, S.M. and Shingler, A.H.: Novel method for the detection of β-lactamases by using a chromogenic cephalosporin substrate, Antimicrob. Agents Chemother. **1:**283-288, 1972.

29. Pien, F.D., and Vosti, K.L.: Variation in performance of the serum bactericidal test, Antimicrob. Agents Chemother. **6:**330-333, 1974.

30. Reller, L.B., Shoenknecht, F.D., Kenny, M.A., and Sherris, J.C.: Antibiotic susceptibility testing of *Pseudomonas aeruginosa:* selection of a control strain and criteria for magnesium and calcium content in media, J. Infect. Dis. **130:**454-463, 1974.

31. Reller, L.B., and Stratton, C.W.: Serum dilution test for bactericidal activity. II. Standardization and correlation with antimicrobial assays and susceptibility tests, J. Infect. Dis. **136:**196-204, 1977.

32. Ryan, K.J., and Sherris, J.C.: Antimicrobial susceptibility testing, Hum. Pathol. **7:**277-286, 1976.

33. Sabath, L.D.: The assay of antimicrobial compounds, Hum. Pathol. **7:**287-295, 1976.

34. Sabath, L.D.: Staphylococcal tolerance to penicillins and cephalosporins. In D. Schlessinger, editor: Microbiology, 1979, Washington, DC, 1979, American Society for Microbiology.

35. Sabath, L.D., Casey, J.I., and Rych, P.A. Rapid microassay of gentamicin, kanamycin, neomycin, streptomycin, and vancomycin in serum or plasma, J. Lab. Clin. Med. **78:**457-463, 1971.

36. Sabath, L.D., and Matsen, J.M. Assay of antimicrobial agents. In Lennette, E.H., Spaulding, E.H., and Truant, J.P., editors: Manual of clinical microbiology, ed. 2, Washington, D.C., 1974, American Society for Microbiology.

37. Sabath, L.D., Wheeler, N., Laverdiere, M., Blazevic, D., and Wilkinson, B.J.: A new type of penicillin resistance of *Staphylococcus aureus,* Lancet **1:**443-447, 1977.

38. Schlichter, J.G., and MacLean, H.: A method of determining the effective therapeutic level in the treatment of subacute bacterial endocarditis with penicillin, Am. Heart J. **34:**209-211, 1947.

39. Schlichter, J.G., MacLean, H., and Milzer, A.: Effective penicillin therapy in subacute bacterial endocarditis and other chronic infections, Am. J. Med. Sci. **217:**600-608, 1949.

40. Smith, D.H., Van Otto, B., and Smith, A.L.: A rapid chemical assay for gentamicin, N. Engl. J. Med. **286:**583-586, 1972.

41. Southern, P.M., Jr., and Bagby, M.K.: Antimicrobial susceptibility patterns (antibiograms) as an aid in identifying *Citrobacter* species, Am. J. Clin. Pathol. **67:**187-189, 1977.

42. Steers, E., Foltz, E.L., and Graves, B.S.: An inocula replicating apparatus for routine testing of bacterial susceptibility to antibiotics, Antibiot. Chemother. **9:**307-311, 1959.

43. Stevens, P., Young, L.S., and Hewitt, W.L.: Radioimmunoassay, acetylating radioenzymatic assay, and microbioassay of gentamicin: a comparative study, J. Lab. Clin. Med. **86:**349-359, 1975.

44. Sutter, V.L., Citron, D.M., and Finegold, S.M.: Wadsworth anaerobic bacteriology manual, ed. 3, St. Louis, 1980, The C.V. Mosby Co.

45. Sutter, V.L., and Finegold, S.M.: Susceptibility of anaerobic bacteria to 23 antimicrobial agents, Antimicrob. Agents Chemother. **10:**736-752, 1976.

46. Thornsberry, C., Gavan, T.L., and Gerlach, E.H. In Sherris, J.C., editor: New developments in antimicrobial agent susceptibility testing, Cumitech 6, Washington, D.C., 1977, American Society for Microbiology.

47. Thornsberry, C., and Kirven, L.A.: Ampicillin resistance in *Haemophilus influenzae* as determined by a rapid test for beta-lactamase production, Antimicrob. Agents Chemother. **6:**653-654, 1974.

48. Thornsberry, C., and Swenson, J.M.: Antimicrobial susceptibility tests for Streptococcus pneumoniae, Lab. Med. **11:**83-86, 1980.

49. Thornton, G.F., and Cramer, J.A.: Antibiotic susceptibility of *Bacteroides* species, Antimicrob. Agents Chemother. **10:**509-513, 1970.

50. Vera, H.D.: Sensitivity plate tests. In BBL manual of products and laboratory procedures, Cockeysville, Md., 1968, Baltimore Biological Laboratory.

51. Washington, J.A., II: Personal communication (E.G.S.), 1973.

52. Washington, J.A., II: Antimicrobial susceptibility of Enterobacteriaceae and nonfermenting gram-negative bacilli, Mayo Clin. Proc. **44:**811-824, 1969.

53. Washington, J.A., II, editor: Laboratory procedures in clinical microbiology, New York, 1981, Springer-Verlag.

54. Washington, J.A., II: Assay techniques. In Current chemotherapy, Proceedings of the Tenth International Congress of Chemotherapy, Washington, D.C., 1978, American Society for Microbiology, pp. 56-59.

55. Washington, J.A., II, Warren, E., and Karlson, A.G.: Stability of barium sulfate turbidity standards, Appl. Microbiol. **24:**1013, 1972.

56. Waterworth, P.M., and Del Piano, M.: Dependability of sensitivity tests in primary culture, J. Clin. Pathol. **29:**179-184, 1976.

57. Wilkins, T.D., and Thiel, T.: Modified broth-disk method for testing the antibiotic susceptibility of anaerobic bacteria, Antimicrob. Agents Chemother. **3:**350-356, 1973.

58. Winters, R.E., Litwack, K.D., and Hewitt, W.L.: Relation between dose and levels of gentamicin in blood, J. Infect. Dis. **124** (Suppl.): S90-S95, 1971.

59. Wold, J.S.: Rapid analysis of cefazolin in serum by high-pressure liquid chromatography, Antimicrob. Agents Chemother. **11:**105-109, 1977.

PART VI

SEROLOGIC METHODS IN DIAGNOSIS

37 SEROLOGIC IDENTIFICATION OF MICROORGANISMS

Wright and colleagues[13] described procedures for preparation of antigens of 14 of the most common clinical bacterial isolates requiring serologic confirmation for identification. These included *Neisseria meningiditis* serogroups A, B, C, D, and Y; *Haemophilus influenzae* type B; *Streptococcus pneumoniae* type 3; *Shigella dysenteriae* serogroup A; *S. flexneri* serogroup B; *S. boydii* serogroup C; *S. sonnei* serogroup D; *Salmonella paratyphi* A serogroup A; *Salmonella typhimurium* serogroup B; *S. cholerae-suis* group C_1; *S. newport* serogroup C_2; *S. typhi* serogroups D and Vi; *S. senftenberg* serogroup E_4; and *Escherichia coli* (alkalescens-dispar group). They described procedures for producing smooth, homogenous bacterial suspensions that were stable for up to 5 months at 4 C. These were as satisfactory as viable cultures in terms of the intensity and rapidity of the agglutination reaction but provided a more uniform suspension and readily available materials.

GROUPING AND TYPING OF BETA-HEMOLYTIC STREPTOCOCCI BY PRECIPITIN TEST

Both the group and the type of a beta-hemolytic streptococcus may be determined by the Lancefield precipitin procedure (Plate 242) using the same antigen. Typing should be carried out soon after isolation of the organism, because the M type-specific protein substance, which determines the type, can be lost on laboratory cultivation. Fresh isolates that have been frozen can be typed successfully later.

LANCEFIELD PROCEDURE
Materials

1. Two sizes of capillary tubing are required: (a) 1.2 to 1.5 mm outside diameter for grouping, and (b) 0.7 to 1 mm outside diameter for typing.* Tube lengths of 7.5 cm should be used.
2. Wooden blocks 12 inches long containing Plasticine are recommended for holding the capillary tubes upright after they are filled with antigen and antiserum.
3. Todd-Hewitt broth at pH 7.8 to 8, dispensed in 40-ml amounts and inoculated 24 hours previously with the culture to be tested.
4. Beta-streptococcus group-specific and type-specific antiserum.†

---

*Kimble Glass Co., Vineland, N.J.
†Difco Laboratories, Detroit, Mich.; Baltimore Biological Laboratory, Cockeysville, Md.; Lee Laboratories, Grayson, Ga.; and others.

5. N/5 hydrochloric acid—1 ml 12 N HCl plus 59 ml of 0.85% saline.
6. Buffer solution—N/5 sodium hydroxide in M/15 phosphate buffer solution at pH 7. To prepare, dissolve 1 g of anhydrous acid sodium phosphate in 100 ml of N/5 sodium hydroxide.
7. Phenol red—0.01%. To prepare, add 0.01 g of phenol red to 60 ml of alcohol and 40 ml of water.
8. Thymol blue—0.01%. To prepare, add 0.01 g of thymol blue to 60 ml of alcohol and 40 ml of water.

Preparation of antigen

1. Grow organisms to be tested for 18 to 24 hours in 40 ml of Todd-Hewitt broth.
2. Centrifuge the culture for 30 minutes and **remove all of the supernatant.**
3. Resuspend sediment in 0.4 ml of N/5 hydrochloric acid pH 2.0 to 2.4.
4. Mix well with a wooden applicator stick.
5. Add 1 drop of thymol blue indicator. A **peach** color will result.
6. Transfer to a 15-ml conical bottom centrifuge tube and heat in a boiling water bath for 3 to 10 minutes, shaking occasionally.

7. Cool in a refrigerator or a cold water bath for 10 minutes.
8. Centrifuge at 3,000 rpm for 10 minutes.
9. Decant the clear supernatant fluid into a clean test tube and add 1 drop of phenol red indicator. The solution will be a distinct **yellow.**
10. Add buffer solution drop by drop until a pale **pink** color develops (pH 7.4 to 7.8). Do not make too strongly alkaline.
11. Centrifuge as described previously and remove the supernatant fluid. This fluid must be **crystal clear** for use as the antigen.
12. The extract may be stored at 4 C for several days to a week.

Another widely used method of preparing the antigen extract is the autoclave method of Rantz and Randall[11]:

1. Inoculate steptococci into 40 ml of Todd-Hewitt broth containing 0.8% glucose and incubate 24 to 48 hours.
2. Centrifuge to completely sediment the bacterial cells; discard the supernatant fluid.
3. Add 0.5 ml of 0.85% NaCl.
4. Transfer the sediment to sterile flocculation tubes and autoclave for 15 minutes at 121 C.
5. Centrifuge to complete sedimentation.
6. Transfer the supernatant fluid to sterile flocculation tubes. This fluid is ready for use as the antigen extract.

Other antigen extraction procedures include the following: *Streptomyces albus* enzyme and *S. albus*–lysozyme enzyme extraction methods, pronase B enzyme method, hot formamide method, and nitrous acid and micro–nitrous acid extraction methods.[4]

Test procedure
For grouping beta-hemolytic streptococci

Clean the outside of a 1.2- to 1.5-mm capillary tube with tissue paper or lens paper. It cannot be overemphasized that all capillary tubes, anti-gen extracts, and antisera must be **perfectly clean.** Antiserum that becomes turbid on storage should be clarified by centrifugation. Dip the capillary tube into group A streptococcus antiserum and permit the serum to rise one third the length of the tube, equivalent to a 2-cm column. Wipe the outside of the tube to remove excess serum and to prevent adulteration of the antigen. Dip the capillary tube into the prepared antigen extract and draw up an equal amount. Wipe the outside of the tube with tissue and invert the tube until there is an air space both above and below the column of liquid. Place the tube upright in the Plasticine in the wooden block.

Repeat the procedure, using groups B, C, D, F, and G antisera, respectively. Immediately after the tests are set up, examine the capillary tubes with a hand lens. This is best done using a strong light in front of a black background. The tubes should be perfectly clear if the test has been correctly performed. Leave the tubes at room temperature and reexamine after 15 to 30 minutes. In the tube containing antigen and homologous antiserum, a **milky ring** will form at the interface of the reactants. A **positive** reaction such as this is sharp and definite and appears in 5 to 10 minutes. After 1 or 2 hours, the ring disappears and a heavy white precipitate settles to the bottom of the liquid. The **negative** tubes should remain perfectly clear.

If the culture tested proves to be group A streptococcus and typing of the strain is desired, the same extract can be used as the antigen; it can be kept in a refrigerator for at least 1 week and still give satisfactory results.

For typing beta-hemolytic streptococci

Clean the outside of a 0.7- to 1-mm capillary tube with tissue or lens paper. Use the same technique as just described, substituting beta-hemolytic streptococcus **type-specific serum** for the group-specific serum, and insert the capillary tube upright in the Plasticine. Incubate the tests for 2 hours, refrigerate overnight, and read as described above. Sometimes it is possible to read the tubes after incubation; in other cases it is necessary to refrigerate them to obtain a reaction.

Cross-reactions may occur with the type-specific antiserum. In such cases these reactions can be largely eliminated by repeating the test, using the antisera in which precipitation has occurred and diluting each one half, one fourth, or one eighth with isotonic salt solution. Incubate for 2 hours, refrigerate overnight, and read as in the regular test.

Attention also is directed to the typing of group A streptococci by the T-agglutination technique. The reproducibility of the procedure has been established. Moody and coworkers[10] were able to T-type 88% of more than 1,300 strains referred to the CDC, compared with 47% typed by the M-precipitin technique. The methods used are described in the report.

Immunofluorescence and CIE are also useful for grouping streptococci, particularly groups A and B (see Chapter 39).

QUELLUNG METHOD FOR TYPING PNEUMOCOCCI

Pneumococcus typing by the **quellung reaction** was formerly one of the most important procedures in a medical diagnostic laboratory. With the advent of antimicrobial therapy for the treatment of pneumococcal infections, serologic typing of pneumococci is no longer necessary as a guide to therapy. However, the quellung test remains one of the most rapid and satisfactory methods for the **direct identification** of the pneumococcal organism in clinical material. For this reason it is still an important laboratory procedure and will be discussed here.

Clinical materials

The quellung test is considered a useful procedure with the following clinical specimens:

1. Sputum in which organisms resembling pneumococci are readily demonstrated in direct smears.

2. CSF sediment that contains organisms suggestive of pneumococci (successful typing of the organisms definitely and immediately establishes their identity).
3. Presumptive fresh pneumococcus colonies obtained from blood agar plates and suspended in a few drops of broth.
4. Positive blood-broth cultures (Plate 50), empyema fluid, and other specimens that show organisms resembling pneumococci on microscopic examination.

Test procedure

1. On a clean glass slide, spread a small loopful of the specimen in a thin film, and **allow to air dry.** Make six of these preparations. If stained smears of the material reveal more than 15 to 25 organisms per oil immersion field, **dilute** the specimen, since too many organisms tend to agglutinate in the antiserum, thereby making the capsular reaction difficult to observe.
2. Place a large loopful of typing serum on a coverglass, and add a small loopful of 1% aqueous methylene blue stain. Invert a No. 1 square coverglass over one of the dried films made previously. When available, the typing sera are individually prepared for pneumococcus types 1 through 34, inclusive. Typing is carried out initially with pools labeled A through F* until a positive quellung reaction is obtained, and then with antisera for the specific types making up that pool. As many as three coverglasses may be used on one slide. These sera are produced by the CDC and are available primarily to public health laboratories and government research agencies. A polyvalent diagnostic antiserum, **Omni serum,** is also available.† This serum can give a capsular swelling reaction with any of the 83 recognized types of pneumococci.

---

*Pools A through F are available from Difco Laboratories, Detroit, Mich.
†Statenserum-Institut, Copenhagen, Denmark.

Also available from the same source are 9 pools (A through I) covering these types and 46 monovalent antisera. All contain methylene blue stain.

3. Examine each preparation under the microscope, using the oil immersion lens with **reduced** illumination. A **positive** reaction is indicated by the appearance of a well-defined and refractile capsule surrounding the blue-stained pneumococcus. There is some variation in the reaction among strains; type 3 pneumococci, for example, possess very large capsules. In general, however, it is the **sharpness** of the capsular outline rather than the size of the capsule that indicates a positive reaction. Capsules that are visible but without adequate swelling are considered a negative reaction. In some negative reactions a thin halo with a definite outline may confuse the inexperienced worker. By focusing above and below such organisms nothing will be observed; in positive reactions the capsules are readily visible in these focal planes. Capsular reactions usually take place in several minutes; negative preparations should be reexamined after 1 hour before discarding. Avoid letting the preparations dry out.

QUELLUNG TEST ON SPINAL FLUID FOR DIAGNOSIS OF HAEMOPHILUS INFLUENZAE MENINGITIS

A rapid diagnosis of meningitis caused by *Haemophilus influenzae* can be made by performing a quellung test on spinal fluid. Gram-stained smears should first be made of the spinal fluid and observed carefully for the presence of small gram-negative coccobacilli; if none are observed, the fluid should be centrifuged and the sediment gram stained. If gram-negative bacilli resembling *H. influenzae* are seen on the smears from either source, quellung tests should be performed using the appropriate specimen. Since almost all cases of *Haemophilus* meningitis are caused by **serotype b** organisms, the use of

homologous antiserum is recommended.* The technique is the same as that described for serotyping the pneumococci. If influenza bacilli of serologic type b are present, a typical quellung reaction will be observed.

QUELLUNG TEST FOR IDENTIFICATION OF SEROTYPES OF KLEBSIELLA PNEUMONIAE

As originally studied by Julianelle,[7] the klebsiellae were serologically categorized into four types: A, B, C, and a heterogeneous group X. More than 70 capsular types are currently recognized. Types 1, 2, and 3 correspond to types A, B, and C of Julianelle. Specific antisera made against most of the capsular serotypes may be used in the performance of the quellung test.† The technique is the same as that described for the typing of pneumoccci.

SEROLOGIC GROUPING OF NEISSERIA MENINGITIDIS

Numerous serologic groups of *Neiseria meningitidis* are currently recognized.[1] However, groups A, B, and C are the most prevalent and therefore the most significant to test for serologically. The serologic grouping of meningococci is primarily one of epidemiologic significance, but if such identification is desired, the following agglutination test can be recommended:

1. Prepare twofold serial dilutions of the group-specific antisera.‡
2. Place 0.1 ml of each serial dilution in a very small test tube.
3. Suspend organisms from a young (5- to 24-hour) culture on solid medium using physiologic saline containing 0.05% potassium

---

*Difco Laboratories, Detroit, Mich., Hyland Laboratories, Los Angeles, Calif.; and Statenserum-Institut, Copenhagen, Denmark.

†Capsular antisera for most serotypes and pooled antisera are available from Difco Laboratories, Detroit, and Lee Laboratories, Grayson, Ga.

‡Central Public Health Laboratories, London; Difco Laboratories, Detroit, Mich.

cyanide not only to enhance smoothness of the bacterial suspension but also to effectively kill the organisms.

4. Filter the suspension by pipetting through a wisp of nonabsorbent cotton or centrifuge for 2 minutes at low speed to remove coarse particles. Clumps will not settle out spontaneously.

5. Dilute the antigen to approximate the No. 8 McFarland standard (see Chapter 44).

6. Add 0.1 ml of the antigen to each serum dilution and shake the rack for 3 minutes at room temperature.

7. Add 0.8 ml of physiologic saline to facilitate reading of the reactions.

8. Read for macroscopic clumping of the organisms.

Typing can also be done by the quellung reaction, using type-specific antisera, as previously described. No quellung reaction is obtained with group B because no morphologic capsule exists.

SLIDE AGGLUTINATION TEST IN SEROLOGIC IDENTIFICATION

Final identification of various members of the Enterobacteriaceae is dependent on serologic analysis. Such analysis is used primarily for the numerous serotypes that make up the genera *Salmonella* and *Shigella*. It may also be applied to other organisms. With the aid of commercially available diagnostic antisera, the identification of many of these bacteria becomes readily obtainable for most laboratories, provided experienced personnel perform and interpret the serologic tests. However, exact antigenic analysis requires the use of specifically absorbed typing sera, which are available primarily through various state health laboratories and at reference centers, such as the CDC, Atlanta, and the Laboratory Center for Disease Control, Ottawa. Recently many of these absorbed typing sera have become available from commercial suppliers.

Test procedure

Mark off a number of squares (¾ inch) on a perfectly clean glass slide with a grease pencil (e.g., Blaisdell, red 169T). Prepare a milky concentration of cells in saline in a tube from the growth on a TSI (or KIA) slant, from an agar slant, or from colonies on an agar plate. Since large numbers of viable cells are involved, extreme caution should be exercised in carrying out this procedure. Place one loopful or a small drop of each antiserum to be tested per square and leave one square blank. Add one drop of 0.85% saline to the blank square. With a Pasteur pipet add one small drop of the cell suspension to each square containing serum and to the blank square (as a control). Tilt the slide back and forth for 1 minute to mix, then observe for agglutination macroscopically. Agglutination is recognized by the prompt formation of fine granules or large aggregates. The control and any negative tests should remain homogeneous.

K antigens, which mask the heat-stable somatic (O) complex, are found in *Salmonella*, *Shigella*, and *Escherichia*. Should the cells fail to agglutinate in O antiserum, the suspension should be heated at 100 C for 10 to 30 minutes, cooled, and retested in the appropriate O antisera. Suspensions of live cells agglutinate in antisera that contain K antibody, for example, *Salmonella* Vi and *E. coli* OB.

For a more thorough discussion of the serologic examination of members of the family Enterobacteriaceae, consult Edwards and Ewing.[3]

The following list of diagnostic antisera* is provided for the reader's convenience.

Salmonella diagnostic sera

Salmonella polyvalent (contains primarily antibody against O antigens 1 through 10, 15, 19, and Vi)

---

*Lederle Laboratories, Pearl River, N.Y.; Baltimore Biological Laboratory, Cockeysville, Md.; Difco Laboratories, Detoit, Mich.; Lee Laboratories, Grayson, Ga.

Salmonella group A (contains primarily antibody against O antigens 1, 2, and 12)

Salmonella group B (contains primarily antibody against O antigens 4, 5, and 12)

Salmonella group C_1 (contains primarily antibody against O antigens 6 and 7)

Salmonella group C_2 (contains primarily antibody against O antigens 6 and 8)

Salmonella group D (contains primarily antibody against O antigens 9 and 12)

Salmonella group E (E_1, E_2) (contains primarily antibody against O antigens 3, 10, and 15)

Salmonella group F

Salmonella group G

Salmonella group H

Salmonella group I

Salmonella Vi

Salmonella H antiserum a (contains primarily antibody against flagellar a antigen)

Salmonella H antiserum b (contains primarily antibody against flagellar b antigen)

Salmonella H antiserum c (contains primarily antibody against flagellar c antigen)

Salmonella H antiserum d (contains primarily antibody against flagellar d antigen)

Salmonella H antiserum i (contains primarily antibody against flagellar i antigen)

Salmonella H antiserum k (contains primarily antibody against flagellar k antigen)

Salmonella H antiserum y (contains primarily antibody against flagellar y antigen)

Salmonella H antisera 1, 2; 1, 5; 1, 6; and 1, 7 (contains primarily antibody against flagellar 1, 2, 5, 6, and 7 antigens)

Shigella grouping sera

Shigella group A (*S. dysenteriae*)
Shigella group B (*S. flexneri*)
Shigella group C (*S. boydii*)
Shigella group D (*S. sonnei*)

COAGGLUTINATION

The Cowan strain of *Staphylococcus aureus* is rich in protein A and binds the Fc portion of IgG subclasses 2 and 4, leaving the Fab portions free to react with any of a series of antibody molecules. The antibodies are coupled via the pro-tein A linkages to dead staphylococci, which serve as carriers. When this reagent is mixed with a sample containing streptococci or other corresponding antigen, the resultant specific antibody-antigen reaction leads to the development of a coagglutination lattice. This is evident as a white precipitate on the slide.

The staphylococcal coagglutination test has been used to identify a variety of bacteria, but most notably groups A, B, C, and G beta-hemolytic streptococci (Plate 244), salmonellae, neisseriae, and *Haemophilus*. A reagent for *S. pneumoniae* is now also available commercially. *Cryptococcus neoformans* may also be identified by coagglutination (Maccani: J. Clin. Microbiol. **13**:828-832, 1981). Inasmuch as this test is used in most laboratories primarily for the identification of streptococci, the coagglutination method described by Facklam for streptococci is presented in detail:

Antigen preparation
4-hour broth suspension

1. Inoculate 2 ml of Todd-Hewitt* broth with several colonies (4 or more) of beta-hemolytic streptococci.
2. Incubate for 4 hours at 35 to 37 C.
3. Mix the suspension thoroughly in a Vortex mixer or by vigorous rotation.
4. Test the suspension as described below. If no reaction occurs, incubate overnight at 35 to 37 C. If multiple reactions occur, centrifuge to sediment cells and retest; if multiple reactions remain, trypsinize (as described below) or reinoculate another broth.

Overnight broth suspension

1. Inoculate 2 ml of broth with 1 or 2 colonies of beta-hemolytic streptococci.
2. Incubate overnight at 35 to 37 C.
3. Mix the suspension thoroughly in a vortex mixer or by vigorous rotation.

---

*BBL Microbiology Systems, Cockeysville, Md.

4. Test the suspension as described below. If no reaction occurs, beta-hemolytic streptococci of group A, B, C, or G are not present. If multiple reactions occur, centrifuge to sediment the cells and retest. If multiple reactions remain, trypsinize as described below.

For direct testing, transfer 5 or more colonies of beta-hemolytic streptococci directly to each of the four reagents.

It has been reported that one can shorten the procedure by using suspensions of colonies from overnight cultures on blood agar plates in small volumes of Todd-Hewitt broth without further incubation (Engel and Silfhout: J. Clin. Microbiol. **14:**252-255, 1981).

Test procedure

1. Label a clean, dry glass slide (50 by 75 mm or larger) with the letters A, B, C, and G. The distance between the labels should be at least 20 mm. (If 25- by 75-mm slides are used, only two coagglutination reagents per slide should be tested.) If the reagents are not placed a sufficient distance apart, the volume is such that they will run together or off the slide.
2. Put one full drop of each of the four reagents on the appropriately labeled slide(s). Because the conjugated cells tend to settle out of solution, shake each reagent well to mix the contents before transferring one drop to the slide.
3. Add one full drop of the antigen (see above) to each of the four reagents on the slide(s).
4. Mix the antigen and coagglutination reagents with an applicator stick, using a separate stick for each reagent.
5. Rock the slide back and forth gently for about 1 minute or until a positive reaction occurs.
6. Examine for agglutination by using transillumination against a dark background. In most instances, only one reagent gives a positive agglutination reaction. However, in instances where more than one reagent shows a positive reaction, the most rapid and strongest reaction is recorded as the correct reaction. When two or more reagents react equally, the test must be repeated with a new antigen preparation or with a trypsin-treated antigen preparation (see below).

Trypsinization

Cell suspensions (antigens) that react in several of the coagglutination reagents can be treated with the proteolytic enzyme trypsin. This enzyme removes the outer surface protein antigens of the streptococcal cell, eliminating most of the cause of the cross-reactions encountered in the coagglutination test. Facklam recommended the following procedure:

1. Prepare a 5% trypsin* solution (1:250) by adding 5 g of trypsin powder to 100 ml of distilled water. Mix for 2 hours on a magnetic stirrer at 4 C. Sterilize by filtration. This solution can be stored at 4 C for as long as 6 months. If left at room temperature for 3 hours, however, it loses as much as 75% of its activity.
2. Add two drops of sterile 5% trypsin to the cell suspension.
3. Adjust the pH of the suspension to about 8.2 with 0.2 N NaOH.
4. Incubate at 35 to 37 C for 30 to 60 minutes.
5. Retest as previously described (see the section on Test Procedure).

It should be noted that the reagents for these coagglutination tests are commercially available. The Phadebact Streptococcus Test† is perhaps the most widely used. Facklam believes that pure cultures of streptococci should be used, because other bacteria may react with the coagglutination reagents and cause erroneous identification. Moreover, to avoid possible "broth reactions," it is recommended that Todd-Hewitt

---

*Difco Laboratories, Detroit, Mich.
†Pharmacia Diagnostics, Piscataway, N.J.

broth be used to prepare the antigens. This so-called broth reaction may occur when the same broth is used to prepare the antigen for the coagglutination test that was used to prepare the streptococcal group-specific antisera. In order to eliminate this potential source of error, each lot of uninoculated broth should be tested with each new lot of coagglutination reagents.

Facklam further believes that the most convenient antigen preparation is the 4-hour broth suspension. However, he has found that about 10% of the suspensions gave multiple reactions; the organisms were eventually grouped by applying the trypsin procedure. In his opinion the overnight broth suspensions gave about the same results as the 4-hour broth suspensions. The overnight broth supernatants were very accurate and nearly free from multiple reactions. Of note were the unfavorable reports he had received from investigators attempting to use the direct test, that is, testing colonies taken directly from an agar plate and mixing them with the coagglutination reagents. Not having had experience with this procedure, he was reluctant to make recommendations concerning its use.

Recently Phadebact has made a reagent available for group D streptococci as well. Because there are serious potential errors in identifying group D streptococci with both the coagglutination and the latex agglutination tests, to be described later in the chapter, Facklam[4] recommended a battery of two physiologic tests to aid in the identification of these organisms. He believes that all suspected group D streptococci should have tests for the bile-esculin reaction and tolerance to 6.5% NaCl broth.

With the use of an extraction procedure with *Streptomyces albus*–lysozyme enzyme mixture, Carlson and McCarthy[2] were able to obtain very good results with the coagglutination technique, using either cell pellets from overnight broth cultures or colonies taken directly from sheep blood agar plates. Slifkin and Interval,[12] employing a micro–nitrous acid extraction method and then the Phadebact streptococcus

test reagents, were able to get specific coagglutination responses using 1 beta-hemolytic streptococcal colony from a blood agar plate or a sweep of an inoculating loop from mixed growth. In contrast with certain other extraction methods, the micro–nitrous acid extraction does not yield cross-reactive antigenic substances from *Streptococcus pneumoniae* that react with group C antibodies.

LATEX AGGLUTINATION

An additional agglutination test procedure that is quite satisfactory for grouping streptococci is latex agglutination.[9] There is a commercial kit—the Streptex test.* This test employs group-specific streptococcal antisera conjugated to latex particles and includes reagents to identify groups A, B, C, D, F, and G. Since the antigens are extracted (by a pronase or autoclaving procedure), broth cross-reactions are not a problem. It seems to be unnecessary to have a pure culture as long as sufficient numbers of beta-hemolytic colonies are present. Since the kit contains a reagent for identifying group D streptococci, the Streptex test has the capability to identify certain non-beta-hemolytic, as well as beta-hemolytic, streptococci. *S. bovis* often does not react with the D reagent in the kit.[5] Results indicate that this latex test is very reliable. Autoclave extraction was somewhat better than extraction with the enzyme provided in the kit. Readers should refer to Facklam's chapter in the *Manual of Clinical Microbiology*[4] for details regarding this test.

The latex agglutination technique also works very well with other organisms, such as meningococci and *Haemophilus influenzae*.[8]

OTHER TESTS

A variety of other serologic tests have been used to identify microorganisms. Oudin gel diffusion has been used to characterize *Escherichia coli* (Plate 243). As noted in Chapter 19, a lectin slide agglutination test has been developed for

---

*Wellcome Reagents Ltd., Beckenham, England.

identification of *Neisseria gonorrhoeae*. This uses wheat germ lectin as an agglutinin. Although radioimmunoassay is widely used for assay of various drugs, hormones, vitamins, and antibiotics, it is not widely used in bacteriology. One problem, applicable to all immunoassays, is that high-titer monospecific antiserum is not widely available at a reasonable cost. Thus, there is a relative lack of antigenic specificity. Radioimmunoassay requires an expensive isotope-counting machine, and although most laboratories have such equipment, it is often difficult for microbiology laboratories to share this with the other facilities using it.

ELISA procedures are based on the assumption that either an antibody or an antigen can be coupled to an enzyme and that the resulting complex will retain both immunologic and enzymatic activity. This type of assay has many of the advantages of radioimmunoassay, such as specificity and sensitivity, but does not require the use of radioisotopes or expensive counting apparatus. ELISA techniques are used more for antigen-antibody determinations on patients' sera and body fluids rather than for identification of organisms. However, an immunoperoxidase method has been described for identification of *Bacteroides fragilis*, as noted in Chapter 27, and immunoperoxidase staining has permitted more rapid detection and identification of rubella virus (Schmidt et al.: J. Clin. Microbiol. **13:**627-630, 1981).

CIE is based on the principle of immunodiffusion, modified by driving the antigen and antibody toward each other electrophoretically. As with the ELISA technique, CIE is used more for detection of antigen or antibody in serum or body fluids of various types of patients, rather than for identification of organisms.

Farmer and Tilton[6] compared the CIE technique with coagglutination and latex agglutination. They indicated that the specificity of the three methods is similar and that known immunologic cross-reactions exist that are independent of the method used. They note that there is varying opinion concerning the relative sensitivity of CIE, coagglutination, and latex agglutination. Some believe that coagglutination and latex agglutination are more sensitive than CIE, whereas others have found coagglutination less sensitive than either CIE or latex agglutination, both of which were of equal sensitivity. The cost per test is primarily related to the cost of the antisera used. Since coagglutination uses much less antibody than the other techniques, it has the lowest reagent costs. Equipment for CIE is relatively expensive; it requires a power supply and an electrophoresis chamber. Nonspecific positive results have been reported for each of the three techniques. The agglutination tests, particularly coagglutination, may be more susceptible to false-positive results because of spontaneous clumping of the sensitized particles, but this is primarily related to the use of these techniques in detecting antigen or antibody in body fluids. It applies to the CIE procedure as well when this is used to detect antigen or antibody in body fluids, inasmuch as antibody protein or protein in the body fluid to be tested may precipitate in a moon-shaped pattern around a well. All of these tests require careful attention to detail and the use of positive and negative controls. CIE requires about 45 minutes per test, as compared with to 2 to 3 minutes for the agglutination tests. However, the time for the agglutination tests may be extended if pretreatment of the specimen is necessary to prevent autoagglutination. All three assays are simple to perform, although CIE is much more complicated than the agglutination tests because of the need to make gel plates, cut holes, adjust voltage and amperage in the chamber, and stain the developed gel. Immunodiffusion (double diffusion in agar) has been used to identify cultures of *Petriellidium boydii* by detection of exoantigen (Morace and Polonelli: J. Clin. Microbiol. **14:**237-240, 1981).

The whole future of serologic identification of microorganisms and of detection of antigen in body fluids of patients is brightened considerably by the prospect of availability of monoclonal antibodies. Few monoclonal antibodies have been studied in this way to date. It was noted in Chapter 17, however, that monoclonal antibody to streptococcal group A carbohydrate gave much better results with the fluorescent antibody technique for identifying group A streptococci than did commercial antibodies. There are a number of inherent limitations in the use of the antisera that are currently available—heteroantisera and alloantisera. It is impossible to produce precisely any given antiserum. Each antiserum is broadly specific and contains antibodies to many determinants on complex antigens. Even small protein molecules present a variety of antigenic sites against which antibodies may be directed. Furthermore, for any well-defined antigenic site a broad variety of antibodies can be raised with differences in affinity, valency, and class, all of which may affect antibody activity. These conventional antisera are also limited by both quantities and the titer of antibody that can be obtained. By fusing antibody-secreting spleen cells from a mouse immunized with a specific antigen to murine myeloma cells and thereby producing hybrid cells called hybridomas, it was possible to grow a continuous tumor line that produced specific antibody. By various manipulations one can grow large quantities of hybridoma cells in culture that have been derived from a single cell. The progeny of such a cloned cell produce a monoclonal antibody—an antibody of a single class and specificity whose physical, chemical, and immunologic properties are constant and immortalized and directed to one antigenic determinant of a complex antigen. Unlimited amounts of antibody can be produced from such hybridoma cells, either in tissue culture or in mice. One cannot be certain that hybridomas will secrete antibody of the specificity sought, since this is a random event. However, one can simply repeat the immunization protocol obtaining multiple fusions of spleen cells and myeloma cells until one obtains the antibody desired. Serologic testing will be vastly improved during the next few years as more reagents of this type become available.

REFERENCES

1. Buchanan, R.E., and Gibbons, N.E.: Bergey's manual of determinative bacteriology, ed. 8, Baltimore, 1974, The Williams & Wilkins Co.
2. Carlson, J.R., and McCarthy, L.R.: Modified coagglutination procedure for the serologic grouping of streptococci, J. Clin. Microbiol. **9:**329-332, 1979.
3. Edwards, P.R., and Ewing, W.H.: Identification of Enterobacteriaceae, ed. 3, Minneapolis, 1972, Burgess Publishing Co.
4. Facklam, R.R.: Streptococci and aerococci. In Lennette, E.H., Balows, A., Hausler, W.J., Jr., and Truant, J.P., editors: Manual of clinical microbiology, ed. 3, Washington, D.C., 1980, American Society for Microbiology.
5. Facklam, R.R., Cooksey, R.C., and Wortham, E.C.: Evaluation of commercial latex agglutination reagents for grouping streptococci, J. Clin. Microbiol. **10:**641-646, 1979.
6. Farmer, S.G., and Tilton, R.C., In Lennette, E.H., Balows, A., Hausler, W.J., Jr., and Truant, J.P., editors: Manual of clinical microbiology, ed. 3, Washington, D.C., 1980, American Society for Microbiology.
7. Julianelle, L.A.: A biological classification of *Encapsulatus pneumoniae* (Friedländer's bacillus), J. Exp. Med. **44:**113, 1926.
8. Leinonen, M., and Sivonen, A.: Serological grouping of meningococci and encapsulated *Haemophilus influenzae* strains by latex agglutination, J. Clin. Microbiol. **10:**404-408, 1979.
9. Lue, Y.A., Howit, I.P., and Ellner, P.D.: Rapid grouping of beta-hemolytic streptococci by latex agglutination, J. Clin. Microbiol. **8:**326-328, 1978.
10. Moody, M.D., Padula, J., Lizana, D., and Hall, C.T.: Epidemiologic characterization of group A streptococci by T-agglutination and M-precipitation tests in the public health laboratory, Health Lab. Sci. **2:**149-162, 1965.
11. Rantz, L.A., and Randall, E.: Use of autoclaved extracts of hemolytic streptococci for serological grouping, Stanford Med. Bull. **13:**290-291, 1955.
12. Slifkin, M., and Interval, G.: Serogrouping single colonies of beta-hemolytic streptococci from primary throat culture plates with nitrous acid extraction and Phadebact streptococcal reagents, J. Clin. Microbiol. **12:**541-545, 1980.
13. Wright, D.N., Welch, D.F., and Matsen, J.M.: Use of preserved organisms for individual test-use quality control of bacterial typing antisera, J. Clin. Microbiol. **11:**305-307, 1980.

38 ANTIGEN-ANTIBODY DETERMINATIONS ON PATIENTS' SERA

Procedures have been developed that permit rapid concentration of bacterial antigens from tissue fluids of patients. Ethanol precipitation at a subzero temperature with albumin added as an antigen coprecipitant made it possible to achieve more than 20-fold concentration of antigen in 15 minutes and a 200-fold concentration in 45 minutes.[7] Antigens that are heat stable can be concentrated from protein-rich fluids, such as serum, after the sample has been deproteinized by boiling (100 C for 3 minutes). The boiling process also liberates bacterial polysaccharides from antibody complexes and eliminates the nonspecific interference of serum in ELISA tests.[7]

Wood and Durham[32] proposed a formula for determining the reproducibility of serologic titers. This is a natural extension of the usual practice of considering a serologic test to be acceptably reproducible if replicate titers remain within a twofold range.

The exciting promise of monoclonal antibodies for all types of serologic studies has been discussed in Chapter 37. This will clearly have tremendous impact as soon as a significant number of monoclonal antibody reagents become available.

DIAGNOSIS OF PNEUMONIA CAUSED BY MYCOPLASMA PNEUMONIAE (PRIMARY ATYPICAL PNEUMONIA)

The differential diagnosis of *Mycoplasma* pneumonia may be clinically difficult and usually necessitates laboratory confirmation. Serologic evidence can be obtained by the use of the cold hemagglutination test or the complement fixation test.

Cold hemagglutination test*

The development of cold hemagglutinins in the serum of patients with primary atypical pneumonia was first reported by Peterson and co-workers in 1943.[22] They observed that these antibodies (now considered macroglobulins) caused human erythrocytes to form visible clumps when incubated at 0 to 10 C but not at 37 C.

Cold agglutinins are found in normal sera in low titers (less than 1:16) but are present in titers of 1:40 to 1:2,048 in a high proportion of patients with *Mycoplasma pneumoniae* infection. However, relatively high titers may be found in other conditions as well. The titer rises during the course of the illness, usually reaching a maximum during the third or fourth week, followed by its rapid disappearance thereafter. The cold agglutinin response is generally related directly to the severity and duration of the illness, although mild cases may also develop a significant titer.[12]

In obtaining serum for the cold hemagglutination test, it is essential that the drawn blood not be refrigerated before separation of the serum. This could result in absorption by the red cells of most or all of the cold agglutinins present, resulting in their removal and thus a valueless test. However, one can elute the antibody from the cells by incubating the patient's clot for 30 minutes in a 37 C water bath. This is followed by

immediate centrifugation and serum separation. It should also be noted that prolonged refrigeration of the serum usually results in the disappearance of the cold agglutinins. Inactivation of the serum by heat to destroy complement, however, does not affect the titer.

Technique

Prepare twofold dilutions of the patient's serum as shown in Table 38-1. A 2% suspension of group O human red cells is used. The red cells are washed in 0.85% saline. Add the saline to the cells, centrifuge the specimen for 5 minutes at 2,000 rpm, decant the supernate, and repeat the process until the supernate is clear. The cells should be centrifuged at least three times. If the supernate is not clear after five washings, discard the suspension and obtain fresh cells. Prepare a 2% suspension by diluting 0.1 ml of packed cells with 5 ml of saline. Add 0.5 ml of the suspension to each tube, including the control tube. The final serum dilutions range from 1:10 to 1:2,560, and the final concentration of red cells is 1%. After mixing the antigen and antiserum by shaking the rack of tubes, refrigerate (4 C) the tubes overnight. **Read the test immediately** for agglutination after refrigeration; do not allow the tubes to stand at room temperature before reading. The titer is the highest dilution of serum showing a 1+ (least amount of visible clumping) or greater agglutination. After reading the test, place the tubes in a 37 C water bath for 2 hours, then reread the test; agglutination caused by cold agglutinins will disappear. A titer of 1:32 or greater is considered significant, although it should be pointed out that the demonstration of a fourfold increase in titer in paired (acute and convalescent) sera is of greater significance.

Complement fixation test

This test, preferably done with the lipid antigen of *M. pneumoniae*, is preferred to the cold agglutinin test, since it is specific. The procedure is detailed elsewhere.[16]

---

*The excellent texts on clinical serology by Bennett[1] and Bryant[3] are recommended for additional reading.

TABLE 38-1

Protocol for single agglutination test by serial dilution system

Tube	1	2	3	4	5	6	7	8	9	10
Amount of saline (ml)	0.8	0.5	0.5	0.5	0.5	0.5	0.5	0.5	0.5	0.5
Amount of serum (ml)	0.2 (Mix)	0.5 of tube 1	0.5 of tube 2	0.5 of tube 3	0.5 of tube 4	0.5 of tube 5	0.5 of tube 6	0.5 of tube 7	0.5 of tube 8	(Discard 0.5 from tube 9)
Initial serum dilution	1:5	1:10	1:20	1:40	1:80	1:160	1:320	1:640	1:1280	Control
Amount of antigen (ml)	0.5	0.5	0.5	0.5	0.5	0.5	0.5	0.5	0.5	0.5
Final serum dilution	1:10	1:20	1:40	1:80	1:160	1:320	1:640	1:1280	1:2560	

DETERMINATION OF ANTISTREPTOLYSIN O AND RELATED TITERS

A significant number of patients who have had a recent infection with group A streptococci develop an antibody response to streptolysin O, a specific hemolysin of these strains (and an occasional group C or G strain). This antibody combines with and neutralizes streptolysin O in vitro, thereby inhibiting its hemolytic activity on erythrocytes. By a parallel tube dilution procedure using the patient's serum and a prestandardized fixed amount of streptolysin O with a red blood cell indicator system, the level of antistreptolysin O can be measured. Since the occurrence of this antibody in the patient's serum is dependent on the production of the streptolysin O by the infecting streptococcus, a **rising antistreptolysin O (ASO) titer** aids in the diagnosis of rheumatic fever, acute hemorrhagic glomerulonephritis, and other complications of group A streptococcal infection.

Because the reagents required for the determination of the ASO titer are readily available commercially,* accompanied by complete directions, the test is not described in detail here. In brief, the test is set up by preparing a series of dilutions of the patient's serum, to which is added a constant volume of streptolysin O reagent. After 15 to 45 minutes' incubation at 37 C, a constant volume of group O human or rabbit erythrocytes is added to each serial dilution, and the test is reincubated. The last tube of the series showing **no hemolysis** is the ASO titer, which is expressed as the reciprocal of that dilution and given in **Todd units.** For example, if the highest dilution showing no hemolysis is 1:250, the ASO titer will be 250 Todd units. A titer of 300 Todd units is considered significant, because most normal adults show titers of up to 200 Todd units. An elevated titer appears from 1 to 3 weeks after onset; a rising titer on repeated weekly specimens is helpful diagnostically.

Ricci and associates[23] have described a sim-

---

*Difco Laboratories, Detroit, Mich.; Baltimore Biological Laboratory, Cockeysville, Md.; and others.

pler technique for determination of ASO that utilizes the patient's own erythrocytes.

In patients with acute rheumatic fever streptococcal antibody tests are generally a more reliable indicator of recent streptococcal infection than are throat cultures. The ASO titer is elevated in 80% to 85% of patients with acute rheumatic fever. Since the rest of such patients have a normal ASO titer, a diagnosis of acute rheumatic fever cannot be ruled out on the basis of the ASO test alone. An additional test, such as the antideoxyribonuclease-B (ADN-B), frequently shows an elevated titer in the latter group of patients.

Furthermore, the ASO test is not as useful as others, such as the ADN-B, for suspected cases of acute glomerulonephritis if this disease follows streptococcal skin infection rather than pharyngitis. The ADN-B test is also useful for Sydenham's chorea and also does not give false-positive results, as may be seen with the ASO test with (1) bacterial growth in the serum specimen, (2) liver disease, and (3) oxidation of the antigen.

Both the ASO and the ADN-B tests have good reproducibility, test for antibody to antigens produced by most strains of group A streptococci, and utilize commercially available antigens.* The ASO test is much better known. The ADN-B titer rise usually occurs later than that of the ASO. Elevated serum DNase levels, such as occur in acute hemorrhagic pancreatitis, can result in a false-negative ADN-B titer. Details for performing the ADN-B test are given by Klein.[18] Klein[17] found that the Wampole Streptonase B ADN-B test correlated quite well with ADN-B titers, although it requires eight times the volume of reagents required by the CDC microtitration test.

Several other procedures for testing antibody response to streptococcal infection are available, but not all of the reagents are available commercially, the reproducibility of some of the tests is not good, and there may be other problems. A multiple antigen test, the Streptozyme test, is also available*; it is a 2-minute slide hemagglutination procedure. Comparative studies by Hederstedt and others[13] showed that the Streptozyme test was distinctly inferior to several other tests, including the ADN-B test. There was a need for stricter control of possible batch-to-batch variation and more careful standardization of the antigen content of the Streptozyme test.

DETERMINATION OF C-REACTIVE PROTEIN

C-reactive protein (CRP) is an abnormal alpha globulin that appears rapidly in the serum of patients who have an inflammatory condition of either infectious or noninfectious origin and is absent in serum from normal persons.

This protein has the capacity for precipitating the somatic C carbohydrate of pneumococci; its presence was first determined by mixing a patient's serum with the purified pneumococcal C polysaccharide. It was subsequently demonstrated that by injecting animals with the C-reactive protein, a specific antibody reacting with the protein could be produced. It is this anti-CRP serum that is used as the sensitive reagent in this precipitin test. The test has proved useful in follow-up of patients with rheumatic fever, since CRP disappears when the inflammation subsides, reappearing only when the disease process becomes reactivated.

The reagents for the test, complete with directions, are available commercially.†

PRECIPITIN TEST ON CEREBROSPINAL FLUID

In the precipitin test CSF and a specific antibacterial serum are allowed to react in a capillary tube. This procedure has proved useful in determining the etiologic agent of meningitis

---

*A microtiter test for both ASO and ADN-B determinations is available from Beckman Instruments, Fullerton, Calif.

*Wampole Diagnostics, Stamford, Conn.
†Difco Laboratories, Detroit, Mich.; Baltimore Biological Laboratory, Cockeysville, Md.; and others.

when negative cultures are obtained. The technique uses various commercial antisera* in individual capillary tubes overlaid with spinal fluid. The mixtures are incubated for 2 hours at 37 C, refrigerated overnight, and read. A positive test is indicated by the formation of a **precipitin ring** at the interface of the reactants. The precipitin test is now largely or entirely replaced by the quellung test, CIE, coagglutination, latex agglutination, and other tests that are simpler and more rapid.

QUELLUNG TEST

The quellung test, described in earlier chapters, uses specific antisera to induce capsular swelling in such organisms as pneumococci and type b *H. influenzae*. The test may be performed on spinal fluid, sputum, and other body fluids.

COUNTERIMMUNOELECTROPHORESIS AND GEL DIFFUSION

Basically, CIE (Plate 247) is the Ouchterlony gel-diffusion technique (Plate 246) with the addition of an electric current to expedite interaction between antigen and antibody. Reactions occur in 30 to 60 minutes. The test has been useful in detecting antigens of pneumococci, meningococci, group B streptococci, and *Haemophilus* in spinal fluid; this provides for rapid specific diagnosis and may be positive in the absence of live (or dead) bacterial cells.[25] In meningitis CIE may also be used to detect staphylococci (teichoic acid), *Klebsiella*, and *Pseudomonas aeruginosa*. Other body fluids, such as serum, urine, empyema fluid, and blood, may be studied effectively in various types of infections. CIE may also be used to detect antibody to agents such as *Candida*.

As noted in Chapter 12, it is important to be certain that all materials used in CIE tests are of high quality. One study utilizing 35 bacterial strains and 76 reference and commercial antisera noted that some of the antisera failed to react with their homologous strains and that there were several cross-reactions between genera as well as within species.[13] The addition of 4% dextran with a mean molecular weight of 70,000 to CIE gels enhanced the clarity of precipitin lines and increased the sensitivity of the procedure with a variety of antigens.[27]

Gel diffusion may sometimes be positive when CIE is negative. It is, of course, a slower procedure. However, a microcapillary immunodiffusion technique required an incubation period of only 2 hours.[30] A microimmunodiffusion test for nocardiosis offers promise as an adjunct to diagnosis.[2] With the use of appropriate reference antisera the test has a high degree of specificity.

Hemolysis in gel, with sheep red blood cells coated with antigen, has been utilized to detect antibody to *Chlamydia*.

COAGGLUTINATION AND LATEX AGGLUTINATION

Antibody-coated staphylococci have been utilized to detect various bacterial cells or antigens, the reaction causing specific agglutination of the staphylococci.

Latex agglutination has been used to detect capsular antigen of *Cryptococcus*, as well as many bacterial antigens.

Some of the tests that have utilized coagglutination and latex agglutination have been described in Chapters 8 and 12. Reagents are available commercially for both of these types of tests. In Chapter 37 coagglutination and latex agglutination tests were compared with CIE and other serologic procedures in terms of sensitivity, specificity, cost, and so on.

RADIOIMMUNOASSAY

Radioimmunoassay is the most specific and sensitive method for detecting hepatitis A antigen and hepatitis B surface antigen and the antibody to them and to core antigen. It has also

---

*Difco Laboratories, Detroit, Mich.; Baltimore Biological Laboratory, Cockeysville, Md.; and others.

been used to detect antibody to *S. aureus* (teichoic acid), *E. coli*, *B. fragilis*,[14] *Staphylococcus* enterotoxins, *C. botulinum* toxin type A, *S. pneumoniae*, *N. meningitidis* groups A and C, *H. influenzae* type b, *P. aeruginosa* in urinary tract infections, varicella-zoster virus, and *Candida* and *Coccidioides*.[10,31]

ENZYME-LINKED IMMUNOSORBENT ASSAY

ELISA, the "double antibody sandwich" method, is utilized to detect and measure antigen. The technique is as follows:

1. Antibody is adsorbed to the well of a microplate; then the plate is washed.
2. Test solution thought to contain antigen is added and incubated in the well and the plate is washed again.
3. Enzyme-labeled specific antibody is added, and the plate is again washed.
4. Specific enzyme substrate is added (chosen to provide a color change on degradation).
5. Color change is assessed visually or with a spectrophotometer; the amount of hydrolysis is proportional to the amount of antigen present.

A modification of this procedure (using enzyme-labeled antiglobulin) may be used for detection of antibody.

The procedure has been used for diagnosis of a wide variety of viral, rickettsial, fungal, parasitic, and bacterial infections.[4,26] A modification of the ELISA technique that yields a fluorescent rather than a colored product has been described; this is known as an enzyme-linked fluorescence assay (ELFA).[33] There are now commercially available multiple-channel photometers for high-speed reading of microplates used in the ELISA assay.[24]

SLIDE AGGLUTINATION TESTS

A simple, rapid, quantitative slide test for the detection of serum agglutinins that develop during certain febrile infections is considered a useful diagnostic procedure in many laboratories. This technique can be as informative as the tube agglutination procedure.

The antigens are standardized and include the following*:

> *Brucella abortus* antigen
> *Proteus* OX-19, OXK, and OX-2
> *Salmonella* group A (O antigens 1, 2, and 12)
> *Salmonella* group B (O antigens 4, 5, and 12)
> *Salmonella* group C (C_1 and C_2) (O antigens 6, 7, 8, and Vi)
> *Salmonella* group D (O antigens 1, 9, 12, and Vi)
> *Salmonella* group E (E_1, E_2, E_3, and E_4) (O antigens 1, 3, 15, 19, and 34)
> Paratyphoid A antigen (flagellar a)
> Paratyphoid B antigen (flagellar b, 1, 2)
> Paratyphoid C antigen (flagellar c, 1, 5)
> Typhoid H antigen (flagellar d)

Technique

1. Using a glass slide 9 by 14 inches ruled in 1½-inch squares,† deliver 0.08-, 0.04-, 0.02-, 0.01-, and 0.005-ml volumes of patient's serum with an 0.2-ml pipet graduated in 0.001 ml to the squares of one row, from left to right. Repeat this for as many rows as there are antigens to be used (usually six).
2. Shake the antigen vials so that the contents are well mixed. By means of the standardized dropper provided with each antigen vial, deliver one drop of antigen (0.03 ml) on each volume of serum in each row, from left to right. When this amount of antigen is mixed with the volumes of serum indicated, the result will be approximately equivalent to a dilution series of 1:20, 1:40, 1:80, 1:160, and 1:320 in a tube test using diluted antigen.

---

*Febrile antigens are available from Lederle Laboratories, Pearl River, N.Y.; Baltimore Biological Laboratory, Cockeysville, Md.; Lee Laboratories, Grayson, Ga.; and others.

†Permanently ruled glass slides are available from Arthur H. Thomas Co., Philadelphia, Pa. These are the Perma Slides, 20-ring 14-mm I.D., No. 6690-M10, or equivalent.

Further dilutions may be prepared by using a 1:10 dilution of serum in physiologic saline and incorporating the volumes described in step 1.

3. Using applicator sticks or toothpicks, mix the serum and antigen, proceeding in each row from **right to left** to minimize the carryover of serum from the low to the high dilutions.

4. Rotate the slide over a surface that is illuminated for maximum visibility for a period of 3 minutes.

5. Read and record the degree of agglutination as follows: 4+, complete agglutination; 3+, 75% agglutination; 2+, 50% agglutination; 1+ or less, 25% or less agglutination.

6. The highest dilution of serum with 2+ agglutination is considered the end point, or **titer.** Therefore, if a serum specimen shows the following pattern:

Serum	Equivalent dilution	Antigen A	Antigen B	Antigen C
0.08 ml	1:20	4+	4+	3+
0.04 ml	1:40	4+	3+	2+
0.02 ml	1:80	4+	2+	2+
0.01 ml	1:160·	2+	+/−	−
0.005 ml	1:320	−	−	−

report it as the following serum titers:

Antigen A = 1:160
Antigen B = 1:80
Antigen C = 1:80

Interpretation of test results is similar to that for tube agglutination tests, described below. Such agglutinin titers are to be considered as **presumptive evidence** (rather than specific evidence) in the diagnosis of disease. Also, the possibility of nonspecific reactions must be considered.

TUBE AGGLUTINATION TESTS

As indicated previously, the examination of a patient's serum for the detection of agglutinins against various organisms is an important diagnostic procedure. In some infections the agglutination test may be the only means of laboratory diagnosis available and, as such, may be of considerable value.

Since agglutinins of variable titer may occur in normal sera, a positive agglutination test on a single specimen of serum has little or no significance. For results to be meaningful, at least a **fourfold rise in titer** must be demonstrated during the course of the infection. This can be determined only by comparing the titers of two or more samples of serum, one during the acute phase and one during convalescence.

When serum is submitted to the laboratory for an agglutination test, the clinician should always provide pertinent case history data to give some indication to the laboratory personnel as to the possible etiology. In cases of suspected **typhoid fever** the patient's serum should be set up against both the H and the O antigens of *Salmonella typhi*. Additional H and O antigens also may be used for the detection of agglutinins against other salmonellae, although the value of these is questionable. For the serologic diagnosis of **rickettsial infections,** antigens prepared from *Proteus* OX-19, *Proteus* OX-2, and *Proteus* OXK should be used. The **typhus fevers** usually give a higher titer with *Proteus* OX-19, whereas the **spotted fevers** may give a higher titer with *Proteus* OX-2 antigens. *Proteus* OXK aids in the diagnosis of tsutsugamushi fever.

Antigens

Standardized suspensions of most bacteria for use as antigens are available commercially.* Readers interested in details of preparation of antigens should refer to Edwards and Ewing[9] particularly with regard to the Enterobacteriaceae.

Technique

Two methods of preparing serial dilutions are available. The first method should be used if a

---

*Excellent standardized antigens are available from Central Public Health Laboratories, London.

TABLE 38-2

Protocol for agglutination test by parallel dilution system

PREPARATION OF MASTER DILUTIONS

	Tube								
	1	2	3	4	5	6	7	8	9
Amount of saline (ml)	8	5	5	5	5	5	5	5	5
Amount of serum (ml)	2	Mix and transfer 5 ml from tube 1 to tube 2. Continue mixing and transferring 5 ml serially through to tube 9, discarding 5 ml from tube 9.								
Serum dilution	1:5	1:10	1:20	1:40	1:80	1:160	1:320	1:640	1:1,280
Volume of serum dilution (ml)	5	5	5	5	5	5	5	5	5

PROCEDURE FOR PARALLEL AGGLUTINATION TESTS

Commencing with the highest dilution in tube 9 of the master dilution series, pipet 0.5 ml of the dilution into the corresponding agglutination tube and proceed in reverse until tube 1 is reached, as indicated, using the same pipet.

	Agglutination tube									
	1	2	3	4	5	6	7	8	9	10
Amount of master dilution (ml)	0.5 of dilution 1	0.5 of dilution 2	0.5 of dilution 3	0.5 of dilution 4	0.5 of dilution 5	0.5 of dilution 6	0.5 of dilution 7	0.5 of dilution 8	0.5 of dilution 9	0.5 of saline
Amount of antigen (ml)	0.5	0.5	0.5	0.5	0.5	0.5	0.5	0.5	0.5	0.5
Final serum dilution	1:10	1:20	1:40	1:80	1:160	1:320	1:640	1:1,280	1:2,560	Control

single test is required; the protocol is given in Table 38-1. When a number of tests are to be performed, such as in the Widal test for typhoid and paratyphoid fevers, the **parallel dilution system** is employed for accuracy and speed. The protocol for this test is shown in Table 38-2.

Single serial dilution test. Set up 10 clean, visually clear agglutination tubes (10 by 100 mm) in a rack. Add physiologic saline (0.85%) as the diluent to the tubes in the amounts shown in Table 38-1. Next, add the patient's undiluted serum with a 1-ml serologic pipet to the first tube, mix, and transfer as indicated. Discard 0.5 ml from tube 9. Tube 10 serves as the control and contains only saline. Add 0.5 ml of the appropriate antigen suspension to each tube of the series.

Parallel dilution method (Bailey, W.R., Unpublished data). Set up nine clean 18- or 20-mm

test tubes in a rack. Add saline to each tube, as indicated in Table 38-2. Add undiluted patient's serum to tube 1 as shown, and, after thorough mixing, serially transfer 5 ml from tube to tube until nine master dilutions have been established. With a 5-ml pipet, transfer 0.5 ml of the highest dilution (tube 9) to the corresponding agglutination tube in each of the test series set up in agglutination racks. By starting with the highest dilution and working backward, the same pipet may be used throughout the procedure with little concern for carrying over any appreciable amount of serum antibody. With the system shown, at least nine parallel series can be established for agglutination tests with different antigens. Adjustments may be made either way in the master series to accommodate the number of agglutination tests planned. The antigen suspensions are added as shown in Table

38-2. Tube 10 serves as the control for each test.

Since antigens used in agglutination tests are subject to variation, it is recommended that **control tests,** using positive antisera of known titer, be routinely carried out as a check on the agglutinability of the test antigens. Such tests are performed by the technique described for the single serial dilution test.

Period of incubation

Febrile antigens are available commercially, accompanied by complete directions. The times and temperatures used for the incubation of tube agglutination tests vary from one manufacturer to another.

Reading of agglutination tests

Observe every tube for clearing of the supernatant fluid and the amount and character of the sediment and agglutinated particles. The pattern of the sediment can be more accurately observed if the tubes are read against a black background using an indirect light source. In the **control** and **negative** test the antigen settles to the bottom of the tube as a small round disk with smooth edges. In the **positive** tubes the cells settle out over a larger area and may even extend up the sides of the tube. The pattern of this sediment is somewhat irregular and varies with the extent of the agglutination. After examining the pattern of the sediment, shake the tube gently. H agglutinins produce large flocular aggregates, which are easily broken up, whereas O agglutinins produce granular or small flaky aggregates. Complete agglutination with complete clearing of the supernatant fluid indicates a 4+ reaction. Decreasing amounts of agglutination and increasing cloudiness of the supernatant fluid are read as 3+, 2+, and 1+ reactions.

Interpretation of results

It is almost impossible to assign positive or negative values to arbitrary titers in any agglutination test. Variable factors, such as past infec-

tion, vaccination, time at which the specimen was taken, and naturally occurring agglutinins, can influence the titer. As mentioned earlier, only a fourfold (two tube) or greater **rise in titer** over a period of time is usually significant. However, the following suggestions may prove helpful in interpreting results.

Negative results. Negative results may be caused by either of the following: (1) obtaining the sample of blood before the appearance of agglutinins in the serum or (2) incorrect diagnosis (patient's not having the infection for which the tests were requested).

Negative results are of particular value for comparing titers that may occur with later samples of serum. Any two-tube increase in titer during the course of an infection is usually significant.

Positive results. Interpretation of positive results obviously varies with the infection and is given only brief mention in this chapter.

1. In **typhoid fever**: (a) Indication of current infection—titer of 1:160 with O antigen— titer rising in subsequent sera; (b) indication of past infection, recent vaccination, or an anamnestic reaction—titer of 1:80 to 1:160 with H antigen only.

2. In **brucellosis**: A titer of 1:160 or greater usually suggests infection, past or present, and 1:320 or greater usually indicates acute brucellosis. As noted in Chapter 23, a modification of the Brucella microagglutination test employing 2-mercaptoethanol (2ME) or dithiothreitol is useful for determining response to therapy. The 2ME disrupts disulfide bonds, rendering IgM antibodies inactive. A negative 2ME titer (only IgG agglutinating antibody) is good evidence against chronic brucellosis and an indication of a favorable response to antimicrobial therapy.

3. In **tularemia**: A titer of 1:80 or greater usually suggests definite infection.

4. In **Rocky Mountain** and **typhus fevers**: Variable results are obtained with *Proteus* OX-19 and *Proteus* OX-2 antigens. In gen-

eral, typhus fever gives a higher titer with OX-19, and Rocky Mountain spotted fever and tick-bite fever may give a higher titer with OX-2. In both instances diagnostic titers are high, over 1:320, and only a rising titer is conclusive. Agglutination with *Proteus* OXK may be diagnostic for tsutsugamushi fever, but it also may be indicative of the spirochetal disease, relapsing fever.

SEROLOGIC TESTS FOR SYPHILIS

Perhaps no other infectious disease process relies so heavily on the serologic test for a diagnosis as syphilis. This situation exists primarily because the etiologic agent, *Treponema pallidum,* cannot be cultured in the laboratory. Although darkfield examination is excellent for demonstrating *T. pallidum* in specimens (particularly in the early stages of the disease), most laboratories do not have the capability or the experience to perform this procedure properly (see Chapter 24).

More than 200 serologic tests for syphilis (STS) have been described, but only a few are in use today. All tests for syphilis depend on the antigen-antibody reaction and are performed on either blood (serum or plasma) or CSF specimens.

Tests are classified according to the type of antigen used. For example, **nontreponemal or reagin tests** are performed with extracts from normal tissue or other sources. **Treponemal tests,** on the other hand, employ treponemes or treponemal extracts to detect antibody. Further details on syphilis serology and its interpretation can be found in three excellent publications cited here.[5,15,20]

Nontreponemal antigen tests

Nontreponemal antigen tests are not immunologically specific for syphilis and are not the most sensitive tests. However, their ease of performance and relatively low cost account for the wide use of these antigen tests, particularly the flocculation tests (below), as screening proce-

dures. The flocculation tests have essentially replaced the more cumbersome and less sensitive Wasserman complement fixation test.[5] Of the nontreponemal antigen tests, the Venereal Disease Research Laboratory (VDRL) and the rapid plasma reagin (RPR) flocculation tests, along with the sometimes used Kolmer complement fixation test, are the most widely used. The RPR card test is quite reliable, and the VDRL is somewhat less specific.[8] The automated reagin test is less sensitive than the others.

Reactive nontreponemal tests confirm the diagnosis in the presence of early or late active syphilis. They offer a diagnostic clue in latent, subclinical syphilis and are effective tools for detecting cases in epidemiologic investigations. Finally, they are superior to the treponemal tests for following the response to therapy. For a thorough discussion on their application, as well as detailed instructions on how to adequately perform these tests, the reader should consult other references.[5,15,19,20,21,28]

Results of **qualitative tests** for syphilis are customarily reported as reactive (or positive, or 4+), weakly reactive (or weakly positive, or 3+, 2+, or 1+), or nonreactive (negative). **Quantitative results** may be obtained by diluting the serum in geometric progression to an end point. The titer is usually expressed as the highest dilution in which the test is fully reactive.

Excessive production of antibody (particularly in the secondary stage of syphilis) occasionally results in a prozone phenomenon because of antibody excess. This is true in both complement fixation and flocculation tests. Undiluted specimens give a nonreactive or weakly reactive test result. Testing at higher dilutions, however, gives reactive test results.

Careful attention must be paid to each reactive or weakly reactive serologic result. Many cases of untreated late latent or late syphilis give only weakly reactive results with undiluted serum. On the other hand, the titer is usually high (>1:16) in secondary syphilis. A high titer does not necessarily mean early syphilis (or even syphilis), but it is strong evidence for the presence of syphilis. Some of the highest titers recorded have been in late visceral or cutaneous syphilis or in nonsyphilitic diseases (e.g., hemolytic anemia or systemic lupus erythematosus).[28]

Treponemal antigen tests

It has been long recognized that the nontreponemal antigen tests are not entirely specific for *T. pallidum* infection. Therefore, antigens for testing also have been made from treponemes. These treponemal antigen tests are primarily used as confirmatory tests, particularly in patients in whom the clinical, historical, or epidemiologic evidence of syphilis is questionable. Three such tests are the *Treponema pallidum* immobilization (TPI) test, the fluorescent treponemal antibody absorption (FTA-ABS) test (Plate 245), and the *Treponema pallidum* hemagglutination test(s).

Although time consuming, technically demanding, and extremely expensive to perform, the TPI test is considered by many to be the standard to which all treponemal antigen tests are compared. The antigen for this test is the Nichols strain of *T. pallidum* and is harvested from testicular syphilomas in artificially infected rabbits. In the TPI test, these harvested live treponemes are combined with the patient's serum and complement. After appropriate incubation, serum that contains treponemal antibodies causes immobilization of the treponemes. Since the TPI antibody develops more slowly, the test is not reactive until later in early syphilis, in contrast with the nontreponemal antigen tests; that is, in some primary syphilitic patients the TPI test may be nonreactive, whereas the VDRL test is reactive. The TPI test is the test of choice for spinal fluids, especially when reagin tests give nonreactive or equivocal results. This test is not available in most serology laboratories.

The most widely used treponemal antigen test is the FTA-ABS test. The antigen in this test consists of nonviable *T. pallidum* (Nichols strain). It is allowed to dry on a glass slide, fixed,

and then combined with serum that has been previously absorbed to remove nonspecific treponemal antibodies. If syphilis antibody is present, it will combine with the nonviable organisms. Fluorescein-labeled antihuman globulin is then added and reacts with the serum that is attached to the organisms. When observed under the fluorescent microscope, this reaction is readily visible (i.e., the organisms **fluoresce** yellow-green). If no syphilis antibodies are present in the test serum, the treponemes will not fluoresce and therefore are nonvisible under the fluorescent microscope.

The FTA-ABS test becomes reactive earlier than the TPI test in early syphilis and is about 5% more sensitive than the TPI in late latent or late syphilis. The FTA-ABS test is now widely available, and because of its increased sensitivity and specificity it is the confirmatory test of choice. A reactive test confirms the presence of treponemal antibodies but does not indicate the stage or activity of infection.

For a more detailed account of these and other treponemal antigen tests, including specific test instructions, the reader should consult the *Manual of Clinical Immunology*[5] and other selected publications.[6,15,19,20,28]

Several *T. pallidum* hemagglutination tests (TPHA) are available. Red cells from one or another animal species and components of the Reiter treponeme are utilized. The microhemagglutination–*Treponema pallidum* (MHA-TP) test is the most popular of these hemagglutination tests. It is simple, rapid, and reproducible and is available in kit form in the United States.* Several studies have shown that the MHA-TP and FTA-ABS tests are comparable in all categories of syphilis except the primary stage, in which the MHA-TP is less reactive than either the FTA-ABS or the VDRL. The MHA-TP is highly specific and compares favorably with the FTA-ABS; it is considered a satisfactory substitute for the FTA-ABS test. The chief advantages of the MHA-TP are its simplic-

---

*Ames Division, Miles Laboratories, Inc., Elkhart, Ind.

ity and economy. It requires three to five times as much time of the technical staff for the FTA-ABS test as for the MHA-TP test. Furthermore, the reading of the FTA-ABS test is more subjective, and quality control is significantly more difficult.

False-positive reactions

All normal sera may contain minute amounts of reagin. The sensitivity of nontreponemal tests is altered by varying the proportion of reagents, temperature, mixing time, and other physicochemical variables. For these reasons about one fourth of all false-positive reactions represent technical errors or day-to-day variability in testing.

Repeatedly reactive nontreponemal tests accompanied by nonreactive treponemal tests (TPI or the more sensitive FTA-ABS) characterize the **false-positive** reactor. The duration of reagin reactivity arbitrarily determines whether the false-positive reaction is **acute** (less than 6 months) or **chronic** (6 months or longer). Though false-positive reactions have been called "biologic," many such reactions are associated with specific diseases or follow vaccination or immunization; therefore, this adjective should be discarded. The terms "acute false-positive" and "chronic false-positive" adequately describe what is observed.[28]

Acute false-positive reactions are found in persons suffering from many viral and bacterial infections or who have had certain vaccinations and immunizations. Pregnancy may also result in a false-positive test. Chronic false-positive reactions are usually less frequent than "technical" or acute false-positive reactions.

Lepromatous leprosy, heroin addiction, lupus erythematosus, and occasionally malaria are associated with chronic false-positive nontreponemal tests for syphilis, whereas the nonvenereal treponematoses (yaws, pinta, and bejel) characteristically give reactive nontreponemal tests as well as treponemal tests and are not serologically distinguishable. It should be pointed out that syphilis and systemic lupus erythematosus or syphilis and leprosy can occur together. In situations such as these a reactive serologic test is not to be considered as a false-positive result.[28]

OTHER DETERMINATIONS

Other types of antigen-antibody determinations and other specific applications of such tests are noted throughout the book in the appropriate areas (e.g., chapters on virus infections, fungal infections, parasitic infections, and so forth). Fluorescent antibody testing is discussed in Chapter 39.

REFERENCES

1. Bennett, C.W.: Clinical serology, rev. ed., Springfield, Ill., 1968, Charles C. Thomas, Publisher.
2. Blumer, S.O., and Kaufman, L.: Microimmunodiffusion test for nocardiosis, J. Clin. Microbiol. **10**:308-312, 1979.
3. Bryant, N.J.: Laboratory immunology and serology, rev. ed., Philadelphia, 1979, W.B. Saunders Co.
4. Buxton, T.B., Crockett, J.K., and Rissing, J.P.: Enzyme-linked immunosorbent assay: available for infectious disease surveillance, Lab. Med. **10**:630-634, 1979.
5. Coffey, E., and Bradford, L.: Serodiagnosis of syphilis. In Rose, N.R., and Friedman, H., editors: Manual of clinical immunology, ed. 2, Washington, D.C., 1980, American Society for Microbiology.
6. Deacon, W.E., Lucas, J.B., and Price, E.J.: Fluorescent treponemal antibody-absorption (FTA-ABS) test for syphilis, J.A.M.A. **98**:624-628, 1966.
7. Doskeland, S.O., and Berdal, B.P.: Bacterial antigen detection in body fluids: methods for rapid antigen concentration and reduction of nonspecific reactions, J. Clin. Microbiol. **11**:380-384, 1980.
8. Dzuik, P.E., Black, D.A., and Therrell, B.L., Jr.: Syphla-check: a qualitative study, J. Clin. Microbiol. **5**:593-595, 1977.
9. Edwards, P.R., and Ewing, W.H.: Identification of Enterobacteriaceae, ed. 3, Minneapolis, 1972, Burgess Publishing Co.
10. Farmer, S.G., and Tilton, R.C.: Immunoserological and immunochemical detection of bacterial antigens and antibodies. In Lennette, E.H., Balows, A., Hausler, W.J., Jr., and Truant, J.P., editors: Manual of clinical microbiology, ed. 3, Washington, D.C., 1980, American Society for Microbiology.

11. Finch, C.A., and Wilkinson, H.W.: Practical considerations in using counterimmunoelectrophoresis to identify the principal causative agents of bacterial meningitis, J. Clin. Microbiol. **10:**519-524, 1979.

12. Hayflick, L., and Chanock, R.M.: *Mycoplasma* species of man, Bacteriol. Rev. **29:**185-221, 1965.

13. Hederstedt, B., Holm, S.E., and Wadström, T.: Discrepancy between results of the Streptozyme test and those of the antideoxyribonuclease B and antihyaluronidase tests, J. Clin. Microbiol. **8:**50-53, 1978.

14. Hoppes, W.L., Rissing, J.P., Smith, J.W., and White, A.C.: Radioimmunoassay for *Bacteroides fragilis* infections, J. Clin. Microbiol. **12:**205-207, 1980.

15. Jaffe, H.W.: The laboratory diagnosis of syphilis, Ann. Intern. Med. **83:**846-850, 1975.

16. Kenny, G.E.: Serology of mycoplasmic infections. In Rose, N.R., and Friedman, H., editors: Manual of clinical immunology, ed. 2, Washington, D.C., 1980, American Society for Microbiology.

17. Klein, G.C.: Evaluation of the Wampole Streptonase B test, J. Clin. Microbiol. **6:**533, 1977.

18. Klein, G.C.: Immune response to streptococcal infection (antistreptolysin O, antideoxyribonuclease B). In Rose, N.R., and Friedman, H., editors: Manual of clinical immunology, ed. 2, Washington, D.C., 1980, American Society for Microbiology.

19. The laboratory aspects of syphilis, Atlanta, 1971, Center for Disease Control.

20. Miller, J.N.: Value and limitations of non-treponemal and treponemal tests in the laboratory diagnosis of syphilis, Clin. Obstet. Gynecol. **18:**191-203, 1975.

21. Nicholas, L., and Beerman, H.: Present day serodiagnosis of syphilis, Am. J. Med. Sci. **249:**466-483, 1965.

22. Peterson, O.L., Ham, T.H., and Finland, M.: Cold agglutinins (autohemagglutinins) in primary atypical pneumonias, Science **97:**167, 1943.

23. Ricci, A., Berti, B., Moauro, C., Porro, M., Neri, P., and Tarli, P.: New hemolytic method for determination of antistreptolysin O in whole blood, J. Clin. Microbiol. **8:**263-267, 1978.

24. Ruitenberg, E.J., Sekhuis, V.M., and Brosi, B.J.M.: Some characteristics of a new multiple-channel photometer for through-the-plate reading of microplates to be used in enzyme-linked immunosorbent assay, J. Clin. Microbiol. **11:**132-134, 1980.

25. Rytel, M.W.: Counterimmunoelectrophoresis in diagnosis of infectious disease, Hosp. Pract. **56:**75-82, 1975.

26. Sever, J.L., and Madden, D.L., editors: Enzyme-linked immunosorbent assay (ELISA) for infectious agents, Proceedings of a meeting at the National Institutes of Health, J. Infect. Dis. **136:**S258-S340, 1977.

27. Siber, G.R., and Skapriwsky, P.: Counterimmunoelectrophoresis for detection of microbial antigens: increased sensitivity with dextran-containing gels, J. Clin. Microbiol. **7:**392-393, 1978.

28. Syphilis: a synopsis, Public Health Service Pub. No. 1660, Atlanta, 1968, U.S. Department of Health, Education, and Welfare, National Communicable Disease Center, pp. 96-108.

29. Voller, A., Bidwell, D., and Bartlett, A.: Enzyme-linked immunosorbent assay. In Rose, N.R., and Friedman, H., editors: Manual of clinical immunology, ed. 2, Washington, D.C., 1980, American Society for Microbiology.

30. Wagstaff, P.A.: Rapid and inexpensive microcapillary immunodiffusion assay technique, J. Clin. Microbiol. **9:**450-452, 1979.

31. Weiner, M.H.: Antigenemia detected in coccidioidomycosis with a new radioimmunoassay, Clin. Res. **28:**832A, 1980.

32. Wood, R.J., and Durham, T.M.: Reproducibility of serological titers, J. Clin. Microbiol. **11:**541-545, 1980.

33. Yolken, R.H. and Stopa, P.J.: Enzyme-linked fluorescence assay (ELFA): a new ultrasensitive method for detection of infectious agents, Abstract 273, Proceedings of the Interscience Conference on Antimicrobial Agents and Chemotherapy, 1979.

39 FLUORESCENT ANTIBODY TECHNIQUES IN DIAGNOSTIC MICROBIOLOGY

The fluorescent antibody method, more properly known as the **immunofluorescence method,** is a rapid, reproducible, and reliable aid, in the hands of experienced workers, for the identification of microorganisms or the antibodies they engender.

Space does not permit a complete review of the vast literature about the method; the interested reader is referred to excellent chapters and technical manuals, including those of Cherry,[1] Jones and associates,[5] Lyerla and Forrester,[9] McKinney,[10] Riggs,[11] Washington and coworkers,[12] and the various manufacturers of reagents.

The fluorescent antibody method is essentially a sophisticated technique for **demonstrating antigen-antibody reactions.** In this technique a film preparation or tissue section is treated with an appropriate serum containing an immune globulin (antibody) that has been labeled (conjugated) with a fluorescent dye, such as fluorescein isothiocyanate. This preparation is then examined against a dark background (darkfield) illuminated by a very bright light source rich in the near-ultraviolet spectrum. This light causes the antigen-antibody complex to become **fluo-**

rescent and appear a bright glowing **yellow-green** (Plate 170) against the dark background (when stained with fluorescein isothiocyanate). Rhodamine-labeled antiglobulins are also available. These fluoresce red. One may simultaneously detect two different organisms quantitatively in a single sample by a dual-label technique.[3]

The diagram in Fig. 39-1 represents the basic optical system utilized in fluorescence microscopy and consists of a high-pressure mercury vapor lamp (Osram HBO 200) that provides light of a very high intensity. This is passed through Schott BG-14 and BG-22 heat-absorbing filters and excited in wavelengths of 350 to 450 mμm by passage through a BG-12 filter, the range in which the fluorescein dye is most brilliant. Since this wavelength is in the ultraviolet spectrum, it must be removed by the insertion of a barrier filter in the eyepiece (usually Schott OG-1) for protection of the observer's eyes. This orange filter holds back wavelengths below 500 mμm and transmits visible wavelengths emitted by the specimen. Corning, Wratten, or an equivalent filter system also may be used, and newer optics and lighting systems are available.

Two important developments in fluorescent microscopy are the introduction of the halogen lamp with the interference filter and the introduction of incident-light, or epi-illumination. (See Cherry[1] for details.)

The choice of the particular fluorescent antibody technique to be used depends largely on the information desired. Generally, the **direct** staining procedure is used in identification of an unknown antigen, such as group A streptococci obtained from throat swabs. The **indirect** method is employed primarily in the detection of antibody, as in the FTA-ABS test for syphilis. Other uses of these basic principles are described in the references previously cited.

To date, a number of fluorescent antibody diagnostic procedures have been evaluated, and thus a number of standardized commercially prepared conjugates have become available.* Fluorescent antibody conjugates are stable for prolonged periods under various conditions.[4]

---

*Baltimore Biological Laboratory, Cockeysville, Md.; Difco Laboratories, Detroit, Mich.; Burroughs Wellcome Reagents Division, Greenville, N.C.; Clinical Sciences, Inc., Whippany, N.J.; and others.

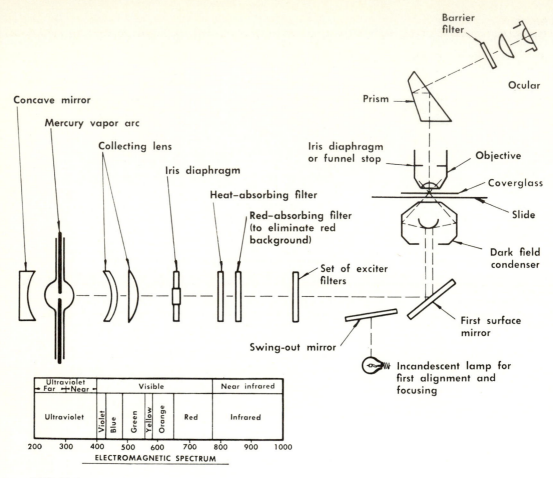

FIG. 39-1

Schematic representation of equipment for fluorescence microscopy. (Prepared with suggestions by Dr. Peter Bartals, E. Leitz, Inc., New York.)

These procedures are in regular use in many public health and hospital microbiology laboratories and include the following: the rapid identification of groups A and B streptococci; the rapid and specific diagnosis of rabies virus in tissue; the identification of enteroviruses and respiratory viruses, herpes simplex, arboviruses, rickettsiae, and so forth in isolates and clinical material; the highly specific FTA-ABS test for syphilis; the rapid identification of *Legionella* species in tissues and exudates; and other tests mentioned in various sections of this text.

The fluorescent antibody tests useful in diagnostic bacteriology and mycology are listed in Tables 39-1 and 39-2. Indirect tests have also been useful in the diagnosis of Legionnaires' disease and chlamydial, viral, and parasitic infec-

TABLE 39-1

List of fluorescent antibody tests most useful in diagnostic bacteriology

Test	Status
A. Group A streptococci. Direct test.	Most highly evaluated and extensively used of all FA tests. Sensitive and specific.
B. Group B streptococci. Direct test.	Good sensitivity. Detection of nonhemolytic group B streptococci. Specific reagent not commercially available.
C. Fluorescent antibody darkfield test (FADF).	Comparable to darkfield for demonstration of *T. pallidum*. As accurate and does not require motile treponemes of specific morphology.
D. Fluorescent treponemal antibody test (FTA-ABS). Indirect test.	Highly specific and sensitive for detection of true antibody to *T. pallidum*. Much easier to perform than treponemal immobilization test.
E. Identification of the gonococcus. Direct test.	A good test, particularly for rapid confirmation of a culture as *N. gonorrhoeae*. Not recommended for diagnosis.
F. Identification of the diphtheria bacillus. Direct test.	Good for use on nasopharyngeal specimens from patients suspected of having diphtheria. Not recommended for carrier surveys, contacts, and so forth. Specificity needs improvement.
G. *Bordetella pertussis*. Direct test. *B. parapertussis*	A rapid, specific, and sensitive test as compared with conventional culture techniques.
H. Incitants of bacterial meningitis. Direct test on spinal fluids. *Haemophilus influenzae* *Neisseria meningitidis* *Streptococcus pneumoniae*	Rapid highly efficient tests to apply to CSF sediments. May detect organisms in partially treated patients.
I. *Listeria monocytogenes*. Direct test.	Excellent for specific detection of organisms in formalin-fixed paraffin-embedded sections, CSF, impression smears of tissue, and so forth, including colonies on plates.
J. *Brucella* (three major species). Direct test.	Sensitive, rapid, and genus specific for detection of smooth strains of *Brucella* in tissues. No advantage over agglutination tests for detection of antibody (IFA).
K. *Yersinia pestis*. Direct test.	Excellent for rapid diagnosis of plague when used on blood, stomach contents of vectors, stored animal tissues, and phagocytic cell preparations. Direct or indirect staining of impression smears or frozen or freeze-dried material may be used. FA technique is method of choice for rapid and specific identification of plaguebacillus in tissues and in culture.

Modified from Jones, Hébert, and Cherry.[5]   *Continued.*

tions. One may use a template method to apply indirect fluorescent antibody (IFA) technique to serial dilutions.[7]

There are numerous pitfalls in the application of immunofluorescence to diagnostic bacteriology; the procedures must be carried out by workers well trained in a meticulous technique and with a strong background in serology and microscopy. The procedures must be monitored at all times by the inclusion of positive and negative controls.[2] Reagents must be standardized, and their specificity must be checked regularly. In short, the fluorescent antibody method should not be used as a substitute for the conventional cultural procedures; rather, it should be utilized as an adjunct to these tests. Its great potential in the field of diagnostic microbiology is well recognized.

TABLE 39-1

List of fluorescent antibody tests most useful in diagnostic bacteriology—cont'd

Test	Status
L. *Francisella tularensis*. Direct test.	Rapid, sensitive, and specific for detection of organisms in culture, impression smears, frozen sections, or formalin-fixed paraffin-embedded sections of specimens from humans or experimental animals or from air. May stain *Erysipelothrix insidiosa* and some pseudomonads.
M. *Bacillus anthracis*. Direct test.	Rapid and sensitive for detection of anthrax organisms in impression smears, formalin-fixed paraffin-embedded tissue, human cutaneous vesicles, and tissues of experimental or naturally infected animals. Test not entirely specific; cross-stains some strains of *B. megaterium* and *B subtilis*.
N. Leptospirae.	Has been used successfully to detect leptospirae in urine sediments, frozen sections, impression smears, formalin-fixed frozen sections and cultures. Not reliable for serotyping.
O. *Salmonella typhi*. Direct test using sorbed Vi conjugate.	Approximately the same sensitivity and specificity as culture on bismuth sulfite agar but very rapid. Excellent when used for detection of chronic typhoid carriers. Culture is more reliable for use on acutely ill and convalescent patients.
P. *Shigella*. Direct test.	
S. sonnei	Sensitive and specific for **screening** of fecal smears. Well evaluated.
S. flexneri	Appears promising for **screening** of fecal smears. Needs further evaluation.
Q. Clostridia. Direct test.	Toxigenic types of *C. botulinum* can be differentiated with absorbed conjugates. Staining of smears from tissues or body fluids is very helpful in diagnosis of animal diseases due to clostridia.
R. *Treponema pallidum*. Direct test.	Procedure may be applied to specimens from lesions, transported either in capillary tubes or on dried slides and mailed to the laboratory.[8]
S. *Actinomyces israelii*. Direct test.	Specific identification for cultures and smears but not tissue sections. Useful for demonstrating organism in tissues or exudates.
T. *Actinomyces naeslundii*. Direct test.	Specific identification for cultures and smears but not tissue sections.
U. *Arachnia (Actinomyces) propionica*. Direct test.	Specific identification for cultures, smears, and tissue sections. Useful for demonstrating organism in exudates.
V. *Chlamydia*. Direct and indirect tests.	Both tests acceptable. IFA reagents available commercially.
W. *Legionella*. Direct and indirect tests.	Direct test is rapid and specific for detecting organisms in tissues and exudates and identifying colonies. Less sensitive than culture. IFA is useful for detecting antibody response (Plate 170).
X. *Bacteroides fragilis* group. Direct and indirect tests.	Potentially valuable for detecting organisms in clinical specimens. Commercially available.
Y. *Bacteroides melaninogenicus* group. Direct test.	Potentially valuable for detecting organisms in clinical specimens. Available commercially. Also stains *B. bivius* and *B. disiens*.

TABLE 39-2

Value and limitations of fluorescent antibody reagents in medical mycology

Conjugate for	Procedure	Staining reaction with fungi in		
		Cultures	Tissue smears, pus, exudates	Tissue sections
Aspergillus species	Direct staining		Conjugate available for differentiating *Aspergillus* species from *Candida* species and phycomycetes[6]	Genus identification[6]
Blastomyces dermatitidis and *Paracoccidioides brasiliensis*	Direct staining	Specific identification of yeast form; no value for identification of mycelial form	Specific (tissue form) identification	Specific identification
Candida species	Direct staining	No specific reactivity for any *Candida* species, but a good rapid screening agent		
Coccidioides immitis, tissue form	Direct staining	No value for identification of mycelial form	Specific identification	Specific identification
Cryptococcus neoformans	Direct staining	Specific identification; does not stain some strains	Specific identification	Specific identification
Histoplasma capsulatum	Direct staining in conjunction with *B. dermatitidis* conjugate	Specific identification; no value for identification of mycelial form	Specific identification	Not optimal
Sporothrix schenckii	Direct staining	Specific identification of yeast form	Specific identification	Specific identification
Trichophyton species	Direct staining	Differentiation of *T. mentagrophytes* from *T. rubrum* only.		

Courtesy Leo Kaufman, Chief, Fungus Immunology Section, Mycology Branch, Centers for Disease Control, Atlanta. Modified.

REFERENCES

1. Cherry, W.B.: Immunofluorescence techniques. In Lennette, E.H., Balows, A., Hausler, W.J., Jr., and Truant, J.P., editors: Manual of clinical microbiology, ed. 3, Washington, D.C., 1980, American Society for Microbiology.
2. Frenkel, J.K., and Piekarski, G.: The demonstration of *Toxoplasma* and other organisms by immunofluorescence: a pitfall, J. Infect. Dis. **138**:265-266, 1978.
3. Gillis, T.P., and Thompson, J.J.: Double-label fluorescence immunoassay of bacteria, J. Clin. Microbiol. **8**:351-353, 1978.
4. Green, J.H., Gray, S.B., Jr., and Harrell, W.K.: Stability of fluorescent antibody conjugates stored under various conditions, J. Clin. Microbiol. **3**:1-4, 1976.
5. Jones, G.L., Hebert, G.A., and Cherry, W.B.: Fluorescent antibody techniques and bacterial applications: CDC laboratory manual, DHEW Pub. No. (CDC) 78-8364, Atlanta, 1978, U.S. Department of Health, Education, and Welfare, Center for Disease Control.
6. Kaplan, W.: Direct fluorescent antibody tests for the diagnosis of mycotic diseases, Ann. Clin. Lab. Sci. **3**:25-29, 1973.
7. Karim, K.A., and Trust, T.J.: Template method for the fluorescent-antibody technique, J. Clin. Microbiol. **5**:543-544, 1977.
8. Kellogg, D.S., Jr.: The detection of Treponema pallidum by a rapid, direct fluorescent antibody darkfield (DFATP) procedure, Health Lab. Sci. **7**:34-41, 1970.
9. Lyerla, H.C., and Forrester, F.T.: Immunofluorescence methods in virology, Course No. 8231-C, Atlanta, 1979, U.S. Department of Health and Human Services, Center for Disease Control.
10. McKinney, R.M.: Immunofluorescence methods and reagents. In Friedman, H., Linna, T.J., and Prier, J.E., editors: Immunoserology in the diagnosis of infectious diseases, Baltimore, 1979, University Park Press.
11. Riggs, J.L.: Immunofluorescent staining. In Lennette, E.H., and Schmidt, N.J., editors: Diagnostic procedures for viral, rickettsial, and chlamydial infections, Washington, D.C., 1979, American Public Health Association, Inc.
12. Washington, J.A., II, Martin, W.J., and Karlson, A.G.: Fluorescent antibody procedures. In Washington, J.A., II, editor: Laboratory procedures in clinical microbiology, Boston, 1974, Little, Brown & Co.

PART VII

AUTOMATION AND RAPID METHODS; QUALITY CONTROL AND SAFETY

40 AUTOMATION AND RAPID METHODS IN THE DIAGNOSTIC MICROBIOLOGY LABORATORY

If we compare the present state of the art in clinical microbiology with that in clinical chemistry in terms of automation and the use of mechanized devices and instruments, we find that we are about 10 to 15 years behind. However, most new techniques are developed over a long period of time and at great expense, and we can benefit from the experience of others.

A great variety of rapid techniques have been applied to diagnosis of infection and to isolation and identification of microorganisms over the years, but few have become commercial successes. Those that have done best, for the most part, are relatively simple variations and adaptations of a technology described some time ago as the "little tube method" by Hartman.[14]

Because of the voluminous literature on this subject, no attempt has been made in this chapter to present a comprehensive review. The data presented relate mainly to the most recently developed instrument systems, with emphasis on instrument capability in detection and identification of organisms. It should be pointed out that there has been no simultaneous critical comparative evaluation of all instrument systems under well-defined clinical laboratory conditions. The interested reader should consult appropriate references for additional information on the respective systems. For a more detailed discussion concerning automation and antimicrobial susceptibility testing, the interested reader should consult Thornsberry.[29]

GAS CHROMATOGRAPHY

In chemistry and toxicology there are a great many applications of gas chromatography, but in microbiology the primary use so far has been to detect metabolic by-products of bacterial growth. For example, gas chromatography has had a major impact on assisting in the identification of anaerobic bacteria[15] (see Chapters 27 to 30). However, this technology has been shown to have other uses,[6,17,25] and one that shows great promise is the direct analysis of body fluids for compounds that indicate the presence of microorganisms.[5,12,18,28] For example, CSF can be analyzed for compounds that can differentiate various types of meningitis.[2,4] Not only is the procedure exceptionally sensitive, but it also can provide a very rapid test result. This may prove useful for the diagnosis of tuberculous meningitis and other meningitides. At the present time,

however, a much larger data base is needed in terms of what compounds might interfere or give similar patterns before we can apply this technique as a routine diagnostic tool. Methods such as frequency pulse-modulated electron capture gas chromatography[4] and pyrolysis gas chromatography[17,24] are under investigation as means to identify various bacteria and fungi (or their metabolic end products) from specimen sources. Mass spectroscopy may be coupled with gas-liquid chromatography. Cell wall fatty acid analysis and whole cell carbohydrate studies by gas-liquid chromatography offer much promise. High-pressure liquid chromatography (HPLC) is extremely useful for assay of antimicrobial agents in serum and body fluids.

ELECTRICAL IMPEDANCE CHANGES

The Bactometer* is an instrument capable of detecting changes in electric impedance as a result of growth and metabolic activity of bacteria in a suitable growth medium.[8] This has been primarily evaluated for use in detecting clinically significant numbers of bacteria in urine[34] and

---

*Bactomatic, Inc., Palo Alto, Calif.

the presence of bacteria in blood.[8] Specimens are inoculated into bottles of appropriate broth medium that contain wire electrodes that have been inserted through the rubber stopper for connection to the instrument. Impedance changes are continuously monitored permitting detection within a matter of hours.

MEASUREMENT OF RADIOLABELED COMPOUNDS

There are a number of automated or semi-automated, usually computerized, instruments available (or soon to be available) that can screen clinical specimens for bacteria, perform antibiotic susceptibility tests, or provide capability for identification; some instruments can do all of these operations. Perhaps the instrument in widest use in the clinical microbiology laboratory is the Bactec system.* This instrument measures the release of $^{14}CO_2$ from ^{14}C-labeled substrates that result from bacterial metabolism. It employs a sampling device and an ionization chamber.[9,10,23,32] Most laboratories employ the Bactec to detect organisms in blood or CSF (see Chapter 7). Specimens are inoculated into bottles of broth medium containing ^{14}C-labeled substrates. Depending on the instrument model, the bottles are monitored either automatically or manually for measurement of $^{14}CO_2$. The instrument converts this into a growth index (GI). This unit of measurement is recorded through lights or on a meter of the instrument as well as on a paper tape. Bactec has a number of other capabilities, including identification and susceptibility testing of *Mycobacterium*, identification of *Neisseria*, and determination of serum aminoglycoside levels.

AUTOBAC

A somewhat more versatile instrument is the Autobac Multi Test (MT) System.† It is

*Johnston Laboratories, Division of Becton Dickinson, Cockeysville, Md.
†General Diagnostics, Morris Plains, N.J.

designed to perform antibiotic susceptibility tests[29,31] and identify fermenting as well as the more commonly encountered nonfermenting bacteria. This instrument consists of an incubator shaker and a photometer system. Also there is a cuvette information device and a remote printer. Each chamber in a disposable cuvette contains a different substrate (or inhibitor) or antibiotic. Identification is based primarily on the pattern of growth and/or substrate utilization in the various chambers, and reaction patterns for various organisms are contained in the computer data base.

A culture obtained from an overnight incubation plate is simply suspended in broth, inoculated into the cuvette, and incubated for 3 hours. Readings are then taken and the results subsequently printed by the instrument. In simple terms, the growth (or lack of growth) in each of the test chambers is monitored by a beam of light passing through the chamber, and the results recorded as percent light transmitted are compared with an uninoculated control. The major advantages of this system are that it provides antibiotic susceptibility results and identification of both fermentative and nonfermentative organisms after a relatively short period of time. In our opinion a major drawback of this instrument is that it requires too much time to manipulate as compared with some of the other instrument systems available. However, it does have the advantage of a wider range of organism identification than most other systems, and, more importantly, a single culture can be tested simultaneously for antibiotic susceptibility and identification by using two different cuvettes.

The use of the Autobac as a rapid screening method for bacteriuria has been described by Hale and colleagues.[13] This collaborative study evaluated 2,720 urine specimens from three laboratories by Autobac and by simultaneous colony counts for evidence of bacteriuria. Of 599 specimens with a colony count of 10^5 colony-forming units (CFU)/ml or more, 93.8% were detected within 6 hours. This rate increased to

97% of 447 positive urine specimens when only specimens from patients not receiving antibiotics were evaluated. The majority (77.9%) of their positive specimens were detected as early as 3 hours. Specimens with 10^5 CFU/ml or more that were negative by Autobac at 6 hours included primarily those organisms considered to be contaminants or were from patients who were being treated with antimicrobial agents. Of 2,121 urine specimens with colony counts of 10^5 or less, 98.1% were correctly determined to be negative by Autobac at 3 hours, and this decreased to 86% at 6 hours. Hale and colleagues believe that the majority of their false-positive specimens were those with colony counts of 10^4 to 10^5 CFU/ml.

MS-2

Another instrument with multifunction capabilities is the Abbott MS-2.* Originally designed for antibiotic susceptibility testing,[3,29,30] the MS-2 is currently being applied also for screening of specimens and for identification.[19] The major components of the system are a control module and an analysis module (several analysis modules can be stacked on top of one another). Besides susceptibility testing, the system presently can identify only the *Enterobacteriaceae*. A disposable cuvette cartridge that contains several chambers and substrates is used. A separate cartridge containing antibiotics is used for susceptibility testing. This cuvette is inoculated and placed into the incubator analysis module. From this point on, everything is done automatically—incubation, reading, and reporting of results. The system scans each chamber once every 5 minutes, and the reaction is compared with an uninoculated control. Results are provided within 5 hours or less. The system does require a pure culture inoculum, but very little other manipulation is required. The MS-2 basic system can also be used for urine screening; for this a special adapter is required that holds 11

glass ampules, or what the manufacturer calls ampvettes. Each of these is inoculated with 0.1 ml of urine and placed in the adapter, which is inserted into the analysis module. The machine scans each ampvette every 5 minutes, and data are put into a computer that compares growth curves with control ampvettes for susceptibility testing and screening of specimens and that utilizes an internal computerized probability matrix for identification. The computer prints out results for all of the ampvettes after 5 hours. Abbott Diagnostics has also designed their system for research use and has made available a variety of accessories for this purpose. In our opinion the major advantage of the Abbott MS-2 system is its level of automation, which we consider quite sophisticated. The nearly constant monitoring of growth chambers, speed of identification and interpreting susceptibility results, and versatility also are pluses. The disadvantage we see at present is its limitation to identification of only the Enterobacteriaceae.

A recent collaborative study revealed the MS-2 to be quite accurate in identifying Enterobacteriaceae.[19] A total of 150 unknown coded organisms and 1,154 clinical isolates were tested both by the MS-2 system and by conventional tube methods. Twenty-six different species were represented. The percentages of strains identified correctly by the MS-2 system and the conventional system were 96% and 94%, respectively. Discrepancies were caused primarily by biochemical variants, expecially among *Enterobacter* species.

DYNATECH MIC-2000

The Dynatech MIC-2000 System* is a semi-automated system for preparing and performing microbroth antibiotic susceptibility and identification tests.[20,29] The system consists of a 96-channel dispenser for accurately delivering a volume of liquid such as antibiotic dilutions from test tubes to a 96-well microtiter plate (the MIC

---

*Abbott Diagnostics Division, Dallas, Tex.

*Dynatech Laboratories, Inc., Alexandria, Va.

Plate*) and an inoculator with 96 pins for accurately transferring liquid inoculum from a disposable inoculum tray* to the 96 wells of the MIC Plate. An illuminated magnifying viewer to assist in discriminating between wells with and without visible growth is also included. The accuracy and reproducibility of both dispenser and inoculator have been verified by McMaster and associates.[20]

Studies conducted in the laboratory of one of us (W.J.M., unpublished data) a few years ago compared the Dynatech with the standard agar dilution method for obtaining minimal inhibitory concentrations from clinical isolates. With 1,200 clinical isolates, the percentage of agreement between the two methods ranged from 91% to 98%, with an overall average of 95.4% agreement.

The Dynatech system is thought to be a time- and media-saving method for obtaining minimal inhibitory concentrations of antibiotics. Moreover, the microbroth method seems to provide an attractive alternative for obtaining minimal inhibitory concentration data within the time and cost range of the disk diffusion method (see Chapter 36).

Another system that is similar in design and function to the Dynatech system is the modular Autotiter System.†

An instrument for automated reading and interpretation of microdilution trays, the auto-SCAN-3, has been introduced and provided 95% agreement with visual reading in identification tests (Ellner and Myers: J. Clin. Microbiol. **14:**326-328, 1981).

REPLISCAN SYSTEM

Inexpensive replicate-plating techniques have been used for many years for agar dilution antibiotic susceptibility testing and are now being employed in a limited way for the identification of microorganisms. The Repliscan System† is a commercially available replica-plating method

for the identification of Enterobacteriaceae. This system consists of a variety of biochemical and antibiotic-containing plated media, a multiple-inoculum replicating device, a viewing table allowing visual inspection and electronic recording of individual reactions, and a computer terminal complete with hard copy printout.

One to three colonies of the bacterium to be identified are inoculated into 2 ml of broth, such as Mueller-Hinton, and grown to a turbidity equal to that of a 0.5 McFarland barium sulfate turbidity standard. Then 0.5 ml of this suspension is placed in an individual well of the replicating device and inoculated onto each of the 23 biochemical and antibiotic plates. The replicating device allows the simultaneous inoculation of up to 36 organisms on a single agar plate. All plates are incubated aerobically at 35 C for 18 to 20 hours. After incubation, the plates are arranged on a loading tray and inserted into the viewing table. The growth of a single isolate on each of the 23 types of media is observed by transmitted light through individual windows in the viewing table. Positive and negative reactions are recorded by using a pen light and photosensitive receptors located directly adjacent to the viewing window for each test plate. When the reactions on all test plates have been recorded, the computer analyzes the information entered and provides the identification of the organism. The limited antibiogram is used by the computer to confirm the biochemical identification of the organism. When a given isolate has been identified, the viewing table automatically advances the plates to the next reading position; the identification cycle is repeated for each of the 36 isolates per plate.

In their evaluation of the Repliscan System for identification of Enterobacteriaceae, Brown and Washington[7] of the Mayo Clinic found it to be an efficient, economical, and effective laboratory tool for identification of these organisms. They tested a total of 1,877 isolates, including 1,712 fermentative and 165 nonfermentative organisms, in parallel with the Repliscan and Enterotube methods of enteric identification. Discrep-

---

*Cook Laboratory Products, Alexandria, Va.
†Cathra International, St. Paul, Minn.

ancies were retested in each system, as well as with conventional methods. The Repliscan method correctly identified 91%, misidentified 2%, and failed to identify 7% of the fermentative organisms tested. The system consistently failed to recognize satisfactorily nonfermentative organisms. Of the genera they studied, *Enterobacter* posed the greatest problem to the system in terms of overall identification rates.

In another recent study, however, the Repliscan System in its present stage of development was considered not reliable for identifying 1,013 isolates of Enterobacteriaceae as compared to API-20E*. Woolfrey and others[33] reported a 62% agreement at the genus level between the two systems. Of the discrepant results, Repliscan classified 22% as "biochemical pattern not on file," 8% as a multiple-genus group that included the API-20E identification, and 8% as a genus other than that designated by API-20E.

AUTOMICROBIC SYSTEM

The AutoMicrobic System (AMS)† was designed for the detection, enumeration, identification, and drug susceptibility testing of microorganisms in clinical specimens, with all of its functions to be performed simultaneously or consecutively by the same instrument.[1,21,26,27] It uses a novel array of highly selective media in which a mixture of substrates and inhibitors is used to permit the growth of one or a group of closely related microorganisms, to concurrently inhibit growth of any other organisms present, and to enumerate the total number of organisms in the sample. The lyophilized media are incorporated in wells of a sealed, disposable, plastic card, which is inoculated and incubated in an automated instrument equipped with an optical system. The optical system monitors light transmission changes in the card wells and transmits optical measurements to a minicomputer, which

compares them with preset thresholds and then displays results in 4 to 13 hours.

The AMS is different from other instrument systems currently on the market in that it was originally designed to screen urine specimens and identify the organisms present without the usual preliminary pure culture technique. The system consists of a diluent dispenser, injector or filling module, incubator reader, computer, and a terminal printer. As with the MS-2 and Autobac, it uses a disposable unit that varies with the type of analysis being made. The card that receives the inoculum is about the size of a playing card and 3 to 4 mm thick. There are 5 wells for quantitating and 15 for identification purposes, of which 13 are actually used. The technician simply pipets undiluted urine into the 2 plastic tubes, with 0.5 µl and 200 µl being diluted respectively to 1:1000 for enumeration and 1:10 for identification with sterile 0.5% saline by the diluent dispenser. This whole unit goes into the injector module, which is a pressurized system that forces the urine into the respective chambers within the card; this procedure takes about 4½ minutes. The technician then puts the card into the incubator reader. From this point on, everything is done automatically. The cards are read hourly with data being fed to the computer. After 13 hours, all results are printed out. Also, one can ask the instrument for results at any time after 1 hour. The system has the capability to identify mixed cultures and report each of the organisms present, but it only provides a total count, not a specific count for each of the various organisms that may be present. Nevertheless, one can obtain a population count and an identification within the same day.

The instrument has many other applications; all all require pure cultures. One such application was the antimicrobial susceptibility card, or "Sensipak." It was basically the same as the urine Identipac card, but the wells contained only antibiotics. Only two cards were developed—an *E. coli* susceptibility card and a *Proteus* species susceptibility card. These two cards

---

*Analytab Products, Plainview, N.Y.
†Vitek Incorporated, McDonnell Douglas Corp., St. Louis, Mo.

have since been discontinued. Another application was the Enterobacteriaceae Biochemical Card (EBC), containing some 30 substrates or reagents for identification of the Enterobacteriaceae. Employing an appropriately diluted culture to reconstitute the medium within the card, the EBC card was inserted in the reader/incubator module. The system monitored all activity within the wells during an 8-hour incubation period, after which the instrument accumulated and interpreted all data and provided a printed identification of the organism, as well as the probability value for the identification. If additional testing was required (as with *Salmonella* or *Shigella*), the message "Serology is Suggested" would appear on the printout with the identification. One well on the EBC card was not used in the identification pattern; that was the positive control well (well No. 3). The medium in this well was designed to support growth of the organism and also to provide a source of pure culture on which serology or an indole test could be performed. Although the EBC has now been replaced with the so-called EBC + , a multicenter collaborative study reported an approximate 93% rate of identification when compared with conventional media against 173 selected and coded isolates supplied by the CDC.[16] The EBC + card that is currently available is designed to identify both the Enterobacteriaceae and a selected number of nonfermenting, gram-negative bacilli. Recent evaluations reveal 97% to 98% accuracy in identification of Enterobacteriaceae in 8 hours (Hasyn et al.: J. Clin. Microbiol. **13**:491-497, 1981; and Freeman et al.: J. Clin. Microbiol. **13**:895-898, 1981).

Another card that has been designed for use with the Vitek instrument is the AMS Gram Negative General Susceptibility Card (GSC), which has been designed for testing the antimicrobial susceptibility of rapidly growing aerobic or facultatively anaerobic gram-negative bacilli and group D enterococci. The card is essentially a miniaturized and abbreviated version of the doubling dilution technique for determination of the minimal inhibitory concentration by the

microtiter broth method and is designed to test 13 antimicrobial agents over appropriate concentration ranges. The GSC contains 30 wells consisting of 12 antimicrobial agents at 2 dilutions each, 1 antimicrobial agent at 3 dilutions, 1 positive control broth, and 2 empty wells for future application. Presently the information with this card indicates a correlation greater than 90% with standard procedures (W.J.M., unpublished data). However, some problems have been noted with carbenicillin and *Pseudomonas aeruginosa*, as well as with tetracycline against a variety of microorganisms. A recent study indicated that good results could be obtained in rapid identification and susceptibility testing of gram-negative bacilli from blood cultures using the EBC+ and GSC cards (Moore et al.: J. Clin. Microbiol. **13**:934-939, 1981).

Another card that has been developed for the AMS system is the Yeast Biochemical Card (YBC). The YBC consists of 30 wells that contain 26 biochemical broths and 4 control broths. The card is inoculated with a McFarland standard No. 2 concentration of yeast prepared from a pure culture on Sabouraud dextrose agar. The filling of the card is accomplished using the filling module cycle designed for all AMS cards, and, once filled, the inoculated YBC is incubated at 30 C for 22 to 23 hours. After the incubation period, the YBC is loaded into the AMS reader/incubator. Final identification is completed following microscopic examination of the morphology of the yeast on corn meal agar.

The current AMS data base contains information on 27 yeast species. The identification of 273 yeasts using the AMS yeast biochemical card and the API-20C system for yeast identification was recently reported by Oblack and colleagues.[22] In this study the YBC data were generated using a preliminary AMS computer program that was subsequently revised following tabulation and examination of these data as they were entered into the AMS data base. For the yeasts that had been tested, overall agreement between the AMS program and the API system was 96%. Good agreement between the two systems was found for nine *Candida* species, *Rhodotorula* species, *Torulopsis candida*, *Cryptococcus* species, *Geotrichum* species, *Saccharomyces cerevisiae*, *Torulopsis glabrata*, and *Trichosporon cutaneum*.

The advantages of the AMS are its versatility, its rapidity of results with urine specimens, its identification potential, and its degree of automation. The system can handle up to 240 specimens simultaneously, and all of the operations (other than initial pipeting and labeling) are automatic. One disadvantage is a high initial instrumentation cost.

OTHER RAPID TESTS

Various other nonautomated systems and tests for rapid identification (e.g., Micro-ID, various API systems, Minitek, Enterotube, Micro Media systems, antibiotic disk identification, rapid fermentation tests, and rapid urease test) have been described in appropriate places in earlier chapters. Computer-aided numerical identification is feasible with some of these. Computerization has many other roles in the microbiology laboratory. Obviously, the many serologic and immunologic approaches to rapid diagnosis of disease and rapid identification of organisms are very important also. These have been discussed in connection with specific disease entities and organisms throughout the book and in Chapters 37, 38, and 39. Microcalorimetry and electronic detection systems (using stainless steel electrodes implanted in blood culture bottles) have been proposed for rapid detection of growth in blood culture bottles, as noted in Chapter 7.

REFERENCES

1. Alridge, C., Jones, P.W., Gibson, S., Lanham, J., Meyer, M., Vannest, R., and Charles, R.: Automated microbiological detection/identification system, J. Clin. Microbiol. **6**:406-413, 1977.
2. Amundson, S., Braude, A.I., and Davis, C.E.: Rapid diagnosis of infection by gas-liquid chromatography: analysis of sugars in normal and infected cerebrospinal fluid, Appl. Microbiol. **28**:298-302, 1974.
3. Barnes, W.G., Green, L.R., and Talley, R.L.: Clinical evaluation of automated antibiotic susceptibility testing with the MS-2 system, J. Clin. Microbiol. **12**:527-532, 1980.
4. Brooks, J.B., Choudhary, G., Craven, R.B., Alley, C.C., Liddle, J.A., Edman, D.C., and Converse, J.D.: Electron capture gas chromatography detection and mass spectrum identification of 3-(2'-ketohexyl) indoline in spinal fluids of patients with tuberculous meningitis, J. Clin. Microbiol. **5**:625-628, 1977.
5. Brooks, J.B., Kellogg, D.S., Alley, C.C., Short, H.B., Handsfield, H.H., and Huff, B.: Gas chromatography as a potential means of diagnosing arthritis. I. Differentiation between staphylococcal, streptococcal, gonococcal, and traumatic arthritis, J. Infect. Dis. **129**:660-668, 1974.
6. Brooks, J.B., Kellogg, D.S., Thacker, L., and Turner, E.M.: Analysis by gas chromatography of hydroxy acids produced by several species of *Neisseria*, Can. J. Microbiol. **18**:157-168, 1972.
7. Brown, S.D., and Washington, J.A., II: Evaluation of the Repliscan system for identification of Enterobacteriaceae, J. Clin. Microbiol. **8**:695-699, 1978.
8. Cady, P.: Progress in impedance measurements in microbiology. In Sharpe, A.N., and Clark, D.S., editors: Mechanizing microbiology, Springfield, Ill., 1978, Charles C Thomas, Publisher.
9. DeBlanc, H.J., Jr., Charache, P., Wagner, H.N., Jr.: Automatic radiometric measurement of antibiotic effect on bacterial growth, Antimicrob. Agents Chemother. **2**:360-366, 1972.
10. DeBlanc, H.J., Jr., Deland, F., and Wagner, H.N., Jr.: Automated radiometric detection of bacteria in 2,967 blood cultures, Appl. Microbiol. **22**:846-849, 1971.
11. Gavin, T.L., and Butler, D.A.: Automated microdilution method for antimicrobial susceptibility testing. In Balows, A., editor: Current techniques for antibiotic susceptibility testing, Springfield, Ill., 1973, Charles C. Thomas, Publisher.
12. Gorbach, S.L., Mayhew, J.W., Bartlett, J.G., Thadepalli, H., and Onderdonk, A.B.: Rapid diagnosis of *Bacteroides fragilis* infections by direct gas liquid chromatography of clinical specimens (Abstract), Clin. Res. **22**:442A, 1974.
13. Hale, D.C., Wright, D.N., McKie, J.E., Isenberg, H.D., Jenkins, R.D., and Matsen, J.M.: Rapid screening for bacteriuria by light scatter photometry (Autobac): a collaborative study, J. Clin. Microbiol. **13**:147-150, 1981.
14. Hartman, P.A.: Miniaturized microbiological methods, Supplement 1 to Advances in Applied Microbiology, New York, 1968, Academic Press, Inc.
15. Holdeman, L.V., Cato, E.P., and Moore, W.E.C., editors: Anaerobe laboratory manual, ed. 4, Blacksburg, Va., 1977, Virginia Polytechnic Institute and State University.

16. Isenberg, H.D., Gavan, T.L., Smith, P.B., Sonnen-wirth, A., Taylor, W., Martin, W.J., Rhoden, D., and Balows, A.: Collaborative investigation of the Auto Microbic System Enterobacteriaceae biochemical card, J. Clin. Microbiol. **11**:694-702, 1980.

17. Larsson, L., and Mårdh, P.: Application of gas chroma-tography to diagnosis of microorganisms and infectious diseases, Acta Pathol. Microbiol. Scand. Sect. B **259**:(Supp.) 5-15, 1977.

18. Mayhew, J.W., Onderdonk, A., Bartlett, J., and Gor-bach, S.L.: Direct gas-liquid chromatographic (GLC) analysis of clinical material for rapid detection of strep-tococci (Abstract M47), Abstracts of the Annual Meeting of the American Society for Microbiology, 1974.

19. McCracken, A.W., Martin, W.J., McCarthy, L.R., Schwab, D.A., Cooper, B.H., Helgeson, N.G.P., Pro-want, S., and Robson, J.: Evaluation of the MS-2 system for rapid identification of Enterobacteriaceae, J. Clin. Microbiol. **12**:684-689, 1980.

20. McMaster, P.R.B., Robertson, E.A., Witebsky, F.G., and MacLowry, J.D.: Evaluation of a dispensing instru-ment (Dynatech MIC-2000) for preparing microtiter antibiotic plates and testing their potency during stor-age, Antimicrob. Agents Chemother. **13**:842-844, 1978.

21. Nicholson, D.P., and Koepka, J.A.: The Automicrobic system for urines, J. Clin. Microbiol. **10**:823-833, 1979.

22. Oblack, D.L., Rhodes, J.C., and Martin, W.J.: Clinical evaluation of the Automicrobic system yeast biochemi-cal card for rapid identification of medically important yeasts, J. Clin. Microbiol. **13**:351-355, 1981.

23. Previte, J.J.: Radiometric detection of some food-borne bacteria, Appl. Microbiol. **24**:535-539, 1972.

24. Reiner, E.: Identification of bacterial strains by pyroly-sis-gas-liquid chromatography, Nature **206**:1272-1273, 1965.

25. Savage, A.M.: Gas liquid chromatography from taxono-my to diagnosis, Chest **77**:506-507, 1980.

26. Smith, P.B., Gavan, T.L., Isenberg, H.D., Sonnen-wirth, A., Taylor, W.I., Washington, J.A., II, and Balows, A.: Multi-laboratory evaluation of an automated microbial detection/identification system, J. Clin. Microbiol. **8**:657-666, 1978.

27. Sonnenwirth, A.C.: Preprototype of an automated microbial detection and identification system: a devel-opment investigation, J. Clin. Microbiol. **6**:400-405, 1977.

28. Thadepalli, H., and Gangopadhyay, P.K.: Rapid diag-nosis of anaerobic empyema by direct gas-liquid chro-matography of pleural fluid, Chest **77**:507-513, 1980.

29. Thornsberry, C.: Automation in antibiotic susceptibility testing. In Lorian, V., editor: Antibiotics in laboratory medicine, Baltimore, Md., 1980, The Williams & Wil-kins Co.

30. Thornsberry, C., Anhalt, J.P., Washington, J.A., II, McCarthy, L.R., Schoenknecht, F.D., Sherris, J.C., and Spencer, H.J.: Clinical laboratory evaluation of the Abbott MS-2 automated antimicrobial susceptibility testing system: report of a collaborative study, J. Clin. Microbiol. **12**:375-390, 1980.

31. Thornsberry, C., Gavan, T., Sherris, J., Balows, A., Matsen, J., Sabath, L., Schoenknecht, F., and Thrupp, L.: Laboratory evaluation of a rapid, automated suscep-tibility testing system: report of a collaborative study, Antimicrob. Agents Chemother. **7**:466-480, 1975.

32. Waters, J.R.: Sensitivity of the $^{14}CO_2$ radiometric meth-od for bacterial detection, Appl. Microbiol. **23**:198-199, 1972.

33. Woolfrey, B.F., Quall, C.O., and Fox, J.M.: Evaluation of the Repliscan system for Enterobacteriaceae identifi-cation, J. Clin. Microbiol. **13**:58-61, 1981.

34. Zafari, Y., and Martin, W.J.: Comparison of the bactom-eter microbial monitoring system with conventional methods for detection of microorganisms in urine spec-imens, J. Clin. Microbiol. **5**:545-547, 1977.

41 QUALITY CONTROL AND SAFETY IN THE MICROBIOLOGY LABORATORY

With the present and continuing reexamination of health care delivery by the medical and allied health professions, it is incumbent on the microbiologist to ensure that the laboratory contributes to the highest quality of patient care by its expertise, its accuracy, its relevance, and the prompt reporting of its findings to the attending physician. It is only by constant self-evaluation of the laboratory's performance through a quality control program that such a level of excellence can be developed and maintained.

It is not the function of this section to detail the methodology for carrying out a quality control program—this is presently available in excellent texts and publications[1,2,5,11,14,19-21]— but to suggest a basic format that can be tailored to individual situations or requirements.

CONTROL OF EQUIPMENT

Generally, equipment is simple to monitor; this consists chiefly of the daily, weekly, or monthly observation and recording of temperatures of incubators (optimal, 35 C), refrigerators, water baths, hot-air ovens, freezers, autoclaves (by temperature-time cycle charts), and so forth. A range of ± 1 C is generally acceptable for heating devices, with a greater range acceptable for refrigerating devices; both should be measured with thermometers that have been calibrated against a Bureau of Standards instrument.* Autoclaves should also be checked at monthly intervals with biologic devices such as the Kilit or Attest spore test ampules or strips.†

In addition to their temperature recordings, CO_2 incubators should also have their CO_2 concentration measured daily by the portable Fyrite CO_2 gas analyzer,‡ which determines the CO_2 level by absorption, with change in level of the absorbent in a graduated tube. Tank pressure also must be monitored, and an extra tank of gas should be kept on hand at all times.

Every laboratory handling material for mycobacteriologic, mycologic, and virologic examination should possess a **biologic safety hood,** which also requires regular recording of the negative pressure within the hood, the interval between the high-efficiency particulate (HEPA) filter changes, the effective output of the UV Sterilamp (measured by a photometric cell),§ and so forth. Directions for these tests are included in the hood operation manual or from the Biological Hazards Control Officer of the CDC.

Other miscellaneous items requiring inspection, calibration or replacement include the standard (0.01- and 0.001-ml) inoculating loops, chipped or cracked glassware, and the presence of residual detergent in glassware. Mechanical devices, such as centrifuges, vacuum pumps, or pipeting machines, require frequent oiling and adjustments. Microscopes and balances should be cleaned semiannually; pH meters and other measuring devices, such as thermometers, graduated cylinders, pipets, and so forth, also should be calibrated periodically.

---

*Thermometers should be in glycerol or tubes of water.
†BBL Microbiology Systems, Cockeysville, Md.
‡Arthur H. Thomas, Co., Philadelphia Pa., catalogue No. 5566-C 10.
§Westinghouse SM-600 meter, Westinghouse Electric Corp., Lamp Division, Bloomfield, N.J.

CONTROL OF CULTURE MEDIA

Most clinical bacteriology laboratories today utilize ready-made, commercially available solid and fluid culture media. These are, in general, of uniformly high quality and good batch-to-batch consistency and are readily obtainable. If, on the other hand, a laboratorian has the good fortune to have on the staff an experienced and dedicated media chef, he or she is assured of a product that is superior in many ways to that available in the marketplace. In this situation, however, strict attention to details of preparation must be adhered to, such as following exact directions of the manufacturer regarding methods of preparation and sterilization (overheating is the most frequent source of error), properly sealing and dating dehydrated media, and so forth. With certain media, such as decarboxylase media or Mueller-Hinton agar, it is also necessary to check the pH of the final product. In certain situations, as in anaerobic bacteriology, freshly made media of certain types are often superior to purchased media.

The foregoing implies the use of a quality control program that is best carried out by **performance testing** for the desired reaction with a number of stock cultures of microorganisms of known stability (Table 41-1). At the Wilmington Medical Center a culture collection of 26 strains of bacteria and 3 strains of fungi is utilized in an ongoing program for the regular testing of culture media, stains, and reagents (Table 41-1).[16] Each new batch of culture media is tested by the quality control technologist, while the stains and reagents are checked in use by the individual technologists performing the procedure. Records are kept on a daily basis and are eventually entered into a master log for monthly review by the microbiologist or laboratory director. A similar program exists at the UCLA Hospital and Clinics.

Stock cultures are preserved in the frozen state at approximately $-70 C$ on glass beads, according to the method of Nagel and Kunz,[10] where they remain viable for many months. When required, a single glass bead is removed

TABLE 41-1

Recommended cultures* for monitoring routine culture media, stains, and reagents†

Medium or test	Control organism	Expected result
Acetate	E. coli	Growth, blue color
	S. flexneri	No growth
Arginine dihydrolase	E. cloacea	Positive
	P. vulgaris	Negative
Bile esculin agar	S. faecalis	Growth, blackening
	Viridans group streptococcus	No growth
Blood culture bottles		
Biphasic (vented)	H. influenzae	Growth on subculture
Anaerobic (unvented)	B. fragilis	Growth on subculture
Brain-heart infusion agar	C. albicans	Growth
with antibiotics	A. fumigatus	Inhibited
Brucella agar with laked blood, vitamin K_1, and hemin	Peptococcus species	Growth (anaerobic)
Catalase test	S. aureus	Positive
	Group A streptococcus	Negative
Chocolate agar	H. influenzae, S. pneumoniae	Growth
Simmons citrate	K. pneumoniae	Positive
	E. coli	Negative
Coagulase test (rabbit plasma)	S. aureus	Clot
	S. epidermidis	No clot
CNA (colistin nalidixic acid) agar	S. faecalis	Growth
	P. aeruginosa	No growth
	S. aureus	Growth
CTA medium		
Glucose	N. gonorrhoeae	Acid (yellow)
Maltose	N. gonorrhoeae	No change
Sucrose	N. gonorrhoeae	No change
Lactose	N. lactamicus	Acid (yellow)
Differential carbohydrates	As indicated[20]	
DNase agar	S. marcescens	Positive
	E. cloacea	Negative
Egg yolk agar (Nagler)	C. perfringens	Positive (anaerobic)
	B. fragilis	Negative (anaerobic)
EMB agar	E. coli	Growth, metallic sheen
	P. mirabilis	Growth, lactose negative (colorless colony)
FA test, group A streptococci	Group A streptococcus	Positive
	Group C streptococcus	Negative
Germ tube test	C. albicans	Positive
GN broth	S. typhimurium	Growth on subculture
	S. flexneri	Growth on subculture
Gram stain	S. aureus	Gram positive
	E. coli	Gram negative

*These stable stocks have been collected from the CDC reference strains, from the ATCC, and from patient isolates confirmed by the CDC. Certain ATCC strains of some of these organisms are available commercially on desiccated disks (Bact-Chek, Roche Diagnostics, Nutley, N.J.; Bactrol Disks,[12] Difco Laboratories, Detroit, Mich.).

†Media are checked on each new batch; sterility tests are performed on 5% of batches of 100 or fewer and 10 randomly selected plates or tubes from larger batches. They are incubated at 35 C or the temperature at which they will be used. Stains and reagents are tested when made or purchased. If they are not used frequently, test before each use. Test working solutions weekly and reagents daily for frequently used stains.

Continued.

TABLE 41-1

Recommended cultures for monitoring routine culture media, stains, and reagents—cont'd

Medium or test	Control organism	Expected result
Hektoen agar	S. typhimurium	Growth, green colony with black center
	E. coli	Growth, orange colony (or no growth)
Hippurate hydrolysis	Group B streptococcus	Positive
	Group A streptococcus	Negative
Indole	E. coli	Positive
	K. pneumoniae	Negative
Kanamycin-vancomycin blood agar	B. fragilis	Growth (anaerobic)
	E. coli	Inhibited (anaerobic)
KCN	C. freundii	Growth
	S. typhimurium	No growth
Kit for identification of Enterobacteriaceae	Directions from manufacturer	
10% Lactose	A. calcoaceticus var. anitratus	Acid
	A. calcoaceticus var. lwoffi	Alkaline
L-J medium	M. tuberculosis (H37-RA strain)	Characteristic colonies
Lysine decarboxylase	S. typhimurium	Positive
	P. vulgaris	Negative
Motility medium	E. coli	Positive
	K. pneumoniae	Negative
Mueller-Hinton agar	S. aureus (ATCC 25923)	Acceptable zone sizes (see Chapter 36)
	E. coli (ATCC 25922)	
	P. aeruginosa (ATCC 27853)	
Nitrate reduction	P. aeruginosa	Positive, N_2
	Acinetobacter calcoaceticus	Negative
	E. coli	Positive
O-F media		
Glucose	P. aeruginosa	Oxidizer (yellow)
Maltose	P. maltophilia	Oxidizer (yellow)
Ornithine decarboxylase	E. cloacea	Positive
	P. vulgaris	Negative
Optochin disk test	S. pneumoniae	≥ 14-mm zone (6-mm disk)
	S. mitis	< 14-mm zone
Oxidase reaction	P. aeruginosa	Positive (blue)
	E. coli	No color change
Rice agar with Tween 80	C. albicans	Characteristic chlamydospores
	C. tropicalis	No chlamydospores
SAB agar with antibiotics	C. albicans	Growth
	A. fumigatus	Inhibited
Sheep blood agar	Group A streptococcus	Growth, beta hemolysis
	S. mitis	Growth, alpha hemolysis
Trypticase soy agar or broth	Group A streptococcus	Growth
TSI agar	P. mirabilis	K/AG, H_2S
	E. coli	A/AG
	P. aeruginosa	K/no reaction
Urea agar (Christensen)	P. vulgaris	Positive (red)
	E. coli	Negative
XLD agar	S. typhimurium	Growth, pink-red with black center
	E. coli	Yellow (or no growth)
Ziehl-Neelsen, fluorochrome stain	M. tuberculosis (H37-RA)	Positive acid-fast
	E. coli	Negative acid-fast

from its reservoir and placed in a tube of trypticase soy broth and incubated until growth is visible. This is then streaked on half of a blood agar plate to obtain isolated colonies. A 1:10 dilution is made in broth from a suspension equivalent to a 0.5 MacFarland standard. This dilution is used to test the plate media.

CONTROL OF REAGENTS AND ANTISERA

The various chemical reagents used in biochemical tests are best monitored, after preparation, by integrating into the daily laboratory work load through the use of a master schedule calendar.[19] Reagents should be dated on preparation and stored in lightproof, tightly stoppered bottles either at room temperature or in the refrigerator as indicated.

Gram-stain reagents are best monitored by staining and examining slides prepared from a suspension of *E. coli* and *S. aureus* that has been grown in broth and sterilized by autoclaving; this procedure should be a part of a **weekly staining schedule.** Acid-fast and special staining reagents should be checked with a suspension of the appropriate killed microorganisms each time the stain is done.

Antisera that have been obtained from reliable sources are dated on receipt and diluted to the manufacturer's specifications. They are then tested with standard stock cultures for sensitivity and specificity with each new lot and every month thereafter. The manufacturer's directions for storage and test performance likewise should be explicitly followed. In a similar manner, bacterial antigens for agglutination tests should be monitored with known positive and negative antisera, if available.

As noted in Chapter 37, Wright and colleagues[22] provided directions for producing smooth, homogeneous bacterial suspensions of 14 bacteria representing the most common clinical isolates that require serologic confirmation for identification. These preserved bacterial antigens are stable for up to 5 months when stored at 4 C.

MONITORING REPORTING ON GRAM-STAINED DIRECT SMEARS

Bartlett and associates[3] stressed the importance of objective criteria for enumeration of cells in identification and quantification of bacteria on direct smears. They suggest two methods for monitoring the accuracy and reproducibility of these examinations: (1) examination of previously examined and reported smears by independent observers, with subsequent review by supervisors, and (2) preparation of suspensions of cells and bacteria to yield identical smears for subsequent examination as unknowns. Both methods provided an economical, practical, and educational approach to assuring quality in preparing and interpreting Gram-stained smears.

PROCEDURE BOOK

The procedure book delineates the current standard procedures employed in the microbiology laboratory and should be comprehensive enough to include all techniques, from the simple preparation of reagents to the methods for identifying isolates of the common genera. It should be easily interpreted by the least experienced bench worker and should not include lengthy descriptions readily found in a standard microbiology text. It should be reviewed at regular intervals, obsolete material deleted and new methods inserted, and initialed and dated by the director of the laboratory. It should be the **working reference standard** for the entire staff. The National Committee for Clinical Laboratory Standards has established guidelines for writing laboratory procedure manuals (NCCLS: Standards for procedure manuals, Villanova, Pa., June, 1980).

QUALITY CONTROL IN SPECIMEN COLLECTION

Until recently one of the least regulated areas of quality control in the microbiology laboratory has been the quality of the clinical specimen itself. Is it representative of the suspected infection site? Has it been collected correctly in a proper container? Were sites of normal flora

TABLE 41-2

Criteria for rejection of requests for microbiologic tests*

Category	Criterion for rejection	Action
Identification	Discrepancy between patient identification on request form and on specimen container	Discuss with sender or return to sender for resolution. If discrepancy is unresolved, specimen is processed but no report issued.
	No identification on container	Do not process unless request form is wrapped around container. Write "Container not identified" on report form in such cases.
	Specimen source or type of culture ordered not on request form	Call physician or service for necessary information.
Specimen	Anaerobic culture request on	Cross anaerobic culture request off form.
	Sputum	Do not perform anaerobic cultures, except with microbiology staff approval. Explain reasoning to requesting physician.
	Midstream urine	
	Catheterized urine	
	Vaginal secretions	
	Prostatic secretions	
	Feces	
	Environmental material	
	Gastric washings	
	Bronchoscopic washings	
	Decubitus ulcer material	
	Throat material	
	Nose material	
	Skin material	
	Mouth material	
	Ileostomy material†	
	Colostomy material†	
	Fistula†	
	Specimen identified by anatomic site only (e.g., chest, leg, etc.)	Request additional information.
	Anaerobic culture request on swab material (unless swab has been submitted in anaerobic transport tube or bag)	Return request form to physician immediately, stamped "This specimen is unacceptable for culture of anaerobic bacteria because it was not transported under anaerobic conditions. Please submit syringe aspirate injected into anaerobic transport tube, or, if necessary, a swab in proper transport setup." Do not perform anaerobic culture unless physician insists it is not feasible to obtain another sample.
	Anaerobic culture request on unacceptable material (specified above) in anaerobic transport tube	Return request form to physician immediately, stamped "This specimen was submitted in an anaerobic transport tube for anaerobic culture. However, since this material is generally contaminated with normal flora anaerobes, no anaerobic culture was performed. Please contact laboratory to discuss obtaining a suitable specimen."

*Adapted from criteria in use at the Mayo Clinic.
†Refers to intraluminal material.

TABLE 41-2

Criteria for rejection of requests for microbiologic tests—cont'd

Category	Criterion for rejection	Action
Specimen—cont'd	Improperly collected sputum (i.e., saliva) for routine culture	Return request form to physician immediately, stamped "Improper specimen; please resubmit." Explain problem.
	Material received in fixative (e.g., formalin)	Notify physician and request new specimen. Stamp "Specimen unsatisfactory; please submit new specimen" on request form and return.
	Gram-stained smear of material from anus or rectum for gonococci	Cross Gram smear request off form.
	Dry swab	Notify physician and request new specimen. Stamp "Specimen unsatisfactory—dry swab; please submit new specimen" on request form and return.
	Blood culture with request for Gram-stained smears or cultures for mycobacteria (TB) or viruses	Cross request off form.
	Foley catheter tips	Discard sample. Explain problem.
	24-hour urine or sputum collections for mycobacteria (TB) or fungi	Notify physician that 24-hour collections are unacceptable and request three single-voided urine specimens or three consecutive, early morning, freshly expectorated sputa.

	Urine
	  Held longer than 2 hours at room temperature
	  Improper container
	  Leaking container
		Return request form to physician immediately, stamped with "Improper specimen; please resubmit." Explain problem.

	Excess barium or oil in stool specimen for ova and parasites	Stamp "Exam for parasites unsatisfactory—oil (or barium) in excess" on report form and return.
	Less than one swab per request for bacterial, mycobacterial (TB), and fungal cultures	Call physician to request additional material. If additional material cannot be obtained, ask physician to state priorities for culture.
	Multiple urine, stool, sputum, and **routine throat specimens** on the same day from the same source (AFB requests excluded). Process all stool specimens received on children younger than 3 years.	One specimen should be processed. Stamp duplicate request forms with "Multiple specimens received; one will be processed. Notify lab within 24 hours if you wish the remaining specimens to be processed and explain circumstances."

avoided in obtaining the specimen, when this is important or feasible? Was it submitted promptly in a proper transport medium or vehicle, when this is important, and cultured without undue delay? These are questions that must be answered affirmatively so that the laboratory results are meaningful and not misleading to the attending physician.

The microbiologist must not be too lenient in acceptance of improperly collected specimens. Too frequently treatment has been initiated on the basis of a report of potential pathogens, including antibiograms, when in reality the isolates represented only colonization of the patient's oropharynx or skin. Examples of the criteria used for rejection of requests for microbiologic tests at the UCLA Hospital and Clinics are shown in Table 41-2.

Murray and Washington[9] have proposed screening all sputum specimens by Gram stain and accepting only those with fewer than 10 squamous epithelial cells per $100\times$ magnification field. These specimens correlated well, on culture, with transtracheal aspirates; the smaller number of epithelial cells indicated less contamination with oropharyngeal flora. Van Scoy[18] has suggested, after reviewing the data of Murray and Washington, that a criterion of more than 25 polymorphonuclear leukocytes per low-power field, regardless of the number of squamous epithelial cells, would be more appropriate. This is discussed in more detail in Chapter 8.

Although we have stressed the importance of obtaining the best possible specimen, it must be appreciated that the physician who has responsibility for the patient must make the final decision regarding what is to be done. The microbiologist should serve as the physician's consultant and adviser. In the event that a physician repeatedly orders inappropriate and meaningless cultures, which may even be misleading, and thus also imposes an unnecessary burden on the laboratory, the microbiologist should sit down with the physician to discuss the situation in depth. If necessary, intercession should be sought from the hospital's infectious disease cli-

nicians, clinical pathologists or laboratory medicine workers, or the hospital staff officers. Obviously, it is always better for the microbiologist and physician to settle things directly.

It is well recognized that a bacterial count of 10^5 or greater in a clean-voided, promptly cultured urine specimen is associated with urinary tract infection, but it should be noted that counts in the range of 10^3 to 10^5 per milliliter also may represent infection; in patients receiving therapy, even lower counts may represent residual infection. Such isolates should be speciated and their antibiotic susceptibilities determined.

Reference has been made to the prime importance of proper specimen collection in the isolation of anaerobic microorganisms (see Chapter 13). The use of "gassed-out" tubes and other appropriate transport devices and proper anaerobic techniques is directly related to the successful isolation of these bacteria.

MISCELLANEOUS MEASURES

Unusual biochemical or other reactions should alert the microbiologist to problems in reagents or media or to the possibility of misidentification or a mixed culture. Thus, for example, an organism identified as a *Proteus* that was found to be sensitive to polymyxin should be rechecked, as should a group A streptococcus resistant to penicillin.

The role of **"blind unknowns,"** that is, simulated clinical specimens (urine, wound, fluids, and so forth) seeded with known bacteria, is well established as an internal quality control procedure. Two such specimens may be introduced each week into the regular laboratory routine. They should be identified in such a way that the worker is not aware of the unknown. More important, a fictitious report should not be routed to the ward or physician indicated on the laboratory request slip. When the report is completed, the microbiologist should discuss the results with the technologist performing the culture, with recommendations for improvement, if indicated. Quality control procedures in antimicrobial susceptibility testing have already been described (see Chapter 36).

Proficiency test specimens, such as those disseminated from state laboratories, the CDC, the College of American Pathologists, and so forth, are not as valuable as quality control devices as are the internal "blind unknowns," in that realistic laboratory conditions are not applicable. The worker is aware of the source, there is usually a prolonged time limit, and the specimen is given a laboratory workup exceeding that normally carried out. However, the proficiency test unknowns can serve an exceedingly useful purpose as an ongoing educational program for the staff, particularly when accompanied by the excellent critiques published regularly by the Proficiency Testing Branch, Licensure and Development Division, Centers for Disease Control. One should keep in mind that these specimens may represent a hazard to personnel.[4,8]

Other miscellaneous methods of quality control are self-evident: an ongoing educational program within the laboratory; weekly departmental conferences with the microbiologist regarding problems, changes, or personnel relations; encouragement and provision for staff members to attend medical conferences, workshops, and seminars; and so forth. It is also necessary to review constantly and correct the performances of night and weekend staff, particularly in plating procedures, relatively simple identification techniques, and especially performance and proper interpretation of a "stat" Gram stain.

In summary, good quality control rests essentially in the conscience of the individual worker, and it is the duty of the microbiologist, by leadership and knowledge, to encourage and nourish this desire for superiority and service at all times.

SAFETY IN THE CLINICAL MICROBIOLOGY LABORATORY

Hazards in the microbiology laboratory may involve chemical or radioactive materials and the laboratory facility itself, in addition to infectious agents. This section, however, will deal primarily with biologic hazards. Nevertheless, a comprehensive safety program must consider questions of storage, use, and disposal of hazardous chemicals and radioactive materials.

Although the primary concern is for people working with specimens and agents in the microbiology laboratory, it is important to realize that there is risk to individuals who do not regularly work in the laboratory but have occasion to come into the facility; there may also be risk to individuals in the area adjacent to the laboratory. For example, Blaser and Feldman[4] noted that 5 of 31 individuals who contracted typhoid fever from proficiency testing specimens did not work in a microbiology laboratory. Two patients were family members of a microbiologist who had worked with *Salmonella typhi*, two were students whose afternoon class was in a laboratory where the organism had been cultured that morning, and one worked in an adjacent chemistry laboratory.

The risk of infection varies not only with the agent itself (virulence, infectious dose, routes of infection, and toxigenicity) but also with the potential host and the type of activity. Risk factors in the host include age, sex, race, pregnancy, level of immunity (if any), and medication or disease that may affect host defense mechanisms. The type of activity influences the type and quantity of agents handled, the manipulations required, and the effectiveness of containment equipment and practices.

With regard to design of the laboratory, the more hazardous organisms encountered in clinical microbiology laboratories belong in class 2 of infectious agents (e.g., hepatitis viruses) and class 3 (e.g., *Mycobacterium tuberculosis*). Organisms of these classes require facilities known as P2 and P3, respectively. Details on laboratory design and operational procedures for laboratories of these grades are provided in "Guidelines for Research Involving Recombinant DNA Molecules"[6] and *Laboratory Safety Monograph*.[17]

Access to microbiology laboratories handling hazardous materials should be restricted to those with legitimate reason for being in or visiting the laboratory. Appropriate warning signs displaying the international biohazard symbol should be posted.

In certain situations prophylactic immunization of personnel may be warranted. Personnel in a laboratory anticipating recovery of *Clostridium botulinum* or working with its toxin should be immunized with botulism toxoid (available from CDC). Richardson and Huffaker[13] listed the various vaccines and toxoids available (not all are licensed) for preventive immunization of laboratory personnel. Clinical laboratory personnel working with measles, rubella, plague, and rabies (in addition to botulism) should be immunized unless it is determined that they are immune. One should remember that immunization should be regarded merely as an adjunct to appropriate microbiologic practices and safe facilities rather than as a substitute for these.

The primary causes of laboratory infection in accidents in which the cause was known were oral aspiration through a pipet, autoinoculation with a needle and syringe, aerosol exposures resulting from spray from needle and syringe, accidents with centrifuges, and animal bites.[13] It is important to realize, however, that only some 20% of laboratory-acquired infections result from known exposures or accidents. It would seem wise to ban mouth pipeting in microbiology laboratories. The use of needles and syringes should be minimized, and only syringes with locking hubs should be used. Personnel should be trained and equipped to handle experimental animals. Centrifuge safety involves proper balancing, acceleration and deceleration procedures, and (where indicated) use of safety cups with sealed covers. Alternatively, one may place a small centrifuge in an exhaust chamber or biologic safety cabinet.

With regard to decontamination, a steam autoclave is generally the most efficient means. However, personnel must be knowledgeable as to proper use and loading of the autoclave, and this equipment must be well maintained and properly monitored. Other decontamination procedures employing either dry heat or boiling may be appropriate and effective. Decontamination employing ultraviolet rays or chemicals is definitely less efficient but practical and appropriate for certain types of contamination. Ethylene oxide sterilizers are very effective, although slow.

It is important that all personnel recognize that every clinical specimen is potentially infectious. The most consistent infection hazard in the widest variety of clinical specimens is the hepatitis virus. A number of precautionary measures against viral hepatitis have been well outlined.[15] A special area should be set aside to receive, open, and record incoming specimens and to serve as a distribution point to other sections of the laboratory. This receiving laboratory should be well lighted and should have work surfaces that are impervious to water and easily cleaned. Personnel should assume that all specimen containers are contaminated on the outside. Definite procedures should be set up for decontamination in the event of obvious leakage or spillage.

Personnel should wash their hands after handling the specimen containers, and eating, drinking, and smoking should be banned in the laboratory. No food should be kept anywhere in the laboratory area.

An emergency plan should be available in all laboratories to cope with potential problems such as fires and spills of infectious materials. This plan should be written, and all personnel should have a copy of it. Personnel should be formally instructed in appropriate procedures, and drills should be conducted at intervals. There should be a system for reporting accidents or emergencies to the supervisor and safety personnel. The Occupational Safety and Health Administration General Industry Standard (Code of Federal Regulations, Title 29, Part 1910) provides regulations or guidelines applicable to fire safety. The appropriate number and type of fire extinguishers should be placed in the laboratories, and personnel should be familiar with their use.

REFERENCES

1. Bartlett, R.C.: Medical microbiology: quality, cost, and clinical relevance, New York, 1974, Wiley-Interscience, Division of John Wiley & Sons, Inc.
2. Bartlett, R.C.: Quality control in clinical microbiology. In Lennette, E.H., Balows, A., Hausler, W.J., Jr., and Truant, J.P., editors: Manual of clinical microbiology, ed. 3, Washington, D.C., 1980, American Society for Microbiology.
3. Bartlett, R.C., Tetreault, J., Evers, J., Officer, J., and Derench, J: Quality assurance of gram-stained direct smears, Am. J. Clin. Pathol. **72:**984-990, 1979.
4. Blaser, M.J., and Feldman, R.A.: Acquisition of typhoid fever from proficiency-testing specimens, N. Engl. J. Med. **303:**1481, 1980.
5. Blazevic, D.J., Hall, C.T., and Wilson, M.E.: Practical quality control procedures for the clinical microbiology laboratory, Cumitech 3, Washington, D.C., 1976, American Society for Microbiology.
6. Department of Health, Education, and Welfare, National Institutes of Health: Guidelines for research involving recombinant DNA molecules, Fed. Reg. **43**(247):60108-60131, 1978.
7. Hall, C.T., and Webb, C.D., Jr.: Proficiency testing: Bacteriology III and IV (July and October 1972), Atlanta, 1973, Center for Disease Control.
8. Holmes, M.B., Johnson, D.L., Fiumara, N.J., and McCormack, W.M.: Acquisition of typhoid fever from proficiency-testing specimens, N. Engl. J. Med. **303:**519-521, 1980.
9. Murray, P.R., and Washington, J.A., II: Microscopic and bacteriologic analysis of expectorated sputum, Mayo Clin. Proc. **50:**339-344, 1975.
10. Nagel, J.G., and Kunz, L.J.: Simplified storage and retrieval of stock cultures, Appl. Microbiol. **23:**837-839, 1972.
11. Prier, J.E., Bartola, J., and Friedman, H.: Quality control in microbiology, Baltimore, 1975, University Park Press.
12. Rhoden, D.L., Tomfohrde, K.M., Swenson, J.M., Smith, P.B., Balows, A., and Thornsberry, C.: Evaluation of the Bactrol disks, a set of quality control cultures, J. Clin. Microbiol. **1:**11-14, 1975.
13. Richardson, J.N., and Huffaker, R.H.: Biological safety in the clinical laboratory. In Lennette, E.H., Balows, A., Hausler, W.J., Jr., and Truant, J.P., editors: Manual of clinical microbiology, ed. 3, Washington, D.C., 1980, American Society for Microbiology.
14. Russell, R.L., Yoshimori, M.A., Rhodes, R.F., Reynolds, J.W., and Jennings, E.R.: A quality control program for clinical microbiology, Am. J. Clin. Pathol. **39:**489-494, 1969.
15. Safety in the clinical laboratory. V. Viral hepatitis, Lab. Med. **11:**589-590, 1980.
16. Scott, E.G.: Personal communication, 1976.
17. U.S. Public Health Service: NIH laboratory safety monograph, Bethesda, Md, 1978, Office of Research Safety, National Cancer Institute.
18. Van Scoy, R.E.: Bacterial sputum cultures: a clinician's viewpoint, Mayo Clin. Proc. **52:**39-41, 1977.
19. Vera, H.D.: Quality control in diagnostic microbiology, Health Lab. Sci. **8:**176-189, 1971.
20. Washington, J.A., II, editor: Laboratory procedures in clinical microbiology, New York, 1981, Springer-Verlag, Inc.
21. Woods, D., and Byers, J.F.: Quality control recording methods in microbiology, Am. J. Med. Technol. **30:**79-85, 1973.
22. Wright, D.N., Welch, D.F., and Matsen, J.M.: Use of preserved organisms for individual test-use quality control of bacterial typing antisera, J. Clin. Microbiol. **11:**305-307, 1980.

PART VIII CULTURE MEDIA, STAINS, REAGENTS, AND TESTS

42 FORMULAS AND PREPARATION OF CULTURE MEDIA

The principles governing the selection, preparation, sterilization, and storage of laboratory culture media have been discussed in Chapter 1; thus, the ensuing chapter will include the media to which reference is made throughout the text, their formulas, and any specific directions that may be needed. Complete directions for the preparation of media from the dehydrated products obtained commercially are provided by the manufacturers.* It should also be noted that there are manufacturers of prepared media in the United States and Canada from whom one can purchase a variety of plated and tubed media suitable for almost every need in the microbiology laboratory.†

Acetate agar

Acetate agar medium is prepared in the same manner as Simmons citrate agar (p. 621), except that 0.25% sodium acetate is used in place of

*Von Riesen (J. Clin. Microbiol. 2:554-555, 1975) has proposed a simple, convenient method of preparing media that are not in daily use.
†BBL Microbiology Systems, Cockeysville, Md.; Difco Laboratories, Detroit, Mich.; Gibco Diagnostics, Madison, Wisc.; Inolex Division, Glenwood, Ill.; and others.

citrate. It is used to determine whether an organism is able to utilize acetate as its sole carbon source. Growth on the slant and development of a **blue** color indicate a positive test. A negative test is no growth or color change.

This test is useful in differentiating *Escherichia coli* from shigellae in that the latter do not utilize acetate.

Alkaline peptone water

See Chapter 9.

Ascospore agar

Potassium acetate	10 g
Yeast extract	2.5 g
Dextrose	1 g
Agar	30 g
Distilled water	1,000 ml

Dissolve, tube, and autoclave at 121 C for 15 minutes. Ascospores are obtained in 2 to 6 days at room temperature (23 to 25 C).

Bacteroides bile esculin agar (BBE agar)

Trypticase soy agar	40 g
Oxgall	20 g
Esculin	1 g

Ferric ammonium citrate	0.5 g
Hemin solution (5 mg/ml)	2 ml
Gentamicin solution (40 mg/ml)*	2.5 ml
Distilled water	1,000 ml

Adjust pH to 7.0, heat to dissolve, dispense in 100-ml bottles, autoclave at 121 C for 15 minutes, and cool to 50 C. Pour plates.

Beef extract agar†

Add 2.5% agar to beef extract broth, dissolve by boiling, adjust to pH 7.6, tube and autoclave at 121 C for 15 minutes, and slant before solidifying.

The medium is used for pure culture preparation of *Candida* species prior to carrying out fermentation tests.

Beef extract broth†

Beef extract	3 g
Peptone	10 g
Sodium chloride	5 g
Distilled water	1,000 ml

*Garamycin injectable (Schering Corp., Kenilworth, N.J.) may be used.
†BBL Microbiology Systems, Cockeysville, Md.; Difco Laboratories, Detroit, Mich.

Dissolve ingredients by boiling, adjust to pH 7.2, tube in 10-ml amounts in 18- by 150-mm tubes, and autoclave at 121 C for 15 minutes. For use as a fermentation base broth, add 100 ml of a 0.04% aqueous solution of bromthymol blue before tubing and sterilizing.

The medium is used for differentiation of *Candida* species by carbohydrate fermentation tests.

Bile esculin agar*

Beef extract	3 g
Peptone	5 g
Oxgall	40 g
Esculin	1 g
Ferric citrate	0.5 g
Agar	15 g
Distilled water	1,000 ml

1. Suspend 64 g of the dehydrated medium in water, heat to boiling to dissolve, and tube in screw-capped tubes.
2. Sterilize by autoclaving at 121 C for 15 minutes.
3. Cool to 55 C, add aseptically 50 ml of filter-sterilized horse serum (optional), and mix well.
4. Dispense in sterile tubes, and cool in a slanted position.

This medium is useful in the selective detection of group D streptococci. After inoculation, these organisms form brownish-black colonies surrounded by a black zone. *Listeria monocytogenes* also reacts positively, as do some other organisms. Other forms of agar and broth media also are available.*

Birdseed agar

Guizottia abyssinica seeds (niger or thistle seeds)	70 g
Creatinine	0.78 g
Dextrose	10 g
Chloramphenicol (one 50-mg capsule)	0.05 g
Agar	20 g
Distilled water	1,000 ml

---

*Pfizer Diagnostics, Flushing, N.Y.; Difco Laboratories, Detroit, Mich.; BBL Microbiology Systems, Cockeysville, Md.; Gibco Diagnostics, Madison, Wisc.

Diphenyl	100 mg
95% Ethyl alcohol	10 ml

1. Grind seed to powder in blender. Add 300 ml of water, and autoclave at 115 C for 10 minutes.
2. Filter through gauze, and bring volume to 1 liter.
3. Add other ingredients except diphenyl, and autoclave at 121 C for 15 minutes.
4. Cool to 50 C.
5. Add diphenyl to 10 ml of 95% ethyl alcohol, and add aseptically to medium.
6. Stir and pour into plates.

Bismuth sulfite agar*

Beef extract	5 g
Peptone	10 g
Dextrose	5 g
Disodium phosphate	4 g
Ferrous sulfate	0.3 g
Bismuth sulfite indicator	8 g
Agar	20 g
Brilliant green	0.025 g
Distilled water	1,000 ml

Bismuth sulfite agar medium is highly recommended for the isolation of *Salmonella typhi*, as well as other salmonellae. It may be used for both streak and pour plates. **Read's modification** of the medium (through the addition of 1% sodium chloride and 1% mannose, the elimination of the brilliant green, and adjustment of the final pH to 9.2) is recommended for the isolation of *Vibrio cholerae*.

Blood agar plates for streaking

Blood agar base medium	500 ml
Sterile blood	20 ml

Sterilize the base medium (trypticase soy agar [BBL] or tryptic soy agar [Difco] are recommended†), cool to 48 or 50 C, and add 5% sterile

---

*BBL Microbiology Systems, Cockeysville, Md; Difco Laboratories, Detroit, Mich.; Gibco Diagnostics, Madison, Wisc.

†Brucella agar is an excellent base for blood agar for anaerobic bacteria (see p. 618). Columbia agar and Schaedler agar have also been recommended for this purpose.

defibrinated sheep, horse, or rabbit blood, aseptically. Rotate to mix thoroughly, and pour into sterile Petri dishes in approximately 20-ml amounts. When agar is set, invert and incubate one or two plates per 100- to 200-ml batch overnight to test for sterility. Discard test plates. Blood agar plates may be refrigerated for 1 week without deterioration, but they should be packaged to minimize water loss, which could amount to 7% per week if unprotected.

The pouring should be done carefully to avoid air bubbles. If bubbles appear in the poured plate, pass a Bunsen flame over the agar before it sets. This causes them to break.

An alternative to pouring media from an Erlenmeyer flask is the use of a Kelly bottle with a release clamp on a piece of rubber tubing connected to a bell device at the other end. This assembly is mounted on a ring stand. Release of pressure on the clamp permits the heated media to flow evenly into the plate. An advantage of this system is that bubbles (when present) rise to the top of the liquid medium in the bottle prior to its being poured into the plate.

Blood agar pour plates
(Brown: Monograph No. 9, The Rockefeller Institute for Medical Research, 1919)

Heat 20-ml tubes of infusion agar in boiling water until the agar is thoroughly melted. Cool the agar to 48 C by standing the tubes in a container of warm water or a 48 C water bath. With a sterile pipet add about 1 ml of sterile blood to each tube. Inoculate the fluid blood agar with a proper dilution of culture or original material. Twirl the tube to mix the blood, inoculum, and agar, taking care not to form bubbles, and pour into a sterile Petri dish.

Blood cystine dextrose agar*
(Francis: J.A.M.A. 91:1155, 1928; Rhamy: Am. J. Clin. Pathol. 3:121, 1933)

Beef heart infusion	500 g

*Available as a dehydrated base from Difco Laboratories, Detroit, Mich.; BBL Microbiology Systems, Cockeysville, Md.; Gibco Diagnostics, Madison, Wisc.

Proteose peptone	10 g
Glucose	10 g
Sodium chloride	5 g
Cystine	1 g
Agar	15 g
Distilled water	1,000 ml

Blood cystine dextrose agar medium may be used satisfactorily for the cultivation of *Francisella tularensis*.

To prepare this medium dissolve 16.8 g of dehydrated product in 300 ml of distilled water. Adjust the reaction to pH 7.3 and autoclave for 20 minutes at 15 pounds pressure. Cool to a temperature of 60 to 70 C, add 18 ml of whole rabbit blood or dehydrated hemoglobin, mix well, and distribute into test tubes aseptically. Cool in a slanting position.

Bordet-Gengou medium*

Potatoes, infusion from	125 g
Sodium chloride	5.5 g
Agar	20 g
Distilled water	1,000 ml

Sterilize at 15 pounds for 15 minutes. Cool to 50 C and add 15% to 20% sterile sheep, rabbit, or human blood aseptically.

The medium is recommended for cultivation of *Bordetella pertussis*.

Brain-heart infusion blood agar (BHIBA)

Brain-heart infusion agar†	26 g
Agar, powdered	2.5 g
Distilled water	500 ml
(Final pH approximately 7.4)	

Suspend the ingredients in the water, and dissolve by boiling. Autoclave for 15 minutes at 121 C. Cool to about 45 C, and add aseptically 30 ml of defibrinated animal blood. Mix well, and distribute aseptically in approximately 20-ml amounts in cotton-plugged and sterilized 25-

*Available as a dehydrated base from Difco Laboratories, Detroit, Mich.; BBL Microbiology Systems, Cockeysville, Md.; Gibco Diagnostics, Madison, Wisc.
†BBL Microbiology Systems, Cockeysville, Md.; Difco Laboratories, Detroit, Mich.; Gibco Diagnostics, Madison, Wisc.; Inolex Division, Glenwood, Ill.

by 150-mm Pyrex test tubes (without lips). Slant, allow to harden, and refrigerate.

This medium is used for the isolation of fastidious fungi.

Brain-heart infusion broth*

Calf brain infusion	200 g
Beef heart infusion	250 g
Proteose peptone	10 g
Dextrose	2 g
Sodium chloride	5 g
Disodium phosphate	2.5 g
Distilled water	1,000 ml

(Reaction of medium pH 7.4)

Brain-heart infusion broth is recommended for cultivating the pneumococcus for the bile solubility test.

Brilliant green agar*

Yeast extract	3 g
Proteose peptone No. 3	10 g
Sodium chloride	5 g
Lactose	10 g
Sucrose	10 g
Phenol red	0.08 g
Brilliant green	0.0125 g
Agar	20 g
Distilled water	1,000 ml

(Final pH 6.9)

Brilliant green agar is a highly selective medium recommended for the isolation of salmonellae other than *Salmonella typhi*. It is not recommended for the isolation of shigellae.

Brucella agar*

Pancreatic digest of casein USP	10 g
Peptic digest of animal tissues USP	10 g
Yeast autolysate	2 g
Dextrose	1 g
Sodium chloride	5 g
Sodium bisulfite	0.1 g
Agar	15 g
Distilled water	1,000 ml

(Final pH 7.0 ± 0.02)

Heat with agitation until dissolved. Dispense and autoclave at 121 C for 15 minutes. Cool to 50 C.

Brucella selective medium (for Brucella)

Heart infusion agar	40 g
Gelatin	1 g
Glucose	2.5 g
Distilled water	1,000 ml

Mix ingredients, autoclave for 15 minutes at 121 C, allow to cool to 50 C, and add 10 ml of sterile sheep blood and the following antibiotics:

1. Cycloheximide—1 ml of a 100-mg/ml stock solution, final concentration = 100µg/ml of agar.
2. Bacitracin*—1 ml of a 25,000-unit/ml stock solution; final concentration = 25 units/ml of agar.
3. Circulin*—1 ml of a 25,000-unit/ml stock solution; final concentration = 25 units/ml of agar.
4. Polymyxin B†—0.6 ml of a 10,000-unit/ml stock solution; final concentration = 6 units/ml of agar.

Brucella–vitamin K_1 blood agar (BRBA)

1. Vitamin K_1 solution (see Chapter 44)
2. Preparation of base:

Brucella agar‡	43 g
Agar	2.5 g
Distilled water	1,000 ml

Sterilize by autoclaving at 121 C for 15 minutes, and cool to 50 C.

3. Add aseptically:

Defibrinated or laked sheep blood	50 ml
Vitamin K_1 solution	1 ml

Mix well and pour plates, using approximately 20 ml per plate. Store at room temperature. The medium is used for the isolation and subculture of anaerobes.

---

*Available in dehydrated form from Difco Laboratories, Detroit, Mich.; BBL Microbiology Systems, Cockeysville, Md.; Gibco Diagnostics, Madison, Wisc.

*The Upjohn Co., Kalamazoo, Mich.
†Burroughs Wellcome Co., Research Triangle Park, N.C.
‡BBL, Gibco, or Difco. The Pfizer product is not recommended for this purpose, as it contains citrate.

Campylobacter media*

The basic plate medium (Campy-BAP) consists of brucella agar base and 5% sheep erythrocytes with the following amounts of antimicrobials per liter: vancomycin, 10 mg; trimethoprim, 5 mg; polymyxin B, 2,500 IU; amphotericin B, 2 mg; and cephalothin, 15 mg. The liquid medium (Campy-thio) is thioglycolate broth with 0.16% agar and the antimicrobials listed above.

Carbohydrate broth

1. Heart infusion broth, 22.5 g, in 900 ml of distilled water.
2. Carbohydrate, 10 g, in 100 ml of distilled water.
3. Indicator, 1 ml (1.6 g of bromcresol purple in 100 ml of 95% ethanol).

Add 1, 2, and 3 together; dispense in 3-ml amounts in 13- by 100-mm screw-capped tubes. Autoclave for 10 minutes at 121 C.

A positive reaction is recorded when the indicator changes from purple to yellow.

Carbohydrate media for fermentation tests

When some carbohydrates are sterilized by heating in alkaline broth, they are more or less broken down into simple carbohydrates. It has been found definitely advantageous to sterilize sugar solutions by filtration through Seitz or membrane filters and to add these aseptically to the broth base in the required amounts. Although several carbohydrates can withstand autoclave temperature and pressure, one is advised to sterilize the following by **filtration**: xylose, lactose, sucrose, arabinose, trehalose, rhamnose, and salicin. These may be prepared as 5% or 10% solutions, depending on solubility, then sterilized by filtration and added aseptical-

ly to the base containing an indicator, to give 0.5% to 1% final concentration.

Other less heat-susceptible carbohydrates may be added to the broth base containing indicator (e.g., bromcresol purple) before autoclaving at 116 to 118 C (10 to 12 pounds pressure) for 15 minutes. Ten Broeck, in 1920, found that unheated serum contains an enzyme that hydrolyzes maltose to glucose. Serum to be added to maltose broth should therefore be heated for 1 hour at 60 C to inactivate the enzyme. Incubate the carbohydrate broth to test sterility.

Casein medium for separation of Nocardia and Streptomyces
(Centers for Disease Control)

Prepare separately:

Skimmed milk (dehydrated or instant nonfat milk)	10 g
Distilled water	100 ml

Autoclave at 121 C for 20 minutes.

Distilled water	100 ml
Agar	2 g

Autoclave as above.

Cool both solutions to approximately 45 C, mix, and pour into sterile Petri dishes.

Test for hydrolysis

Streak or make point inoculations of each culture on casein plates, using half of a plate for each organism. Incubate at 25 C (or 35 C if it does not grow at room temperature). Observe for clearing of casein in 7 and 14 days. *Nocardia asteroides* does not hydrolyze casein. *N. brasiliensis* and *Streptomyces* species hydrolyze casein.

Cetrimide agar*
(Lowbury and Collins: J. Clin. Pathol. 8:47, 1955)

Peptone	20 g
Magnesium chloride	1.4 g
Potassium sulfate	10 g

---

*These media are available commercially from BBL Microbiology Systems, Cockeysville, Md.; Regional Media Laboratories, Lenexa, Kan.; and Gibco Diagnostics, Madison, Wisc.

*Pseudosel agar (BBL Microbiology Systems, Cockeysville, Md.)

Agar, dried	13.6 g
Cetrimide*	0.3 g
Distilled water	1,000 ml
Glycerol	10 ml

(Final pH 7.2±)

Suspend the powder in the water, add 10 ml of glycerol, heat with frequent agitation, and boil for 1 minute.

Dispense in 5-ml amounts in 15- by 125-mm screw-capped tubes, autoclave at 118 to 121 C for 15 minutes, and slant to give a generous slant.

This medium is used for the selective isolation or identification of *Pseudomonas aeruginosa*, whose growth is not inhibited by the cetrimide. Other members of the genus (except *P. fluorescens*) and related nonfermentative organisms are inhibited.

Chlamydospore agar

Chlamydospore agar†	18.5 g
Distilled water	500 ml

Suspend the dehyrated product in a 1-liter Erlenmeyer flask, dissolve by heating, and tube in approximately 15-ml amounts in screw-capped, 20- by 150-mm test tubes. Autoclave at 121 C for 15 minutes with caps loosened. When cool, tighten caps and store at room temperature. When needed, melt a tube in a water bath, pour into a sterile Petri plate, and allow to solidify.

Chocolate agar

Chocolate agar is agar to which blood or hemoglobin has been added and then heated until the medium becomes brown or chocolate colored. The recommended method of preparing this is as follows.

Suspend sufficient proteose No. 3 agar,* Eugonagar,† or GC agar base‡ in distilled water to make a double-strength base. Mix thoroughly, and heat to boiling for 1 minute with frequent agitation. Autoclave at 121 C for 15 minutes. At the same time, autoclave an equal volume of 2% hemoglobin,‡ which is made by the gradual addition of distilled water to the dehydrated hemoglobin, to obtain a **smooth suspension.** Cool both solutions to approximately 50 C, add the supplement (Iso-VitaleX enrichment† or Supplement B or C* is recommended), combine with bacteriologic precautions, and then pour into sterile, disposable Petri plates. Best results are obtained when plates are **freshly prepared.** One or two plates per 100- to 200-ml batch should be incubated at 35 C overnight to determine sterility and later discarded.

Thayer-Martin agar (see p. 643) for the selective isolation of *Neisseria gonorrhoeae* and *N. meningitidis* may be prepared from the aforementioned chocolate agar by adding an antimicrobial agent inhibitor (V-C-N, BBL, or Difco). The use of Thayer-Martin medium results in a higher recovery of neisseriae from clinical specimens likely to be contaminated with other bacteria.

Chocolate agar slants may be prepared individually by the method just described, slanting the medium after it has been tubed in 5- to 10-ml amounts in sterile screw-capped tubes. To prepare a large number of slants, use a flask containing 50 to 100 ml of agar, proceeding as before.

Chopped meat glucose (CMG)

Ground beef, fat-free	500 g
Distilled water	1,000 ml
Sodium hydroxide, 1 N	25 ml

---

*Cetyl trimethyl ammonium bromide.
†Available in dehydrated form from Difco Laboratories, Detroit, Mich.; BBL Microbiology Systems, Cockeysville, Md.; Gibco Diagnostics, Madison, Wisc.

---

*Difco Laboratories, Detroit, Mich.
†BBL Microbiology Systems, Cockeysville, Md.
‡BBL Microbiology Systems, Cockeysville, Md.; Difco Laboratories, Detroit, Mich.; Gibco Diagnostics, Madison, Wisc.

1. Mix ingredients, bring to boil, and simmer with frequent stirring for 20 minutes.
2. Cool to room temperature, skim off fat, and filter through three layers of gauze. Squeeze out gauze, retaining both meat particles and filtrate (filtered through coarse and fine paper).
3. Restore filtrate to 1 liter with distilled water, and add:

Trypticase	30 g
Yeast extract	5 g
Dipotassium phosphate	5 g
Resazurin solution (25 mg/100 ml water)	4 ml

4. Boil, cool, adjust to pH 7.8, and add 0.5% glucose and 0.5 g of cystine.
5. Dispense 6- to 7-ml amounts into tubes containing meat particles (step 2), 1 part meat to 4 or 5 parts broth, and autoclave at 121 C for 20 minutes.

This medium is recommended as a "backup" medium for the primary isolation of anaerobes and also for growing pure cultures for gas-liquid chromatographic analysis.* It may also be obtained as a dehydrated medium, cooked meat phytone.†

Chopped-meat medium*‡

To 1 pound of finely ground beef heart and other muscle (fat free) add 500 ml of boiling sodium hydroxide (N/15 to N/20) and boil for 20 minutes. Cool, strain off the fat, and filter through muslin. Adjust the fluid to pH 7.5, and add 1% peptone. Add approximately 2 inches of meat and a small ball of steel wool to each tube, and add enough broth to overlay the meat by about 1 inch. Heat tubes for 30 minutes in boiling water, and sterilize by autoclaving at 121 C for 15 minutes. The medium should be boiled for a few minutes to drive off dissolved oxygen if it is not to be used the same day, unless the prereduced tubed media are used. Incubation in an anaerobic jar or under a petrolatum seal may be required for cultivation or maintenance of certain *Clostridium* species, except in the case of prereduced tubed media.

Citrate agar*

*(Simmons: J. Infect. Dis. **39**:209, 1926)*

Agar	20 g
Sodium chloride	5 g
Magnesium sulfate	0.2 g
Ammonium dihydrogen phosphate	1 g
Dipotassium phosphate	1 g
Sodium citrate	2 g
Bromthymol blue	0.08 g
Distilled water	1,000 ml
(Final pH 6.9±)	

Citrate agar is used to determine the utilization of citrate as the sole carbon source. Development of a blue color indicates a positive test.

Columbia agar base†

Polypeptone or Pantone	10 g
Biosate or Bitone	10 g
Myosate or tryptic digest of beef heart	3 g
Cornstarch	1 g
Sodium chloride	5 g
Agar	13.5 g
Distilled or demineralized water	1,000 ml
(Final pH 7.3 ± 0.2)	

Heat with agitation until the medium boils. Dispense and autoclave at 121 C for 15 minutes.

Columbia CNA agar†

Polypeptone peptone	10 g
Biosate peptone	10 g
Myosate peptone	3 g
Cornstarch	1 g

---

*Available in prereduced tubes from Scott Laboratories, Fiskeville, R.I.
†BBL Microbiology Systems, Cockeysville, Md.; Gibco Diagnostics, Madison, Wisc.
‡Available in dehydrated form from BBL Microbiology Systems, Cockeysville, Md.

*BBL Microbiology Systems, Cockeysville, Md.; Difco Laboratories, Detroit, Mich.; Gibco Diagnostics, Madison, Wisc.
†Available in dehydrated form from BBL Microbiology Systems, Cockeysville, Md., and others.

Sodium chloride	5 g
Agar, dried	13.5 g
Colistin	10 mg
Nalidixic acid	15 mg
Distilled water	1,000 ml

(Final pH 7.3±)

1. Suspend 42.5 g of dehydrated medium in water, heat with frequent agitation, and boil for 1 minute.
2. Sterilize by autoclaving at 121 C for 15 minutes.
3. Cool to 50 C, add 5% defibrinated sheep blood, and pour plates.

This medium is excellent for the selective growth of gram-positive cocci, particularly streptococci, when gram-negative bacilli, especially *Proteus* species, tend to overgrow on conventional blood agar plates. This medium may be inhibitory for certain strains of staphylococci.

Cornmeal agar*

Yellow cornmeal	125 g
Distilled water	3,000 ml

Heat the cornmeal in water at 60 C for 1 hour, filter through paper, make up to volume, and add 50 g of agar. Expose to flowing steam for 1 hour, filter through absorbent cotten, dispense in tubes, and autoclave at 121 C for 30 minutes. Cornmeal agar suppresses vegetative growth of many fungi while stimulating sporulation. With the addition of 1% Tween 80, it is useful in stimulating production of chlamydospores of *Candida albicans*.†

Cycloserine-cefoxitin fructose agar (CCFA)

Prepare 1 liter of egg yolk agar base, substituting 6 g of fructose for the glucose and adding 3 ml of 1% neutral red in ethanol. This base is dispensed in 100-ml quantities and sterilized at 121 C for 15 minutes. After cooling to 50 C,

cycloserine base is added to a final concentration of 500 mg/ml, and cefoxitin base is added at a final concentration of 16 mg/ml. The egg yolk suspension is added as indicated for egg yolk agar. Alternatively, one may leave out the egg yolk suspension (the medium is effective without the egg yolk, but the lecithinase and lipase reactions cannot be determined directly, of course). This is a highly selective and differential medium for *Clostridium difficile*.

Cystine tellurite blood agar
*(Frobisher: J. Infect. Dis. **60**:99, 1937)*

1. Melt 100 ml of sterile 2% infusion agar in a flask, and cool to 45 to 50 C. Care should be taken to maintain this temperature throughout the following steps in the preparation of the medium.
2. Add aseptically 15 ml of sterile 0.3% solution of potassium tellurite in distilled water. The tellurite solution may be sterilized by autoclaving.
3. Add aseptically 5 ml of sterile blood, and mix well.
4. Add 3 to 5 mg of cystine. The dry powder is used and need not be sterilized. Since different lots of cystine vary, the optimal amount necessary to produce the best growth of *Corynebacterium diphtheriae* may vary from 3 to 5 mg/100 ml.
5. Thoroughly mix the medium, and pour into sterile Petri dishes. Since the cystine does not go entirely into solution, shake the flask frequently while pouring the plates.

This medium is used for the isolation of *Corynebacterium diphtheriae*.

Cystine trypticase agar (CTA)*
*(Vera: J. Bacteriol. **55**:531, 1948)*

Cystine	0.5 g
Trypticase	20 g
Agar	3.5 g
Sodium chloride	5 g

---

*Available in dehydrated form from BBL Microbiology Systems, Cockeysville, Md., and others.
†Some workers find that "homemade" media give more consistent results.

*Available in dehydrated form from BBL Microbiology Systems, Cockeysville, Md.

Sodium sulfite	0.5 g
Phenol red	0.017 g
Distilled water	1,000 ml

(Final pH, 7.3±)

CTA is an excellent all-purpose medium for the growth of pathogenic organisms. It can be used for the maintenance of cultures (including fastidious organisms, held at 25 C), the determination of motility, and (with the addition of carbohydrates) the determination of fermentation reactions of fastidious organisms, including *Neisseria*. Sterilize at 115 to 118 C (no more than 12 pounds pressure) for 15 minutes.

Decarboxylase test media

(Moeller: Acta Pathol. Microbiol. Scand. 36:161, 1955)

BASAL MEDIUM*

Peptone (Orthana special†)	5 g
Beef extract	5 mg
Bromcresol purple (1.6%)	0.625 ml
Cresol red (0.2%)	2.5 ml
Glucose	0.5 g
Pyridoxal	5 mg
Distilled water	1,000 ml

(Adjust to pH 6)

Divide the basal medium into four 250-ml amounts; one portion is tubed without addition of any of the amino acids (control). To another portion add 1% L-lysine dihydrochloride,‡ to a third add 1% L-arginine monohydrochloride, and to the fourth add 1% L-ornithine dihydrochloride. Adjust the ornithine portion to pH 6 with N/1 NaOH before sterilization. Tube the media in 3- to 4-ml amounts in small (13- by 100-mm) screw-capped tubes. Autoclave at 121 C for 10 minutes.

Inoculate all four tubes from an agar slant culture, and overlay each tube with 4 to 5 mm of sterile mineral oil.* If oil is not added, the reactions are not valid after 24 hours. Some workers recommend the addition of 0.3% agar to the basal medium in place of an oil overlay.

Incubate all four tubes at 35 C, and read daily for not more than 4 days (most positive reactions with the enteric bacilli occur in 1 to 2 days). A **positive** reaction is indicated by alkalinization of the medium with a change in color from yellow (caused by the initial fermentation of glucose) to **violet** (caused by the decarboxylation of the amino acid). Therefore, a **yellow** color after several days' incubation indicates a **negative** test, or the absence of the enzymes decarboxylase or dihydrolase. All positive tests should be compared with the control tube, which remains yellow.

These media are used primarily for differentiating members of the Enterobacteriaceae.

DNase test medium†

DNA	2 g
Phytone	5 g
Sodium chloride	5 g
Trypticase	15 g
Agar	15 g
Distilled water	1,000 ml

(Approximate final pH 7.3)

This medium may be sterilized in the autoclave at 15 pounds pressure for 15 minutes at 121 C, cooled, and poured into Petri dishes. The dry surface may be streaked in several places (½-inch streaks) with strains of staphylococci to be tested for DNase activity. Flooding of the plate after 24 hours of growth with N/1 hydrochloric acid reveals **clear zones** around the growth of the DNase-positive strains. Some workers prefer flooding the plate with 0.1% toluidine blue; a bright **rose pink** color is produced around the growth of DNase-positive organisms.

---

*BBL Microbiology Systems, Cockeysville, Md.; Difco Laboratories, Detroit, Mich.; Gibco Diagnostics, Madison, Wisc.

†Proteose peptone No. 3, 0.3%, has been found to be a suitable alternative.

‡Amino acids are available from Nutritional Biochemicals Corp., Cleveland, Ohio.

---

*Sterilize in test tubes at 121 C for 45 minutes.

†BBL Microbiology Systems, Cockeysville, Md.; Difco Laboratories, Detroit, Mich.; Gibco Diagnostics, Madison, Wisc.

Desoxycholate agar*

(Leifson: J. Pathol. Bacteriol. 40:581, 1935)

Peptone	10 g
Lactose	10 g
Sodium citrate	1 g
Ferric citrate	1 g
Sodium chloride	5 g
Dipotassium phosphate	2 g
Sodium desoxycholate	1 g
Agar	16 g
Neutral red	0.033 g
Distilled water	1,000 ml

(Final pH 7.2±)

Desoxycholate agar is used for the isolation of gram-negative enteric bacilli and the differentiation of lactose-fermenting and non-lactose-fermenting species.

Desoxycholate citrate agar*

(Leifson: J. Pathol. Bacteriol. 40:581, 1935)

Meat, infusion from	350 g
Peptone	10 g
Lactose	10 g
Sodium citrate	20 g
Ferric citrate	1 g
Sodium desoxycholate	5 g
Agar	17 g
Neutral red	0.02 g
Distilled water	1,000 ml

(Final pH 7.3±)

Desoxycholate citrate agar is used for the isolation of salmonellae and shigellae from stool and other specimens.

Dextrose ascitic fluid semisolid agar for spinal fluid cultures

Phenol red broth base	4 g
Agar, powdered (weigh accurately)	0.5 g
Distilled water	250 ml

Suspend the ingredients in a 1-liter Erlenmeyer flask, plug with cotton, and autoclave at 121 C for 15 minutes. At the same time sterilize a rack of 18- by 125-mm screw-capped test tubes and a wrapped Cornwall automatic pipet.* Cool the medium, and add the following aseptically:

Ascitic fluid†	50 ml
Dextrose, sterile 20% solution	15 ml

Using the sterile pipet, tube in 5-ml amounts in screw-capped tubes, incubate overnight for sterility, and store at room temperature. This medium is poured over remaining spinal fluid sediment after smears and plate cultures have been made.

Drug-containing media for susceptibility testing of mycobacteria

See Chapter 31.

Egg yolk agar

Add 10 ml of sterile yolk emulsion‡ to 90 ml of melted and cooled blood agar base, and pour the plates.

Proteose peptone No. 2	40 g
Sodium orthophosphate (Na_2HPO_4)	5 g
Potassium dihydrophosphate (KH_2PO_4)	1 g
Sodium chloride	2 g
Magnesium sulfate	0.1 g
Glucose	2 g
Hemin solution (see Chapter 44) (5mg/ml)	1 ml
Agar	25 g
Distilled water	1,000 ml

(Adjust to pH 7.6)

Autoclave at 121 C for 15 minutes. This medium is used for the isolation and identification of members of the genus *Clostridium* and certain other anaerobes.

Eosin–methylene blue agar (EMB)§

Peptone	10 g
Lactose	5 g
Sucrose	5 g

---

*Beckton-Dickinson's Cornwall Pipetting Unit with 5-ml syringe.

†Bacto-Ascitic Fluid, 10-ml ampules, Difco Laboratories, Detroit, Mich.

‡Colab Laboratories, Inc., Glenwood, Ill.

§Available in dehydrated form from BBL Microbiology Systems, Cockeysville, Md.; Difco Laboratories, Detroit, Mich.; Gibco Diagnostics, Madison, Wisc.; Inolex Division, Glenwood, Ill.

---

*BBL Microbiology Systems, Cockeysville, Md.; Difco Laboratories, Detroit, Mich.; Gibco Diagnostics, Madison, Wisc.

Dipotassium phosphate	2 g
Agar	13.5 g
Eosin Y	0.4 g
Methylene blue	0.065 g
Distilled water	1,000 ml

The agar concentration may be increased to 5% (use an additional 3.65 g of agar) to inhibit the spreading of *Proteus*. The Levine EMB agar, preferred by some workers, does not contain sucrose.

Lactose-fermenting, gram-negative bacteria may be distinguished from non-lactose-fermenting types by their appearance. Colonies of *Escherichia coli* usually have a characteristic metallic sheen. If the sucrose-containing medium is used, *Proteus* colonies also show this characteristic, provided they are inhibited from spreading by the higher agar concentration.

Esculin agar, modified

Esculin	1 g
Ferric citrate	0.5 g
Heart infusion agar (blood agar base)	40 g
Distilled water	1,000 ml

Heat to dissolve. Cool to 55 C, and adjust pH to 7.0. Dispense in 5-ml amounts in 16- by 125-mm cotton-plugged tubes. Autoclave at 121 C for 15 minutes. Cool in a slanted position.

Esculin hydrolysis is indicated when the medium turns black.

Fermentation broth for Listeria

Proteose peptone No. 3*	10 g
Beef extract	1 g
Sodium chloride	5 g
Bromcresol purple	0.1 g
Distilled water	1,000 ml

Dissolve with the aid of heat, and sterilize at 121 C for 20 minutes. Add aseptically 0.5% of the following carbohydrates: glucose, salicin, rhamnose, dulcitol, and raffinose.

These carbohydrate broths are helpful in the biochemical studies of *Listeria*.

Fermentation media for neisseriae

1. Suspend 4.3 g of dehydrated CTA medium (see pp. 622-623) in 150 ml of distilled water, and heat to boiling with frequent agitation.
2. Adjust to pH 7.4 to 7.6 with 1 N NaOH, dispense in 50-ml amounts in 250-ml Erlenmeyer flasks, and sterilize at no more than 118 C (12 pounds) for 15 minutes.
3. Prepare 20% solutions of glucose, lactose, maltose, and sucrose in distilled water; tube and sterilize by membrane filtration.
4. Add 2.5 ml of each carbohydrate to separate flasks of the 50-ml cooled CTA medium.
5. Mix and dispense in 2.0-ml amounts in sterile screw-capped tubes (13 by 100 mm) and refrigerate at 4 C.

Fermentation medium for differentiating Staphylococcus and Micrococcus
(Facklam and Smith: Human Pathol. 7:187 1976)

Difco tryptone	1 %
Difco yeast extract	0.1 %
Bromcresol purple	0.004 %
Glucose or mannitol	1 %
Agar	0.22 %
(pH 7.0)	

Tube in 16- by 120-mm tubes to a depth of 7 to 8 cm. Before use, steam for 10 minutes, cool rapidly, and inoculate heavily by stabbing to the bottom. Incubate under anaerobic conditions.

Fildes enrichment* agar†

Sodium chloride (0.85% solution)	150 ml
Hydrochloric acid	6 ml
Defibrinated sheep blood	50 ml
Pepsin, granular	1 g

1. Mix well, and heat in 56 C water bath for 4 hours, with occasional agitation.
2. Adjust to pH 7 with 20% NaOH (approximately 12 ml).
3. Readjust to pH 7.0 to 7.2 with HCl.
4. Add 0.25 ml of chloroform, mix thoroughly, stopper tightly, and refrigerate at 4 C.

---

*Difco Laboratories, Detroit, Mich.

*Fildes enrichment, itself, is also available commercially.
†Difco Laboratories, Detroit, Mich.

5. After heating 4 to 10 ml of this enrichment mixture in a sterile container in a 56 C water bath for 30 minutes to eliminate the chloroform, add to 200 ml of melted nutrient agar cooled to 56 C, and pour into Petri dishes.

This is an excellent medium for the isolation of *Haemophilus influenzae*.

Fletcher's semisolid medium for Leptospira*

1. Sterilize 1.76 liters of distilled water by autoclaving at 121 C for 30 minutes.
2. Cool to room temperature, and add 240 ml of sterile normal rabbit serum.
3. Inactivate by incubation at 56 C for 40 minutes.
4. Add 120 ml of melted and cooled (no greater than 56 C) 2.5% meat extract agar at pH 7.4.
5. Dispense 5-ml amounts in sterile, 16- by 130-mm, screw-capped test tubes and 15-ml amounts in sterile, 25-ml, diaphragm-type, rubber-stoppered vaccine bottles.
6. Inactivate at 56 C for 60 minutes on 2 successive days.

Gelatin medium*

To extract or infusion broth add 12% gelatin. Heat in an Arnold sterilizer or a double boiler until the gelatin is thoroughly dissolved. Adjust reaction to pH 7. Tube and autoclave at 121 C (15 pounds pressure) for 15 minutes. Sodium thioglycollate, 0.05%, may be added for cultivation of certain species of clostridia in an external aerobic environment.

Gelatin medium (dilute) for differentiation of Nocardia and Streptomyces
(Centers for Disease Control)

Gelatin	4 g
Distilled water	1,000 ml
(Adjust to pH 7)	

---

*Difco Laboratories, Detroit, Mich.; BBL Microbiology Systems, Cockeysville, Md.; Gibco Diagnostics, Madison, Wisc.

Dispense in tubes, approximately 5 ml per tube. Autoclave at 121 C for 5 minutes. Inoculate with a small fragment of growth from a Sabouraud dextrose agar slant. Incubate at room temperature for 21 to 25 days. Examine for quantity and type of growth.

Nocardia asteroides exhibits no growth or very sparse, thin, flaky growth. *N. brasiliensis* shows good growth and round compact colonies. *Streptomyces* species show poor to good growth (stringy or flaky).

GN broth*
(Hajna: Pub. Health Lab. 13:83, 1955)

Peptone	20 g
Glucose	1 g
D-Mannitol	2 g
Sodium citrate	5 g
Sodium desoxycholate	0.5 g
Dipotassium phosphate	4 g
Monopotassium phosphate	1.5 g
Sodium chloride	5 g
Distilled water	1,000 ml
(Final pH 7±)	

Dissolve the dehydrated medium in distilled water and autoclave at 116 C (10 pounds steam pressure) for 15 minutes or steam for 30 minutes at 100 C.

This broth medium is used as an enrichment for isolating salmonellae and shigellae in fecal specimens.

Haemophilus ducreyi media

See Chapter 11.

Hektoen enteric agar†*

Proteose peptone	12 g
Bile salts	9 g
Yeast extract	3 g
Lactose	12 g
Salicin	2 g

---

*Difco Laboratories, Detroit, Mich.; BBL Microbiology Systems, Cockeysville, Md.; Gibco Diagnostics, Madison, Wisc.
†Difco Laboratories, Detroit, Mich; BBL Microbiology Systems, Cockeysville, Md.; Gibco Diagnostics, Madison, Wisc.; Inolex Division, Glenwood, Ill.

Sucrose	12 g
Sodium chloride	5 g
Sodium thiosulfate	5 g
Ferric ammonium citrate	1.5 g
Agar	14 g
Acid fuchsin	0.1 g
Bromthymol blue	0.065 g
Distilled water	1,000 ml

Suspend 76 g of dehydrated medium, if using the commercial product, in 1,000 ml of distilled water. Heat to boiling, and continue until the medium dissolves. **Do not autoclave.** Cool to 50 C, and pour into Petri dishes.

This medium is useful for the isolation and differentiation of gram-negative enteric pathogens. The coliforms are usually salmon to orange, whereas the salmonellae and shigellae are bluish-green.

Indole-nitrite medium

See p. 647, Trypticase nitrate broth.

Kanamycin-vancomycin blood agar (KVBA)

1. Preparation of base:

Trypticase soy agar	40 g
Agar	2.5 g
Distilled water	1,000 ml
Kanamycin base*	100 mg

Sterilize by autoclaving at 121 C for 15 minutes, and cool to 50 C.
2. Add aseptically†:

Defibrinated sheep blood	50 ml
Vancomycin‡	7.5 mg
Vitamin K₁ solution (see Chapter 44)	1 ml

Mix well, pour plates (approximately 20 ml per plate), and store at room temperature.

This medium is extremely useful for primary inoculation of clinical specimens for selective isolation of anaerobes, particularly *Bacteroides,* but a nonselective medium (Brucella blood agar plate) should always be used as well.

*Bristol Laboratories, Syracuse, N.Y.
†Hemin may also be added (1 ml of hemin solution) (see Chapter 44).
‡Eli Lilly and Co., Indianapolis, Ind.

Kanamycin-vancomycin laked blood agar (KVLBA)

KVLBA is the same as KVBA, except that the final concentration of kanamycin is 75 μg/ml and the blood is laked (hemolyzed) by freezing whole blood overnight and then thawing. This medium is particularly useful for isolating the *Bacteroides melaninogenicus* group.

Kligler's iron agar

See p. 646, triple sugar iron (TSI) agar.

LD Presumpto Plate

See Chapter 13.

Legionella pneumophila media
*Charcoal-yeast extract diphasic blood culture medium (CYE-DBCM)**

(Feeley, Gorman, and Gibson. In Jones and Hebert, editors: "Legionnaires": the disease, the bacterium, and methodology, Atlanta, 1979, Center for Disease Control, pp. 77-84)

AGAR PHASE

Activated charcoal (Norit SG)†	2 g
Agar	17 g
Distilled water	500 ml

BROTH PHASE

Yeast extract	20 g
L-Cysteine HCl · H₂O	0.40 g
Fe (NO₃)₃ · 9H₂O	0.10 g
Distilled water	500 ml

Prepare agar first. Combine ingredients, boil, and dispense as 20-ml aliquots into each of a series of 125-ml Wheaton serum bottles. Stopper each bottle loosely with both a rubber stopper and a metal cap. Autoclave the bottles at 121 C for 20 minutes, cool to 50 C, remix the warm charcoal and agar thoroughly, and place the bottles at an angle so that an agar slant with a

*Available in individual blood culture bottles from Remel Labs, Lenexa, Kan.
†Sigma Chemical Co., St. Louis, Mo. (catalogue No. C5510). Activated charcoal, washed with phosphoric and sulfuric acids.

vertical height of 6 cm is formed. This procedure should leave a portion of the agar protruding above the 25 ml of liquid—broth plus specimen—that is added later.

Prepare the broth by first autoclaving the yeast extract and water at 121 C for 15 minutes. Allow to cool, and then add fresh sterile solutions of L-cysteine-HCl and ferric nitrate, in that order. Adjust the pH to 6.9 by adding 6 ml of 1 N KOH. Dispense the broth in 20-ml aliquots into the Wheaton bottles of charcoal agar slants. Seal the bottles by crimping the metal caps over the rubber stoppers. Check for sterility by preincubation at 35 C for 2 days.

It is recommended that Difco ingredients be used.

Charcoal-yeast extract (CYE) agar
(Feeley et al.: J. Clin. Microbiol. 10:437-441, 1979)

Yeast extract	10 g
Activated charcoal (Norit SG)	2 g
L-Cysteine HCl · H$_2$O	0.4 g
Ferric pyrophosphate, soluble*	0.25 g
Agar	17 g
Distilled water	1,000 ml

Add all other ingredients of CYE agar except L-cysteine HCl and soluble ferric pyrophosphate to 980 ml of distilled water. Dissolve by boiling, autoclave at 121 C for 15 minutes, and cool to 50 C in a water bath.

Prepare separate fresh solutions of L-cysteine HCl (0.40 g in 10 ml of distilled water) and soluble ferric pyrophosphate (0.25 g in 10 ml of distilled water). Filter sterilize each solution separately. Add the L-cysteine HCl to the basal medium first, and then add the ferric pyrophosphate.

Adjust the pH with 4 to 4.5 ml of 1 N KOH, so that the final pH of the medium is 6.90 ± 0.05. Use 1 N HCl when necessary.

It is recommended that Difco ingredients be used.

Feeley-Gorman (F-G) agar
(Feeley et al.: J. Clin. Microbiol. 8:320-325, 1978)

Casein (acid hydrolysis)	17.5 g
Beef extractives	3 g
Starch	1.5 g
Agar	17 g
L-Cysteine HCl · H$_2$O	0.4 g
Ferric pyrophosphate, soluble*	0.25 g
Distilled water	1 liter

Mueller-Hinton agar contains all the ingredients of F-G agar, except for L-cysteine HCl and ferric pyrophosphate, soluble, and provides a source of casein, beef extractives, starch, and agar. **Note:** Some lots of Mueller-Hinton agar may vary too widely in formulation and stability to serve as the base for satisfactory F-G agar.

Add the casein (acid hydrolysate), beef extractives, starch, and agar (or their equivalent, 38 g of Mueller-Hinton agar) to 980 ml of distilled water, autoclave at 121 C for 15 minutes, cool to 50 C in a water bath, and hold until L-cysteine HCl and soluble ferric pyrophosphate are added.

Prepare separate fresh solutions of L-cysteine HCl (0.4 g in 10 ml of distilled water) and soluble ferric pyrophosphate (0.25 g in 10 ml of distilled water). Filter sterilize each solution separately. Add the L-cysteine HCl to the agar mixture first, and then add the ferric pyrophosphate. Adjust the pH with either 1 N KOH or 1 N HCl, so that the final pH of the medium is 6.90 ± 0.05.

Feeley-Gorman (F-G) broth

F-G broth has the same formulation as F-G agar, except that it lacks agar, and the concentration of soluble ferric pyrophosphate is 100 mg/liter (w/v). Tube broth in 2-ml aliquots in screw-capped tubes (13 by 100 mm).

---

*Available on request from Biological Products Division, Centers for Disease Control, Atlanta, Ga. This reagent must be kept dry and stored in the dark. Do not use if its color changes from green to yellow or brown.

*Biological Products Division, Centers for Disease Control, Atlanta, Ga. This reagent must be kept dry and stored in the dark. Do not use if its color changes from green to yellow or brown.

MH-IH agar

(Feeley et al.: J. Clin. Microbiol. 8:320-325, 1978)

COMPONENT A

Mueller-Hinton agar	38 g
Distilled water	490 ml

COMPONENT B

Hemoglobin powder	10 g
Distilled water	490 ml

COMPONENT C

IsoVitaleX	20 ml

Prepare components A and B separately, and autoclave at 121 C for 15 minutes. Cool to 50 C, combine A and B, and hold at 50 C in a water bath. Prepare component C by adding 10 ml of sterile distilled water to each of two vials containing lyophilized IsoVitaleX. Add the contents of both vials to the A-B mixture. Adjust the pH with either 1 N KOH or 1 N HCl, so that the final pH of the medium is 6.90 ± 0.05.

Buffered charcoal yeast extract agar (BCYE)*

(Modified from Pasculle et al.: J. Infect. Dis. 441:727, 1980)

Yeast extract	10 g
Activated charcoal (Norit A or SG)	2 g
L-Cysteine HCl · H$_2$O	0.4 g
Ferric pyrophosphate, soluble	0.25 g
ACES buffer (Calbiochem, Behring, or Sigma)	10 g
Agar	17 g
α-Ketoglutarate,† monopotassium salt (Sigma)	1 g
Purified water	980 ml

1. Dissolve the cysteine and ferric pyrophosphate separately in 10 ml of purified water. Place in a 37 C water bath for about 15 minutes to aid dissolution.
2. Add the ACES to 200 ml of purified water, and heat stir at lowest temperature for 30 minutes. Membrane filter sterilize, and store in a sterile container.

---

*Available in prepared plates from Remel Labs, Lenexa, Kan.
†Use of α-ketoglutarate was suggested by Feeley. This compound significantly improves results with this medium (Edelstein, P.H.: Personal communication, 1981).

3. Add yeast extract, agar, and Norit to a flask containing 750 ml purified water.
4. Boil, add a stir bar, and sterilize by autoclaving for 15 minutes at 121 C.
5. Place the sterilized agar in a 50 to 52 C water bath for 1 hour.
6. Place the melted agar on a heated stirrer, and rotate the stir bar slowly to avoid frothing.
7. Add filtered ACES slowly to stirring agar. **Note:** Preheat ACES in a 50 C water bath before adding.
8. Add the cysteine and then the ferric pyrophosphate to the stirred agar, using a syringe with an attached disk filter (e.g., Gelman Acrodisc 0.20 μm) in order to filter sterilize the small volume added.
9. Check the pH, and adjust it to 6.9 ± 0.05 using 1 N KOH. **Note:** 35 to 40 ml of KOH is required.
10. Pour into plates (15 to 20 ml per plate). **Note:** Swirl the bulk agar after pouring each plate to keep charcoal in suspension.
11. Incubate plates at room temperature for 24 to 48 hours, and store packaged at 2 to 8 C for a maximum of 8 weeks.

Differential buffered charcoal yeast extract agar (DIFF/BCYE)

(Vickers et al.: J. Clin. Microbiol. 13:380, 1981)

Yeast extract	10 g
Activated charcoal (Norit A or SG)	1.5 g
L-Cysteine HCl	0.4 g
Ferric pyrophosphate (soluble)	0.25 g
ACES buffer	10 g
Agar	17 g
Bromcresol purple	0.01 g
Bromthymol blue	0.01 g
Polymyxin B (optional)	50,000 units
Vancomycin (optional)	0.001 g
Purified water	approx. 1,000 ml

1. Dissolve the cysteine and ferric pyrophosphate separately in 10 ml of purified water. Place in a 37 C water bath for about 15 minutes to aid dissolution.
2. Add the ACES to 200 ml of purified water,

and heat stir at lowest temperature for 30 minutes. Membrane filter sterilize, and store in a sterile container.

3. Prepare separately 1% solutions (w/v) of bromcresol purple and bromthymol blue in 0.1 N KOH (1 gm in 100 ml 0.1 N KOH). Membrane filter sterilize, and store at 2 to 8 C.

4. Prepare a sterile solution of polymyxin B (50,000 units/ml) and vancomycin (1,000 μg/ml), and store in aliquots at −20 C.

5. Add yeast extract, agar, and Norit to a flask containing 750 ml of purified water.

6. Boil, add a stir bar, and sterilize by autoclaving for 15 minutes at 121 C.

7. Place the sterilized agar in a 50-52 C water bath for 1 hour.

8. Place the melted agar on a heated stirrer, and rotate the stir bar slowly to avoid frothing.

9. Add filtered ACES slowly to stirring agar. **Note:** Preheat ACES in a 50 C water bath before adding.

10. Add the cysteine and then the ferric pyrophosphate to the stirring agar using a syringe with an attached disk filter (e.g., Gelman Acrodisc 0.20 μm) to filter sterilize the small volume added.

11. Check the pH, and adjust it to 6.9 ± 0.05 using 1 N KOH. **Note:** 35 to 40 ml of KOH is required.

12. Add 1 ml each of the sterile 1% bromcresol purple and 1% bromthymol blue dye solutions to the adjusted agar.

13. Optional: Add the polymyxin B and vancomycin agents to the adjusted agar at final concentrations of 50,000 units and 1,000 μg, respectively, per liter of medium.

14. Pour into plates (15 to 20 ml per plate). **Note:** Swirl the bulk agar after pouring each plate to keep charcoal in suspension.

15. Incubate the plates at room temperature for 24 to 48 hours, and store packaged at 2 to 8 C for a maximum of 8 weeks.

Semiselective medium for Legionella pneumophila (BMPA-α)
(Edelstein: J. Clin. Microbiol. 14:298-303, 1981)

Charcoal yeast extract agar (see p. 628)	
ACES buffer	1 %
α-Ketoglutarate	0.1 %
Anisomycin	80 μg/ml
Polymyxin B	80 units/ml
Cefamandole	4 μg/ml

Loeffler coagulated serum slants*
(Zentralbl. Bakt. 2:105, 1887)

Add 3 volumes of beef, hog, or horse serum (collected as cleanly as possible) to 1 volume of glucose infusion broth (1% glucose). Dispense in tubes, slant, and inspissate for about 2 hours at 75 to 85 C on each of 3 successive days. The medium also may be sterilized in a slanted position in a horizontal autoclave. Close the autoclave tightly, and without allowing the air to escape, autoclave at 15 pounds pressure for 15 minutes to coagulate the medium. Then allow the air to escape slowly, and admit steam so that the pressure is maintained at 15 pounds. When an atmosphere of pure steam has been obtained, close the outlet valve tightly, and sterilize the medium with steam under 15 pounds pressure (121 C) for 15 or 20 minutes.

Lowenstein-Jensen (L-J) medium†
(Holm and Lester: Public Health Rep. [abstr.]

Salt solution	
Monopotassium phosphate	2.4 g
Magnesium sulfate (7H$_2$O)	0.24 g
Magnesium citrate	0.6 g
Asparagin	3.6 g
Glycerol, reagent grade	12 ml
Distilled water	600 ml

---

*Available in tube form from BBL Microbiology Systems, Cockeysville, Md.; Difco Laboratories, Detroit, Mich.

†Prepared tubed media are available from Difco Laboratories, Detroit, Mich.; BBL Microbiology Systems, Cockeysville, Md.; Gibco Diagnostics, Madison, Wisc.; and many others.

Potato flour	30 g
Homogenized whole eggs	1,000 ml
Malachite green (2% aqueous)	20 ml

Add the potato flour to the flask of salt solution, and autoclave the mixture at 121 C for 30 minutes. Clean fresh eggs, no more than 1 week old, by vigorous scrubbing in 5% soap solution, and allow them to remain in it for 30 minutes. Place the eggs in running cold water until the water becomes clear. Immerse the washed eggs in 70% alcohol for 15 minutes, remove, and break into a sterile flask; homogenize completely by shaking with glass beads. Then filter the homogenate through four layers of sterile gauze.

Add 1 liter of the homogenized egg suspension to the flask of cooled potato flour–salt solution. Add the malachite green to this emulsion, and mix thoroughly. Dispense the medium aseptically with a sterile aspirator bottle in 6-ml amounts into sterile, screw-capped 150-mm glass tubes. Inspissate the tubes at 85 C for 50 minutes, and check for sterility by incubating at 35 C for 48 hours. Store in a refrigerator, where the medium will keep for at least 1 month if the tubes are tightly sealed to prevent loss of moisture.

This medium is used for the cultivation of *Mycobacterium tuberculosis*.

Lysine-iron agar*
(Edwards and Fife: Appl. Microbiol. 9:478, 1961)

Peptone	5 g
Yeast extract	3 g
Glucose	1 g
L-Lysine	10 g
Ferric ammonium citrate	0.5 g
Sodium thiosulfate	40 mg
Bromcresol purple	20 mg
Agar	15 g
Distilled water	1,000 ml
(Adjust to pH 6.7)	

Dispense 4-ml amounts into 13- by 100-mm tubes, and sterilize at 121 C for 12 minutes. Slant tubes to obtain a deep butt and a short slant. This medium is inoculated by using a straight wire to stab the butt twice and to streak the slant. Incubation is at 35 C for 18 to 24 hours. If necessary, incubate for 48 hours.

This medium is useful for determining whether members of the family Enterobacteriaceae can decarboxylate or deaminate lysine. However, this medium is not to be considered as a substitute for the Moeller method. A **positive** reaction is indicated by an alkaline or **purple** reaction in the butt of the tube. The absence of lysine decarboxylase is indicated by an acidic or **yellow (negative)** reaction in the butt of the tube caused by fermentation of glucose. Lysine deaminase is indicated by the formation of a **red** slant and is characteristic of the tribe Proteeae. It should be noted that H_2S-producing *Proteus* species do not blacken this medium. Furthermore, *M. morganii* does not consistently produce a red slant after 24 hours' incubation.

MacConkey agar*

Peptone	17 g
Proteose peptone	3 g
Lactose	10 g
Bile salts	1.5 g
Sodium chloride	5 g
Agar	13.5 g
Neutral red	0.03 g
Crystal violet	0.001 g
Distilled water	1,000 ml

The agar concentration may be increased to 5% (use an additional 3.65 g of agar) to inhibit the spreading of *Proteus*. The medium is inhibitory for gram-positive bacteria and differential rather than selective. Coliforms (lactose fermenting) produce red colonies on the medium, whereas nonlactose fermenters produce colorless colonies.

---

*Available in dehydrated form from BBL Microbiology Systems, Cockeysville, Md.; Difco Laboratories, Detroit, Mich.; Gibco Diagnostics, Madison, Wisc.; Inolex Division, Glenwood, Ill.

*Available in dehydrated form from BBL Microbiology Systems, Cockeysville, Md.; Difco Laboratories, Detroit, Mich.; Gibco Diagnostics, Madison, Wisc.

Malonate (sodium) broth*

(Leifson: J. Bacteriol. 26:329, 1933; Ewing et al.: Pub. Health Lab. 15:153, 1957)

Yeast extract	1 g
Ammonium sulfate	2 g
Dipotassium sulfate	0.6 g
Monopotassium phosphate	0.4 g
Sodium chloride	2 g
Sodium malonate	3 g
Glucose	0.25 g
Bromthymol blue	0.025 g
Distilled water	1,000 ml

(Final pH 6.7±)

Sterilize in small tubes in 3-ml amounts at 121 C for 15 minutes. Inoculate from TSI slants or broth cultures; incubate cultures at 35 C for 48 hours.

The medium is used to test for utilization of sodium malonate by members of the Enterobacteriaceae. A **positive** test is shown by a change of the indicator from green to a **Prussian blue.**

Mannitol salt agar*

Beef extract	1 g
Proteose peptone No. 3	10 g
Sodium chloride	75 g
Mannitol	10 g
Agar	15 g
Phenol red	0.025 g
Distilled water	1,000 ml

Sterilize the medium at 15 pounds pressure for 15 minutes, cool to 48 C, and pour into sterile Petri dishes. Use 15 to 20 ml per plate.

This medium is used for the selective isolation of pathogenic staphylococci, since many other bacteria are inhibited by the high salt concentration. Colonies of potentially pathogenic staphylococci are surrounded by a **yellow** halo, indicating mannitol fermentation.

Martin-Lewis agar

See Chapter 11.

---

*Available in dehydrated form from BBL Microbiology Systems, Cockeysville, Md.; Difco Laboratories, Detroit, Mich.; Gibco Diagnostics, Madison, Wisc.

McBride medium, modified

(J. Lab. Clin. Med. 55:153, 1960)

Phenylethanol agar*	35.5 g
Glycine, anhydride	10 g
Lithium chloride	0.5 g
Distilled water	1,000 ml

Dissolve with the aid of heat and sterilize at 121 C for 20 minutes.

This medium is recommended for the cultivation of *Listeria*.

Methyl red–Voges-Proskauer medium (MR-VP) (Clark and Lubs medium)*

Buffered peptone	7 g
Glucose	5 g
Dipotassium phosphate	5 g
Distilled water	1,000 ml

(Final pH 6.9±)

This medium is used for the methyl red test and the Voges-Proskauer test (production of acetylmethylcarbinol).

Middlebrook 7H10 agar with OADC enrichment

The preparation of 7H10 oleic acid–albumin agar as originally described is extremely tedious and complicated. Its preparation may be simplified by the use of a combination of six stock solutions prepared in advance, as described in the handbook *Tuberculosis Laboratory Methods of the Veterans Administration*.† However, for the average diagnostic microbiology laboratory, it is strongly recommended that **commercially prepared** 7H10-OADC complete medium be used whenever possible.‡ For purposes of orientation, the ingredients of each medium are listed, but the directions are intended solely for prepa-

---

*Available in dehydrated form from BBL Microbiology Systems, Cockeysville, Md.; Difco Laboratories, Detroit, Mich.; Gibco Diagnostics, Madison, Wisc.

†Obtainable from the Superintendent of Documents, U.S. Government Printing Office, Washington, D.C.

‡BBL Microbiology Systems, Cockeysville, Md.; Difco Laboratories, Detroit, Mich.; Gibco Diagnostics, Madison, Wisc.

ration from dehydrated medium and prepared enrichment.

Middlebrook 7H10 agar*

Ammonium sulfate	0.5 g
D-Glutamic acid	0.5 g
Sodium citrate	0.4 g
Disodium phosphate	1.5 g
Monopotassium phosphate	1.5 g
Ferric ammonium phosphate	0.04 g
Magnesium sulfate	0.05 g
Pyridoxine	0.001 g
Biotin	0.0005 g
Malachite green	0.001 g
Agar	15 g

Middlebrook OADC enrichment*

Oleic acid	0.5 g
Bovine albumin, fraction V	50 g
Glucose	20 g
Beef catalase	0.04 g
Sodium chloride	8.5 g
Distilled water	1,000 ml

To rehydrate the 7H10 agar, suspend 20 g in 1 liter of cold distilled water containing 0.5% reagent grade glycerol and heat to boiling to dissolve completely. Distribute in 180-ml amounts in flasks; sterilize by autoclaving at 121 C for 10 minutes; cool to 50 to 55 C; add 20 ml of OADC enrichment aseptically to each flask; and dispense in sterile plastic Petri dishes. Store at 4 C in the dark for no longer than 2 months in a plastic bag to prevent dehydration.

Milk media
Skimmed milk

Fresh, clean, skimmed cow's milk may be used. This is dispensed in tubes and sterilized either by tyndallization (flowing steam for 30 minutes on 3 successive days) or in the autoclave at 10 pounds pressure for 10 minutes.

Commercial dehydrated skimmed milk is also completely satisfactory. The concentration used is 10% in distilled water. The method of sterilization is as before.

Litmus milk

Skimmed milk powder	100 g
Litmus	5 g
Distilled water	1,000 ml

Autoclave at 10 pounds pressure for 10 minutes.

Reactions in litmus milk. Pink color of litmus indicates an acid reaction caused by fermentation of lactose. A purple or blue color (alkaline) indicates no fermentation of lactose. White color (reduction) results when litmus serves as an electron acceptor and is reduced to its leuco base. Coagulation (clot) is caused by precipitation of casein by the acid produced from lactose. Coagulation may also be caused by the conversion of casein to paracasein by the enzyme rennin.

Peptonization (dissolution of the clot) indicates digestion of the curd or milk proteins by proteolytic enzymes.

Milk medium with a reducing agent*

Skimmed milk powder	100 g
Peptone	10 g
Sodium thioglycollate	0.5 g
Litmus	5 g
Distilled water	1,000 ml

Methylene blue milk

Skimmed milk powder	10 g
Methylene blue (1% aqueous)	10 ml
Distilled water	90 ml

Methylene blue milk is used in the identification of the enterococci.

---

*BBL Microbiology Systems, Cockeysville, Md.; Difco Laboratories, Detroit, Mich.; Gibco Diagnostics, Madison, Wisc.

---

*This medium has been found satisfactory for the cultivation of *Clostridium* species and allows observation of their reactions in litmus milk. Autoclave at 10 pounds pressure for 10 minutes, and stopper tightly.

Moeller potassium cyanide broth*
(Acta Pathol. Microbiol. Scand. 34:115, 1954)

Peptone (Orthana special†)	10 g
Sodium chloride	5 g
Monobasic potassium phosphate	0.225 g
Dibasic sodium phosphate (2 H₂O)	5.64 g
Distilled water	1,000 ml

(Adjust reaction to pH 7.6)

Autoclave the medium in flasks. Dissolve 0.5 g of potassium cyanide in 100 ml of **cold sterile broth.** Place 1 ml of the cyanide broth in 12- by 100-mm tubes. Immediately stopper with paraffined corks, and store at 4 to 5 C. The medium remains stable for 2 to 3 weeks.

Inoculate medium with one small loopful of a 24-hour broth culture. Incubate at 35 C, and observe daily for 2 days for **growth,** which is recognized by turbidity of the medium.

Motility test medium‡§

Beef extract	3 g
Gelysate peptone	10 g
Sodium chloride	5 g
Agar	4 g
Distilled water	1,000 ml

(Final pH 7.3±)

1. Suspend 22 g of dehydrated medium in water, and add 0.05 g triphenyltetrazolium. Heat with frequent agitation; boil 1 minute to dissolve ingredients.
2. Dispense in screw-capped tubes, and sterilize by autoclaving at 121 C for 15 minutes.
3. Tighten caps when cool; store at room temperature.

This medium is stabbed once and read after 1 to 2 days' incubation at 35 C. Motile organisms spread out from the line of inoculation; nonmotile organisms grow only along the stab.

If the results are negative, follow with further incubation at 21 to 25 C for 5 days. For special purposes, such as enhancement of the motility and flagellar development in poorly motile cultures, it is often advisable to pass cultures first through a semisolid medium containing 0.2% agar tubed in Craigie tubes or in U tubes. Subsequent passages may be made in 0.4% agar medium.

Motility media containing concentrations higher than 0.3% produce gels through which many motile organisms cannot spread. Spreading in a semisolid medium is judged by macroscopic examination of the medium for a diffuse zone of growth emanating from the line of inoculation. Many aerobic pseudomonads fail to grow deep in semisolid medium in a test tube. Organisms possessing "paralyzed" flagella are nonmotile and cannot spread in the medium. Some filamentous organisms spread in or on semisolid medium but are nonmotile and nonflagellated. Although cultures may grow at 37 C or higher temperatures, the flagellar proteins of some organisms are not synthesized optimally at this temperature; hence, motility medium should be incubated at temperatures near 18 to 20 C. These observations require judicious interpretation of motility and limit, to some extent, the reliability of using spreading in semisolid agar as the sole taxonomic criterion to delineate related species.

Motility test semisolid agar for Listeria

Bacto-tryptose*	10 g
Sodium chloride	5 g
Agar	5 g
Glucose	1 g
Distilled water	1,000 ml

Dissolve with the aid of heat, distribute in tubes, and sterilize at 121 C for 20 minutes.

---

*The base medium is available from BBL Microbiology Systems, Cockeysville, Md.; Difco Laboratories, Detroit, Mich.; Gibco Diagnostics, Madison, Wisc.
†Proteose peptone No. 3, 0.3%, has been found to serve as a satisfactory substitute.
‡BBL Microbiology Systems, Cockeysville, Md.
§Discussion adapted from Paik. In Lennette, Balows, Hausler, and Truant, editors: Manual of clinical microbiology, ed. 3, Washington, D.C., 1980, American Society for Microbiology.

---

*Difco Laboratories, Detroit, Mich.

Inoculate by stabbing with a 24-hour broth culture. Incubate the tubes at 25 and 35 C, and observe for growth away from the stab line (motile).

This medium is useful for demonstrating the motility of *Listeria*.

Mueller-Hinton agar*
(Proc. Soc. Exp. Biol. Med. 48:330, 1941)

Beef, infusion from	300 g
Peptone	17.5 g
Starch	1.5 g
Agar	17 g

(Final pH 7.4±)†

Suspend the medium in distilled water, mix thoroughly, and heat with frequent agitation. Boil for about 1 minute, dispense, sterilize by autoclaving at 116 to 121 C (12 to 15 pounds steam pressure) for **no longer than 15 minutes,** and cool by placing immediately in a 50 C water bath before pouring.

The medium is used primarily for the disk-agar diffusion method of testing for antimicrobial susceptibility of microorganisms. It has also been used to detect starch hydrolysis by *S. bovis* (Lee: J. Clin. Microbiol. 4:312, 1976) and for culturing the Legionnaires' disease agent.

Five percent defibrinated animal blood may be added as enrichment; this may be chocolatized in the testing of *Haemophilus* species.

Mycoplasma (PPLO) isolation media
Mycoplasma isolation (PPLO) agar‡

Beef heart, infusion from fresh tissue	50 g
Peptone	10 g
Sodium chloride	5 g
Agar	14 g

(Final pH 7.8)

1. Suspend 34 g of dry medium in 1,000 ml of distilled water, mix, and boil for 1 minute. Dispense in 70- to 75-ml amounts. Autoclave at 121 C for 15 minutes.
2. Cool to approximately 50 C, and add aseptically:

Horse serum*	20 ml
Yeast extract (25%) (see below)	10 ml
Penicillin G solution (100,000 units/ml)	2 ml

3. Mix gently, pour approximately 20 ml per plate into sterile Petri dishes (100 by 15 mm). The smaller (60- by 15-mm) dishes accommodate 8-ml amounts and are used for subculture.
4. If bacterial contamination is excessive, add 5 ml of a 1:2,000 dilution of thallium acetate; reduce fungal contamination by adding 0.7 ml of a 0.05% solution of amphotericin B.
5. Seal plates with parafilm, and store in the refrigerator.

Mycoplasma isolation broth†

Mycoplasma isolation broth medium is identical to PPLO agar medium with the agar omitted. It is prepared by dissolving 21 g of dry medium in 1,000 ml of distilled water, dispensing in 70-ml volumes, and sterilizing in the autoclave at 121 C for 15 minutes. After cooling to about 50 C, the horse serum, yeast extract, and penicillin are added as described previously.

Preparation of 25% yeast extract

1. Suspend 125 g of Fleischmann's pure dry yeast (Type 20-40)‡ in 500-ml distilled/deionized water in a 1-liter beaker. Boil for 2 minutes with constant stirring.
2. Dispense in centrifuge tubes, and refrigerate overnight to settle the yeast cells.

---

*BBL Microbiology Systems, Cockeysville, Md.; Difco Laboratories, Detroit, Mich.; Gibco Diagnostics, Madison, Wisc.; Inolex Division, Glenwood, Ill.
†Check by using a surface electrode, if available, after gelling.
‡Difco Laboratories, Detroit, Mich.; BBL Microbiology Systems, Cockeysville, Md.

---

*BBL Microbiology Systems, Cockeysville, Md.
†Difco Laboratories, Detroit, Mich.; BBL Microbiology Systems, Cockeysville, Md.; Gibco Diagnostics, Madison, Wisc.
‡Standard Brands, Inc., New York, N.Y.

3. Centrifuge at 3,000 rpm for 30 minutes, and carefully remove the supernate.
4. Adjust to pH 8.0 with 1 N NaOH.
5. Dispense in 2.5-ml amounts in screw-capped tubes or small bottles, and autoclave at 121 C for 15 minutes.
6. Store in frozen state at −20 C. Use within 3 months. When thawing, the extract becomes quite turbid but clears after standing at room temperature.

Biphasic isolation medium for M. pneumoniae

1. Prepare basal broth medium as described previously.
2. Add 1 ml of a 0.1% phenol red solution and 2 ml of a 0.1% methylene blue solution to 70 ml of broth.
3. Sterilize by autoclaving at 121 C for 15 minutes.
4. Cool to approximately 50 C, and add aseptically the horse serum, yeast extract, and penicillin as described previously.
5. Add aseptically about 3 ml to tubes containing the isolation agar (2-ml amounts in screw-capped tubes), and seal tightly.

Growth of *M. pneumoniae* is indicated by a change in color of the indicator.

E agar

Papaic digest of soy meal USP	20 g
Sodium chloride	5 g
Purified water	1,000 ml
Agar	10 g

1. Heat with agitation to obtain solution.
2. Cool and adjust pH to 7.4 with 1 N sodium hydroxide.
3. Dispense and autoclave at 121 C · for 15 minutes. Cool to 50 C.
4. To 65 ml of solution add 10 ml of yeast dialysate, 25 ml of horse serum, 2 ml of penicillin (10,000 units/ml), and 1 ml of 3.3% aqueous thallium acetate.
5. Dispense in 5-ml amounts in 10- by 35-mm Petri dishes, and incubate overnight at room temperature.

Note: Prepare yeast dialysate as follows. Suspend 450 g of active dried yeast (e.g., Fleischmann) in 1,250 ml of water at 40 C. Heat in an autoclave at 121 C for 5 minutes. Place in dialysis casing, and dialyze against 1 liter of water at 4 C for 2 days. Discard casing and contents. Autoclave dialysate at 121 C for 15 minutes. Store frozen.

MES agar

Papaic digest of soy meal USP	20 g
Sodium chloride	5 g
2-(N-Morpholino) ethanesulfonic acid (MES, Calbiochem)	4.25 g
Water	1,000 ml
Agarose	10 g

1. Dissolve, adjust pH to 6.0 at 37 C, autoclave at 121 C for 15 minutes and cool to 50 C.
2. To 65 ml of solution add 10 ml of yeast dialysate, 25 ml of horse serum, and 2 ml of penicillin (10,000 units/ml).
3. Dispense in plates as for E agar.

Nitrate broth for nitrate reduction test

Tryptone	5 g
Neopeptone	5 g
Distilled water	1,000 ml
Potassium nitrate (reagent grade)	1 g
Glucose	0.1 g

Before adding the potassium nitrate and glucose, boil the other ingredients in the water and adjust pH to 7.3 to 7.4. Dispense 5 ml per tube and sterilize at 15 pounds pressure for 15 minutes. The reagents and tests for nitrate reduction are listed in Chapter 44.

Nutrient agar*

Beef extract	3 g
Peptone or Gelysate pancreatic digest of gelatin	5 g
Agar	15 g
Distilled water	1,000 ml
(Final pH 6.8)	

---

*Difco Laboratories, Detroit, Mich.; BBL Microbiology Systems, Cockeysville, Md.; Gibco Diagnostics, Madison, Wisc.; Inolex Division, Glenwood, Ill.

Autoclave at 121 C for 15 minutes.

NYC medium, modified NYC medium

See Chapter 11.

ONPG (beta-galactosidase) test

The ability of certain gram-negative bacilli to ferment lactose is a useful criterion for identifying certain members of the family Enterobacteriaceae. Since some coliform organisms, the so-called paracolon bacteria, ferment this carbohydrate slowly or not at all, they have been confused with the enteric pathogens.

Lactose fermentation is dependent on two enzymes: **permease,** which allows lactose to enter the bacterial cell, and **beta-galactosidase,** which splits lactose into glucose and galactose. The slow lactose fermenters are deficient in permease, and the demonstration of beta-galactosidase in such organisms permits more rapid identification of a lactose fermenter. This enzyme can be detected conveniently by the use of a tablet of ortho-nitrophenyl-beta-galactopyranoside (ONPG)* dissolved in distilled water and inoculated with a heavy suspension of the organism to be tested. The test is incubated at 35 C for 6 hours; hydrolysis of ONPG is detected by the liberation of ortho-nitrophenol, with its characteristic **yellow** color, often within 30 minutes. Thus, a **positive** ONPG test indicates that the organism contains lactose-fermenting enzymes and may be classed as a lactose fermenter.

Oxidative-fermentative (O-F) basal medium†
(Hugh and Leifson: J. Bacteriol. 66:24-26, 1953)

Trypticase or tryptone	2 g
Sodium chloride	5 g
Dipotassium phosphate	0.3 g
Agar, dried	2.5 g
Bromthymol blue (3 ml of 1% aqueous [not alcoholic] solution)	0.03 g
Distilled water	1,000 ml
(Final pH 7.1 ±0.2)	

---

*Key Scientific Products Co., Los Angeles, Calif.
†Available in dehydrated form from BBL Microbiology Systems, Cockeysville, Md.; Difco Laboratories, Detroit, Mich.; Gibco Diagnostics, Madison, Wisc.

Suspend the material in 1 liter of distilled water, and heat to dissolve with frequent agitation; adjust reaction to a pH of approximately 7.1. Sterilize by autoclaving at 121 C for 15 minutes. To 100 ml of sterile base add 10 ml sterile 10% glucose solution (10% lactose, mannitol, and sucrose also may be added to separate 100-ml portions if required). The completed medium should be **green.** Proceed as follows:

Inoculate (stab) lightly two tubes of medium from a young agar slant culture. Cover one of the tubes with a layer (about 5 mm) of sterile melted petrolatum or sterile paraffin oil. Incubate at 37° C and observe daily for 3 or 4 days. Acid formation in the open tube only indicates oxidative utilization of dextrose. Acid formation in both the open and the sealed tubes is indicative of a fermentative reaction. Lack of acid production in either tube indicates that the organism does not utilize dextrose by either method.

O-F basal medium is used for differentiating organisms such as *Acinetobacter, Alcaligenes,* and *Pseudomonas* from members of the Enterobacteriaceae.

Peptic digest agar

Add 5% Fildes enrichment to trypticase soy agar base. This is a very good medium for demonstrating *H. influenzae.* Colonies are translucent blue.

Phenol red broth base*

Trypticase	10 g
Sodium chloride	5 g
Phenol red	0.018 g
(Final pH 7.4±)	

Phenol red broth base can be used as a base for determining carbohydrate fermentation reactions. Carbohydrates can be added to the

---

*Available in dehydrated form from BBL Microbiology Systems, Cockeysville, Md., and Gibco Diagnostics, Madison, Wisc. Similar media with bromcresol purple indicator can be obtained either from BBL Microbiology Systems or Difco Laboratories. If bromcresol purple is preferred to phenol red indicator, purple broth base is also available in dehydrated form from these laboratories.

medium in 0.5% to 1% concentrations before dispensing and sterilization. Durham tubes should be inserted into the tubed medium for detection of gas formation.

Phenylalanine agar*

(Ewing et al.: Pub. Health Lab. 15:153, 1957)

Yeast extract	3 g
DL-Phenylalanine	2 g
(or L-phenylalanine)	1 g
Disodium phosphate	1 g
Sodium chloride	5 g
Agar	12 g
Distilled water	1,000 ml

Dispense 3-ml amounts in small tubes, and sterilize at 121 C for 10 minutes. Allow to solidify in a slanted position.

This medium is used to test for deamination of phenylalanine to phenylpyruvic acid by members of the Enterobacteriaceae.

After incubation of the culture for 18 to 24 hours at 35 C, allow 4 to 5 drops of fresh 10% ferric chloride solution to run down over the growth on the slant. If acid has been formed, a **green** color immediately develops on the slant and in the fluid at the base of the slant.

Phenylethyl alcohol agar*

(Lilley and Brewer: J. Am. Pharm. Assoc. [Scient. Ed.] 42:6-8, 1953)

Trypticase	15 g
Phytone	5 g
Sodium chloride	5 g
Beta-phenylethyl alcohol	2.5 g
Agar	15 g
Distilled water	1,000 ml
(Final pH 7.3±)	

Suspend the powder in the water, mix thoroughly, heat with agitation, and boil 1 minute. Dispense in 16- by 150-mm screw-capped tubes. Sterilize at 118 to 121 C (12 to 15 pounds pressure) for 15 minutes. If desired, 5% blood may be added to the cooled medium (45 to 50 C) before pouring plates.

Phenylethyl alcohol agar is useful for the isolation of gram-positive cocci and the inhibition of gram-negative bacilli (particularly *Proteus*) when these are found in mixed culture.

Polymyxin staphylococcus medium

(Finegold and Sweeney: J. Bacteriol. 81:636-641, 1961)

Nutrient agar	23 g
Tween 80	10.2 ml
Lecithin	0.7 g
Polymyxin*	75 mg
Distilled water	1,000 ml

Autoclave at 15 pounds pressure for 15 minutes. Pour plates.

Coagulase-negative staphylococci, micrococci, and most gram-negative rods are inhibited. In addition to *S. aureus*, *Proteus* will grow; the latter can be recognized by translucent colonies. *Proteus* does not swarm on this medium.

Potato-carrot agar

Carrots, peeled	20 g
Potatoes, peeled	20 g
Distilled water	1,000 ml
Agar	15 g
Tween 80	5 ml

Wash potatoes and carrots, mash them, and place them in distilled water for 1 hour. Boil for 5 minutes, filter through paper, make up to 1,000 ml of volume, and add 15 g of agar and 5 ml of Tween 80. Dispense in tubes, autoclave at 121 C for 20 minutes, slant, and cool. Potato-carrot agar is an excellent medium for demonstrating color characteristics of a fungal colony.

Potato-dextrose agar†

Potatoes, infusion from	200 g
Glucose	20 g
Agar	20 g
Distilled water	1,000 ml

---

*Difco Laboratories, Detroit, Mich.; BBL Microbiology Systems, Cockeysville, Md.; Gibco Diagnostics, Madison, Wisc.

*75 mg = 75,000 μg or 750,000 units of activity.
†Available in prepared tubes from BBL Microbiology Systems, Cockeysville, Md.; Difco Laboratories, Detroit, Mich.; Gibco Diagnostics, Madison, Wisc.

Boil potatoes in water for 15 minutes, filter through cotton, and make up to volume with water. Add dry ingredients, and dissolve agar with heat. No pH adjustment is required. Dispense as desired, and autoclave at 121 C for 10 minutes. The agar is used to stimulate spore production of fungi.

Purple broth base*

Peptone: Proteose or peptic digest of animal tissue USP	10 g
Beef extract	1 g
Sodium chloride	5 g
Bromcresol purple	0.015 g
Distilled water	1,000 ml
(Final pH 6.8)	

Autoclave at 121 C for not more than 15 minutes. Add sugars and alcohols to 1% (w/v).

Rice grain medium

White rice	8 g
Distilled water	25 ml

Place in a 125-ml Erlenmeyer flask, and autoclave at 121 C for 15 minutes.

Rice grain medium is used for differentiation of *Microsporum* species. *M. canis* and *M. gypseum* grow and sporulate well in this medium; *M. audouini* grows poorly. Conidial formation is stimulated in some of the *Trichophyton* species.

Sabhi agar†

(Gorman: Am. J. Med. Technol. 33:151, 1967)

Calf brain, infusion from	100 g
Beef heart, infusion from	125 g
Proteose peptone	5 g
Neopeptone	5 g
Glucose	21 g
Sodium chloride	2.5 g
Disodium phosphate	1.25 g
Agar	15 g
Distilled water	1,000 ml
(Final pH 7.0)	

---

*Difco Laboratories, Detroit, Mich.; BBL Microbiology Systems, Cockeysville, Md.; Gibco Diagnostics, Madison, Wisc.

†Difco Laboratories, Detroit, Mich. (No. 0797).

1. Suspend 59 g in 1,000 ml of distilled water, and heat to boiling to completely dissolve medium.
2. Sterilize by autoclaving at 121 C for 15 minutes.
3. Cool to 50 to 55 C, and add 1 ml sterile chloramphenicol solution (100 mg/ml).
4. Mix well, and dispense in sterile, cotton-plugged 25- by 150-mm Pyrex test tubes.
5. Slant, allow to harden, and refrigerate.

Sabhi is an equal mixture of Sabouraud dextrose agar and brain-heart infusion agar and has proved useful for isolation of clinically significant fungi, particularly from specimens containing bacteria, such as sputum.

Sabouraud dextrose agar (SAB)

Sabouraud dextrose agar*	32.5 g
Agar, powdered	2.5 g
Distilled water	500 ml

Suspend ingredients in water, dissolve by heating to boiling, and dispense in approximately 20-ml amounts in cotton-plugged, 25- by 150-mm Pyrex test tubes (without lips). If antimicrobial agents are to be added, this may be done after heating the medium and before autoclaving. The following amounts are recommended (CDC):

Cycloheximide† (0.5 mg/ml)	250 mg
Chloramphenicol‡ (0.05 mg/ml)	25 mg

Add the chloramphenicol dissolved in 5 ml of 95% ethanol and the cycloheximide dissolved in 5 ml of acetone. Mix well, and distribute into tubes or bottles as indicated. Autoclave at 118 C for **no longer than 10 minutes.** Slant, allow to harden, and refrigerate. This selective medium

---

*This medium and also media containing the antimicrobial agents are available from BBL Microbiology Systems, Cockeysville, Md.; Difco Laboratories, Detroit, Mich.; Gibco Diagnostics, Madison, Wisc.

†Available in 4-g amounts from The Upjohn Co., Kalamazoo, Mich., as Actidione.

‡Available from Parke, Davis & Co., Detroit, Mich., as Chloromycetin.

is used for the isolation of fungi when contaminating microorganisms may be present.

Sabouraud dextrose broth

Dextrose	40 g
Peptone	10 g
Distilled water	1,000 ml

Dissolve ingredients, dispense in 10-ml amounts in 18- by 150-mm tubes, and autoclave at 121 C for 10 minutes. Sabouraud dextrose broth is useful for differentiation of *Candida* species.

Salmonella-Shigella (SS) agar*

Beef extract	5 g
Peptone	5 g
Lactose	10 g
Bile salts mixture	8.5 g
Sodium citrate	8.5 g
Sodium thiosulfate	8.5 g
Ferric citrate	1 g
Agar	13.5 g
Brilliant green	0.33 g
Neutral red	0.025 g
Distilled water	1,000 ml

Dissolve by boiling. **Do not autoclave.**

Salmonella-Shigella agar is used primarily as a selective medium for isolation of salmonellae and shigellae, while inhibiting coliform bacilli. It can also differentiate lactose-fermenting from nonlactose-fermenting strains.

Schneider's Drosophila medium†

(Supplemented with 30% v/v fetal calf serum)

Schneider's Drosophila medium is used for primary isolation as well as routine maintenance of a wide variety of leishmanial and trypanosomal species.

---

*Available in dehydrated form from Difco Laboratories, Detroit, Mich.; BBL Microbiology Systems, Cockeysville, Md.; Gibco Diagnostics, Madison, Wisc.; Inolex Division, Glenwood, Ill.

†Gibco Diagnostics, Madison, Wisc.

Scott's modified Castañeda media and thioglycollate broth for blood culture

AGAR BOTTLE—SLANT

Trypticase soy agar*	40 g
Agar, granulated	15 g
Distilled water	1,000 ml

Heat in autoclave at 121 C for 5 minutes to melt agar or heat on a hot plate with a magnetic stirring bar.

AGAR BOTTLE—BROTH

Trypticase soy broth*	30 g
Sodium polyanethol sulfonate (SPS)	5 ml
("Grobax," 5% sterile solution SPS)†	
Distilled water	1,000 ml

THIOGLYCOLLATE MEDIUM (135 C)‡

	30 g
Sucrose	100 g
Sodium polyanethol sulfonate (SPS)	5 ml
Distilled water	1,000 ml
(pH of all media after autoclaving should be 7.2 ± 0.2)	

1. Dispense agar medium (slant) in the melted state in approximately 20-ml amounts into each of 50 clean, nonchipped, 4-ounce, square, clear-glass, screw-capped bottles (10 ml in 2-ounce bottles).§
2. Insert the disposable rubber diaphragms in the special screw caps, which are then applied loosely on the bottle tops.
3. Dispense the thioglycollate medium into 50 clean bottles, approximately 75 ml per bottle (30 ml in 2-ounce bottles), and apply screw caps as noted earlier.
4. Make up trypticase broth in a 2-liter flask and plug. Prepare a dispensing buret (a 300-ml Salvarsan tube‖ or satisfactory substitute)

---

*Available in dehydrated form from Difco Laboratories, Detroit, Mich.; BBL Microbiology Systems, Cockeysville, Md.; Gibco Diagnostics, Madison, Wisc.

†Roche Diagnostics, Nutley, N.J. (No. 43000).

‡BBL Microbiology Systems, Cockeysville, Md.

§Blood culture bottles (St. Louis Health Dept. type) with special screw caps and disposable rubber diaphragms, 4-ounce and 2-ounce sizes, can be obtained from Curtin Scientific Co., Rockville, Md., and others.

‖Arthur H. Thomas Co., Philadelphia.

to the end of which are attached a 2-foot length of rubber tubing, a needle holder, and a 1½-inch, 21-gauge needle, in that order. Insert the attached needle, together with a portion of the rubber tubing, in the top of the buret, and make fast by plugging, thus assuring a closed unit during sterilization.

5. Autoclave all media and equipment at 118 C to 121 C for 12 to 15 minutes.
6. As soon as the pressure reaches zero, open the autoclave, remove all bottles rapidly, and tightly fasten the screw caps. The hands must be protected from the hot bottles by asbestos gloves.
7. Place the bottles containing the agar on their sides on a cool table top to permit hardening of the agar layer. After about 1 hour, place bottles upright, and sterilize tops with alcohol sponges.* (The agar does not become detached from the sides of the bottles.)
8. Clamp the sterile dispensing buret to a ring stand. Using aseptic technique, fill the buret with sterile trypticase broth.
9. To each agar slant bottle add 60 ml of broth (25 ml in 2-ounce bottles) by puncturing the rubber diaphragm with the sterile needle. The partial vacuum in each bottle will readily permit addition of this amount.
10. Incubate agar slant bottles at 35 C for 48 hours to ensure sterility. The thioglycollate bottles do not need incubation for a sterility check.
11. Inspect bottles, label, and store at room temperature (shelf life is 6 months).

*At the Wilmington Medical Center the use of a loose application of a piece of steam autoclave tape (No. 1222-3M) to the bottle top, which is then fastened down after sterilization, obviates the need for disinfection of the diaphragm when filling with broth (step 8) or when collecting the blood culture.

Selenite-F enrichment medium*
(Leifson: Am. J. Hyg. 24:423, 1936)

Sodium hydrogen selenite (anhydrous)	0.4%
Sodium phosphate (anhydrous)	1%
Peptone	0.5%
Lactose	0.4%

(Final pH 7)

Dissolve ingredients in distilled water. Sterilize gently; 30 minutes in flowing steam in an autoclave is sufficient. It is important to note that the medium should not be autoclaved. This medium is used for the selective isolation of *Salmonella* and some strains of *Shigella*.

Sellers differential agar†
(Bact. Proc. 1963, p. 65)

Yeast extract	1 g
Peptone	20 g
L-Arginine	1 g
D-Mannitol	2 g
Bromthymol blue	0.04 g
Phenol red	0.008 g
Sodium chloride	2 g
Sodium nitrate	1 g
Sodium nitrite	0.35 g
Magnesium sulfate	1.5 g
Dipotassium phosphate	1 g
Agar	15 g

To rehydrate the medium suspend 45 g in 1,000 ml of cold distilled water, and heat to boiling to dissolve the medium completely. Dispense into test tubes, and stopper with cotton plugs or loosely fitting caps. Sterilize in the autoclave for 10 minutes at 15 pounds pressure (121 C). Allow the tubes to cool in the slanted position to give approximately 1½-inch butts and 3-inch slants. **Immediately before inoculating,** add 2 large drops or 0.15 ml of a sterile 50% glucose solution to each tube by letting it run down the **side of the tube opposite the slant.**

*Available in dehydrated form from BBL Microbiology Systems, Cockeysville, Md.; Difco Laboratories, Detroit, Mich.; Gibco Diagnostics, Madison, Wisc.
†Difco Laboratories, Detroit, Mich.; BBL Microbiology Systems, Cockeysville, Md.; Gibco Diagnostics, Madison, Wisc.

TABLE 42-1

Reactions produced on Sellers medium by nonfermentative gram-negative bacilli

Organism	Slant color	Butt color	Band color	Fluorescent slant	Nitrogen gas
Pseudomonas aeruginosa	Green	Blue or no change	Sometimes blue	Yellow-green	Produced
Acinetobacter calcoaceticus var. *anitratus*	Blue	No change	Yellow	Absent	Absent
A. calcoaceticus var. *lwoffii*	Blue	No change	Absent	Absent	Absent
Alcaligenes faecalis	Blue	Blue or no change	Absent	Absent	Produced

Inoculate the tubes by stabbing deep into the butt and streaking the slant. Incubate for 24 hours at 35 C. The final reaction of the medium will be pH 6.7 at 25 C.

Sellers differential agar is useful for differentiating and identifying nonfermentative gram-negative bacilli that produce an alkaline reaction on TSI agar (or KIA). The dehydrated medium is prepared according to the formula of Sellers and is recommended. This medium is particularly useful in differentiating *Pseudomonas aeruginosa*, *Acinetobacter calcoaceticus*, and *Alcaligenes faecalis* (Table 42-1).

Sodium chloride broth (6.5%)

Heart infusion broth*	100 ml
Sodium chloride	6 g

Brain-heart infusion broth contains 0.5% sodium chloride. Thus, by adding an additional 6%, the desired concentration is obtained. The medium is selective for enterococci and other salt-tolerant organisms and is useful in identification as well.

*Available in dehydrated form from BBL Microbiology Systems, Cockeysville, Md.; Difco Laboratories, Detroit, Mich.; Gibco Diagnostics, Madison, Wisc.; Inolex Division, Glenwood, Ill.

Sodium-gelatin-phosphate enrichment broth

See Chapter 9.

Starch agar medium

Bacto-agar	20 g
Bacto-peptone	5 g
Beef extract	3 g
Sodium chloride	5 g
Soluble starch	20 g
Distilled water	1,000 ml

(Final pH 7.2±)

1. Dissolve the agar in 300 ml of water with heat.
2. Dissolve the beef extract and peptone in 200 ml of water.
3. Mix the solutions in steps 1 and 2, and make up to 1,000 ml volume.
4. To this mixture add the starch, dissolve, and autoclave at 121 C for 15 minutes.

The medium may be dispensed in tubes (15- to 20-ml amounts) or flasks convenient for pouring plates and should be stored in a refrigerator. For pouring of plates, melt the medium in tubes or flasks as required. **If poured plates of starch agar are refrigerated, the medium becomes opaque.**

Starch agar is useful in developing smooth cultures by streaking borderline rough strains on the surface of the medium. It also may be used for testing cultures for starch hydrolytic activity.

Stock culture and motility medium
(Hugh. In ASM Man. Clin. Microbiol. ed. 2, 1974, p. 263)

Casitone	10 g
Yeast extract	3 g
Sodium chloride	5 g
Agar	3 g
Distilled water	1,000 ml

1. Suspend the ingredients in distilled water; heat to boiling to completely dissolve agar.
2. Dispense in 13- by 100-mm screw-capped tubes, 4 ml per tube.
3. Sterilize by autoclaving at 121 C for 15 minutes; store as butts.

This medium is used for motility testing by stabbing the inoculum once into the agar and incubating overnight at 35 C. Motility is indicated by growth spreading out from the line of stab.

The medium is also excellent for preserving stock cultures of non-fermenting and fermenting gram-negative rods (up to 6 months). After inoculation and overnight incubation, the caps are sealed with tape and the tubes refrigerated.

Sucrose (5%) broth or agar

Prepare a 50% aqueous solution of sucrose, sterilize in an autoclave at 10 pounds pressure for 10 minutes, and refrigerate.

To prepare broth add aseptically 0.5 ml of the stock sucrose solution to 5 ml of tubed sterile infusion broth.

To prepare agar plates add aseptically 1.5 ml of the stock sucrose solution to 15 ml of sterile melted agar. Mix well, and pour into a sterile Petri dish.

Tellurite reduction test medium
Medium

1. Suspend 4.7 g of Middlebrook 7H9 dehy-

drated base* in 900 ml of distilled water, and add 0.5 ml of Tween 80.
2. Autoclave at 121 C for 15 minutes, cool to 55 C, and add aseptically 100 ml ACD enrichment.*
3. Dispense aseptically in 5-ml amounts in 20- by 150-mm screw-capped tubes, check for sterility, and refrigerate.

Tellurite solution

1. Dissolve 0.2 g of potassium tellurite in 100 ml of distilled water.
2. Dispense in 2- to 5-ml amounts, and sterilize by autoclaving at 121 C for 10 minutes.

This medium is used to test the ability of certain mycobacteria of Runyon group III nonphotochromogens to reduce tellurite rapidly to the **black,** metallic tellurium.

Tetrathionate broth†

Proteose peptone‡	5 g
Bile salts	1 g
Calcium carbonate	10 g
Sodium thiosulfate	30 g
Distilled water	1,000 ml

Dispense the medium in 10-ml amounts, and heat to boiling. **Before use** add 0.2 ml of iodine solution (6 g of iodine crystals and 5 g of potassium iodide in 20 ml of water) to each tube.

This is a selective liquid enrichment medium for use in the isolation of *Salmonella*, except *S. typhi*. The sterile base **without iodine** may be stored in a refrigerator indefinitely.

Thayer-Martin (TMF) agar

GC agar base† (double strength)	72 g
Agar	10 g
Distilled water	1,000 ml

*Difco Laboratories, Detroit, Mich.; BBL Microbiology Systems, Cockeysville, Md.
†Available in dehydrated form from Difco Laboratories, Detroit, Mich.; BBL Microbiology Systems, Cockeysville, Md.; Gibco Diagnostics, Madison, Wisc.
‡Difco Laboratories, Detroit, Mich.

1. Suspend the dehydrated medium in water, mix well, and heat with agitation. Boil for 1 minute.
2. Sterilize by autoclaving at 121 C for 15 minutes.
3. At the same time, autoclave a suspension of 20 g of dehydrated hemoglobin in 1,000 ml water for 15 minutes (suspension must be **smooth** before sterilizing).
4. Cool both to 50 C, mix aseptically, then add 20 ml IsoVitaleX enrichment (BBL) and 20 ml V-C-N inhibitor (BBL). Pour plates, using 20 ml per plate. Refrigerate.

This medium is recommended for the isolation of *Neisseria gonorrhoeae* from all sites that might contain a mixed flora, as well as for the recovery of *N. meningitidis* from nasopharyngeal and throat cultures.

Modified Thayer-Martin medium (MTM) has 2% agar, 0.25% glucose, and trimethoprim lactate, which is inhibitory to *Proteus*.

Thioglycollate medium without indicator* (THIO)
(Brewer: J. Bacteriol. 39:10, 1940; and 46:395, 1943)

Peptone	20 g
L-Cystine	0.25 g
Glucose	6 g
Sodium chloride	2.5 g
Sodium thioglycollate	0.5 g
Sodium sulfite	0.1 g
Agar	0.7 g
Distilled water	1,000 ml
(Final pH 7.2±)	

Dispense the medium in 15-ml amounts in 6- by ¾-inch test tubes, making a column of medium 7 cm high. Autoclave for 15 minutes at 121 C. **Store at room temperature.**

---

*Available in dehydrated form from BBL Microbiology Systems, Cockeysville, Md. (No. 11720); Difco Laboratories, Detroit, Mich. (No. 0430); Gibco Diagnostics, Madison, Wisc. (No. B6434). It is also available with indicator. This may be enriched by the addition of 10% normal rabbit or horse serum when cool.

Enriched THIO is prepared by adding to the freshly prepared and autoclaved medium (or to previously prepared medium that has been boiled for 10 minutes and then cooled) vitamin K_1 solution (see Chapter 44), 0.1 µg/ml; sodium bicarbonate, 1 mg/ml; and hemin (see Chapter 44), 5 µg/ml. Rabbit or horse serum (10%) or Fildes enrichment (5%) may also be added.

Thionine or basic fuchsin agar
(Huddleson et al.: Brucellosis in man and animals, New York, 1939, The Commonwealth Fund)

Trypticase soy agar may be used as a base for differential media containing thionine and basic fuchsin.

Prepare the dyes, thionine and basic fuchsin, in 0.1% stock solutions in sterile distilled water. These stock solutions may be stored indefinitely. Before adding to the media, heat the dye solutions in flowing steam in an autoclave for 20 minutes, shake well, and while still hot, add to melted agar. In trypticase soy agar the final concentration of the dye should be 1:100,000 (10 ml/liter of medium). Thoroughly mix the dyes (added individually) and the melted agar, and pour immediately into Petri dishes, one set containing thionine and one containing basic fuchsin. Place the plates in a 35 C incubator until the water of condensation disappears, at which time they are ready for use. Inoculate plates within 24 hours of preparation.

Streak the surface of plates with a heavy suspension of *Brucella* prepared from a 48- to 72-hour trypticase soy agar slant culture. It is advisable to streak plates in duplicate, incubating one set aerobically and the other in 10% CO_2. Incubate plates for 72 hours, and observe for **inhibition of growth** by thionine or basic fuchsin or both.

Tinsdale agar, Moore and Parsons, modified*

Proteose No. 3 or Thiotone peptic digest of animal tissue USP	20 g

---

*Difco Laboratories, Detroit, Mich.

L-Cystine	0.24 g
Sodium chloride	5 g
Sodium thiosulfate	0.43 g
Agar, dried or	14 g
not dried	20 g
Distilled water	1,000 ml

(Final pH 7.4)

1. Heat with agitation, and boil for 1 minute. Dispense.
2. Autoclave at 121 C for 15 minutes. Cool to 56 C, and to each 100 ml of base add:

Sterile serum (e.g., bovine)	10 ml
Potassium tellurite, 1% aqueous	3 ml

3. Alternatively, the thiosulfate may be dissolved in 1.7 ml of water and added separately. It must be prepared fresh each time the medium is prepared. The cystine may be dissolved in 6 ml of 0.1 N HCl and added separately, in which case it may be necessary to add 6 ml of 0.1 N NaOH to make sure that the final pH is correct.

Todd-Hewitt broth, modified*
(J. Pathol. Bacteriol. 35:973, 1932)

Beef heart infusion	1,000 ml
Neopeptone	20 g

Adjust to pH 7 with normal sodium hydroxide and add:

Sodium chloride	2 g
Sodium bicarbonate	2 g
Disodium phosphate	0.4 g
Glucose	2 g

(Final pH 7.8±)

Mix the chemicals in broth, and bring to a slow boil. Boil for 15 minutes, filter through paper, dispense in tubes, and autoclave at 115 C for 10 minutes.

Modified Todd-Hewitt broth is used for growing streptococci for serologic identification.

Transport media
Buffered glycerol-saline base* (Sachs' modification)

Sodium chloride	4.2 g
Potassium dihydrophosphate (KH_2PO_4)	1 g
Potassium orthophosphate (K_2HPO_4)	3.1 g
Phenol red	0.003 g
Distilled water	700 ml
Glycerol	300 ml

(Adjust final pH to 7.2)

Dispense in 10-ml amounts in 30-ml screw-capped bottles. Sterilize for 10 minutes at 116 C.

This solution serves as an excellent stool specimen preservative and transport medium for fecal material.

Cary and Blair transport medium*

Disodium phosphate	1.1 g
Sodium chloride	5 g
Sodium thioglycollate	1.5 g
Agar	5 g
Distilled water	991 ml

Add the ingredients to a chemically clean flask rinsed with Sorensen's 0.067 M buffer (pH 8.1). Heat with frequent agitation until the solution just becomes clear. Cool to 50 C. Add 9 ml of freshly prepared aqueous 1% $CaCl_2$, and adjust the pH to 8.4.

Distribute 7 ml into previously rinsed and sterilized 9-ml screw-capped vials. Steam for 15 minutes, cool, and tighten caps.

Specimen preservative medium†
(Hajna: Public Health Lab. 13:83, 1955

Sodium desoxycholate	0.5 g
Yeast extract	1 g
Sodium chloride	5 g
Sodium citrate · 2 H_2O	5 g
Potassium dihydrophosphate (KH_2PO_4)	2 g
Magnesium sulfate · 7 H_2O	0.4 g
$(NH_4)_2 HPO_4$	4 g
Distilled water	700 ml

(Final pH 7)

---

*Available in dehydrated form from BBL Microbiology Systems, Cockeysville, Md.; Difco Laboratories, Detroit, Mich:, Gibco Diagnostics, Madison, Wisc.

*BBL Microbiology Systems, Cockeysville, Md.
†BBL Microbiology Systems, Cockeysville, Md.; Difco Laboratories, Detroit, Mich.

Dissolve ingredients by heating. Add 300 ml of glycerol, mix well, dispense into tubes (or vials), and sterilize at 116 C for 10 minutes.

This medium is useful as a stool specimen preservative and to transport fecal material.

Amies transport medium*
(Amies: Can. J. Public Health 58:296-300, 1967)

1. Add 4 g of agar to 1 liter of distilled water, heat until dissolved, and while hot add:

Sodium chloride	3 g
Potassium chloride	0.2 g
Sodium thioglycollate	1 g
Disodium phosphate, anhydrous	1.15 g
(or disodium phosphate · 12 H₂O)	2.9 g
Monopotassium phosphate	0.2 g
Calcium chloride, 1% aqueous, freshly prepared	10 ml
Magnesium chloride · 6 H₂O, 1% aqueous	10 ml

(Final pH 7.3)

2. Stir until dissolved, and then add 10 g of pharmaceutical neutral charcoal. Dispense 5 to 6 ml per 13- by 100-mm screw-capped tube (or vial), with frequent stirring to keep the charcoal in suspension. Avoid cooling or gelling.
3. Sterilize at 121 C for 20 minutes. **Prior to solidification,** invert tubes to distribute the charcoal evenly. Store in refrigerator.
4. It should be emphasized that prolonged heating in open flasks should be avoided, since the reducing agent (sodium thioglycollate) is volatile.

Transport media for Chlamydia

See Chapter 11.

Triple sugar iron (TSI) agar*
(Hajna: J. Bacteriol. 49:516, 1945)

Peptone	20 g
Sodium chloride	5 g
Lactose	10 g
Sucrose	10 g
Glucose	1 g
Ferrous ammonium sulfate	0.2 g
Sodium thiosulfate	0.2 g
Phenol red	0.025 g
Agar	13 g
Distilled water	1,000 ml

(Final pH 7.3±)

TSI agar is used for determining carbohydrate fermentation and hydrogen sulfide production as a first step in the identification of gram-negative bacilli.

This medium is considered to be a modification of KIA. The only difference between the two is that sucrose is not included in KIA. It should be stressed that pH changes in the butt and in the slant of the medium must be recorded only after 18 to 24 hours of incubation.

Trypticase dextrose agar†

Trypticase	20 g
Dextrose	5 g
Agar	3.5 g
Bromthymol blue	0.01 g
Distilled water	1,000 ml

(Final pH 7.3±)

Trypticase dextrose agar can be used to determine motility and dextrose fermentation of aerobic and anaerobic organisms.

Prepare according to the directions on the label.

Trypticase lactose iron agar†

Trypticase	20 g
Lactose	10 g

---

*Difco Laboratories, Detroit, Mich.; Gibco Diagnostics, Madison, Wisc.

---

*Available in dehydrated form from BBL Microbiology Systems, Cockeysville, Md.; Difco Laboratories, Detroit, Mich.; Gibco Diagnostics, Madison, Wisc.; Inolex Division, Glenwood, Ill.

†Available in dehydrated form from BBL Microbiology Systems, Cockeysville, Md.

Ferrous sulfate	0.2 g
Agar	3.5 g
Sodium sulfite	0.4 g
Sodium thiosulfate	0.08 g
Phenol red	0.02 g
Distilled water	1,000 ml

(Final pH 7.3±)

This medium can be used for the determination of motility, lactose fermentation, and production of hydrogen sulfide by aerobes and anaerobes.

Trypticase nitrate broth*†

Trypticase	20 g
Disodium phosphate	2 g
Glucose	1 g
Agar	1 g
Potassium nitrate	1 g
Distilled water	1,000 ml

(pH 7.2)

This medium is used to demonstrate indole production and nitrate reduction by aerobes and anaerobes.

Trypticase soy agar*

Trypticase	15 g
Phytone	5 g
Sodium chloride	5 g
Agar	15 g
Distilled water	1,000 ml

(Final pH 7.3±)

Trypticase soy agar is an excellent **blood agar base** and can be used for the isolation and maintenance of all organisms, except some with very special nutritional requirements.

Trypticase soy broth*

Trypticase	17 g
Phytone	3 g
Sodium chloride	5 g
Dipotassium phosphate	2.5 g
Glucose	2.5 g
Distilled water	1,000 ml

(Final pH 7.3±)

*Available in dehydrated form from BBL Microbiology Systems, Cockeysville, Md.
†Indole nitrate medium (No. 11298).

Trypticase soy broth is excellent for the rapid (6 to 8 hours) growth of most organisms and supports growth of pneumococci and streptococci without the addition of blood or serum. It also supports growth of *Brucella*. However, fermentation of the glucose present will cause a drop in pH, and acid-sensitive organisms, particularly pneumococci, may die in 18 to 24 hours.

Trypticase sucrose agar*

Trypticase	20 g
Sucrose	10 g
Agar	3.5 g
Phenol red	0.02 g
Distilled water	1,000 ml

(Final pH 7.2±)

This medium can be used to determine motility and sucrose fermentation by aerobes and anaerobes.

Tryptophane broth

Tryptophane broth is a popular medium for the detection of indole production. Trypticase (BBL) or tryptone (Difco) is recommended, in 1% aqueous solution. Follow label directions for preparation.

Tyrosine or xanthine agar

Nutrient agar	23 g
Tyrosine or	5 g
Xanthine	4 g
Demineralized water	1,000 ml

1. Dissolve the nutrient agar in the water.
2. Add tyrosine or xanthine, and mix to distribute the crystals evenly.
3. Adjust to pH 7.0, and autoclave at 121 C for 15 minutes.
4. Dispense in plates, 20 ml per plate, with the crystals evenly distributed.

Tyrosine or xanthine agar is recommended for differentiation of species of aerobic actinomycetes. Its use is similar to that of casein agar.

*Available in dehydrated form from BBL Microbiology Systems, Cockeysville, Md.

Urea agar—urease test medium*
(Christensen: J. Bacteriol. 52:461, 1946)

Peptone	1 g
Glucose	1 g
Sodium chloride	5 g
Monopotassium phosphate	2 g
Phenol red	0.012 g
Agar	20 g
Distilled water	1,000 ml

(Final pH 6.8 to 6.9)

Prepare the agar base, and sterilize in the autoclave at 121 C for 15 minutes in flasks containing 100- to 200-ml amounts. Store until needed. Prepare a 29% solution of urea. Sterilize by filtering through a sterile bacteriologic filter. Add the sterile urea solution in a final concentration of 10% to a flask of the agar base that has been melted and cooled to a temperature of 50 C. Mix well, and distribute aseptically into sterile small tubes in amounts of 2 to 3 ml. Allow the medium to solidify in a slanting position in such a way as to obtain an agar butt of ½ inch and an agar slant of 1 inch.

Urea agar can be used to demonstrate **urease production** by species of *Proteus*. It also detects the small amounts of urease produced by other enteric bacilli, thus differentiating them from urease-negative *Salmonella* and *Shigella*. It also may be used to detect urease production by *Cryptococcus* species.

Urease test broth†
(Rustigian and Stuart)

See Chapter 44.

Xanthine agar

See p. 647.

Xylose lysine desoxycholate (XLD) agar*
(Taylor: Am. J. Clin. Pathol. 44:471, 1965)

This medium may be prepared by using the dehydrated xylose lysine agar base* and adding the sodium thiosulfate, ferric ammonium citrate, and sodium desoxycholate (procedure recommended by some workers) or by utilizing the complete (XLD) agar.

Xylose	3.5 g
L-Lysine	5 g
Lactose	7.5 g
Sucrose	7.5 g
Sodium chloride	5 g
Yeast extract	3 g
Phenol red	0.08 g
Agar, dried	13.5 g
Sodium desoxycholate	2.5 g
Sodium thiosulfate	6.8 g
Ferric ammonium citrate	0.8 g
Distilled water	1,000 ml

(Final pH 7.4±)

Suspend the medium in distilled water, and heat with frequent agitation just to the boiling point. **Do not boil.** Transfer immediately to a 50 C water bath, and pour plates as soon as the medium has cooled. The medium should be red-orange and clear, or nearly so. Excessive heating or prolonged holding at 50 C may cause precipitation, which could lead to some differences in colony morphology.

This medium is useful for the isolation of enteric pathogens, especially shigellae.

---

*Available in dehydrated form from BBL Microbiology Systems, Cockeysville, Md.; Difco Laboratories, Detroit, Mich.; Gibco Diagnostics, Madison, Wisc.; Inolex Division, Glenwood, Ill.

†BBL Microbiology Systems, Cockeysville, Md.; Difco Laboratories, Detroit, Mich.; Gibco Diagnostics, Madison, Wisc.; Inolex Division, Glenwood, Ill.

---

*BBL Microbiology Systems, Cockeysville, Md.; Difco Laboratories, Detroit, Mich.; Gibco Diagnostics, Madison, Wisc.; Inolex Division, Glenwood, Ill.

43 STAINING FORMULAS AND PROCEDURES

STAINS

Although a number of the more important staining formulas and procedures are presented in this chapter, space does not permit a comprehensive review of the subject. Further details are available in the *Manual of Clinical Microbiology*.[3] The solubilities of the more widely used stains and dyes, in water and in alcohol, are shown in Table 43-1.

Acid-fast stain

See also Fluorochrome stain, pp. 653-655.

Kinyoun carbolfuchsin method
(Kinyoun: Am. J. Pub. Health 5:867, 1915)

Basic fuchsin	4 g
Phenol	8 ml
Alcohol (95%)	20 ml
Distilled water	100 ml

Dissolve the basic fuchsin in the alcohol, and add the water slowly while shaking. Melt the phenol in a 56 C water bath, and add 8 ml to the stain, using a pipet with a rubber bulb.

Stain the fixed smear for 3 to 5 minutes (no heat necessary), and continue as with Ziehl-Neelsen stain.

TABLE 43-1

Solubility of stains

Stain	Percent soluble at 26 C	
	In water	In 95% ethanol
Bismarck brown	1.36	1.08
Congo red	0	0.19
Crystal violet (chloride)	1.68	13.87
Eosin Y	44.2	2.18
Fuchsin, basic (chloride)	0.26	5.93
Malachite green (oxalate)	7.60	7.52
Methylene blue (chloride)	3.55	1.48
Neutral red (chloride)	5.64	2.45
Safranin O	5.45	3.41
Thionin	0.25	0.25

Data from Conn.[2]

By the addition of a detergent or wetting agent the staining of acid-fast organisms may be accelerated. Tergitol No. 7* may be used. Add 1 drop of Tergitol No. 7 to every 30 to 40 ml of the Kinyoun carbolfuchsin stain. Stain the smears for 1 minute, decolorize, and counterstain as described in the following section.

The technique and interpretation of the acid-fast stain are given in Chapter 3.

Ziehl-Neelsen method

CARBOLFUCHSIN STAIN

Basic fuchsin	0.3 g
Ethanol (95%)	10 ml

Mix these with the following:

Phenol, melted crystals	5 ml
Distilled water	95 ml

ACID ALCOHOL*

Hydrochloric acid, concentrated	3 ml
Ethanol (95%)	97 ml

COUNTERSTAIN

Methylene blue	0.3 g
Distilled water	100 ml

Some workers may prefer 0.5% aqueous brilliant green or a saturated solution of picric acid as a counterstain; the latter is pale and does not selectively stain cellular material.

1. Prepare a smear of appropriate thickness; dry and fix as described previously.
2. Place a strip of filter paper slightly smaller than the slide over the smear.
3. Flood the slide with carbolfuchsin stain; heat to steaming with a low Bunsen flame or electrically heated slide warmer. **Do not boil,** and do not allow to dry out.
4. Allow to stand 5 minutes without further heating; then remove the paper, and wash the slide in running water.
5. Decolorize to a faint pink with acid alcohol while continuously agitating the slide until no more stain comes off in the washings (approximately 1 minute for films of average thickness). Thoroughness in decolorization is essential to prevent the possibility of a false-positive reading.
6. Wash with water; counterstain with methylene blue for 20 to 30 seconds.
7. Wash with water, dry in air, and examine under the oil immersion lens.

Auramine-rhodamine stain

See Fluorochrome stain, pp. 653-655.

Capsule stain

The principles of capsule stains are discussed in Chapter 3.

---

*Carbide and Carbon Chemical Corporation, New York, N.Y.

*Use a 1% aqueous solution of sulfuric acid or 0.5% acid alcohol as a decolorizer when staining smears of suspected acid-fast *Nocardia*, such as *N. asteroides*.

Anthony method

1. Make a thin even smear of a culture in skimmed milk or litmus milk by spreading with a glass slide or an inoculating needle bent at a right angle. If it is not a milk culture, a loopful of the material may be mixed with a loopful of skimmed milk and then spread to give a uniform background.
2. Air dry. Do not fix with heat.
3. Stain with 1% aqueous crystal violet for 2 minutes.
4. Wash with a solution of 20% copper sulfate.
5. Air dry in a vertical position, and examine under the oil immersion lens. The capsule is unstained against a purple background; the cells are deeply stained.

Hiss method

Mix a loopful of physiologic saline suspension of growth with a drop of normal serum on a glass slide. Allow the smear to air dry and heat fix. Flood the smear with crystal violet (1% aqueous solution). Steam the preparation gently for 1 minute, and rinse with copper sulfate (20% aqueous solution). Capsules appear as faint blue halos around dark blue to purple cells.

India ink method*

In the India ink method, the capsule displaces the colloidal carbon particles of the ink and appears as a clear halo around the microorganism. The procedure is especially recommended for demonstrating the capsule of *Cryptococcus neoformans*.

1. To a small loopful of saline, water or broth on a clean slide, add a **minute amount of growth** from a young agar culture, using an inoculating needle. Spinal fluid may be used directly.
2. Mix well; then add a small loopful of India

---

*Not all India inks are suitable. Pelikan India ink made by Gunther Wagner of Hanover, Germany, is recommended; add about 0.3% tricresol as a preservative.

ink and immediately cover with a thin coverglass, allowing the fluid to spread as a thin film beneath the coverglass.
3. Examine immediately under the oil immersion objective, reducing the light considerably by lowering the condenser. Capsules, when present, stand out as **clear halos** against a dark background.

Muir method

MUIR MORDANT

Tannic acid, 20% aqueous solution	2 parts
Saturated aqueous solution of mercuric chloride	2 parts
Saturated aqueous solution of potassium alum	5 parts

1. Prepare a thin even film of bacteria; allow to dry in air.
2. Cover the film with a piece of filter paper the size of the smear, and flood the slide with Ziehl-Neelsen carbolfuchsin.
3. Heat to steaming with a low Bunsen flame for 30 seconds.
4. Rinse gently with 95% ethanol and then with water.
5. Add the mordant for 15 to 30 seconds; wash well with water.
6. Decolorize with ethanol to a faint pink; wash with water.
7. Counterstain with 0.3% methylene blue for 30 seconds.
8. Air dry and examine under the oil immersion lens. The cells are stained red and the capsules blue.

Carbolfuchsin counterstain for Legionella pneumophila

SOLUTION A

Basic fuchsin	0.3 gm
Ethyl alcohol	10 ml

SOLUTION B

Phenol (melted crystals)	5 ml
Distilled water	95 ml

Prepare the counterstain by mixing solutions A and B together. Stain the smears according to the procedure generally practiced for other bacteria. Counterstain with carbolfuchsin solution for 1 minute. Examine the smears microscopically, using an oil immersion objective ($\times$100).

Dieterle stain (modified)

The Dieterle stain is a silver impregnation stain and is used for demonstrating *Legionella* in paraffin-embedded tissue sections. The complicated procedure is described in detail by Van Orden and Greer.[5]

Flagella stain

(Gray: J. Bacteriol. 12:273, 1926)

MORDANT

Potassium alum, saturated aqueous solution	5 ml
Tannic acid, 20% aqueous solution	2 ml
Mercuric chloride, saturated aqueous solution	2 ml

Mix and add 0.4 ml of a saturated alcoholic solution of basic fuchsin. Make up fresh mordant for use each day.

Gray method

1. Using a grease-free, well-cleaned slide that has been flamed and cooled, spread a drop of distilled water on the slide to cover an area of approximately 2 sq cm.
2. Select part of a colony from a young agar culture or take a small amount of growth from a slant with an inoculating needle and **touch gently** into the drop of water at several places on the slide; then gently rotate the slide.
3. Allow to **air dry. Do not heat.**
4. Add the mordant, and allow it to act for 10 minutes.
5. Wash gently with distilled water or clean tap water.
6. Add Ziehl-Neelsen carbolfuchsin, and leave it on for 5 to 10 minutes.
7. Wash with tap water, air dry, and examine under oil.

Recently a simplified version of the Leifson flagella stain was reported by Clark.[1] Employing scrupulously clean slides and organisms taken directly from 24- and 48-hour blood agar plates, this method proved to be a simple and reliable procedure. Readers interested in this procedure should consult the original paper.

Silver stain for flagella

SOLUTION A (MORDANT OR PRESTAIN)

Saturated aqueous solution of aluminum potassium sulfate (approximately 14 g/ 100 ml of water) (maintain as stock)	25 ml
Tannic acid, 10%	50 ml
Ferric chloride solution, 5% (maintain as stock)	5 ml

Combine and store in dark bottle at room temperature. The solution will remain stable for several months.

SOLUTION B (SILVER STAIN)

1. Prepare 100 ml of 5% silver nitrate solution.
2. Add concentrated ammonium hydroxide (2 to 5 ml) dropwise to 90 ml of the 5% silver nitrate solution until the brown precipitate formed just redissolves.
3. Add some of the remaining 5% silver nitrate dropwise to the solution until a faint cloudiness persists.
4. Store the solution in a dark bottle at room temperature. The solution will remain stable for several months.

STAINING PROCEDURE

1. Label and flame commercially cleaned slides to burn off any residue. While the slides are hot, a heavy line may be drawn with wax pencil to reduce the amount of stain needed (optional).
2. Using growth from 18- to 24-hour cultures on heart infusion or trypticase soy agar slants incubated at 35 C, prepare a light suspension of organisms in 3 ml of sterile distilled water.* Suspension should be only slightly cloudy and less than 0.5 McFarland standard.

---

*Note: Do not use any fluid for suspension other than distilled water or nutrient broth.

3. Place one large loopful of culture suspension on the flamed slide, and allow it to run to the end. Allow to air dry. Do not fix.
4. Place the slide on staining rack, and flood with Solution A. Leave it for 4 minutes, and then rinse with distilled water.
5. Flood the slide with solution B, and heat just until steam is emitted by running a burner under the slide on a rack. Remove the burner, allow the slide to stain 4 minutes, rinse with distilled water, and slant to dry.

Fluorochrome stain (Truant method)

By staining a smear with fluorescent dyes, such as auramine and rhodamine, and examining by fluorescence microscopy using an ultraviolet light source, acid-fast bacilli, when present, appear to glow with a **yellow-orange** color. They are visible under lower magnifications of the microscope; thus, a stained smear can be examined in much less time than is required by conventional methods. Numerous modifications of the procedure have been introduced; that reported by Truant and co-workers[4] is recommended.

Auramine O*	1.5 g
Rhodamine B†	0.75 g
Glycerol	75 ml
Phenol	10 ml
Distilled water	50 ml

Combine the solutions, mix well (using a magnetic stirring device for 24 hours or heating until warm and stirring vigorously for 5 minutes), filter through glass wool, and store in a glass-stoppered bottle at 4 C. The stain is stable for several months under refrigeration.

1. Heat fix on a slide warmer‡ at 65 C for 2 hours or overnight.

---

*Chroma 1B339, Chroma Gesselschaft, Schmid GMBH and Co., available from Roboz Surgical Instrument Co., Inc., Washington, D.C.
†Matheson, Coleman, and Bell, Norwood, Ohio, CI 45170.
‡Microslide staining and drying bath are available from Scientific Products, Division of American Hospital Supply Corp., McGaw Park, Ill.

2. Cover the smear with the auramine-rhodamine solution.
3. Stain for 15 minutes at room temperature or at 35 C.
4. Rinse off with distilled water.
5. Decolorize with 0.5% hydrochloric acid in 70% ethanol for 2 to 3 minutes, then rinse thoroughly with distilled water.
6. Flood the smear with counterstain, a 0.5% solution of potassium permanganate (filter and store in amber bottle), for 2 to 4 minutes (no longer—excessive exposure results in loss of brilliance).
7. Rinse with distilled water, dry, and examine.

Ultraviolet light source

The smears are examined under a binocular microscope using an ultraviolet light source. The Leitz, Zeiss, and Reichert fluorescent microscopy units are highly recommended and are equipped with Osram HBO 200 maximum pressure mercury vapor lamps as light sources, BG 12 (3- or 4-mm) or C 5113 (2-mm) violet exciter filters, and OG 1 deep yellow barrier filters in the eyepieces. This recommended filter combination results in **bright yellow-orange** staining bacilli against a dark background; nonspecific background debris fluoresces a pale yellow, quite distinct from the yellow-orange bacilli.

It is suggested that a drop of immersion oil be placed on the darkfield condenser, the slide inserted, and the microscope first focused under bright light until a clear central area is seen on the slide. The microscope should then be switched over to the ultraviolet source. Smears may be rapidly examined under low- or high-power objective (25× or 40×) with a 10× eyepiece; after a little practice, all smears may be examined at these magnifications or lower in a matter of seconds. Occasionally, it may be necessary to switch to the oil immersion objective to confirm typical morphologic characteristics, such as beading and cording. It is recommended that microscopic examination be carried out in a darkened room for maximum efficiency.

Quartz-halogen illuminator

(Runyon et al. In Lennette, Balows, Hausler, and Truant, editors: Manual of clinical microbiology, ed. 3, Washington, D.C., 1980, American Society for Microbiology)

Excellent demonstration of fluorochrome-stained mycobacteria is obtained by use of a microscope equipped with a quartz-halogen illuminator and the proper combinations of primary (exciter) and secondary (barrier) filters. This system provides the same benefits as ultraviolet apparatus with the added advantages that the **blue light apparatus** does not require a special dark room (although subdued lighting is recommended), does not require oil on the condenser or slide, is simpler and more economical, and does not present radiation hazards. The following recommendations based on use of the Zeiss RA 38 microscope and attachments are applicable to other equipment having comparable features.

The equipment needed is a standard binocular microscope with an illuminator containing a collector lens and a 12-V, 100-W quartz-halogen lamp or high-intensity tungsten bulb, front-surface reflecting mirrors, brightfield condenser, low-power objectives (10× or 25×) for scanning and high-dry (63×) planachromat (flat field; if the high-dry objective is corrected for coverslip, then a coverslip must be placed, not mounted, over the smear), a 100× oil immersion objective for more critical examination of acid-fast (fluorescent) bodies, and 10× compensating eyepieces. A turret or intermediate tube with holder for secondary filters located in the tube body between the objectives and the eyepieces facilitates filter changing. The optics and light path must be precisely aligned to avoid loss of light intensity. The light source is adjusted for Koehler illumination by centering and focusing the lamp filament on the closed iris diaphragm of the condenser. Maximal intensity is obtained by making small adjustments of the condenser while viewing an auramine-stained mycobacterial smear.

Combinations of primary and secondary filters are selected to provide good contrast between a dark background and the fluorescing, yellow bacillus. However, the background must be sufficiently light that nonfluorescing debris can be seen for maintaining focus while scanning the slide. A BG 12 primary filter transmitting only wavelengths less than about 500 nm (peak 404 nm) in combination with secondary filters that transmit only wavelengths above 500 nm or 530 nm, as Zeiss No. 50 or No. 53, respectively, provides satisfactory demonstration of fluorescing mycobacteria. The particular combination of complementary exciter and barrier filters determines the color of the background. The greater the overlap of transmission curves, the lighter the background, and vice versa. Therefore, the user should have on hand BG 12 filters of various thicknesses (1.0, 1.5, 2, 3 mm*) for neutral density purposes and secondary filters having transmission cutoffs at 500, 515, and 530 nm to determine which combinations provide optimal background-contrast qualities. The following exciter and barrier filter combinations have been found to be excellent for demonstrating fluorochrome-stained mycobacteria: 3-mm BG 12 and No. 50—light green background; 4-mm BG 12 and No. 50—dark green; 3-mm BG 12 and No. 53—light brown; 3.5-mm BG 12 and No. 53—dark brown. Another primary filter, the fluorescein isothiocyanate (FITC) interference filter, used in combination with a 3-mm BG 12 and a No. 50 or 53 barrier filter, results in excellent dark green and dark red-brown backgrounds, respectively. The FITC laminated to a BG 38 (to reduce red transmission) and in combination with a 1.5-mm BG 12 produces a reddish-tinged gray background with the No. 50 and a red field with the No. 53.

---

*Fish-Schurman Corp., New Rochelle, N.Y.

All positive smears should be confirmed with a Kinyoun or Ziehl-Neelsen stain. This may be done without removing the auramine-rhodamine stain. The reverse of this procedure is not satisfactory.

Giemsa stain for chlamydiae

(Schachter. In Lennette, Balows, Hausler, and Truant, editors: Manual of clinical microbiology, ed. 3, Washington, D.C., 1980, American Society for Microbiology)

Giemsa stain is prepared by dissolving 0.5 g of powder in 33 ml of glycerol at 55 to 60 C for 1½ to 2 hours. To this is added 33 ml of absolute methanol, acetone free. The solution is mixed thoroughly and allowed to sediment and then is stored at room temperature as stock. Dilutions of the stock stain are made with neutral distilled water or buffered water in a ratio of 1 part of stock Giemsa solution to 40 or 50 parts of diluent.

The smear is air dried, fixed with absolute methanol for at least 5 minutes, and again dried. It is then covered with the diluted Giemsa stain (freshly prepared each day) for 1 hour. The slide is then rinsed rapidly in 95% ethyl alcohol to remove excess dye, dried, and examined for the presence of the typical basophilic intracytoplasmic inclusion body.

Giemsa stain for malaria

See Chapter 35.

Giménez stain for chlamydiae and Legionella

(Schachter. In Lennette, Balows, Hausler, and Truant, editors: Manual of clinical microbiology, ed. 3, Washington, D.C., 1980, American Society for Microbiology)

Stock carbol fuchsin contains 100 ml of 10% (w/v) fuchsin in 95% ethyl alcohol, 250 ml of 4% (v/v) aqueous phenol, and 650 ml of distilled water. This stock solution should be held at 37 C for 48 hours before use; for the "working" solution, the stock is diluted 1:2.5 with phosphate buffer, pH 7.45 (3.5 ml of 0.2 M NaH_2PO_4, 15.5

ml of 0.2 M Na_2HPO_4, and 19 ml of distilled water). This working solution is immediately filtered and is filtered again before every stain. It is usable for 3 to 4 days.

Malachite green is used as 0.8% aqueous malachite green oxalate.

The smear should be heat fixed. Stain the smear as follows: stain with fuchsin for 1 to 2 minutes, wash with tap water; stain with malachite green for 6 to 9 seconds, wash with tap water; restain with malachite green for 6 to 9 seconds, wash thoroughly with tap water, and blot dry. In yolk sac smears, most elementary bodies stain red against a greenish background.

Gram stain (Hucker modification)

REAGENTS

Stock crystal violet	
Crystal violet (85% dye)	20 g
Ethanol (95%)	100 ml
Stock oxalate solution	
Ammonium oxalate	1 g
Distilled water	100 ml

Working solution. Dilute the stock crystal violet solution 1:10 with distilled water, and mix with 4 volumes of stock oxalate solution. Store in a glass-stoppered bottle.

Gram iodine solution	
Iodine crystals	1 g
Potassium iodide	2 g

Dissolve these completely in 5 ml of distilled water; then add:

Distilled water	240 ml
Sodium bicarbonate, 5% aqueous solution	60 ml

Mix well; store in an amber-glass bottle.

Decolorizer	
Ethanol (95%)	250 ml
Acetone	250 ml

Mix; store in a glass-stoppered bottle.

Counterstain (Stock safranin)	
Safranin O	2.5 g
Ethanol (95%)	100 ml

Working solution. Dilute stock safranin 1:5 or 1:10 with distilled water; store in a glass-stoppered bottle.

The principles of the Gram stain are discussed in Chapter 3. The following procedure is for the **rapid method:**

1. Prepare a thin film of the material to be examined; dry and fix as previously described.
2. Flood the slide with crystal violet stain, and allow it to remain on the slide for 10 seconds.
3. Pour off the stain, and wash off the remainder with the iodine solution.
4. Flood with iodine solution, and allow to mordant for 10 seconds.
5. Rinse off with running water. Shake off excess.
6. Decolorize with alcohol-acetone solution or 95% alcohol (an alcohol-acetone solution may prove to be too rapid) until no further color flows from the slide. This usually takes from 10 to 20 seconds, depending on the thickness of the smear. Care should be taken not to overdecolorize the film, since this may result in an incorrect reading of the stain.
7. Counterstain with safranin for 10 seconds; then wash off with water.
8. Blot between clean sheets of bibulous paper and examine under oil immersion.

Grocott-Gomori methenamine–silver nitrate stain for actinomycetes and fungi in tissue sections

SOLUTION A

Borax, 5%	8 ml
Distilled water	100 ml

SOLUTION B

Silver nitrite, 10%	7 ml
Methenamine, 3%	100 ml

Add equal parts of solutions A and B to make a working methenamine–silver nitrate solution. These solutions should be made up fresh.

STOCK LIGHT GREEN SOLUTION

Light green SF (yellow)	0.2 g
Distilled water	100 ml
Glacial acetic acid	0.2 ml

Deparaffinize and bring to distilled water. Oxidize in 5% chromic acid for 1 hour. Wash in running tap water for a few seconds. Rinse in 1% sodium bisulfite for 1 minute to remove residual chromic acid. Wash in tap water for 5 to 10 minutes. Wash in three or four changes of distilled water. Place in working methenamine–silver nitrate solution in oven (58 to 60 C) for 30 to 60 minutes. When the section turns yellowish-brown, use paraffin-coated forceps to remove the slide from the silver nitrate solution. Dip the slide in distilled water, and check with a microscope for adequate silver impregnation. Fungi should be dark brown at this stage. Rinse in six changes of distilled water. Tone in 0.1% gold chloride for 2 to 5 minutes. Rinse in distilled water. Remove the unreduced silver with 2% sodium thiosulfate for 2 to 5 minutes. Wash in tap water. Counterstain for 1 minute with fresh 1:5 dilution in distilled water of stock light green solution. Dehydrate, clear, and mount.

Iron-hematoxylin stain

See Chapter 35.

Metachromatic granule stain
Albert stain

The Albert stain is a differential stain and is recommended for its simplicity in staining *Corynebacterium diphtheriae*.

1. Prepare the smear and fix with heat.
2. Flood the smear with Albert stain for 3 to 5 minutes.
3. Wash in tap water, and drain off excess.
4. Flood with Gram's iodine. Allow to react for 1 minute.
5. Wash, blot dry, and examine.

Granules appear blue-black; the bands appear blue to blue-green; and the cytoplasm appears green.

Methylene blue stain

Methylene blue	0.3 g
Ethyl alcohol (95%)	30 ml

When dissolved add:

Distilled water	100 ml

Cover the fixed smear with staining solution, and stain for 1 minute. Wash with water, and blot dry with blotting paper.

Loeffler methylene blue stain, as formerly used, was prepared by adding alkali to the foregoing solution. Current commercial preparations of methylene blue do not require the addition of alkali. The older preparations contained acid impurities.

This is a simple stain. Prepare a smear of the organism, and fix with heat. Flood smear with Loeffler methylene blue, and allow to react for 1 minute. Wash and blot dry. The granules readily absorb the dye and appear deep blue. Overstaining lessens the contrast.

PPLO (Mycoplasma) stain

*(Dienes and Weinberger: Bacteriol. Rev. **15**:245, 1951)*

REAGENTS

Methylene blue	2.5 g
Azure II	1.25 g
Maltose	10 g
Sodium carbonate	0.25 g
Distilled water	100 ml

Dissolve the ingredients in the water.
1. Spread a drop of stain on a grease-free coverglass, and allow it to dry.
2. With a sterile scalpel, cut out a small block of agar medium containing a few *Mycoplasma* colonies and place, with colonies up, on a clean glass slide.
3. Lay coverglass, stain side down, carefully on the agar block, without rubbing.
4. Seal the preparation with a mixture of 3 parts petrolatum and 1 part of paraffin to prevent drying.
5. Examine under low-power objective.

6. *Mycoplasma* colonies are quite distinct with dense blue centers and light blue peripheries.

Relief stain (Dorner)

REAGENTS

Nigrosin	10 g
Distilled water	100 ml

Boil for 30 minutes, add 0.5 ml of formalin when cool, filter through paper, and store in 2-ml amounts in sterile, corked tubes.
1. Place a loopful of the bacterial suspension on a grease-free slide, and immediately add a loopful of the nigrosin solution.
2. Spread out in a thin film.
3. Dry slide in air or hasten drying with gentle heat.
4. Examine under an oil immersion lens.
5. Cells are unstained against the dark background.

Rickettsial stains
Castañeda stain

REAGENTS

Solution A	
Potassium phosphate (KH_2PO_4) (1% aqueous)	100 ml
Sodium phosphate ($Na_2HPO_4 \cdot 12H_2O$) (25% aqueous)	100 ml

Mix and add 1 ml of formalin.

Solution B	
Methyl alcohol	100 ml
Methylene blue	1 g

Mix 20 ml of solution A with 0.15 ml of solution B and add 1 ml of formalin.

Solution C (counterstain)	
Safranin O (0.2% aqueous)	25 ml
Acetic acid (0.1%)	75 ml

1. Prepare a homogeneous film, and dry in air.
2. Cover film with stain (mixture of solutions A and B).
3. Drain off stain. Do not wash.

4. Counterstain with safranin O (solution C) for 1 to 4 seconds.
5. Wash with tap water. Blot dry.
6. Examine under oil immersion lens.
7. The rickettsiae stain blue, whereas the cellular elements stain red.

Giemsa method*

1. Prepare a homogeneous film on a clean glass slide. Air dry.
2. Flood with methyl alcohol for 1 minute.
3. Drain off alcohol, and allow to dry.
4. Cover film with Giemsa stain (15 drops), and allow to react for 1 minute.
5. Add distilled water (30 drops), and continue staining for 5 minutes. Drain off.
6. Wash with distilled water.
7. Place slide on end, and allow to dry in air.
8. Examine under oil immersion lens. The rickettsiae stain a bluish-purple.

Spore stain
Dorner method

1. Make a heavy suspension of organisms in distilled water in a test tube, and add an equal volume of freshly filtered carbolfuchsin.
2. Place tube in boiling water bath for 5 to 10 minutes.
3. Mix a loopful of the aforementioned combination with a loopful of boiled and filtered 10% aqueous solution of nigrosin on a clean slide.
4. Spread out and dry film quickly with gentle heat.
5. Examine under oil. The spores stain red, and the bacterial cells are almost colorless against a dark gray background.

A modification of the Dorner method may be employed, whereby a smear of the culture is prepared and fixed. The smear is then covered with a strip of filter paper, to which carbolfuchsin is added. The dye is heated to steaming for 5

---

*This stain may also be used for spirochetes, which stain blue.

to 7 minutes with a Bunsen burner, and the filter paper is removed. Wash with water, blot dry, and cover with a thin film of nigrosin using a second slide or a needle. The appearance of the cells is as previously described.

Wirtz-Conklin method
(Paik. In Lennette, Balows, Hausler, and Truant, editors: Manual of clinical microbiology, ed. 3, Washington, D.C., 1980 American Society for Microbiology)

Flood the entire slide with 5% aqueous malachite green. Steam for 3 to 6 minutes, and rinse under running tap water. Counterstain with 0.5% aqueous safranin for 30 seconds. Spores are seen as green spherules in red-stained rods or with red-stained debris.

Sudan black B fat stain
(Burdon: J. Bacteriol. 52:665-678, 1946)

Sudan black B	0.3 g
Ethyl alcohol, 70%	100 ml

Shake the solution thoroughly at intervals during the day, and allow it to stand overnight before use. Dry and fix the smear with heat. Stain the slide with Sudan black for 10 minutes, drain, and blot dry. Wash and clear the smear with xylol. Counterstain with a 0.5% aqueous solution of safranin for 10 to 15 seconds. Wash in tap water; blot dry. The cells stain red; the highly refractile poly-beta-hydroxybutyrate granules are blue-black. For *Legionella pneumophila* counterstain for 1 minute.

Trichrome stain for intestinal protozoa

See Chapter 35.

Wayson stain for smears of pus

Dissolve 0.2 g of basic fuchsin and 0.75 g of methylene blue in 20 ml of absolute ethanol. Add the dye solution to 200 ml of a 5% solution of phenol in distilled water. Filter. Stain smears for a few seconds. Wash, blot, and dry. This stain is useful in detecting polar staining morphology.

Wright stain for malaria

See Chapter 35.

Wright-Giemsa method for staining conjunctival scrapings

The Wright-Giemsa stain, along with a Gram stain of the scrapings, gives immediate information to the ophthalmologist regarding conjunctivitis of bacterial origin, inclusion body conjunctivitis and trachoma, or eosinophilia of allergic conjunctivitis.

1. Two slide preparations of scrapings are made; one is stained by the Gram method and one by the Wright-Giemsa technique.
2. To carry out staining by the Wright-Giemsa technique, apply Wright stain to the slide for 1 minute. Add an equal volume of neutral distilled water, and stain for 4 minutes.
3. Shake off stain; then apply dilute Giemsa stain (1 drop to 1 ml of neutral distilled water), and allow to stain for 15 minutes.
4. Shake off, decolorize lightly with ethanol, and air dry (do not blot).

MOUNTING FLUIDS
Chloral lactophenol

Chloral lactophenol may be used in place of 10% potassium hydroxide, in the same manner.

Chloral hydrate	2 parts
Phenol crystals	1 part
Lactic acid	1 part

Dissolve the ingredients by gentle heating over a steam bath.

Lactophenol cotton blue

Phenol crystals	20 g
Lactic acid	20 g
Glycerin	40 g
Distilled water	20 ml

Dissolve these ingredients by heating gently over a steam bath. Add 0.05 g of cotton blue dye (Poirrier's blue). This may be used for yeasts as well as molds and serves as both a mounting fluid and a stain.

1. Place a drop of fluid on a clean slide.
2. Place a small amount of culture in this drop. If the culture is on agar, remove a piece of the medium with the embedded growth.
3. Cover with a coverglass, and press down gently to flatten.
4. Warm gently to remove air bubbles if necessary.
5. Examine under the microscope with high-dry or oil immersion objectives.
6. Ring edges of coverglass with nail polish if a permanent mount is required.

Sodium hydroxide–glycerin

Glycerin	10 ml
Sodium hydroxide*	20 g
Distilled water	90 ml

This mounting fluid is used in moist preparations when examining clinical material for fungi.

---

*Potassium hydroxide may be substituted for sodium hydroxide.

REFERENCES

1. Clark, W.A.: A simplifed Leifson flagella stain, J. Clin. Microbiol. **3**:632-634, 1976.
2. Conn, J.G.: Biological stains, Commission on Standardization of Biological Stains, Geneva, N.Y., 1928, W.F. Humphrey Press.
3. Lennette, E.H., Balows, A., Hausler, W.J., Jr., and Truant, J. P., editors: Manual of clinical microbiology, ed. 3, Washington, D.C., 1980, American Society for Microbiology.
4. Truant, J.P., Brett, W.A., and Thomas, W., Jr.: Fluorescence microscopy of tubercle bacillus stained with auramine and rhodamine, Henry Ford Hosp. Med. Bull. **10**:287-296, 1962.
5. Van Orden, A.E., and Greer, P.W. In Jones, G.L., and Hebert, G.A., editors: "Legionnaires": the disease, the bacterium, and methodology, Atlanta, 1978, Center for Disease Control, pp. 147-154.

44 REAGENTS AND TESTS

Acetate utilization

See Chapter 42.

Anaerobe identification disks

See Chapter 13.

Andrade's indicator

Distilled water	100 ml
Acid fuchsin	0.5 g
1 N NaOH	16 ml

Dissolve the fuchsin in distilled water, and add the sodium hydroxide. If the fuchsin is not sufficiently decolorized after several hours, an additional 1 or 2 ml of sodium hydroxide is added.

Arylsulfatase color standards

1. Prepare a stock solution of 0.1 g of phenolphthalein in 10 ml of ethyl alcohol.
2. Prepare a 2 N sodium carbonate solution by adding 10.6 g of sodium carbonate to 100 ml of distilled water.
3. Prepare standards according to the chart on p. 662.
4. Mix each dilution, and dispense in 2-ml

quantities in 16- by 125-mm screw-capped tubes.

5. Add 6 drops of 2 N sodium carbonate to each tube.
6. Solutions without added sodium carbonate may be stored in the refrigerator for several months; tubes containing sodium carbonate fade in 2 to 4 weeks and must be freshly prepared as indicated.
7. A more stable set of standards, valid for 6 months, can be prepared using M/15 Na_2HPO_4 as a reagent and 0.1% phenol red as a color indicator.[12]

Arylsulfatase test reagent

STOCK SUBSTRATE

Dissolve 2.6 g of tripotassium phenolphthalein* in 50 ml of distilled water (0.08 M); sterilize by filtration and refrigerate.

STOCK SOLUTION OF SUBSTRATE

Prepare a 0.001 M substrate solution by adding 2.5 ml of the 0.08 M stock substrate to 200 ml of Dubos Tween-albumin broth.* Dispense

aseptically in 2-ml amounts in 16- by 125-ml screw-capped tubes.

Bacitracin disk identification test

See Chapter 17.

Benzidine test solutions
(Deibel and Evans: J. Bacteriol. 79:356, 1960)

Partially dissolve 1 g of benzidine dihydrochloride or benzidine base† in 20 ml of glacial acetic acid. Add 30 ml of distilled water, and heat the solution gently. Cool; then add 50 ml of 95% ethyl alcohol. The reagent is stable for at least 1 month at refrigerator temperature (a slight yellow color does not affect the reagent's sensitivity).

Fresh 5% hydrogen peroxide solution is prepared each week by diluting 30% reagent grade hydrogen peroxide.

---

*BBL Microbiology Systems, Cockeysville, Md.; Difco Laboratories, Detroit, Mich.
†This may not continue to be available, since it is considered to be carcinogenic.

---

*Nutritional Biochemicals Corp., Cleveland, Ohio; L. Light & Co., Colinbrook, Bucks, England.

Arylsulfatase color chart

Tube	Phenolphthalein	Distilled water	Amount	2 N Na₂CO₃	Reading
1	1 ml of stock	50 ml	2 ml	6 drops	5+
2	5 ml of tube 1	25 ml	2 ml	6 drops	4+
3	2 ml of tube 1	25 ml	2 ml	6 drops	3+
4	1.5 ml of tube 1	50 ml	2 ml	6 drops	2+
5	0.5 ml of tube 1	50 ml	2 ml	6 drops	1+
6	0.5 ml of tube 1	100 ml	2 ml	6 drops	±

Beta-lactamase tests

See Chapters 19, 23, and 36.

Bile solubility

See Chapter 18.

Bile test for identification of anaerobes

Inoculate a tube of thioglycollate medium (BBL 135 C) containing 2% commercial dehydrated oxgall (equivalent to 20% bile) and 0.1% sodium desoxycholate, as well as a control tube without bile. Incubate and compare growth in the two tubes. Observe bile broth for inhibition (less growth than in control; not necessarily total inhibition), no inhibition, or stimulation of growth.

Buffer solutions
Buffered glycerol-saline solution
(Teague and Clurman, 1916; modified by Sachs, 1939)

Sodium chloride	4.2 g
Dipotassium phosphate, anhydrous	3.1 g
Monopotassium phosphate, anhydrous	1 g
Glycerol	300 ml
Distilled water	700 ml

Dispense in bottles with tightly fitting screw caps in approximately 10-ml amounts; autoclave for 15 minutes at 116 C. Add sufficient phenol red to give a distinct red color; if the solution becomes yellow (acid), it should be discarded. The solution is used for preserving fecal specimens.

Sorensen pH buffer solutions

Buffer solutions may be added to culture media to prevent a significant change in hydrogen ion concentration. Sorensen buffers, prepared from potassium and sodium phosphates, are readily prepared from the anhydrous salts or purchased from commercial sources.

REAGENTS

Solution A
  M/15 Na₂PO₄

Dissolve 9.464 g of the anhydrous salt, previously dried at 130 C, in distilled water, to make 1 liter of solution.

Solution B
  M/15 KH₂PO₄

Dissolve 9.073 g of the anhydrous salt, previously dried at 110 C, in distilled water to make 1 liter of solution. Mix solutions A and B as indicated.

pH	Solution A	Solution B
5.29	0.25 ml	9.75 ml
5.59	0.5 ml	9.5 ml
5.91	1 ml	9 ml
6.24	2 ml	8 ml
6.47	3 ml	7 ml
6.64	4 ml	6 ml
6.81	5 ml	5 ml
6.98	6 ml	4 ml
7.17	7 ml	3 ml
7.38	8 ml	2 ml
7.73	9 ml	1 ml
8.04	9.5 ml	0.5 ml

Camp test

See Chapter 17.

Catalase test

Use an 18- to 24-hour agar slant culture* incubated at 35 C. Pour 1 ml of a 3% solution of hydrogen peroxide over the growth, and set the tube in an inclined position. The reaction is **positive** if there is a rapid ebullition of gas. Micrococci and staphylococci are catalase positive; streptococci and pneumococci are catalase negative; *Bacillus* species are catalase positive.

The test may also be carried out with a 24- to 48-hour culture in broth or thioglycollate medium (microaerophiles and anaerobes). Add approximately 1 ml of the hydrogen peroxide to the culture and observe for gas as before.

The test is not recommended for cultures grown on blood agar because of the catalase present in the red blood cells.

It may be done on egg yolk agar for anaerobes. Expose to air for at least 30 minutes before testing. Growth may be removed to a drop of H_2O_2 on a glass slide and observed for evolution of bubbles. If subcultures are to be made, this should be done prior to exposure of plate to air.

A color streak catalase test has also been described.[5]

Citrate utilization†

(Simmons: J. Infect. Dis. 39:209-214, 1926)

Prepare Simmons' citrate according to manufacturer's directions.
1. Inoculate the surface of the slant lightly, using a saline suspension of the organism and a straight wire.
2. Incubate for 24 to 28 hours (maximum 7 days) at 35 C.

---

*The agar slant should be inoculated quite heavily. An old slant culture will not give a proper test.
†Adapted from Blazevic, D. N., and Ederer, G. M.: Biochemical tests in diagnostic microbiology, New York, 1975, John Wiley & Sons, Inc.

Positive: growth, alkaline reaction. **Negative:** no growth, no change of indicator.

Coagulase test

See Chapter 16.

Decarboxylase (lysine and ornithine) and dihydrolase (arginine)

See Chapter 42 (decarboxylase test media and lysine iron agar).

Deoxyribonuclease (DNase) test

See Chapter 42.

Digesting and decontaminating solutions for culturing of sputum for Mycobacterium tuberculosis
N-acetyl-L-cysteine-alkali method
(Kubica et al.: Am. Rev. Respir. Dis. 89:284, 1964)

1. Prepare the necessary volume of digestant as shown in Table 44-1. The solution is self-sterilizing but should be used within 24 hours, since it deteriorates on standing.
2. In a well-ventilated safety cabinet, transfer no more than 10 ml of sputum to a sterile 50-ml screw-capped, aerosol-free centrifuge tube. Smaller volumes may be used in smaller tubes, but in no case should the volume of sputum exceed one fifth of the volume of the tube.
3. Add an equivalent volume of the acetyl cysteine-sodium hydroxide digestant (Table 44-1) to the specimen; mix well in a Vortex mixer. Digestion is generally effected in 5 to 30 seconds. Avoid extreme agitation, which may inactivate the acetyl cysteine by oxidation. Proceed as described in Chapter 31.

Trisodium phosphate–benzalkonium chloride method

1. Dissolve 1,000 g of trisodium phosphate 12H_2O in 4,000 ml of hot distilled water. Add 7.4 ml of 17% aqueous benzalkonium chloride concentrate.*

---

*17% Zephiran chloride is available from Winthrop Laboratories, New York, N.Y.

TABLE 44-1

Preparation of acetyl cysteine–sodium hydroxide digestant

	Volume of digestant needed				
Reagent	50 ml	100	200	500	1,000
1 N (4%) sodium hydroxide	25 ml	50	100	250	500
0.1 M (2.94%) sodium citrate · 2H$_2$O	25 ml	50	100	250	500
N-acetyl-L-cysteine powder*	0.25 g	0.5 g	1 g	2.5 g	5 g

*Powdered N-acetyl-L-cysteine is available from Mead Johnson Laboratories, Evansville, Ind.; Sigma Chemcial Co., St. Louis; BBL Microbiology Systems, Cockeysville, Md.

2. M/15 phosphate neutralizing buffer, pH 6.6

SOLUTION A

Sodium monohydrogen phosphate (anhydrous)	9.47 g
Distilled water	1,000 ml

SOLUTION B

Potassium dihydrophosphate	9.08 g
Distilled water	1,000 ml

Mix 625 ml of solution B with 375 ml of solution A. Check the reaction, and adjust the pH to 6.6 if required; dispense in small volumes in appropriate containers, and sterilize at 121 C for 15 minutes. This is used to wash and neutralize the sediment.

Egg yolk plate reactions
Lecithinase

A positive lecithinase reaction is indicated by an **opaque zone** in the medium around the colonies.

Lipase

A positive lipase reaction is indicated by an **iridescent** ("oil on water") sheen on the surface of the growth (observed under oblique light). This reaction may be delayed. Therefore, plates should be kept 1 week before being discarded as negative.

Nagler reaction

Prior to inoculating an egg yolk agar plate, swab one half of the plate with *Clostridium perfringens* type A antitoxin, and allow it to dry. Streak the inoculum across both halves of the plate, starting on the half without antitoxin. Incubate anaerobically 24 to 48 hours, and observe. Inhibition of lecithinase production on the half of the plate containing the antitoxin indicates a positive reaction. This antitoxin is not specific for *C. perfringens*, but is an alpha-toxin inhibitor. Other species that produce alpha-toxin (a lecithinase) also give a positive Nagler reaction. These are *C. bifermentans*, *C. sordellii*, and *C. paraperfringens*.

Esculin hydrolysis—anaerobes

Inoculate a tube of esculin broth (heart infusion broth with 0.1% esculin and 0.1% agar), and after good growth is obtained, add a few drops of 1% ferric ammonium citrate solution. A positive reaction is indicated by the development of a **black** color. Alternatively, the tube may be observed under long-wave ultraviolet light (365 nm). Loss of fluorescence indicates a positive reaction.

Ethanol for selecting sporeformers

See Chapter 13.

Fermentation of carbohydrates—anaerobes

Tubes of Bacto CHO base broth (Difco) containing various carbohydrates are inoculated.* After good growth is obtained, pH is determined using a pH meter equipped with a long, thin electrode. Interpretation is as follows: pH 5.5 and below, acid; 5.6 to 6.0, weak acid; and above 6.0, negative, providing the pH in the control broth is 6.2 or higher. If the pH in the control broth is 6.1 or less, lower the values for interpretation accordingly. Uninoculated tubes from each batch of medium should be incubated along with the inoculated tubes. Ordinarily the pH of such uninoculated tubes is 6.2 to 6.4. Occasionally carbohydrate broths, such as arabinose and xylose, have a pH of 5.8 or 5.9. Therefore, a pH of less than 5.4 would be acid and 5.4 to 5.6 or 5.7 would be weak acid production.

Ferric ammonium citrate

Use as a 1% aqueous solution to test for esculin hydrolysis. Keep in a dark bottle.

Fildes enrichment†

Use as a supplement for thioglycollate and other media. It is added just prior to using the medium.

Gastric mucin (5%)
(Strauss and Klegman: J. Infect. Dis. 88:151, 1951)

Emulsify 5 g of gastric hog mucin (granular type)‡ in 95 ml of distilled water in a blender for 5 minutes. Autoclave for 15 minutes at 121 C. Cool to room temperature; adjust to pH 7.3 with sterile sodium hydroxide. Check for sterility, and store in a refrigerator.

Mix equal parts of 5% gastric mucin and a fungus suspension; inject 1 ml intraperitoneally into the appropriate laboratory animal.

Gelatin liquefaction*
Method 1: stab method
(Edwards and Ewing: Identification of Enterobacteriaceae, ed. 3, Minneapolis, 1972, Burgess Publishing Co., p. 345; Lennette et al.: Manual of clinical microbiology, ed. 3, Washington, D.C, 1980, American Society for Microbiology)

Prepare 12% gelatin in nutrient broth. Dispense into tubes as deeps. Autoclave at 121 C for 12 minutes.
1. Inoculate gelatin deeps by stabbing to the bottom of the tube. Incubate the inoculated tube and uninoculated negative control tube at 20 C to 22 C for 30 days.
2. To detect liquefaction, place the tubes in a refrigerator for 30 minutes. Remove and observe for liquefaction. Continue to incubate until liquefaction occurs or until the 30-day period is over.

Strong positive: liquefaction within 3 days.
Weak positive: liquefaction after 3 days.

Method 2
(Frazier: J. Infect. Dis. 39:302-309, 1926; Cowan and Steel: Manual for the identification of medical bacteria, New York, 1970, Cambridge University Press, p. 156)

Prepare 12% gelatin in nutrient broth. Autoclave at 121 C for 12 minutes; pour into plates.
1. Inoculate plate in one spot. Incubate at 30 C for 3 days.
2. Flood plate with mercuric chloride solution:

$HgCl_2$	12 g
Distilled water	80 ml
Concentrated HC1	16 ml

Positive: clear zone around growth.

---

*Thioglycollate medium without dextrose or indicator, supplemented with vitamin K_1 (0.1 µg/ml), hemin (5 µg/ml), and sodium bicarbonate (1 mg/ml) can also be used as a base.

†BBL Microbiology Systems, Cockeysville, Md. (No. 20810); Difco Laboratories, Detroit, Mich.

‡Wilson Laboratories, Chicago, Ill.

*Adapted from Blazevic, D.N., and Ederer, G.M.: Biochemical tests in diagnostic microbiology, New York, 1975, John Wiley & Sons, Inc.

Rapid method

(Blazevic et al.: Appl. Microbiol. 25:107-110, 1973)

1. Inoculate 0.5 ml of saline with a heavy loopful of growth.
2. Insert a strip of exposed, undeveloped x-ray paper (approximately 1 by 1¼ inches) into the saline suspension.
3. Incubate in a heating block or water bath at 37 C. Observe at 1, 2, 3, 4, and 24 hours for removal of the green gelatin emulsion from the strip.

Positive: transparent blue-gray appearance of the strip. **Negative:** strip remains green.

Gelatin liquefaction—anaerobes (Thiogel medium, BBL)

Test after good growth is observed by refrigerating an inoculated gelatin tube along with an uninoculated tube of gelatin until the uninoculated tube has solidified (usually ½ to 1 hour). Remove the tubes to room temperature, and invert. A positive reaction is indicated if the inoculated tube fails to solidify. A weak reaction is indicated when the inoculated tube begins to become liquid in approximately one half the time required for the control (uninoculated) tube to liquefy.

Gluconate oxidation test

(Haynes: J. Gen. Microbiol. 5:939, 1951)

Pseudomonas aeruginosa is able to oxidize glucose or gluconate to ketogluconate, which in turn is detected by the reduction of copper salts, as found in Benedict's solution. This test is helpful in identifying nonpigmented strains of *P. aeruginosa*.

The use of gluconate substrate tablets* is recommended for this test. A single tablet is added to 1 ml of distilled water, which is then heavily inoculated with the test organism. After 12 to 18 hours' incubation at 35 C, test the culture for reducing substances with Benedict's solution.* A positive test is indicated by a change from blue to green-yellow.

Growth tests—anaerobes

The growth of some anaerobic isolates is enhanced by the addition of supplements, such as bile, Fildes enrichment, or Tween 80. After 48 to 72 hours' incubation, growth in the tubes containing supplements is compared with growth in the conventional medium (Bacto CHO base with glucose). If one of the supplements enhances growth, it should be added to each tube required for biochemical tests before inoculation.

Hemin solution

Hemin solution is used as a medium supplement in a final concentration of 5 μg/ml. To prepare, dissolve 0.5 g of hemin† in 10 ml of commercial ammonia water (or 1 N sodium hydroxide), bring volume to 100 ml with distilled water, and autoclave at 121 C for 15 minutes. A stock solution is 5 mg/ml.

Hippurate hydrolysis

(Ayers and Rupp: J. Infect. Dis. 30:388, 1922)

Hippurate hydrolysis (rapid)‡

(Hwang and Ederer: J. Clin. Microbiol. 1:114-115, 1975)

Prepare a 1% aqueous solution of sodium hippurate, and dispense it in 0.4-ml aliquots. Cork and store at −20 C.

1. Thaw tubes of sodium hippurate substrate.
2. Emulsify several small colonies or one large colony of beta-hemolytic streptococci

---

*Key Scientific Products Co., Los Angeles, Calif.

*A Clinitest tablet from Ames Co., Elkhart, Ind., may be substituted.
†Sigma Chemical Co., St. Louis, Mo.
‡Adapted from Blazevic, D.N., and Ederer, G.M.: Biochemical tests in diagnostic microbiology, New York, 1975, John Wiley & Sons, Inc.

in a tube of substrate. The suspension should be very cloudy.

3. Inoculate positive and negative control organisms, group B and group A streptococci, respectively.

4. Incubate the tubes in a heating block at 37 C for 2 hours.

5. Add approximately 0.2 ml (5 drops) of ninhydrin reagent (3.5 g of ninhydrin in 100 ml of a 1:1 mixture of acetone and butanol) to each tube. **Do not shake tube.**

6. Continue incubation for 10 minutes. **Do not incubate longer than ½ hour: false-positive results could occur.**

7. Remove tubes and immediately record results.

Positive: deep purple. **Negative:** no change or a very faint purple.

Hydrogen sulfide production
Lead acetate paper test

Saturate filter paper strips (5 by 1 cm) with 5% lead acetate solution. Air dry, then autoclave at 15 pounds pressure for 15 minutes.

Inoculate a sulfur-containing liquid medium and insert a lead acetate strip between the plug and inner wall of tube and above the liquid. Hydrogen sulfide production is evidenced by the **blackening** of the lower portion of the strip.

A negative test may be checked by adding a small amount of 2 N hydrochloric acid to the tube and closing the tube as before. Any dissolved sulfide will be liberated and will combine with the lead in the strip to form the black lead sulfide.

Note: The lead acetate paper test may be positive when the butt reaction in TSI agar (or KIA) is negative or only weakly positive. It is more sensitive.

Triple sugar iron (TSI) agar or Kligler's iron agar (KIA) method

The butts of these media are stabbed with the culture. Hydrogen sulfide production is de-

tected by the blackening of the butt. Lead acetate paper may also be used by inserting a strip between the loosened cap and inner wall of the tube.

Immunofluorescence (direct) procedure for Neisseria gonorrhoeae

1. Prepare a **thin film** of a suspected colony from a Thayer-Martin plate (may be made up to 15 minutes after performing the oxidase test) on a slide containing a 6-mm diameter etched circle.

2. Thoroughly dry the film in air.

3. Overlay with adsorbed (with antimeningococcus group B serum) fluorescein-labeled *N. gonorrhoeae* antiserum,* keeping within the 6-mm diameter circle.

4. Incubate the slide at 35 C in a moist chamber for 30 minutes (alternatively for 5 minutes at room temperature).

5. Rinse with pH 7.2 phosphate buffer, dry, mount in buffered glycerine with a coverglass, and examine under fluorescence microscopy. Gonococci appear as **yellow-green** diplococci of typical size and shape.

6. Include a positive urethral smear or one prepared from a known **fresh** isolate of *N. gonorrhoeae*, along with one of a boiled suspension of *Enterobacter cloacae* and one of *Neisseria meningitidis*, as positive, negative, and nonspecific staining controls.

Indicators for anaerobiosis
Fildes and McIntosh indicator

Prepare the following solutions:
1. 6% aqueous glucose (add a small crystal of thymol as a preservative).
2. 0.1 N sodium hydroxide; 6 ml to 94 ml of distilled water.
3. Aqueous methylene blue (0.5%); 3 to 100 ml of distilled water.

For use, mix 1 ml of each solution in a test tube, boil the mixture until colorless, then place

---

*Difco Laboratories, Detroit, Mich. (No. 2361).

in a loaded anaerobic jar before sealing. A blue color at the end of incubation indicates that anaerobiosis was not achieved.

Smith modified methylene blue indicator
(Smith: ASM meeting, Washington, D.C., 1964)

Mix thoroughly 1 pound of sodium bicarbonate (commercial grade is satisfactory) with 50 g of glucose and 20 mg of methylene blue. For use, add about 1 inch to a 16- by 100-mm test tube, half fill with tap water, invert to mix, and place within the anaerobic jar. The solution will slowly become colorless during incubation at 35 C; if more rapid decolorization is required, the solution may be heated to boiling and cooled rapidly immediately before placing in the jar. The indicator should be **colorless** at the end of incubation if anaerobiosis was maintained.

Indole tests
Ehrlich indole test for nonfermenters and miscellaneous gram-negative bacteria
(Modification of Bohme: Zentralbl. Bakt., Orig. 40:129, 1906)

REAGENT

Paradimethylaminobenzaldehyde	2 g
Ethyl alcohol (95%)	190 ml
Hydrochloric acid (concentrated)	40 ml

Add 1 ml of xylene to a 48-hour culture of organisms in tryptone or trypticase broth or other appropriate medium. Shake the tube well, and allow it to stand for a few minutes until the solvent rises to the surface.

Gently add about 0.5 ml of the reagent down the sides of the tube, so that it forms a ring between the medium and the solvent. If indole has been produced by the organisms, it will, being soluble in solvent, be concentrated in the solvent layer, and on addition of the reagent, a brilliant **red ring** will develop just below the solvent layer. If no indole is produced, no color will develop.

Kovacs indole test for Enterobacteriaceae

REAGENT

Pure amyl or isoamyl alcohol	150 ml
Paradimethylaminobenzaldehyde	10 g
Concentrated hydrochloric acid (A.R.)	50 ml

Dissolve the aldehyde in the alcohol, and add the acid slowly. Prepare in small quantities, and refrigerate when not in use.

Inoculate tryptophane broth, and incubate for 48 hours at 35 C. Add 5 drops of Kovacs reagent. A **deep red** color indicates the presence of indole.

Indole spot test
(Vracko and Sherris: Am. J. Clin. Pathol. 39:429, 1963)

The indole spot test utilizes a Whatman No. 1 filter paper moistened with 1 to 1.5 ml of a 5% solution of paradimethylaminobenzaldehyde in 10% aqueous HCl placed inside the cover of a Petri dish. Colonies to be tested are picked carefully with a sterile loop from overnight growth on a sheep blood agar plate and smeared on a small area of the moistened filter paper. Development of a **brown-red** or **purple-red** color within 20 seconds indicates the presence of indole.

It should be emphasized that this procedure is to be used only with pure cultures of colonies that produce a metallic sheen on eosin–methylene blue agar. It can also be used on pure cultures of swarming colonies of *Proteus* (*P. mirabilis* does not produce indole).

Another spot test of significance is useful for detection of indole produced by anaerobic bacteria.[11] As above, growth obtained from a single, pure culture on a blood agar plate is smeared on filter paper that has been saturated with 1% paradimethylaminocinnamaldehyde in 10% (v/v) concentrated HCl. Immediate formation of a **blue** color around the growth indicates a **positive** reaction. Negative reactions give no color change or a pinkish color. Late color development should be ignored. The reagent should be stored in a dark bottle and refrigerated when not in use.

Iodine solutions for wet mount preparations

Iodine solutions are used to stain protozoan cysts in wet mounts. A weak rather than a strong iodine solution is best. The strong iodine tends to coagulate the fecal particles and to destroy the refractile nature of the organism.

Several iodine solutions can be used satisfactorily. The two described below have been widely used and are simply prepared. The one recommended by Dobell and O'Connor[2] is a weak iodine that should be prepared fresh about every 10 days for best results. Lugol iodine must be diluted about five times with distilled water, since the full-strength solution is too strong. Lugol iodine should be prepared fresh about every 3 weeks. Gram iodine used for bacteriologic work is not satisfactory for staining protozoan cysts.

Dobell and O'Connor iodine solution

(Dobell and O'Connor: Intestinal protozoa of man, New York, 1921, William Wood)

Iodine (powdered crystals)	1 g
Potassium iodide	2 g
Distilled water	100 ml

The KI is dissolved in the distilled water, and the iodine crystals are added slowly and shaken thoroughly. Filter or decant.

Lugol iodine solution

Iodine (powdered crystals)	5 g
Potassium iodide	10 g
Distilled water	100 ml

The KI is dissolved in the distilled water, and the iodine crystals are added slowly and shaken until dissolved. Filter, and place in tightly stoppered bottle. Dilute to 1:5 with distilled water for use in staining protozoan cysts.

A small portion of feces is comminuted in a drop of the iodine solution, mounted with a coverslip, and sealed with a heated paraffin-petrolatum mixture.

In a correctly stained cyst the glycogen appears reddish-brown, the cytoplasm appears yellow, and the nuclei stand out as lighter refractile bodies. The location of the karyosomes may be more easily determined, but the chromatoid bodies are less visible than in saline solution. Since glycogen is a reserve food, it does not usually appear in older cysts.

D'Antoni's solution

See Chapter 35.

Kanamycin stock solution

Dissolve 1 g of kanamycin (base activity) in 10 ml of sterile phosphate buffer, pH 8.0. The final concentration is 100,000 µg/ml. Refrigerate for up to 1 year. The solution can be autoclaved.

KOH solution

Potassium hydroxide	10 or 20 g
Distilled water	100 ml

1. Mix the specimen (pus, exudate, tissue) with a drop of 10 or 20% solution on a clean slide, cover with a No. 2, 22- by 40-mm coverslip, and press gently to make a thin mount. Gentle warming may aid in clearing the mount. Viscid specimens may require overnight storage in a moist chamber. (Place slide on applicator stick supports over moist filter paper in a Petri dish, or place in a screw-capped Coplin jar laid on its side.)
2. Scan under low power with reduced lighting. Switch to high power to check presence of suspected fungal elements.

KOH test for Gram stain reaction

See Chapter 3.

Lecithinase

See Egg yolk plate reactions, p. 664.

Lipase

See Egg yolk plate reactions, p. 664.

Malonate utilization*
Rapid method
(Blazevic: Laboratory procedures in diagnostic microbiology, ed. 2, St. Paul, 1974, Telstar Products, Inc., p. 111)

Prepare modified malonate broth according to manufacturer's directions. Dispense in 0.5-ml aliquots.

1. Inoculate the broth with a heavy loopful of an overnight growth from TSI agar or sheep blood agar (do not use growth from MacConkey agar, as false-negative results may occur from this medium).
2. Incubate in a heating block at 37 C for 3 hours.
   Positive: blue. **Negative:** green or yellow.

McFarland nephelometer standards

1. Set up 10 test tubes or ampules of equal size and of good quality. Use new tubes that have been thoroughly cleaned and rinsed.
2. Prepare 1% chemically pure sulfuric acid.
3. Prepare 1% aqueous solution of chemically pure barium chloride.
4. Add the designated amounts of the two solutions to the tubes as shown in Table 44-2 to make a total of 10 ml per tube.
5. Seal the tubes or ampules. The suspended barium sulfate precipitate corresponds approximately to homogeneous *Escherichia coli* cell densities per milliliter throughout the range of standards, as shown in Table 44-2.

Meat digestion—anaerobes

The test is read in chopped meat–glucose. A positive reaction is indicated by disintegration and gradual disappearance of meat particles, leaving a flocculent sediment in the tube.

Methyl red test
(Clark and Lubs: J. Infect. Dis. 17:160, 1915)

To 5 ml of culture in MR-VP broth, add 5 drops of methyl red solution. A positive reaction is indicated by a distinct **red** color, showing the presence of acid (pH < 4.5). A negative reaction is indicated by a **yellow** color. *Escherichia coli* and other methyl red–positive organisms produce high acidity from the dextrose in this medium within 48 hours, which turns the indicator red.

The solution of methyl red is prepared by dissolving 0.1 g of the indicator in 300 ml of 95% alcohol and diluting to 500 ml with distilled water.

Rapid method*
(Barry et al.: Appl. Microbiol. 20:866-870, 1970)

1. Inoculate 0.5 ml of MR-VP broth in a 13- by 100-mm test tube with one colony. Incubate at 35 C for 18 hours.
2. Add 1 drop of methyl red reagent.
   Positive: bright red. **Negative:** yellow or orange.
   METHYL RED REAGENT
   Dissolve 0.5 g of methyl red in 300 ml of 95% ethanol. Add 200 ml of distilled water.

Micromethods

Micromethods are available commercially (API, Analytab Products, Inc.; Enterotube, Roche Diagnostics; R-B, Flow Laboratories; Minitek, BBL, and others) for both aerobic and facultative bacteria and anaerobes. Results with the Enterobacteriaceae are good, averaging better than 90% correlation with conventional procedures. Evaluation with the anaerobes is less complete; the selection of tests is still inadequate for these organisms.

---

*Adapted from Blazevic, D. N., and Ederer, G. M.: Biochemical tests in diagnostic microbiology, New York, 1975, John Wiley & Sons, Inc.

*Adapted from Blazevic, D. N., and Ederer, G. M.: Biochemical tests in diagnostic microbiology, New York, 1975, John Wiley & Sons, Inc.

TABLE 44-2

McFarland nephelometer standards

	Tube number									
	1	2	3	4	5	6	7	8	9	10
Barium chloride (ml)	0.1	0.2	0.3	0.4	0.5	0.6	0.7	0.8	0.9	1
Sulfuric acid (ml)	9.9	9.8	9.7	9.6	9.5	9.4	9.3	9.2	9.1	9
Approx. cell density ($\times 10^8$/ml)	3	6	9	12	15	18	21	24	27	30

Milk reactions

See Chapter 42.

Motility

See Chapter 42, motility test medium. Alternatively for anaerobes, prepare a hanging drop slide from a 4- to 6-hour thioglycollate medium culture. Observe under high-dry magnification.

Nagler reaction

See Egg yolk plate reactions, p. 664.

Niacin test

See Chapter 31.

Nitrate reduction test

REAGENTS

Solution A	
Sulfanilic acid	8 g
Acetic acid (5 N)	1,000 ml
Solution B	
Alpha-naphthylamine	5 g
Acetic acid (5 N)	1,000 ml

Inoculate nitrate reduction broth containing the inverted Durham tube and incubate at 35 C. Examine at 24 and 48 hours for the presence of nitrogen gas, which accumulates in the Durham tube. After 48 hours, add 5 drops of each reagent to the tube. A positive test for nitrites is revealed by the development of a **red** color in 1 to 2 minutes.

Some organisms can reduce nitrate beyond the nitrite stage to nitrogen gas or ammonia. **A negative test for nitrite, therefore, should not necessarily be construed as a negative nitrate reduction test without first testing for the presence of unreduced nitrate.**

Add a very small amount of zinc dust to the broth medium, which has shown a negative reduction test with the foregoing reagents. The presence of unreduced nitrate is revealed by the development of a red color, thus confirming a negative nitrate reduction test. If no color develops, nitrate was reduced beyond nitrite.

Rapid method*

(Blazevic et al.: Appl. Microbiol. 25:107-110, 1973; Schreckenberger and Blazevic: Appl. Microbiol. 28:759-762, 1974)

1. Inoculate 0.5 ml of nitrate broth with a heavy loopful of growth from an appropriate medium (e.g., TSI, blood agar, chocolate agar).
2. Incubate in a heating block or water bath at 35 C for 2 hours.
3. Add 1 drop of solution A and 1 drop of solution B. Shake.
   Positive: red.
   If the test is **negative,** add a minute amount of zinc dust. Shake.
   Positive: absence of red color.

*Adapted from Blazevic, D. N., and Ederer, G. M.: Biochemical tests in diagnostic microbiology, New York, 1975, John Wiley & Sons, Inc.

Disk method for anaerobes

A simplified disk test for nitrate reduction by anaerobes has been described.[11]

Nitrate reduction test for mycobacteria (nitrite standards)

1. Prepare a M/100 sodium nitrite solution by dissolving 0.14 g of sodium nitrite in 200 ml of distilled water.
2. Carry out twofold serial dilutions of the foregoing in 2 ml-volumes in 13 marked tubes.
3. To tubes 6, 7, 8, 10, 11, and 13 add 1 drop of 1:2 dilution of hydrochloric acid, 2 drops of 0.2% aqueous solution of sulfanilamide, and 2 drops of 0.1% aqueous solution of N-naphthylethylenediamine dihydrochloride.
4. Nitrite standards **fade rapidly** and must be freshly prepared each time.

Tube	Dilution	Reading
6	1:64	5+
7	1:128	4+
8	1:256	3+
10	1:1024	2+
11	1:2048	1+
13	1:8192	+/−

ONPG test

See Chapter 42.

Optochin disk test

See Chapter 18.

Oxgall (40%)

Dissolve 40 g oxgall in 100 ml of distilled water, autoclave at 121 C for 15 minutes, and refrigerate.

Oxidase test for detecting colonies of Neisseria

(Steel: J. Gen. Microbiol. 25:297-306, 1961)

A 1% aqueous solution of tetramethylparaphenylenediamine dihydrochloride is used (see pp. 672-673). It gives the colonies a lavender color that eventually turns purple. The reagent sometimes colors the surrounding medium. The reagent is prepared fresh daily or refrigerated for no longer than 1 week.

Indophenol method*

(Ewing and Johnson: Int. Bull. Bact. Nomencl. Taxon. 10:223-230, 1960)

1. Inoculate a nutrient agar slant; incubate at 35 C for no longer than 18 to 24 hours. Also inoculate an agar slant with *Aeromonas* for a positive control.
2. Add 2 to 3 drops of reagent A and reagent B to the growth on the slant. Tilt the tube so that reagents are mixed and flow over the growth.

Positive: blue color in the growth within 2 minutes. Weak or doubtful reactions that occur after 2 minutes should be ignored.

REAGENT A

Dissolve 1 g of alpha-napthol in 100 ml of 95% ethanol.

REAGENT B

Dissolve 1 g of para-aminodimethylaniline HCl (or oxalate) in 100 ml of distilled water. Reagent B should be refrigerated and should be freshly prepared each month.

Oxidase test for Pasteurella.

See Chapter 23.

Oxidase test for Pseudomonas

(Kovacs: Nature 178:703, 1956)

REAGENTS	
Tetramethylparaphenylenediamine dihydrochloride	0.1 g
Distilled water	10 ml

Add the dye to the water, and allow it to stand for 15 minutes before using. Prepare freshly for use each time. The dye loses its activity after 2 hours.†

---

*Adapted from Blazevic, D. N., and Ederer, G. M.: Biochemical tests in diagnostic microbiology, New York, 1975, John Wiley & Sons, Inc.

†A stable reagent in a dropper is available commercially and is recommended (Cepti-seal oxidase test reagent, Marion Scientific Corp., Rockford, Ill.).

Place 2 or 3 drops of the reagent on a piece of Whatman No. 1 filter paper (6 sq cm). Remove a colony* (colonies should be no older than 24 hours to avoid false-negative reactions) from plate,† or some growth from an agar slant, and smear with a loop on the reagent-saturated paper. A positive reaction (oxidase-positive), recognized by a **dark purple** color, develops in 5 to 10 seconds.

Penicillinase test

See Chapter 19.

Phenylalanine deaminase‡

See also Chapter 42.

Method 1
*(Ewing et al.: Public Health Lab. **15**:153-167, 1957)*

Prepare phenylalanine agar in long slants according to the manufacturer's directions.

1. Inoculate the phenylalanine agar slant by streaking heavily. Incubate it at 35 C for 4 hours or 18 to 24 hours.
2. Allow 4 to 5 drops of 10% (w/v) ferric chloride to run over the growth.

Positive: dark green color in the fluid and slant surface.

Method 2
*(Ederer et al.: Appl. Microbiol. **21**:545, 1971)*

Prepare phenylalanine-urea (PU) medium:

Yeast extract	1 g
$(NH_4)_2SO_4$	2 g
NaCl	3 g
K_2HPO_4	1.2 g

KH_2PO_4	0.8 g
DL-Phenylalanine	5 g
(or L-phenylalanine)	2.5 g
Distilled water	975 ml

Dissolve all ingredients; autoclave at 121 C for 15 minutes. Aseptically add 25 ml of urea agar concentrate (Difco). Mix well, and aseptically dispense 0.5 ml into 13- by 100-mm sterile tubes. If the medium is to be kept for a long time, store at −20 C.

1. Inoculate 0.5 ml of PU medium with a colony of organism to be tested. Incubate overnight at 35 C. **Positive urease:** definite pink. **Negative urease:** yellow or faint tinge of pink.
2. Add 1 to 2 drops of 1% (v/v) HCl to adjust the medium to an acid pH (yellow).
3. Add 2 drops of 10% (w/v) ferric chloride. **Positive phenylalanine deaminase:** dark green. **Negative phenylalanine deaminase:** yellow. The phenylalanine deaminase reaction must be read within 10 seconds after adding the ferric chloride, as the green color fades rapidly.

With this method *Proteus*, most *Klebsiella*, some *Enterobacter*, and *Yersinia* will be positive for urease. All other Enterobacteriaceae will be negative.

Rapid method

1. Inoculate 0.5 ml of PU medium with a large loopful of growth from TSI or other solid medium.
2. Incubate in a heating block or water bath at 37 C for 2 hours.
3. Read urease and phenylalanine deaminase reactions as under Method 2.

Polyvinyl alcohol fixative technique for parasitologic specimens

See Chapter 35.

Porphyrin test for Haemophilus

See Chapter 23.

---

*Use a platinum wire loop, as nichrome may cause a false-positive reaction.

†Not satisfactory for colonies growing on selective media or media containing glucose. Fermentation inhibits oxidase enzyme activity and leads to a false-negative result.

‡Adapted from Blazevic, D.N., and Ederer, G.M.: Biochemical tests in diagnostic microbiology, New York, 1975, John Wiley & Sons, Inc.

Preservation of fungal cultures*

Obtain a good grade of **heavy mineral oil,†** and dispense it in approximately 125-ml amounts in 250-ml Erlenmeyer flasks (cotton plugged). Autoclave at 121 C for 45 minutes. Using sterile technique, pour the oil over a small but actively growing fungus culture on a short slant of Sabouraud agar. It is essential that the oil cover not only the fungus colony but also the whole agar surface (about 1 inch above the top of the slant), otherwise the exposed agar or colony will act as a wick and in time cause the medium to dry out.

The stock culture is stored upright at room temperature and remains viable without further attention for several years.

In transferring from oiled cultures, remove a bit of the fungus with a long inoculating needle, drain off the oil by touching it on the inside of the tube, and inoculate to a fresh slant. Rinse off the needle in xylol before flaming.

Quellung reaction

See Chapters 18 and 37.

Resazurin

Use as an Eh indicator in PRAS media. Dissolve one tablet (Difco) in 44 ml of distilled water. Store the stock solution at room temperature.

Ringer's solution

Sodium chloride	8.5 g
Potassium chloride	0.2 g
Calcium chloride · 2H₂O	0.2 g
Sodium carbonate	0.01 g
Distilled water	1,000 ml

(pH 7)

Sterilize by autoclaving at 121 C for 15 minutes. To use in dissolving calcium alginate swabs, prepare in one-quarter strength, and add 1% sodium hexametaphosphate. Approximately 10 minutes of shaking usually suffices for complete dissolution of the swab.

Sereny test

See Chapter 20.

Sodium bicarbonate

Sodium bicarbonate is used as a medium supplement for anaerobes in a final concentration of 1 mg/ml. To prepare, dissolve 2 g in 100 ml of distilled water, and filter sterilize. The stock solution is 20 mg/ml. For use, add 0.5 ml to 10 ml of medium.

Sodium chloride tolerance

See Chapter 17.

Spores—anaerobes

Spores can be observed in stained preparations (Gram or spore stain) made from solid or broth medium. Some commonly encountered species, such as *C. perfringens* and *C. ramosum*, sporulate poorly, and spores are rarely seen. Heat tests are often used if spores cannot be demonstrated in stained smears. One should suspend growth from chopped meat slant or other solid medium in two tubes of starch broth, being careful not to touch the loop to the sides of the tubes above the level of the medium; at the same time, subculture to BAP for anaerobic incubation to check viability. Place one tube of starch broth in a water bath at 80 C with water level above the level of the medium in the tube. Place the tube, containing an equal amount of water, and a thermometer in the water bath at the same time. Leave the starch tube in the bath for 10 minutes after the tube of water has reached 80 C. Remove the starch tube, and incubate with the unheated tube. Observe for growth (up to 10 days). Growth in both tubes indicates a positive test. If growth is questionable on visual inspection, both tubes should be subcultured. (See also Ethanol for selecting sporeformers).

---

*Recommended by the Mycology Branch of the CDC.
†Parke-Davis Co., Detroit, Mich.

SPS disk test

Inhibition zones at least 12mm in diameter about disks impregnated with 20 µl of 5% sodium polyanethol sulfonate (SPS)* on brucella blood agar provide good presumptive evidence that an anaerobic gram-positive coccus is *Peptostreptococcus anaerobius*.

Starch hydrolysis†
(Allen: J. Bacteriol. 3:15-17, 1918)

Prepare broth or agar (appropriate to the type of organism being tested) with 0.2% soluble starch added. Prepare either slants or plates from the agar.
1. Inoculate the starch medium. Incubate in an appropriate atmosphere at 35 C overnight or until sufficient growth has occurred.
2. To a broth add a few drops of Gram's iodine. Read immediately. **Positive:** no change in color. **Negative:** blue (may fade after a while).
3. For plates or slants, flood with Gram's iodine. **Positive:** medium is blue with colorless area around growth. **Negative:** medium is blue even around growth.

String of pearls test

See Chapter 25.

Sulfamethoxazole-trimethoprim susceptibility test

See Chapter 17.

Tween 80 hydrolysis substrate

M/15 phosphate buffer, pH 7	100 ml
Tween 80	0.5 ml
Neutral red (0.1% aqueous solution)	2 ml

1. Mix the foregoing solutions, and dispense in 16- by 125-mm screw-capped tubes in 2-ml amounts.
2. Sterilize by autoclaving at 121 C for 10 minutes.
3. Check for sterility by incubating overnight at 35 C. Final color is amber or straw.
4. Refrigerate in the dark for no longer than 2 weeks.

This substrate is used to test the ability of certain strains of mycobacteria to rapidly degrade the Tween 80 to oleic acid, which is detected by a change in color of the indicator.

Tyrosine degradation

See Chapter 28.

Urease—anaerobes

See also Chapter 42.

Scrape the growth from egg yolk agar or other solid medium. Make a heavy suspension in 0.5 ml of sterile urea broth. Incubate and observe for up to 24 hours aerobically. A bright red color indicates a positive reaction. With a heavy inoculum, urease production usually is evident within 15 to 30 minutes. If the indicator has been reduced, add Nessler's reagent to determine ammonia production. The presence of ammonia indicates a positive reaction.

Urease test broth

Urea	20 g
Monopotassium phosphate	9.1 g
Disodium phosphate	9.5 g
Yeast extract	0.1 g
Phenol red	0.01 g
(Final pH 6.8±)	

Use 3.87 g/100 ml of distilled water. **Do not heat.** When the powder has dissolved, filter the medium through a sterile bacteriologic filter. Distribute the broth in 0.5- to 2-ml amounts in small sterile tubes. Large amounts may be used if desired, but reactions are slower. If a filter is not available, it is possible to sterilize the medi-

---

*Harleco, Philadelphia, Pa.
†Adapted from Blazevic, D.N., and Ederer, G.M.: Biochemical tests in diagnostic microbiology, New York, 1975, John Wiley & Sons, Inc.

um in an autoclave, if the tubes are not tightly packed and the steam pressure is held at 5 pounds for 7 minutes or at 8 pounds for 20 minutes.[7]

In addition, the medium generally gives reliable results without sterilization, if prepared and inoculated immediately.

Urease test broth is prepared according to the formula of Rustigian and Stuart.[9,10] It may be used for identification of bacteria on the basis of urea utilization and is particularly recommended for the differentiation of members of the genus *Proteus* from those of *Salmonella* and *Shigella* in the diagnosis of enteric infections.

Urease test broth may be inoculated from TSI agar (or KIA), trypticase soy agar, or other agar slants having heavy growth. It is recommended that large inocula be employed when it is desirable to obtain results rapidly. Incubate at 35 C. Normally the finished medium has a pale pink or pinkish-yellow color and a neutral pH of about 6.8 to 7.0. In cultures that attack urea ammonia is formed during incubation and makes the reaction of the medium alkaline, with a **deep purple** or bluish-red color. In the medium described by the above investigators no other organism of the family Enterobacteriaceae has been found that gives evidence of urease production.

For a **rapid urease test,** Ewing recommends inoculation of 3 ml of broth with three loopfuls of an agar slant culture. After shaking, tests are incubated in a 37 C water bath and read after 10, 60, and 120 minutes.[3]

Urease test broth may be used in the same manner for the detection of urease activity of such organisms as members of the genera *Brucella*, *Bacillus*, *Sarcina*, and *Mycobacterium*.[4] Incubation usually should be longer than for enteric bacilli.

Note: Both prepared broth and dehydrated base should be stored in the refrigerator. If the seal on the bottle has been broken, the bottle should preferably be stored with desiccant in a sealed container.

Vancomycin stock solution

Dissolve 75 mg of vancomycin base activity in 5 ml N/20 HCl; add 5 ml of sterile distilled water. The final concentration is 7,500 μg/ml. Store in refrigerator for up to 1 month or in a freezer (-20 C) for up to 1 year.

Vitamin K$_1$ solution

Vitamin K$_1$ solution is used as a medium supplement in a final concentration of 0.1 μg/ml for liquid media and 10 μg/ml for agar media. To prepare, weigh out 0.2 g of vitamin K$_1$* on a small piece of sterile aluminum foil, and aseptically add it to 20 ml of absolute ethanol in a sterile tube or bottle. The stock solution is 10 mg/ml. The stock solution can be further diluted for use in sterile distilled water. Refrigerate in a tightly closed container protected from light.

Voges-Proskauer test for acetyl-methylcarbinol or acetoin
(*Coblentz: Am. J. Pub. Health 33:315,1943*)

Barritt's test

REAGENTS

Alpha-naphthol (5%) in absolute ethyl alcohol
Potassium hydroxide (40%) containing 0.3% creatine

1. Pipet 1 ml of a 48-hour culture grown in MR-VP broth into a clean Wassermann tube.
2. Add 0.6 ml of 5% alpha-naphthol in absolute ethyl alcohol.
3. Add 0.2 ml of a 40% potassium hydroxide-creatine solution.
4. Shake well, and allow it to stand for 10 to 20 minutes. If acetylmethylcarbinol has been produced, a bright **orange-red** color will develop at the surface of the medium and will gradually extend throughout the broth. The development of a copperlike color in some tubes is not considered a positive reaction.

---

*Nutritional Biochemical Corp., Cleveland, Ohio.

O'Meara's test (modified)

REAGENTS

KOH	40 g
Creatine	0.3 g
Distilled water	100 ml

Dissolve the KOH in the distilled water, and add the creatine.

1. O'Meara's (modified) reagent should be added in equal volume to a 48-hour culture.
2. Incubate mixture at 35 C or at room temperature.
3. Final readings are made after 4 hours. Tests should be aerated by shaking the tubes.
4. Positive reactions are indicated by the formation of a **red-pink** color. If equivocal results are obtained, repeat the tests with broth cultures incubated at 25 C for 48 hours.
5. O'Meara's reagent should be prepared frequently and should be refrigerated when not in use. It should not be kept longer than 2 to 3 weeks, since it deteriorates rapidly beyond this time.

Note: Both the methyl red (modified) and the Voges-Proskauer (modified) tests can be run at 24 hours if the volume of the broth is reduced to 0.5 ml. The broth-reagent mixture should be frequently shaken. A positive result is the appearance of a red color, usually within 15 minutes.

Zinc sulfate solution for concentration of parasitologic stool specimens

See Chapter 35.

REFERENCES

1. Blazevic, D.N., and Ederer, G.M.: Biochemical tests in diagnostic microbiology, New York, 1975, John Wiley & Sons, Inc.
2. Dobell, C., and O'Connor, F.W.: Intestinal protozoa of man, New York, 1921, William Wood.
3. Ewing: Enterobacteriaceae, U.S. Public Health Service Pub. No. 734, Washington, D.C., 1960, U.S. Government Printing Office.
4. Gordon, R.E., and Mihm, J.M.: A comparison of four species of mycobacteria, J. Gen. Microbiol. **21:**736-748, 1959.
5. Hanker, J.S., and Rabin, A.N.: Color reaction streak test for catalase-positive micro-organisms, J. Clin. Microbiol. **2:**463-464, 1975.
6. MacFaddin, J.F.: Biochemical tests for identification of medical bacteria, Baltimore, 1976, The Williams & Wilkins Co.
7. McKay, J., Edwards, C.E., and Leonard, H.B.: Genitourinary infection: bacteriologic study of 150 cases, Am. J. Clin. Pathol. **17:**479-482, 1947.
8. Paik, G.: Reagents, stains, and miscellaneous test procedures. In Lennette, E.G., Balows, A., Hausler, W.J., Jr., and Truant, J.P., editors: Manual of clinical microbiology, ed. 3, Washington, D.C., 1980, American Society for Microbiology.
9. Rustigian, R., and Stuart, C.A.: Decomposition of urea by *Proteus,* Proc. Soc. Exp. Biol. Med. **47:**108-112, 1941.
10. Stuart, C.A., Van Stratum, E., and Rustigian, R.: Further studies on urease production by *Proteus* and related organisms, J. Bacteriol. **49:**437-444, 1945.
11. Sutter, V.L., Citron, D.M., and Finegold, S.M.: Wadsworth anaerobic bacteriology manual, ed. 3, St. Louis, 1980, The C.V. Mosby Co.
12. Vestal, A.L.: Procedures for the isolation and identification of mycobacteria, DHEW Pub. No. (CDC) 75-8230, Washington, D.C., 1975, Dept. of Health, Education, and Welfare.

GLOSSARY

TERMS

abscess Localized collection of pus.

accolé Early ring form of *Plasmodium falciparum* found at margin of red cell.

acid-fast Characteristic of certain bacteria, such as mycobacteria, that involves resistance to decolorization by acids when stained by an aniline dye, such as carbol fuchsin.

aerobe, obligate Microorganism that lives and grows freely in air and cannot grow anaerobically.

aerogenic Producing gas (in contrast to anaerogenic—non-gas-producing).

aerotolerant Ability of an anaerobic microorganism to grow in air, usually poorly, especially after anaerobic isolation.

alopecia Baldness.

aminoglycosides Group of related antibiotics including streptomycin, kanamycin, neomycin, tobramycin, gentamicin, and amikacin.

amniotic Pertaining to the innermost fetal membrane forming a fluid-filled sac.

anaerobe, obligate Microorganism that grows only in complete or nearly complete absence of air or molecular oxygen.

anergy Absence of reaction to antigens or allergens.

antibiotic Substance, produced by a microorganism, that inhibits or kills other microorganisms. A broad-spectrum antibiotic is therapeutically effective against a wide range of bacteria.

antibody Substance, (immunoglobulin) formed in the blood or tissues, that interacts only with the antigen that induced its synthesis (e.g., agglutinin).

antigen Molecular structure that is capable of stimulating production of antibody.

antimicrobial Chemical substance, either produced by a microorganism or by synthetic means, that is capable of killing or suppressing the growth of microorganisms.

analytic reagent (AR) Grade of chemical.

arthroconidium A spore formed by septation of a hypha and subsequent separation at the septa.

ascitic fluid Serous fluid in peritoneal cavity.

autotroph Organism that can utilize inorganic carbon sources (CO_2).

auxotroph Differing from the wild strain (prototroph) by an additional nutritional requirement.

bacteremia Presence of viable organisms in the blood.

bacteriocins Antibioticlike substances, produced by bacteria, that exert a lethal effect on other bacteria.

bacteriuria Presence of bacteria in urine.

benign tertian malaria Malaria caused by *Plasmodium vivax*.

beta-lactamases Enzymes that destroy penicillins and/or cephalosporins and are produced by a variety of bacteria.

biopsy Removal of tissue from a living body for diagnostic purposes (e.g., lymph node biopsy).

blackwater fever Condition in which the diagnostic symptom is passage of reddish or red-brown urine, which indicates massive intravascular hemolysis (*Plasmodium falciparum*).

blastoconidium A spore formed by budding, as in yeasts.

bronchoscopy Examination of the bronchi through a bronchoscope, a tubular illuminated instrument introduced through the trachea (windpipe).

bubo Inflammatory enlargement of lymph node, usually in the groin or axilla.

buffy coat Layer of white blood cells and platelets above red blood cell mass when blood is sedimented.

bullae Large blebs or blisters, filled with fluid, in or just beneath the epidermal layer of skin.

bursitis Inflammation of a bursa, which is a small sac lined with synovial membrane and filled with fluid interposed between parts that move upon each other.

capneic incubation Incubation under increased CO_2 tension, as in a candle extinguishing jar (approximately 3% CO_2).

capsule Gelatinous material surrounding bacterial cell wall, usually of polysaccharide nature.

caseation necrosis Tissue death with loss of cell outlines and a cheeselike, amorphous appearance.

catalase Bacterial enzyme that breaks down peroxides with liberation of free oxygen.

catheter Flexible tubular (rubber or plastic) instrument used for withdrawing fluids from (or introducing fluids into) a body cavity or vessel (e.g., urinary bladder catheter).

cellulitis Inflammation of subcutaneous tissue.

cerebriform With brainlike folds.

cervical Pertaining either to the neck or to the cervix of the uterus.

Charcot-Leyden crystals Slender crystals shaped like a double pyramid with pointed ends, formed from the breakdown products of eosinophils and found in feces, sputum, and tissues; indicative of an immune response that may have parasitic or nonparasitic causes.

chemotherapeutic Chemical agent used in the treatment of infections (e.g., sulfonamides).

chlamydospore Thick-walled spore formed from a vegetative cell.

chromatography Method of chemical analysis by which a mixture of substances is separated by fractional extraction or adsorption or ion exchange on a porous solid.

chromogen Bacterial species whose colonial growth is pigmented (e.g., *Flavobacterium* species, yellow).

clavate Club shaped.

colitis Inflammation of the mucosa of the colon.

colony Macroscopically visible growth of a microorganism on a solid culture medium.

commensal Microorganism living on or in a host but causing the host no harm.

conjunctivitis Inflammation of the conjunctivae or membranes of the eye and eyelid.

culdocentesis Aspiration of fluid from the cul-de-sac by puncture of the vaginal vault.

definitive host Host in which the sexual reproduction of a parasite occurs.

dermatophyte A fungus parasitic on skin, hair, or nails.

desquamation Shedding or scaling of skin or mucous membrane.

dichotomous Branching in two directions.

dimorphic fungi Fungi with both a mold phase and a yeast phase.

DNase Deoxyribonuclease, an enzyme that depolymerizes DNA, an essential component of all living matter, which contains the genetic code.

dysentery Inflammation of the intestinal tract, particularly the colon, with frequent bloody stools (e.g., bacillary dysentery).

dysgonic Growing poorly (bacterial cultures).

ectoparasite Organism that lives on or within skin.

ectothrix Outside of hair shafts.

edema Excessive accumulation of fluid in tissue spaces.

effusion Fluid escaping into a body space or tissue (e.g., pleural effusion).

elephantiasis Condition caused by inflammation and obstruction of the lymphatic system, resulting in hypertrophy and thickening of the surrounding tissues, usually involving the extremities and external genitalia (filariasis).

elution Process of extraction by means of a solvent.

empyema Accumulation of pus in a body cavity, particularly empyema of the thorax or chest.

encephalitis Inflammation of the brain.

endocervix The mucous membrane of the cervical canal.

endogenous Developing from within the body.

endoparasite Parasite that lives within the body.

endothrix Within the hair shaft.

enterotoxigenic Producing an enterotoxin (e.g., enterotoxigenic *E. coli*).

enterotoxin Toxin affecting the cells of the intestinal mucosa.

erythema Redness of the skin from various causes.

erythrocytic cycle Developmental cycle of malarial parasites within red blood cells.

eugonic Growing luxuriantly (bacterial cultures).

exanthem Skin eruption as a symptom of an acute disease, usually viral.

exoerythrocytic cycle Portion of the malarial life cycle occurring in the vertebrate host in which sporozoites, introduced by infected mosquitoes, penetrate the parenchymal liver cells and undergo schizogony, producing merozoites, which then initiate the erythrocytic cycle.

exogenous From outside the body.

exudate Fluid that has passed out of blood vessels into adjacent tissues or spaces; high protein content.

facultative anaerobe Microorganism that grows under either anaerobic or aerobic conditions.

favus Dermatophyte infection of the scalp produced by *Trichophyton schoenleinii*.

fermentation Anaerobic decomposition of carbohydrate.

filamentous Threadlike.

fistula Abnormal communication between two surfaces or between a viscus or other hollow structure and the exterior.

floccose Cottony, in tufts.

fluorescent Emission of light by a substance (or a microscopic preparation) while acted on by radiant energy, such as ultraviolet rays, as in the immunofluorescent procedure.

fungemia The presence of viable fungi in the blood.

fusiform Spindle shaped, as in the anaerobe *Fusobacterium nucleatum*.

gangrene Death of a part or tissue resulting from disease, injury, or failure of blood supply.

gastroenteritis Inflammation of the mucosa of the stomach and intestines.

germ tube Tubelike process, produced by a germinating spore, that develops into mycelium.

glabrous Smooth.

granuloma Aggregation and proliferation of macrophages to form small (usually microscopic) nodules.

halophilic Preferring high salt content.

hemagglutination Agglutination of red blood cells caused by certain antibodies, virus particles, or high molecular weight polysaccharides.

hematogenous Disseminated by the bloodstream.

herpes Inflammation of the skin characterized by clusters of small vesicles (e.g., herpes simplex).

heterotroph Organism that requires an organic carbon source.

hyaline Colorless, transparent.

hyperemia Increased blood in a part, resulting in distention of blood vessels.

hypertrophy Increased size of an organ resulting from enlargement of individual cells.

hypha Tubular cell making up the vegetative portion or mycelium of fungi.

immunofluorescence Microscopic method of determining the presence or location of an antigen (or antibody) by demonstrating fluorescence when the preparation is exposed to a fluorescein-tagged antibody (or antigen) using ultraviolet radiation.

immunoglobulin Synonymous with antibody; five distinct classes have been isolated: IgG, IgM, IgA, IgE, and IgD.

immunosuppression Depression of the immune response caused by disease, irradiation, or administration of antimetabolites, antilymphocyte serum, or corticosteroids.

impetigo Acute inflammatory skin disease, caused by streptococci or staphylococci, characterized by vesicles and bullae that rupture and form yellow crusts.

inclusion bodies Microscopic bodies, usually within body cells; thought to be virus particles in morphogenesis.

indigenous flora Normal or resident flora.

induced malaria Malaria infection acquired by parenteral inoculation (e.g., blood transfusion or sharing of needles by drug addicts).

induration Abnormal hardness of a tissue or part resulting from hyperemia or inflammation, as in a reactive tuberculin skin test.

infection Invasion by and multiplication of microorganisms in body tissue resulting in disease.

intermediate host Required host in the life cycle in which essential larval development must occur before a parasite is infective to its definitive host or to additional intermediate hosts.

intertrigo Erythematous skin eruption of adjacent skin parts.

intramuscular (intraperitoneal, intravenous) Within the muscle (peritoneum, vein), as in intramuscular injection.

in vitro Literally, within a glass (i.e., in a test tube, culture plate, or other nonliving material).

in vivo Within the living body.

involution forms Abnormally shaped bacterial cells occurring in an aging culture population.

keratitis Inflammation of the cornea.

lag phase Period of slow microbial growth that occurs following inoculation of the culture medium.

Leishman-Donovan body Small, round intracellular form (called amastigote or leishmanial stage) of *Leishmania* species and *Trypanosoma cruzi*.

leukocytosis Elevated white blood cell count.

leukopenia Low white blood cell count.

logarithmic phase Period of maximal growth rate of a microorganism in a culture medium.

lysis Disintegration or dissolution of bacteria or cells.

malignant tertian malaria Malaria caused by *Plasmodium falciparum*.

meconium Pasty greenish mass in intestine of fetus; made up of mucus, desquamated cells, bile, and such.

meningitis Inflammation of the meninges, the membranes that cover the brain and spinal cord (e.g., bacterial meningitis).

merozoite Product of schizogonic cycle in malaria that will invade red blood cells.

mesenteric adenitis Inflammation of mesenteric lymph nodes.

mesentery A fold of the peritoneum that connects the intestine with the posterior abdominal wall.

metastatic Spread of an infectious (or other) process from a primary focus to a distant one via the bloodstream or lymphatic system.

microaerophile, obligate Microorganism that grows only under reduced oxygen tension and cannot grow aerobically or anaerobically.

microfilaria Embryos produced by filarial worms and found in the blood or tissues of individuals with filariasis.

mixed culture (pure culture) More than one organism growing in or on the same culture medium, as opposed to a single organism in pure culture.

mucopurulent Material containing both mucus and pus (e.g., mucopurulent sputum).

mucosa A mucous membrane.

mycelium Mass of hyphae making up a colony of a fungus.

mycetoma Chronic infection, usually of feet, caused by various fungi or by *Nocardia* or *Streptomyces*, resulting in swelling and sinus tracts; pulmonary mycetoma is a mass of fungal hyphae ("fungus ball") growing in a cavity from previous tuberculosis or other pathologic condition.

mycoses Diseases caused by fungi (e.g., dermatomycosis, fungal infection of the superficial skin).

myocarditis Inflammation of the heart muscle.

nares External openings of nose (i.e., nostrils).

nasopharyngeal Pertaining to the part of the pharynx above the level of the soft palate.

necrosis Pathologic death of a cell or group of cells.

neonatal First 4 weeks after birth.

neurotrophic Having a selective affinity for nerve tissue. Rabies is caused by a neurotrophic virus.

nonsporulating Does not produce spores.

nosocomial Pertaining to or originating in a hospital, as nosocomial infection.

operculated ova Ova possessing a cap or lid.

osteomyelitis Inflammation of the bone and the marrow.

otitis Inflammation of the ear from a variety of causes, including bacterial infection. Otitis media, inflammation of the middle ear.

pandemic Epidemic over a wide geographic area, or even worldwide.

paracentesis fluid Fluid obtained by tapping the peritoneal cavity.

parasite Organism that lives on or within and at the expense of another organism.

paronychia Purulent inflammation about margin of a nail.

paroxysm Rapid onset (or return) of symptoms; term usually applies to cyclic recurrence of malaria symptoms, which are chills, fever, and sweating.

pathogenic Producing disease.

pathologic Caused by or involving a morbid condition, as a pathologic state.

penicillinase (beta-lactamase I) Enzyme produced by some bacterial species that inactivates the antimicrobial activity of certain penicillins (e.g., penicillin G).

percutaneous Performed through the skin (e.g., percutaneous bladder aspiration).

pericarditis Inflammation of the covering of the heart (pericardium).

peritoneal cavity The space between the visceral and parietal layers of the peritoneum, the serous membrane lining the abdominal cavity and surrounding the contained viscera.

plasma Fluid portion of blood; obtained by centrifuging anticoagulated blood.

plasmids Extrachromosomal DNA elements of bacteria carrying a variety of determinants that may permit survival in an adverse environment or successful competition with other microorganisms of the same or different species.

pleomorphic Having more than one form, usually widely different forms, as in pleomorphic bacteria.

pleura The serous membrane enveloping the lung and lining the internal surface of the thoracic cavity.

pleuropulmonary Pertaining to the lungs and pleura.

prodromal Early manifestations of a disease before specific symptoms become evident.

proglottid Segments of the tapeworm containing male and female reproductive systems; may be immature, mature, or gravid.

prognosis Forcast as to the possible outcome of a disease.

prophylaxis Preventive treatment (e.g., the use of drugs to prevent infection).

prototroph Naturally occurring or wild strain.

pseudomembrane Necrosis of mucosal surface simulating a membrane.

psychrophilic Cold loving (e.g., microorganisms that grow best at low [4 C] temperatures).

purulent Consisting of pus.

pus Product of inflammation, consisting of fluid and many white blood cells; often bacteria, cellular debris, and such are also present.

pyogenic Pus producing.

quartan malaria Malaria caused by *Plasmodium malariae*.

rhizoid Rootlike absorbing organ.

saprophytic Nonpathogenic.

schizogony Stage in the asexual cycle of the malaria parasite that takes place in the red blood cells of humans.

sclerotic Hard, indurated.

scolex (plural, scolices) Head portion of a tapeworm; may attach to the intestinal wall by suckers or hooklets.

septate Having cross walls.

septicemia (**sepsis**) Systemic disease associated with the presence of pathogenic microorganisms or their toxins in the blood.

sequestrum A detached or dead piece of bone within a cavity, abscess, wound, or area of osteomyelitis.

serum Cell and fibrinogen-free fluid after blood clots.

sinus Suppurating tract; paranasal sinus, hollows or cavities near the nose (e.g., frontal and maxillary sinuses).

somatic Pertaining to the body (of a cell) (e.g., the somatic antigens of *Salmonella* species).

spore Reproductive cell of bacteria, fungi, or protozoa; in bacteria may be inactive, resistant forms within the cell.

sporogony Stage in the sexual cycle in the malarial parasite that takes place in the mosquito.

sporozoite Slender, spindle-shaped organism that is the infective stage of the malarial parasite; it is inoculated into humans by an infected mosquito and is the result of the sexual cycle of the malarial parasite in the mosquito.

sputum Material discharged from the surface of the lower respiratory tract air passages and expectorated (or swallowed).

stab culture Culture in which the inoculation of a tube of solid medium is made by stabbing with a needle to encourage anaerobic growth in the bottom.

stat (Do) immediately.

stationary phase Stage in the growth cycle of a bacterial culture in which the vegetative cell population equals the dying population.

sterile (**sterility**) Free of living microorganisms (the state of being sterile).

strobila Entire chain of tapeworm proglottids, excluding the scolex and neck.

sulfur granule Small colony of organisms with surrounding clublike material. Yellow-brown. Resembles grain of sulfur.

suppuration Formation of pus.

suprapubic bladder aspiration Obtaining urine by direct needle puncture of the full bladder through the abdominal wall above the pubic bone.

syndrome Set of symptoms occurring together (e.g., nephrotic syndrome).

synergism Combined effect of two or more agents that is greater than the sum of their individual effects.

synovial fluid Sterile viscid fluid secreted by the synovial membrane; found in joint cavities, bursae, and so forth.

therapy, antimicrobial Treatment of a patient for the purpose of combating an infectious disease.

thermolabile Adversely affected by heat (as opposed to thermostable, not affected by heat).

thoracentesis Drainage of fluid from the pleural space.

thoracic Pertaining to the chest cavity.

tinea Dermatophyte infection (tinea capitis, tinea of scalp; tinea corporis, tinea of the smooth skin of the body; tinea cruris, tinea of the groin; tinea pedis, tinea of the foot).

tolerance A form of resistance to antimicrobial drugs; of uncertain clinical importance.

transtracheal aspiration Passage of needle and plastic catheter through the trachea for obtaining lower respiratory tract secretions.

transudate Similar to exudate, but with low protein content.

trophozoite Feeding, motile stage of protozoa.

typing Methods of grouping organisms, primarily for epidemiologic purposes (e.g., biotyping, serotyping, bacteriophage typing, and the antibiogram).

urethritis Inflammation of the urethra, the canal through which urine is discharged (e.g., gonococcal urethritis).

vesicle A small bulla or blister containing clear fluid.

virulence Degree of pathogenicity or disease-producing ability of a microorganism.

viscera Internal organs, particularly of abdominal cavity.

xenodiagnosis Procedure involving the feeding of laboratory-reared triatomid bugs on patients suspected of having Chagas' disease; after several weeks, the feces of the bugs are checked for intermediate stages of *Trypanosoma cruzi*.

zoonoses Diseases of lower animals transmissable to humans (e.g., tularemia).

ABBREVIATIONS

A Acid.

AFB Acid-fast bacilli.

Alk or K Alkaline.

ART Automated reagin test for syphilis.

ATCC American Type Culture Collection.

B cells Lymphocytes involved in antibody production.

BAP Blood agar plate.

BCG Bacillus Calmette-Guerin (for tuberculosis immunization).

BFP Biological false-positive.

CAMP Lytic factor named after Christie, Atkins, and Munch-Peterson.

CAP Chocolate agar plate.

C & S Culture and sensitivity.

CDC Centers for Disease Control.

CF Complement fixation.

CFU Colony-forming unit (i.e., colony count).

CIE Counterimmunoelectrophoresis.

CNS Central nervous system.

CPC Clinical pathologic conference.

CPE Cytopathogenic effect.

CRP C-reactive protein.

CSF Cerebrospinal fluid.

CYE Charcoal yeast extract (agar plate).

DFA Direct fluorescent antibody test.

DNA Deoxyribonucleic acid.

DNAse Deoxyribonuclease.

Dx Diagnosis.

ELISA Enzyme-linked immunosorbent assay.

EMB Eosin–methylene blue (agar plate).

FTA Fluorescent treponemal antibody.

FUO Fever of unknown origin.

GC Gonococcus.

GN Gram-negative (broth).

HAA Hepatitis-associated antigen.

HAI Hemagglutination inhibition.

ID Infectious disease; identification.

IFA Indirect fluorescent antibody; immunofluorescent antibody.

Ig, IgG, etc. Immunoglobulin, immunoglobulin G, etc.

KIA Kligler's iron agar (tube).

KOH Potassium hydroxide.

MAC MacConkey (agar plate).

MBC Minimum bactericidal concentration.

MIC Minimum inhibitory concentration.

NFB Glucose non-fermenting gram-negative bacteria.

NGU Nongonococcal urethritis.

O-F Oxidation-fermentation medium.

O & P Ova and parasites.

ONPG O-nitrophenol-β-galactopyranoside (β-galactosidase test).

PID Pelvic inflammatory disease.

PPD Purified protein derivative (skin test antigen - tuberculosis).

PPNG Penicillinase-producing (i.e., penicillin-resistant) gonococcus.

PRAS Prereduced, anaerobically sterilized.

QC Quality control.

QNS Quantity nonsufficient.

RNA Ribonucleic acid.

SBE Subacute bacterial endocarditis.

SBA Suprapubic bladder aspiration.

STD Sexually transmitted disease.

Stat Statim (Latin), immediately.

T cells Lymphocytes involved in cellular immunity.

TTA Transtracheal aspiration.

TB Tuberculosis.

T-M Thayer-Martin (agar plate).

TSI Triple sugar iron (agar tube).

TSS Toxic shock syndrome.

URI Upper respiratory tract infection.

UTI Urinary tract infection.

VD Venereal disease.

V-P Voges-Proskauer.

INDEX